NCLEX-RN
Review

made
Incredibly
Easy!®

Sixth Edition

NCLEX-RN® Review

made Incredibly Easy!®

Sixth Edition

Clinical Editor
Candice Rome, DNP, RN
Chair, Digital Learning Programs
Associate Professor of Nursing
Hunt School of Nursing
Gardner-Webb University
Boiling Springs, North Carolina

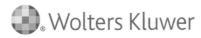

Wolters Kluwer

Philadelphia • Baltimore • New York • London
Buenos Aires • Hong Kong • Sydney • Tokyo

Vice President and Publisher: Julie K. Stegman
Director, Nursing Education Content Publishing Health Learning, Research & Practice: Renee Gagliardi
Director of Product Development: Jennifer K. Forestieri
Content Strategist: Dawn Lagrosa
Editorial Coordinator: Emily Buccieri
Editorial Assistant: Arielle Dameshghi
Marketing Manager: Sarah Schuessler
Production Project Manager: Sadie Buckallew
Design Coordinator: Elaine Kasmer
Art Director, Illustration: Jennifer Clements
Manufacturing Coordinator: Kathleen Brown
Prepress Vendor: SPi Global

Sixth Edition

Cataloging in Publication data available on request from publisher

ISBN: 978-1-9751-1690-3

RRS1908

Dr. Candice Rome is a tenured Associate Professor of Nursing and Chair of Digital Learning Programs in the Hunt School of Nursing at Gardner-Webb University in Boiling Springs, North Carolina. She earned her ASN from Foothills Nursing Consortium in Shelby, North Carolina; her BSN from Winston-Salem State University in Winston-Salem, North Carolina; and her MSN with a concentration in education and DNP from Gardner-Webb University in Boiling Springs, North Carolina. She also serves as an NCLEX-RN review course instructor, an NCLEX-style item writer, and a member of the Wolters Kluwer Adaptive Quizzing Editorial Advisory Board. She teaches at the undergraduate and graduate levels and leads students on international medical mission trips. Dr. Rome's awards include being named one of the 2017–2018 Highest Ranking Professors Among Undergraduate Student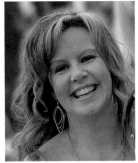
Opinion of Instruction, the 2015 Outstanding Scholar Award, and the 2014 Meg Meccariello Session Presenter at the INACSL conference. Throughout her career, she has published a nursing simulation book, has contributed to textbooks, and has presented at multiple regional and national conferences.

Contributors

Abby Garlock, RN, LCCE
Chair, Pre-Licensure Programs
Associate Professor
Hunt School of Nursing
Gardner-Webb University
Boiling Springs, North Carolina

Melissa McNeilly, MSN, RN
BSN Licensure and Program Coordinator
Instructor
Hunt School of Nursing
Gardner-Webb University
Boiling Springs, North Carolina

Cynthia Short, DNP, CCRN
Associate Dean
Jersey College
Fort Lauderdale, Florida

Linda Turchin, MSN, RN, CNE
Professor Emeritus/Adjunct Faculty
School of Nursing
Fairmont State University
Fairmont, West Virginia

Cynthia J. Young, MSN, RN, CMSRN
Adjunct Faculty
Hunt School of Nursing
Gardner-Webb University
Boiling Springs, North Carolina

Reviewers

Faculty

Mary Bjorklund, MSN, RN, CPN
Lone Star College–Kingwood
Kingwood, Texas

Sherrilyn Coffman, PhD, RN
Nevada State College
Henderson, Nevada

Linda Carman Copel, PhD, RN, PMHCNS, BC, CNE, ANEF, NCC, FAPA
Villanova University
Villanova, Pennsylvania

Karen R. Ferguson, PhD, RNC
Martin Methodist College
Pulaski, Tennessee

Nora James, DNP, RN
Lee College
Baytown, Texas

Laura Bevlock Kanavy, MSN, RN
Career Technology Center of
Lackawanna County Practical
Nursing Program
Scranton, Pennsylvania

Nicole de Bosch Kemper, MSN, RN
University of British Columbia
Okanagan
Kelowna, British Columbia

Christine Krause, MSN, CPNP
Jefferson Health-Aria School of
Nursing
Trevose, Pennsylvania

Donald A. Laurino, MSN, CCRN, CMSRN, PHN, RN-BC
Charles Drew University
Los Angeles, California

Kathleen Lehmann, EdD(c), EdSp, MEd, BSN, BA, RN-BC, PMHN
Boston Healthcare System/Edith
Nourse Rogers Memorial VA
Medical Center
Bedford, Massachusetts

J. Mari Beth Linder, PhD, MSN, RN, BC
Missouri Southern State University
Joplin, Missouri

Marisue Rayno, EdD, RN
Luzerne County Community College
Nanticoke, Pennsylvania

Chad Rogers, APRN, FNP-BC, MSN
Morehead State University
Morehead, Kentucky

Lynn Scussel, MSN, RN
Nursing Exam Development and
Analysis Consulting LLC
Longwood, Florida

Stephen VanSlyke, RN, BN, MN, PMHN(c)
University of New Brunswick
Fredericton, New Brunswick,
Canada

Sherylyn Watson, PhD, MSN, RN, CNE
Sacred Heart University
Fairfield, Connecticut

Kathleen Williamson, PhD, MSN, RN
Midwestern State University
Wichita Falls, Texas

Students

Robert Casna
Rock Valley College
Rockford, Illinois

Louise Gustafson
College of Lake County
Grayslake, Illinois

Rebecca Hilhorst
McMaster University
Hamilton, Ontario

Kelsey Knolhoff
Maryville University
St. Louis, Missouri

Travis Navarro
The College of St. Scholastica
Duluth, Minnesota

Elizabeth Pugh
Jefferson Davis Community
College
Brewton, Alabama

Jennifer Torrey
Fresno City College
Fresno, California

Morgan Ziegler
University of Regina
Saskatoon, Saskatchewan

Preface

I began as a nurse educator in 2008 teaching labs and clinicals part-time for both PN and RN programs, while working on a women's and children's unit at a hospital. I realized that my calling and passion was serving as a nursing educator. After earning an MSN, I transitioned into a full-time nurse educator position at a university, working with both undergraduate and graduate nursing students. My teaching methods include multiple classroom activities to promote student engagement and facilitate concept comprehension and incorporating NCLEX-style practice question discussions.

It is essential to practice NCLEX-style questions throughout your nursing program not simply prior to taking NCLEX. I recommend you set aside a few blocks of time each week to complete NCLEX-style practice questions related to concepts currently being discussed in your class(es). After completing the questions, begin the most important step, which is to remediate each question to ensure you have an understanding of why you got the question right or why you did not get it right. Read each question stem thoroughly to determine what the question is asking. Read the rationale for each answer choice to determine your understanding of the concepts. This will promote a deeper knowledge and in turn facilitate your ability to apply the concept to various scenarios. This resource is developed to provide practice questions and tests to assist you in achieving your goal of NCLEX success and a nursing career. It is also designed to give you a brief overview of information you may have covered in your nursing program. The explanations will help you understand not only why the answer is correct, but also why the distractors are incorrect. Few questions are written at the understanding level, with most at the applying and analyzing levels of Bloom's revised taxonomy—just like the NCLEX. And, the many alternate format questions will allow you to practice for whatever questions your NCLEX contains.

I wish you success on your journey throughout your nursing program, the NCLEX, and your nursing career. The nursing profession is truly rewarding as you will serve clients during the best and worst times of their lives. You will make impacts your clients will remember always. Strive for those impacts to be positive and reflect a caring profession.

—Candice Rome, DNP, RN

NCLEX-RN® Review Made Incredibly Easy! will improve your knowledge while building your ability to apply that knowledge to real nursing scenarios. It also will strengthen your preparation for your licensure experience. Let's cut right to the chase! Here's how:

1. It will teach you all the important things you need to know about preparing for and passing the NCLEX (and it will leave out all the fluff that wastes your time).
2. It will direct your eye to the alternate-format questions.
3. It will help you remember what you've learned.
4. It will make you smile as it enhances your knowledge and skills.

Don't believe it? Try these features on for size:

- Reliable NCLEX preparation guidelines and hundreds of test-taking hints and strategies
- 3,000 NCLEX-style questions within the book to test your knowledge in all areas tested on the real examination
- Two-column format with questions on the left and answers and rationales on the right
- Bookmark for you to hide the answers while reading the question
- Red font for alternate-format questions, and full color photographs and illustrations for graphic and hot spot questions
- Accompanying Web site with these questions in an interactive format—including graphic, hot spot, and audio questions

Plus, check out these updates:

- Alignment of all information with the 2019 NCLEX-RN test plan and NCSBN standards
- Full four-color design and art program integrated throughout
- Thorough content revision based on feedback from nursing faculty and recent graduates across the United States to ensure the most up-to-date practices, highest quality questions, and appropriateness of content for review by students
- Free 7-day trial of *Lippincott NCLEX-RN PassPoint*

Plus, look for Joy, Jake, and friends in the margins throughout this book. As always, they will be there to explain key concepts, provide important hints, and offer reassurance. And, if you don't mind, they'll be spicing up the pages with a bit of humor along the way, to teach and entertain in a way that no other resource can.

Contents

Part I

Surviving the NCLEX®

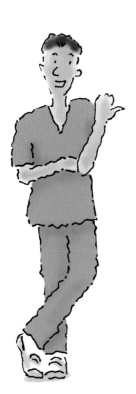

Preparing for the NCLEX®

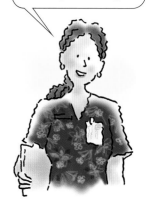

Just the facts

In this chapter, you will learn:

◆ why you must take the NCLEX
◆ what you need to know about taking the NCLEX by computer
◆ strategies to use when answering NCLEX questions
◆ how to recognize and answer NCLEX alternate-format questions
◆ how to avoid common mistakes when taking the NCLEX.

NCLEX basics

Passing the National Council Licensure Examination (NCLEX®) is an important landmark in your career as a nurse. The first step on your way to passing the NCLEX is to understand what it is and how it is administered.

Exam structure

The NCLEX is a test developed by registered nurses with a master's degree and clinical expertise in a particular area of nursing. Only one small difference distinguishes nurses who write NCLEX questions from those who are similarly qualified: They are trained to write questions in a style particular to this examination.

If you have completed an accredited nursing program, you have already taken numerous tests developed by nurses with backgrounds and experiences similar to those of the nurses who write for the NCLEX. Therefore, the test-taking knowledge you have already gained will help you pass the NCLEX and your NCLEX review should be just that—a review of what you have already learned and should know.

What is the point?

The NCLEX is designed for one purpose: to determine whether it is appropriate for you to receive a license to practice as a nurse. By passing this exam, you demonstrate that you possess the minimum level of knowledge, understanding, and skills necessary to practice nursing safely.

Mix 'em up

In nursing school, you probably took courses either organized according to the medical model or that were concept-based. Courses were separated into subjects such as medical-surgical, pediatric, maternal-neonatal, and psychiatric nursing or by concepts such as oxygenation, inflammation, and managing care. In contrast, the NCLEX is integrated, which means that different subjects are mixed together.

As you answer NCLEX questions, you may encounter clients in any stage of life, from neonatal to geriatric. These clients may be of any background, may be completely well or extremely ill, and may have any of a variety of disorders.

Client needs, front and center

The NCLEX draws questions from four categories of client needs that were developed by the National Council of State Boards of Nursing (NCSBN), the organization that sponsors and manages the NCLEX. Client needs categories ensure that a wide variety of topics appear on every NCLEX.

Client needs categories

Each question on the NCLEX is assigned a category based on client needs. This chart lists client needs categories and subcategories and the percentages of each type of question that appear on the NCLEX.

Category	Subcategories	Percentage of questions
Safe and effective care environment	• Management of care • Safety and infection control	17% to 23% 9% to 15%
Health promotion and maintenance	—	6% to 12%
Psychosocial integrity	—	6% to 12%
Physiological integrity	• Basic care and comfort • Pharmacological and parenteral therapies • Reduction of risk potential • Physiological adaptation	6% to 12% 12% to 18% 9% to 15% 11% to 17%

The NCSBN developed client needs categories after conducting a work-study analysis of new nurses. All aspects of nursing care observed in the study were broken down into four main categories, some of which were broken down further into subcategories. (See *Client needs categories*.)

The whole kit and caboodle

The categories and subcategories are used to develop the NCLEX test plan, the content guidelines for the distribution of test questions. Question writers and the people who put the NCLEX together use the test plan and client needs categories to make sure that a full spectrum of nursing activities is covered in the examination. Client needs categories appear in most NCLEX review and question-and-answer books, including this one. As a test-taker, you do not have to concern yourself with client needs categories. You will see those categories for each question and answer in this book, but they will be invisible on the actual NCLEX.

Testing by computer

Like many standardized tests today, the NCLEX is administered by computer. That means you will not be filling in empty circles, sharpening pencils, or erasing frantically. It also means that you must become familiar with computerized tests, if you are not already. Fortunately, the skills required to take the NCLEX on a computer are simple enough to allow you to focus on the questions, not the keyboard.

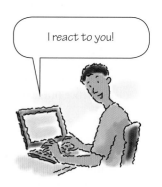

I react to you!

Q&A formats—mixing them up

When you take the test, depending on the question format, you will be presented with a question and four or more possible answers, a blank space in which to enter your answer, a figure on which you use your mouse to select the correct area, a series of charts or exhibits you will use to select the correct response, or items you must rearrange in priority order by dragging and dropping them in place.

Feeling smart? Think hard!

The NCLEX is a computer-adaptive test (CAT). When you respond to a question on the test, the computer supplies more difficult questions if you answer correctly and slightly easier questions if you answer incorrectly. This means each test is uniquely adapted to the individual test-taker.

A matter of time

You have a maximum of 6 hours to complete the test. That gives you the flexibility to spend extra time on more challenging questions. Just the same, it is important to keep an appropriate pace. Most students have plenty of time to finish the test. However, if you run out of time, the computer will look at your last 60 questions to determine if you are competent. To pass, your last 60 questions must be above the competency level.

Most students have plenty of time to complete the test, so take as much time as you need to get the question right without wasting time. Keep moving at a decent pace to help maintain concentration.

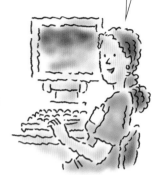

The harder it gets, the better I'm doing.

Difficult items = good news

As you progress through the test, you may notice that the questions seem to be increasingly difficult. That is a good sign. The more questions you answer correctly, the more difficult the questions become.

Some students, knowing that questions get progressively harder, focus on the degree of difficulty of subsequent questions to figure out if they are answering questions correctly. Avoid this temptation and stay focused on selecting the best answer for each question.

Free at last!

The computer test ends when one of the following events occurs:
- You demonstrate minimum competency, according to the computer program.
- You demonstrate a lack of minimum competency, according to the computer program.
- You answer the maximum number of questions (265).
- You use the maximum time allowed (6 hours).

NCLEX® questions

Many questions on the NCLEX are standard four-option, multiple-choice questions with only one correct answer. However, some questions are presented in other formats. Being able to identify the different types of questions you might find on the NCLEX can help you understand them and answer them correctly.

Alternate formats

The types of alternate-format questions are multiple-response, fill-in-the-blank, hot spot, chart/exhibit, ordered response, graphic option, and audio.

Multiple, multiple: it is all or nothing

The first type of alternate-format question is the multiple-response question. Each multiple-response question has, at a minimum, one correct answer. These questions do not have a maximum amount of correct answers, so all the choices may be correct. You will recognize this type of question because it will ask you to select all of the correct answers that apply—not just the best answer.

Keep in mind that for each multiple-response question, you must select all of the correct answers for the item to be counted as correct. On the NCLEX, you do not receive partial credit in the scoring of these items.

Do not go blank!

The second type of alternate-format question is the fill-in-the-blank. In this type of question, you perform a calculation and type your answer (a number, without any words, commas, or spaces) in the blank space provided after the question. No answer options are presented.

Feeling hot, hot, hot

The third type of alternate-format question is one that asks you to identify an area on an illustration or graphic. For these so-called "hot-spot" questions, the computerized exam will ask you to place your cursor and click over the correct area on an illustration. Try to be as precise as possible when marking the location. As with the fill-in-the-blanks, these questions require extremely precise answers.

Take a look at that!

The fourth alternate-format type is the chart/exhibit format. For this question type, you will be given a problem and then a series of small screens with additional information you will need to answer the question. By clicking on the tabs on screen, you can access each chart or exhibit item. After viewing the chart or exhibit, you select your answer from four multiple-choice options.

Keep things in order!

Ordered response, the fifth type of alternate-format question, involves prioritizing actions or placing a series of statements in correct order using a drag-and-drop technique. To move an answer option from a list of unordered options into the correct sequence, click on it using the mouse. While still holding down the mouse button, drag the option to the ordered response part of the screen. Release the mouse button to "drop" the option into place. Repeat this process until you have moved all the available options into the correct order.

Now hear this

The sixth alternate-format item type is the audio item format. You will be given a set of headphones and asked to listen to an audio clip and select the correct answer from four options. You will need to select the correct answer on the computer screen as you would with traditional multiple-choice questions.

Picture perfect

The final alternate-format item type is the graphic option question. This varies from the exhibit format type because in the graphic option, your answer choices will be graphics, such as electrocardiography (ECG) strips. You will have to select the appropriate graphic to answer the question presented.

The standard is still the standard

The number of alternate-format questions will vary for each candidate. In fact, your exam may contain only one or may contain several. Keep in mind that standard four-option, multiple-choice questions constitute the bulk of the test. (See *Sample NCLEX® questions*, pages 7 and 8)

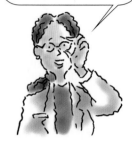

Focusing on what the question is really asking can help you choose the correct answer.

Understanding the question

NCLEX® questions are commonly long. As a result, it is easy to become overloaded with information. To focus on the question and avoid becoming overwhelmed, apply these proven strategies for answering NCLEX questions.
- Determine what the question is asking.
- Determine relevant facts about the client.
- Rephrase the question in your mind.
- Choose the best option(s) before entering your answer.

Determine what the question is asking

Read the question twice. If the answer is not apparent, rephrase the question in simpler, more personal terms. This strategy may help you to focus more effectively to determine the correct answer.

Give it a try

For example, a question might be, "An older adult client with a history of a myocardial infarction (MI) is admitted to the telemetry unit with heart failure and placed on 6 L of oxygen per minute and given furosemide. Which parameter will the nurse watch closely to monitor the client's response to furosemide?"

The answer options for this question might include:
1. Daily weight
2. 24-hour intake and output
3. Serum sodium levels
4. Hourly urine output

Hocus, focus on the question

Read the question again, ignoring all details except what is being asked. Focus on the last line of the question. It asks you to select the appropriate parameter for monitoring a client who received furosemide.

Sample NCLEX® questions

Sometimes, getting used to the format is as important as knowing the material. Try your hand at these sample questions, and you will have a leg up when you take the real test!

Four-option, multiple-choice question

The nurse is assessing a client 4 days after abdominal surgery. When assessing the incision, the nurse notes part of the client's intestine is protruding. Which action will the nurse take?

1. Cover the incision and protruding intestine with sterile gauze.
2. Immediately irrigate the incision with a normal saline solution.
3. Cover the incision and protruding intestine with saline-soaked gauze.
4. Attempt to reinsert the protruding intestine and cover with an abdominal binder.

Correct answer: 3

Multiple-response question

A client is admitted with chronic obstructive pulmonary disease (COPD). The nurse understands which finding(s) is characteristic of COPD? Select all that apply.

1. Decreased respiratory rate
2. Dyspnea on exertion
3. Barrel chest
4. Shortened expiratory phase
5. Clubbed fingers
6. Fever

Correct answers: 2, 3, 5

Fill-in-the-blank, calculation question

The health care provider prescribes 600 mg of ceftriaxone oral suspension to be given daily to a client diagnosed with pneumonia. The nurse obtains the suspension from the pharmacy and reads the label, which indicates the dosage strength is 125 mg/5 mL. How many milliliters of the medication will the nurse administer with each dose? Record your answer using a whole number.

_____ milliliters

Correct answer: 24

Hot-spot question

Orders for a client with cirrhosis request a daily measurement of abdominal girth. Identify the anatomical landmark where the nurse will place the tape measure to obtain this measurement.

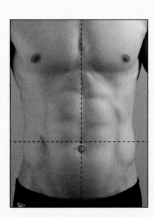

Correct answer:

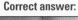

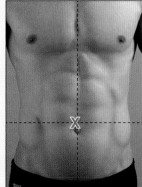

Chart/Exhibit question

A child is being admitted to the hospital and isolation precautions are prescribed. Based on the chart exhibit below, which isolation precautions will the nurse use when caring for this client?

Sample NCLEX® questions *(continued)*

Progress notes	
5/15	5-year-old with varicella admitted with high fever, dehydration, and pruritic rash on face and trunk with lesions in all stages. See graphic record for vital signs. IV started in L arm. Isolation precautions instituted. —J. Jefferson, RN

1. Standard precautions
2. Airborne precautions
3. Droplet precautions
4. Contact precautions

Correct answer: 2

Ordered response question

The nurse suspects a client is in cardiac arrest. Arrange the steps for cardiopulmonary resuscitation in the order the nurse will perform them. Use all options once.

Unordered options:

	Correct answer:
1. Activate the emergency response system.	**2.** Assess responsiveness.
2. Assess responsiveness.	**1.** Activate the emergency response system.
3. Call for a defibrillator.	**3.** Call for a defibrillator.
4. Provide two breaths.	**5.** Assess pulse.
5. Assess pulse.	**6.** Begin cycles of 30 compressions.
6. Begin cycles of 30 chest compressions.	**4.** Provide two breaths.

Graphic option question

The nurse is assessing a client's respiratory pattern. Which graphic illustrates Kussmaul's respirations?

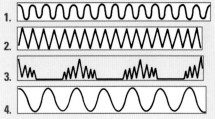

1.

2.

3.

4.

Correct answer: 2

Audio question (sample audio questions are available on thePoint)

Listen to the audio clip. What sound, heard in the lung bases of this client with heart failure, will the nurse document in the client's medical record?

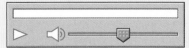

1. Crackles
2. Rhonchi
3. Wheezes
4. Pleural friction rub

Correct answer: 1

Determine what facts about the client are relevant

Next, sort out the relevant client information. Identify any irrelevant information provided about the client. For instance, do you need to know the client has been admitted to the telemetry unit? Probably not; the client's reaction to furosemide will not be affected by location in the hospital.

Determine what you do know about the client. In the example, you know that:

- the client just received a dose of the diuretic furosemide, a crucial fact
- the client has heart failure, the most fundamental aspect of the client's underlying condition
- the client is receiving oxygen at 6 L/minute, which suggests heart failure is moderately severe
- the client is an older adult who has had an MI, a fact that may or may not be relevant.

Rephrase the question

After you have determined relevant information about the client and the question being asked, consider rephrasing the question to make it easier to understand what is being asked. Eliminate jargon and put the question in simpler, more personal terms. Here is how you might rephrase the question in the example: "My client has heart failure and requires 6 L/minute of oxygen. The client is an older adult and has had an MI. The client received a dose of furosemide. What parameter should I monitor?"

Choose the best option

Armed with all this information, it is time for you to select an option. You know the client received a dose of furosemide. You know that monitoring fluid intake and output is a key nursing intervention for a client taking a diuretic, a fact that eliminates options 1 and 3 (daily weight and serum sodium levels) and narrows the answer down to options 2 and 4 (24-hour intake and output or hourly urine output).

Can I use a lifeline?

Monitoring the client's 24-hour intake and output would be appropriate for monitoring the effects of repeated doses of furosemide. However, hourly urine output is most appropriate in this situation because it monitors the more immediate effect of this drug.

Key strategies

Regardless of the type of question, four key strategies will help you determine the correct answer for each question. (See *Strategies for success.*) These strategies include:

- considering the nursing process
- referring to Maslow's hierarchy of needs
- reviewing client safety
- reflecting on principles of therapeutic communication.

Nursing process

One of the ways to answer a question is to apply the nursing process. Steps in the nursing process are implemented in this order:

- assessing
- planning
- implementation
- evaluation.

First things first

The nursing process may provide insights that help you analyze a question. According to the nursing process, data collection comes before planning, which comes before implementation, which comes before evaluation.

You are halfway to the correct answer when you encounter a four-option, multiple-choice question that asks you to collect data and then provides two assessment options and two implementation options. You can immediately eliminate the implementation

Strategies for success

Keeping a few main strategies in mind as you answer each NCLEX question can help ensure greater success. These four strategies are critical for answering NCLEX questions correctly.

- If the question asks what you will do in a situation, use the nursing process to determine which step in the process will be next.
- If the question asks what the client needs, use Maslow's hierarchy to determine which need to address first.
- If the question indicates the client does not have an urgent physiological need, focus on the client's safety.
- If the question involves communicating with a client, use the principles of therapeutic communication.

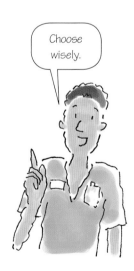

Choose wisely.

options. This gives you, at worst, a 50–50 chance of selecting the correct answer. Apply the nursing process to the following sample question:

A client returns from an endoscopic procedure that required sedation. Before offering the client food, which action will the nurse take?
1. Monitor the client's respiratory status.
2. Check the client's gag reflex.
3. Place the client in a side-lying position.
4. Have the client drink a few sips of water.

Collect data before intervening

According to the nursing process, the nurse must collect client data before performing an intervention. Does the question indicate that data have been properly collected? No, it does not. Therefore, you can eliminate options 3 and 4 because they are both interventions.

That leaves options 1 and 2, both of which demonstrate data collection. Your nursing knowledge should tell you the correct answer—in this case, option 2. The sedation required for an endoscopic procedure may impair the client's gag reflex, so you would check the gag reflex before giving food to the client to reduce the risk of aspiration and airway obstruction.

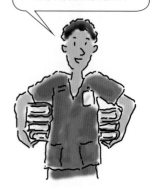

Say it 1,000 times: Studying for the NCLEX is fun…studying for the NCLEX is fun…

Final elimination

Why not select option 1, monitoring the client's respiratory status? The question is specifically asking about offering the client food, an action that would not be taken if the client's respiratory status was at all compromised. In this case, you are making a judgment based on the phrase, "before offering the client food." If the question was designed to test your knowledge of respiratory depression following an endoscopic procedure, it probably would not mention a function such as feeding a client. This option clearly occurs only after the client's respiratory status has been stabilized.

Maslow's hierarchy

Knowledge of Maslow's hierarchy of needs can be a vital tool for answering questions on the NCLEX that require you to establish priorities. Maslow's theory states that physiological needs are the most basic human needs of all. Only after physiological needs have been met can safety concerns be addressed. Only after safety concerns are met can concerns involving love and belonging be addressed. Once concerns of love and belonging are met, an individual may explore the needs of self-esteem, then, ultimately, the needs of self-actualization. Apply the principles of Maslow's hierarchy of needs to the following sample question:

A client reports severe pain 2 days after surgery. Which action will the nurse perform **first**?
1. Tell the client the pain will be less tomorrow.
2. Allow time for the client to verbalize feelings.
3. Check the client's vital signs.
4. Administer an analgesic.

Phys before psych

In this example, options 3 and 4 address physiological needs. Options 1 and 2 address psychosocial concerns. According to Maslow, physiological needs must be met before psychosocial needs, so you can eliminate options 1 and 2.

Final elimination

Now, use your nursing knowledge to choose the best answer from the two remaining options. In this case, option 3 is correct because the client's vital signs should be checked before administering an analgesic (assessment before intervention). When prioritizing according to Maslow's hierarchy, remember your ABCs—airway, breathing, circulation—to help you further prioritize. Check for a patent airway before addressing breathing. Check breathing before checking the health of the cardiovascular system.

One caveat…

Always examine your choice in light of your knowledge and experience. Ask yourself, "Does this choice make sense for this client?" Allow yourself to eliminate choices—even ones that might normally take priority—if they do not make sense for a particular client's situation.

Client safety

As you might expect, client safety takes a high priority on the NCLEX. You will encounter many questions that can be answered by asking yourself, "Which answer will best ensure the safety of this client?" Use client safety criteria for situations involving laboratory values, drug administration, or nursing care procedures.

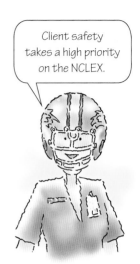

Client safety takes a high priority on the NCLEX.

Client first, equipment second

You may encounter a question in which some options address the client and others address the equipment. When in doubt, select an option relating to the client; never place equipment before a client.

For instance, suppose a question asks what the nurse will do first when entering a client's room where an infusion pump alarm is sounding. If two options deal with the infusion pump, one with the infusion tubing, and another with the client's catheter insertion site, select the one relating to the client's catheter insertion site. Always check the client first; the equipment can wait.

Therapeutic communication

Some NCLEX questions focus on the nurse's ability to communicate effectively with the client. Therapeutic communication incorporates verbal or nonverbal responses and involves:
* listening to the client
* understanding the client's needs
* promoting clarification
* gaining insight into the client's condition.

Room for improvement

Like other NCLEX questions, those dealing with therapeutic communication commonly require choosing the best response. First, eliminate options that indicate the use of poor therapeutic communication techniques, such as those where the nurse:
* tells the client what to do without regard to the client's feelings or desires (the "do this" response)
* asks a question that can be answered with a one-word response, such as "yes" or "no"
* seeks reasons for the client's behavior
* implies disapproval of the client's behavior
* offers false reassurances
* attempts to interpret the client's behavior rather than allow the client to verbalize feelings
* offers a response that focuses on the nurse, not the client.

Ah, that is better!

When answering NCLEX questions, look for responses that:
* allow the client time to think and reflect
* encourage the client to talk
* encourage the client to describe a particular experience
* reflect that the nurse has listened to the client through paraphrasing the client's response or another communication technique.

Avoiding pitfalls

Even the most knowledgeable students can be tripped up by certain NCLEX questions. Students commonly cite three areas that can be difficult for unwary test-takers:
1. knowing the difference between the NCLEX and the "real world"
2. delegating care
3. knowing laboratory values.

NCLEX® examination versus the real world

Some students who take the NCLEX have extensive practical experience in health care. For example, many test-takers have worked as nursing assistants. In that capacity, test-takers might have been exposed to less than optimal clinical practice and may carry those experiences over to the NCLEX.

However, the NCLEX is a textbook examination—not a test of clinical skills. Take the NCLEX with the understanding that what happens in the real world may differ from what the NCLEX and your nursing school recommend.

Do not take shortcuts

If you have had experience in health care, you may know a quicker way to perform a procedure or tricks to help you get by when you do not have the right equipment. Situations such as staff shortages may force you to improvise. On the NCLEX, such scenarios can lead to trouble. Always check your practical experiences against textbook nursing care and be sure to select the response that follows the textbook.

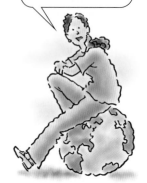

Remember, this is an exam, not the real world.

Delegating care

On the NCLEX, you may encounter questions that assess your ability to delegate care. Delegating care involves managing the efforts of other health care workers to provide effective care for your client. On the NCLEX, you may be asked to assign duties to other registered nurses, licensed practical nurses, nurses from other units, assistive personnel, and other support staff.

In addition, you will be asked to decide when to notify a health care provider (physician or practitioner), a social worker, or another hospital staff member. In each case, you will have to decide when, where, and how to delegate.

Shoulds and should nots

As a general rule, it is okay to delegate actions that involve stable clients or standard procedures. Bathing, feeding, dressing, and transferring clients are examples of procedures that can be delegated.

Be careful not to delegate complicated or complex activities. In addition, do not delegate activities that involve assessment, evaluation, teaching, or your own nursing judgment to someone with less training. On the NCLEX and in the real world, these duties fall squarely on your shoulders. Make sure that you take primary responsibility for assessment, evaluation, education, and making decisions about the client's care. Never hand off those responsibilities to someone with less training.

Calling in reinforcements

Notifying a health care provider, a social worker, or another hospital staff member is an important element of nursing care. On the NCLEX, choices that involve notifying the health care provider are usually incorrect. Remember that the NCLEX tests you, the nurse, at work.

When you are sure the correct answer is to notify the health care provider, first make sure the client's safety has been addressed. On the NCLEX, the client's safety has a higher priority than notifying other health care providers.

Knowing laboratory values

Some NCLEX questions supply laboratory results without indicating normal levels. As a result, answering questions involving laboratory values requires you to have the normal range of the most common laboratory values memorized in order to make an informed decision. (See *Normal laboratory values*)

Normal laboratory values

- Blood urea nitrogen: 8 to 25 mg/dL (0.444 to 1.3875 mmol/L)
- Creatinine: 0.6 to 1.5 mg/dL (53.0 to 132.6 μmol/L)
- Sodium: 135 to 145 mEq/L (135 to 145 mmol/L)
- Potassium: 3.5 to 5 mEq/L (3.5 to 5 mmol/L)
- Chloride: 97 to 110 mmol/L
- Glucose (fasting plasma): 70 to 100 mg/dL (3.89 to 5.55 mmol/L)
- Hemoglobin
  - *Male:* 13.8 to 17.2 g/dL (138 to 172 g/L)
  - *Female:* 12.1 to 15.1 g/dL (121 to 151 g/L)
- Hematocrit
  - *Male:* 40.7% to 50.3% (0.407 to 0.503)
  - *Female:* 36.1% to 44.3% (0.361 to 0.443)

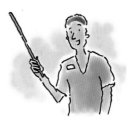

Chapter 2

Passing the NCLEX®

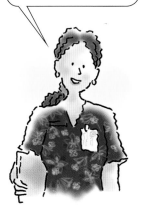

Pssst! Here's my secret formula for passing the NCLEX: Develop a creative study plan that includes sufficient scheduled study time, get plenty of rest and regular exercise, and believe in yourself!

Just the facts

In this chapter, you will review how:
◆ to properly prepare for the NCLEX
◆ to concentrate during difficult study times
◆ to make more effective use of your time
◆ creative strategies can enhance study.

Study preparations

If you are like most people preparing to take the NCLEX®, you are probably feeling nervous, anxious, or concerned. Keep in mind that most test-takers pass the first time.

Passing the test will not happen by accident, though; you will need to prepare carefully and efficiently. You should start studying sooner rather than later. To help jump-start your preparations:
• determine your strengths and weaknesses
• create a study schedule
• set realistic goals
• find an effective study space
• think positively.

Determine strengths and weaknesses

Most students recognize by the end of their nursing studies that they know more about some topics than others. Because the NCLEX covers a broad range of material, you should make some decisions about how intensively you will review each subject.

Make a review list

Decide what to include in a comprehensive list of topics you need to study. Start with the contents page in the front of this book, which summarizes the information you covered in school. Divide a sheet of paper in half vertically. Label one side "know well" and label the other side "needs review." List each topic from the contents page in the appropriate column. Do not worry if one list is longer than the other. After you have studied, you will feel strong in every area. Separating content areas this way helps you allocate your study time.

Schedule study time

Study when you are most alert. If you feel most alert and energized in the morning, for example, set aside sections of time early in the day for topics that need a lot of review. Then you can use the evening, a time you are less alert, to refresh your memory about more familiar topics. The opposite is true as well; if you are more alert in the evening, study difficult topics at that time.

What you will do when

Set up a basic schedule for studying. Using a calendar or an organizer, determine how much time remains before you will take the NCLEX. (See *2 to 3 months before the NCLEX®*, page 14.) Fill in the remaining days with specific times and topics to study.

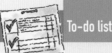

To-do list

2 to 3 months before the NCLEX®

Take these steps 2 to 3 months before you plan to take the examination:

• Establish a study schedule. Set aside ample time to study but leave time for social activities, exercise, family and personal responsibilities, and other matters.

• Become knowledgeable about the NCLEX: its content, the types of questions it asks, and the testing format by visiting the National Council of State Boards of Nursing (NCSBN) website at ncsbn.org.

• Begin reviewing and studying your notes, Web sites, texts, and other appropriate materials.

• Take some NCLEX practice questions and online examinations to help you diagnose your strengths and weaknesses as well as to become familiar with NCLEX questions and computerized testing.

For example, you might schedule the respiratory system on a Tuesday morning and the gastrointestinal system that afternoon. Remember to schedule difficult topics during your most alert times.

Keep in mind that you should not fill each day with studying. Be realistic and set aside time for breaks and activities. Try to create ample study time before the NCLEX and then stick to the schedule.

Set realistic goals

Part of creating a schedule means setting goals you can accomplish. You no doubt studied a great deal in nursing school, and by now you have a sense of your own capabilities. Ask yourself, "How much can I cover in a day?" Set aside that amount of time and then stay on task. You will feel better about yourself—and your chances of passing the NCLEX—when you meet your goals regularly.

Find an effective study space

Find a space to study that is conducive to effective learning. Whatever you do, do not study with videos playing in the room or in an environment with multiple sources of distraction. Instead, find an inviting, quiet, convenient place, away from normal traffic patterns. Sit in a solid chair that encourages good posture. (Avoid studying in bed; you will be more likely to fall asleep and not accomplish your goals.) The room should have comfortable, soft lighting with which you can see clearly without straining, a temperature between 65°F (18.3°C) and 70°F (21.1°C), and a comfortable environment.

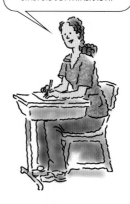

Approach your studying with enthusiasm, sincerity, and determination.

Accentuate the positive

Consider taping positive messages around your study space. Make signs with words of encouragement, such as "I CAN do it!" and "I WILL PASS!" These upbeat messages can help keep you going when your attention begins to waver.

Maintaining concentration

When you are faced with reviewing the amount of information covered by the NCLEX, it is easy to become distracted and lose your concentration. When you lose concentration, you make less effective use of valuable study time. To stay focused, keep these tips in mind.

• Alternate the order of the subjects you study to add variety to your day. Try alternating between topics you find more interesting and those you find less interesting.

• Approach your study with enthusiasm, sincerity, and determination.

- Begin studying on a schedule and do not let anything interfere with your thought processes after you have begun.
- Concentrate on accomplishing one task at a time, to the exclusion of everything else, such as going online and conversing with friends.
- Work continuously without interruption for a while but do not study for such a long period that the whole experience becomes grueling or boring.
- Take breaks to give yourself a change of pace. These breaks can ease your transition into studying a new topic.
- When studying in the evening, wind down from your studies slowly. Do not go directly from studying to sleeping.

Taking care of yourself

Never neglect your physical and mental well-being in favor of longer study hours. Maintaining physical and mental health is critical for success in taking the NCLEX. (See *4 to 6 weeks before the NCLEX®*.)

A few simple rules

You can increase your likelihood of passing the test by following simple health rules listed below.

- Get plenty of rest. You cannot think deeply or concentrate for long periods when you are tired.
- Eat nutritious meals and snacks. Maintaining your energy level is impossible when you are undernourished.
- Exercise regularly. Regular exercise helps you work harder and think more clearly. As a result, you will study more efficiently.

Memory power!

If you are having trouble concentrating but would rather push through than take a break, try making your studying more active by reading out loud. Active studying can renew your powers of concentration. By reading review material out loud, you are engaging your ears as well as your eyes—and making your study a more active process. Hearing the material out loud fosters memory and subsequent recall.

You can also rewrite in your own words a few of the more difficult concepts you are reviewing. Explaining these concepts in writing forces you to think through the material and can jump-start your memory.

Study schedule

When you were creating your schedule, you might have asked yourself, "How long should I study? One hour at a stretch? Two hours? Three?" To make the best use of your study time, you will need to answer those questions.

Optimal study time

Experts are divided about the optimal duration of study time. Some say you should study no more than 1 hour at a time several times per day. Their reasoning: You tend to only remember the material you study at the beginning and end of a longer session and are less likely to remember material studied in the middle of the session.

Other experts say you should hold longer study sessions because you lose time in the beginning, when you are just warming up, and again at the end, when you are cooling down. That means a long, concentrated study period will allow you to cover more material.

To thine own self be true

So what is the best plan? It does not matter as long as you determine what is best for you. At the beginning of your NCLEX study schedule, try study periods of varying lengths. Pay close attention to those that seem more successful.

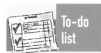

4 to 6 weeks before the NCLEX®

Take these steps 4 to 6 weeks before you plan to take the examination:

- Focus on your areas of weakness, identified through online and book review. Keep in mind that you will have time to review these areas again before the test date.
- Find a study partner or form a study group if you study well with others.
- Take practice tests to gauge your skill level early. Use remediation tools offered through online resources and book rationales to address your learning gaps.
- Take time to eat, sleep, exercise, and socialize to avoid burnout.

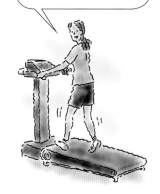

Regular exercise helps you work harder and think more clearly.

Remember that you are a trained nurse who competently collects data. Think of yourself as a client and collect data about your own progress. Then implement the strategy that works best for you.

Finding time to study

Regardless of the study plan you have chosen, remember that we all have periods in our day that might otherwise be dead time. These are perfect times to review for the NCLEX. However, you should not cover new material because you may not have enough time to get deeply into it. Always keep your mobile device or tablet, flash cards, or a small notebook handy for situations when you have a few extra minutes. (See *1 week before the NCLEX*.)

You will be amazed by how many short sessions you can find in a day and how much review you can do in 5 minutes. For example, the following occasions offer short stretches of time you can use for studying:
- eating breakfast
- waiting for a train or bus
- standing in line at the bank, post office, or store

Creative studying

Even when you study in a perfect place and concentrate better than ever, preparing for the NCLEX can get a little, well, dull. Even people with great study habits occasionally feel bored or sluggish. That is why it is important to have some creative tricks in your study bag to liven up those down times.

Creative studying does not have to be hard work. It involves making efforts to alter your study habits a bit. Some techniques that might help include alternating traditional book review with online adaptive quizzing programs, studying with a partner or group, and creating flash cards or other audiovisual study tools.

Online adaptive quizzing

Adaptive quizzing programs such as *Lippincott NCLEX-RN PassPoint* can help keep you engaged with learning because the quizzes and exams are individualized to your level of understanding. The more correct knowledge you demonstrate, the more challenging the learning experience becomes. PassPoint gives ongoing feedback about your strengths and weaknesses so you know how to prioritize your study plan. It gives you an opportunity to take NCLEX-style exams of varying lengths to help you build your endurance and become more familiar with a simulated computer adaptive testing environment. By alternating your book review and quizzing with online learning, you can stay energized and prepare for the NCLEX using the different media available to you.

Study partners

Studying with a partner or group of students can be an excellent way to energize your studying. It allows you to test each other on the material you have reviewed and share ways of studying. You can also encourage and help each other to stay motivated. Perhaps most important, working with a partner can provide a welcome break from solitary studying.

What to look for in a partner

Exercise care when choosing a study partner or assembling a study group. A partner who does not fit your needs will not help you make the most of your study time. Look for a partner who:
- has similar goals as yours—for example, someone taking the NCLEX at approximately the same date as you will likely feel the same sense of urgency as you and might make an excellent partner

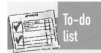

1 week before the NCLEX®

One week before the NCLEX, take these steps:
- Take a review test to measure your progress.
- Record key ideas and principles on your mobile device, tablet, note cards, or audiotapes.
- Rest, eat well, and avoid thinking about the examination during nonstudy times.
- Treat yourself to one special event. You have been working hard, and you deserve it!

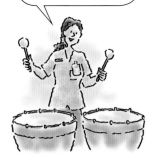

Studying getting dull? Get creative and liven it up.

- possesses about the same level of knowledge as you—tutoring someone can help you learn, but each partner should add to the other's knowledge
- studies without excessive chatting or interruptions—socializing is an important part of creative study, but you have to pass the NCLEX, so stay serious!

Audiovisual tools

Using flash cards and other audiovisual tools fosters retention and makes learning and reviewing fun.

Flash cards!

Flash cards can be an excellent study tool. The process of writing material on a flash card will help you remember it. In addition, flash cards are small and portable, perfect for those 5-minute slivers of time during the day.

Creating flash cards should be fun. Use magic markers, highlighters, and other colorful tools to make them visually stimulating. The more effort you put into creating your flash cards, the better you will remember the material contained on them.

Other visual tools

Flowcharts, drawings, diagrams, and other image-oriented study aids can also help you learn material more effectively. Substituting images for text can be a great way to give your eyes a break and recharge your brain. Use vivid colors to make your creations visually engaging.

Hear is the thing

If you learn more effectively when you hear information rather than see it, consider recording key ideas using a voice memo–type app on your phone or tablet. Recording information helps promote memory because you say the information aloud and then listen to it as it plays back. Like flash cards, these portable recordings are perfect for those short study periods during the day. (See *The day before the NCLEX®*.)

Practice questions

Practice questions should be an important part of your NCLEX study strategy. Practice questions can improve your studying by helping you review material and familiarize yourself with the exact style of questions you will encounter on the test. Remember to remediate all questions to ensure you understand rationales for the correct and *incorrect* answer choices. This will help you to apply the concept in other similar questions.

Practice at the beginning

Consider working through some practice questions as soon as you begin studying for the NCLEX. For example, you might try a few of the questions that appear at the end of each chapter in this book.

If you do well, you probably understand that topic and can spend less time reviewing it. If you have trouble with the questions, spend extra study time on that topic.

I am getting there

Practice questions can also provide an excellent means of marking your progress. Do not worry if you have trouble answering the first few practice questions; you will need time to learn how the questions are asked. Eventually, you will become accustomed to the question format and begin to focus more on the questions themselves.

If you make practice questions a regular part of your study regimen, you will be able to recognize areas in which you are improving. You can then adjust your study time accordingly.

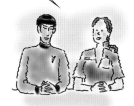

It isn't easy to find a partner who has the same study habits I do.

To-do list

The day before the NCLEX®

One day before the NCLEX, take these steps:
- Drive to the test site to check traffic patterns and find out where to park. If your drive occurs during heavy traffic or if you are expecting bad weather, set aside extra time to ensure your prompt arrival.
- Do something relaxing during the day.
- Avoid thinking too much about the test.
- Rest and eat well.
- Do not study.
- Call a supportive friend or relative for some last-minute words of encouragement.

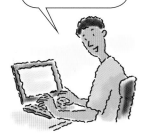

Taking lots of practice tests will help you succeed on the real exam!

Practice makes perfect

As you near the examination date, you should increase the number of NCLEX practice questions you answer at one sitting. This will enable you to approximate the experience of taking the actual NCLEX. Using thePoint Web site that accompanies this resource (the code for which is found on this inside cover of this book), you can take practice tests with varying numbers of questions. Additionally, this code offers you a free 7-day trial of *Lippincott NCLEX-RN PassPoint*, which allows you to take adaptive quizzes across the curriculum as well as to take practice exams of 75 to 265 questions. These practice exams simulate the real NCLEX in every way. Note that 75 questions is the minimum number of questions you will be asked on the actual NCLEX. Experts recommend doing a minimum of 75 questions at a time when practicing to closely mimic NCLEX. Then, gradually tackle larger practice tests to increase your confidence, build test-taking endurance, and strengthen the concentration skills that will enable you to succeed. (See *The day of the NCLEX®*.)

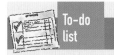

The day of the NCLEX®

On the day of the NCLEX:

* Eat a nutritious breakfast.
* Wear comfortable clothes, preferably with layers you can add and remove to adjust to the room temperature.
* Leave your house early so you can arrive at the test site with plenty of spare time.
* Do not study.
* Listen carefully to the instructions given before entering the test room.

Part II

Care of the Adult

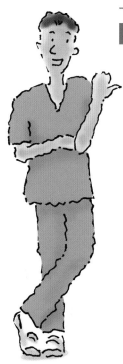

Chapter 3

Cardiovascular Disorders

Cardiovascular refresher

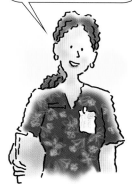

Abdominal aortic aneurysm

Stretched and bulging section of the wall of the aorta

Key signs and symptoms
- Commonly produces no symptoms

Key test results
- Abdominal x-ray shows an aneurysm.
- Computed tomography (CT) scan reveals size.

Key treatments
- Abdominal aortic aneurysm resection or repair
- Blood administration, as needed

Key interventions
- Assess, record, and monitor vital signs.
- Assess and monitor intake, output, and laboratory studies.
- Observe for signs of hypovolemic shock from aneurysm rupture, such as:
  - anxiety and restlessness
  - severe back pain
  - decreased pulse pressure
  - increased thready pulse
  - pale, cool, moist, clammy skin.

Angina

Chest pain caused by reduced blood flow to heart muscle

Key signs and symptoms
- Pain may be substernal, crushing, or compressing; may radiate to the arms, jaw, or back; usually lasts 3 to 5 minutes; usually occurs after exertion, emotional excitement, or exposure to cold but can also develop when at rest.

Key test results
- Electrocardiogram (ECG) shows ST-segment depression and T-wave inversion during anginal pain.

Key treatments
- Percutaneous transluminal coronary angioplasty (PTCA) or coronary artery stent placement

Key interventions
- Administer medications as prescribed.
- Withhold nitrates and notify health care provider if systolic blood pressure is less than 90 mm Hg.
- Withhold beta-blockers and notify health care provider if heart rate is less than 60 beats/minute.
- Assess and monitor for chest pain; if present, evaluate its characteristics.
- Obtain 12-lead ECG during an acute attack.

Arrhythmias

Abnormal heart rhythm

Key signs and symptoms

Atrial fibrillation
- Commonly produces no symptoms
- Irregular pulse with no pattern to the irregularity

Asystole
- Apnea
- Cyanosis
- No palpable blood pressure
- Pulselessness

Ventricular fibrillation
- Apnea
- No palpable blood pressure
- Pulselessness

Ventricular tachycardia
- Diaphoresis
- Hypotension
- Weak pulse or pulselessness
- Dizziness

Key test results

Atrial fibrillation
- ECG shows:
  - irregular atrial rhythm
  - atrial rate greater than 400 beats/minute
  - irregular ventricular rhythm
  - QRS complexes of uniform configuration and duration
  - no discernible PR interval
  - no P waves, or P waves that appear as erratic, irregular baseline fibrillation waves.

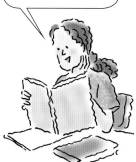

Asystole

- ECG shows no atrial or ventricular rate or rhythm, nor any discernible P waves, QRS complexes, or T waves.

Ventricular fibrillation

- ECG shows ventricular activity that appears as fibrillatory waves with no recognizable pattern.
- Atrial rate and rhythm and ventricular rhythm cannot be determined because no pattern or regularity occurs.
- The P wave, PR interval, QRS complex, T wave, and QT interval cannot be determined.

Ventricular tachycardia

- ECG shows ventricular rate of 100 to 250 beats/minute, wide and bizarre QRS complexes, and no discernible P waves.
- May start or stop suddenly.

Key treatments

Atrial fibrillation

- Antiarrhythmics: amiodarone, digoxin, diltiazem, procainamide
- Synchronized cardioversion (if client is unstable)

Asystole

- Cardiopulmonary resuscitation (CPR)
- Advanced cardiac life support (ACLS) protocol for endotracheal (ET) intubation and possible transcutaneous pacing
- Atropine, epinephrine per ACLS protocol

Ventricular fibrillation

- CPR
- Defibrillation
- ACLS protocol for ET intubation
- Amiodarone, epinephrine, lidocaine, magnesium sulfate, procainamide, vasopressin per ACLS protocol

Ventricular tachycardia

- CPR, if pulseless
- Defibrillation
- ACLS protocol for ET intubation
- Amiodarone, epinephrine, lidocaine, magnesium sulfate, procainamide

Key interventions

- Assess and monitor ECG to detect arrhythmias and ischemia.
- If pulse is abnormally rapid, slow, or irregular, watch for signs of hypoperfusion, such as hypotension and altered mental status.
- When life-threatening arrhythmias develop, rapidly assess the level of consciousness (LOC), respirations, and pulse.
- Initiate CPR, if indicated.
- Administer medications as needed, and prepare for medical procedures (e.g., cardioversion) if indicated.

- Monitor pulse oximetry. Provide adequate oxygen to reduce the heart's workload while carefully maintaining metabolic, neurologic, respiratory, and hemodynamic status.

Arterial occlusive disease

Narrowing of the arteries that leads to decreased blood supply to muscles and tissues

Key signs and symptoms

Femoral, popliteal, or innominate arteries

- Mottling of the affected extremity
- Pallor
- Paralysis and paresthesia in the affected arm or leg
- Pulselessness distal to the occlusion
- Sudden and localized pain in the affected arm or leg (most common symptom)
- Temperature change distal to the occlusion

Internal and external carotid arteries

- Transient ischemic attacks (TIAs) that produce transient monocular blindness, dysarthria, hemiparesis, possible aphasia, confusion, decreased mentation, headache

Subclavian artery

- Subclavian steal syndrome (SSS) (characterized by the backflow of blood from the brain through the vertebral artery on the same side as the occlusion into the subclavian artery distal to the occlusion; clinical effects of vertebrobasilar occlusion and exercise-induced arm claudication)

Vertebral and basilar arteries

- TIAs that produce binocular vision disturbances, vertigo, dysarthria, and falling without loss of consciousness

Key test results

- Arteriography demonstrates the type (thrombus or embolus), location, degree of obstruction, and the status of collateral circulation.
- Doppler ultrasonography shows decreased blood flow distal to the occlusion.

Key treatments

- Surgery (for acute arterial occlusive disease): atherectomy, balloon angioplasty, bypass graft, embolectomy, laser angioplasty, patch grafting, stent placement, thromboendarterectomy, amputation
- Thrombolytic agents: alteplase

Key interventions

Preoperatively (during an acute episode)

- Assess distal pulses and inspect skin color and temperature.

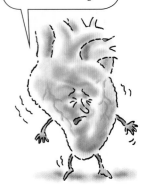

I'm sounding a little irregular. What could be wrong?

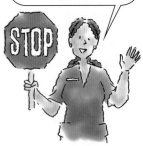

Your client is having a transient ischemic attack during an office visit. What signs and symptoms do you expect to assess?

- Assess pain and provide pain relief as needed.
- Initiate heparin infusion per protocol; monitor activated partial thromboplastin time (aPTT) and partial thromboplastin time (PTT).
- Assess for signs of fluid and electrolyte imbalance, and monitor intake and output for signs of renal failure (urine output less than 30 mL/hour).

Postoperatively
- Assess and monitor vital signs. Continuously assess circulatory function by inspecting skin color, taking temperature, and checking for distal pulses. While charting, compare earlier findings and observations. Watch closely for signs of hemorrhage (tachycardia, hypotension), and check dressings for excessive bleeding.
- Assess neurologic status frequently for changes in LOC, muscle strength, or pupil size.
- With mesenteric artery occlusion, connect a nasogastric tube to low intermittent suction. Monitor intake and output. Assess abdominal status.
- With saddle block occlusion, check distal pulses for adequate circulation. Assess for signs of renal failure and mesenteric artery occlusion (severe abdominal pain).
- With iliac artery occlusion, monitor urine output for signs of renal failure from decreased perfusion to the kidneys as a result of surgery. Provide meticulous catheter care.
- With femoral and popliteal artery occlusion, assist with early ambulation and discourage prolonged sitting.

Cardiac tamponade

Accumulation of blood or fluids in space between the sac encasing the heart and the heart muscle

Key signs and symptoms
- Muffled heart sounds on auscultation
- Narrow pulse pressure
- Jugular vein distention
- Pulsus paradoxus (abnormal inspiratory drop in systemic blood pressure greater than 15 mm Hg)
- Restlessness
- Upright, leaning forward posture

Key test results
- Chest x-ray shows slightly widened mediastinum and cardiomegaly.
- Echocardiography identifies pericardial effusion with signs of right ventricular and atrial compression.

- ECG may reveal:
  - low-amplitude QRS complex and electrical alternans
  - alternating beat-to-beat change in the amplitude of the P wave, QRS complex, and T wave
  - generalized ST-segment elevation in all leads.

Key treatments
- Supplemental oxygen
- Surgery: pericardiocentesis (needle aspiration of the pericardial cavity) or surgical creation of an opening to drain fluid (thoracotomy)
- Inotropic agent: dopamine

Key interventions
Pericardiocentesis
- Keep a pericardial aspiration needle attached to a 50-mL syringe by a three-way stopcock, an ECG machine, and an emergency cart with a defibrillator at the bedside. Keep the equipment turned on to be prepared for immediate use.
- Position the client at a 45- to 60-degree angle.
- Assess blood pressure during and after pericardiocentesis to watch for complications such as hypotension, which may indicate cardiac chamber puncture.
- Be alert for complications of pericardiocentesis, such as ventricular fibrillation, vasovagal response, or coronary artery or cardiac chamber puncture.

Thoracotomy
- Explain the procedure and what to expect after the operation (chest tubes, drainage bottles, administration of oxygen). Teach how to turn, deep-breathe, and cough.
- Setup and maintain the chest drainage system, and assess for complications, such as hemorrhage and arrhythmias.

Cardiogenic shock

Heart damaged so severely that it cannot supply enough blood to organs of the body

Key signs and symptoms
- Cold, clammy skin
- Hypotension (systolic pressure below 90 mm Hg)
- Narrow pulse pressure
- Tachycardia or other arrhythmias

Key test results
- ECG shows myocardial infarction (MI), as indicated by an enlarged Q wave and elevated ST segment.

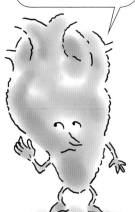

I'm sounding a little muffled. I wonder what that means?

Key treatments
- Intra-aortic balloon pump
- Adrenergic agent: epinephrine
- Cardiac glycoside: digoxin
- Cardiac inotropic agents: dopamine, dobutamine, milrinone
- Diuretics: furosemide, bumetanide, metolazone
- Vasodilators: nitroprusside sodium, nitroglycerin
- Vasopressor: norepinephrine

Key interventions
- Assess and monitor vital signs, heart sounds, capillary refill, skin temperature, and peripheral pulses.
- Assess and monitor ECG.
- Assess and monitor respiratory status, including breath sounds and arterial blood gas (ABG) levels.
- Administer oxygen and medications as prescribed.
- Maintain IV fluids.

Cardiomyopathy
Progressive heart muscle disease related to decreased contractility

Key signs and symptoms
- Murmur
- S3 and S4 heart sounds

Key test results
- ECG shows left ventricular hypertrophy and nonspecific changes.
- Echocardiogram shows dilated cardiomyopathy.

Key treatments
- Dual chamber pacing (for hypertrophic cardiomyopathy)
- Beta-blockers: atenolol, propranolol, nadolol, metoprolol for hypertrophic cardiomyopathy
- Calcium channel blockers: amlodipine, diltiazem for hypertrophic cardiomyopathy
- Diuretics: furosemide, bumetanide, metolazone for dilated cardiomyopathy
- Inotropic agents: dobutamine, milrinone, digoxin for dilated cardiomyopathy
- Oral anticoagulant: warfarin for dilated or hypertrophic cardiomyopathy

Key interventions
- Monitor ECG.
- Monitor vital signs.
- Administer oxygen and medications, as prescribed.

Coronary artery disease (CAD)
Plaque buildup in the arteries that supply blood to the heart

Key signs and symptoms
- Chest pain that may be substernal, crushing, or compressing; may radiate to the arms, jaw, or back; usually lasts 3 to 5 minutes; usually occurs after exertion, emotional excitement, or exposure to cold but can also develop when at rest

Key test results
- Blood chemistry tests show increased cholesterol (decreased high-density lipoproteins [HDL] and increased low-density lipoproteins [LDL]).
- ECG or Holter monitor shows ST-segment depression and T-wave inversion during an anginal episode.

Key treatments
- Activity changes, including weight loss, if necessary
- Dietary changes, including establishing a low-sodium, low-cholesterol, low-fat diet with increased dietary fiber (low-calorie only if appropriate)
- Oxygen therapy
- Antilipemic agents: cholestyramine, lovastatin, simvastatin, nicotinic acid, gemfibrozil, colestipol
- Antiplatelet aggregation: clopidogrel, aspirin
- Beta-blockers: atenolol, metoprolol

Key interventions
- Obtain ECG during anginal episodes.
- Assess vital signs.
- Continually monitor ECG.
- Monitor intake and output.
- Administer nitroglycerin for anginal episodes.

Endocarditis
Inflammation of the inside of the heart chambers and heart valves

Key signs and symptoms
- Chills
- Fatigue
- Fever
- Loud, regurgitant murmur

Key test results
- Echocardiography may identify valvular damage

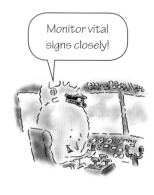

Monitor vital signs closely!

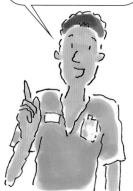

A client has been diagnosed with cardiomyopathy. What medications do you anticipate being prescribed?

- ECG may show atrial fibrillation and other arrhythmias that accompany valvular disease
- Three or more blood cultures in a 24- to 48-hour period identify the causative organism in up to 90% of clients

Key treatments
- Maintaining sufficient fluid intake
- Antibiotics: based on causative organism
- Antiplatelet agent: aspirin

Key interventions
- Obtain and monitor ECG.
- Assess and monitor cardiovascular status.
- Assess for signs of embolization (hematuria, pleuritic chest pain, left-upper-quadrant pain, and paresis), a common occurrence during the first 3 months of treatment.
- Assess and monitor the client's renal status (blood urea nitrogen [BUN] level, creatinine clearance, and urine output).
- Assess for signs of heart failure, such as dyspnea, tachypnea, tachycardia, crackles, jugular vein distention, edema, and weight gain.

Heart failure
Physiologic state when heart muscle is weakened and cannot pump enough blood to meet body's need of blood and oxygen

Key signs and symptoms
Left-sided failure
- Crackles
- Dyspnea
- Gallop rhythm: S3, S4 heart sounds

Right-sided failure
- Dependent edema
- Jugular vein distention
- Weight gain

Key test results
Left-sided failure
- B-type natriuretic peptide (BNP) levels elevated
- Chest x-ray shows increased pulmonary congestion and left ventricular hypertrophy

Right-sided failure
- BNP levels elevated
- Chest x-ray reveals pulmonary congestion, cardiomegaly, and pleural effusion

Key treatments
- Diuretics: furosemide, bumetanide, metolazone
- Human B-type natriuretic peptide: nesiritide
- Angiotensin-converting enzyme (ACE) inhibitors: captopril, enalapril, lisinopril
- Cardiac glycoside: digoxin

- Inotropic agents: dopamine, dobutamine
- Nitrates: isosorbide dinitrate, nitroglycerin
- Vasodilator: nitroprusside sodium

Key interventions
- Administer oxygen.
- Obtain ECG.
- Assess vital signs.
- Assess and monitor respiratory status.
- Keep the client in semi-Fowler's position.
- Weigh the client daily.

Hypertension
Blood pressure in arteries is elevated; also known as high blood pressure

Key signs and symptoms
- Produces no symptoms

Key test results
- Blood pressure measurements result in sustained readings greater than 130/80 mm Hg

Key Treatments
- Weight reduction
- Increased physical activity
- Dietary changes
- Reducing sodium intake
- Limiting alcohol intake
- ACE inhibitors: captopril, enalapril, lisinopril

Key interventions
- Assess and monitor vital signs. Take two or more blood pressure readings rather than relying on a single, possibly abnormal reading.

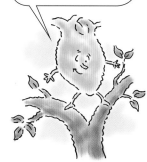
Exercise can help alleviate arterial blood pressure that is too high.

Hypovolemic shock
Severe blood and fluid loss making the heart unable to pump enough blood to the body

Key signs and symptoms
- Cold, pale, clammy skin
- Decreased sensorium
- Hypotension with narrow pulse pressure
- Reduced urine output (less than 25 mL/hour)
- Tachycardia

Key test results
- Blood tests show:
  - elevated serum potassium, serum lactate, and blood urea nitrogen (BUN) levels
  - increased urine specific gravity (greater than 1.020) and urine osmolality
  - decreased hemoglobin and hematocrit
  - decreased blood pH.
- ABG analysis reveals metabolic acidosis.

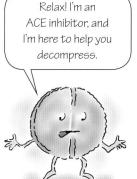
Relax! I'm an ACE inhibitor, and I'm here to help you decompress.

Key treatments

- Supplemental oxygen
- Blood and fluid replacement
- Control of bleeding

Key interventions

- Record blood pressure, pulse rate, peripheral pulses, respiratory rate, and pulse oximetry readings every 15 minutes, and monitor ECG continuously. A systolic blood pressure lower than 80 mm Hg usually results in inadequate coronary artery blood flow, cardiac ischemia, arrhythmias, and further complications of low cardiac output. When blood pressure drops below 80 mm Hg, increase the oxygen flow rate and notify the charge nurse or health care provider immediately.
- Initiate and maintain IV lines with normal saline or lactated Ringer's solution.
- Indwelling urinary catheter may be inserted to measure urine output. If less than 30 mL/hour in adults, increase the fluid infusion rate but watch for signs of fluid overload. Notify the charge nurse or health care provider if urine output does not improve. An osmotic diuretic such as mannitol may be prescribed.
- During therapy, assess skin color and temperature; note any changes.

Myocardial infarction

Irreversible necrosis of heart muscle secondary to prolonged ischemia; also known as a heart attack

Key signs and symptoms

- Crushing substernal chest pain that may:
  - radiate to the jaw, back, and arms
  - last longer than anginal pain
  - not be relieved by rest or nitroglycerin
  - not be present (in silent MI—present atypically in women, people with diabetes, and older adults).

Key test results

- ECG shows an enlarged Q wave, an elevated or a depressed ST segment, and T-wave inversion.
- Elevated cardiac biomarkers (myoglobin, troponin) confirm the diagnosis.

Key treatments

- Morphine sulfate
- Antiplatelet aggregation: aspirin, abciximab, clopidogrel, eptifibatide
- Thrombolytic agents: reteplase (tissue plasminogen activator [t-PA]); given within 6 hours of onset of symptoms but most effective when started within 3 hours

Key interventions

- Monitor respiratory status.
- Obtain an ECG reading during acute pain.

Myocarditis

Inflammation of the heart muscle

Key signs and symptoms

- Arrhythmias (S3 and S4 gallops, faint S1)
- Dyspnea
- Fatigue
- Fever

Key test results

- ECG typically shows diffuse ST-segment and T-wave abnormalities (as in pericarditis), conduction defects (prolonged PR interval), and other supraventricular arrhythmias.
- Endomyocardial biopsy confirms the diagnosis, but a negative biopsy *does not exclude* the diagnosis; repeat biopsy may be needed.

Key treatments

- Bed rest
- Antiarrhythmics: amiodarone, procainamide
- Antibiotics according to sensitivity of causative organism
- Cardiac glycoside: digoxin to increase myocardial contractility
- Diuretic: furosemide

Key interventions

- Assess and monitor breathing pattern and pulmonary status.
- Stress the importance of bed rest. Assist the client with bathing as needed; provide a bedside commode. Reassure the client that activity limitations are temporary.

Pericarditis

Inflammation of the sac covering the heart

Key signs and symptoms

Acute pericarditis
- Pericardial friction rub (grating sound heard as the heart moves)
- Sharp and (commonly) sudden pain that usually starts over the sternum and radiates to the neck, shoulders, back, and arms (unlike the pain of MI, pericardial pain is commonly pleuritic, increasing with deep inspiration and decreasing when the client sits up and leans forward, pulling the heart away from the diaphragmatic pleurae of the lungs)

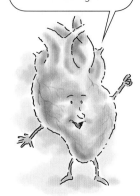

ECG and other tests can help to confirm a diagnosis.

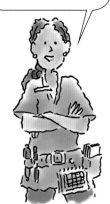

What key interventions do you need in your tool belt when caring for a client who's had a heart attack?

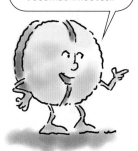

We antibiotics come in handy when your pericardium becomes infected.

Chronic pericarditis
- Pericardial friction rub
- Symptoms similar to those of chronic right-sided heart failure (fluid retention, ascites, hepatomegaly)

Key test results
- Echocardiography confirms the diagnosis when it shows an echo-free space between the ventricular wall and the pericardium (in cases of pleural effusion).
- ECG shows the following changes in acute pericarditis: elevation of ST segments in the standard limb leads and most precordial leads without significant changes in QRS morphology that occur with MI; atrial ectopic rhythms such as atrial fibrillation; and diminished QRS voltage in pericardial effusion.

Key treatments
- Bed rest
- Surgery: pericardiocentesis (for cardiac tamponade), partial pericardiectomy (for recurrent pericarditis), and total pericardiectomy (for constrictive pericarditis)
- Antibiotics according to sensitivity of causative organism

Key interventions
- Provide complete bed rest.
- Assess pain related to respiration and body position.
- Place client in an upright position.
- Provide analgesics and oxygen, and reassure the client with acute pericarditis that condition is temporary and treatable.

Pulmonary edema
Collection of excess fluid in the lungs

Key signs and symptoms
- Dyspnea, orthopnea, tachypnea

Key test results
- Chest x-ray shows pulmonary congestion.

Key treatments
- Diuretics: furosemide, bumetanide, metolazone
- Cardiac glycoside: digoxin
- Inotropic agents: dobutamine, milrinone, nesiritide
- Nitrates: isosorbide dinitrate, nitroglycerin
- Vasodilator: nitroprusside sodium

Key interventions
- Administer oxygen.
- Assess and monitor vital signs and breathing pattern.

- Place in high-Fowler's position if blood pressure remains stable; if hypotensive, maintain in semi-Fowler's position if tolerated.
- Obtain and monitor ECG.
- Monitor pulse oximetry readings.

Raynaud's disease
Reduced blood flow to fingers or toes in response to cold or emotional stress

Key signs and symptoms
- Numbness and tingling that are relieved by warmth
- Blanching of the skin on the fingers, which then become cyanotic before changing to red; typically occurs after exposure to cold or stress

Key test results
- Arteriography reveals vasospasm

Key treatments
- Activity changes: avoidance of cold
- Smoking cessation (if appropriate)
- Surgery (used in less than 25% of clients): sympathectomy
- Calcium channel blockers: diltiazem, nifedipine

Key interventions
- Educate client to avoid exposure to the cold, and to wear mittens/gloves in cold weather and when handling cold items

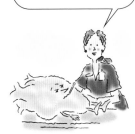

Wow—a temperature of 102°F (38.9°C), reports of pain and swelling in the joints, and recent history of strep throat. What is your diagnosis?

Rheumatic fever and rheumatic heart disease
Arises from complication of strep throat and can cause pain and swelling of joints and heart damage

Key signs and symptoms
- Temperature of 100.4°F (38°C) or higher
- Migratory joint pain or polyarthritis

Key test results
- Blood tests show elevated white blood cell count and erythrocyte sedimentation rate, as well as slight anemia during periods of inflammation.
- Cardiac enzyme levels may increase in severe carditis.
- C-reactive protein test is positive (especially during the acute phase).

Key treatments
- Bed rest (in severe cases)
- Surgery: corrective valvular surgery (in cases of persistent heart failure)

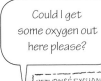

Could I get some oxygen out here please?

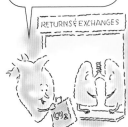

RETURNS & EXCHANGES

- Antibiotics: erythromycin, penicillin
- Nonsteroidal anti-inflammatory drugs (NSAIDs): aspirin, indomethacin

Key interventions

- Before giving penicillin, ask if client has ever had a hypersensitive reaction to it. Even if client has never had a reaction to penicillin, warn that such a reaction is possible.
- Warn client to watch for, and immediately report signs of, recurrent streptococcal infection:
  - diffuse throat redness and oropharyngeal exudate
  - swollen and tender cervical lymph glands
  - pain on swallowing
  - temperature of 101°F to 104°F (38.3°C to 40°C).
  - Urge client to avoid people with respiratory tract infections.

Thoracic aortic aneurysm

Stretched and bulging area in the wall of the aorta

Key signs and symptoms

Ascending aneurysm
- Pain (described as severe, penetrating, and ripping; extending to the neck, shoulders, lower back, or abdomen)
- Unequal intensities of the right carotid pulse and left radial pulse

Descending aneurysm
- Pain (described as sharp and tearing, usually starting suddenly between the shoulder blades and possibly radiating to the chest)

Transverse aneurysm
- Dyspnea
- Pain (described as sharp and tearing and radiating to the shoulders)

Key test results

- Aortography, the definitive test, shows the lumen of the aneurysm, its size and location, and the false lumen in a dissecting aneurysm.
- Chest x-ray shows widening of the aorta.
- Computed tomography (CT) scan confirms and locates the aneurysm and may be used to monitor its progression.

Key treatments

- Surgery: resection of aneurysm with a synthetic polymer graft replacement; possible replacement of aortic valve
- Blood product administration

- Oxygen therapy and possibly ET intubation and mechanical ventilation
- Analgesic: morphine
- Antihypertensives: nitroprusside sodium, labetalol
- Negative inotropic agent: propranolol

Key interventions

- Assess and monitor blood pressure. Also evaluate pain; breathing; and carotid, radial, and femoral pulses.
- Insert an indwelling urinary catheter. Maintain IV infusion of normal saline or lactated Ringer's solution and antibiotics as needed.
- When the health care provider suspects that an aneurysm is leaking, give any prescribed whole-blood transfusion.
- After repair of thoracic aneurysm:
  - evaluate the client's LOC. Monitor vital signs, pulse rate, urine output, and pain.
  - assess respiratory function. Carefully observe and record the type and amount of chest tube drainage, and frequently assess heart and breath sounds.
  - monitor IV therapy to prevent fluid excess, which may occur with rapid fluid replacement.
  - administer medications as appropriate.

Thrombophlebitis

Blood clot blocking one or more veins usually in legs

Key signs and symptoms

- Deep vein thrombosis
- Cramping calves
- Edema
- Tenderness to touch
- Superficial vein thrombosis
- Redness along vein
- Warmth and tenderness along vein

Key test results

- Photoplethysmography (PPG) shows venous-filling defects.
- Ultrasound reveals decreased blood flow.

Key treatments

- Activity changes: maintaining bed rest and elevating the affected extremity
- Anticoagulants: warfarin, heparin, dalteparin, enoxaparin sodium
- Antiplatelet aggregation agent: aspirin
- Fibrinolytic agent: reteplase (t-PA)

Key interventions

- Assess breathing pattern and breath sounds.

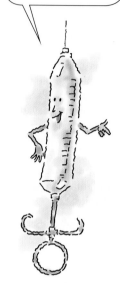

Make sure the client is not allergic to me before administering me!

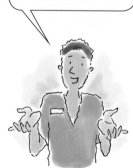

Thoracic aortic aneurysms can be extremely painful. What analgesic would be appropriate to administer?

- Maintain bed rest and elevate the affected extremity.
- Apply warm, moist compresses to improve circulation.
- Perform neurovascular checks.
- Monitor laboratory values.

Valvular heart disease

Any disease involving one of four valves of the heart

Key signs and symptoms

Aortic insufficiency
- Angina
- Cough
- Dyspnea
- Fatigue
- Palpitations

Mitral insufficiency
- Angina
- Dyspnea
- Fatigue
- Orthopnea
- Peripheral edema

Mitral stenosis
- Dyspnea on exertion
- Fatigue
- Orthopnea
- Palpitations
- Peripheral edema
- Weakness

Mitral valve prolapse
- May produce no symptoms
- Palpitations
- Tricuspid insufficiency
- Dyspnea
- Fatigue

Key test results

Aortic insufficiency
- Echocardiography shows left ventricular enlargement.
- Chest x-ray shows left ventricular enlargement and pulmonary vein congestion.

Mitral insufficiency
- Cardiac catheterization shows mitral regurgitation and elevated atrial and pulmonary artery wedge pressures

Mitral stenosis
- Cardiac catheterization shows diastolic pressure gradient across valve, and elevated left atrial and pulmonary artery wedge pressures.
- Echocardiography shows thickened mitral valve leaflets.
- ECG shows left atrial hypertrophy.
- Chest x-ray shows left atrial and ventricular enlargement.

Mitral valve prolapse
- ECG shows prolapse of the mitral valve into the left atrium
- Tricuspid insufficiency
- Echocardiography shows systolic prolapse of the tricuspid valve
- ECG shows right atrial or right ventricular hypertrophy
- Chest x-ray shows right atrial dilation and right ventricular enlargement

Key treatments

- Surgery: open-heart surgery using cardiopulmonary bypass for valve replacement (in severe cases)
- Anticoagulant: warfarin to prevent thrombus formation around diseased or replaced valves

Key interventions

- Assess closely for signs of heart failure or pulmonary edema; evaluate for adverse effects of drug therapy.
- Place in an upright position.
- Maintain bed rest; provide assistance with bathing, if necessary.
- If client undergoes surgery, assess for hypotension, arrhythmias, and thrombus formation. Assess and monitor vital signs, intake, output, daily weight, and blood chemistry values.

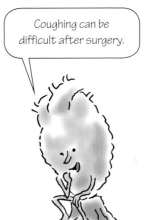

Coughing can be difficult after surgery.

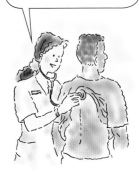

Listening to the client's heart and breathing can help you detect valvular heart disease.

Cardiovascular questions, answers, and rationales

1. An adult client is admitted to an acute care floor with the diagnosis of heart failure. Upon further workup the health care provider informs the nurse that the client has right-sided heart failure. Which symptom(s) does the nurse expect to assess in this client? Select all that apply.
1. Dependent edema
2. Jugular vein distention
3. Weight loss
4. Crackles
5. Weight gain

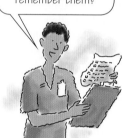

Right-sided heart failure has different symptoms from left-sided heart failure. Can you remember them?

1. **1, 2, 5.** Signs of right-sided heart failure include dependent edema, jugular vein distention, and weight gain. Crackles are a sign of left-sided heart failure. Weight loss is not an indication of heart failure.
CN: Physiological integrity; CNS: Physiological adaptation; CL: Apply

2. A client is seen in the emergency department and the health care provider suspects an abdominal aortic aneurysm. Which action(s) is **priority** for the nurse to perform? Select all that apply.
1. Monitor and record vital signs.
2. Monitor intake, output, and laboratory values.
3. Observe client for signs of hypovolemic shock.
4. Apply a non-rebreather oxygen mask.
5. Prepare the client for an abdominal ultrasound.

2. **1, 2, 3, 5.** The nurse should monitor and record vital signs, monitor input and output as well as laboratory values, observe the client for hypovolemic shock in case the aneurysm has ruptured, prepare for testing. An abdominal ultrasound is commonly used to diagnose an abdominal aortic aneurysm. There is no indication in the scenario that the client needs oxygen at this time.
CN: Safe, effective care environment; CNS: Management of care; CL: Apply

3. The nurse identifies which client to be at **greatest** risk for developing hypertension (HTN)?
1. A 45-year-old Caucasian woman who has diabetes mellitus and drinks a glass of wine once a month
2. A 58-year-old Caucasian man who works in a factory and does not eat gluten or dairy products
3. A 49-year-old woman of African decent who is moderately overweight and birthed four children
4. A 52-year-old man of African decent who has a sedentary lifestyle and drinks beer daily

3. **4.** Clients of African decent are two to three times more likely to develop hypertension than Caucasian clients. Men are more likely to have HTN than women until age 65. The older a person is, the more likely the person is to be diagnosed with HTN. Modifiable risk factors include sedentary lifestyle, poor diet high in sodium, overweight/obese, excessive alcohol consumption, hypercholesterolemia, diabetes, stress, sleep apnea, and smoking/tobacco use. Consuming a glass of wine monthly is not excessive; however, daily consumption of beer is. Factory work, a diet free of gluten and dairy, and parity are not related to HTN.
CN: Health promotion and maintenance; CNS: None; CL: Analyze

4. The nurse is caring for a client who is symptomatic for coronary artery disease (CAD). Which symptom(s) does the nurse expect to find when assessing this client? Select all that apply.
1. Chest pain
2. Arm pain
3. Jaw pain
4. Renal failure
5. Liver failure

4. **1, 2, 3.** Chest pain, arm pain, jaw pain, and back pain are key signs and symptoms of CAD. These can occur after exertion, emotional stress, or exposure to cold, but can also develop when the client is at rest. Renal and liver failure are not expected symptoms.
CN: Physiological integrity; CNS: Physiological adaptation; CL: Apply

5. A client calls the nurse and states, "I think I am having bad indigestion because my chest hurts." Which response by the nurse is **most** appropriate?
1. "Immediately go to the hospital."
2. "Have you ever felt this way before?"
3. "What did you eat yesterday?"
4. "Take an antacid and see if it subsides."

5. **1.** The most common symptom of an myocardial infarction is chest pain resulting from deprivation of oxygen to the heart. The nurse would inform the client to seek medical help immediately. All other responses are inappropriate as postponing care could lead to serious complication or even death.
CN: Safe, effective care environment; CNS: Management of care; CL: Apply

CN: Client needs category   CNS: Client needs subcategory   CL: Cognitive level

6. A client with a family history of heart disease is diagnosed with coronary artery disease (CAD). The client asks the nurse, "How might this affect my future health status?" Which nursing response(s) is appropriate? Select all that apply.
1. "It can lead to hypertension."
2. "It can lead to angina."
3. "It can lead to a myocardial infarction (MI)."
4. "It can lead to gastritis."
5. "It can lead to heart failure."

7. The nurse is obtaining a health history from a client who has just been diagnosed with coronary artery disease (CAD). Which finding(s) will the nurse report **immediately** to the health care provider? Select all that apply.
1. Normal findings during asymptomatic progression
2. Chest pain
3. Palpitations
4. Confusion
5. Syncope
6. Excessive fatigue

8. Which intervention is **best** for the nurse to suggest to a client who has a serum total cholesterol level of 250 mg/dL (6.47 mmol/L)?
1. Limit fats and carbohydrates.
2. Eat more animal meat and dairy.
3. Limit consumption of raw fruits.
4. Increase fresh vegetables each day.

9. Which nursing action is **priority** when caring for a client exhibiting manifestations of coronary artery disease?
1. Decrease anxiety level.
2. Enhance myocardial oxygenation.
3. Administer sublingual nitroglycerin.
4. Educate the client about symptoms.

10. The nurse is caring for a client newly diagnosed with coronary artery disease (CAD). Which prescription will the nurse anticipate the health care provider prescribing for this client?
1. Cardiac catheterization
2. Coronary artery bypass surgery
3. Lovastatin orally
4. Percutaneous transluminal coronary angioplasty (PTCA)

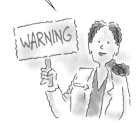
Warn your client that coronary artery disease can lead to many serious complications.

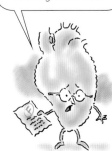
What do you mean I failed my cholesterol test? I thought 250 was a great score!

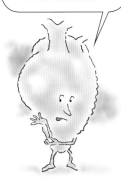
My arteries are feeling "gummed up" recently. What do you think I could do?

6. 1, 2, 3, 5. Coronary artery disease causes decreased perfusion of myocardial tissue and inadequate myocardial oxygen supply. This can cause hypertension, angina, MI, heart failure, and even death. Causes of gastritis, the inflammation of the stomach lining, include infection, injury, regular use of NSAIDs, and excessive alcohol consumption.
CN: Physiological integrity; CNS: Physiological adaptation; CL: Apply

7. 4. Confusion is associated with decreased blood flow to the brain, not the heart. This finding is not expected and should be immediately reported to the health care provider. Symptoms of CAD occur when the artery is occluded to the point that inadequate blood supply to the cardiac muscle occurs. Assessment findings include: potential normal findings during asymptomatic progression, chest pain, palpitations, syncope, and excessive fatigue.
CN: Safe, effective care environment; CNS: Management of care; CL: Apply

8. 1. A change in diet would be the best intervention and should include limited fats and carbohydrates. Total cholesterol levels above 240 mg/dL (6.22 mmol/L) are considered high; they require dietary restriction and, perhaps, medication. Eating more protein or limiting fruits will not help decrease the level. Easting more vegetables could be a good thing but does not guarantee a decrease in cholesterol.
CN: Physiological integrity; CNS: Reduction of risk potential; CL: Apply

9. 2. Enhancing myocardial oxygenation is always the priority when a client exhibits manifestations of cardiac compromise. Without adequate oxygen, the myocardium suffers damage. Sublingual nitroglycerin dilates the coronary vessels to increase blood flow, but its administration is not the priority. Although educating the client and decreasing anxiety are important, neither are priority for a compromised client.
CN: Safe, effective care environment; CNS: Management of care; CL: Apply

10. 3. Oral medication administration is a noninvasive medical treatment for CAD and is usually the initial treatment for coronary artery disease. Antilipemic agents such as lovastatin are generally prescribed. Cardiac catheterization is not a treatment but rather a diagnostic tool. Coronary artery bypass surgery and PTCA are invasive, surgical treatments.
CN: Physiological integrity; CNS: Pharmacological and parenteral therapies; CL: Apply

11. A client diagnosed with acute arterial occlusive disease is scheduled to undergo an atherectomy. What is the **priority** nursing intervention for this client **immediately** after the procedure?
1. Monitor vital signs every hour.
2. Closely monitor the site for bleeding.
3. Ambulate the client as soon as possible.
4. Teach client about the importance of exercise.

11. 2. Atherectomy is a surgical treatment used for acute arterial occlusive disease. After the procedure, the client should be monitored frequently for bleeding at the catheter site and vital signs should be taken every 15 minutes times four, and then every hour for the first few hours. Ambulation should be delayed for the first 12 hours, and exercise is not a priority at this time.
CN: Safe, effective care environment; CNS: Management of care; CL: Apply

12. A client with coronary artery disease (CAD) comes to the clinic with a total serum cholesterol level of 240 mg/dL (6.22 mmol/L). Which medication(s) does the nurse anticipate the health care provider will prescribe? Select all that apply.
1. Cholestyramine
2. Lovastatin
3. Atenolol
4. Propranolol
5. Metoprolol

12. 1, 2. Cholestyramine and lovastatin help to lower total cholesterol. Atenolol, propranolol, and metoprolol are not used to lower cholesterol, but prescribed to lower blood pressure and decrease tachycardia.
CN: Physiological integrity; CNS: Pharmacological and parenteral therapies; CL: Apply

13. Which area(s) on the precordium will the nurse use for auscultation of heart sounds. Select all that apply.
1. Aortic area
2. Pulmonic area
3. Erb's point
4. Mitral area
5. Tricuspid area
6. Bronchial area

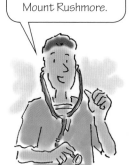

When auscultating, remember your landmarks—and I'm not talking about Mount Rushmore.

13. 1, 2, 3, 4, 5. The correct landmarks that can be used for auscultation of heart sounds are the aortic area, pulmonic area, Erb's point, tricuspid area and mitral area. Bronchial area is not appropriate.
CN: Physiological integrity; CNS: Physiological adaptation; CL: Apply

14. A client is hospitalized to rule out an acute myocardial infarction (MI). Laboratory results are: lactate dehydrogenase (LDH) level 140 U/L (2.34 µkat/L) and troponin I level 0.5 ng/mL (0.5 µg/L). The nurse enters the client's room and finds the client pacing the floor. Which statement by the nurse is **most** appropriate in this situation?
1. "You had a heart attack. Get back in bed now."
2. "You seem upset. Let us sit and talk for a while."
3. "You sure have a lot of energy; do you want to play cards?"
4. "Your health care provider does not want you up. Please get into bed."

14. 2. Given the laboratory data, especially the elevated troponin I level, the nurse should realize that the client probably had an MI and needs to lie down and rest the heart. However, the nurse should also realize the need to respond to the client's emotional distress by acknowledging the client's feelings and offering to discuss the situation. Stating the client had a heart attack would be giving a medical diagnosis that has not yet been made and would also be practicing outside the scope of nursing. A comment about the energy level acknowledges the client's pacing but not the underlying concerns. Stating the health care provider's preferences attempts to impose authority to control the client's behavior. It does not acknowledge the client's distress.
CN: Safe, effective care environment; CNS: Management of care; CL: Apply

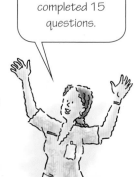

Hooray! You've completed 15 questions.

15. The nurse is admitting a client for suspected myocardial infarction (MI). The nurse will prepare the client for which laboratory test **first**?
1. Arterial blood gas (ABG) levels
2. Complete blood count (CBC)
3. Complete chemistry
4. Creatine kinase isoenzymes (CK-MB)

15. 4. CK-MB isoenzymes are present in the blood after a MI. These enzymes spill into the plasma when cardiac tissue is damaged. ABG levels are obtained to review respiratory function, a CBC is obtained to review blood counts, and a complete chemistry is obtained to review electrolytes. Other testing may be indicated depending on the results of the CK-MB.
CN: Health promotion and maintenance; CNS: None; CL: Apply

CN: Client needs category   CNS: Client needs subcategory   CL: Cognitive level

16. A client is having an acute myocardial infarction (MI). Which prescription(s) will the emergency room nurse complete? Select all that apply.
1. Prepare the client for an angioplasty.
2. Administer intravenous morphine.
3. Apply a 12-lead electrocardiogram.
4. Administer aspirin orally.
5. Provide oxygen therapy.

16. **1, 2, 3, 4, 5.** An angioplasty may be done to unblock the arteries. Morphine is administered as analgesia because chest pain stimulates the sympathetic nervous system, leading to an increase in heart rate and vasoconstriction. In addition, morphine will reduce anxiety and the workload of the heart; however, the primary indication to administer morphine is to relieve chest pain. An EKG will assist in determining which area of the heart was affected and to monitor the heart. Aspirin is given to prevent platelet aggregation. Oxygen is given to assist in tissue perfusion.
CN: Safe, effective care environment; CNS: Management of care; CL: Apply

17. When educating a client about the importance of smoking cessation, which statement(s) made by the client indicates to the nurse the education is understood? Select all that apply.
1. "It causes platelets in the blood to clump together and become sticky."
2. "It causes spasms in the coronary arteries to occur."
3. "Clients who smoke have lower high-density lipoprotein levels."
4. "Smoking causes vasodilatation of the arteries."
5. "It reduces the amount of oxygen carried by red blood cells."

17. **1, 2, 3, 5.** Smoking is the leading modifiable risk factor for developing coronary heart disease. Smoking causes the platelets of the blood to clump together, causes spasms in the coronary arteries, lowers good cholesterol, causes vasoconstriction, and reduces the amount of oxygen carried in the red blood cells.
CN: Physiological integrity; CNS: Physiological adaptation; CL: Apply

18. An adult client with heart failure and 2+ pitting edema is prescribed furosemide. Which supplemental medication does the nurse expect will be prescribed for this client?
1. Chloride
2. Digoxin
3. Potassium
4. Sodium

18. **3.** Supplemental potassium is given with furosemide because potassium loss occurs as a result of this diuretic. Chloride and sodium are not lost during diuresis. Digoxin acts to increase contractility but is not given routinely with furosemide.
CN: Physiological integrity; CNS: Pharmacological and parenteral therapies; CL: Apply

19. A client recently had a myocardial infarction (MI). Which finding does the nurse identify to be a normal metabolic change occurring after an MI?
1. Slowing of impulses through the atrioventricular (AV) node
2. Increased platelet aggregation
3. Decreased left ventricular ejection fraction
4. Increased serum glucose and free fatty acid protein levels

19. **4.** Glucose and fatty acids are metabolites whose levels increase after an MI. Slow conduction of impulses through the AV node is an electrophysiologic change. Hematologic changes affect the blood cells and platelets. Ejection fraction measures the mechanical pumping action of the heart.
CN: Physiological integrity; CNS: Physiological adaptation; CL: Apply

20. The nurse is auscultating a client's heart and identifies a third heart sound. Which additional finding(s) will the nurse expect to assess? Select all that apply.
1. Dyspnea while supine
2. Bradycardia
3. Persistent cough with pink sputum
4. Nocturnal polydipsia
5. Increased hunger
6. Rapid weight gain

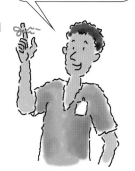
Can you remember what the third heart sound indicates— other than the fact that you're alive?

20. **1, 3, 4, 6.** An S3 sound occurs when the ventricles are resistant to filling and is heard just after S2 when the atrioventricular valves open. The most common cause is congestive heart failure, which the nurse would expect to assess in this client is dyspnea while supine or with exertion. Tachycardia, not bradycardia, is expected. A persistent cough with white or blood-tinged sputum, nocturnal polydipsia, and rapid weight gain are expected. A lack of appetite is common.
CN: Physiological integrity, CNS: Physiological adaptation; CL: Apply

CN: Client needs category   CNS: Client needs subcategory   CL: Cognitive level

21. The nurse is caring for a client who had an anterior wall myocardial infarction (MI). During assessment, the nurse notes crackles in the client's lungs. What nursing action is **priority**?
1. Notify the health care provider.
2. Reassess the client in 1 hour.
3. Apply oxygen via nasal cannula.
4. Document the finding in the medical record.

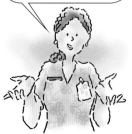

I'm hearing some crackles and galloping. What condition do you suspect?

21. 1. The nurse would suspect the client is experiencing left-sided heart failure. The left ventricle is responsible for most of the cardiac output. An anterior wall MI may result in a decrease in left ventricular function. When the left ventricle does not function properly, resulting in left-sided heart failure, fluid accumulates in the interstitial and alveolar spaces in the lungs and causes crackles. The health care provider needs to be notified to confirm the nurse's suspicion. There are no indications the client needs oxygen therapy at this time. The nurse would assess respiratory rate and oxygen saturation level to determine if oxygen is needed. The nurse would document the finding and reassess the client; however, these are not priority as they provide no assistance to the client at this time.
CN: Safe, effective care environment; CNS: Management of care; CL: Analyze

22. A client is admitted to the emergency department with chest discomfort, diaphoresis, and nausea. Suspecting possible myocardial infarction (MI), the nurse prepares the client for which test **first**?
1. Cardiac catheterization
2. Cardiac enzymes
3. Echocardiogram
4. Electrocardiogram (ECG)

22. 4. ECG is the quickest, most accurate, and most widely used tool to diagnose a MI. Cardiac enzymes also are used to diagnose MI, but the results cannot be obtained as quickly. An echocardiogram is used most widely to view myocardial wall function after an MI has been diagnosed. Cardiac catheterization is an invasive study for determining coronary artery disease.
CN: Safe, effective care environment; CNS: Management of care; CL: Analyze

23. What is the nurse's **first** intervention for a client experiencing a myocardial infarction (MI)?
1. Give morphine intravenously.
2. Apply oxygen via a facemask.
3. Provide sublingual nitroglycerin.
4. Administer aspirin.

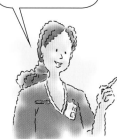

*Remember— Question 23 is asking what you should do **first**.*

23. 2. Administering supplemental oxygen to the client is the first priority of care. The myocardium is deprived of oxygen during an infarction, so additional oxygen is administered to assist in oxygenation and prevent further damage. Next, the nurse will give nitroglycerin, followed by aspirin, and last is morphine. Remember the acronym ONAM (oxygen, nitroglycerin, aspirin, morphine) for clients experiencing a MI.
CN: Safe, effective care environment; CNS: Management of care; CL: Analyze

24. Which symptom(s) will the nurse report to the health care provider if assessed in a client diagnosed with left-sided heart failure? Select all that apply.
1. Syncope
2. Orthopnea
3. Jugular vein distention
4. Peripheral edema
5. S3 heart gallop
6. Ascites

24. 3, 4, 6. The nurse would report unexpected findings to the health care provider. Jugular vein distention, peripheral edema, and ascites are expected in clients with right-sided heart failure. Right-sided heart failure often results from left-sided heart failure. When the left ventricle fails, increased pressure in the lungs can result in right-sided damage. Symptoms result when the right side no longer pumps effectively, leading to venous congestion. Left-sided heart failure causes decreased cardiac output and increases pulmonary congestion. Decreased cardiac output may cause a decrease in cerebral perfusion, resulting in syncope. Orthopnea is caused by pulmonary congestion. Development of an S3 gallop is caused by the left atria attempting to fill the distended left ventricle.
CN: Safe, effective care environment; CNS: Management of care; CL: Apply

25. The nurse is discharging a client diagnosed with hypertension after having a myocardial infarction (MI). The nurse will question which prescription?
1. Metolazone
2. Metolazone
3. Losartan
4. Amiodarone

26. A client treated for a myocardial infarction (MI) in the emergency room is admitted to the hospital. The nurse will complete which prescription **first**?
1. Give metolazone 2.5 mg daily.
2. Administer aspirin 160 mg daily.
3. Apply cardiac monitor.
4. Consult cardiac rehabilitation.

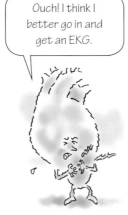

Ouch! I think I better go in and get an EKG.

27. The nurse is assessing a client and observes jugular vein distention (JVD). The nurse will assess the client for which condition?
1. Abdominal aortic aneurysm
2. Heart failure
3. Myocardial infarction (MI)
4. Deep vein thrombosis

28. The client is prescribed amlodipine. Which primary action(s) will the nurse discuss with the client? Select all that apply.
1. Dilation of arteries
2. Decreases peripheral vascular resistance
3. Increases overload
4. Reduces afterload
5. Promotes calcium influx

29. Which symptom(s) does the nurse expect a client with right-sided heart failure to exhibit? Select all that apply.
1. Jugular vein distention (JVD)
2. Peripheral edema
3. Hepatomegaly
4. Fatigue
5. Crackles

25. 4. The nurse would question amiodarone being prescribed for this client. Antiarrhythmics such as amiodarone are used to treat life-threatening recurrent ventricular fibrillation and hemodynamically unstable tachycardia. Beta-blockers, such as metoprolol, work by decreasing catecholamines and sympathetic nerve stimulation. They protect the myocardium, helping to reduce the risk of another infarction by decreasing the heart's workload. Thiazide diuretics, such as metolazone, work by limiting the body's ability to absorb sodium, resulting in fluid excretion. Angiotensin II receptor blockers, such as losartan, work by reducing the effect of angiotensin II in the body. This results in vasodilation, which lowers blood pressure.
CN: Physiological integrity; CNS: Pharmacological and parenteral therapies; CL: Apply

26. 3. The nurse would first apply cardiac monitors to assess for arrhythmias. Arrhythmias, caused by oxygen deprivation to the myocardium, are the most common complication of an MI. Metolazone and aspirin are long-term medications used to prevent another MI. Aspirin may be prescribed in conjunction with another antiplatelet medication; this is known as dual antiplatelet therapy (DAPT). Consulting cardiac rehabilitation assists a client to recover from a MI and is not priority.
CN: Safe, effective care environment; CNS: Management of care; CL: Analyze

27. 2. Elevated venous pressure, exhibited as JVD, indicates the heart's failure to pump. This is not a symptom of abdominal aortic aneurysm or deep vein thrombosis. A MI, if severe enough, can progress to heart failure; however, in and of itself, a MI does not cause JVD.
CN: Physiological integrity; CNS: Physiological adaptation; CL: Apply

28. 1, 2, 4. Amlodipine is a calcium channel blocker, which inhibits calcium influx through the coronary arteries, causing arterial dilation and decreasing peripheral vascular resistance, which reduces afterload. Impulse conduction is slowed when calcium flow into cardiac cells is inhibited and contractility is decreased.
CN: Physiological integrity; CNS: Pharmacological and parenteral therapies; CL: Apply

29. 1, 2, 3, 4. During right-sided heart failure, the right ventricle fails to empty adequately, causing a backup of blood into systemic blood vessels. This can lead to jugular vein distention, peripheral edema, fatigue, and hepatomegaly. Crackles are a symptom of left-sided heart failure.
CN: Physiological integrity; CNS: Physiological adaptation; CL: Apply

CN: Client needs category   CNS: Client needs subcategory   CL: Cognitive level

30. An adult client is newly diagnosed with left-sided heart failure. Which sign, **most** commonly associated with this type of heart failure, will the nurse expect to note when assessing this client?
1. Crackles
2. Arrhythmias
3. Hepatic engorgement
4. Hypotension

30. 1. Crackles in the lungs are a classic sign of left-sided heart failure. These sounds are caused by fluid backing up into the pulmonary system. Arrhythmias can be associated with right- and left-sided heart failure. Hepatic engorgement is associated with right-sided heart failure. Left-sided heart failure causes hypertension, not hypotension, secondary to an increased workload on the system.
CN: Physiological integrity; CNS: Physiological adaptation; CL: Apply

31. The nurse is preparing to administer digoxin to a client. What will the nurse do **before** administering digoxin?
1. Assess an apical pulse.
2. Monitor the blood pressure.
3. Weigh the client.
4. Check the respiratory rate.

31. 1. An apical pulse is essential for accurately assessing the client's heart rate before administering digoxin. The apical pulse is the most accurate pulse point in the body. An apical pulse should be checked for 1 minute prior to administration. The nurse will withhold digoxin and notify the health care provider if the pulse is <60 bpm in an adult. Blood pressure is monitored periodically, as it usually is only affected if the heart rate is too low, in which case the nurse would withhold digoxin. The client is generally weighed daily but does not have to be weighed at the time of medication administration. Digoxin has no effect on respiratory function.
CN: Physiological integrity; CNS: Pharmacological and parenteral therapies; CL: Apply

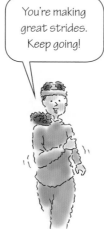

You're making great strides. Keep going!

32. A client is admitted to the hospital displaying sinus bradycardia, nausea, anorexia, and blurred vision. The nurse anticipates treating the client for which condition?
1. Digoxin toxicity
2. Myocardial infarction
3. Hypertensive crisis
4. Cor pulmonale

32. 1. Digoxin toxicity typically causes bradycardia, nausea, anorexia, and vision disturbances. A MI, hypertensive crisis, and cor pulmonale usually do not cause vision disturbance.
CN: Physiological integrity; CNS: Physiological adaptation; CL: Apply

33. The nurse receives report on a client who has been diagnosed with an abdominal aortic aneurysm (AAA). The nurse will expect the client to have which underlying disease?
1. Atherosclerosis
2. Type 1 diabetes
3. Chronic obstructive pulmonary disease (COPD)
4. Renal failure

33. 1. Atherosclerosis is linked to 75% of all AAAs. Plaque damages the wall of the artery and weakens it, causing an aneurysm. Although the other conditions are related to the development of aneurysm, none is a direct cause.
CN: Health promotion and maintenance; CNS: None; CL: Apply

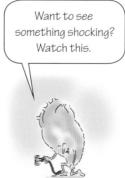

Want to see something shocking? Watch this.

34. A client demonstrates signs of cardiogenic shock. Which medication(s) will the nurse expect the health care provider to prescribe for this client? Select all that apply.
1. Digoxin
2. Dopamine
3. Furosemide
4. Clopidogrel
5. Nitroprusside sodium

34. 1, 2, 3, 5. Medications given for cardiogenic shock include a cardiac glycoside (digoxin), a cardiac inotropic agent (dopamine), a diuretic (furosemide), and a vasodilator (nitroprusside sodium). The client does not indicate a need for an antiplatelet aggregate such as clopidogrel.
CN: Physiological integrity; CNS: Pharmacological and parenteral therapies; CL: Analyze

35. The nurse is monitoring a client with asthma taking atenolol. Which finding **most** concerns the nurse?
1. Baseline blood pressure 166/88 mm Hg; blood pressure 138/74 mm Hg after two doses of medication
2. Baseline resting heart rate 106 beats/minute; resting heart rate 88 beats/minute after two doses of medication
3. Development of audible expiratory wheezes the nurse can hear from anyplace in the client's room
4. A serum potassium level of 4.2 mEq/L (4.2 mmol/L) taken this morning prior to the start of the shift

36. A client is placed on epinephrine to stimulate the sympathetic nervous system. Which finding indicates to the nurse the client is responding appropriately to this medication?
1. Heart rate decreased from 78 to 56 beats/minute
2. Heart rate increased from 60 to 88 beats/minute
3. Blood pressure decreased from 120/80 to 100/56 mm Hg
4. Decrease of myocardial contractility

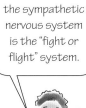
Remember— the sympathetic nervous system is the "fight or flight" system.

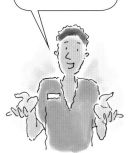

37. The nurse notes dependent edema, weight gain, shortness of breath, and jugular vein distention (JVD) while assessing a 62-year-old client. The client's brain natriuretic peptide (BNP) level is 950 pg/mL (950 ng/L). Which nursing intervention is **priority**?
1. Administer furosemide IV.
2. Complete chest x-ray as prescribed.
3. Notify the health care provider.
4. Apply oxygen to the client.

38. The nurse is caring for a client with a diagnosis of an abdominal aortic aneurysm (AAA). Locate the area in which this is found.

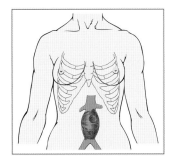

35. 3. Audible wheezing may indicate serious bronchospasm, especially in clients with asthma or obstructive pulmonary disease. Decreases in blood pressure and heart rate are expected outcomes when beta-blockers are administered. A serum potassium level of 4.2 mEq/L (4.2 mmol/L) is within normal limits.
CN: Physiological integrity; CNS: Pharmacological and parenteral therapies; CL: Analyze

36. 2. Epinephrine is a vasopressor, which belongs to a category of drugs called adrenergic drugs. Adrenergic drugs stimulate the sympathetic nervous system, causing tachycardia, increased blood pressure, vasoconstriction, and bronchodilation. This response causes an increase in contractility, which compensates for the response. The other symptoms listed are related to the parasympathetic nervous system, which is responsible for slowing the heart rate.
CN: Physiological integrity; CNS: Physiological adaptation; CL: Apply

37. 4. The nurse would first apply oxygen to the client having shortness of breath. The BNP level indicates unstable heart failure (>900 pg/mL [>900 ng/L] in clients age 50 or older); therefore, the nurse would notify the health care provider. Dependent edema, weight gain, and JVD are secondary effects of right-sided heart failure. A chest x-ray may be done to assess for pulmonary congestion. Furosemide would be given to promote fluid excretion.
CN: Safe, effective care environment; CNS: Management of care; CL: Analyze

38. The portion of the aorta distal to the renal arteries is more prone to aneurysm formation due to increased pressure as it divides into the iliac arteries. The aorta is proximal to the iliac arteries. There is no area adjacent to the aortic arch, which bends into the thoracic (descending) aorta. Aortic aneurysms proximal to the renal arteries are uncommon.

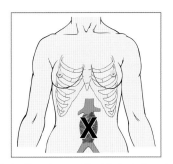

CN: Physiological integrity; CNS: Physiological adaptation; CL: Apply

39. The nurse is administering digoxin to a client with pulmonary edema. Which finding will cause the nurse to hold the medication?
1. The client states, "I feel very sleepy."
2. The client's pulse is 69 beats/minute.
3. Urine output is 940 mL over the past 24 hours.
4. Digoxin level is 3.5 ng/mL (4.48 nmol/L).

40. A client is admitted with acute pulmonary edema. Which signs and symptoms will the nurse expect this client to exhibit?
1. Weight gain, abdominal distention, peripheral edema, jugular vein distention (JVD), tachycardia, and restlessness
2. Apprehension and restlessness, cough with frothy pink sputum, moist gurgling respirations with tachypnea, and orthopnea
3. Exertional dyspnea, cough with mucopurulent sputum, prolonged expiration with wheezing and crackles, and orthopnea
4. Sharp chest pain that worsens on inspiration, dyspnea, cyanosis, light-headedness, and tachycardia

41. The nurse is providing discharge education to a client diagnosed with unilateral, lower extremity deep vein thrombophlebitis (DVT). Which client statement indicates to the nurse additional discharge education is needed?
1. "I will elevate my legs when sitting and get up and walk around periodically."
2. "I need to take my warfarin exactly the way my health care provider prescribed it."
3. "If my compression hose roll down behind my knees, I will pull them up."
4. "I will contact my health care provider immediately if I have unusual bleeding."

42. A client is admitted to the emergency department with a pulsating sensation in the abdomen and an audible bruit. Which test will the nurse expect to prepare the client for **first**?
1. Abdominal x-ray
2. Arteriogram
3. Computed tomography (CT) scan
4. Ultrasound

43. Which finding(s) **most** concerns the nurse caring for a preoperative adult client with an abdominal aortic aneurysm (AAA)? Select all that apply.
1. Clammy skin
2. Sudden back pain
3. Pulsation near the umbilicus
4. Pulse 88 bpm
5. Blood pressure 84/46 mm Hg
6. Intermittent, dull abdominal pain

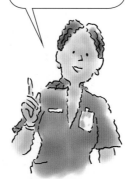

Don't be apprehensive about question #43. I'm sure you can figure it out.

39. 4. The nurse would withhold digoxin for a serum level of 3.5 ng/mL (4.48 nmol/L). Therapeutic digoxin levels range from 0.5 to 2 ng/mL (0.64 to 2.56 nmol/L). Feeling sleepy is not an indication to hold digoxin. The pulse rate and urine output are both within normal limits.
CN: Physiological integrity; CNS: Pharmacological and parenteral therapies; CL: Apply

40. 2. Apprehension, restlessness, frothy pink sputum, and moist breath sounds are typical findings in clients with acute pulmonary edema. Weight gain, edema, and JVD are signs and symptoms of right-sided heart failure. Exertional dyspnea and mucopurulent sputum are typical of emphysema. Chest pain that worsens with inspiration, dyspnea, cyanosis, light-headedness, and tachycardia are typical signs of acute pulmonary embolism.
CN: Physiological integrity; CNS: Physiological adaptation; CL: Apply

41. 3. Hose that roll down behind the knee indicates improperly fitting hose that will impede venous return and cause venous stasis. Support hose should be smooth from the toes to the end of the hose. Elevating the legs while sitting promotes venous return. Warfarin must be taken exactly as prescribed, and the client must monitor for potential bleeding.
CN: Physiological integrity; CNS: Reduction of risk potential; CL: Apply

42. 4. Ultrasound is a noninvasive, cost-effective method of determining the presence of an abdominal aortic aneurysm (AAA) with 95% accuracy. Arteriograms and CT scans are more expensive, require the use of contrast agents and radiation, and are riskier to the client. An AAA would only be visible on an x-ray if it were calcified.
CN: Safe, effective care environment; CNS: Management of care; CL: Analyze

43. 1, 2, 5. Clammy skin; sudden, intense, and persistent abdominal or back pain that is described as a tearing sensation; hypotension; and tachycardia are indications that an AAA has ruptured. Rupture of the aneurysm is a life-threatening emergency. A pulsation and dull, intermittent, or constant abdominal or back pain are expected findings with an AAA. A heart rate of 88 bpm is within normal range.
CN: Physiological integrity; CNS: Reduction of risk potential; CL: Apply

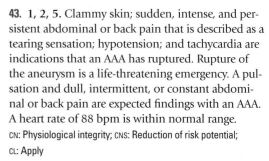

44. A client comes to the emergency department with symptoms of a myocardial infarction. The health care provider prescribes reteplase. The nurse will administer reteplase to the client at which time?
1. Within 3 hours of onset of symptoms
2. Within 6 hours of onset of symptoms
3. Within 8 hours of onset of symptoms
4. Within 12 hours of onset of symptoms

44. 1. Thrombolytic agents such as reteplase can be given within 6 hours of the onset of symptoms but will be most effective when started within 3 hours. CN: Physiological integrity; CNS: Pharmacological and parenteral therapies; CL: Apply

45. Which precaution will the nurse take when caring for a client with a myocardial infarction who has received a thrombolytic agent?
1. Avoid puncture wounds.
2. Monitor potassium level.
3. Maintain a supine position.
4. Restrict fluid intake.

45. 1. Thrombolytic agents are declotting agents that place the client at risk for hemorrhage from puncture wounds. All unnecessary needle sticks and invasive procedures should be avoided. The potassium level should be monitored in all cardiac clients, not just those receiving a thrombolytic agent. Although no specific position is required, most cardiac clients seem more comfortable in semi-Fowler's position. The client's fluid balance must be carefully monitored, but it is inappropriate to restrict fluid intake. CN: Physiological integrity; CNS: Reduction of risk potential; CL: Apply

46. The nurse knows which client is at **highest** risk of developing an abdominal aortic aneurysm (AAA)?
1. A 54-year-old female client who has an infection of the aorta and a family history of heart failure.
2. A 69-year-old male client who has smoked for 55 years and whose blood pressure is 144/92 mm Hg
3. A 75-year-old female client with new onset type 1 diabetes mellitus and a history of alcohol use disorder
4. A 60-year-old male client whose father died suddenly from a ruptured abdominal aortic aneurysm

46. 2. Risk factors for AAA include age 65 and older, tobacco use, Caucasian ethnicity, male gender, family history, atherosclerosis, hypertension, and a history of large vessel aneurysms. Aorta infections are rarely associated with AAAs. A family history of heart failure, diabetes, and alcohol use disorder are not associated with AAAs. CN: Health promotion and maintenance; CNS: None; CL: Apply

47. The nurse is caring for a client whose cardiac monitor suddenly shows fibrillatory waves with no recognizable pattern. Which nursing intervention is **priority**?
1. Notify the health care provider.
2. Begin cardiopulmonary resuscitation (CPR).
3. Intubate the client.
4. Administer epinephrine.

47. 2. The nurse would recognize the client was experiencing ventricular fibrillation (VF), which is the arrhythmia most commonly associated with sudden cardiac death. The nurse would begin CPR first. The nurse would notify the health care provider. If VF persisted, intubation, defibrillation, and medications would be initiated. CN: Physiological integrity; CNS: Reduction of risk potential; CL: Analyze

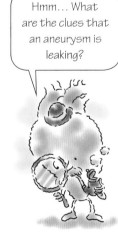

Hmm… What are the clues that an aneurysm is leaking?

48. The nurse is caring for a client with a 7-cm infrarenal abdominal aortic aneurysm (AAA). The computed tomography (CT) scan indicates the aneurysm may be leaking. When performing an assessment on the client, the nurse will expect which finding(s)? Select all that apply.
1. Constant, severe lower back pain
2. Constant, "tearing" abdominal sensation
3. Blood pressure 86/52 mm Hg
4. Decreased red blood cell (RBC) count
5. Weak or absent bilateral leg pulses
6. Intermittent, mild epigastric pain

48. 1, 2, 3, 4, 5. Severe, constant lower back pain or constant "tearing" abdominal pain indicates a leaking or ruptured aneurysm as blood enters the abdominal cavity and retroperitoneal space. The client's blood pressure and RBC count will fall as the client becomes hypovolemic from hemorrhage. Diminished blood flow through the iliac and femoral arteries causes weak or absent bilateral leg pulses. Pain from a leaking or ruptured aneurysm is constant. CN: Physiological integrity; CNS: Reduction of risk potential; CL: Apply

CN: Client needs category   CNS: Client needs subcategory   CL: Cognitive level

49. The nurse is caring for a client just diagnosed with a 3-cm infrarenal abdominal aortic aneurysm (AAA). Which nursing statement(s) will be included when educating this client? Select all that apply.
1. "AAAs occur more commonly above the level of the renal artery origins."
2. "AAAs occur more commonly in men than they do in women."
3. "AAAs are rarely linked to genetic factors."
4. "A client with an AAA may also have 'blue toe syndrome'."
5. "A 3-cm AAA rarely causes symptoms such as back pain."

49. 2, 4, 5. An AAA is more than twice as common in men as women and up to 28% of these clients have a first-degree family member with an AAA. Small AAAs (less than 4 cm) are commonly identified coincidentally and are usually asymptomatic. Larger AAAs may be lined with an intraluminal thrombus, and "blue toe syndrome" occurs when the thrombus from the aneurysm microembolizes to the foot.
CN: Physiological integrity; CNS: Reduction of risk potential; CL: Apply

50. The nurse reviews the medical record of a client who recently underwent an abdominal aortic aneurysm (AAA) resection. Which finding will the nurse expect in the client's medical record?
1. Cystic fibrosis
2. Lupus erythematosus
3. Marfan syndrome
4. Myocardial infarction (MI)

50. 3. Marfan syndrome results in the degeneration of the elastic fibers of the aortic media. Therefore, clients with the syndrome are more likely to develop an aneurysm. Cystic fibrosis, lupus erythematosus, and MIs are not linked to AAAs.
CN: Health promotion and maintenance; CNS: None; CL: Apply

51. A client is diagnosed with a ruptured aortic aneurysm. Which nursing action is appropriate?
1. Give captopril orally.
2. Transport the client for an aortogram.
3. Administration propranolol.
4. Prepare the client for surgery.

51. 4. When the vessel ruptures, surgery is the only intervention that can repair it. Administration of angiotensin-converting enzyme (ACE) inhibitors and beta-blockers can help control hypertension, reducing the risk of rupture. An aortogram is a diagnostic tool used to detect an aneurysm.
CN: Physiological integrity; CNS: Reduction of risk potential; CL: Apply

52. A client is diagnosed with a 4.5-cm infrarenal abdominal aortic aneurysm (AAA). Which statement(s) will the nurse include when teaching the client? Select all that apply.
1. "Controlling blood pressure and lipid levels helps to slow aneurysm expansion."
2. "An AAA will be monitored for expansion every 6 to 12 months."
3. "Smoking has no effect on the rate of aneurysm expansion."
4. "Genetic factors influence the development of AAA."
5. "All AAAs need to be repaired as soon as they are identified."

52. 1, 2, 4. Multiple factors lead to arterial wall damage and aneurysm formation. These include heredity, atherosclerosis, infection, smoking, and hypertension; therefore, controlling these factors help to slow progression. Clients with AAAs of 4 to 5.4 cm should be monitored for expansion of the aneurysm using ultrasound or computed tomography (CT) scan every 6 to 12 months. The average aneurysm expansion rate is 10% per year but the rate of expansion is highly individual; many AAAs remain stable without expansion for many years.
CN: Safe, effective care environment; CNS: Management of care; CL: Apply

What complication is most likely to occur with cardiomyopathy?

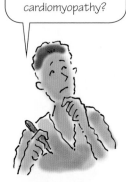

53. The nurse is caring for a client with cardiomyopathy. For which condition will the nurse closely assess the client?
1. Heart failure
2. Diabetes
3. Myocardial infarction (MI)
4. Pericardial effusion

53. 1. Because the structure and function of the heart muscle is affected, heart failure most commonly occurs in clients with cardiomyopathy. MI results from atherosclerosis. Pericardial effusion is most predominant in clients with pericarditis. Diabetes is unrelated to cardiomyopathy.
CN: Physiological integrity; CNS: Physiological adaptation; CL: Apply

54. The nurse is teaching a client newly diagnosed with hypertrophic cardiomyopathy (HCM). Which statement by the client **best** demonstrates an understanding of this disease process?
1. "I should participate in a vigorous aerobic exercise program to strengthen my heart function."
2. "Since this is a hereditary disorder, my family members should be evaluated for similar symptoms."
3. "Exercise or exertion could kill me. I should have a caretaker to perform my activities of daily living."
4. "I should keep a journal of my symptoms and take my prescribed medications only when I have symptoms."

55. The nurse is caring for a client newly diagnosed with hypertrophic cardiomyopathy (HCM). Which health care provider prescription will the nurse question?
1. Activity as tolerated
2. Administer atenolol daily
3. Give diltiazem daily
4. Consult cardiologist on call

56. The nurse is providing education to a client about warfarin. Which statement by the client **best** indicates to the nurse an understanding of warfarin?
1. "I should use a soft toothbrush."
2. "I can expect to have bruising."
3. "I will adjust my diet to eat less protein."
4. "I should use a safety razor to shave."

57. The nurse is caring for a client with cardiac tamponade. Which findings(s) will the nurse expect to assess on this client? Select all that apply.
1. Paradoxical chest movement
2. Tracheal deviation
3. Pulsus paradoxus
4. Light-headedness
5. Narrowing pulse pressure
6. Muffled heart sounds

54. 2. Hypertrophic cardiomyopathy is a hereditary disease in which the heart muscle is abnormally thick and asymmetrical. In young clients, especially athletes, the first symptom may be sudden death during strenuous exercise. Strenuous physical exertion is restricted because it may precipitate arrhythmias or sudden cardiac death. The client is usually encouraged to perform normal activities of daily living after discussing restrictions with the health care provider. Medications, such as beta-blockers, calcium channel blockers, and antiarrhythmics, are usually prescribed and should be taken daily to help prevent complications.
CN: Physiological integrity; CNS: Reduction of risk potential; CL: Apply

55. 1. The nurse would question unrestricted activity. Hypertrophic cardiomyopathy involves abnormal thickening of the heart muscle, particularly affecting the muscle of the heart's main pumping chamber (left ventricle). The thickened heart muscle can make it harder for the heart to pump blood. Restricting physical activity limits aggravating the heart. Atenolol and diltiazem are commonly used to control symptoms such as tachycardia and hypertension. A cardiologist would be consulted for treatment management.
CN: Safe, effective care environment; CNS: Management of care; CL: Apply

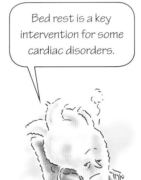

Bed rest is a key intervention for some cardiac disorders.

56. 1. A soft toothbrush will help prevent bleeding from friable gum tissue. Increased bruising should be reported to the health care provider. Dietary adjustments include consuming consistent amounts of dark green, leafy vegetables, which are high in vitamin K, but do not include protein restriction. Electric razors are recommended to reduce the risk of cutting the skin.
CN: Physiological integrity; CNS: Pharmacological and parenteral therapies; CL: Apply

57. 3, 4, 5, 6. Pulsus paradoxus is a symptom of cardiac tamponade caused by a marked decrease in cardiac output, which results in a diminished pulse and decreased blood pressure during inspiration. Light-headedness, narrowing pulse pressure, and muffled heart sounds are additional signs of cardiac tamponade. Paradoxical chest movement occurs with flail chest. Tracheal deviation is seen with tension pneumothorax.
CN: Physiological integrity; CNS: Physiological adaptation; CL: Apply

58. A client diagnosed with pulmonary edema is prescribed furosemide. Which statement made by the nurse is appropriate?
1. "Furosemide may cause hyperkalemia."
2. "Do not take with an aminoglycoside antibiotic."
3. "You should avoid eating bananas."
4. "If you develop a rash, apply topical diphenhydramine."

58. 2. Furosemide may increase the ototoxic potential of aminoglycoside antibiotics and should be avoided. Furosemide can cause hypokalemia. Clients should eat foods high in potassium, such as spinach, yogurt, navy beans, and bananas, to limit the risk for hypokalemia. A rash could indicate a life-threatening complication and should be reported to the health care provider.
CN: Physiological integrity; CNS: Pharmacological and parenteral therapies; CL: Apply

59. The nurse is caring for a client diagnosed with myocardial infarction (MI) who is prescribed a nitrate. What does the nurse identify as the purpose of giving a nitrate to this client?
1. Relieve pain.
2. Dilate coronary arteries.
3. Relieve secondary headaches.
4. Calm and relax the client.

59. 2. Nitrates dilate the arteries, allowing oxygen to continue flowing to the myocardium. Nitrates can cause headaches but do not relieve pain, and they do not calm or relax the client.
CN: Physiological integrity; CNS: Pharmacological and parenteral therapies; CL: Understand

60. The nurse administers atenolol to a client diagnosed with cardiomyopathy. What finding(s) indicates to the nurse that atenolol is appropriate for this client? Select all that apply.
1. Improved cardiac output
2. Improved myocardial filling
3. Increasing contractility
4. Increased blood pressure
5. Increased heart rate

60. 1, 2. The health care provider may prescribe medications to improve the heart's pumping ability and function, improve blood flow, lower blood pressure, slow the heart rate, remove excess fluid from the body, or keep blood clots from forming. By decreasing the heart rate and contractility, beta-blockers, such as atenolol, improve myocardial filling and cardiac output, which are primary goals in the treatment of cardiomyopathy.
CN: Physiological integrity; CNS: Pharmacological and parenteral therapies; CL: Apply

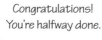
Congratulations! You're halfway done.

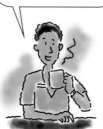

61. A client who is very anxious often comes to the emergency department with reports of chest pain rated a "5" on a scale of 0 to 10. The nurse will assess this client for which condition?
1. Anxiety
2. Stable angina
3. Unstable angina
4. Variant angina

61. 2. The pain of stable angina is predictable in nature, builds gradually, and quickly reaches maximum intensity. Anxiety generally is not described as painful. Unstable angina does not always need a trigger, is more intense, and lasts longer than stable angina. Variant angina usually occurs at rest, not as a result of exertion or stress.
CN: Physiological integrity; CNS: Physiological adaptation; CL: Apply

62. The telemetry monitor technician notifies the nurse a client has sinus bradycardia with a heart rate of 42 beats/minute. What is the **priority** nursing intervention?
1. Administer a calcium channel blocker.
2. Obtain a 12-lead electrocardiogram (ECG).
3. Notify the client's health care provider.
4. Check the client's level of consciousness (LOC) and vital signs.

62. 4. The priority is to assess the client's LOC, obtain vital signs, and determine the presence or absence of symptoms. Administering a calcium channel blocker and calling the health care provider are not priorities. Obtaining a 12-lead ECG may be necessary but is not the priority.
CN: Safe, effective care environment; CNS: Management of care; CL: Analyze

63. Which characteristic will the nurse expect to see on a normal cardiac rhythm strip obtained from an adult client?
1. PR interval of greater than 0.24 second
2. Heart rate of 88 beats/minute
3. Two P waves preceding each QRS complex
4. QRS complexes greater than 0.16 second that vary in configuration

63. 2. The normal adult heart rate is between 60 and 100 beats/minute. The normal PR interval is 0.12 to 0.20 second. In a normal cardiac cycle, there should be one P wave preceding each QRS complex. A normal QRS complex should be less than 0.10 second.
CN: Physiological integrity; CNS: Reduction of risk potential; CL: Apply

CN: Client needs category CNS: Client needs subcategory CL: Cognitive level

64. A client, 1 hour after undergoing a cardiac catheterization through a percutaneous femoral access site, reports, "There is something wet under my buttocks." Upon entering the client's room, what is the **priority** nursing action?
1. Reinforce the groin dressing.
2. Obtain the client's vital signs.
3. Reposition the client in bed.
4. Assess the femoral access site.

65. A client comes to the emergency department reporting chest pain. Upon further assessment the client is diagnosed with unstable angina. The nurse understands additional education is needed if the client makes which statement regarding measures to prevent a common complication associated with unstable angina?
1. "I will take aspirin 325 mg with each meal."
2. "I will not drink alcohol while I take aspirin."
3. "I will stop eating fried foods and limit red meat intake."
4. "I need to work on managing my stress level."

66. When a client experiences chest pain during an acute anginal episode, the nurse will expect to administer which form of nitroglycerin **first**?
1. Nitroglycerin IV drip at 10 mcg/minute
2. Application of 2 in (5 cm) of nitroglycerin paste to the chest wall
3. Metered buccal nitroglycerin spray, 0.4 mg/spray
4. Transdermal nitroglycerin patch, 0.2 mg/hour

67. Which statement made by a client who had a fasting lipoprotein profile indicates to the nurse that additional education is needed?
1. "Changing my diet has really helped lower my cholesterol. Now my LDL cholesterol level is 98 mg/dL (2.5 mmol/L)."
2. "My total cholesterol level is optimal. It used to be 350 mg/dL (9.1 mmol/L) and now it is 250 mg/dL (6.5 mmol/L)."
3. "My HDL cholesterol level is 60 mg/dL (1.6 mmol/L) so my risk for coronary heart disease is lower."
4. "Even though my lipoprotein profile is normal this year, I know I will need another one in 5 years."

68. The nurse identifies which intervention as **priority** for a client experiencing chest pain while walking?
1. Sitting the client down
2. Getting the client back to bed
3. Obtaining an electrocardiogram (ECG)
4. Administering sublingual nitroglycerin

Looks like things are on the upswing. Great work!

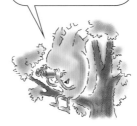

Have a seat and take a look. I'm sure you'll spot the right answer.

64. 4. Assessing the femoral access site for potential bleeding is the priority. Reinforcing the groin dressing may be necessary after the site is assessed. Obtaining vital signs is not the priority at this time. After a femoral puncture, the client is usually prescribed complete bed rest with the affected leg straight and immobilized for 2 to 4 hours to reduce the risk of bleeding.
CN: Physiological integrity; CNS: Reduction of risk potential; CL: Analyze

65. 1. Unstable angina progressively increases in frequency, intensity, and duration and is related to an increased risk of MI within 3 to 18 months. The nurse would educate the client on measures to decrease the risk of a future MI. It is recommended to take a blood thinner, such as aspirin for angina, to promote blood flow. The client should take 81 to 325 mg aspirin once daily, not TID. It is recommended to eat healthy; reduce stress; exercise; stop smoking; and monitor blood pressure, glucose, and cholesterol levels to reduce a client's risk of having an MI.
CN: Physiological integrity; CNS: Physiological adaptation; CL: Apply

66. 3. Sublingual or buccal nitroglycerin is the route of choice to quickly reduce myocardial oxygen demand and dilate coronary arteries. IV nitroglycerin is usually begun after a trial of sublingual or buccal spray nitroglycerin has proved unsuccessful in relieving the client's symptoms. Nitroglycerin paste and transdermal patches may be administered later because they have slower actions.
CN: Physiological integrity; CNS: Pharmacological and parenteral therapies; CL: Apply

67. 2. The National Cholesterol Education Program classifies a total cholesterol of 240 mg/dL (6.2 mmol/L) or more as high, levels of 200 to 239 mg/dL (5.2 to 6.2 mmol/L) as borderline high, and levels less than 200 mg/dL (5.2 mmol/L) as desirable. LDL cholesterol levels of 100 mg/dL (2.6 mmol/L) or less and HDL cholesterol levels 60 mg/dL (1.6 mmol/L) or more are optimal. Adults should have a fasting lipoprotein profile performed every 5 years beginning at age 20.
CN: Physiological integrity; CNS: Reduction of risk potential; CL: Analyze

68. 1. The priority is to decrease the oxygen consumption; this would be achieved by sitting the client down. An ECG can be obtained after the client is sitting down. After the ECG, sublingual nitroglycerin would be administered. The client can return to bed once stabilized.
CN: Physiological integrity; CNS: Basic care and comfort; CL: Analyze

CN: Client needs category   CNS: Client needs subcategory   CL: Cognitive level

69. The nurse is reviewing the diagnostic test results for a client with reports of chest pain. Which test result is **most** consistent with a diagnosis of angina?
1. Troponin level greater than 1.5 mg/mL
2. Creatine kinase isoenzymes (CK-MB) level of 45%
3. 12-lead electrocardiogram with abnormal T waves
4. Left ventricular ejection fraction of 30%

69. 3. The 12-lead ECG with depressed, inverted, or downward slope to the T waves indicates ischemia. Elevated troponin and CK-MB levels indicate myocardial infarction, not ischemia. A decreased ejection fraction indicates heart failure.
CN: Physiological integrity; CNS: Reduction of risk potential; CL: Apply

70. A client arrives in the emergency department and is diagnosed with unstable angina. Which nursing intervention(s) is **priority** for this client? Select all that apply.
1. Apply oxygen.
2. Administer aspirin.
3. Give nitroglycerin.
4. Apply cardiac monitor.
5. Provide nutrition counseling.
6. Provide smoking cessation education.

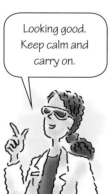

Looking good. Keep calm and carry on.

70. 1, 2, 3, 4. The initial treatment consists of administration of oxygen, aspirin, nitroglycerin, and a beta-blocker, and application of a cardiac monitor. Given an altered, yet nondiagnostic ECG and no contraindications, further treatment with heparin (low molecular weight or unfractionated), clopidogrel, or other antiplatelet agents may be initiated. Most often, an additional abnormal marker (e.g., an elevated serum troponin, myoglobin, or CPK level) will be verified prior to antiplatelet therapy. Education on nutrition and smoking cessation would be provided once the client is stabilized.
CN: Safe, effective care environment; CNS: Management of care; CL: Analyze

71. A client is experiencing chest pain at rest that is unresponsive to nitroglycerin. The health care provider diagnoses unstable angina and prescribes immediate surgical intervention. For which treatment will the nurse prepare the client?
1. Cardiac catheterization
2. Echocardiogram
3. Heart transplantation
4. Percutaneous transluminal coronary angioplasty (PTCA)

71. 4. PTCA can alleviate the blockage and restore blood flow and oxygenation. An echocardiogram is a noninvasive diagnostic test. Heart transplantation involves replacing the client's heart with a donor heart and is the treatment for end-stage cardiac disease. Cardiac catheterization is a diagnostic tool, not a treatment.
CN: Physiological integrity; CNS: Physiological adaptation; CL: Apply

72. A client with heart failure is experiencing symptoms of cardiogenic shock. Which symptom(s) will the nurse expect this client to exhibit? Select all that apply.
1. Tachycardia
2. Hypotension
3. Bradycardia
4. Decreased peripheral pulses
5. Tachypnea

72. 1, 2, 4, 5. Cardiogenic shock is related to ineffective pumping of the heart and is an acute and serious complication of heart failure. Symptoms include tachycardia, decreased blood pressure, tachypnea, and decreased peripheral pulses. Bradycardia is not associated with this disease process.
CN: Physiological integrity; CNS: Physiological adaptation; CL: Apply

73. Which client does the nurse identify as having the **greatest** chance of developing cardiogenic shock?
1. A client who had an acute myocardial infarction (MI)
2. A client diagnosed with coronary artery disease (CAD)
3. A client whose hemoglobin level is 10 g/dL (100 g/L)
4. A client with a blood pressure of 92/56 mm Hg

73. 1. Of all clients with an acute MI, 15% suffer cardiogenic shock secondary to the myocardial damage and decreased function. CAD causes MI. Hypotension is the result of a reduced cardiac output produced by the shock state. A decreased hemoglobin level is a result of bleeding.
CN: Physiological integrity; CNS: Reduction of risk potential; CL: Apply

74. The nurse is monitoring laboratory results for a client admitted with a possible myocardial infarction (MI). Which laboratory result will the nurse flag for the health care provider to review?
1. White blood cell (WBC) count 15,000 mm^3 (15×10^9/L)
2. Troponin level less than 0.2 ng/mL (0.2 µg/L)
3. Red blood cell (RBC) count of 4.7 mm^3 (4.7×10^{12}/L)
4. Mean corpuscular hemoglobin (MCH) of 27 pg/cell

74. 2. Cardiac troponins are proteins that exist in cardiac muscle and are released with cardiac muscle injury. A troponin level of less than 0.2 ng/mL is considered normal and rules out an MI for this client. An elevated WBC count is seen in many disease processes and with severe necrosis but does not specifically indicate MI. An RBC count of 4.7 mm^3 (4.7×10^{12}/L) is within normal limits for males and females but is not used to rule out an MI. MCH is an RBC index providing information about the hemoglobin concentration of RBCs and is not used to rule out an MI.
CN: Physiological integrity; CNS: Reduction of risk potential; CL: Apply

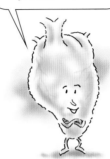

I've been feeling a little off my rhythm lately. What assessment do you recommend?

75. While the nurse is assessing a client, the client states, "Sometimes my heart seems to race." The nurse will be especially vigilant to assess this client for which cardiac arrhythmia?
1. Ventricular fibrillation
2. Sinus tachycardia
3. Atrial fibrillation
4. Atrial flutter

75. 1. Ventricular fibrillation is a life-threatening arrhythmia. It occurs when the ventricle fibrillates, failing to fully contract and pump blood through the heart. Sinus tachycardia, atrial fibrillation, and atrial flutter are arrhythmias that may require treatment but are not considered life-threatening.
CN: Physiological integrity; CNS: Physiological adaptation; CL: Understand

76. Which factor does the nurse determine is **most** useful in detecting a client's risk of developing cardiogenic shock?
1. Monitoring the client's heart rate
2. Determining the client's cardiac index
3. Blood pressure fluctuations over the past month
4. Symptoms associated with decreased cerebral blood flow

76. 2. The cardiac index, a figure derived by dividing the cardiac output by the client's body surface area, is used to identify whether the cardiac output is meeting a client's needs. Decreased cerebral blood flow, blood pressure, and heart rate are less useful in detecting the risk of cardiogenic shock.
CN: Physiological integrity; CNS: Physiological adaptation; CL: Apply

77. A client arrives in the emergency department with tachycardia, decreased urination, restlessness, and confusion. Auscultation reveals a fourth heart sound. What does the nurse suspect is occurring?
1. Myocardial infarction
2. Cardiogenic shock
3. Peripheral vascular disease
4. Abdominal aortic aneurysm (AAA)

77. 2. In cardiogenic shock, initially the nurse would see a decrease in cardiac output resulting in a decrease in cerebral blood flow, which causes restlessness, agitation, or confusion. Tachycardia, decreased urine output, and an S4 heart sound are all later signs of shock. Peripheral vascular disease, AAA, and MI do not have these same signs.
CN: Physiological integrity; CNS: Basic care and comfort; CL: Analyze

78. The nurse is educating a client on the initial treatment goal of increasing myocardial oxygen supply for cardiogenic shock. The client demonstrates an understanding of this by making which statement?
1. "Increasing my oxygen will cause me to become acidotic."
2. "If I get less oxygen it will be easier on my body and I will get better quicker."
3. "If my body is in a shock state, it will actually need less oxygen."
4. "A balance must be maintained between oxygen supply and demand."

78. 4. A balance must be maintained between oxygen supply and demand. In a shock state, the myocardium requires more oxygen. If it cannot get more oxygen, the shock worsens. Increasing the oxygen will also help correct metabolic acidosis and hypoxia. Infarction typically causes the shock state, so prevention is not an appropriate goal for this condition.
CN: Physiological integrity; CNS: Physiological adaptation; CL: Apply

CN: Client needs category   CNS: Client needs subcategory   CL: Cognitive level

79. A client with a history of chronic obstructive pulmonary disease (COPD) arrives in the emergency department with an oxygen saturation of 84% on room air. Which procedure does the nurse anticipate preparing the client for **next**?
  1. Arterial blood gas (ABG)
  2. Complete blood count (CBC)
  3. Electrocardiogram (ECG)
  4. Lung scan

79. 1. ABG levels reflect cellular metabolism and indicate hypoxia. A CBC is performed to determine various constituents of venous blood. An ECG shows the electrical activity of the heart. A lung scan is performed to view the lungs' function.
CN: Physiological integrity; CNS: Reduction of risk potential; CL: Apply

80. A client is suspected of having cardiogenic shock. Which medication does the nurse anticipate administering to the client?
  1. Dopamine
  2. Enalapril
  3. Furosemide
  4. Metoprolol

80. 1. Dopamine, a sympathomimetic drug, improves myocardial contractility and blood flow through vital organs by increasing perfusion pressure. Enalapril is an angiotensin-converting enzyme (ACE) inhibitor that directly lowers blood pressure. Furosemide is a diuretic and does not have a direct effect on contractility or tissue perfusion. Metoprolol is a beta-blocker that slows the heart rate and lowers blood pressure, neither of which is a desired effect in the treatment of cardiogenic shock.
CN: Physiological integrity; CNS: Pharmacological and parenteral therapies; CL: Apply

81. During a local wellness fair, the nurse assesses several clients' blood pressures. The nurse will refer which client for further evaluation for primary hypertension?
  1. A 35-year-old pregnant woman with a blood pressure of 126/80 mm Hg
  2. A 72-year-old woman with a blood pressure of 142/88 mm Hg
  3. A 44-year-old man with end-stage renal failure and a blood pressure of 130/70 mm Hg
  4. A 76-year-old man with a systolic blood pressure of 136 mm Hg

My favorite treatment for high blood pressure is napping.

81. 2. Hypertension is defined as a sustained systolic blood pressure of 140 mm Hg or a diastolic blood pressure of 90 mm Hg. Secondary hypertension is attributed to an identifiable medical diagnosis, such as gestational hypertension or renovascular disease. The 76-year-old man has prehypertension, which is defined as systolic blood pressure of 120 to 139 mm Hg or a diastolic pressure of 80 to 89 mm Hg.
CN: Physiological integrity; CNS: Reduction of risk potential; CL: Analyze

82. A client is admitted to the emergency department with a suspected diagnosis of shock. The nurse will anticipate preparing the client for which procedure?
  1. Arterial line placement
  2. Indwelling urinary catheter insertion
  3. Intra-aortic balloon pump (IABP) placement
  4. Pulmonary artery (PA) catheterization

82. 4. A PA catheterization is performed to obtain accurate pressure measurements within the heart, which aids in diagnosing and determining the course of treatment. An arterial line is used to directly assess blood pressure continuously. An indwelling urinary catheter is used to drain the bladder. An IABP is an assistive device used to rest the damaged heart.
CN: Physiological integrity; CNS: Reduction of risk potential; CL: Apply

83. The nurse is obtaining a client's blood pressure and hears a faint, clear tapping sound. What will the nurse do **next**?
  1. Continue obtaining the blood pressure.
  2. Call the health care provider.
  3. Notify the rapid response team.
  4. Determine if the client recently had a MI.

83. 1. Initially, auscultation produces a faint, clear tapping sound that gradually increases in intensity. Therefore, the nurse should continue to listen. It is not necessary to call the health care provider, call a rapid response, or determine if the client has had a MI at this time.
CN: Physiological integrity; CNS: Basic care and comfort; CL: Apply

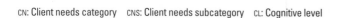

CN: Client needs category   CNS: Client needs subcategory   CL: Cognitive level

84. The nurse has provided education about angina to a client who has pain from angina. Which statement made by the client indicates a need for further teaching?
1. "Angina pain is relieved with nitroglycerin."
2. "Angina pain can develop slowly or quickly."
3. "I may feel angina pain in my shoulders, neck, arms or back."
4. "Angina pain usually lasts less than 5 minutes."

85. The emergency room nurse assesses a client and notes: clammy skin, blood pressure 68/42 mm Hg, labored breathing, and pulse 134 beats/minute. What will the nurse do **next**?
1. Apply oxygen.
2. Monitor vital signs.
3. Obtain arterial blood gas (ABG) levels.
4. Prepare for an angioplasty.

86. The nurse is educating a client with a blood pressure of 140/92 mm Hg on treatments. Which health care provider prescription will the nurse question?
1. Enalapril once daily
2. Limit physical activity
3. Limit alcohol and sodium intake
4. Decrease consumption of saturated fats

87. A client is placed on lisinopril to reduce blood pressure. The nurse understands which hormone(s) is associated with this medication and is responsible for preventing peripheral vasoconstriction? Select all that apply.
1. Angiotensin I
2. Angiotensin II
3. Epinephrine
4. Norepinephrine
5. Aldosterone

88. A client is newly diagnosed with hypertension of unknown origin. During assessment, the client's blood pressure is 152/94 mm Hg and the client is asymptomatic. How will the nurse document this condition?
1. Accelerated hypertension
2. Malignant hypertension
3. Primary hypertension
4. Secondary hypertension

89. When assessing a client admitted with a blood pressure of 154/96 mm Hg, the nurse will expect the client to report which symptom?
1. Blurred vision
2. Epistaxis
3. Headache
4. Peripheral edema

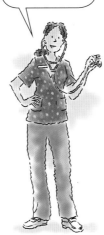

I see your baroreceptors are working just fine.

84. 1. Angina pain, if unstable, may or may not be relieved by nitroglycerin. It can develop slowly or quickly, and it can radiate to arms, neck, shoulders and back. Angina pain usually lasts only 5 minutes but can last up to 15 to 20 minutes. It also can be described as mild or moderate.
CN: Physiological integrity; CNS: Physiological adaptation;
CL: Apply

85. 1. The nurse will first apply oxygen to the client as this client is exhibiting signs of cardiogenic shock. The nurse will monitor vital signs and ABG levels. An angioplasty may be needed for stent placement. However, these actions are not priority.
CN: Physiological integrity; CNS: Reduction of risk potential;
CL: Analyze

86. 2. The nurse would question limiting physical activity for a client with hypertension. Treatments include weight reduction, exercise, dietary alterations, limiting alcohol intake, and ACE inhibitors.
CN: Safe, effective care environment; CNS: Management of care;
CL: Apply

87. 1, 2. An ACE inhibitor inhibits the renin–angiotensin–aldosterone system by blocking conversion of angiotensin I to angiotensin II and helps to prevent vasoconstriction. ACE inhibitors do not have an effect on epinephrine, norepinephrine, or aldosterone.
CN: Physiological integrity; CNS: Pharmacological and parenteral therapies; CL: Apply

88. 3. Characterized by a progressive, usually asymptomatic blood pressure increase over several years, primary hypertension is the most common type. Malignant hypertension, also known as accelerated hypertension, is rapidly progressive and uncontrollable and causes a rapid onset of complications. Secondary hypertension occurs secondary to a known, potentially correctable cause.
CN: Physiological integrity; CNS: Reduction of risk potential;
CL: Apply

89. 3. An occipital headache is typical of hypertension owing to increased pressure in the cerebral vasculature. Blurred vision (due to arteriolar changes in the eye) and epistaxis (nosebleed) are far less common than headache but can also be diagnostic signs. Peripheral edema can occur from an increase in sodium and water retention, but it is usually a latent sign.
CN: Physiological integrity; CNS: Physiological adaptation;
CL: Apply

CN: Client needs category   CNS: Client needs subcategory   CL: Cognitive level

90. The nurse is educating a client with a history of diabetes who has been prescribed furosemide for new onset hypertension. Which statement made by the client indicates to the nurse additional education is needed?
1. "If I miss a pill, I will take two when the next dose is scheduled."
2. "I will closely monitor my glucose levels while taking furosemide."
3. "If I have trouble swallowing this pill, I can crush it and take with food."
4. "I will move slowly when I am changing my position."

91. The registered nurse (RN) delegates obtaining a client's blood pressure to the assistive personnel (AP). Which action by the AP warrants immediate intervention by the RN?
1. Applies clean gloves before applying the blood pressure cuff
2. Placing the stethoscope over the brachiocephalic artery
3. Uses the diaphragm of the stethoscope for auscultation
4. Washes hands before taking the blood pressure

92. The nurse will recommend which activity for a client at risk of developing hypertension? Select all that apply.
1. Maintain a healthy weight for height.
2. Attend smoking cessation classes.
3. Participate in physical activity once per week.
4. Eat a diet low in sodium and high in potassium.
5. Drink less than three alcoholic beverages per day.

93. The client diagnosed with hypertension asks the nurse, "Will this condition affect my eye sight?" Which statement by the nurse is **most** appropriate?
1. "If you keep your hypertension controlled, you do not need to worry about your vision."
2. "Yes, you need to have your eyes checked every 6 months."
3. "To assess for changes, you need to have your eyes checked annually."
4. "You will be referred to an ophthalmologist who can detect changes in your eyes."

94. A client with varicose veins is admitted for right leg vein ligation and stripping. The nurse will perform which intervention postoperatively?
1. Have the client elevate the legs when sitting.
2. Have the client remain inactive until healed.
3. Apply knee-high stockings over the dressing.
4. Apply ice packs to the client's dressings.

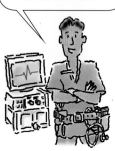

Ready for an adventure in assessment? First make sure you have all your tools and know how to use them.

90. 1. Furosemide is a loop diuretic that inhibits sodium and water reabsorption in the loop of Henle, thereby causing a decrease in blood pressure. If a dose is missed, it should be taken as soon as possible, but the dose should not be doubled. Furosemide can cause glucose levels to increase in clients with diabetes. Furosemide can be crushed and taken with food. It can cause orthostatic hypotension; therefore, slow movements are best.
CN: Physiological integrity; CNS: Pharmacological and parenteral therapies; CL: Apply

91. 2. The brachiocephalic artery is not accessible for blood pressure measurement. The brachial artery is typically used because of its easy accessibility and location. Gloves are not required when assessing a client's blood pressure unless the nurse expects to come in contact with blood or body fluids. However, immediate intervention is not required for using gloves. The AP uses standard precautions by washing hands whenever performing skills, and the diaphragm is the correct part of stethoscope to use when taking a blood pressure.
CN: Physiological integrity; CNS: Basic care and comfort; CL: Apply

92. 1, 2, 4. Risk factors for hypertension include obesity, smoking, heredity, diabetes, and a lack of exercise, among other factors. Activities to help the client decrease risk factors include maintaining a healthy weight, stopping smoking, participating in physical activity at least three times per week, not once, eating a diet low in sodium and high in potassium (helps keep blood pressure low), and limiting alcohol consumption. Three alcoholic beverages per day is excessive.
CN: Health promotion and maintenance; CNS: None; CL: Apply

93. 3. Because hypertension can negatively affect eye sight, annual eye exams are recommended to allow for early intervention. Biannual exams are not currently recommended. Telling the client not to worry or that he or she will receive a referral does not address the client's concern.
CN: Health promotion and maintenance; CNS: None; CL: Apply

94. 1. Postoperative nursing interventions must focus on maintaining peripheral circulation and venous return. Elevating the legs and early ambulation are encouraged to facilitate venous return. Applying knee-high stockings and ice would constrict circulation.
CN: Physiological integrity; CNS: Reduction of risk potential; CL: Apply

CN: Client needs category   CNS: Client needs subcategory   CL: Cognitive level

95. A healthy, pregnant woman is diagnosed with varicose veins. What education will the nurse provide to this client? Select all that apply.
1. Elevate legs periodically.
2. Change positions often.
3. Monitor weight daily.
4. Wear ankle-high socks.
5. Drink 64 oz of water per day.

95. 1, 2, 3. Primary varicose veins have a gradual onset and progressively worsen. To help prevent or lessen the effects of varicose veins during pregnancy, the client should elevate legs to help promote circulation, change position frequently, and monitor weight, as a large weight gain in a short period of time is hard on the veins. The client should use support panty hose or stockings, not ankle socks, to help prevent varicose veins, and should take steps to avoid constipation as this can lead to hemorrhoids. The pregnant client should drink at least 96 oz of water daily.
CN: Health promotion and maintenance; CNS: None; CL: Apply

96. The nurse is admitting a client to the medical unit. Which client statement indicates to the nurse the client may have varicose veins?
1. "When I walk or stand for a long time, my legs feel tired and have a dull ache."
2. "My foot pain gets better if I dangle my foot off the edge of the bed."
3. "My legs become numb and get weaker the farther I walk."
4. "After I walk 1/2 mile (800 m) I get severe calf pain that goes away when I rest."

96. 1. Fatigue, aching, and pressure are classic symptoms of varicose veins, secondary to increased blood volume and edema. Severe foot pain that is relieved by dangling from the bed or chair, as well as severe calf pain after walking that is relieved with rest, are symptoms of decreased peripheral arterial blood flow. Numbness and weakness that increase as the client walks are consistent with spinal stenosis.
CN: Physiological integrity; CNS: Physiological adaptation; CL: Analyze

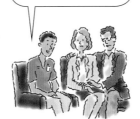
Remember to keep the client's family in the loop about the client's prognosis and treatment.

97. A client is admitted with suspected cardiac tamponade. Which symptom(s) will the nurse expect to assess in this client? Select all that apply.
1. Muffled heart sounds
2. Wide pulse pressure
3. Jugular vein distention
4. Restlessness
5. Pulsus paradoxus

97. 1, 3, 4, 5. Key signs and symptoms of cardiac tamponade are muffled heart sounds upon auscultation, narrow pulse pressure, jugular vein distention, pulsus paradoxus (an abnormal inspiratory drop in systemic blood pressure greater than 15 mm Hg), restlessness, and sitting upright or leaning forward.
CN: Physiological integrity; CNS: Reduction of risk potential; CL: Apply

98. The nurse is caring for a client with increased hydrostatic pressure and chronic venous stasis. The nurse will monitor this client for which condition?
1. Venous occlusion
2. Cool extremities
3. Nocturnal calf muscle cramps
4. Diminished blood supply to the feet

98. 3. Calf muscle cramps result from increased pressure and venous stasis secondary to varicose veins. An occlusion is a blockage of blood flow. Cool extremities and diminished blood supply to the feet are symptoms of decreased arterial blood flow.
CN: Health promotion and maintenance; CNS: None; CL: Apply

99. The nurse is providing discharge education for a client with varicose veins. Which statement by the client indicates a need for further instruction?
1. "Exercise will make me feel better."
2. "I have to elevate my legs."
3. "Lying down can relieve my symptoms."
4. "Wearing tight clothes will not affect me."

99. 4. Tight clothing, especially below the waist, increases vascular volume and impedes blood return to the heart. Exercise, leg elevations, and lying down usually relieve symptoms of varicose veins.
CN: Health promotion and maintenance; CNS: None; CL: Apply

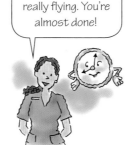
Wow—time is really flying. You're almost done!

100. A client is diagnosed with valvular heart disease with a primary symptom of fatigue. Which disease process does the nurse suspect the client is experiencing? Select all that apply.
1. Aortic insufficiency
2. Mitral insufficiency
3. Mitral valve prolapse
4. Mitral stenosis
5. Tricuspid insufficiency

100. 1, 2, 4, 5. A key symptom of aortic insufficiency, mitral insufficiency, mitral stenosis, and tricuspid insufficiency is fatigue. Palpitations are usually the only symptom for mitral valve prolapse.
CN: Physiological Integrity; CNS: Physiological adaptation; CL: Apply

CN: Client needs category   CNS: Client needs subcategory   CL: Cognitive level

101. A client is admitted with a diagnosis of post-thrombotic deep vein changes in both legs. Which assessment findings will the nurse expect to assess in this client?
1. Edema and pigmentation
2. Pallor and severe pain
3. Severe pain and edema
4. Absent hair growth and pigmentation

102. A client has undergone ligation of stripping of veins in the lower extremities. Which intervention will the nurse complete for this client?
1. Have the client sit for most of the day.
2. Maintain the client on strict bed rest.
3. Apply ice packs to the lower extremities.
4. Apply thigh-high elastic leg compressions.

103. The nurse is preparing a client for surgery. Which statement by the client **best** indicates understanding of the surgical procedure to remove varicose veins?
1. "The surgeon will tie off a large vein in my leg and then remove it."
2. "The surgeon will use a laser to prevent further varicose veins."
3. "A piece of vein will be removed and then used to replace my blocked artery."
4. "A cold solution will be infused to shrink the vein."

104. Which task will the registered nurse (RN) delegate to the assistive personnel (AP)?
1. Obtaining a blood pressure on a client being admitted for new onset hypertension
2. Applying oxygen to a client experiencing a myocardial infarction
3. Increasing the intravenous fluid rate for a client with hypovolemic shock
4. Taking the temperature on a client admitted yesterday for pericarditis

105. The nurse understands which client is at **highest** risk for developing deep vein thrombosis (DVT)?
1. A 62-year-old woman recovering from a total hip replacement
2. A 35-year-old woman who is 2 days' postpartum
3. A 33-year-old male runner with Achilles tendonitis
4. An ambulatory 70-year-old man who is recovering from pneumonia

106. An adult client has a potassium level of 3.2 mEq/L (3.2 mmol/L). Which dietary recommendation is **best** for the nurse to provide for this client?
1. Increase consumption of bananas and oranges.
2. Avoid intake of sweet potatoes and mushrooms.
3. Increase consumption of oatmeal and apples.
4. Avoid intake of spinach and broccoli.

101. 1. Blood clots in the deep veins of the leg typically cause permanent damage to the venous valves. Incompetent valves lead to impaired venous return, and edema and pigmentation result from venous stasis. Severe pain, pallor, and absent hair growth are symptoms of an altered arterial blood flow.
CN: Physiological integrity; CNS: Physiological adaptation; CL: Apply

102. 4. Thigh-high elastic leg compressions helps venous return to the heart, thereby decreasing venous stasis. Prolonged sitting and bed rest are contraindicated because both promote decreased blood return to the heart and venous stasis. Although ice packs would help reduce edema, they would also cause vasoconstriction and impede blood flow.
CN: Physiological integrity; CNS: Basic care and comfort; CL: Apply

103. 1. Ligation and stripping surgically removes varicose veins. The use of laser ablation therapy will not prevent further varicose veins from developing. Veins can be used to create bypasses for blocked arteries, but this is not a treatment for varicose veins. Infusion of a cold solution is not used to treat varicose veins.
CN: Safe, effective care environment; CNS: Management of care; CL: Understand

104. 4. The RN will delegate taking a temperature to the AP. The AP cannot obtain initial admission vital signs as this is part of the RN's initial assessment. The AP cannot apply oxygen or titrate IV fluids.
CN: Safe, effective care environment; CNS: Management of care; CL: Analyze

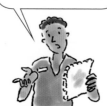
Do you remember the major contributor to DVT?

105. 1. DVT is more common in immobilized clients who have had surgical procedures such as total hip replacement. Pregnancy can cause varicose veins, which can lead to venous stasis, but it is not a primary cause of DVT. Clients who are recovering from an injury or pneumonia may have decreased mobility, but these clients do not have the highest risk of developing DVT.
CN: Physiological integrity; CNS: Reduction of risk potential; CL: Apply

106. 1. A normal serum potassium blood level is 3.5 to 5 mEq/L (3.5 to 5 mmol/L) in adult clients. Bananas, oranges, sweet potatoes, spinach, broccoli, and mushrooms are high in potassium. Oatmeal and apples are high in fiber.
CN: Physiological integrity; CNS: Basic care and comfort; CL: Apply

CN: Client needs category   CNS: Client needs subcategory   CL: Cognitive level

107. A client diagnosed with deep vein thrombosis (DVT) reports dyspnea, chest pain, and has diminished breath sounds. For which condition does the nurse prepare treatment?
1. Hemothorax
2. Pneumothorax
3. Pulmonary embolism
4. Pulmonary hypertension

108. The nurse is educating a client recently diagnosed with a deep vein thrombosis (DVT). Which statement made by the client indicates to the nurse a need for further education?
1. "I will wear compression stockings at night."
2. "I will elevate my legs if I note swelling."
3. "I will be sure to walk every hour."
4. "I will not wear tight-fitting pants."

109. A client with a deep vein thrombosis (DVT) is admitted to the hospital for treatment. The nurse anticipates a prescription for which oral medication for this client?
1. Warfarin
2. Heparin
3. Furosemide
4. Metoprolol

110. The nurse educates a client with acute pulmonary edema that high Fowler's position is best to aid breathing. Which statement made by the client indicates an understanding of this concept?
1. "This position will allow for better access if you need to do an assessment."
2. "It will cause constriction of all of my arteries that will help my breathing."
3. "This position reduces venous return and thus will help my breathing."
4. "It will increase my heart's workload and thus make breathing easier."

111. A postoperative client in ICU begins exhibiting signs of hypovolemic shock. During assessment, which symptom(s) will the nurse expect to see? Select all that apply.
1. Cold, pale, clammy skin
2. Decreased sensorium
3. Hypertension
4. Oliguria
5. Bradycardia

107. 3. The most common complication of a DVT is a pulmonary embolus. A pulmonary embolism is a thrombus that forms in a vein, travels to the lungs, and lodges in the pulmonary vasculature. Hemothorax refers to blood in the pleural space. Pneumothorax is caused by an opening in the pleura. Pulmonary hypertension is an increase in pulmonary artery pressure, which increases the workload of the right ventricle.
CN: Physiological integrity; CNS: Physiological adaptation; CL: Analyze

108. 1. Compression stockings should be worn during the day and removed at night. The client should elevate lower extremities to promote circulation and decrease edema. If the sitting for extended times, the client should ambulate hourly. Tight clothing can restrict circulation.
CN: Physiological integrity; CNS: Physiological adaptation; CL: Apply

109. 1. Warfarin prevents vitamin K from synthesizing certain clotting factors. This oral anticoagulant can be given long term. Heparin is a parenteral anticoagulant that interferes with coagulation by readily combining with antithrombin; it cannot be given by mouth. Neither furosemide nor metoprolol affect anticoagulation.
CN: Physiological integrity; CNS: Pharmacological and parenteral therapies; CL: Apply

110. 3. High Fowler's position facilitates breathing by reducing venous return. It does not cause constriction of the arteries and it will not increase the workload of the heart. It may allow for better access, but this is not the reason for the position.
CN: Physiological integrity; CNS: Basic care and comfort; CL: Apply

111. 1, 2, 4. Key signs and symptoms of hypovolemic shock are cold, pale, and clammy skin; decreased sensorium; hypotension; reduced urine output; and tachycardia.
CN: Physiological integrity; CNS: Physiological adaptation; CL: Apply

112. The nurse is caring for an older adult client with sick sinus syndrome who is awaiting permanent pacemaker placement. Which assessment findings indicate to the nurse the client is experiencing an initial drop in cardiac output?
1. Decreased blood pressure
2. Altered level of consciousness (LOC)
3. Decreased blood pressure and diuresis
4. Increased blood pressure and fluid volume

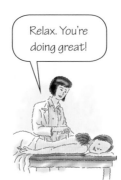

Relax. You're doing great!

113. Which nursing action is **priority** for a client coughing up pink, frothy sputum?
1. Initiate the rapid response team.
2. Notify the health care provider.
3. Obtain intravenous access.
4. Suction the client's oropharynx.

114. An adult client has experienced an episode of acute pulmonary edema. Fearful of a repeat episode, the client asks what precautions should be taken. The nurse will include which statement when providing this client education?
1. "It will be best if you limit your daily caloric intake."
2. "It is currently recommended that you restrict carbohydrates."
3. "You need to measure your weight daily in the morning and at night."
4. "Call your health care provider if you gain more than 3 lb (1.4 kg) in a day."

115. The nurse recognizes a client with severe hypertension will experience increased workload that can be attributed to which process?
1. Increased afterload
2. Increased cardiac output
3. Increased preload
4. Overload of the heart

116. A client recovers from an episode of acute pulmonary edema and is prescribed enalapril. The nurse determines which outcome is **most** important for this client?
1. To decrease overload by promoting diuresis
2. To increase contractility of the heart
3. To decrease contractility of the heart
4. To decrease workload of the heart

112. 4. The body compensates for a decrease in cardiac output with a rise in blood pressure (due to the stimulation of the sympathetic nervous system) and an increase in fluid volume as the kidneys retain sodium and water. Blood pressure does not initially drop in response to the compensatory mechanism of the body. Alteration in LOC will occur only if decreased cardiac output persists.
CN: Physiological integrity; CNS: Physiological adaptation; CL: Apply

113. 1. Production of pink, frothy sputum is a classic sign of acute pulmonary edema. Because the client is at high risk for decompensation, the nurse should call for help but not leave the room. The other three interventions should immediately follow.
CN: Safe, effective care environment; CNS: Management of care; CL: Analyze

114. 4. Gaining 3 lb (1.4 kg) in 1 day is indicative of fluid retention that would increase the heart's workload, thereby putting the client at risk for acute pulmonary edema. Restricting carbohydrates would not affect fluid status. The body needs carbohydrates for energy and healing. Limiting calorie intake does not influence fluid status. The client must only be weighed in the morning after the first urination. If the client is weighed later in the day, the finding would not be accurate because of fluid intake during the day.
CN: Physiological integrity; CNS: Reduction of risk potential; CL: Apply

115. 1. Afterload refers to the resistance normally maintained by the aortic and pulmonic valves, the condition and tone of the aorta, and the resistance offered by the systemic and pulmonary arterioles. Hypertension increases afterload as the left ventricle has to work harder to eject blood against vasoconstriction. Cardiac output is the amount of blood expelled from the heart per minute. Preload is the volume of blood in the ventricle at the end of diastole. Overload refers to an abundance of circulating volume and can contribute to hypertension.
CN: Physiological integrity; CNS: Physiological adaptation; CL: Understand

116. 4. Enalapril maleate is an angiotensin-converting enzyme (ACE) inhibitor that reduces blood pressure and decreases the workload of the heart. Diuretics are given to decrease circulating fluid volume. Inotropic agents increase cardiac contractility. Negative inotropic agents decrease cardiac contractility.
CN: Physiological integrity; CNS: Pharmacological and parenteral therapies; CL: Apply

117. Which task will the registered nurse (RN) delegate to the assistive personnel (AP)?
1. Take a client diagnosed with Raynaud's disease to radiology for testing.
2. Insert an indwelling catheter in a client with heart failure.
3. Explain a thoracotomy to a client diagnosed with cardiac tamponade.
4. Monitor a client with cardiomyopathy for a murmur.

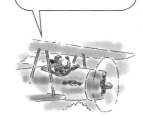

118. A client has been hospitalized with a diagnosis of acute arterial occlusive disease. After surgery the health care provider prescribes heparin IV therapy for the client. The nurse anticipates monitoring which test for this client?
1. Partial prothrombin time (PTT)
2. Complete blood count (CBC)
3. Prostate specific antigen (PSA)
4. Blood urea nitrogen (BUN)

119. A client with a history of hypertension had a total hip replacement. The health care provider prescribes hydrochlorothiazide 35 mg oral solution by mouth once per day. The label on the solution reads hydrochlorothiazide 50 mg/5 mL. How many milliliters will the nurse administer to the client? Record your answer using one decimal place.

_____ mL

120. The nurse is assessing a client at risk for cardiac tamponade due to chest trauma sustained in a motorcycle accident. What is the client's pulse pressure if the blood pressure is 108/82 mm Hg? Record your answer using a whole number.

_____ mm Hg

121. A client is admitted with a diagnosis of new onset atrial fibrillation. To obtain an accurate pulse, the nurse counts the apical heart rate. Identify the area where the nurse will place the stethoscope to **best** hear the apical rate.

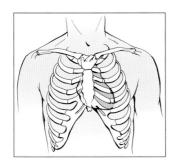

117. 1. The RN would delegate taking a stable client to another department. The AP cannot perform sterile procedures (indwelling catheter), provide education (explain procedure), or assessment (assess for a murmur).
CN: Safe, effective care environment; CNS: Management of care; CL: Analyze

118. 1. PTT is used to monitor a client's response to heparin therapy and is used to evaluate all the clotting factors of the intrinsic pathway. Both are monitored whenever a client is on heparin. CBC is used to determine infection or inflammation. PSA is used to screen for prostate cancer in men. BUN is used to evaluate kidney function.
CN: Physiological integrity; CNS: Reduction of risk potential; CL: Apply

119. 3.5.
The correct formula to calculate a drug dosage is:
$$Dose\ on\ hand = \frac{Dose\ desired}{X}$$
In this example, the equation is:
$$50mg/5mL = \frac{35mg}{X}$$
$$X = 3.5mL$$
CN: Physiological integrity; CNS: Pharmacological and parenteral therapies; CL: Analyze

120. 26.
Pulse pressure is the difference between systolic and diastolic pressures.
$$108 - 82 = 26.$$
Normally, systolic pressure exceeds diastolic pressure by about 40 mm Hg (30–50 mm Hg is normal range). Narrowed pulse pressure, a difference of less than 30 mm Hg, is a sign of cardiac tamponade.
CN: Physiological integrity; CNS: Physiological adaptation; CL: Apply

121. The apical heart rate is best heard at the point of maximal impulse, which is generally in the fifth intercostal space at the midclavicular line.

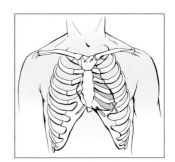

CN: Health promotion and maintenance; CNS: None; CL: Apply

Chapter 4

Hematologic & Immune Disorders

Hematologic & immunologic refresher

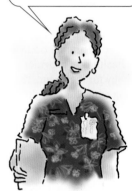

This challenging chapter covers HIV infection, AIDS, rheumatoid arthritis, DIC, and lots of other complex disorders. You can handle it, though; I know you can.

Acquired immunodeficiency syndrome (AIDS)

Immunologic disorder caused by human immunodeficiency virus (HIV) that lowers CD4+ T-cell count, increases susceptibility to opportunistic infections, and is the end stage of HIV infection

Key signs and symptoms

- Anorexia, weight loss, recurrent diarrhea, generalized lymphadenopathy
- Disorientation, confusion, dementia
- History of night sweats
- History of opportunistic infections (e.g., tuberculosis, candidiasis)

Key test results

- CD4+ T-cell level is less than 200 cells/µL.
- Enzyme-linked immunosorbent assay shows positive HIV antibody titer.
- Western blot test is positive.

Key treatments

- Transfusion therapy: fresh frozen plasma, platelets, and packed red blood cells (RBCs)
- Antibiotic: sulfamethoxazole and trimethoprim
- Antiprotozoal agent: pentamidine
- Combination therapy
- Non-nucleoside reverse transcriptase inhibitors: delavirdine, nevirapine, efavirenz
- Nucleoside reverse transcriptase inhibitors: lamivudine, zidovudine, abacavir, didanosine, emtricitabine, stavudine, tenofovir
- Protease inhibitors: indinavir, nelfinavir, ritonavir, atazanavir
- Fusion inhibitor: enfuvirtide

Key interventions

- Monitor for opportunistic infections.
- Maintain the client's diet.
- Provide mouth care.
- Maintain standard precautions.
- Make referrals to community agencies for support.
- Monitor respiratory status.

Anaphylaxis

Severe and life-threatening allergic reaction with massive release of histamine from the damaged cells

Key signs and symptoms

- Cardiovascular symptoms (hypotension, shock, cardiac arrhythmias) that may precipitate circulatory collapse if untreated
- Sudden physical distress within seconds or minutes after exposure to an allergen (may include feeling of impending doom or fright, weakness, sweating, sneezing, shortness of breath, nasal pruritus, urticaria, and angioedema, followed rapidly by symptoms in one or more target organs)
- Respiratory symptoms (nasal mucosal edema; profuse, watery rhinorrhea; itching; nasal congestion; sudden sneezing attacks; edema of the upper respiratory tract that causes hoarseness, stridor, and dyspnea [early sign of acute respiratory failure])

Key test results

- Rapid onset of severe respiratory or cardiovascular symptoms after an insect sting or after ingestion or injection of a drug, vaccine, diagnostic agent, food, or food additive

Key treatment

- Immediate subcutaneous (SQ) injection of epinephrine 1:1,000 aqueous solution, 0.1 to 0.5 mL, repeated every 10 to 15 minutes as necessary

Key interventions

- In early stages, give epinephrine intramuscularly (IM) or SQ and help it move into the circulation faster by massaging the injection site.
- In severe reactions, epinephrine should be given intravenously (IV).
- Maintain airway patency.
- Observe for early signs of laryngeal edema (stridor, hoarseness, and dyspnea).
- Prepare for endotracheal tube insertion or a tracheotomy and oxygen therapy.
- Monitor blood pressure and urine output.

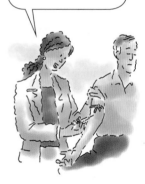

In anaphylaxis, epinephrine can be a life saver.

Ankylosing spondylitis

Inflammation of the spine causing abnormal fusion of vertebrae

Key signs and symptoms

- Intermittent lower back pain (the first indication), usually most severe in the morning or after a period of inactivity
- Mild fatigue, fever, anorexia, or weight loss; unilateral acute anterior uveitis
- Stiffness and limited motion of the lumbar spine

Key test results

- Typical symptoms, a family history, and the presence of HLA-B27 strongly suggest ankylosing spondylitis.
- Confirmation requires characteristic x-ray findings:
  - Blurring of the bony margins of joints in the early stage
  - Bilateral sacroiliac involvement
  - Patchy sclerosis with superficial bony erosions
  - Eventual squaring of vertebral bodies
  - "Bamboo spine" with complete ankylosis

Key treatments

- Good posture, stretching, and deep-breathing exercises; in some clients, braces and lightweight supports to delay further deformity
- Anti-inflammatory agents: aspirin, ibuprofen, indomethacin, naproxen, sulfasalazine to control pain and inflammation
- Tumor necrosis factor blockers: adalimumab, etanercept, infliximab, golimumab

Key interventions

- Offer support and reassurance; keep in mind that the client's limited range of motion makes simple tasks difficult.
- Administer medications as needed.
- Apply local heat and provide massage; assess mobility and degree of discomfort frequently.

Aplastic anemia

Decrease in production of RBCs and other blood elements due to bone marrow suppression

Key signs and symptoms

- Dyspnea, tachypnea
- Epistaxis
- Melena
- Palpitations, tachycardia
- Purpura, petechiae, ecchymosis, pallor

Key test results

- Bone marrow biopsy shows decrease in activity or no cell production.

Key treatments

- Transfusion of platelets and packed RBCs
- Antithymocyte globulin
- Hematopoietic growth factor: epoetin alfa

Key interventions

- Monitor for infection, bleeding, and bruising.
- Administer oxygen.
- Monitor transfusion therapy as prescribed.
- Maintain protective precautions.
- Avoid giving the client IM injections.

Calcium imbalance

Hypocalcemia
- Decrease in blood calcium level

Hypercalcemia
- Increase in blood calcium level

Key signs and symptoms

Hypocalcemia
- Cardiac arrhythmias
- Chvostek sign
- Tetany
- Trousseau sign

Hypercalcemia
- Anorexia
- Decreased muscle tone
- Lethargy
- Muscle weakness
- Nausea
- Polydipsia
- Polyuria

Key test results

Because approximately one half of serum calcium is bound to albumin, changes in serum protein must be considered when interpreting serum calcium levels.

Hypocalcemia
- Serum calcium level is less than 4.5 mEq/L.
- Electrocardiogram reveals a lengthened QT interval, a prolonged ST segment, and arrhythmias.

Hypercalcemia
- Serum calcium level is greater than 5.5 mEq/L.
- Electrocardiogram reveals a shortened QT interval and heart block.

Key treatments

Hypocalcemia
- Diet: adequate intake of calcium, vitamin D, and protein

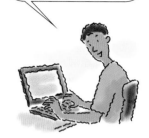

Let's refresh your memory on hematologic and immune disorders.

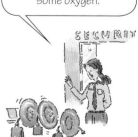

We're just carrying some oxygen.

- Ergocalciferol (vitamin D_2), cholecalciferol (vitamin D_3), calcitriol, dihydrotachysterol (synthetic form of vitamin D_2) for severe deficiency
- Immediate correction by IV calcium gluconate or calcium chloride for acute hypocalcemia (an emergency)

Hypercalcemia
- Calcitonin
- Loop diuretics: ethacrynic acid and furosemide to promote calcium excretion (thiazide diuretics are contraindicated in hypercalcemia because they inhibit calcium excretion)

Key interventions

Hypocalcemia
- Monitor serum calcium levels every 12 to 24 hours. When giving calcium supplements, frequently check the pH level. Check for Trousseau and Chvostek signs.

Hypercalcemia
- Monitor serum calcium levels frequently.
- Increase fluid intake.

Chloride imbalance

Hypochloremia
- Decrease in blood chloride level

Hyperchloremia
- Increase in blood chloride level

Key signs and symptoms

Hypochloremia
- Muscle hypertonicity (in conditions related to loss of gastric secretions)
- Muscle weakness
- Shallow, depressed breathing
- Twitching

Hyperchloremia
- Agitation
- Deep, rapid breathing
- Diminished cognitive ability
- Hypertension
- Pitting edema
- Tachycardia
- Weakness

Key test results

Hypochloremia
- Serum chloride level is less than 98 mEq/L.
- Supportive values with metabolic alkalosis include a serum pH greater than 7.45 and a serum carbon dioxide level greater than 32 mEq/L.

Hyperchloremia
- Serum chloride level is greater than 108 mEq/L.

- With metabolic acidosis, serum pH is less than 7.35 and the serum carbon dioxide level is less than 22 mEq/L.

Key treatments

Hypochloremia
- Acidifying agent: ammonium chloride
- Diet: salty broth
- Saline solution IV

Hyperchloremia
- Alkalinizing agent: sodium bicarbonate IV
- Lactated Ringer's solution

Key interventions

Hypochloremia
- Monitor electrolyte levels.
- Watch for excessive or continuous loss of gastric secretions.

Disseminated intravascular coagulation (DIC)

- Overactivity of clotting cascade related to a triggering factor (sepsis, trauma, cancer, shock, toxins, etc.), resulting in widespread formation of clots in microcirculation with subsequent reduction of clotting factors

Key signs and symptoms

- Abnormal bleeding without an accompanying history of serious hemorrhagic disorder
- Oliguria
- Shock

Key test results

- Blood tests show a prothrombin time (PT) greater than 15 seconds; a partial thromboplastin time (PTT) greater than 60 seconds; fibrinogen levels less than 150 mg/dL; platelet levels less than 100,000/μL; and fibrin degradation product levels commonly greater than 100 μg/mL.
- A positive D-dimer test is specific for DIC.

Key treatments

- Treat the underlying cause (e.g., sepsis requires antibiotics).
- Bed rest
- Transfusion therapy: fresh frozen plasma, platelets, packed RBCs
- Anticoagulant: heparin IV (heparin sodium injection) is a controversial treatment used to interrupt the thrombosis activity; however, this places the client at increased risk of bleeding.

Key interventions

- Enforce complete bed rest during bleeding episodes; pad the side rails if the client becomes agitated.

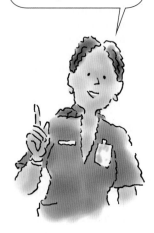

Encourage clients with hypocalcemia to increase their intake of calcium, vitamin D, and protein.

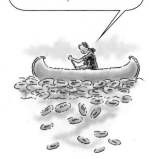

Excessive clotting and insufficient clotting are both problematic.

- Check all IV and venipuncture sites frequently for bleeding. Apply pressure to injection sites for at least 10 minutes. Alert other personnel to the client's tendency to hemorrhage.
- Watch for transfusion reactions and signs of fluid overload.
- Weigh the client daily, particularly in renal involvement.
- Monitor the results of serial blood studies (particularly hematocrit [HCT], hemoglobin [Hb] level, and coagulation times).

Hemophilia

Group of hereditary bleeding disorders caused by lack of coagulation factor

Key signs and symptoms

- Hematuria
- Joint tenderness
- Pain and swelling in a weight-bearing joint
- Prolonged bleeding after major trauma or surgery (in mild hemophilia)
- Spontaneous or severe bleeding after minor trauma (in severe hemophilia)
- SQ and IM hematomas (in moderate hemophilia)
- Tarry stools

Key test results

- Factor VIII assay reveals 0% to 25% of normal factor VIII (hemophilia A)
- Factor IX assay shows deficiency (hemophilia B)

Key treatments

- Administration of factor VIII or lyophilized cryoprecipitate antihemophilic factor (AHF) and lyophilized (dehydrated) AHF to encourage normal hemostasis (for hemophilia A)
- Administration of purified factor IX to promote hemostasis (for hemophilia B)
- Administration of analgesics to control joint pain (for both types)

Key interventions

- During bleeding episodes, monitor clotting factor or plasma administration; also administer analgesics.
- Avoid IM injections.
- Aspirin and aspirin-containing medications are contraindicated.
- If the client has bled into a joint, immediately elevate the joint.

Iron deficiency anemia

Anemia caused by inadequate intake of iron, malabsorption, and blood loss, which depletes iron stores

Key signs and symptoms

- Pallor
- Sensitivity to cold
- Weakness and fatigue

Key test results

- Hematology shows decreased levels of Hb, HCT, iron, ferritin, reticulocytes, red cell indices, transferrin, and saturation; absent hemosiderin; and increased iron-binding capacity.

Key treatments

- Diet: high in iron, fiber, and protein with increased fluids; avoid teas and coffee, which reduce absorption of iron
- Vitamins: pyridoxine (vitamin B_6), ascorbic acid (vitamin C)
- Iron supplements: ferrous sulfate, iron dextran

Key interventions

- Monitor cardiovascular and respiratory status.
- Monitor stool, urine, and vomitus for occult blood.
- Administer medications as prescribed; administer iron injection deep into muscle using Z-track technique.
- Provide mouth, skin, and foot care.

Kaposi sarcoma

Red-brown to purplish skin lesion seen mainly in clients with AIDS

Key signs and symptoms

- One or more obvious lesions in various shapes, sizes, and colors (ranging from red-brown to dark purple) that appear most commonly on the skin, buccal mucosa, hard and soft palates, lips, gums, tongue, tonsils, conjunctivae, and sclerae
- Pain (if the sarcoma advances beyond the early stages or if the lesion breaks down or impinges on nerves or organs)

Key test results

- Tissue biopsy identifies the lesion's type and stage

Key treatments

- High-calorie, high-protein diet
- Radiation therapy
- Antineoplastics: doxorubicin, etoposide, vinblastine, vincristine
- Antiemetics: dolasetron

Key interventions

- Inspect the client's skin every shift. Look for new lesions and skin breakdown. Help

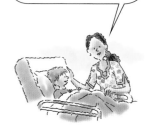

Use extra care when working with clients with hemophilia, as they bruise and bleed easily.

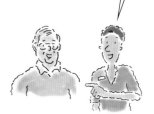

Encourage clients with iron deficiency anemia to consume plenty of protein.

the client into a more comfortable position if lesions are painful.

- Administer pain medications. Suggest distractions and help the client with relaxation techniques.
- Urge the client to share his or her feelings; provide encouragement.
- Supply the client with high-calorie, high-protein meals. Provide the client with frequent, smaller meals if regular meals are not tolerated. Consult with a dietitian and plan meals around the client's treatment.
- Be alert for adverse reactions to radiation therapy or chemotherapy, such as anorexia, nausea, vomiting, and diarrhea. Take steps to prevent or alleviate these reactions.
- Explain infection-prevention techniques; if necessary, demonstrate basic hygiene measures. Advise the client not to share his or her toothbrush, razor, or other items that may be contaminated with blood (especially if the client also has HIV or AIDS).

Leukemia

Hematologic malignant disorder, resulting in an overproduction and overcrowding of immature leukocytes in the bone marrow

Key signs and symptoms

- Enlarged lymph nodes, spleen, and liver
- Frequent infections
- Bone pain
- Weakness and fatigue

Key test results

- Bone marrow biopsy shows large numbers of immature leukocytes.

Key treatments

- Antimetabolites: fluorouracil, methotrexate
- Vinca alkaloids: vinblastine, vincristine
- Antineoplastic antibiotics: doxorubicin
- Hematopoietic growth factor: epoetin alfa
- Granulocyte-colony stimulating factor: filgrastim

Key interventions

- Monitor for bleeding.
- Place a client with epistaxis in an upright position, leaning slightly forward.
- Monitor for infection; promptly report any temperature over 101 °F (38.3 °C) and decreased white blood cell (WBC) counts.
- Monitor transfusion therapy for adverse reactions.
- Provide gentle mouth and skin care.

Lymphoma

Type of cancer of lymphoid tissue, consisting of two main types: Hodgkin lymphoma and non-Hodgkin lymphoma (malignant lymphoma)

Key signs and symptoms

- Predictable pattern of spread (Hodgkin lymphoma)
- Enlarged, nontender, firm, and movable lymph nodes in lower cervical regions (Hodgkin lymphoma)
- Less predictable pattern of spread (malignant lymphoma)
- Prominent, painless, generalized lymphadenopathy (malignant lymphoma)

Key test results

- Lymph node biopsy is positive for Reed-Sternberg cells (Hodgkin lymphoma).
- Bone marrow aspiration and biopsy reveal small, diffuse, lymphocytic cells or large, follicular-type cells (malignant lymphoma).

Key treatments

- Radiation therapy
- Transfusion of packed RBCs
- Chemotherapy for Hodgkin lymphoma: vincristine, procarbazine, doxorubicin, bleomycin, vinblastine, dacarbazine
- Chemotherapy for malignant lymphoma: cyclophosphamide, vincristine, doxorubicin

Key interventions

- Monitor for bleeding, infection, jaundice, and electrolyte imbalance.
- Provide mouth and skin care.
- Encourage fluids.
- Administer medications as prescribed and monitor for adverse effects.
- Maintain transfusion therapy as prescribed and monitor for adverse reactions.

Magnesium imbalance

Hypomagnesemia
- Decrease in blood magnesium level

Hypermagnesemia
- Increase in blood magnesium level

Key signs and symptoms

Hypomagnesemia
- Arrhythmias
- Neuromuscular irritability
- Chvostek sign
- Mood changes
- Confusion

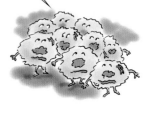

Overcrowding of the "good guys" can be an indicator of trouble brewing.

We're ready to spring into action!

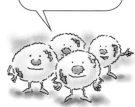

Hypermagnesemia
- Diminished deep tendon reflexes
- Weakness
- Confusion
- Heart block
- Nausea
- Vomiting

Key test results
Hypomagnesemia
- Serum magnesium levels less than 1.5 mEq/L

Hypermagnesemia
- Serum magnesium levels greater than 2.5 mEq/L

Key treatments
Hypomagnesemia
- Daily magnesium supplements IM or by mouth
- High-magnesium diet
- Magnesium sulfate IV (10 to 40 mEq/L diluted in IV fluid) for severe cases

Hypermagnesemia
- Diet: low magnesium with increased fluid intake
- Loop diuretic: furosemide
- Magnesium antagonist: calcium gluconate (10%)
- Peritoneal dialysis or hemodialysis if renal function fails, or if excess magnesium cannot be eliminated

Key interventions
Hypomagnesemia
- Monitor serum electrolyte levels (including magnesium, calcium, and potassium) daily for mild deficits (every 6 to 12 hours during replacement therapy).
- Measure intake and output frequently (urine output should not fall below 25 mL/hour or 600 mL/day).
- Monitor vital signs during IV therapy. Infuse magnesium replacement slowly. Watch for bradycardia, heart block, and decreased respiratory rate.
- Have calcium gluconate IV available to reverse hypermagnesemia from overcorrection.

Hypermagnesemia
- Frequently check level of consciousness (LOC), muscle activity, and vital signs.
- Keep accurate intake and output records; provide sufficient fluids.
- Correct abnormal serum electrolyte levels immediately.
- Monitor the client receiving cardiac glycosides and calcium gluconate simultaneously.

Metabolic acidosis
Accumulation of excess hydrogen ions in the body or excessive loss of bicarbonate from the body

Key signs and symptoms
- Central nervous system depression
- Kussmaul respirations
- Lethargy

Key test results
- Arterial blood gas (ABG) analysis: pH below 7.35; bicarbonate level less than 24 mEq/L

Key treatments
- Correction of underlying cause
- Sodium bicarbonate IV or orally

Key interventions
- Keep sodium bicarbonate ampules handy.
- Frequently monitor vital signs, laboratory results, and LOC.
- Record intake and output.

Metabolic alkalosis
- Accumulation of excess bicarbonate in the body or excessive removal of acid from the body

Key signs and symptoms
- Atrial tachycardia
- Confusion
- Diarrhea
- Hypoventilation
- Twitching
- Vomiting

Key test results
- ABG analysis: pH greater than 7.45; bicarbonate level above 29 mEq/L

Key treatments
- Treatment of underlying cause
- Acidifying agent: ammonium chloride IV

Key interventions
- Monitor ammonium chloride 0.9% infusion.
- Monitor vital signs and record intake and output.

Multiple myeloma
Proliferation of malignant plasma cells in the bone marrow

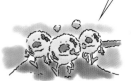

Your immune response team is on the way!

Key signs and symptoms

- Anemia, thrombocytopenia, hemorrhage
- Constant, severe bone pain
- Pathologic fractures, skeletal deformities of the sternum and ribs, loss of height

Key test results

- Bence Jones protein assay is positive.
- X-ray shows diffuse, round, punched-out bone lesions; osteoporosis; osteo-lytic lesions of the skull; and widespread demineralization.
- Bone marrow biopsy confirms diagnosis with the presence of sheets of plasma cells.

Key treatments

- Orthopedic devices: braces, splints, casts
- Alkylating agents: melphalan, cyclophosphamide
- Antibiotics: doxorubicin
- Antigout agent: allopurinol
- Antineoplastics: vinblastine, vincristine
- Glucocorticoid: prednisone
- Proteasome inhibiting agent: bortezomib

Key interventions

- Monitor renal status.
- Evaluate bone pain.
- Maintain IV fluids.

Pernicious anemia

Vitamin B_{12} deficiency caused by lack of the intrinsic factor produced by gastric mucosa

Key signs and symptoms

- Paresthesia of hands and feet
- Weight loss, anorexia, dyspepsia
- Smooth, sore, bright red tongue
- Cheilosis

Key test results

- Bone marrow aspiration shows increased megaloblasts, few maturing erythrocytes, and defective leukocyte maturation.
- Schilling test is positive.
- Peripheral blood smear reveals oval, macro-cytic, hyperchromic erythrocytes.

Key treatment

- Vitamins: pyridoxine (vitamin B_6), ascorbic acid (vitamin C), cyanocobalamin (vitamin B_{12}), folic acid (vitamin B_9)

Key interventions

- Monitor cardiovascular status.
- Administer medications as prescribed.
- Provide mouth care before and after meals.
- Prevent the client from falling.

Phosphorus imbalance

Hypophosphatemia
- Decrease in blood phosphorus level

Hyperphosphatemia
- Increase in blood phosphorus level

Key signs and symptoms

Hypophosphatemia
- Muscle weakness
- Paresthesia
- Tremor

Hyperphosphatemia
- Usually produces no symptoms

Key test results

Hypophosphatemia
- Serum phosphorus level is less than 1.7 mEq/L (or 2.5 mg/dL).
- Urine phosphorus level greater than 1.3 g/24 hours supports this diagnosis.

Hyperphosphatemia
- Serum phosphorus level is greater than 2.6 mEq/L (or 4.5 mg/dL).
- Supportive values include decreased levels of serum calcium (less than 9 mg/dL) and urine phosphorus (less than 0.9 g/24 hours).

Key treatments

Hypophosphatemia
- High-phosphorus diet
- Phosphate supplements

Hyperphosphatemia
- Low-phosphorus diet
- Calcium supplement: calcium acetate

Key interventions

Hypophosphatemia
- Record intake and output accurately. Assess renal function. Be alert for hypocalcemia when giving phosphate supplements.
- Advise the client to follow a high-phosphorus diet containing milk and milk products, kidney, liver, turkey, and dried fruits.

Hyperphosphatemia
- Monitor intake and output; notify the health care provider immediately if urine output falls below 25 mL/hour or 600 mL/day.
- Watch for signs of hypocalcemia (e.g., muscle twitching, tetany), which commonly accompany hyperphosphatemia.
- Advise the client to eat foods low in phosphorus (e.g., vegetables); obtain dietary consultation if the condition results from chronic renal insufficiency.

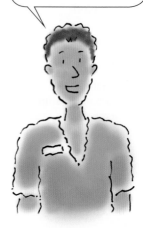

A deficiency of B_{12} is only pernicious without medical intervention.

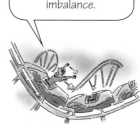

Hyper, hypo— with all these ups and downs, I must be experiencing an imbalance.

Polycythemia vera

Overproduction of erythrocytes in the bone marrow

Key signs and symptoms

- Clubbing of the digits
- Dizziness
- Headache
- Hypertension
- Ruddy cyanosis of the nose
- Thrombosis of smaller vessels
- Visual disturbances (blurring, diplopia, engorged veins of fundus and retina)

Key test results

- Elevated Hb level, RBC count, WBC count, platelet count, and leukocyte alkaline phosphatase, serum B_{12}, and uric acid levels; low levels of erythropoietin

Key treatments

- Phlebotomy: 350 to 500 mL of blood (typically) removed every other day until the client's HCT is reduced to the low-to-normal range
- Antimetabolites: hydroxyurea
- Antiplatelet aggregation: anagrelide
- Plasmapheresis
- Antineoplastics: melphalan
- Antigout agent: allopurinol

Key interventions

- Check blood pressure, pulse rate, and respirations before and during phlebotomy.
- During phlebotomy, make sure the client is lying down comfortably.
- Stay alert for tachycardia, clamminess, or reports of vertigo; stop the procedure if these occur.
- Check blood pressure and pulse rate after phlebotomy. Have the client sit up for about 5 minutes before allowing him or her to walk. Administer 24 oz (710 mL) of juice or water.
- Tell the client to watch for and report symptoms of iron deficiency (pallor, weight loss, weakness, glossitis).
- Give additional fluids, administer allopurinol, and alkalinize the urine.
- Warn outpatients who develop leukopenia that their resistance to infection is low; advise them to avoid crowds and watch for symptoms of infection.
- Tell the client about possible adverse effects of alkylating agents (nausea, vomiting, risk of infection).
- Have the client lie down during IV administration of alkylating agents and for 15 to 20 minutes afterward.

Rheumatoid arthritis

Chronic, systemic, autoimmune disease causing inflammation of the joints and related structures

Key signs and symptoms

- Painful, swollen joints; crepitus; morning stiffness
- Symmetrical joint swelling (mirror image of affected joints)

Key test results

- Antinuclear antibody test: Positive
- Rheumatoid factor test: Positive

Key treatments

- Cold therapy during acute episodes
- Heat therapy to relax muscles and relieve pain in chronic disease
- Disease-modifying antirheumatic drugs: etanercept, adalimumab, abatacept, methotrexate, tofacitinib, hydroxychloroquine
- Cyclo-oxygenase-2 inhibitor: celecoxib
- Glucocorticoids: prednisone, hydrocortisone
- Immunosuppressant: cyclophosphamide
- Nonsteroidal anti-inflammatory drugs (NSAIDs): indomethacin, ibuprofen, naproxen, diflunisal

Key interventions

- Check joints for swelling, pain, and redness.
- Splint inflamed joints.
- Provide warm or cold therapy as prescribed.

Scleroderma

Progressive, systemic, autoimmune disease involving fibrosis of the skin and connective tissue

Key signs and symptoms

- Pain
- Signs and symptoms of Raynaud phenomenon (e.g., blanching, cyanosis, erythema of the fingers and toes) in response to stress or exposure to cold
- Stiffness
- Swelling of fingers and joints
- Taut, shiny skin over the entire hand and forearm
- Tight and inelastic facial skin, causing a masklike appearance and "pinching" of the mouth
- Signs and symptoms of renal involvement, usually accompanied by malignant hypertension, the main cause of death

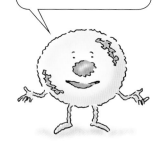

We immune cells sometimes get a little confused and attack your body ... sorry about that.

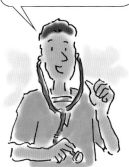

Blanching, cyanosis, and reddening of fingers and toes in the cold—what condition does this sound like?

Key test results

- Erythrocyte sedimentation rate (ESR) is slightly elevated. A positive rheumatoid factor occurs in 25% to 35% of clients. The antinuclear antibody test is positive.
- Skin biopsy may show changes consistent with progress of the disease (e.g., marked thickening of the dermis, occlusive vessel changes).

Key treatments

- Physical therapy to maintain function and promote muscle strength
- Immunosuppressants: cyclosporine, cyclophosphamide, azathioprine, mycophenolate

Key interventions

- Evaluate the client's motion restrictions, pain, vital signs, intake and output, respiratory function, and daily weight.
- Teach the client to monitor blood pressure at home and report any increases above baseline.
- Whenever possible, let client participate in treatment.

Septic shock

Type of shock that occurs in severe infection and sepsis

Key signs and symptoms

Early stage
- Chills
- Oliguria
- Sudden fever (over 101°F [38.3°C])

Late stage
- Altered LOC
- Anuria
- Hyperventilation
- Hypotension
- Hypothermia
- Restlessness
- Tachycardia
- Tachypnea

Key test results

- Blood cultures isolate the organism.
- Decreased platelet count and leukocytosis (15,000 to 30,000/μL), increased blood urea nitrogen and creatinine levels, decreased creatinine clearance, and abnormal PT and PTT are present.

Key treatments

- Removing and replacing any IV or urinary drainage catheters that may be the source of infection

- Oxygen therapy (may require endotracheal intubation and mechanical ventilation)
- Colloid or crystalloid infusion to increase intravascular volume
- Diuretic: furosemide after sufficient fluid volume has been replaced to maintain urine output above 20 mL/hour
- Antibiotics: according to the sensitivity of the causative organism
- Vasopressors: dopamine, norepinephrine, or phenylephrine, if fluid resuscitation fails to increase blood pressure

Key interventions

- Remove any IV or urinary drainage catheters and send to the laboratory; new catheters can be reinserted.
- Maintain IV infusion with normal saline solution or lactated Ringer's solution, usually using a large-bore (14G to 18G) catheter.
- If systolic blood pressure drops below 80 mm Hg, increase oxygen flow rate and call the health care provider immediately.
- Keep accurate intake and output records.
- Administer antibiotics IV and monitor drug levels.

Sickle cell anemia

Chronic, severe, genetic type of anemia characterized by crescent-shaped RBCs, causing a decrease in tissue perfusion

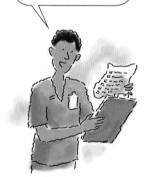

Sickle cell anemia—it's all in the genes.

Key signs and symptoms

- Aching bones
- Jaundice (worsens during painful crisis), pallor
- Unexplained dyspnea or dyspnea on exertion
- Tachycardia
- Severe pain (during sickle cell crisis)

Key test results

- Low RBC counts, elevated WBC and platelet counts, decreased ESR, increased serum iron levels, decreased RBC survival, and reticulocytosis are present.
- Hb electrophoresis shows Hb S.

Key treatments

- Iron and folic acid supplements to prevent anemia
- IV fluid therapy to prevent dehydration and vessel occlusion
- Analgesics: meperidine or morphine (to relieve pain from vaso-occlusive crises)

Key interventions
- Apply warm compresses to painful areas; cover the client with a blanket.
- Maintain the client on bed rest.
- Encourage fluid intake and maintain prescribed IV fluids.

Sodium imbalance
Hyponatremia
- Decrease in blood sodium level

Hypernatremia
- Increase in blood sodium level

Key signs and symptoms
Hyponatremia
- Abdominal cramps
- Cold, clammy skin
- Cyanosis
- Hypotension
- Oliguria or anuria
- Seizures
- Tachycardia

Hypernatremia
- Dry, sticky mucous membranes
- Excessive weight gain
- Flushed skin
- Hypertension
- Intense thirst
- Oliguria
- Pitting edema
- Rough, dry tongue
- Tachycardia

Key test results
Hyponatremia
- Serum sodium level less than 135 mEq/L

Hypernatremia
- Serum sodium level greater than 145 mEq/L

Key treatments
Hyponatremia
- IV infusion of saline solution
- Potassium supplement: potassium chloride

Hypernatremia
- Diet: sodium restrictions
- Salt-free solution (such as dextrose in water), followed by infusion of 0.45% sodium chloride to prevent hyponatremia

Key interventions
Hyponatremia
- Watch for extremely low serum sodium and accompanying serum chloride levels. Monitor urine specific gravity and other laboratory results. Record fluid intake and output accurately. Weigh the client daily.
- During administration of isosmolar or hyperosmolar saline solution, watch closely for signs of hypervolemia (dyspnea, crackles, engorged neck or hand veins).

Hypernatremia
- Measure serum sodium levels every 6 hours or at least daily. Monitor vital signs for changes, especially for rising pulse rate. Watch for signs of hypervolemia, especially in a client receiving IV fluids.
- Record fluid intake and output accurately, checking for body fluid loss; weigh the client daily.

Systemic lupus erythematosus
Chronic, systemic, inflammatory, autoimmune disease that can cause multiorgan failure

Key signs and symptoms
- Butterfly rash on the face (the rash may vary in severity from malar erythema to discoid lesions)
- Fatigue
- Migratory pain, joint stiffness, and swelling

Key test result
- Lupus erythematosus cell preparation is positive.

Key treatments
- Cytotoxic drug: methotrexate to delay or prevent deteriorating renal status
- Immunosuppressants: azathioprine, cyclophosphamide
- NSAIDs: indomethacin, ibuprofen, diclofenac sodium, naproxen, diflunisal

Key interventions
- Evaluate musculoskeletal status.
- Monitor renal status.
- Provide prophylactic skin, mouth, and perineal care.
- Maintain seizure precautions.
- Minimize environmental stress, and provide rest periods.

Vasculitis
Group of disorders that can cause inflammation of the blood vessels

Key signs and symptoms
- Wegener granulomatosis
- Cough
- Fever
- Malaise

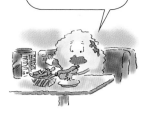

Diet can have an impact on blood sodium levels.

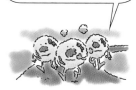

Immune cells of the body, charge! What do you mean we're going the wrong way?

- Signs and symptoms of pulmonary congestion
- Weight loss
- Temporal arteritis
- Headache (associated with polymyalgia rheumatica syndrome)
- Jaw claudication
- Myalgia
- Visual changes
- Takayasu arteritis
- Arthralgias
- Bruits
- Loss of distal pulses
- Malaise
- Pain or paresthesia distal to affected area
- Syncope
- Weight loss

Key test results
- Wegener granulomatosis is present.
- Tissue biopsy shows necrotizing vasculitis with granulomatous inflammation.
- Temporal arteritis is present.
- Tissue biopsy shows panarteritis with infiltration of mononuclear cells, giant cells within

the vessel wall, fragmentation of internal elastic lamina, and proliferation of intima.
- Takayasu arteritis is present.
- Arteriography shows calcification and obstruction of affected vessels.
- Tissue biopsy shows inflammation of adventitia and intima of vessels and thickening of vessel walls.

Key treatments
- Removal of the identified environmental antigen
- Diet: elimination of antigenic food, if identifiable
- Corticosteroid: prednisone
- Antineoplastic: cyclophosphamide

Key interventions
- Regulate environmental temperature.
- Monitor vital signs. Use a Doppler ultrasonic flowmeter, if available.
- Monitor intake and output. Check daily for edema. Keep the client well hydrated (3 L daily).

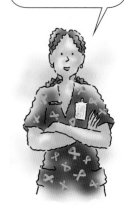

The word "-itis" refers to inflammation; so, what does "vasculitis" mean?

thePoint® You can download tables of drug information to help you prepare for the NCLEX®! View Generic Drug Names, Drug Classifications, Drug Actions, and Nursing Implications for the drugs discussed in this refresher at **http://thePoint.lww.com**

Hematologic & immunologic questions, answers, and rationales

1. Which nutritional education will the nurse include while teaching a client with acquired immunodeficiency syndrome (AIDS)? Select all that apply.
1. Thoroughly cook meats.
2. Choose foods low in fat.
3. Choose low-calorie foods.
4. Weigh yourself weekly.
5. Eat small, frequent meals.

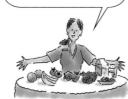

Let's get this chapter started with some good nutrition!

1. **1, 2, 5.** To prevent foodborne illness, all meat and poultry should be cooked thoroughly. It is necessary to avoid foods high in fats because drugs used to treat AIDS may cause hyperlipidemia. Consuming small, frequent meals consisting of high-calorie, nutrient-dense food helps improve overall nutrition. Daily, not weekly, weighing is important in determining patterns of weight loss.
CN: Physiological integrity; CNS: Basic care and comfort; CL: Apply

2. The nurse is reviewing a client's complete blood count (CBC) and notes an erythrocyte count of $8.2 \times 10^6/\mu L$ ($8.20 \times 10^{12}/L$), leukocytes of $12,100/\mu L$ ($12.10 \times 10^9/L$), and thrombocytes of $400,000/\mu L$ ($400 \times 10^9/L$). The nurse will suspect the client has which condition?
1. Pernicious anemia
2. Aplastic anemia
3. Sickle cell anemia
4. Polycythemia vera

2. **4.** Polycythemia vera is an overproduction of erythrocytes in the bone marrow. Clients with polycythemia vera may have elevated levels of hemoglobin, red blood cells (RBCs), white blood cells (WBCs), and platelets. The normal erythrocyte (RBC) count for an adult male is $4.6 \times 10^6/\mu L$ ($4.60 \times 10^{12}/L$) to $6.2 \times 10^6/\mu L$ ($6.20 \times 10^{12}/L$) and female is $4.2 \times 10^6/\mu L$ ($4.20 \times 10^{12}/L$) to $5.4 \times 10^6/\mu L$ ($5.40 \times 10^{12}/L$). The normal leukocyte (WBC) is $4,500/\mu L$ ($4.50 \times 10^9/L$) to $11,000/\mu L$ ($11.00 \times 10^9/L$), and the normal thrombocyte (platelet) count is $150,000/\mu L$ ($150 \times 10^9/L$) to $400,000/\mu L$ ($400 \times 10^9/L$).
CN: Physiological integrity; CNS: Reduction of risk potential; CL: Analyze

CN: Client needs category   CNS: Client needs subcategory   CL: Cognitive level

3. Immediately after giving an injection, a nurse is inadvertently stuck with the needle. When is the **best** time to test the nurse for human immunodeficiency virus (HIV) antibodies?
1. Immediately, and then again in 6 weeks
2. Immediately, and then again in 3 months
3. In 2 weeks, and then again in 6 months
4. In 2 weeks, and then again in 1 year

4. A nurse is assigned to a medical-surgical floor. Which client will the nurse see **first**?
1. A client with systemic lupus erythematosus (SLE) reporting fatigue and stiffness
2. A client with scleroderma reporting blanching and erythema of fingers while eating
3. A client with vasculitis reporting malaise and is taking prednisone daily
4. A client with hemophilia reporting joint pain after bumping into the bed

5. A client with human immunodeficiency virus (HIV) experiences frequent bouts of diarrhea. The nurse determines that dietary teaching is effective when the client chooses which food?
1. Coffee
2. Cheese pizza
3. Chicken soup
4. Hot chocolate

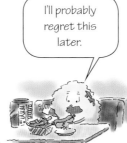

I'll probably regret this later.

6. A disease-modifying antirheumatic drug (DMARD) is prescribed by the health care provider to a client with rheumatoid arthritis. Which medication will the nurse anticipate administering?
1. Aspirin
2. Methotrexate
3. Ferrous sulfate
4. Prednisone

7. A client is admitted with rheumatoid arthritis. Which dietary recommendation will the nurse make to help reduce the client's inflammation?
1. Consume more salmon.
2. Drink vitamin D–fortified milk.
3. Increase red meat consumption.
4. Consume more spinach.

3. 2. The nurse should be tested immediately to determine whether a preexisting infection is present, and then again in 3 months to detect seroconversion as a result of the needlestick. Waiting 2 weeks to perform the first test is too late to detect preexisting infection. Retesting sooner than 3 months may yield false-negative results.
CN: Safe, effective care environment; CNS: Safety and infection control; CL: Remember

4. 4. The nurse should see the client with hemophilia first because an injury that causes joint pain after coming into contact with an object can also cause bleeding in a client with hemophilia. Therefore, the nurse should see this client first to evaluate for signs of bleeding and elevate the extremity. Fatigue and joint stiffness are commonly seen in clients with SLE. A client with scleroderma who reports blanching, erythema, and cyanosis of fingers may have Raynaud phenomenon, which is expected with scleroderma. A client with vasculitis is expected to have malaise and to take prednisone to decrease inflammation.
CN: Safe, effective care environment; CNS: Management of care; CL: Analyze

5. 3. The client may consume chicken soup and broiled meat. Clients with chronic diarrhea may develop intolerance to lactose, which may worsen the diarrhea. Other foods that the client should avoid include fatty foods, other lactose-containing foods, caffeine, and sugar.
CN: Physiological integrity; CNS: Reduction of risk potential; CL: Apply

6. 2. Methotrexate is considered the first-line disease-modifying antirheumatic drug (DMARD) for most clients with rheumatoid arthritis. Ferrous sulfate is not used to treat rheumatoid arthritis. Prednisone may be used to control inflammation when NSAIDs such as aspirin cannot be tolerated.
CN: Physiological integrity; CNS: Pharmacological and parenteral therapies; CL: Apply

7. 1. Salmon is high in omega-3 fatty acids. The therapeutic effect of fish oil is to suppress inflammatory mediator production (such as prostaglandins); how it works is unknown. Iron-rich foods, such as spinach and red meats, are recommended to decrease the anemia associated with rheumatoid arthritis. Calcium and vitamin D found in milk may help reduce bone resorption.
CN: Physiological integrity; CNS: Physiological adaptation; CL: Apply

CN: Client needs category   CNS: Client needs subcategory   CL: Cognitive level

8. A client is admitted with human immunodeficiency virus (HIV). Which statement by the client indicates to the nurse the need for further education regarding safer sex practices?
  1. "I should use plenty of oil-based lubricant when using a latex condom."
  2. "I should inspect the condom for damage or defects before I use it."
  3. "I must check the expiration date on the package before using the condom."
  4. "Latex condoms are the best choice for preventing the spread of HIV."

8. **1.** Water-based lubricants should be used; oil- or petroleum-based products can damage latex condoms and lead to holes or tearing. Latex condoms, as well as polyurethane condoms, which are a good option if the client has a latex allergy, have been proven to decrease the spread of HIV. Checking for damaged, defective, or expired condoms ensures the integrity of the condoms and decreases the likelihood of HIV transmission.
CN: Health promotion and maintenance; CNS: None; CL: Apply

9. The nurse prepares to start an intravenous access site in a client with Kaposi sarcoma. Which action(s) will the nurse perform? Select all that apply.
  1. Wear gloves.
  2. Apply shoe covers.
  3. Don a surgical mask.
  4. Use aseptic technique.
  5. Wash hands prior to performing the procedure.

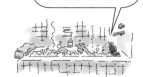

Now this is my idea of preparing for clients on precautions.

9. **1, 4, 5.** Kaposi sarcoma is a type of skin cancer seen in clients with acquired immunodeficiency syndrome (AIDS). It is a red-brown to purplish skin lesion. The nurse should use standard precautions when caring for clients with AIDS, which include washing hands, wearing gloves, and using aseptic (sterile) technique when starting an intravenous line. Surgical masks are used for droplet precaution. Shoe covers are not necessary.
CN: Safe, effective care environment; CNS: Safety and infection control; CL: Apply

10. Which instruction is appropriate for the nurse to include when providing education to a client with human immunodeficiency virus (HIV) who is at high risk for altered oral mucous membranes?
  1. "Brush your teeth frequently with a firm toothbrush."
  2. "Use mouthwash that contains an astringent agent."
  3. "You always have to heat the foods you consume."
  4. "It is important for you to lubricate your lips."

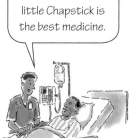

Sometimes a little Chapstick is the best medicine.

10. **4.** Lubricating the lips keeps them moist and prevents cracking. A firm toothbrush would damage already sensitive gums. An astringent would be painful, as would foods that are too hot.
CN: Physiological integrity; CNS: Reduction of risk potential; CL: Apply

11. The nurse is caring for a client with leukemia who is receiving chemotherapy. Which client need will the nurse consider a **priority**?
  1. Discussing self-image
  2. Planning appropriate nutrition
  3. Encouraging family support
  4. Enhancing mobility

11. **2.** The priority should be the client's nutritional needs because chemotherapy may cause nausea, vomiting, stomatitis, and diarrhea. All the other needs are also important but not the priority. According to Maslow's hierarchy of needs, physiologic needs should be met first before psychosocial needs.
CN: Physiological integrity; CNS: Basic care and comfort; CL: Analyze

12. The nurse is assessing a client who has been experiencing black stools for the past month. The client suddenly reports chest and stomach pain. Which action will the nurse perform **first**?
  1. Give nasal oxygen.
  2. Take vital signs.
  3. Begin cardiac monitoring.
  4. Draw blood for laboratory analysis.

12. **2.** Taking vital signs would determine hemodynamic stability, and monitoring heart rhythm may be indicated based on assessment findings. Giving nasal oxygen and drawing blood are not part of a screening assessment.
CN: Safe, effective care environment; CNS: Management of care; CL: Apply

CN: Client needs category   CNS: Client needs subcategory   CL: Cognitive level

13. Which information will the nurse include in the discharge instruction(s) for a client diagnosed with hemophilia? Select all that apply.
1. "Swimming is an appropriate form of exercise for you."
2. "Playing basketball is a great way for you to socialize with others."
3. "You should immediately elevate your extremity if you start bleeding."
4. "Take acetaminophen if you experience pain or fever."
5. "If you eat healthy foods, you should not have to worry about bleeding."

14. A client with rheumatoid arthritis is receiving oral prednisone. Which side effect(s) will the nurse expect to see from prolonged use of this medication? Select all that apply.
1. Weight loss
2. Hyperglycemia
3. Osteoporosis
4. Hirsutism
5. Cataract

15. A client with multiple myeloma is admitted with a calcium level of 14.6 mg/dL (3.65 mmol/L). Which finding(s) will the nurse anticipate in this client on assessment? Select all that apply.
1. Tetany
2. Renal calculi
3. Positive Chvostek sign
4. Decreased bowel sounds
5. Hyperactive deep tendon reflexes (DTRs)

16. The nurse assesses a client diagnosed with human immunodeficiency virus (HIV) infection. Which scenario suggests to the nurse the client has acquired immunodeficiency syndrome (AIDS) wasting syndrome?
1. A 34-year-old male with oral pain, dysphagia, and yellow-white plaques in his mouth and throat
2. A 42-year-old female with recurrent vaginitis causing intense itching and white, thick vaginal discharge
3. A 52-year-old male with impaired memory, hallucinations, loss of balance, and personality changes
4. A 46-year-old female who has lost 12% of her body weight, with weakness, fever, and chronic diarrhea for the past 35 days

13. 1, 3, 4. A client with hemophilia should avoid contact sports such as basketball because of the risk of bleeding with injury. The client can safely participate in noncontact sports such as swimming. The nurse should instruct the client to elevate extremities if bleeding occurs. The client with hemophilia may take acetaminophen for pain or fever but should avoid aspirin because of the increased risk of bleeding. Because hemophilia is a genetic disorder, eating healthy foods does not alter the client's diagnosis of hemophilia.
CN: Safe, effective care environment; CNS: Safety and infection control; CL: Analyze

14. 2, 3, 4, 5. Prednisone is a corticosteroid used for inflammation. Prolonged use of this drug causes hyperglycemia, osteoporosis, hirsutism, and cataract formation. Clients taking this medication experience weight *gain*, not weight loss, due to fluid retention.
CN: Physiological integrity; CNS: Pharmacological and parenteral therapies; CL: Apply

15. 2, 4. The client has hypercalcemia. Normal calcium level is 8.5 to 10.5 mg/dL (2.1 to 2.6 mmol/L). Calcium acts like a sedative; therefore, too much calcium causes sedative effects such as lethargy, confusion, muscle weakness, decreased DTRs, and decreased bowel sounds. Renal calculi are formed because most kidney stones are calcium stones, usually in the form of calcium oxalate. Tetany and Chvostek sign are both signs of hypocalcemia, in which the muscles are becoming tight due to a decrease in calcium. Chvostek sign is the twitching of the facial muscles in response to gentle tapping over the facial nerve in front of the ear.
CN: Physiological integrity; CNS: Physiological adaptation; CL: Analyze

16. 4. AIDS wasting syndrome is diagnosed when there is a loss of 10% or more of body weight and the presence of one or more of the following for more than 30 days: fever, weakness, and at least two loose stools daily. Oral pain with visible yellow-white plaques and vaginitis with a white, cottage cheese–like discharge suggest infection with *Candida albicans*. Impaired intellect and motor functioning indicate HIV infection of the central nervous system with AIDS dementia complex.
CN: Physiological integrity; CNS: Physiological adaptation; CL: Analyze

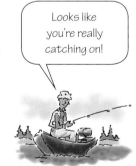

Looks like you're really catching on!

17. The nurse is making assignments for the assistive personnel (AP). Which task(s) can the nurse safely assigned to AP? Select all that apply.
 1. Providing information on dietary changes for a client with anemia
 2. Assisting the client with hyperphosphatemia in choosing a meal
 3. Teaching a client with rheumatoid arthritis how to use the cane
 4. Bathing a client who is diagnosed with ankylosing spondylitis
 5. Turning a client diagnosed with AIDS who is poorly nourished

18. The nurse cares for a client reporting chest and stomach pain with a history of black, tarry stools for the past 2 months. Which client lab value is **priority** for the nurse to review?
 1. Complete blood count (CBC)
 2. Prothrombin time (PT)
 3. Fecal occult blood test
 4. Serum metabolic panel

19. While the nurse is teaching a client about the adverse effects of filgrastim, which adverse effect will the nurse tell the client to **immediately** report to the health care provider?
 1. Nausea
 2. Bone pain
 3. Petechiae
 4. Fatigue

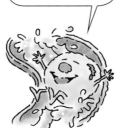

Leukocytes are delivered quickly to the site of an infection.

20. A client is scheduled for a magnetic resonance imaging (MRI). Which situation will require further assessment by the nurse?
 1. The client has history of leukemia.
 2. The client is allergic to barium.
 3. The client is afraid of using elevators.
 4. The client is experiencing phototherapy.

21. The nurse understands that which client is at the **highest** risk of developing anemia?
 1. A client with a colostomy following colon resection
 2. A client with gastroesophageal reflux disease (GERD)
 3. A client who has had a gastrectomy
 4. A client diagnosed with dumping syndrome

17. 4, 5. Assistive personnel (AP) can safely perform bathing and turning a client. The registered nurse (RN) should only delegate routine, unchanging tasks and tasks with lower priority. Teaching a client how to use the cane and providing education on dietary choices that are high in iron or low in phosphorus are not within the scope of AP's practice.
CN: Safe, effective care environment; CNS: Management of care; CL: Apply

18. 1. A CBC determines anemia (hemoglobin) and is priority for the nurse to review based on the client's history. The test for occult blood determines blood in the stool and is helpful to determine the site of bleeding, but knowing the hemoglobin level first helps determine whether the client needs a blood transfusion immediately. A serum metabolic panel includes assessment of glucose, electrolytes, blood urea nitrogen, and creatinine levels. PT is measured to verify bleeding dyscrasias.
CN: Physiological integrity; CNS: Reduction of risk potential; CL: Analyze

19. 3. Filgrastim is a leukocyte growth factor used to stimulate the production of white blood cells (WBCs). It is used to decrease the incidence of infection in clients with neutropenia. Adverse effects include petechiae, related to thrombocytopenia, which indicates bleeding. The other conditions are side effects of filgastrim use that do not need to be immediately reported. Fatigue is a common client report with chemotherapy.
CN: Physiological integrity; CNS: Pharmacological and parenteral therapies; CL: Apply

20. 3. During an MRI, the client is confined in a small, enclosed, tube-shaped machine. The client who is afraid of using an elevator needs further data collection because this fear may indicate claustrophobia. The other findings are not associated with an MRI.
CN: Physiological integrity; CNS: Reduction of risk potential; CL: Apply

21. 3. Lack of intrinsic factor following gastrectomy would cause pernicious anemia due to the client's inability to absorb vitamin B_{12}. The presence of a colostomy, GERD, or dumping syndrome would not place a client at risk for developing anemia.
CN: Physiological integrity; CNS: Physiological adaptation; CL: Apply

CN: Client needs category   CNS: Client needs subcategory   CL: Cognitive level

22. The nurse in a family health clinic is caring for a client with a hemoglobin level of 9 g/dL (90 g/L). Which instruction will the nurse provide to the client?
1. Restrict activity as much as possible.
2. Eat foods that are high in calcium.
3. Space activities to allow time to rest.
4. Be supervised when ambulating.

22. 3. The normal hemoglobin level for males is 14 to 18 g/dL (140 to 180 g/L) and for females is 12 to 16 g/dL (120 to 160 g/L). Clients with anemia become fatigued easily and need rest between activities to conserve energy. Activities do not need to be severely restricted for clients with anemia. The client needs to eat food that is high in iron (not calcium), such as lean red meat and fortified breakfast cereal. The client does not need close supervision when walking.
CN: Physiological integrity; CNS: Physiological adaptation; CL: Apply

23. A nurse is caring for a client with leukemia who has had a bone marrow transplant. Which nursing intervention is **priority**?
1. Assisting the client with daily hygiene needs
2. Listening to the breath sounds every 2 hours
3. Palpating the client's pedal pulse every 2 hours
4. Administering pain medication as necessary

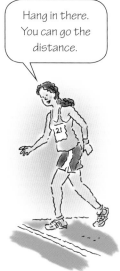

Hang in there. You can go the distance.

23. 2. The two major complications of bone marrow transplantation are bleeding and infection. Listening to the client's breath sounds frequently, comparing them with the baseline, and immediately reporting any congestion helps prevent complications due to infection. Although hygiene and comfort needs should be addressed, they do not take priority over assessing for infection. Collecting data for potentially impaired peripheral circulation is not a priority for clients after a bone marrow transplant.
CN: Physiological integrity; CNS: Reduction of risk potential; CL: Apply

24. A nurse is educating a group of student nurses on disease prevalence in community health and epidemiologic nursing. The nurse knows the students have an understanding of disease prevalence when they make which statement?
1. "It is the number of individuals affected by a particular disease at a specific time."
2. "It is the rate at which individuals without a specific disease develop that disease."
3. "It is the proportion of individuals affected by the disease who live for a specific period."
4. "It is the amount of individuals without the disease who ultimately develop the disease."

24. 1. Prevalence is the number of individuals affected by the disease at a specific time. Risk is the proportion of individuals without the disease who develop the disease within a particular period. Incidence rate is the rapidity with which individuals without the disease contract it. Survival is the proportion of individuals affected by the disease who live for a particular length of time.
CN: Health promotion and maintenance; CNS: None; CL: Understand

25. A client with scleroderma is prescribed a combination of medications that includes steroids and cyclosporine. Which client education will the nurse provide?
1. Avoid eating home-canned foods.
2. Avoid being in crowded places.
3. Stop the medications if bleeding occurs.
4. Take acetaminophen for a fever.

25. 2. The client should avoid situations in which infections can be transmitted because the ability to resist pathogens is diminished. Steroids impair the immune system, and cyclosporine is given to suppress the immune response. Home-canned foods should be boiled for 20 minutes and inspected before being consumed but generally pose no greater risk of infection than commercially canned foods. Steroids and cyclosporine are not associated with bleeding tendencies and should never be stopped abruptly. Even mild febrile episodes should be reported immediately because the client's immune system is impaired, and taking medications such as acetaminophen could mask the presence of serious infections.
CN: Physiological integrity; CNS: Pharmacological and parenteral therapies; CL: Apply

26. A nurse is teaching a client with iron-deficiency anemia about proper dietary choices. Which food(s) will the nurse advise the client to avoid? Select all that apply.
1. Iced tea
2. Yogurt
3. Coffee
4. Steak
5. Broccoli

26. 1, 2, 3. Clients with iron-deficiency anemia should choose foods high in iron, high in fiber, and high in protein. Tea, coffee, and calcium (in yogurt) block iron absorption and thus should be avoided.
CN: Physiological integrity; CNS: Basic care and comfort; CL: Analyze

27. A nurse has provided education to a client about taking ferrous sulfate liquid preparation. Which statement by the client indicates to the nurse that additional education is needed?
1. "I should take the iron with an antacid to prevent gastric distress."
2. "I can expect my stools to be dark green or black."
3. "I should rinse my mouth with water after taking the iron."
4. "I should add the iron to juice and drink it with a straw."

27. 1. Antacids interfere with absorption of iron and should be avoided. Dark green or black stools are a common adverse effect of iron supplements. Rinsing the mouth after swallowing liquid iron and drinking the liquid iron through a straw help the client prevent teeth discoloration from contact with the iron preparation.
CN: Physiological integrity; CNS: Pharmacological and parenteral therapies; CL: Apply

28. A nurse is caring for a client with rheumatoid arthritis. When is the **best** time for the nurse to schedule the client for ambulation?
1. Each morning when the client first awakens
2. After returning from physical therapy
3. After the client has taken a bath
4. Daily, just before the noontime meal

28. 3. Warmth and the movement of the extremities during a bath ease the stiffness and pain of rheumatoid arthritis. When the client first awakens is the worst time for ambulation because pain and stiffness are greatest after long periods of immobility. The client may be too tired to walk soon after returning from therapy. There is no relationship between eating and ease of ambulation in rheumatoid arthritis.
CN: Physiological integrity; CNS: Basic care and comfort; CL: Understand

29. The nurse is caring for a client who has just had a total hip replacement. It is **priority** for the nurse to monitor the client closely for the development of which condition?
1. Anemia
2. Polycythemia
3. Purpura
4. Thrombocytopenia

29. 1. Surgery is a risk factor for anemia. Polycythemia can occur from severe hypoxia due to congenital heart and pulmonary disease. Purpura and thrombocytopenia may result from decreased bone marrow production of platelets, but not from surgery.
CN: Physiological integrity; CNS: Reduction of risk potential; CL: Apply

30. The nurse is preparing to administer medications to four clients. Which prescription will the nurse question?
1. Indomethacin to a client with lymphoma being prepped for a lung biopsy
2. Magnesium sulfate to a client with a current serum magnesium level of 1.2 mEq/L
3. Filgrastim to a client with a low white blood cell count and neutropenia
4. Emtricitabine to a client with acquired immunodeficiency syndrome (AIDS)

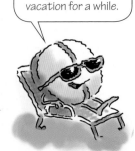

Before major surgery, you may need to give your medications a vacation for a while.

30. 1. Indomethacin is an NSAID that may inhibit platelet aggregation. The administration of indomethacin should be questioned prior to invasive procedures because it can increase the risk of bleeding. Magnesium sulfate is given to clients with hypomagnesemia (serum magnesium level less than 1.5 mEq/L). Filgrastim is given to a client with a low white blood cell (WBC) count and neutropenia. Emtricitabine is a non-nucleoside reverse transcriptase inhibitor (NNRTI) drug used for clients with HIV/AIDS.
CN: Physiological integrity; CNS: Pharmacological and parenteral therapies; CL: Analyze

31. A client is admitted with a platelet count of 75,000/µL (75 × 10⁹/L). Which finding(s) will the nurse anticipate during the assessment? Select all that apply.
1. Nausea
2. Dizziness
3. Vomiting
4. Purpura
5. Fever

31. 4. The normal thrombocytes (platelet) count is 150,000/µL (150 × 10⁹/L) to 400,000/µL (400 × 10⁹/L). The client has thrombocytopenia or low platelet count. Platelets are necessary for clot formation, so purpura is a sign of a decreased number of platelets. Petechiae is also a sign of low platelets. Nausea, dizziness, fever, and vomiting are *not* usual signs of thrombocytopenia.
CN: Physiological integrity; CNS: Reduction of risk potential; CL: Analyze

32. The nurse has instructed the client on self-administration of heparin injections. The nurse determines that teaching is effective when the client makes which statement?
1. "Heparin slows the time it takes for my blood to clot."
2. "Heparin works by stopping my blood from clotting."
3. "Heparin will cause my blood to become thin."
4. "Heparin will dissolve any clots in my blood."

32. 1. Heparin prolongs the time needed for blood to clot; however, it does not thin the blood. If given in large doses, heparin may stop the blood from clotting; however, this is not why heparin is usually given. Heparin does not dissolve clots.
CN: Physiological integrity; CNS: Pharmacological and parenteral therapies; CL: Understand

33. The health care provider prescribes a bone marrow biopsy and a platelet transfusion for a client with a bleeding disorder. When will the nurse anticipate the platelets will be administered?
1. Immediately following the bone marrow biopsy
2. One to two hours before the bone marrow biopsy
3. Immediately before the start of the bone marrow biopsy
4. Slowly, while the client is undergoing the bone marrow biopsy

33. 3. Administering platelets immediately before beginning an invasive procedure increases the number of circulating platelets, thereby providing the greatest protection from potential hemorrhage. Administering platelets following the procedure may have some benefit but is not as effective and may not prevent hemorrhage. Administering platelets too early may result in fewer circulating platelets during the procedure. Platelets are fragile and are administered as rapidly as the client can tolerate to minimize their destruction.
CN: Physiological integrity; CNS: Reduction of risk potential; CL: Analyze

34. A client with thrombocytopenia, secondary to leukemia, begins bleeding around the intravenous (IV) site. What will the nurse do **first**?
1. Discontinue the IV.
2. Attempt to flush the IV.
3. Elevate the client's arm.
4. Apply pressure to the site.

34. 4. The initial action for a client with thrombocytopenia who is bleeding is to apply pressure to the site to stop bleeding. After applying pressure, the nurse can elevate the arm and discontinue the IV. If the IV site is bleeding, it is not appropriate to flush the IV.
CN: Physiological integrity; CNS: Reduction of risk potential; CL: Analyze

35. A client is receiving epoetin alfa. Which laboratory value indicates to the nurse the treatment is effective for this client?
1. Hemoglobin of 14 g/dL (140 g/L)
2. Hematocrit of 30% (0.30)
3. White blood cell count of 7,000/µL (7.00 × 10⁹/L)
4. Platelet of 350,000/µL (350 × 10⁹/L)

35. 1. Epoetin alfa is given to a client to stimulate the production of red blood cells. The normal hemoglobin level for males is 14 to 18 g/dL (140 to 180 g/L) and for females is 12 to 16 g/dL (120 to 160 g/L). The normal hematocrit level for males is 40% to 54% (0.40 to 0.54) and for females is 37% to 47% (0.37 to 0.47). The other findings are unrelated to the drug's effectiveness.
CN: Physiological integrity; CNS: Pharmacological and parenteral therapies; CL: Apply

36. A pregnant woman arrives at the emergency department with abruptio placentae at 34 weeks' gestation. The nurse will closely monitor the client for which blood dyscrasia?
1. Thrombocytopenia
2. Idiopathic thrombocytopenic purpura (ITP)
3. Disseminated intravascular coagulation (DIC)
4. Heparin-associated thrombocytopenia and thrombosis (HATT)

37. Which statement by a client with sickle cell disease indicates to the nurse that further education is needed?
1. "I should avoid vacationing or traveling in areas of high altitude."
2. "Cigarette smoking can cause me to have a sickle cell crisis."
3. "I should drink 4 to 6 liters of fluids every day."
4. "Taking an aspirin daily will help prevent a sickle cell crisis."

38. Which client laboratory test(s) does the nurse recognize as **best** for confirming the diagnosis of essential thrombocytopenia? Select all that apply.
1. Bleeding time
2. Platelet count
3. Complete blood count (CBC)
4. Immunoglobulin (Ig) G level
5. Prothrombin time (PT) and international normalized ratio (INR)

39. The nurse is reviewing the client's chart exhibit noted below. Based on the results, which intervention(s) will the nurse include in the client's care plan? Select all that apply.

Test	Result
Sodium	133 mEq/L (133 mmol/L)
Potassium	4.1 mEq/L (4.1 mmol/L)
Chloride	94 mEq/L (94 mmol/L)
Calcium	11.2 mg/dL (2.79 mmol/L)
Magnesium	1.2 mEq/L (0.49 mmol/L)
Phosphorus	3.1 mg/dL (1 mmol/L)

1. Give daily hydrochlorothiazide per the health care provider's prescription.
2. Encourage the client to eat yogurt, milk, cheese, and almonds.
3. Administer magnesium sulfate per the health care provider's prescription.
4. Observe for muscle cramps and hyperactive deep tendon reflexes.
5. Limit fluid intake and monitor for jugular vein distension (JVD).

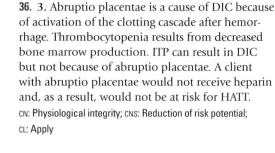

Sir—you are just begging for a sickle cell crisis.

Can you spot which laboratory result is abnormal? That's the key to getting this one right.

36. 3. Abruptio placentae is a cause of DIC because of activation of the clotting cascade after hemorrhage. Thrombocytopenia results from decreased bone marrow production. ITP can result in DIC but not because of abruptio placentae. A client with abruptio placentae would not receive heparin and, as a result, would not be at risk for HATT.
CN: Physiological integrity; CNS: Reduction of risk potential; CL: Apply

37. 4. Aspirin inhibits platelet aggregation and will not help prevent sickle cell crisis. Hydroxyurea is prescribed for some people to help prevent sickle cell crisis. High altitudes increase oxygen demand and therefore can also precipitate a crisis. Tobacco, alcohol, and dehydration can precipitate a sickle cell crisis and should be avoided.
CN: Physiological integrity; CNS: Reduction of risk potential; CL: Apply

38. 1, 2. A platelet count and bleeding time are the best tests to determine thrombocytopenia. The platelet count is decreased and bleeding time prolonged in a client with thrombocytopenia. IgG assays are nonspecific but may help determine the diagnosis. A CBC shows the hemoglobin levels, hematocrit, and white blood cell values. PT and INR evaluate the effect of warfarin therapy.
CN: Physiological integrity; CNS: Physiological adaptation; CL: Apply

39. 3, 5. The client has hypercalcemia, hypomagnesemia, hyponatremia, and hypochloremia. The normal calcium level is 8.5 to 10.5 mg/dL (2.1 to 2.6 mmol/L). Normal sodium level is 135 to 145 mEq/L (135 to 145 mmol/L). Normal chloride level is 98 to 107 mEq/L (98 to 107 mmol/L). Normal magnesium level is 1.5 to 2.5 mEq/L (0.62 to 1.03 mmol/L). The nurse should encourage the client to avoid foods high in calcium, such as dairy products and almonds. The nurse should monitor for signs of fluid volume overload related to hyponatremia and hypochloremia by assessing for JVD and should limit fluid intake. The nurse should administer magnesium sulfate because the magnesium level is low. Hydrochlorothiazide is a thiazide diuretic that is contraindicated with hypercalcemia because it inhibits calcium secretion. Signs and symptoms of hypocalcemia, which include muscle cramps, tetany, positive Chvostek sign, positive Trousseau sign, arrhythmias, and hyperactive deep tendon reflexes, would not be expected. All the other laboratory results are normal.
CN: Physiological integrity; CNS: Reduction of risk potential; CL: Analyze

40. The nurse is educating a client on about atazanavir. Which adverse effect will the nurse include in the teaching?
1. Hyperglycemia
2. Thrombocytopenia
3. Leukocytosis
4. Hypolipidemia

41. The nurse provides education to a group of clients about types of immunity. Which statement will the nurse provide as an example of passive acquired immunity?
1. "A toddler receives the necessary immunizations before beginning preschool."
2. "After having chickenpox, a teenager is unlikely to get the disease again."
3. "A nurse exposed to hepatitis B virus from a needlestick receives hepatitis B immune globulin."
4. "An adult with a history of having varicella zoster as a child develops shingles."

42. The registered nurse (RN) is making assignments for the next shift. Which client(s) will the RN assign to the licensed practical nurse (LPN)? Select all that apply.
1. A client scheduled for initial chemotherapy treatment
2. A client admitted with generalized petechiae and bruising
3. A client ready to be discharged home after surgery
4. A client with hypocalcemia receiving calcitrol orally
5. A client with hemophilia who needs pain medication

43. A client is receiving 1 liter of 0.9% sodium chloride intravenously (IV), to be infused for 12 hours. The IV infusion set has a drop factor of 15 drops per milliliter. How many drops per minute will the nurse set the IV to infuse at? Record your answer using a whole number.

_____ gtts/min

40. 1. Atazanavir is an antiretroviral-protease inhibitor drug used in combination with other antiretroviral medications to help manage human immunodeficiency virus (HIV) infection. Adverse effects include hyperglycemia, new-onset or worsened diabetes, and lactic-acidosis syndrome but do not include thrombocytopenia, leukocytosis, or hypolipidemia.
CN: Physiological integrity; CNS: Pharmacological and parenteral therapies; CL: Apply

41. 3. Immune globulin provides a temporary immunity that is passively acquired. Antibodies from one person are recovered and administered to another person to help prevent infection. Because the recipient's immune system did not make the antibodies, the immunity is considered to be passively acquired. Immunizations and actual disease processes, such as chickenpox, cause the body to manufacture antibodies against future exposure to these specific antigens; this is called active immunity. Active immunity produces antibodies that are either permanent or longer lasting than passively acquired immunity. Shingles develops when latent varicella zoster virus is activated. Varicella zoster is the virus that causes chickenpox.
CN: Physiological integrity; CNS: Reduction of risk potential; CL: Understand

42. 4, 5. An LPN can administer pain medication and oral calcitrol (vitamin D). A client scheduled for initial chemotherapy treatment requires education and needs to be monitored by an RN. The initial admission assessment of a client admitted with petechiae and bruising should be performed by an RN. A client who is ready to be discharged home after surgery requires discharge education by the RN.
CN: Safe, effective care environment; CNS: Management of care; CL: Apply

43. 21.

$$Drops\ per\ minute = \frac{mL/hr}{60\ min/hr} \times Drop\ Factor$$

$$1,000\ mL \times 12\ hr = 83\ mL/hr$$

$$Drops\ per\ minute = \frac{83\ mL/hr}{60\ min/hr} \times 15\ gtts$$

$$Drops\ per\ minute = 21\ gtts/min$$

CN: Physiological integrity; CNS: Pharmacological and parenteral therapies; CL: Apply

44. The nurse is caring for an older adult client. Based on the chart exhibit below, which intervention(s) will the nurse include in the client's plan of care? Select all that apply.

Laboratory Results

Test	Result
Hematocrit	61% (0.61)
BUN	32 mg/dL (11.4 mmol/L)
Sodium	159 mEq/L (159 mmol/L)

1. Check for a distended neck vein.
2. Test urine for specific gravity.
3. Weigh the client daily.
4. Record input and output.
5. Limit fluid intake.

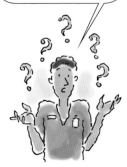

This question has a lot of moving parts. Here's a hint—the client is dehydrated.

44. 2, 3, 4. The client is experiencing dehydration. Signs and symptoms of dehydration include thirst, poor skin turgor, flat neck veins, weight loss, confusion, decreased urine output, increased heart rate, thready pulse, and postural hypotension. Fluid volume deficit causes hemoconcentration. Hematocrit, blood urea nitrogen (BUN), and sodium levels increase when the blood is concentrated. The normal hematocrit level for males is 40% to 54% (0.40 to 0.54) and for females is 37% to 47% (0.37 to 0.47). The normal BUN level is from 8 to 23 mg/dL (2.9 to 8.2 mmol/L). The normal range for sodium level is from 135 to 145 mEq/L (135 to 145 mmol/L). The kidneys compensate by conserving the remaining fluid in the body, leading to a decrease in urine output. Urine specific gravity increases because the urine is concentrated. The nurse should encourage the client to increase fluid intake.

CN: Physiological integrity; CNS: Physiological adaptation; CL: Analyze

45. The nurse expects a client admitted with *Pneumocystis jirovecii* pneumonia (PJP) to have a history of which condition?
1. Type 2 diabetes mellitus
2. Right-sided heart failure
3. Chronic obstructive pulmonary disease (COPD)
4. Acquired immunodeficiency syndrome (AIDS)

45. 4. PJP is a type of pneumonia caused by the fungus *P. jirovecii*. It is one of the opportunistic infections seen in clients who are immunocompromised, particularly in clients with HIV/AIDS. PJP is not associated with type 2 diabetes mellitus, right-sided heart failure, or COPD.

CN: Safe, effective care environment; CNS: Safety and infection control; CL: Analyze

46. A client diagnosed with ankylosing spondylitis is newly prescribed indomethacin. The nurse will notify the health care provider if the client states he or she is are also taking which medication?
1. Heparin
2. Gabapentin
3. Adalimumab
4. Etanercept

46. 1. Indomethacin is a nonsteroidal anti-inflammatory drug (NSAID) used for clients with ankylosing spondylitis. NSAIDs are aspirin and aspirin-like medications that may increase the risk of bleeding when taken with an anticoagulant such as heparin. An anticonvulsant drug (gabapentin) or a tumor necrosis factor inhibitor (adalimumab or etanercept) would not cause a serious drug interaction when taken with indomethacin.

CN: Physiological integrity; CNS: Pharmacological and parenteral therapies; CL: Apply

47. A client who received massive packed red blood cell blood transfusions now reports feeling heart palpitations and weakness. Which nursing action is **priority**?
1. Administer insulin.
2. Apply a cardiac monitor.
3. Assess the client's pain level.
4. Reassess hemoglobin and hematocrit levels.

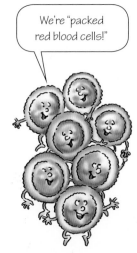

We're "packed red blood cells!"

47. 2. The client is experiencing symptoms of transfusion-associated hyperkalemia. Storing packed red blood cells increases the potassium concentration. The priority nursing action would be to apply a cardiac monitor to assess for cardiac arrhythmias. Intravenous regular insulin pushes potassium from the blood into the cell, decreasing the serum potassium level; however, the nurse would first need to assess the potassium level to determine whether hyperkalemia is present. Severe cases of hyperkalemia require hemodialysis. Reassessing the hemoglobin and hematocrit levels and asking the client about pain can be done after verifying the cardiac rhythm.

CN: Physiological integrity; CNS: Reduction of risk potential; CL: Analyze

48. A client undergoing colon cancer treatment has developed thrombocytopenia. The nurse will assess the client for which manifestation(s)? Select all that apply.
   1. Diarrhea
   2. Hematuria
   3. Ecchymosis
   4. Melena
   5. Epistaxis

48. 2, 3, 4, 5. With thrombocytopenia, there is an abnormal decrease in the number of blood platelets, which can result in bleeding. Hematuria, ecchymosis, melena, and epistaxis are all signs of bleeding. The client may have constipation but usually not diarrhea.
CN: Physiological integrity; CNS: Reduction of risk potential; CL: Analyze

49. The nurse cares for a client brought to the emergency department for a gunshot wound to the abdomen. The nurse obtains the client's vital signs and notes that the client's pulse is 120 beats/min, respirations 22 breaths/min, and blood pressure 76/42 mm Hg. The client is unresponsive. Which action will the nurse perform **first**?
   1. Give 1 U of O negative packed red blood cells (RBCs).
   2. Begin infusion of fresh frozen plasma.
   3. Reassess the client's vital signs.
   4. Obtain blood for a type and crossmatch.

49. 1. In a trauma situation, the first blood product given is unmatched (O negative) packed RBCs. Fresh frozen plasma is commonly used to replace clotting factors. Reassessment of the client's vital signs can be done after the nurse has intervened. A type and crossmatch for blood is not needed in an emergency situation.
CN: Physiological integrity; CNS: Physiological adaptation; CL: Analyze

50. A nurse is monitoring a client receiving a blood transfusion for volume replacement. The client reports itching about 20 minutes after the infusion begins. Which nursing action is **priority**?
   1. Stop the blood transfusion.
   2. Call the health care provider.
   3. Give oral diphenhydramine.
   4. Continue to monitor the client.

50. 1. Itching is a sign of an adverse reaction, so the nurse must stop the infusion. The health care provider should be called but only after the infusion has been stopped and the client is assessed. No medications should be administered without first reporting the symptom and having the infusion stopped. The nurse should continue to monitor the client after intervening.
CN: Physiological integrity; CNS: Reduction of risk potential; CL: Analyze

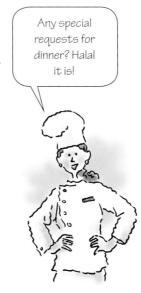

Any special requests for dinner? Halal it is!

51. A nurse is assigned to a client who is a practicing Muslim. Which cultural consideration(s) will the nurse take into account when caring for the client? Select all that apply.
   1. Administration of blood and blood products is forbidden.
   2. An individual should be treated by a health care provider of the same sex.
   3. Meat products not ritually slaughtered are forbidden.
   4. The right hand should be used in handing over items.
   5. Any combination of meat and milk is forbidden.
   6. Organ donation and transplantation is not allowed.

51. 2, 3, 4. Muslim clients prefer same-gender health care providers to take care of them. Muslims only eat "halal," or ritually slaughtered, meat products. Eating pork is prohibited in Islam. The left hand is reserved for bodily hygiene and is considered unclean. The nurse should always use the right hand in handing over items. Organ donation is allowed for the purpose of saving life. Administration of blood and blood products is prohibited in Jehovah's Witnesses. Eating meat with milk is prohibited in Judaism.
CN: Psychosocial integrity; CNS: None; CL: Apply

52. Which symptom reported by a client with systemic lupus erythematosus (SLE) alerts the nurse that the client may be experiencing a life-threatening complication?
   1. Joint pain
   2. Foamy urine
   3. Butterfly rash
   4. Fever

52. 2. Foamy urine indicates proteinuria and is associated with kidney damage, which is a life-threatening complication of SLE. Joint pain, rashes, and fever are all common symptoms of SLE but are not life-threatening.
CN: Physiological integrity; CNS: Physiological adaptation; CL: Apply

53. A nurse is reviewing the laboratory results of a client with anemia. Which laboratory value requires the nurse to contact the health care provider **immediately**?
1. Erythrocyte count of 3.1 × 10⁶/μL (3.10 × 10¹²/L)
2. Neutrophil count of 500/μL (0.5 × 10⁹/L)
3. Leukocyte count of 2,300/μL (2.30 × 10⁹/L)
4. Platelet count of 115,000/μL (115 × 10⁹/L)

54. Which finding(s) will the nurse expect to assess in a client diagnosed with systemic lupus erythematosus (SLE)? Select all that apply.
1. Rash on the face
2. A client report of feeling tired
3. Swollen joints bilaterally
4. Petechiae on the chest and back
5. A client report of arthralgia

55. The nurse is providing education about the adverse reactions of doxorubicin. Which side effect(s) will the nurse include in the teaching for the client? Select all that apply.
1. Chest pain
2. Nausea
3. Dehydration
4. Liver failure
5. Bone damage

56. The nurse is providing teaching about what to expect during bone marrow aspiration. Place the following nursing actions in chronological order according to how the nurse will assist the client during the procedure. Use all of the options.
1. Apply direct pressure over the puncture site.
2. Explain the procedure and obtain consent.
3. Monitor the puncture site for bleeding.
4. Help the client maintain position.
5. Check coagulation studies.
6. Position the client on the lateral decubitus or prone.

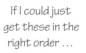
If I could just get these in the right order …

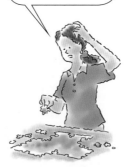

57. A client diagnosed with human immunodeficiency virus (HIV) is receiving zidovudine. Which laboratory data will the nurse monitor closely for this client? Select all that apply.
1. White blood cell count
2. Hemoglobin level
3. Liver function tests results
4. Lactate level
5. Glucose level

53. 2. Anemia is defined as a decreased number of erythrocytes (red blood cells) and is an expected finding for a client with anemia. Leukopenia is a decreased number of leukocytes (white blood cells [WBCs]). Neutropenia is a decreased number of neutrophils (a type of WBC) and is not expected with anemia, indicating that the client may have another hematological disorder. Thrombocytopenia is a decreased number of thrombocytes (platelets).
CN: Physiological integrity; CNS: Reduction of risk potential; CL: Analyze

54. 1, 2, 3, 5. Common signs and symptoms of SLE include a butterfly rash on the face, fatigue, swollen joints, and painful joints (arthralgia). Petechiae is not associated with SLE and would indicate decreased platelets resulting in minor bleeding from broken capillaries.
CN: Physiological integrity; CNS: Physiological adaptation; CL: Apply

55. 1, 2, 3, 4. Doxorubicin is an antineoplastic antibiotic. Adverse reactions to doxorubicin include cardiac changes, liver changes, nausea, and dehydration. Bone damage is not considered an adverse effect of this medication.
CN: Physiological integrity; CNS: Pharmacological and parenteral therapies; CL: Apply

56. Ordered Response:
2. Explain the procedure and obtain consent.
5. Check coagulation studies.
6. Position the client on the lateral decubitus or prone.
4. Help the client maintain position.
1. Apply direct pressure over the puncture site.
3. Monitor the puncture site for bleeding.
CN: Physiological integrity; CNS: Reduction of risk potential; CL: Apply

57. 1, 2, 3, 4. Zidovudine (AZT), which is used to treat HIV infection, can cause agranulocytosis, anemia, hepatomegaly, and lactic acidosis. Glucose changes are not common with AZT, although the nurse may see hyperglycemia with other HIV medications.
CN: Physiological integrity; CNS: Pharmacological and parenteral therapies; CL: Analyze

58. The nurse is reviewing the chart exhibit noted below. Based on the findings, which disorder will the nurse suspect?

Test	Result
White blood cells	3.500/µL (3.50 × 10⁹/L)
Red blood cells	3.8 × 10⁶/µL (3.80 × 10¹²/L)
Platelets	90,000/µL (90 × 10⁹/L)
Antinuclear antibody	Positive

1. Aplastic anemia
2. Rheumatoid arthritis
3. Ankylosing spondylitis
4. Systemic lupus erythematosus (SLE)

58. 4. Laboratory findings for clients with SLE usually show pancytopenia and a positive antinuclear antibody (ANA) titer. The normal erythrocyte (red blood cell) count for an adult male is $4.6 \times 10^6/\mu L$ ($4.60 \times 10^{12}/L$) to $6.2 \times 10^6/\mu L$ ($6.20 \times 10^{12}/L$) and for an adult female is $4.2 \times 10^6/\mu L$ ($4.20 \times 10^{12}/L$) to $5.4 \times 10^6/\mu L$ ($5.40 \times 10^{12}/L$). The normal leukocyte (white blood cell) count is $4.500/\mu L$ ($4.50 \times 10^9/L$) to $11,000/\mu L$ ($11.00 \times 10^9/L$), and the normal thrombocyte (platelet) count is $150,000/\mu L$ ($150 \times 10^9/L$) to $400,000/\mu L$ ($400 \times 10^9/L$). A client with rheumatoid arthritis is expected to have a positive ANA titer, but pancytopenia is not expected. Pancytopenia is expected with aplastic anemia, but a positive ANA titer is not. Neither pancytopenia nor a positive ANA titer is expected with ankylosing spondylitis.

CN: Physiological integrity; CNS: Physiological adaptation; CL: Analyze

59. The nurse suspects enlarged upper chest and neck lymph nodes in a client with Hodgkin lymphoma if which symptoms are noted during assessment?

1. Fever, weight loss, and night sweats
2. Bone pain and jaundice
3. Cough, dysphagia, and stridor
4. Weight loss and malaise

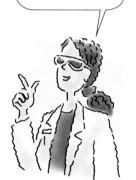

I love your swagger. Stay confident.

59. 3. Enlarged lymph nodes of the neck and upper chest can produce such symptoms as cough, dysphagia, and stridor due to pressure and obstruction of the structures of the respiratory system and esophagus. Although fever, weight loss, night sweats, and malaise are also seen with Hodgkin lymphoma, these symptoms are not directly related to enlargement of neck and chest lymph nodes. Bone pain and jaundice may indicate bone and liver metastasis.

CN: Physiological integrity; CNS: Physiological adaptation; CL: Apply

60. A client is prescribed aspirin. Which other medication prescription will cause the nurse to notify the health care provider?

1. Acetaminophen
2. Furosemide
3. Pyridoxine
4. Heparin

60. 4. Aspirin, also known as acetylsalicylic acid, is used for mild-to-moderate pain, fever, inflammation, and atrial fibrillation stroke prevention. Aspirin may increase the risk of bleeding when taken with heparin. Acetaminophen, furosemide, and pyridoxine do not increase the risk of bleeding.

CN: Physiological integrity; CNS: Pharmacological and parenteral therapies; CL: Analyze

61. An anemic client is admitted with pallor, fatigue, dry lips, and a smooth, bright red tongue. Which diagnostic test will the nurse anticipate preparing the client for to confirm the client's specific type of anemia?

1. Bone marrow examination
2. Ventilation-perfusion scan
3. Schilling test
4. Tensilon test

61. 3. A smooth, bright red tongue is a sign of vitamin B_{12} deficiency. The Schilling test is performed to evaluate vitamin B_{12} absorption and to diagnose pernicious anemia. Pernicious anemia is caused by a lack of intrinsic factor produced by gastric mucosa, which is necessary for vitamin B_{12} absorption. In the Schilling test, radioactive vitamin B_{12} is given orally and then urine is collected over the next 24 hours to measure whether the vitamin B_{12} is normally absorbed. Bone marrow examination is used for aplastic anemia. A ventilation-perfusion scan is used to help diagnose a client with pulmonary embolism. The Tensilon test is a test for myasthenia gravis.

CN: Physiological integrity; CNS: Reduction of risk potential; CL: Apply

62. A nurse receives the laboratory results below for a hospitalized adult client who has acute leukemia. Which result will the nurse **immediately** report to the health care provider?

Test	Result
White blood cells	12,000/µL (12.0 × 10⁹/L)
Red blood cells	4.2 × 10⁶/µL (4.20 × 10¹²/L)
Hemoglobin	12 g/dL (120 g/L)
Hematocrit	30% (0.30)
Platelets	15,000/µL (15 × 10⁹/L)

1. Red blood cell (RBC) count
2. Hemoglobin level
3. Hematocrit level
4. Platelet count

63. Which activity will the nurse recommend for a client receiving chemotherapy who is not on protective isolation?
1. Continuous bed rest
2. Activity as tolerated
3. Walking to the bathroom only
4. Brief periods in a recliner

64. Which nursing intervention is **most** appropriate for a client diagnosed with multiple myeloma?
1. Monitoring respiratory status
2. Balancing rest and activity
3. Restricting fluid intake
4. Preventing bone injury

65. A nurse is providing discharge education to a client who had an anaphylactic reaction. Which nursing recommendation is **most** appropriate for this client?
1. Dry-mop hardwood and ceramic floors.
2. Wear a medical identification bracelet at all times.
3. Have carpet installed in every room of the house.
4. Advise family and friends not to visit during the winter.

66. Which food will the nurse inform a client with a leukocyte count of 2,500/µL (2.50 × 10⁹/L) to avoid?
1. Breakfast cereal
2. Chicken pot pie
3. Steamed broccoli
4. Soft boiled eggs

62. 4. A platelet count below 20,000/µL (20 × 10⁹/L) is considered a life-threatening situation and generally requires medical treatment of immediate platelet transfusions. The RBC count, hemoglobin level, and hematocrit level are lower than normal but do not require immediate intervention if the client is asymptomatic. The white blood cell count is slightly elevated and would be expected in a client with leukemia.
CN: Physiological integrity; CNS: Physiological adaptation; CL: Analyze

63. 2. It is important that the client be able to engage in activities that are of interest and to maintain as much independence and autonomy as possible. Bed rest is not necessary, nor is it necessary to limit the client's activity to just walks to the bathroom or brief periods out of the bed to a recliner.
CN: Health promotion and maintenance; CNS: None; CL: Apply

64. 4. When caring for a client with multiple myeloma, the nurse should focus on relieving pain, preventing bone injury and infection, and maintaining hydration. Monitoring respiratory status and balancing rest and activity are appropriate interventions for any client. To prevent such complications as pyelonephritis and renal calculi, the nurse should keep the client well hydrated, not restrict the client's fluid intake.
CN: Safe, effective care environment; CNS: Safety and infection control; CL: Apply

65. 2. If the client becomes unconscious or cannot report allergies, medical identification jewelry could provide that information and help health care providers intervene and treat anaphylaxis as soon as possible. The client should wet-mop hardwood and ceramic floors because dry-mopping scatters dust, which can trigger allergies. The client should minimize the amount of carpet in the home because carpet traps allergens, such as dust and dirt. Unless the client is ill, the nurse may encourage visits by family and friends to promote healthy social interaction.
CN: Health promotion and maintenance; CNS: None; CL: Apply

66. 4. The normal leukocyte (WBC) count is 4,500/µL (4.50 × 10⁹/L) to 11,000/µL (11.00 × 10⁹/L). A WBC count of 2,500/µL (2.50 × 10⁹/L) is low, making the client prone to infection. A low-bacteria diet is indicated, which excludes consuming raw fruits and vegetables or undercooked meat and eggs.
CN: Health promotion and maintenance; CNS: None; CL: Apply

67. A client with leukemia has neutropenia. Which assessment finding will require the nurse to contact the health care provider **immediately**?
   1. Self-report of fatigue
   2. Bowel sounds hypoactive
   3. A heart rate of 105 beats/min
   4. Crackles bilaterally in the lungs

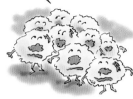

I'm feeling a little out of breath here. Maybe I should get checked out.

67. **4.** Pneumonia—viral and fungal—is a common cause of death in clients with neutropenia, so frequent assessment of respiratory rate and breath sounds is required. Signs and symptoms of pneumonia should be reported to the health care provider immediately. Although fatigue, tachycardia, and hypoactive bowel sounds could be reported to the health care provider, the priority is to report infection.
CN: Physiological integrity; CNS: Physiological adaptation; CL: Apply

68. The nurse is assessing a client with suspected pernicious anemia. Which finding(s) suggest to the nurse that the client has this diagnosis? Select all that apply.
   1. Cracked corners of the mouth
   2. Smooth, bright red tongue
   3. Hemoglobin level of 14 g/dL (140 g/L)
   4. Sensitivity to cold air
   5. Dyspnea when walking

68. **1, 2, 4, 5.** Pernicious anemia is a vitamin B_{12} deficiency due to a lack of the intrinsic factor produced by gastric mucosa. Intrinsic factor is necessary for the absorption of vitamin B_{12}. Clinical manifestations include pallor, fatigue, dyspnea on exertion, cheilosis (scaling of the surface of lips and fissures in the corner of the mouth), and sensitivity to cold. The client also has a smooth, sore, bright red tongue because of the atrophy of the papillae of the tongue due to vitamin B_{12} deficiency. A hemoglobin level of 14 g/dL (140 g/L) is normal.
CN: Physiological integrity; CNS: Physiological adaptation; CL: Analyze

69. A nurse is reviewing the health care provider's prescription for a client admitted with fatigue, photosensitivity, and a "butterfly" rash on the face. Which medication will the nurse expect to find in the client's medication administration record?
   1. Meperidine
   2. Azathioprine
   3. Phenylephrine
   4. Acyclovir

Taking the right meds can help you do your happy dance.

69. **2.** Fatigue, photosensitivity, and a "butterfly" rash on face are all signs and symptoms of systemic lupus erythematosus (SLE). Azathioprine is an immunosuppressant used in the treatment of SLE. Pharmacologic treatment of SLE also involves nonsteroidal anti-inflammatory drugs, corticosteroids, and other immunosuppressive agents. Meperidine is an opioid analgesic, phenylephrine is a vasopressor, and acyclovir is an antiviral drug.
CN: Physiological integrity; CNS: Pharmacological and parenteral therapies; CL: Analyze

70. A client with multiple myeloma has developed hypercalcemia. Which nursing intervention is **priority**?
   1. Protecting the client from trauma
   2. Elevating the head of bed 45 degrees
   3. Monitoring fluid intake and output
   4. Providing a quiet, darkened room

70. **3.** Hypercalcemia may lead to renal dysfunction. By carefully monitoring fluid intake and output, the nurse would be alerted to decreased urine output. All clients should be protected from trauma. Elevating the head of the bed is an intervention for impaired ventilation, gastroesophageal reflux disease, and increased intracranial pressure. A quiet, dark room is commonly used to decrease sensory stimulus for clients who have meningitis or preeclampsia.
CN: Physiological integrity; CNS: Reduction of risk potential; CL: Apply

71. A client is admitted with a serum calcium level of 6 mg/dL (1.5 mmol/L). The nurse will monitor the client for which finding(s)? Select all that apply.
   1. Fatigue
   2. Muscle weakness
   3. Confusion
   4. Diarrhea
   5. Bradycardia

71. **1, 2, 3.** The normal serum calcium level is 8.5 to 10.5 mg/dL (2.1 to 2.6 mmol/L). Common signs and symptoms of hypocalcemia include fatigue, muscle weakness, confusion, and constipation. Diarrhea and bradycardia are not associated with hypocalcemia.
CN: Physiological integrity; CNS: Physiological adaptation; CL: Apply

CN: Client needs category   CNS: Client needs subcategory   CL: Cognitive level

72. The nurse is caring for a client with multiple myeloma. Which laboratory value will the nurse anticipate for this client?
1. Serum calcium of 10.9 mg/dL (2.72 mmol/L)
2. Serum potassium of 5.8 mEq/L (5.8 mmol/L)
3. Serum sodium of 150 mEq/L (150 mmol/L)
4. Serum magnesium of 3.0 mEq/L (1.5 mmol/L)

72. 1. Calcium is released when bone is destroyed. This causes an increase in serum calcium levels. Normal serum calcium level is 8.5 to 10.5 mg/dL (2.1 to 2.6 mmol/L). The normal serum potassium level is 3.5 to 5.3 mEq/L (3.5 to 5.3 mmol/L). The normal sodium level ranges from 135 to 145 mEq/L (135 to 145 mmol/L). The normal magnesium level is 1.5 to 2.5 mEq/L (0.75 mmol/L to 1.25 mmol/L). Multiple myeloma does not affect potassium, sodium, or magnesium levels.
CN: Physiological integrity; CNS: Physiological adaptation; CL: Apply

73. A client is admitted with multiple myeloma. Which finding will the nurse tell the client to **immediately** report?
1. Increased appetite
2. Back pain
3. Weight gain
4. Decreased thirst

73. 2. Back pain or paresthesia in the lower extremities may indicate impending spinal cord compression from a spinal tumor. This should be recognized and treated promptly because progression of the tumor may result in paraplegia. The other sings and symptoms are unrelated to multiple myeloma.
CN: Physiological integrity; CNS: Physiological adaptation; CL: Apply

74. The nurse cares for a client experiencing a health crisis. Which nursing action is **most** important after stabilizing the client?
1. Provide education to the family.
2. Assess the client's emotional status.
3. Determine the client's dietary preference.
4. Offer the client assistance with bathing.

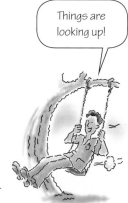

Things are looking up!

74. 2. Although all of the answers are important in the care of the client, it is most important to determine the individual's ability to cope with the emotional, spiritual, and psychological aspects of the crisis. This will make further care easier to provide.
CN: Psychosocial integrity; CNS: None; CL: Analyze

75. The nurse is providing education to a group of older adult clients about avoiding infection. Which information will the nurse include in the teaching? Select all that apply.
1. "Decreased cardiac output is a common physiologic cause of infection in older adults."
2. "Void frequently to prevent bladder infections as your bladder may not empty completely."
3. "The ability of your skin to heal decreases as you age, so monitor any wounds carefully."
4. "Your visual acuity may improve if you avoid becoming sick during the winter months."
5. "Wash your hands often because as you age your immune system has decreased resistance."

75. 2, 3, 5. Although decreased cardiac output is a common physiologic change of aging, this is not a common cause of infection. There is an increase in residual volume of the urine due to the decrease in muscle tone of bladder during aging, which can increase the risk of urinary tract infections. Older adult clients should monitor wounds carefully because the ability for the skin to heal diminishes with aging. Visual acuity loss is a common change with aging, and avoiding illness during the winter months does not improve the loss. Washing hands is recommended to prevent illness, as a decreased resistance to infection is a common physiologic change during aging.
CN: Health promotion and maintenance; CNS: None; CL: Apply

76. Which action will the nurse perform when caring for a client with multiple myeloma?
1. Maintain the client on strict bed rest.
2. Encourage dairy products in the diet.
3. Ensure that intravenous fluids are infusing.
4. Assess the client's platelet level.

76. 3. Ensuring fluids are infusing is necessary to dilute calcium and uric acid, and thereby reduce the risk of renal dysfunction for the client with multiple myeloma. Walking, not strict bed rest, is encouraged to prevent further bone demineralization. Clients should avoid dairy products because of high calcium levels. Platelets are not typically affected in multiple myeloma.
CN: Physiological integrity; CNS: Basic care and comfort; CL: Apply

77. A client is admitted with a serum potassium level of 6.5 mEq/L (6.5 mmol/L). Which medication will the nurse anticipate administering to the client?
1. Potassium chloride
2. Sodium polystyrene
3. Lisinopril
4. Spironolactone

78. An older adult client has a wound on the lower leg that is not healing normally. Which intervention will the nurse include in the plan of care?
1. Assess blood urea nitrogen (BUN) and creatinine levels.
2. Administer an influenza vaccination.
3. Elevate the client's leg on a pillow.
4. Encourage ambulation around the unit.

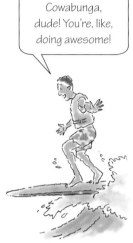

Cowabunga, dude! You're, like, doing awesome!

79. A client is admitted with a platelet count of 98,000/μL (98 × 10⁹/L). Which instruction(s) will the nurse provide during client education? Select all that apply.
1. Do not use dental floss.
2. Use an electric razor to shave.
3. Do not go to crowded places.
4. Avoid eating crusty or rough foods.
5. Eat fresh, uncooked vegetables.

80. Which action is the **priority** for the nurse to perform for a client infected with human immunodeficiency virus (HIV)?
1. Monitor viral load and CD4 count.
2. Encourage the client to eat high-protein foods.
3. Administer prescribed medications as scheduled.
4. Educate the client about receiving a pneumonia vaccine.

77. 2. The client has an elevated serum potassium level. The normal serum potassium level is 3.5 to 5.3 mEq/L (3.5 to 5.3 mmol/L). Sodium polystyrene is used to lower serum potassium in clients with hyperkalemia. Giving potassium chloride, an angiotensin-converting enzyme inhibitor (such as lisinopril), or a potassium-sparing diuretic (such as spironolactone) would further increase the serum potassium level.

CN: Physiological integrity; CNS: Pharmacological and parenteral therapies; CL: Apply

78. 4. Immune function is important in the healing process, and diminished response may slow or prevent the healing process from taking place. Although immune function declines with age, there are healthy behaviors that will enhance the older adult's response to tissue trauma (e.g., exercise). Reviewing BUN and creatinine levels is important but does not improve the client's wound. Although elevation of the leg may improve edema, it could decease circulation, which could prevent wound healing. Older adults should be encouraged to receive vaccinations, including the influenza vaccine, but this does not improve wound healing of the leg.

CN: Physiological integrity; CNS: Physiological adaptation; CL: Analyze

79. 1, 2, 4. The normal thrombocyte (platelet) count is 150,000/μL (150 × 10⁹/L) to 400,000/μL (400 × 10⁹/L). The client has thrombocytopenia or low platelet count, which predisposes the client to bleeding. The client should avoid using dental floss because it may injure the gums and cause bleeding. Eating crusty or rough foods such as crackers, nuts, and chips may cut the inside of the mouth and cause bleeding. The use of an electric razor rather than a blade is recommended to avoid cuts. Avoiding crowded places and avoiding eating fresh vegetables are precautionary measures for a client with a low white blood cell count.

CN: Physiological integrity; CNS: Reduction of risk potential; CL: Apply

80. 3. Compliance with the prescribed medications is a priority intervention in delaying the onset of acquired immunodeficiency syndrome (AIDS). Eating a diet high in protein to assist with cellular repair, preventative vaccinations, and monitoring viral load and CD4 count is important to assist in the management of HIV. However, administering prescribed medications (antiretrovirals) is priority to delaying or preventing the progression of HIV to AIDS.

CN: Health promotion and maintenance; CNS: None; CL: Analyze

81. A client is receiving dabigatran. Which medication instruction will the nurse include during client education?
1. "We will monitor your partial thromboplastin (PT) time and international normalized ratio."
2. "Avoid consuming green leafy vegetables while you are taking dabigatran."
3. "If you experience an upset stomach, immediately report it to your health care provider."
4. "To avoid unwanted side effects, take this medication with food or milk."

82. A client is placed on neutropenic precautions. Which nursing action(s) is appropriate? Select all that apply.
1. Placing the client in a private room
2. Asking the client to wear a mask during transport
3. Limiting the number of visitors allowed in the room
4. Placing the client on reverse isolation precautions
5. Brushing the client's teeth with a soft toothbrush

83. Which nursing action is **priority** when caring for a client who has been prescribed corticosteroids?
1. Obtain a finger-stick glucose.
2. Perform strict intake and output monitoring.
3. Assess a daily chemistry panel.
4. Promote a nighttime sleeping schedule.

84. The nurse assesses a client with a history of bacterial infection and notes the following vital signs: a blood pressure reading of 80/54 mm Hg, a heart rate of 128 beats/minute, a respiratory rate of 26 breaths/minute, cool and clammy skin, and a decreased level of consciousness. Which nursing action is **priority**?
1. Obtain a temperature.
2. Ask about pain.
3. Initiate intravenous (IV) line access.
4. Assess urine output.

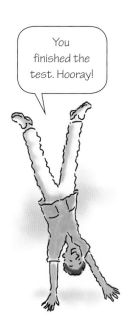

You finished the test. Hooray!

81. 3. Dabigatran is a direct thrombin inhibitor, which reduces the risk of stroke, atrial fibrillation, deep vein thrombosis, and pulmonary embolism. The major side effect of this medication is bleeding. Stomach upset should be immediately reported because it may be a sign of gastric ulcer, which would cause bleeding. Unlike with warfarin, monitoring PT and INR and avoiding green leafy vegetables are not necessary while taking dabigatran. This medication can be taken with or without food.
CN: Physiological integrity; CNS: Pharmacological and parenteral therapies; CL: Apply

82. 1, 2, 3, 4, 5. A client with neutropenia has a low white blood cell count, which makes it easier for the client to get an infection. Neutropenic precautions involve placing the client in a private room, using reverse isolation (the nurse wears a mask when entering the client's room to prevent infecting the client and the client wears a mask during transport), and avoiding crowds around the client by limiting the number of visitors. A soft toothbrush should be used to prevent damaging the gums, which could lead to an infection.
CN: Health promotion and maintenance; CNS: None; CL: Apply

83. 1. Corticosteroids cause elevated blood glucose levels, which increases the client's chance of infection; because insulin may be necessary to maintain normal blood glucose levels, it is priority to assess glucose level. Corticosteroids can cause edema, but strict intake and output is generally unnecessary unless the client also has renal or cardiac disease. Although corticosteroids can cause changes in potassium levels, it is usually not necessary to monitor a daily chemistry panel in clients undergoing corticosteroid therapy. Corticosteroids can alter a client's sleeping pattern, but promoting sleep is not the priority.
CN: Physiological integrity; CNS: Pharmacological and parenteral therapies; CL: Analyze

84. 3. Signs and symptoms of septic shock would include a change in the level of consciousness; cool, clammy, and pale skin; hypotension; tachycardia; and tachypnea. The priority intervention for a client in septic shock is to initiate IV access to begin an infusion. Although obtaining a temperature, asking about pain, and assessing urinary output are important, the nurse has enough information about this client to begin a life-saving intervention before continuing to assess the client.
CN: Physiological integrity; CNS: Physiological adaptation; CL: Analyze

Chapter 5

Respiratory Disorders

Respiratory refresher

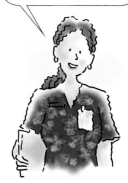

Looking for the latest information about respiratory disorders? Check out the American Association for Respiratory Care's Web site at www.aarc.org. It'll respire—er, inspire—you!

Acute respiratory distress syndrome

Sudden failure of the respiratory system, in which adequate oxygen is prevented from getting to the lungs or into blood

Key signs and symptoms
- Anxiety, restlessness
- Crackles, rhonchi, decreased breath sounds
- Dyspnea, tachypnea

Key test results
- Arterial blood gas (ABG) levels indicate:
  - respiratory acidosis
  - metabolic acidosis
  - hypoxemia that does not respond to increased fraction of inspired oxygen
- Chest x-ray indicates:
  - bilateral infiltrates (in early stages)
  - lung fields with a "ground-glass" appearance
  - massive consolidation of both lung fields (in later stages)

Key treatments
- Intubation and mechanical ventilation using positive end-expiratory pressure (PEEP) or pressure-controlled inverse ratio ventilation
- Antibiotics most effective in treating causative organism
- Analgesic: morphine
- Neuromuscular blocking agents: pancuronium, vecuronium
- Steroids: hydrocortisone, methylprednisolone

Key interventions
- Monitor respiratory, cardiovascular, and neurologic status.
- Monitor electrocardiogram (ECG).
- Maintain bed rest, with alternating supine and prone positioning if possible.
- Perform turning, chest physiotherapy, and postural drainage.

Acute respiratory failure

Inadequate gas exchange by the respiratory system, resulting in levels of arterial oxygen or carbon dioxide (or both) that cannot be maintained within normal limits

Key signs and symptoms
- Decreased respiratory excursion, accessory muscle use, retractions
- Difficulty breathing, dyspnea (shortness of breath), tachypnea, orthopnea
- Fatigue

Key test results
- ABG levels indicate:
  - hypoxemia
  - acidosis
  - alkalosis
  - hypercapnia

Key treatments
- Supplemental oxygen (O_2) therapy, intubation, and mechanical ventilation (possibly with PEEP)
- Analgesic: morphine
- Antianxiety agent: lorazepam
- Bronchodilators: terbutaline theophylline; via nebulizer: albuterol, ipratropium bromide
- Neuromuscular blocking agents: pancuronium, vecuronium, atracurium besylate
- Steroids: hydrocortisone, methylprednisolone

Key interventions
- Monitor respiratory status.
- Administer O_2.
- Provide suctioning; assist with turning, coughing, and deep breathing; perform chest physiotherapy and postural drainage.
- Maintain bed rest.

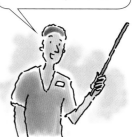

Quick—what are three key treatments for acute respiratory distress syndrome?

Asbestosis

Serious and fatal lung disease resulting from inhaling, over time, a group of minerals with thin microscopic fibers

Key signs and symptoms
- Dry crackles at lung bases
- Dry cough

- Dyspnea on exertion (usually first symptom)
- Pleuritic chest pain

Key test results
- Chest x-rays:
  - show fine, irregular, and linear diffuse infiltrates; extensive fibrosis results in "honeycomb" or "ground-glass" appearance
  - show pleural thickening and calcification, with bilateral obliteration of costophrenic angles
  - in later stages, show an enlarged heart with a classic "shaggy" heart border
- Antibiotics most effective in treating causative organism

Key treatments
- Chest physiotherapy
- Fluid intake up to 3,000 mL/day
- O_2 therapy or mechanical ventilation (with advanced cases)
- Antibiotics most effective in treating causative organism (for treatment of respiratory tract infections)
- Mucolytic inhalation therapy: acetylcysteine

Key interventions
- Perform chest physiotherapy techniques (controlled coughing and segmental bronchial drainage) with chest percussion and vibration.
- Administer O_2 by cannula or mask (1 to 2 L/minute); use mechanical ventilation if arterial oxygen saturation cannot be maintained above 40 mm Hg.

Asphyxia

Lack of oxygen or excess of carbon dioxide that results in state of unconsciousness or death

Key signs and symptoms
- Agitation
- Altered respiratory rate (apnea, bradypnea, occasionally tachypnea)
- Anxiety
- Central and peripheral cyanosis (cherry-red mucous membranes in late-stage carbon monoxide poisoning)
- Altered mental status
- Decreased breath sounds
- Dyspnea

Key test results
- Pulse oximetry reveals decreased oxygen saturation
- ABG measurement indicates:
  - decreased partial pressure of arterial oxygen (PaO_2) < 60 mm Hg
  - increased partial pressure of arterial carbon dioxide ($PaCO_2$) > 50 mm Hg

Key treatments
- O_2 therapy, which may include endotracheal (ET) intubation and mechanical ventilation
- Bronchoscopy (for extraction of a foreign body)
- Opioid antagonist: naloxone (for opioid overdose)

Key interventions
- Monitor cardiac and respiratory status.
- Position the client upright, if tolerable.
- Suction carefully, as needed, and encourage deep breathing.

Asthma

Reactive airway disease in which airways narrow and swell, producing extra mucus and making breathing difficult

Key signs and symptoms
- Usually produces no symptoms between attacks
- Wheezing, primarily on expiration but sometimes on inspiration

Key test results
- Pulmonary function tests (PFTs) during attacks show:
  - decreased forced expiratory volumes that improve with therapy
  - increased residual volume
  - increased total lung capacity.

Key treatments
- Fluid intake up to 3,000 mL/day as tolerated
- Beta-adrenergic drugs: epinephrine, salmeterol, formoterol
- Bronchodilators: terbutaline, theophylline; via nebulizer: albuterol, ipratropium bromide
- Mast cell stabilizer: cromolyn, nedocromil
- Anti-immunoglobulin E agent: omalizumab
- Inhaled corticosteroids: fluticasone, budesonide, mometasone, flunisolide

Key interventions
- Administer low-flow humidified O_2.
- Monitor respiratory status and pulse oximetry values.
- Keep the client in high Fowler's position.

Atelectasis

Collapse or closure of lung tissue, preventing normal oxygen absorption to healthy tissues

Key signs and symptoms
- Diminished or bronchial breath sounds
- Dyspnea

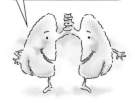

It feels great to breathe easy!

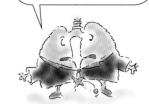

Relax or we'll start to come apart like a cheap suit!

- Low-grade fever
- In severe cases:
  - anxiety
  - cyanosis
  - diaphoresis
  - severe dyspnea
  - substernal or intercostal retractions
  - tachycardia

Key test results
- Chest x-ray shows:
  - characteristic horizontal lines in the lower lung zones and, with segmental or lobar collapse, characteristic dense shadows often associated with hyperinflation of neighboring lung zones (in widespread atelectasis)

Key treatments
- Bronchoscopy
- Chest physiotherapy
- Bronchodilators: albuterol
- Mucolytic inhalation therapy: acetylcysteine
- Pain control

Key interventions
- Encourage postoperative and other high-risk clients to cough and deep breathe every hour during their waking hours.
- Postoperatively:
  - teach client to hold a pillow tightly over the incision while deep breathing or moving
  - gently reposition these clients often, and help them walk as soon as possible.
- Administer adequate analgesics.
- Teach client how to use an incentive spirometer and encourage client to use it hourly during waking hours.
- Humidify inspired air.
- Encourage adequate fluid intake.
- Perform postural drainage and chest percussion.
- Monitor breath sounds and ventilatory status frequently and be alert for any changes.

Bronchiectasis

Condition in which airways are abnormally stretched and widened

Key signs and symptoms
- Chronic cough that produces copious, foul-smelling, mucopurulent secretions, possibly totaling several cupfuls daily
- Coarse crackles during inspiration over involved lobes or segments

- Dyspnea
- Hemoptysis
- Weight loss

Key test results
- Chest x-ray shows:
  - peribronchial thickening
  - areas of atelectasis
  - scattered cystic changes
- Sputum culture and Gram stain identify predominant organisms

Key treatments
- Bronchoscopy (to mobilize secretions)
- Chest physiotherapy
- O_2 therapy
- Antibiotics most effective in treating the causative organism
- Bronchodilator: albuterol

Key interventions
- Monitor respiratory status and pulse oximetry values.
- Provide supportive care.
- Help client adjust to permanent changes in lifestyle that irreversible lung damage makes necessary.
- Perform chest physiotherapy, including postural drainage and chest percussion designed for involved lobes.
  - Perform several times a day; best times are early morning and just before bedtime
  - Instruct client to maintain each position for 10 minutes.
  - Perform percussion and tell client to cough.

Chronic bronchitis

Inflammation of bronchial tubes causing daily cough, which:
- produces mucus
- persists at least 3 months per year
- persists for at least 2 years consecutively.

Key signs and symptoms
- Cyanosis
- Dyspnea
- Increased sputum production
- Productive cough

Key test results
- Chest x-ray shows:
  - hyperinflation
  - increased bronchovascular markings
- PFTs may reveal:
  - increased residual volume, decreased vital capacity and forced expiratory volumes, and normal static compliance and diffusion capacity

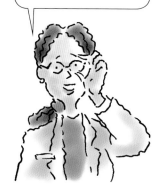

A client is suspected of having bronchiectasis. What signs should you look for?

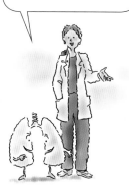

O_2 therapy is used to treat many respiratory disorders.

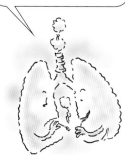

I wonder if there's any connection between this and our chronic bronchitis? Oh well— my turn.

Key treatments

- Fluid intake up to 3,000 mL/day, if not contraindicated by other conditions
- Intubation and mechanical ventilation, if respiratory status deteriorates
- Antibiotics most effective in treating causative organism
- Bronchodilators: terbutaline, theophylline; via nebulizer: albuterol, ipratropium bromide
- Influenza and pneumococcal vaccines
- Steroids: hydrocortisone, methylprednisolone
- Steroids (via nebulizer): beclomethasone, triamcinolone

Key interventions

- Administer low-flow O_2.
- Monitor respiratory status and pulse oximetry values.
- Assist with diaphragmatic and pursed-lip breathing.
- Monitor and record the color, amount, and consistency of sputum.
- Provide chest physiotherapy, postural drainage, incentive spirometry, and suction.

Cor pulmonale

Increase in size of right ventricle caused by a disorder of the respiratory system

Key signs and symptoms

- Dyspnea on exertion
- Edema
- Fatigue
- Orthopnea
- Tachypnea
- Weakness

Key test results

- ABG analysis: decreased PaO_2 (less than 70 mm Hg)
- Chest x-ray:
  - shows large central pulmonary arteries
  - suggests right ventricular enlargement by rightward enlargement of cardiac silhouette on an anterior chest film
- Pulmonary artery pressure measurements:
  - show increased right ventricular and pulmonary artery pressures because of increased pulmonary vascular resistance

Key treatments

- O_2 therapy as necessary by mask or cannula in concentrations of 24% to 40%, depending on PaO_2 and, in acute cases, mechanical ventilation
- Cardiac glycoside: digoxin

- Diuretic: furosemide
- Vasodilators: hydralazine, nitroprusside, prostaglandins (in primary pulmonary hypertension)
- Calcium channel blocker: diltiazem
- Angiotensin-converting enzyme (ACE) inhibitor: captopril

Key interventions

- Monitor respiratory status and pulse oximetry values.
- Monitor cardiovascular status.
- Limit the client's fluid intake to 1,000 to 2,000 mL/day, and provide a low-sodium diet.
- Reposition bedridden clients often.
- Provide meticulous respiratory care, including O_2 therapy.
- For clients with chronic obstructive pulmonary disease, teach pursed-lip breathing exercises.
- Watch for signs of respiratory failure (change in pulse rate, increased fatigue from exertion, deep and labored respirations).

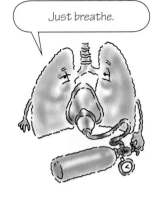

Just breathe.

Emphysema

Long-term progressive disease of lungs, causing shortness of breath due to overinflation of the alveoli

Key signs and symptoms

- Barrel chest
- Dyspnea
- Pursed-lip breathing

Key test results

- Chest x-ray of clients in advanced disease stage reveals:
  - flattened diaphragm
  - reduced vascular markings in lung periphery
  - enlarged anteroposterior chest diameter
  - vertical heart
- PFTs show:
  - increased residual volume
  - total lung capacity and compliance
  - decreased vital capacity
  - diffusing capacity
  - expiratory volumes

Key treatments

- Chest physiotherapy, postural drainage, and incentive spirometry
- Fluid intake up to 3,000 mL/day, if not contraindicated by heart failure
- O_2 therapy at 2 to 3 L/minute, transtracheal therapy for home O_2 therapy
- Antibiotics most effective in treating causative organism

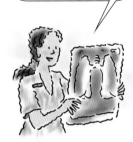

Hmm. I see some barrel chest here. Do you know what that means?

- Bronchodilators: terbutaline, theophylline; via nebulizer: albuterol, ipratropium bromide
- Influenza and pneumococcal vaccines
- Steroids: hydrocortisone, methylprednisolone
- Steroids (via nebulizer): beclomethasone, triamcinolone

Key interventions

- Monitor respiratory status, pulse oximetry values.
- Assist with diaphragmatic and pursed-lip breathing.
- Monitor and record color, amount, and consistency of sputum.
- Perform chest physiotherapy, postural drainage, incentive spirometry, suction.

Legionnaires' disease

Serious type of lung infection or pneumonia caused by *Legionella* bacterium

Key signs and symptoms

- Cough, initially nonproductive, that eventually produces grayish, nonpurulent, blood-streaked sputum
- Fever
- Generalized weakness
- Malaise
- Recurrent chills

Key test results

- Chest x-ray shows patchy, localized infiltration, which progresses to multilobar consolidation (usually involving the lower lobes); pleural effusion; and, in fulminant disease, opacification of the entire lung
- Direct immunofluorescence of *Legionella pneumophila* and indirect fluorescent serum antibody testing compare findings from initial blood studies with findings from those done at least 3 weeks later; convalescent serum sample showing a 4-fold or greater rise in antibody titer for *L. pneumophila* confirms the diagnosis

Key treatments

- Antibiotics: erythromycin, rifampin, tetracycline
- Antipyretics: acetaminophen, aspirin

Key interventions

- Closely monitor client's respiratory status.
- Evaluate chest wall expansion, depth and pattern of respirations, cough, and chest pain.
- Monitor client's vital signs, pulse oximetry values, level of consciousness (LOC), and

dryness and color of the lips and mucous membranes.
- Watch for signs of shock (decreased blood pressure, thready pulse, diaphoresis, clammy skin).
- Administer IV fluids.
- Provide respiratory therapy as needed.
- Give antibiotics as necessary and observe carefully for adverse effects.

Lung cancer

Carcinoma of the lung, characterized by uncontrollable cell growth in tissues of the lung

Key signs and symptoms

- Cough, hemoptysis
- Weight loss, anorexia

Key test results

- Chest x-ray shows lesion or mass

Key treatments

- Resection of the affected lobe (lobectomy) or lung (pneumonectomy)
- Antineoplastics: cyclophosphamide, doxorubicin, cisplatin, vincristine, vinorelbine, gemcitabine, paclitaxel, docetaxel, irinotecan

Key interventions

- Monitor client's pain level.
- Administer analgesics as prescribed.
- Perform suctioning and assist with turning, coughing, and deep breathing.
- Monitor for bleeding, infection, and electrolyte imbalance caused by effects of chemotherapy.

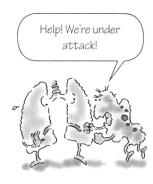

Help! We're under attack!

Pleural effusion and empyema

Excess fluid that accumulates in the pleural cavity (pleural effusion); accumulation of pus in the pleural cavity (empyema)

Key signs and symptoms

- Decreased breath sounds
- Dyspnea
- Fever
- Pleuritic chest pain

Key test results

- Chest x-ray shows radiopaque fluid in dependent regions.
- Thoracentesis results include:
  - lactate dehydrogenase (LD) levels less than 200 U/L (3.34 μkat/L)
  - protein levels less than 3 g/dL (30 g/L) (in transudative effusions)

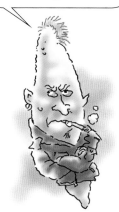

Keep us pink and healthy—put down that cigarette!

○ ratio of protein in pleural fluid to protein in serum greater than or equal to 0.5
○ LD in pleural fluid greater than or equal to 200 U/L (3.34 μkat/L)
○ ratio of LD in pleural fluid to LD in serum greater than 0.6 (in exudative effusions)
○ acute inflammatory white blood cells and microorganisms (in empyema)

Key treatments

- Supplemental O_2 therapy
- Thoracentesis to remove fluid
- Thoracotomy if thoracentesis is not effective
- Antibiotics most effective in treating the organism that causes empyema

Key interventions

- Explain thoracentesis to the client.
- Before the procedure, tell the client to expect a stinging sensation from the local anesthetic and a feeling of pressure when the needle is inserted.
- Instruct the client to tell you immediately if he feels uncomfortable or has trouble breathing during the procedure.
- Administer O_2.
- Administer antibiotics.
- Use care when inspecting chest tube so as not to dislodge it.
- Ensure chest tube patency by watching for bubbles in the underwater seal chamber.
- Record amount, color, and consistency of any tube drainage.

Pleurisy

Inflammation of the pleura (lining of the lungs)

Key signs and symptoms

- Pleural friction rub (a coarse, creaky sound heard during late inspiration and early expiration)
- Sharp, stabbing pain that increases with respiration

Key test results

- Diagnosis generally rests on client's history and respiratory assessment
- Diagnostic tests help rule out other causes and pinpoint underlying disorder

Key treatments

- Bed rest
- Analgesic: acetaminophen with oxycodone
- Anti-inflammatory: indomethacin

Key interventions

- Stress the importance of bed rest.

- Allow client as much uninterrupted rest as possible.
- Administer antitussives and pain medication as needed.
- Encourage client to cough.
- During coughing exercises, apply firm pressure at the pain site.

Pneumocystis pneumonia (PCP)

Form of pneumonia caused by the yeast-like fungus pneumocystis; usually found in those with a weakened immune system

Key signs and symptoms

- Generalized fatigue
- Low-grade, intermittent fever
- Nonproductive cough
- Dyspnea
- Weight loss

Key test results

- Chest x-ray may show slowly progressing, fluffy infiltrates, and occasionally nodular lesions or a spontaneous pneumothorax
- Findings must be differentiated from findings associated with other types of pneumonia or acute respiratory distress syndrome
- Histologic study results confirm *Pneumocystis jirovecii*. In clients with human immunodeficiency virus (HIV) infection, initial examination of a first morning sputum specimen (induced by inhaling an ultrasonically dispersed saline mist) may be sufficient; however, this technique is usually ineffective in clients without HIV infection

Key treatments

- O_2 therapy, which may include ET intubation and mechanical ventilation

Key interventions

- Monitor the client's respiratory status and pulse oximetry values.
- Administer O_2 therapy as needed.
- Encourage client to ambulate.
- Encourage client to perform deep-breathing exercises and incentive spirometry.
- Administer antipyretics as needed.
- Monitor intake and output and weigh the client daily. Replace fluids as needed.
- Administer antimicrobial drugs as prescribed:
  ○ Never give pentamidine IM.
  ○ Administer the IV form slowly over 60 minutes.
- Monitor the client for adverse reactions to antimicrobial drugs:
  ○ If receiving sulfamethoxazole and trimethoprim, watch for nausea, vomiting,

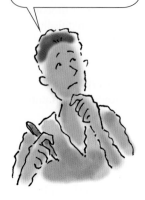

Let's see ... pleurisy is inflammation of the ...

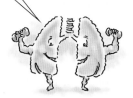

"One! Two! Three! Four!" Physical exercise is a lifestyle factor that can affect oxygenation.

rash, bone marrow suppression, thrush, fever, hepatotoxicity, and anaphylaxis.
  o If receiving pentamidine, watch for cardiac arrhythmias, hypotension, dizziness, azotemia, hypocalcemia, and hepatic disturbances.
- Supply nutritional supplements as needed.
- Encourage client to eat a high-calorie, protein-rich diet.
- Offer small, frequent meals if client cannot tolerate large amounts of food.

Pneumonia

Lung infection that can be caused by bacteria, fungi, or virus

Key signs and symptoms
- Chills, fever
- Crackles, rhonchi, and pleural friction rub on auscultation
- Dyspnea, tachypnea, and accessory muscle use
- Sputum that is rusty, green, or bloody with pneumococcal pneumonia and yellow-green with bronchopneumonia

Key test results
- Chest x-ray shows pulmonary infiltrates
- Sputum study identifies the causative organism

Key treatments
- Antibiotics most effective in treating causative organism
- Supplemental O_2 therapy; intubation and mechanical ventilation if condition deteriorates

Key interventions
- Monitor and record intake and output.
- Monitor pulse oximetry values.
- Monitor respiratory status.
- Force fluids to 3 to 4 L/day and maintain IV fluids.

Pneumothorax and hemothorax

Abnormal collection of air or gas in the pleural space (pneumothorax); pocket of blood in pleural space (hemothorax)

Key signs and symptoms
- Diminished or absent breath sounds unilaterally
- Dyspnea, tachypnea, subcutaneous emphysema, and cough
- Sharp chest pain that increases with exertion

Key test results
- Chest x-ray confirms diagnosis

Key treatments
- Chest tube to water-seal drainage

Key interventions
- Monitor and record vital signs.
- Monitor respiratory status and pulse oximetry values.
- Monitor chest tube site for subcutaneous emphysema.
- Monitor chest tube drainage.
- Evaluate cardiovascular status.
- Maintain chest tube to water-seal drainage; the water seal chamber prevents air from entering the chest tube when the client inhales.

Pulmonary embolism

Sudden blockage of a major blood vessel in the lung, usually by a blood clot

Key signs and symptoms
- Sudden onset of dyspnea, tachypnea, and crackles

Key test results
- ABG levels typically show decreased PaO_2 and $PaCO_2$.
- Lung scan shows ventilation-perfusion mismatch.

Key treatments
- Vena cava filter insertion
- Anticoagulants: heparin (heparin sodium injection), warfarin
- Fibrinolytics: tissue plasminogen activator

Key interventions
- Monitor respiratory status and pulse oximetry values.
- Evaluate cardiovascular status and monitor ECG.
- Administer O_2.

Respiratory acidosis

Inability of lungs to remove all of the carbon dioxide produced by body; usually accompanied by hypoventilation

Key signs and symptoms
- Cardiovascular abnormalities (tachycardia, hypertension, atrial and ventricular arrhythmias and, in severe acidosis, hypotension with vasodilation)

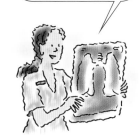

This x-ray confirms your diagnosis.

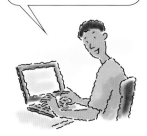

What actually causes pneumonia? My mom always said it was going outside without a coat on in winter.

Key test results

- ABG measurements confirm presence of respiratory acidosis
  - $PaCO_2$ exceeds the normal level of 45 mm Hg
  - pH is usually below the normal range of 7.35 to 7.45
  - client's bicarbonate level is normal in the acute stage and elevated in the chronic stage

Key treatments

- Correction of the underlying cause
- Sodium bicarbonate in severe cases

Key interventions

- Closely monitor client's blood pH level.
- Be alert for critical changes in the client's respiratory, central nervous system (CNS), and cardiovascular functions.
- Maintain adequate hydration.
- If acidosis requires mechanical ventilation:
  - maintain patent airway
  - provide adequate humidification
  - perform tracheal suctioning regularly and vigorous chest physiotherapy if needed.

Respiratory alkalosis

Low levels of carbon dioxide due to hyperventilation

Key signs and symptoms

- Agitation
- Cardiac arrhythmias that fail to respond to conventional treatment (severe respiratory alkalosis)
- Circumoral or peripheral paresthesia (a prickling sensation around the mouth or extremities)
- Deep, rapid breathing, possibly exceeding 40 breaths/minute (cardinal sign)
- Light-headedness or dizziness (from decreased cerebral blood flow)

Key test results

- ABG analysis confirms respiratory alkalosis and rules out respiratory compensation for metabolic acidosis:
  - $PaCO_2$ is below 35 mm Hg
  - pH is elevated in proportion to the fall in $PaCO_2$ in acute stage
  - pH drops toward normal in chronic stage
  - bicarbonate level is normal in acute stage
  - bicarbonate level is below normal in chronic stage

Key treatments

- Instruct client to breathe into a paper bag:
  - helps relieve acute anxiety

- increases CO_2 levels (for severe respiratory alkalosis).

Key interventions

- Watch for and report any changes in neurologic, neuromuscular, or cardiovascular function.
- Monitor respiratory status.

Sarcoidosis

Abnormal collection of inflammatory cells that form as nodules in different body organs

Key signs and symptoms

Initial
- Arthralgia in the wrists, ankles, and elbows
- Fatigue
- Malaise
- Weight loss

Respiratory
- Breathlessness
- Substernal pain

Cutaneous
- Erythema nodosum
- Subcutaneous skin nodules with maculopapular eruptions

Ophthalmic
- Anterior uveitis (common)

Musculoskeletal
- Muscle weakness
- Pain

Hepatic
- Granulomatous hepatitis (usually produces no symptoms)

Genitourinary
- Hypercalciuria (excessive calcium in the urine)

Cardiovascular
- Arrhythmias (premature beats, bundle-branch block, or complete heart block)

Central nervous system
- Cranial or peripheral nerve palsies
- Basilar meningitis (inflammation of the meninges at the base of the brain)

Key test results

- Positive Kveim-Siltzbach skin test supports the diagnosis; in this test, client receives an intradermal injection of an antigen prepared from human sarcoidal spleen or lymph nodes from clients with sarcoidosis; if client has active sarcoidosis, granuloma develops at the injection site in 2 to 6 weeks; reaction is considered positive when biopsy of the skin at the injection site shows discrete epithelioid cell granuloma

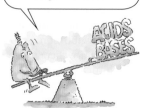

Keeping that acid–base balance in the lungs in critical.

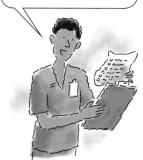

Your client is breathing at a rate of 45 breaths/minute. What respiratory condition will this lead to?

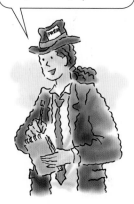

Word on the street is that sarcoidosis is a real pain in the joints. Care to comment on any other symptoms?

Key treatments
- Low-calcium diet
- Avoidance of direct exposure to sunlight (in clients with hypercalcemia)
- O_2 therapy
- Corticosteroid: prednisone
- Cytotoxic agents: methotrexate, azathioprine

Key interventions
- Provide nutritious, high-calorie diet and plenty of fluids.
- If client has hypercalcemia, suggest low-calcium diet.
- Weigh client regularly.

Severe acute respiratory syndrome (SARS)
Serious form of pneumonia caused by a virus

Key signs and symptoms
- High fever (usually greater than 100.4°F [38°C])
- Dry cough
- Dyspnea

Key test results
- History reveals recent travel to an area with documented SARS cases or close contact with a person suspected of having SARS
- Chest x-ray shows atypical pneumonia
- Reverse transcription polymerase chain reaction (RT-PCR) test detects ribonucleic acid of the SARS virus

Key treatments
- Supplemental O_2; may require ET intubation and mechanical ventilation
- Droplet precautions

- Antiviral agents: oseltamivir, ribavirin, interferon beta-1a

Key interventions
- Monitor respiratory status.
- Administer supplemental O_2 as prescribed.
- Maintain droplet precautions.

Tuberculosis
Infection caused by mycobacterium that usually attacks the lungs but can spread to any part of the body

Key signs and symptoms
- Fever
- Night sweats

Key test results
- Mantoux skin test is positive.
- Sputum study results are positive for:
  - acid-fast bacillus
  - *Mycobacterium tuberculosis.*

Key treatments
- Standard and airborne precautions:
  - while client is contagious, everyone entering client's room must wear a respirator with a high-efficiency particulate air filter
- Antitubercular agents: isoniazid (INH), ethambutol, rifampin, pyrazinamide

Key interventions
- Monitor respiratory status and pulse oximetry values.
- Maintain infection-control precautions.
- Instruct the client to cover nose and mouth when sneezing.
- Provide a room with negative-pressure ventilation.

"Hold on tight, partner, we're in this together!"

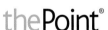

Respiratory questions, answers, and rationales

1. The nurse knows which client is at the highest risk for developing pneumonia?
1. A 45-year-old client admitted for malnutrition secondary to alcohol use disorder who smokes one pack per day
2. A 56-year-old client who is recovering from a left arthroplasty and attends physical therapy weekly
3. A 69-year-old client with chronic obstructive pulmonary disease (COPD) who lives in a group home
4. A 75-year-old client who refuses both the pneumonia and influenza vaccines and has hypokalemia

1. 3. Risk factors for the development of pneumonia include: weakened immune system, hospitalization, residing in a group living situation, chronic condition, smoking, and being older than 65 years of age. The client with advanced age, COPD, and living in a group home is at greatest risk, with three risk factors. The client admitted with malnutrition has two risk factors (hospitalization, smoker). The client who had an arthroplasty has no risk factors. The client with hypokalemia is at increased risk due to age and refusal of the vaccination.
CN: Physiological integrity; CNS: Physiological adaptation; CL: Analyze

CN: Client needs category   CNS: Client needs subcategory   CL: Cognitive level

2. A client is admitted with signs and symptoms of early pneumonia. The nurse will monitor the client for which complication?
  1. Atelectasis
  2. Bronchiectasis
  3. Effusion
  4. Inflammation

2. **4.** The common feature of all types of pneumonia is an inflammatory pulmonary response to the offending organism or agent. Atelectasis and bronchiectasis indicate a collapse of a portion of the airway that does not occur in pneumonia. An effusion is an accumulation of excess pleural fluid in the pleural space, which may be a secondary response to pneumonia.
CN: Physiological integrity; CNS: Physiological adaptation; CL: Apply

3. An older adult client has just been admitted with pneumonia. The client tells the nurse, "I have never had pneumonia before and nobody in my family has ever suffered from pneumonia. I do not understand how I contracted this disease." Which statement by the nurse is **most** appropriate?
  1. "You should not worry about how you contracted pneumonia."
  2. "You could have had it in the past and not know it."
  3. "Advanced age is a risk factor for developing pneumonia."
  4. "Immobility can help to prevent this disease."

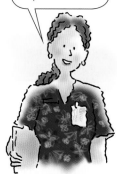
Older clients are much more susceptible to contracting pneumonia.

3. **3.** Advanced age, due to the possibility of depressed cough and glottis reflexes and nutritional depletion, is a risk factor for developing pneumonia. Telling the client not to worry is incorrect as pneumonia can be deadly. Saying that the client might have contracted pneumonia in the past is not really helpful or therapeutic. Immobility is a risk factor and not a factor that would prevent pneumonia.
CN: Physiological integrity; CNS: Reduction of risk potential; CL: Apply

4. The nurse is caring for an older adult client newly diagnosed with pneumonia. Which symptoms will the nurse monitor this client for **first**?
  1. Altered mental status and dehydration
  2. Fever and chills
  3. Hemoptysis and dyspnea
  4. Pleuritic chest pain and cough

4. **1.** Fever, chills, hemoptysis, dyspnea, cough, and pleuritic chest pain are the common symptoms of pneumonia, but older adult clients are more likely to *first* exhibit only an altered mental status and dehydration due to a blunted immune response.
CN: Safe, effective care environment; CNS: Management of care; CL: Apply

5. During admission, the nurse is auscultating the chest of a client with pneumonia and notes bronchial sounds. Which nursing action is **most** appropriate?
  1. Continue to assess the client.
  2. Obtain a sputum culture.
  3. Notify the health care provider.
  4. Apply oxygen via a facemask.

5. **1.** Chest auscultation reveals bronchial breath sounds over areas of consolidation, which is expected in a client with pneumonia. The nurse would continue to assess the client to determine appropriate interventions and obtain baseline data. A sputum culture will be used to determine the causative agent, but the culture is not priority over completing the initial respiratory assessment. The nurse would not notify the health care provider for an expected finding. There are no indications oxygen is needed at this time.
CN: Safe, effective care environment; CNS: Management of care; CL: Apply

6. A client is admitted with a fever, cough with copious secretions, and chest pain. Which test will the nurse ensure is performed prior to giving an antibiotic?
  1. Arterial blood gas (ABG) analysis
  2. Chest x-ray
  3. Blood cultures
  4. Sputum culture and sensitivity

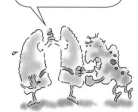
Don't let pneumonia pummel your client's lungs. Get that antibiotic started STAT!

6. **4.** Sputum culture and sensitivity can help identify the organism causing the pneumonia and should be done prior to giving an antibiotic. A chest x-ray can show the presence of lung infiltrates, confirming the diagnosis, but should be done after starting an antibiotic. ABG analysis helps determine the extent of hypoxia present due to the pneumonia, and blood cultures help determine if the infection is systemic, but these also may be done after starting the antibiotic.
CN: Physiological integrity; CNS: Physiological adaptation; CL: Apply

7. A client with pneumonia has a nonproductive cough and copious secretions. Which action will the nurse encourage the client to perform to facilitate effective coughing?
1. Lying in semi-Fowler's position
2. Sipping water, hot tea, or coffee
3. Inhaling and exhaling from pursed lips
4. Using thoracic breathing

8. An older adult client with pneumonia has copious secretions but is having difficulty coughing them up. Which nursing action is **most** appropriate?
1. Monitor the client's need for suctioning every hour.
2. Encourage the client to cough every 10 minutes.
3. Teach the client how to use an incentive spirometer.
4. Notify the client's primary health care provider.

9. On entering the room of a client with chronic obstructive pulmonary disease (COPD), the nurse notes the client is receiving oxygen at 4 L/minute via nasal cannula. Which action will the nurse complete?
1. Decrease the oxygen flow rate.
2. Monitor the oxygen saturation level.
3. Ask whether the client uses oxygen at home.
4. Remove the nasal cannula and apply a face mask.

10. A client has been treated with antibiotic therapy for right lower lobe pneumonia for 10 days and will be discharged today. Which finding will the nurse report to the primary health care provider **immediately**?
1. Continued dyspnea
2. Temperature of 99°F (37.2°C)
3. Respiratory rate of 20 breaths/minute
4. Vesicular breath sounds in right base

11. The right forearm of a client who had a purified protein derivative (PPD) test for tuberculosis (TB) is reddened and raised about 3 mm where the test was given. What will the nurse do **next**?
1. Document the findings.
2. Place the client on isolation.
3. Check to see if client had an x-ray.
4. Notify the health care provider.

7. 2. Sips of water, hot tea, or coffee may stimulate coughing. The best position is sitting in a chair with the knees flexed and the feet placed firmly on the floor. The client should inhale through the nose and exhale through pursed lips. Diaphragmatic, not thoracic, breathing helps to facilitate coughing.
CN: Physiological integrity; CNS: Basic care and comfort; CL: Apply

8. 1. Suctioning should be performed only when necessary, based on the client's condition at the time of assessment. Suctioning is a nursing procedure and does not require a health care provider's prescription. It is not appropriate to ask the client to cough every 10 minutes. Incentive spirometry would not help move the secretions.
CN: Physiological integrity; CNS: Basic care and comfort; CL: Apply

9. 1. The administration of oxygen at 1 to 2 L/minute by way of a nasal cannula is recommended for clients with COPD; therefore, a rate of 4 L/minute is too high. The normal mechanism that stimulates breathing is a rise in blood carbon dioxide. Clients with COPD retain blood carbon dioxide, so their mechanism for stimulating breathing is a low blood oxygen level. High levels of oxygen may cause hypoventilation and apnea. Oxygen delivered at 1 to 2 L/minute should aid in oxygenation without causing hypoventilation. Whether the client uses oxygen at home has no bearing on the priority nursing action in this situation. The nurse should monitor the oxygen saturation level after correcting the flow rate. It is not appropriate to switch the client to a face mask.
CN: Safe, effective care environment; CNS: Safety and infection control; CL: Apply

10. 1. Continued dyspnea indicates the client is still having difficulty breathing and should be assessed by the health care provider before being discharged. The client's temperature is slightly elevated; however, dyspnea is most concerning. The client's respiratory rate is within normal range. If the client still had pneumonia, the breath sounds in the right base would be bronchial, not the normal vesicular breath sounds.
CN: Safe, effective care environment; CNS: Management of care; CL: Analyze

11. 1. This test would be classed as negative; therefore, the nurse would document the findings and continue to monitor the client. A 3 mm raised area would be a positive result if a client had recent close contact with someone diagnosed with, or suspected of having, infectious TB. The remaining options are not appropriate for this client.
CN: Physiological integrity; CNS: Reduction of risk potential; None; CL: Apply

12. A client who is being treated for pneumonia has a persistent cough and reports severe pain on coughing. Which instruction will the nurse provide to the client?
1. "You need to hold in your cough as much as possible."
2. "Splint your chest wall with a pillow when you cough."
3. "Place the head of your bed flat to help with coughing."
4. "Restrict fluids to help decrease the amount of sputum."

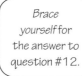

Brace yourself for the answer to question #12.

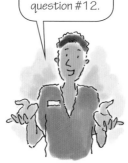

13. The nurse working in a walk-in clinic has been alerted of an outbreak of tuberculosis (TB). Which client does the nurse identify as having the **highest** risk for developing TB?
1. A 16-year-old high school student
2. A 33-year-old day care worker with asthma
3. A 43-year-old who is homeless with a history of alcoholism
4. A 54-year-old business professional who travels a few times a year

14. A client comes to the clinic and is diagnosed with active tuberculosis (TB). Which medication(s) does the nurse expect the health care provider to prescribe initially for this client? Select all that apply.
1. Isoniazid
2. Ethambutol
3. Clindamycin
4. Rifampin
5. Pyrazinamide

15. A client is being screened in the clinic for tuberculosis. The client reports having negative purified protein derivative (PPD) test results in the past. The nurse performs a PPD test on the client's right forearm. Which statement made by the client indicates a need for further education?
1. "I need to return to the clinic to assess the results."
2. "I can return to the clinic in 48 hours for the results."
3. "I do not have to return to the clinic if the area stays flat."
4. "A health care provider has to read the results."

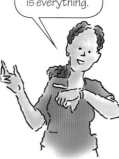

In question #15, timing is everything.

16. The nurse will monitor a client suspected of having a primary tuberculosis (TB) infection for which finding?
1. Secondary pneumonia
2. Active TB within 1 month
3. A fever requiring hospitalization
4. A positive skin test

12. 2. Showing this client how to splint the chest wall should help decrease discomfort when coughing. Holding in coughs would only increase pain. Placing the head of the bed flat may increase the frequency of coughing and require more respiratory effort; a 45-degree angle may help the client cough more efficiently and with less pain. Increasing fluid intake would help thin secretions, making it easier for the client to clear them. Promoting fluid intake is appropriate in this situation.
CN: Physiological integrity; CNS: Basic care and comfort; CL: Apply

13. 3. Clients who are economically disadvantaged, malnourished, and have reduced immunity, such as a homeless client with a history of alcoholism, are at extremely high risk for developing TB. A high school student, a business professional, and a day care worker have a much lower risk of contracting TB, regardless of their age.
CN: Physiological integrity; CNS: Physiological adaptation; CL: Analyze

14. 1, 2, 4, 5. The TB bacillus is airborne and carried in droplets exhaled by an infected person. Key treatments include the antitubercular medications isoniazid, ethambutol, rifampin, and pyrazinamide. Clindamycin is an antibiotic used to treat acne and other infections but not TB.
CN: Physiological integrity; CNS: Pharmacological and parenteral therapies; CL: Apply

15. 3. It is very important to have the results read accurately and clients should return to the clinic for this. PPD tests should be read in 48 to 72 hours. If read too early or too late, the results will not be accurate. The client cannot self-read the results; it is also important that a health care provider (physician, nurse, etc.) read the results.
CN: Health promotion and maintenance; CNS: None; CL: Apply

16. 4. A primary TB infection occurs when the bacillus has successfully invaded the entire body after entering through the lungs. At this point, the bacilli are walled off and skin tests read positive. However, all but infants and immunosuppressed people would remain asymptomatic. The general population has a 10% risk of developing active TB over their lifetime often because of a break in the body's immune defenses. The active stage shows the classic symptoms of TB: fever, hemoptysis, and night sweats.
CN: Physiological integrity; CNS: Physiological adaptation; CL: Apply

17. A client was infected with tuberculosis (TB) bacillus 10 years ago but never developed the disease. The client is now being treated for cancer and begins to develop signs of TB. Which statement by the nurse is **most** accurate?
1. "Some people carry dormant TB infections that develop into active disease."
2. "You should be all right since it has been 10 years since you were infected."
3. "There is a really good chance that you will now develop a superinfection."
4. "It is not unusual to develop another infection when you have cancer."

18. A client comes to the clinic with chills, a low-grade fever, night sweats, and hemoptysis. Which intervention(s) will the nurse perform at this time? Select all that apply.
1. Encouraging airway clearance
2. Advocating adherence to treatment regimen
3. Promoting activity and nutrition
4. Prescribing medication therapy
5. Preventing transmission

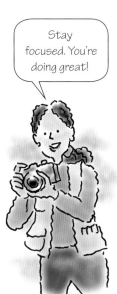

Stay focused. You're doing great!

19. The nurse will prepare a client who has recently been exposed to a family member diagnosed with active tuberculosis and has had several false-positive skin tests in the past for which test?
1. Chest x-ray
2. Mantoux skin test
3. Sputum culture
4. Tuberculin skin test

20. The nurse is referring a client with a positive Mantoux skin test result for a chest x-ray. The client is confused and asks the nurse why the extra radiation is necessary. Which response by the nurse is **best**?
1. "The x-ray is to confirm the suspected diagnosis."
2. "The x-ray is to determine whether a repeat skin test is needed."
3. "The x-ray is to determine the extent of lesions."
4. "The x-ray will show whether this is a primary or secondary infection."

21. The nurse is caring for a client experiencing acute exacerbation of asthma. Which symptom(s) will the nurse expect to assess? Select all that apply.
1. Wheezing
2. Tachycardia
3. Hoarseness
4. Agitation
5. Chest tightness
6. Dyspnea

17. 1. Some people carry dormant TB infections that may develop into active disease. In addition, primary sites of infection containing TB bacilli may remain latent for years and then activate when the client's resistance is lowered, as when a client is being treated for cancer. The nurse should not tell the client that he will be all right. Superinfection does not apply in this case. This is not a usual development for a client who has cancer.
CN: Safe, effective care environment; CNS: Safety and infection control; CL: Apply

18. 1, 2, 3, 5. Typical signs and symptoms of active TB are chills, fever, night sweats, and hemoptysis. Clients with TB typically have low-grade fevers not higher than 102°F (38.9°C). When active TB is diagnosed it is important for the nurse to help promote airway clearance, advocate for adherence to treatment regimen, promote the importance of good nutrition and activity, and instruct the client in ways to prevent transmission. The primary health care provider, not the nurse, should prescribe the necessary medications.
CN: Physiological integrity; CNS: Physiological adaptation; CL: Analyze

19. 3. Skin tests may be false-positive or false-negative. Lesions in the lung may not be big enough to be seen on x-ray. The sputum culture for *Mycobacterium tuberculosis* is the only method of confirming the diagnosis.
CN: Physiological integrity; CNS: Physiological adaptation; CL: Apply

20. 3. If the lesions are large enough, the chest x-ray will show their presence in the lungs. Sputum culture, not an x-ray or additional skin test, confirms the diagnosis, as false-positive and false-negative skin test results may occur. A chest x-ray cannot determine whether this is a primary or secondary infection.
CN: Physiological integrity; CNS: Physiological adaptation; CL: Apply

21. 1, 2, 4, 5, 6. Asthma exacerbations are episodes characterized by progressive increasing in one or more typical asthma symptoms accompanied by a decrease in expiratory flow. Typical symptoms include wheezing, tachycardia, agitation, dyspnea, and chest tightness, but not hoarseness.
CN: Physiological integrity; CNS: Physiological adaptation; CL: Apply

CN: Client needs category   CNS: Client needs subcategory   CL: Cognitive level

22. A client with a productive cough, chills, and night sweats is suspected of having active tuberculosis (TB). Which action will the nurse take **first**?
1. Place the client on airborne precautions.
2. Administer isoniazid and have the client rest.
3. Give a tuberculin skin test.
4. Assess for adventitious breath sounds.

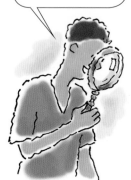

In question #22, which action will the safe nurse take **first**?

23. A client with a positive result on a skin test for tuberculosis (TB) is not showing signs of active disease. Still, the client is worried and asks the nurse what can be done to help prevent the development of active TB. The nurse will anticipate educating the client on which medication regimen?
1. Metronidazole therapy for 10 to 14 days
2. Metronidazole therapy for 2 to 4 weeks
3. Isoniazid therapy for 3 to 6 months
4. Isoniazid therapy for 9 to 12 months

24. A client diagnosed with active tuberculosis is started on triple antibiotic therapy. Which findings indicate to the nurse the client's therapy is inadequate?
1. Decreased shortness of breath and absent cough
2. Improved chest x-ray and no reports of chest pain
3. Nonproductive cough and decreased night sweats
4. Acid-fast bacilli in a sputum sample after 2 months of treatment

25. Which instruction is **priority** for the nurse to provide to a client regarding therapy for active tuberculosis (TB)?
1. "It is okay to miss a dose of your medication every day or two."
2. "If adverse effects occur, stop taking the medication."
3. "Only take the medication until you feel better."
4. "You must comply with the medication regimen to treat TB."

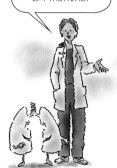

Let's discuss your medication. Treatment for TB lasts for 24 months.

26. The nurse auscultates inspiratory and expiratory wheezes with a decreased forced expiratory volume in a client with asthma. Which class of medication will the nurse administer **first**?
1. Beta-blockers
2. Bronchodilators
3. Inhaled steroids
4. Oral steroids

22. **1.** This client is showing signs and symptoms of active TB and, because of the productive cough, is highly contagious. The client should be placed on airborne precautions immediately, and three sputum cultures should be obtained to confirm the diagnosis. The client would then most likely be given isoniazid and two or three other antitubercular antibiotics until the diagnosis is confirmed, and then isolation and treatment would continue if the cultures were positive for TB. The client does not need a skin test. The nurse should perform a respiratory assessment after placing the client on isolation.
CN: Safe, effective care environment; CNS: Safety and infection control; CL: Analyze

23. **4.** Because of the increasing incidence of resistant strains of TB, the disease must be treated for up to 24 months in some cases, but treatment typically lasts for 9 to 12 months. Isoniazid is the most common medication used for the treatment of TB, but other antibiotics are added to the regimen to obtain the best results. Metronidazole is an antibiotic but is not normally used in the treatment of TB.
CN: Physiological integrity; CNS: Pharmacological and parenteral therapies; CL: Apply

24. **4.** Continuing to have acid-fast bacilli in the sputum after 2 months indicates continued infection. The other choices indicate improvement.
CN: Physiological integrity; CNS: Pharmacological and parenteral therapies; CL: Apply

25. **4.** The treatment regimen for TB may last up to 24 months. It is essential that the client comply with therapy during that time or resistance will develop. At no time should the client stop taking the medications without the primary health care provider's approval.
CN: Safe, effective care environment; CNS: Safety and infection control; CL: Apply

26. **2.** Bronchodilators are the first line of treatment for asthma because bronchoconstriction is the cause of reduced airflow. Inhaled or oral steroids may be given to reduce the inflammation but are not used for emergency relief. Beta-blockers are not used to treat asthma and can cause bronchoconstriction.
CN: Physiological integrity; CNS: Pharmacological and parenteral therapies; CL: Apply

27. A client diagnosed with active tuberculosis (TB) asks the nurse, "Why do I have to be hospitalized?" Which nursing response is **most** appropriate?
1. "To evaluate the severity of your current condition."
2. "To prevent you from spreading of the disease to others."
3. "To determine whether you will be compliant with treatment."
4. "To determine which antibiotic therapy will work best for you."

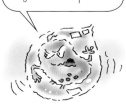

Watch out for those sneezes. TB germs like to travel by water droplets.

28. A client is admitted with chronic obstructive pulmonary disease (COPD). Which action(s) will the nurse perform for this client? Select all that apply.
1. Maintain an adequate airway.
2. Educate on smoking and other triggers.
3. Teach the pursed-lips breathing technique.
4. Decrease the calories in the diet.
5. Assess pulse oximetry.

29. A client is exhibiting signs of asthma. Which finding(s) provides the nurse with confirmation of this diagnosis? Select all that apply.
1. Circumoral cyanosis
2. Increased forced expiratory volume
3. Chest tightness
4. Normal breath sounds
5. Expiratory and inspiratory wheezing

30. A client is experiencing a new-onset asthma attack. Which position will the nurse **immediately** place the client in?
1. High Fowler's
2. Left side-lying
3. Right side-lying
4. Supine

31. A client has symptoms of acute asthma every time the family eats at a Chinese restaurant. Which instruction will the nurse provide for this client?
1. "Only eat Chinese food once per month."
2. "Use your inhalers before eating Chinese food."
3. "Avoid Chinese food because it is a trigger for you."
4. "Next time, order different food to see if that helps."

27. 2. The client with active TB is highly contagious until three consecutive sputum cultures are negative, so the client is put on airborne precautions in the hospital. Assessment of the client's physical condition, need for antibiotic therapy, and likely compliance are not considered primary reasons for hospitalization in this case.
CN: Safe, effective care environment; CNS: Safely and infection control; CL: Apply

28. 1, 2, 3, 5. Typical findings for clients with COPD include dyspnea on exertion, a barrel chest, and clubbed fingers and toes. Clients with COPD are usually tachypneic with a prolonged expiratory phase. It is important for the nurse to maintain an adequate airway and breathing pattern for this client as well as to educate the client on the importance of avoiding any triggers that increase mucus production, such as smoking. The pursed-lips breathing technique helps the client in expelling carbon dioxide; because these clients expend many calories, the calories in their diet should be increased and not decreased. Monitoring pulse oximetry is important to maintain a normal level of oxygen throughout the body.
CN: Physiological integrity; CNS: Physiological adaptation; CL: Apply

29. 3, 5. Inspiratory and expiratory wheezes and chest tightness are typical findings in asthma. Circumoral cyanosis may be present in extreme cases of respiratory distress. The nurse would expect the client to have a decreased forced expiratory volume because asthma is an obstructive pulmonary disease. Breath sounds would be "tight" sounding or markedly decreased; they would not be normal.
CN: Physiological integrity; CNS: Physiological adaptation; CL: Apply

30. 1. The best position is high Fowler's, which helps lower the diaphragm and facilitates passive breathing and thereby improves air exchange. A side-lying position would not facilitate the client's breathing. A supine position increases the breathing difficulty of a client with asthma.
CN: Safe, effective care environment; CNS: Safety and infection control; CL: Apply

31. 3. If the trigger of an acute asthma attack is known, this trigger should always be avoided. Food is typically a trigger for an acute asthma attack, and using an inhaler before eating would not prevent an attack.
CN: Physiological integrity; CNS: Reduction of risk potential; CL: Apply

CN: Client needs category   CNS: Client needs subcategory   CL: Cognitive level

32. An adolescent client comes to the emergency department with acute asthma. The nurse notes a respiratory rate of 44 breaths/minute and severe respiratory distress. What is the **priority** nursing action?
1. Take a full medical history.
2. Give a bronchodilator by nebulizer.
3. Apply an apneic monitor to the client.
4. Provide emotional support to the client.

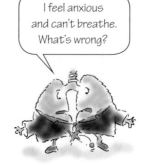

I feel anxious and can't breathe. What's wrong?

32. **2.** The client having an acute asthma attack needs to increase oxygen delivery to the lungs and body. Nebulized bronchodilators open airways and increase the amount of oxygen delivered. The priority at this time is the respiratory status, and the client will be anxious until this is resolved. First, resolve the acute phase of the attack; afterward, obtain a full medical history to determine the cause of the attack and how to prevent attacks in the future. Application of an apneic monitor is not a priority at this point in the treatment plan.
CN: Safe, effective care environment; CNS: Management of care; CL: Analyze

33. Which intervention requires the nurse to frequently monitor a client with chronic obstructive pulmonary disease (COPD)?
1. Administering opioids for pain relief
2. Increasing the client's fluid intake
3. Monitoring the client's cardiac rhythm
4. Assisting the client with coughing and deep breathing

33. **1.** Opioids suppress the respiratory center in the medulla. Both COPD and pneumonia cause alterations in gas exchange; any further problems with oxygenation could result in respiratory failure and cardiac arrest. Increasing the fluid intake would help to thin the client's secretions. Although the nurse would need to monitor the intake and output and watch for signs of heart failure, this is not as critical as administering opioids. The cardiac rhythm provides an indication of the client's myocardial oxygenation; it should be a part of the nurse's regular assessment. Assisting the client in coughing and with deep breathing should be included in the plan of care. The only caution would be to assess for possible rupture of emphysematous alveolar sacs and pneumothorax.
CN: Physiological integrity; CNS: Reduction of risk potential
CL: Apply

34. A client admitted with a diagnosis of pneumonia asks the nurse, "I heard the nurse at the clinic say I was a 'blue bloater.' What does that mean?" Which response from the nurse is **best**?
1. "This means you are exhaling too much oxygen."
2. "This means you are producing a lot of sputum."
3. "This means you are retaining more carbon dioxide."
4. "This means you are coughing more frequently than normal."

34. **3.** Clients with chronic obstructive bronchitis appear bloated; they have large barrel chests and peripheral edema, cyanotic nail beds and, at times, circumoral cyanosis. Retaining more carbon dioxide, not exhaling more oxygen, is the reason for the blue color. Producing more sputum and coughing more frequently do not contribute to the overall color of the client. Clients with emphysema appear pink and cachectic.
CN: Physiological integrity; CNS: Physiological adaptation;
CL: Apply

35. The nurse is caring for a client with emphysema. Which finding(s) will the nurse report to the primary health care provider **immediately**? Select all that apply.
1. Increased residual lung capacity
2. Dyspnea and pink color
3. Prolonged expiratory phase
4. Decreased expiratory flow rate
5. Cyanosis

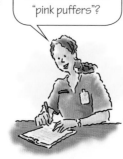

Why are clients with emphysema sometimes called "pink puffers"?

35. **5.** The nurse would report cyanosis. Because of the large amount of energy it takes to breathe, clients with emphysema are usually pink, not cyanotic, and they usually breathe through pursed lips. Clients with emphysema usually have an increased residual lung capacity and volume, as well as decreased elastic recoil. They also have a prolonged expiratory phase and decreased expiratory flow rate. They also suffer from dyspnea.
CN: Safe, effective care environment; CNS: Management of care;
CL: Apply

36. A client has marked dyspnea at rest, is thin, and uses accessory muscles to breathe. The client is tachypneic with a prolonged expiratory phase but has no cough. The nurse observes the client leaning forward with arms braced on the knees to support the chest and shoulders for breathing. Based on these findings, the nurse anticipates which diagnosis?
   1. Acute respiratory distress syndrome (ARDS)
   2. Asthma
   3. Chronic obstructive bronchitis
   4. Emphysema

37. A 72-year-old client who has chronic respiratory disease comes to the clinic for a follow-up appointment. The nurse informs the client it is time for the pneumococcal and flu vaccines. What is the nurse's **best** explanation to the client for these injections?
   1. "All clients are recommended to have these vaccines annually."
   2. "These vaccines produce bronchodilation and improve oxygenation."
   3. "These vaccines help reduce tachypnea in clients with chronic diseases."
   4. "Getting these vaccines may help prevent life-threatening complications."

38. A client with chronic bronchitis asks the nurse, "Why is it important for me to exercise?" Which nursing response is **best**?
   1. "It enhances cardiovascular fitness."
   2. "It improves respiratory muscle strength."
   3. "It reduces the number of acute attacks."
   4. "It worsens respiratory function and is discouraged."

39. A client who has chronic obstructive bronchitis is prescribed furosemide. Which explanation will the nurse give the client regarding the beneficial effects of taking this medication?
   1. Furosemide helps improve clients' mobility
   2. Furosemide helps reduce oxygen demand
   3. Furosemide helps reduce sputum production
   4. Furosemide helps improve respiratory function

40. A client underwent an open cholecystectomy. Which complication will the nurse monitor the client for over the next 24 hours?
   1. Atelectasis
   2. Bronchitis
   3. Pneumonia
   4. Pneumothorax

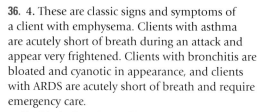

Always model excellent hand hygiene for your clients.

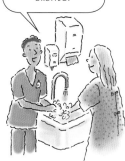

We love exercise. Get out there and get moving!

36. 4. These are classic signs and symptoms of a client with emphysema. Clients with asthma are acutely short of breath during an attack and appear very frightened. Clients with bronchitis are bloated and cyanotic in appearance, and clients with ARDS are acutely short of breath and require emergency care.
CN: Physiological integrity; CNS: Physiological adaptation;
CL: Apply

37. 4. It is highly recommended that clients with respiratory disorders be given vaccines to protect against respiratory infection. Infections can cause respiratory failure, and these clients may need to be intubated and mechanically ventilated. The vaccines have no effect on respiratory rate or bronchodilation. The influenza vaccine is recommended for all clients older than 6 months of age annually. The pneumococcal vaccine is recommended for clients older than 65 years of age.
CN: Health promotion and maintenance; CNS: None; CL: Apply

38. 1. Exercise can improve cardiovascular fitness, which helps the client to better tolerate periods of hypoxia, perhaps reducing the risk of heart attack. Most exercise has little effect on respiratory muscle strength, and these clients cannot tolerate the type of exercise necessary to do this. Exercise will not reduce the number of acute attacks. In some instances, exercise may be contraindicated. The client should check with the health care provider before starting any exercise program.
CN: Health promotion and maintenance; CNS: None; CL: Apply

39. 2. Reducing fluid volume reduces the workload of the heart, which reduces oxygen demand and, in turn, reduces the respiratory rate. Sputum may get thicker and make it harder to clear airways. Reducing fluid volume will not improve respiratory function but may improve oxygenation. Reducing fluid volume may reduce edema and improve mobility slightly, but exercise tolerance would still be poor.
CN: Physiological integrity; CNS: Physiological adaptation;
CL: Apply

40. 1. Atelectasis develops when there is interference with the normal negative pressure that promotes lung expansion. Clients in the postoperative phase typically guard their breathing because of pain and positioning, which causes hypoxia. It is uncommon for any of the other respiratory disorders to develop after surgery.
CN: Physiological integrity; CNS: Physiological adaptation;
CL: Apply

CN: Client needs category   CNS: Client needs subcategory   CL: Cognitive level

41. A client diagnosed with pleural effusion has been on supplemental oxygen for 24 hours and is still having dyspnea with decreased breath sounds on the left side of the chest. The nurse will anticipate preparing the client for which procedure?
1. Thoracotomy
2. Thoracentesis
3. CT scan
4. Bronchoscopy

42. When explaining the hypoxic drive to a client with emphysema, which statement by the nurse is **best**?
1. "This is when your body does not notice you need to breathe."
2. "This is when you only breathe when your oxygen levels climb above a certain point."
3. "This is when you only breathe when your oxygen levels dip below a certain point."
4. "This is when you only breathe when your carbon dioxide level dips below a certain point."

43. A client is diagnosed with chronic obstructive pulmonary disease (COPD). Which statement will the nurse include when discharging this client?
1. "Check your oxygen saturation levels daily."
2. "You need to decrease your oral fluid intake."
3. "You can use home remedies to treat respiratory infections."
4. "Let's review how to recognize signs of a respiratory infection."

44. A client returns to the acute care unit after abdominal surgery. Which intervention will the nurse perform for the client?
1. Chest physiotherapy
2. Mechanical ventilation
3. Reduce oxygen requirements
4. Use of an incentive spirometer

45. The nurse knows which client is at the **highest** risk for respiratory failure?
1. A client with breast cancer
2. A client with a cervical sprain
3. A client with a fractured hip
4. A client with Guillain-Barré syndrome

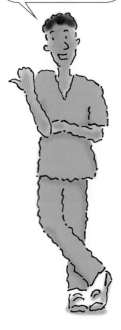
Hypoxic drive? This question sounds like it should be on a mechanic's exam.

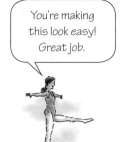
You're making this look easy! Great job.

41. 2. Pleural fluid normally seeps continually into the pleural space from the capillaries, lining the parietal pleura; the fluid is reabsorbed by the visceral pleural capillaries and lymphatics. Any condition that interferes with either the secretion or drainage of this fluid leads to a pleural effusion. Key treatments include supplemental oxygen and a thoracentesis to remove the fluid. If this is not successful, then a thoracotomy is performed. The client is also placed on antibiotics to treat the organism that causes empyema. A CT scan and bronchoscopy are not indicated for this client and would not address the client's dyspnea.
CN: Physiological integrity; CNS: Physiological adaptation; CL: Apply

42. 3. Clients with emphysema breathe when their oxygen levels drop to a certain level; this is known as the hypoxic drive. Clients with emphysema and chronic obstructive pulmonary disease take a breath when they have reached this low oxygen level. They do not take a breath when their levels of carbon dioxide are higher than normal, as do those with healthy respiratory physiology. If too much oxygen is given, the client has little stimulus to take another breath. The client's carbon dioxide levels climb, the client loses consciousness, and respiratory arrest occurs.
CN: Physiological integrity; CNS: Physiological adaptation; CL: Understand

43. 4. Respiratory infection in clients with a respiratory disorder can be fatal. It is important for the client to understand how to recognize an impending respiratory infection. Oxygen saturation assessment would not prevent complications. The client should be taught to increase fluid intake to help thin secretions. If the client has signs and symptoms of an infection, the client should contact the health care provider at once to obtain prompt treatment, not rely on home remedies.
CN: Physiological integrity; CNS: Reduction of risk potential; CL: Apply

44. 4. Using an incentive spirometer requires the client to take deep breaths and promotes lung expansion. Chest physiotherapy helps mobilize secretions but will not prevent atelectasis. Reducing oxygen requirements or placing someone on mechanical ventilation does not affect the development of atelectasis.
CN: Physiological integrity; CNS: Basic care and comfort; CL: Apply

45. 4. Guillain-Barré syndrome is a progressive neuromuscular disorder that can affect the respiratory muscles and cause ascending paralysis and potential for respiratory failure. The other conditions typically do not affect the respiratory system.
CN: Physiological integrity; CNS: Physiological adaptation; CL: Analyze

CN: Client needs category   CNS: Client needs subcategory   CL: Cognitive level

46. The nurse is caring for a client who begins experiencing status asthmaticus. Which medication does the nurse prepare to administer this client?
  1. Inhaled levalbuterol
  2. Inhaled fluticasone
  3. Intravenous albuterol
  4. Oral prednisone

46. 1. Inhaled beta-adrenergic agents, such as levalbuterol, help promote bronchodilation, which improves oxygenation. IV beta-adrenergic agents, such as albuterol, can be used but have to be monitored because of their greater systemic effects. They are typically used when the inhaled beta-adrenergic agents do not work. Corticosteroids, such as fluticasone and prednisone, are slow-acting, so their use will not reduce hypoxia in the acute phase.
CN: Physiological integrity; CNS: Pharmacological and parenteral therapies; CL: Apply

47. An adult client who is being treated in the emergency department with a diagnosis of status asthmaticus is prescribed albuterol and intravenous (IV) prednisone. Which finding indicates to the nurse the client's treatment was not effective?
  1. The client's lips have a bluish tint.
  2. The client's legs are shaking.
  3. The client's heart rate is 120 beats/minute.
  4. The client reports flushing of the face.

47. 1. Lips with a bluish tint are a sign of respiratory distress indicating ineffective treatment. Shaking of the extremities is a common side effect of albuterol. A rapid heart rate is a common side effect of both albuterol and IV prednisone. Flushing is a common side effect of IV prednisone. These side effects do not indicate treatment was not effective.
CN: Physiological integrity; CNS: Pharmacological and parenteral therapies; CL: Apply

48. A client was given intravenous morphine sulfate for pain as prescribed. The client is sleeping and has a respiratory rate of 6 breaths/minute. What will the nurse do **next**?
  1. Notify the health care provider.
  2. Begin cardiopulmonary resuscitation (CPR).
  3. Attempt to arouse the client.
  4. Administer naloxone.

48. 3. The nurse would first attempt to arouse the client. Opioids suppress the respiratory center in the medulla and can cause respiratory arrest. The nurse will notify the health care provider after arousing and assessing the client. CPR is needed if the client is not breathing and does not have a heart rate. Naloxone would be needed if the client cannot be aroused or continues to decline.
CN: Physiological integrity; CNS: Pharmacological and parenteral therapies; CL: Apply

49. Which data will the nurse gather **immediately** to determine the status of a client with a respiratory rate of 4 breaths/minute?
  1. Arterial blood gas (ABG) levels and breath sounds
  2. Level of consciousness (LOC) and a pulse oximetry value
  3. Breath sounds and reflexes
  4. Pulse oximetry value and heart sounds

49. 2. First, the nurse should attempt to rouse the client because this should increase the client's respiratory rate. Then a spot pulse oximetry check should be done and breath sounds should be checked. The health care provider should be notified immediately of the findings and is likely to prescribe an ABG to determine specific carbon dioxide and oxygen levels. Heart sounds and reflexes should be checked after these initial actions are completed.
CN: Safe, effective care environment; CNS: Management of care; CL: Apply

50. A client, following the administration of meperidine, has a $PaCO_2$ value of 80 mm Hg. How will the nurse interpret this finding?
  1. A mild case of hyperventilation
  2. Perfectly normal
  3. At risk for developing mild pneumonia
  4. At risk for respiratory arrest

50. 4. A client about to go into respiratory arrest would have inefficient ventilation and would be retaining carbon dioxide. The $PaCO_2$ value expected would be around 80 mm Hg. It is not indicative of hyperventilation, as the CO_2 is high, or pneumonia, as this value does not rise in pneumonia.
CN: Physiological integrity; CNS: Physiological adaptation; CL: Apply

51. A client requires a chest tube to be inserted in the right upper chest. Which action will the nurse perform during the procedure?
1. Injecting local anesthetic to prevent pain
2. Preparing the chest tube drainage system
3. Bringing the chest x-ray to the client's room
4. Inserting the chest tube

52. A client has been prescribed a new drug for hypertension. Thirty minutes after taking the drug, the client develops chest tightness, becomes short of breath and tachypneic, and exhibits an altered level of consciousness. Which complication does the nurse expect?
1. The client is having an asthma attack
2. The client is having a pulmonary embolism
3. The client is experiencing medication hypersensitivity
4. The client is suffering from rheumatoid arthritis

53. A client is suspected of impending anaphylaxis secondary to a hypersensitivity to a medication. Which nursing action is **priority**?
1. Administer oxygen.
2. Insert an IV catheter.
3. Obtain a complete blood count (CBC).
4. Take vital signs.

54. The nurse is caring for a client exhibiting signs of impending anaphylaxis from a medication hypersensitivity. The client has a history of asthma. Which action by the nurse is **priority**?
1. Give a beta-blocker.
2. Administer albuterol.
3. Obtain serum electrolyte levels.
4. Lay the client flat in the bed.

55. A critically ill client's chest x-ray shows fluid in the alveolar spaces. The nurse notes the client is severely short of breath. Which prescription will the nurse anticipate?
1. Give albuterol.
2. Administer ibuprofen.
3. Prepare client for intubation.
4. Initiate airborne precautions.

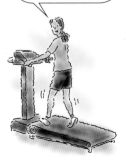

Hey! You've made it through 51 questions. Way to go.

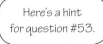

Here's a hint for question #53.

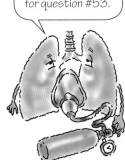

51. 2. The nurse must anticipate a drainage system is required and assemble it before the insertion, so the tube can be directly connected to the drainage system. The chest x-ray does not need to be brought to the client's room. The health care provider should administer the local anesthetic and insert the chest tube.
CN: Physiological integrity; CNS: Physiological adaptation; CL: Apply

52. 3. These signs indicate a hypersensitivity to the new medication, leading to anaphylaxis and respiratory failure. An asthma attack is characterized by wheezing. A client with pulmonary embolism typically has chest pain with inspiration and hypoxemia. Rheumatoid arthritis does not cause respiratory symptoms.
CN: Physiological integrity; CNS: Pharmacological and parenteral therapies; CL: Analyze

53. 1. Giving oxygen would be the best first action in this case. Vital signs then should be checked and the health care provider immediately notified. If the client does not already have an IV catheter, one may be inserted now if anaphylactic shock is developing. Obtaining a CBC would not help the emergency situation.
CN: Physiological integrity; CNS: Pharmacological and parenteral therapies; CL: Apply

54. 2. A bronchodilator, such as albuterol, would help open the client's airway and improve oxygenation status. Beta-blockers are not indicated in the management of asthma because they may cause bronchospasm. Obtaining laboratory values would not be done on an emergency basis, and having the client lie flat in bed could worsen the client's ability to breathe.
CN: Safe, effective care environment; CNS: Management of care; CL: Apply

55. 3. The nurse would suspect the client has acute respiratory distress syndrome (ARDS), where the alveolar membranes are more permeable and the alveolar spaces are filled with fluid. The fluid interferes with gas exchange and reduces perfusion. Treatment for ARDS includes intubation, mechanical ventilation, vasoconstrictors, norepinephrine, and an induced coma. Albuterol is a bronchodilator given to asthma clients. Ibuprofen, a nonsteroidal anti-inflammatory drug (NSAID), is given to relieve pain, decrease inflammation, and reduce fever. Standard precautions are needed for clients with ARDS.
CN: Physiological integrity; CNS: Physiological adaptation; CL: Analyze

56. An unconscious client is brought to the emergency department. The client's friend states, "We went to a party, took some pills, and drank beer." Which finding will the nurse expect when assessing the client?
1. Hyper-reflexive reflexes
2. Muscle spasms
3. Shallow respirations
4. Tachypnea

57. An unconscious client has been diagnosed with a probable drug overdose complicated by alcohol ingestion. What is the **priority** nursing intervention?
1. Administer IV fluids.
2. Give IV naloxone.
3. Monitor vital signs.
4. Draw blood for a drug screen.

> Question #58 sounds like an opportunity for some teaching.

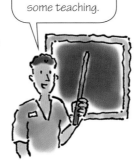

58. An unconscious client who overdosed on an opioid receives naloxone. After the client awakens, what is the **priority** action by the nurse?
1. Feed the client a well-balanced meal.
2. Educate on the effects of mixing opioids with alcohol.
3. Discharge the client from the hospital.
4. Admit the client to an inpatient psychiatric facility.

59. A client arrives in the emergency department with smoke inhalation due to a house fire. What is the **priority** nursing action for this client?
1. Checking the oral mucous membranes
2. Checking for any burned areas
3. Obtaining a medical history
4. Ensuring a patent airway

60. After a motor vehicle crash, a client has a chest tube inserted that begins to drain a large amount of dark red fluid. Which response by the nursing is **best**?
1. "The chest tube was inserted improperly."
2. "It is normal for the drainage to be dark red."
3. "An artery was nicked during insertion."
4. "We are going to treat you for a hemothorax."

56. 3. The client has taken a combination of pills and alcohol and cannot be roused. This has probably caused the client to breathe shallowly, which, if action is not taken immediately, could lead to respiratory arrest. The nurse would not expect to find tachypnea and does not have enough information about which drugs the client took to expect muscle spasms or hyperreflexia.
CN: Physiological integrity; CNS: Physiological adaptation; CL: Apply

57. 2. If the client took opioids, giving naloxone could reverse the effects and awaken the client. IV fluids would then most likely be administered, and the nurse would closely monitor the client over a period of several hours to several days. A drug screen should be drawn in the emergency department, but results may not come back for several hours, making it of lower priority than administering the naloxone.
CN: Safe, effective care environment; CNS: Management of care; CL: Analyze

58. 2. This client needs information about the dangers of combining opioids and alcohol. Discharge at this point is inappropriate. Unless the client was trying to commit suicide, admission to a psychiatric facility is not necessary. It may not be advisable to feed the client at first; the level of consciousness could drop again, increasing the possibility of aspiration.
CN: Safe, effective care environment; CNS: Management of care; CL: Apply

59. 4. The nurse's priority is to make sure the airway is open and the client is breathing. Checking the mucous membranes and burned areas is important, but not as vital as maintaining a patent airway. Obtaining a medical history can be pursued after ensuring a patent airway.
CN: Safe, effective care environment; CNS: Management of care; CL: Apply

60. 4. Because of the traumatic cause of injury, the client most likely has a hemothorax, in which blood collection causes the collapse of the lung. The placement of the chest tube would drain the blood from the space and re-expand the lung. There is a slight chance of nicking an intercostal artery during insertion, but it is fairly unlikely if the person placing the chest tube has been trained. The initial chest x-ray would help confirm whether there was blood in the pleural space or just air. It is not normal for chest tube drainage to be dark red, and it is not likely that the chest tube was inserted improperly.
CN: Safe, effective care environment; CNS: Management of care; CL: Analyze

CN: Client needs category   CNS: Client needs subcategory   CL: Cognitive level

61. The nurse is assessing a client with smoke inhalation. When auscultating the lungs, which breath sound(s) will the nurse expect to hear? Select all that apply.
1. Crackles
2. Diminished breath sounds
3. Inspiratory and expiratory wheezing
4. Upper airway rhonchi
5. Stridor

62. The nurse is caring for a client receiving oxygen via a nasal cannula at a rate of 2 L/minute. How will the nurse facilitate breathing in this client? Select all that apply.
1. Position client in Fowler's position.
2. Decrease anxiety in the client.
3. Set the line marked "2" so it cuts the ball in half.
4. Set any part of the ball so it touches the line marked "2."
5. Give the client an extra dose of a narcotic to allow for rest.

63. An older adult client who recently had surgery for a fractured right femur develops acute shortness of breath and progressive hypoxia requiring mechanical ventilation. The nurse knows that what is the **most** likely cause of this client's hypoxia?
1. Asthma attack
2. Atelectasis
3. Bronchitis
4. Fat embolism

64. The nurse is caring for a client with a fracture of the right femur caused by a skiing accident. Which clinical manifestation will the nurse suspect is a complication of the fracture?
1. Abdominal cramping
2. Fatty stools
3. Confusion
4. Numbness in the right foot

65. The nurse is caring for a client with a fat embolism after a fractured femur. Following respiratory therapy, the client continues to be hypoxic. What is the **best** intervention by the nurse?
1. Administer furosemide.
2. Give neuromuscular blockers.
3. Place the head of the bed flat.
4. Provide albuterol.

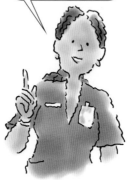

Snap, crackle, pop. Listening to breath sounds can tell you a lot about a client's respiratory function.

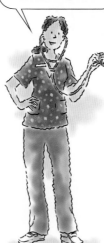

Don't be confused by question #64. I'm sure the answer will come to you.

61. 1. When treating smoke inhalation, the most frequently heard sounds are crackles throughout the lung fields. Decreased breath sounds or inspiratory and expiratory wheezing are associated with asthma, and rhonchi are heard when there is sputum in the airways. Stridor indicates upper airway obstruction.
CN: Physiological integrity; CNS: Physiological adaptation; CL: Apply

62. 1, 2, 3. Positioning client in Fowler's position would allow for maximum chest expansion, which eases respirations. Decreasing anxiety in the client would also ease the respiratory effort. The oxygen flow rate is set by centering the indicator on the line marked "2." Having any part of the ball touching the line marked "2" is not the correct dose; giving a client an extra dose of narcotic is not safe and is considered to be a medication error.
CN: Safe, effective care environment; CNS: Safety and infection control; CL: Apply

63. 4. Long bone fractures are correlated with fat emboli, which cause shortness of breath and hypoxia. It is unlikely the client has developed asthma or bronchitis without a previous history. The client could have atelectasis, but it typically does not produce progressive hypoxia.
CN: Physiological integrity; CNS: Physiological adaptation; CL: Apply

64. 3. Confusion and irritability are signs of hypoxia, which is caused by the fat emboli traveling to the lungs and producing an inflammatory response in the lung tissue. Abdominal cramping may be a sign of abdominal distention and constipation caused by immobility, not by the fracture itself. Fatty stools occur with pancreatitis, not secondary to fracture of the femur. Numbness may be secondary to neurovascular impairment.
CN: Physiological integrity; CNS: Physiological adaptation; CL: Apply

65. 2. Neuromuscular blockers cause skeletal muscle paralysis, reducing the amount of oxygen used by the restless skeletal muscles. This should improve oxygenation. Bronchodilators may be used, but they typically do not have enough of an effect to reduce the amount of hypoxia present. The head of the bed should be partially elevated to facilitate diaphragm movement, and diuretics can be administered to reduce pulmonary congestion. However, bronchodilators, diuretics, and head elevation would improve oxygen delivery, not reduce oxygen demand.
CN: Safe, effective care environment; CNS: Management of care; CL: Apply

66. A client arrives in the emergency department displaying apnea, altered mental status, dyspnea, and central cyanosis. The client was found inside a car in the garage by neighbors while the motor was still running. Which findings will the nurse expect to observe while assessing this client?
1. Dilated pupils
2. Chest pains
3. Increased breath sounds
4. Cherry-red mucous membranes

66. **4.** In a client with late-stage carbon monoxide poisoning, the nurse would see cherry-red mucous membranes. Key signs of asphyxia are agitation, altered respiratory rate, anxiety, altered mental status, decreased breath sounds, dyspnea, and central and peripheral cyanosis. The client would not experience chest pains or dilated pupils as a result of carbon monoxide poisoning.
CN: Physiological integrity; CNS: Physiological adaptation; CL: Apply

67. A client experiencing acute respiratory distress is lying flat in bed. When entering the room, the nurse suggests to the client a change in position would be beneficial. Which position will the nurse recommend?
1. Lying prone
2. Side-lying on the left side
3. Alternating prone and supine
4. Lying supine

67. **3.** Alternating supine and prone positioning (if possible) is recommended for clients with acute respiratory distress. Turning the client to the prone position may recruit new alveoli in the posterior region of the lung and improve oxygenation status.
CN: Physiological integrity; CNS: Physiological adaptation; CL: Apply

68. The emergency room nurse will assess which client **first**?
1. A 20-year-old client in moderate pain due to probable appendicitis
2. A 32-year-old client thrown from the car during a motor vehicle accident
3. A 40-year-old client reporting nasal congestion for 2 weeks
4. A 55-year-old client who has pneumonia and an unproductive cough

68. **2.** In a client with massive trauma, the tissues lining the alveoli and pulmonary capillaries are injured directly or indirectly, increasing the permeability of protein and fluid and leading to the development of hypoxemia and ARDS, making this client the most emergent and in need of assessment. A client with appendicitis, unless it causes overwhelming sepsis, is not as emergent as one with massive trauma and impending ARDS. Pneumonia and nasal congestion are not emergent in this situation.
CN: Safe, effective care environment; CNS: Management of care; CL: Analyze

69. The nurse is monitoring the progress of a client with acute respiratory distress syndrome (ARDS). Which finding **best** indicates to the nurse the client's condition is improving?
1. Arterial blood gas (ABG) values are normal
2. The bronchoscopy results are negative
3. The client's blood pressure has stabilized
4. The sputum and sensitivity culture shows no growth in bacteria

69. **1.** Normal ABG values would indicate that the client's oxygenation has improved. ARDS is characterized by hypoxia, so the bronchoscopy and sputum culture results have no bearing on the improvement of ARDS. Increased blood pressure is not relative to the client's respiratory condition.
CN: Physiological integrity; CNS: Physiological adaptation; CL: Apply

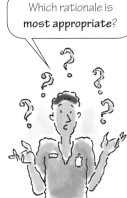

Which rationale is **most appropriate?**

70. The nurse has advised a client's family not to increase the client's oxygen flow rate. Which rationale is **most** appropriate for to nurse to provide the family?
1. Extra oxygen may cause the client to breathe too rapidly
2. Oxygen toxicity may reduce the amount of functional alveolar surface area
3. Increased oxygen may decrease carbon dioxide levels and cause apnea
4. Increasing the oxygen level may cause pulmonary barotrauma

70. **2.** Oxygen toxicity causes direct pulmonary trauma, reducing the amount of alveolar surface area available for gaseous exchange, which results in increased carbon dioxide levels and decreased oxygen uptake. Excessive oxygen therapy may eliminate hypoxic respiratory drive, causing the client to breathe too slowly or even to stop breathing. Pulmonary barotrauma is caused by high lung pressures, not excessive oxygenation.
CN: Safe, effective care environment; CNS: Management of care; CL: Apply

71. Which client will the nurse monitor **most closely** for the development of a complication with lung function?
1. A client scheduled for an appendectomy
2. A client with a meniscus tear
3. A client with sleep apnea
4. A client with thoracic kyphoscoliosis

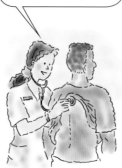

Let's take a listen to your breathing.

72. A client arrives in the clinic reporting right-sided chest pain and shortness of breath that started suddenly. Which intervention will the nurse complete **first**?
1. Auscultation of breath sounds
2. A chest x-ray
3. An echocardiogram
4. An electrocardiogram

73. A client is treated in the emergency department with reports of dyspnea, cough, and sharp pain that increases with exertion. The nurse auscultates diminished breath sounds, and the health care provider prescribes a chest x-ray. What does the nurse suspect this will indicate?
1. Asthma
2. Pulmonary embolism
3. Spontaneous pneumothorax
4. Tuberculosis

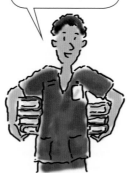

All your studying is paying off. This test is a breeze for you.

74. A client is receiving emergency care following a motor vehicle accident. The nurse notes absent breath sounds over the left lung field, shortness of breath, and tachypnea. Which primary health care provider prescription will the nurse question?
1. Prepare client for intubation.
2. Gather chest tube insertion equipment.
3. Administer oxygen.
4. Apply a continuous oxygen saturation monitor.

75. The nurse is reviewing data on a client suspected of having a pneumothorax. Which intervention will the nurse use to confirm the diagnosis?
1. Auscultation of breath sounds
2. Review of chest x-ray results
3. Incentive spirometer use
4. Assessment of the client for signs of dyspnea

71. 4. Thoracic kyphoscoliosis causes lung compression, restricts lung expansion, and results in more rapid and shallow respiration. An otherwise healthy client who is scheduled for an appendectomy or has a meniscus tear would not experience any problems with lung function due to either of these illnesses. Clients with sleep apnea also would not normally have problems with lung function.
CN: Physiological integrity; CNS: Physiological adaptation; CL: Apply

72. 1. Auscultation of the lungs would indicate whether the breath sounds are normal or abnormal and thus help determine the cause of the shortness of breath. Depending on the results of auscultation and on the cause of the shortness of breath, the client may need a chest x-ray and an electrocardiogram. An echocardiogram may be necessary if a pulmonary embolus is suspected.
CN: Safe, effective care environment; CNS: Management of care; CL: Apply

73. 3. Spontaneous pneumothorax is characterized by diminished or absent breath sounds with dyspnea, a cough, and tachypnea. Sharp chest pain that increases with exertion is a key sign of this condition. Asthma is usually accompanied by wheezes and produces no symptoms between attacks. Pulmonary embolism would have sudden onset of dyspnea and crackles in the lungs. TB is demonstrated by fever, night sweats, and, at times, a cough.
CN: Physiological integrity; CNS: Physiological adaptation; CL: Apply

74. 1. The nurse would suspect the client has a left pneumothorax. A pneumothorax can occur as a result of trauma in which the pleurae separating the lung from the chest wall are damaged, allowing air to enter the pleural space. This air causes the lung to collapse, resulting in absent breath sounds. Treatment includes a chest tube, oxygen, and continuous monitoring. The client does not require intubation at this time.
CN: Safe, effective care environment; CNS: Management of care; CL: Apply

75. 2. A chest x-ray would show the area of collapsed lung if pneumothorax is present, as well as the volume of air in the pleural space. Listening to breath sounds would not confirm a diagnosis. The client would not do well with an incentive spirometer at this time. A client may experience dyspnea for many reasons besides a pneumothorax.
CN: Physiological integrity; CNS: Physiological adaptation; CL: Apply

76. A client presents with shortness of breath and absent breath sounds on the right side, from the apex to the base. The nurse prepares to provide the client care for which condition?
1. Acute asthma
2. Chronic bronchitis
3. Pneumonia
4. Spontaneous pneumothorax

76. **4.** Spontaneous pneumothorax occurs when the client's lung collapses, causing an acute decrease in the amount of functional lung used in oxygenation; this results in shortness of breath with absent breath sounds. A client with an asthma attack would present with wheezing breath sounds, and bronchitis would be indicated by auscultating rhonchi. Bronchial breath sounds over the area of consolidation would indicate pneumonia.
CN: Physiological integrity; CNS: Physiological adaptation; CL: Apply

77. A hospitalized client needs a central venous access device inserted. The health care provider places the device in the subclavian vein. Shortly afterward, the client develops shortness of breath and appears restless. Which action will the nurse take **first**?
1. Administer a sedative.
2. Advise the client to calm down.
3. Auscultate breath sounds.
4. Start an intravenous line.

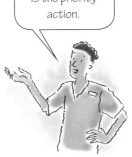

Remember, the first action is the priority action.

77. **3.** Because this is an acute episode, the nurse should listen to the client's lungs to see whether anything has changed. The nurse should not give this client medication, especially sedatives, because the client is having trouble breathing; the medication may further decrease respirations. The nurse should give the client emotional support and contact the health care provider who placed the central venous access after auscultation, but should not advise the client to calm down as this is not therapeutic. Starting an intravenous line is not indicated at this time.
CN: Safe, effective care environment; CNS: Management of care; CL: Analyze

78. Which prescription will the nurse expect for a client who recently had a central venous access device inserted and is now short of breath and anxious?
1. Chest x-ray
2. Electrocardiogram
3. Laboratory tests
4. Sedation

78. **1.** Inserting an IV catheter in the subclavian vein can result in a pneumothorax, so a chest x-ray should be done. If it is negative, then other tests should be done, but they are not appropriate as the first intervention.
CN: Physiological integrity; CNS: Reduction of risk potential; CL: Apply

79. A client with acute respiratory failure has just been admitted to the acute care unit. The nurse will prepare to administer which treatment(s) to the client? Select all that apply.
1. Supplemental oxygen
2. An analgesic
3. A bronchodilator
4. An antibiotic
5. A steroid

79. **1, 2, 3, 5.** Key treatments for a client with acute respiratory failure include supplemental oxygen, an analgesic such as morphine, an antianxiety agent, a bronchodilator such as albuterol, and a steroid such as hydrocortisone. Antibiotics are not necessarily needed for this client.
CN: Physiological integrity; CNS: Physiological adaptation; CL: Apply

80. When monitoring the closed-chest drainage system of a client who has just returned from a lobectomy, what will the nurse be sure is occurring?
1. The fluid in the water seal chamber rises from inspiration and falls with expiration
2. The tubing remains looped below the level of the bed
3. The drainage chamber does not drain more than 100 mL in 8 hours
4. The suction-control chamber bubbles vigorously when connected to suction

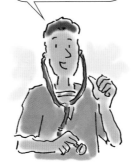

Congrats! You've finished 80 questions. You're over halfway done.

80. **1.** Rise and fall of the water seal chamber immediately after surgery indicates patency of the chest tube drainage system. The tubing should be coiled on the bed, without dependent loops, to promote drainage. Up to 500 mL of drainage can occur in the first 24 hours after surgery. Gentle, not vigorous, bubbling is indicated after surgery to prevent excessive evaporation.
CN: Physiological integrity; CNS: Physiological adaptation; CL: Understand

CN: Client needs category   CNS: Client needs subcategory   CL: Cognitive level

81. When a chest tube is inadvertently dislodged from a client, what will be the nurse's **first** action?
1. Notify the health care provider.
2. Wipe the chest tube with alcohol and reinsert.
3. Apply a petroleum gauze over the site.
4. Auscultate the lung fields for breath sounds.

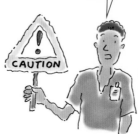

A dislodged chest tube is a serious concern. What is the **priority** nursing response?

81. **3.** If a chest tube is unintentionally dislodged, the nurse would immediately cover the insertion site opening with petroleum gauze and apply pressure to prevent air from entering the chest and causing a tension pneumothorax. Next, notify the health care provider. It is not appropriate to attempt to reinsert the chest tube. Auscultation of the lungs may be important but is not the priority.
CN: Safe, effective care environment; CNS: Management of care; CL: Apply

82. Which intervention will the nurse complete before a client's chest tube is removed?
1. Provide the results of the most recent chest x-ray for the health care provider.
2. Ensure the health care provider prescribes arterial blood gas analysis before removal.
3. Disconnect the drainage system from the chest tube before removal.
4. Sedate the client to limit the amount of discomfort the client will experience.

82. **1.** A chest x-ray should be done before chest tube removal to ensure the client's lung has remained expanded after suction was discontinued. Pulse oximetry would be sufficient and is more commonly used than arterial blood gas analysis to track oxygenation. Disconnecting the drainage system before the chest tube is removed could cause a tension pneumothorax. Client cooperation during chest tube removal is desirable; if the client can hold his or her breath while the chest tube is removed, there is less chance that air will be drawn back into the pleural space during removal. Therefore, the client should not be sedated.
CN: Physiological integrity; CNS: Reduction of risk potential; CL: Apply

83. A client is placed on oxygen therapy via a nasal cannula. Which action will the nurse complete **first**?
1. Make sure all electronic monitoring devices in use are properly grounded.
2. Know the location of the O₂ turn-off valve on the nursing unit.
3. Instruct the client and family, as well as visitors, not to smoke.
4. Confirm the health care provider's prescription for oxygen.

83. **4.** The priority when administering oxygen is to check the health care provider's prescription because this is considered a medication. The nurse also should make sure all electronic monitoring devices are grounded, instruct everyone not to smoke, and know the location of the turn-off valve for the O₂, but these actions should be taken after confirming the health care provider's prescription for oxygen.
CN: Safe, effective care environment: CNS: Safety and infection control; CL: Apply

84. The nurse is preparing to educate a client who has recently been diagnosed with squamous cell carcinoma of the left lung. Which statement by the nurse is **best**?
1. "You have a slow-growing cancer that rarely spreads."
2. "In terms of prognosis, you may have only a few months to live."
3. "Squamous cell cancer is a very rapid-growing cancer."
4. "The cancer has generally metastasized by the time the diagnosis is made."

84. **1.** Squamous cell carcinoma of the lung is a slow-growing, rarely metastasizing type of cancer. It has the best prognosis of all lung cancer types.
CN: Physiological integrity; CNS: Physiological adaptation; CL: Understand

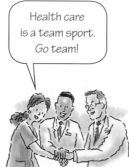

Health care is a team sport. Go team!

85. A client has been admitted with an exacerbation of emphysema. Which classification of medication(s) will the nurse expect to administer? Select all that apply.
1. Antibiotics
2. Bronchodilators
3. Steroids
4. Diuretics
5. Calcium channel blockers

85. **1, 2, 3.** Key treatments for the client with emphysema in regard to medications include antibiotics to treat the causative agent, bronchodilators to assist in ventilation, and steroids to decrease inflammation. Diuretics and calcium channel blockers are not prescribed unless there is an underlying problem.
CN: Physiological integrity; CNS: Pharmacological and parenteral therapies; CL: Apply

CN: Client needs category   CNS: Client needs subcategory   CL: Cognitive level

86. A client is admitted to the acute care unit due to a chronic cough with copious, foul-smelling secretions. The nurse identifies dyspnea, hemoptysis, and recent weight loss. What is the **priority** action(s) by the nurse for this client? Select all that apply.
1. Monitor respiratory status.
2. Check oxygen saturation levels.
3. Provide supportive care.
4. Give intravenous penicillin.
5. Administer albuterol.

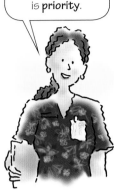

The key word in question #86 is **priority**.

87. A client who is a longtime smoker receives lab results that indicate an elevated carcinoembryonic antigen level. Which action will the nurse take in response to these results?
1. Inform the client it means lung cancer is definitely present.
2. No action is needed; this level is usually elevated in a smoker.
3. Inform the client cancer is present and has now spread to other organs.
4. Inform the client death is imminent due to some cancer in the body.

88. A client arrives in the local clinic and reports a chronic cough and fatigue. The client admits to smoking two packs of cigarettes daily for 10 years and also informs the nurse of a 19.8 lb (9 kg) weight loss over the last 2 months. The health care provider suspects cancer. The nurse will anticipate preparing the client for which test?
1. Bronchoscopy
2. Chest x-ray
3. Chest computed tomography
4. Surgical biopsy

89. The nurse is caring for a client newly diagnosed with lung cancer. The primary health care provider is now determining the stage of the client's cancer. Which prescription(s) will the nurse question? Select all that apply.
1. Magnetic resonance imaging (MRI)
2. Computerized tomography (CT) scan
3. Obtain sputum specimen
4. Position emission tomography (PET) scan
5. Bone scans

90. A client with a long history of smoking is suspected of having lung cancer. The nurse knows which intervention is **most** important at this point to increase the client's chances of survival, should the client prove to have lung cancer?
1. Bronchoscopy, with hopes of early detection
2. Chest x-ray, with hopes of early detection
3. High-dose chemotherapy, should the client be shown to have cancer
4. Smoking cessation, should the client be shown to have cancer

CN: Client needs category   CNS: Client needs subcategory   CL: Cognitive level

86. 1, 2. The client most likely has bronchiectasis. The priority intervention would be to monitor respiratory status and pulse oximetry. Providing supportive care is also important, but not as important as monitoring values to ensure adequate oxygenation. Antibiotics and bronchodilators are part of the overall treatment but are not priority.
CN: Safe, effective care environment; CNS: Management of care; CL: Analyze

87. 2. Because the level of carcinoembryonic antigen is elevated in clients who smoke, it cannot be used as a general indicator of cancer. This test by itself cannot confirm cancer of any kind in a smoker. However, the carcinoembryonic antigen level is helpful in monitoring cancer treatment because it usually falls to normal within 1 month if treatment is successful.
CN: Physiological integrity; CNS: Physiological adaptation; CL: Apply

88. 4. Only surgical biopsy with cytologic examination of the cells can give a definitive diagnosis of the type of cancer. Bronchoscopy gives positive results in only 30% of the cases. Chest x-ray and computed tomography can identify the location of cancer but not diagnose the type.
CN: Physiological integrity; CNS: Physiological adaptation; CL: Apply

89. 3. Staging describes the extent and severity of the cancer and helps the health care provider determine the most appropriate therapy. Staging systems continue to evolve as cancer is better understood. Multiple data collection methods, including laboratory testing, physical examinations, and imaging, are used to determine the stage of a cancer. A sputum specimen would be needed to diagnose the cancer, not stage the disease.
CN: Physiological integrity; CNS: Physiological adaptation; CL: Apply

90. 2. Detecting cancer early when the cells may be premalignant and potentially curable would be most beneficial. However, a tumor must be 1 cm in diameter before it is detectable on a chest x-ray, so this is difficult. If the cancer is detected early, a bronchoscopy may help identify cell type. High-dose chemotherapy has minimal effect on long-term survival. Smoking cessation will not reverse the process but may prevent further decompensation.
CN: Health promotion and maintenance; CNS: None; CL: Apply

91. The nurse is assigned to care for a client with a chest tube and observes constant bubbling in the water seal chamber of the closed drainage system. Which nursing action will be performed **first**?
1. Document the finding in the medical record.
2. Check the system's connections.
3. Continue to monitor the client.
4. Preform a comprehensive pulmonary assessment.

92. A client has been diagnosed with lung cancer and is told a wedge resection is required. The client appears confused and asks the nurse for an explanation. What is the nurse's **best** response?
1. "The health care provider will remove one entire lung."
2. "The lobe of the lung involved will be removed."
3. "A small, localized area near the surface of the lung will be removed."
4. "A segment of the lung, including a bronchiole and alveoli, will be removed."

93. A client has been diagnosed with cor pulmonale. Which test result(s) will the nurse expect to see in this client? Select all that apply.
1. Large central pulmonary arteries upon x-ray
2. Increased right pulmonary artery pressure
3. Decreased pulmonary vascular resistance
4. Decreased right ventricular pressure
5. Increased pulmonary vascular resistance

94. During a pneumonectomy, the phrenic nerve on the surgical side is typically cut to cause hemidiaphragm paralysis. What is the **best** explanation for the nurse to use when teaching the client about this procedure?
1. Paralyzing the diaphragm reduces oxygen demand
2. Cutting the phrenic nerve is a mistake during surgery
3. The client is no longer using that lung to breathe
4. Paralyzing the diaphragm reduces the space left by the pneumonectomy

95. A client who has just had a right arthroscopy is back on the acute care unit. What action does the nurse identify as **best** to prevent a pulmonary embolism in this client?
1. Early ambulation
2. Frequent chest x-rays
3. Frequent lower extremity venous scans
4. Intubation of the client

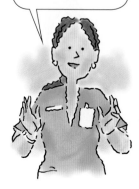

Bubbling is never a good thing when chest tubes are involved.

91. 2. Constant bubbling in the water seal chamber indicates a leak or loose connection between the client and the water seal chamber. The nurse would assess the system first. The nurse will document the findings, continue monitoring the client, and preform pulmonary assessments after determining the cause of the bubbling.
CN: Safe, effective care environment; CNS: Management of care; CL: Analyze

92. 3. A very small area of tissue close to the surface of the lung is removed in a wedge resection. A segment of the lung is removed in a segmental resection, a lobe is removed in a lobectomy, and an entire lung is removed in a pneumonectomy.
CN: Physiological integrity; CNS: Physiological adaptation; CL: Apply

93. 1, 2, 5. An arterial blood gas analysis in a client with cor pulmonale would exhibit decreased PaO_2. Chest x-ray would show large central pulmonary arteries and suggest right ventricular enlargement by rightward enlargement of cardiac silhouette. Pulmonary artery pressure measurements would show increased right ventricular and pulmonary artery pressures because of increased pulmonary vascular resistance.
CN: Physiological integrity; CNS: Physiological adaptation; CL: Apply

94. 4. Because the hemidiaphragm is a muscle that does not contract when paralyzed, an uncontracted hemidiaphragm remains in an "up" position, which reduces the space left by the pneumonectomy. Serous fluid has less space to fill, thus reducing the extent and duration of mediastinal shift after surgery. Although it is true that the client no longer needs the hemidiaphragm on the operative side to breathe, this alone would not be sufficient justification for cutting the phrenic nerve. Paralyzing the hemidiaphragm does not significantly decrease total-body oxygen demand.
CN: Physiological integrity; CNS: Physiological adaptation; CL: Apply

95. 1. Early ambulation helps reduce pooling of blood, which reduces the tendency of the blood to form a clot that could then dislodge. None of the other measures would prevent a pulmonary embolism from forming.
CN: Safe, effective care environment; CNS: Safety and infection control; CL: Apply

96. A client with lung cancer is experiencing excruciating pain due to the size of the tumor and is scheduled for a lung resection the next morning. What education will the nurse provide regarding lung resection?
1. The surgery will remove the tumor and all surrounding tissue
2. The surgery will remove the tumor and as little surrounding tissue as possible
3. A biopsy of the tumor will be done as well as removal of the whole tumor
4. A biopsy of the tumor will be done and half of the tumor will be removed

97. A client who has just undergone a pneumonectomy asks the nurse which position is best when lying in bed. What is the nurse's **best** response?
1. "Always lie on the nonoperative side."
2. "It does not matter. Any position is fine."
3. "Always lie prone when you are in bed."
4. "Lie on the operative side or on the back."

98. What is the rationale(s) for the nurse providing preoperative education for a client who will be undergoing lung surgery? Select all that apply.
1. Deciding whether the client should have surgery
2. Offering emotional support
3. Giving detailed explanations of the surgery
4. Providing general information
5. Answering questions

99. A client with a benign lung tumor is scheduled for removal of the tumor. Which statement made by the client demonstrates to the nurse a proper understanding of the reason for the procedure?
1. "It will facilitate pain control."
2. "It will prevent further lung compression."
3. "It will help to prevent metastatic cancer."
4. "It is for cosmetic purposes."

100. What is the **primary** intervention by the nurse while caring for a client with terminal lung cancer?
1. Offering emotional support
2. Ensuring pain control
3. Providing nutritional support
4. Preparing the client's will

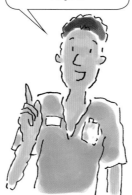

The answer to question #97 might be counterintuitive to you.

96. 2. The goal of surgical lung resection is to remove the cancerous lung tissue that has tumor in it while preserving as much surrounding tissue as possible. It may be necessary to remove alveoli and bronchioles, but care is taken to remove only what is absolutely necessary.
CN: Physiological integrity; CNS: Physiological adaptation; CL: Apply

97. 4. A client who has undergone a pneumonectomy does not have a chest tube in place; therefore, the client can lie on the operative side. In fact, the best position for this client is to lie on the operative side or on the back to prevent fluid from draining into the unaffected lung and to promote maximum ventilation. The client should not lie on the nonoperative side, which would allow unwanted drainage.
CN: Physiological integrity; CNS: Reduction of risk potential; CL: Apply

98. 2, 4, 5. The nurse's role is to provide general, not detailed, information about the client's surgery, explain preoperative and postoperative care, answer the client's questions, and offer emotional support. The nurse's role is not to decide whether the client should have surgery. If the client has questions that require detailed explanations of the surgery, the client should be referred to the surgeon.
CN: Physiological integrity; CNS: Physiological adaptation; CL: Apply

99. 2. The tumor is removed to prevent further compression of lung tissue as the tumor grows, which could lead to respiratory decompensation. If for some reason the tumor cannot be removed, then chemotherapy or radiation may be used to try to shrink it. At this point pain is not a problem; preventing cancer and cosmetics are not issues in this case.
CN: Physiological integrity; CNS: Physiological adaptation; CL: Apply

100. 2. The client with terminal lung cancer may have extreme pleuritic pain and should be treated to reduce discomfort. Preparing the client and family for the impending death is also important but should not be the primary focus until pain is under control. Nutritional support may be provided, but as the terminal phase advances, the client's nutritional needs greatly decrease. Nursing care does not focus on helping the client prepare a will.
CN: Physiological integrity; CNS: Basic care and comfort; CL: Apply

CN: Client needs category   CNS: Client needs subcategory   CL: Cognitive level

101. A client has been diagnosed with lung cancer. When the family members are informed of the diagnosis, they begin crying and shouting. Which statement by the nurse to the family is **best**?
1. "I understand this is shocking and not the news you wanted to hear."
2. "Please remain calm. You need to be strong for your loved one."
3. "If you do not calm down, I will have to have you removed from the unit."
4. "I can tell you are very upset. Please sit and talk with me about your feelings."

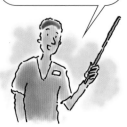

Remember— family members need to be cared for too.

101. 4. Lung cancer is a devastating diagnosis for family members to hear. The nurse would acknowledge and discuss the family's feelings. Stating this is not what the family wanted to hear or to remain calm does not address the family's immediate need. Telling the family they may be removed could lead to confrontation.
CN: Psychosocial integrity; CNS: None; CL: Apply

102. The nurse provides education for a pregnant woman who is scheduled for a cesarean birth regarding prevention of complications that can develop after the birth. Which statement by the client indicates a need for further education?
1. "At least one complication I do not have to worry about is blood clots."
2. "I will be sure to drink plenty of fluids so my milk will come in."
3. "I will cough and take deep breaths so I do not develop pneumonia."
4. "I will need to be active as soon as possible so I do not get muscle atrophy."

102. 1. Although venous thrombi in the thigh and pelvis are the most common sources for pulmonary emboli, clients who have undergone a cesarean birth are prone to develop clots in the amniotic fluid, leading to pulmonary embolus and possible death. Increasing fluids, coughing, and deep breathing—as well as being active—are all components that would help to prevent complications following a cesarean birth.
CN: Physiological integrity; CNS: Physiological adaptation; CL: Apply

103. The nurse recognizes which client is at **highest** risk for developing a pulmonary embolism?
1. An ambulatory client with an inflammatory joint disease
2. An ambulatory client who has type 1 diabetes
3. A healthy client who is 6 months' pregnant
4. A client who has fractures of the pelvis and right femur

103. 4. Thrombosis formation is caused by abnormalities in blood flow, vein wall integrity, and blood coagulation. The client with pelvic and femur fractures would be immobilized and probably have edema, which leads to venous stasis and predisposes the client to the development of deep vein thrombosis. A pulmonary embolus commonly arises from clots in the deep veins of the legs that break off and travel to the pulmonary arteries. The risk of developing venous thrombosis is not as high with the other conditions.
CN: Physiological integrity; CNS: Physiological adaptation; CL: Apply

104. At 0800, the nurse assesses a client scheduled for surgery at 1000. The nurse observes dyspnea, nonproductive cough, and back pain. What is the nurse's **priority** action?
1. Ensure the chest x-ray was done yesterday, as prescribed.
2. Check the serum electrolyte levels and complete blood count (CBC).
3. Immediately notify the health care provider of these findings.
4. Sign the preoperative checklist for this client.

104. 3. The nurse should make sure that the health care provider is immediately notified of the findings because dyspnea, a nonproductive cough, and back pain may signal a change in the client's respiratory status. The nurse should check any prescribed tests (such as chest x-ray, serum electrolyte levels, and CBC) after notifying the health care provider because they may help explain the change in the client's condition. The nurse should sign the preoperative checklist after notifying the health care provider of the client's condition and learning the health care provider's decision on whether to proceed with surgery.
CN: Safe, effective care environment; CNS: Management of care; CL: Apply

105. When a client is placed on oxygen therapy, the nurse will follow protocol. Place the following steps in the correct order the nurse will complete them. Use all options.

1. Attach the flow meter to a wall outlet, fill the humidifier with water, and attach the delivery system and tubing.

2. Explain the procedure to the client.

3. Check the health care provider's prescription.

4. Place the face mask or cannula on the client.

5. Re-assess the client and document the procedure.

106. The nurse is caring for a client who has a pulmonary embolism. What is the nurse's **best** explanation for this client's potential to develop chest pain?
1. It is the same as costochondritis
2. It is a result of a myocardial infarction
3. It is pleuritic pain due to inflammation
4. It is caused by referred pain from the pelvis

107. Which symptom will the nurse expect to observe **first** in a client with an acute pulmonary embolism?
1. Distended jugular veins
2. Bradycardia
3. Dyspnea
4. Nonproductive cough

108. The client who has a pulmonary embolus is also experiencing hemoptysis. When educating the client, what is the nurse's **best** explanation for the cause of hemoptysis?
1. Alveolar damage in the infarcted area
2. Involvement of major blood vessels in the occluded area
3. Loss of lung parenchyma
4. Loss of massive lung tissue

109. Following a pulmonary embolism, a client is placed on IV heparin. The client asks the nurse about the purpose of the heparin. Which statement by the nurse is appropriate?
1. "Heparin will dissolve the clot in your lungs."
2. "Heparin will slow the development of any more clots."
3. "Heparin will prevent pieces of the clot from breaking off and going to your lung."
4. "Heparin will dissolve any circulating clots."

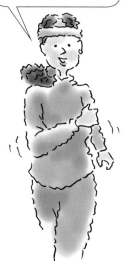

Taking the NCLEX is more like running a marathon than a sprint. Hang in there!

105. Ordered Response:

3. Check the health care provider's prescription.

2. Explain the procedure to the client.

1. Attach the flow meter to a wall outlet, fill the humidifier with water, and attach the delivery system and tubing.

4. Place the face mask or cannula on the client.

5. Re-assess the client and document the procedure.

CN: Safe, effective care environment; CNS: Safety and infection control; CL: Apply

106. 3. Pleuritic pain is caused by the inflammatory reaction of the lung parenchyma to the pulmonary embolism. The pain is not associated with myocardial infarction, costochondritis, or referred pain from the pelvis to the chest.
CN: Physiological integrity; CNS: Physiological adaptation; CL: Apply

107. 3. Dyspnea is usually the first symptom of pulmonary embolus because the thrombus prevents gas exchange in the pulmonary arterial bed. If the embolus is large enough, the client may then develop right ventricular failure, with such symptoms as distended jugular veins, tachycardia, and circulatory collapse. The client may also have hemoptysis.
CN: Safe, effective care environment; CNS: Management of care; CL: Analyze

108. 1. The infarcted area produces alveolar damage that can lead to the production of bloody sputum, sometimes in large amounts. There is a loss of lung parenchyma and subsequent scar tissue formation, and blood vessels may be involved, but these do not cause hemoptysis.
CN: Physiological integrity; CNS: Physiological adaptation; CL: Apply

109. 2. Heparin is an anticoagulant and is administered to slow thrombus formation. Fibrinolytic medications dissolve clots. Heparin will not prevent clots from embolizing or dissolve circulating clots.
CN: Physiological integrity; CNS: Pharmacological and parenteral therapies; CL: Apply

CN: Client needs category   CNS: Client needs subcategory   CL: Cognitive level

110. A client with a large pulmonary embolism has results from an arterial blood gas analysis indicating respiratory alkalosis. What will the nurse determine is the potential cause of this finding?
1. Hypoventilation
2. Alveolar damage
3. Large amount of bloody sputum
4. Large region of lung tissue unavailable for perfusion

111. The nurse is caring for a client diagnosed with a pulmonary embolism prescribed a ventilation-perfusion scan. The client asks what this test can show. Which use(s) does the nurse correctly identify for this test to the client? Select all that apply.
1. To detect poor blood flow in the lungs and blood vessels
2. To examine the lungs before different types of surgeries
3. To detect air trapping in the lungs
4. To determine the location and size of the pulmonary embolism
5. To determine the location of all the peripheral arteries

112. A client is suspected of having a pulmonary embolus. Which definitive test will the nurse prepare the client for?
1. Arterial blood gas (ABG) analysis
2. Computed tomography scan
3. Pulmonary angiogram
4. Ventilation-perfusion scan

113. A client with a pulmonary embolism has received a thrombolytic medication. What is the **most** important concept for the nurse to educate this client and family on at this time?
1. The medication was given to break apart the blood clot blocking the pulmonary artery
2. The medication is taken orally and will thin the blood
3. The medication will prevent future clots from forming
4. The medication will help the client to breathe by dilating bronchial tubes

110. 4. A client with a large pulmonary embolism would have a large region of lung tissue unavailable for perfusion. This causes the client to hyperventilate and blow off large amounts of carbon dioxide, which crosses the unaffected alveolar-capillary membrane more readily than does oxygen, resulting in respiratory alkalosis. A client with respiratory alkalosis would hyperventilate and not hypoventilate. Alveolar damage and a large amount of bloody sputum can be present with a pulmonary embolus, but they do not cause respiratory alkalosis.
CN: Physiological integrity; CNS: Physiological adaptation; CL: Apply

111. 1, 2, 3. The ventilation-perfusion scan provides information on the extent of occlusion caused by the pulmonary embolism and the amount of lung tissue involved in the area not perfused. It does not tell the size of the pulmonary embolism or the location of all the peripheral arteries. There are other reasons for doing this test: to detect poor blood flow, to detect air trapping, and to examine the lungs before different surgeries.
CN: Physiological integrity; CNS: Reduction and risk potential; CL: Understand

112. 3. A pulmonary angiogram is used to definitively diagnose a pulmonary embolism. A catheter is passed through the circulation to the region of the occlusion; the region can be outlined with an injection of contrast medium and viewed by fluoroscopy. This shows the location of the clot, as well as the extent of the perfusion defect. A computed tomography scan can show the location of infarcted or ischemic tissue but cannot be used for a definitive diagnosis. ABG levels can define the amount of hypoxia present but cannot be used for a definitive diagnosis. The ventilation-perfusion scan can report whether there is a ventilation-perfusion mismatch present and define the amount of tissue involved but cannot be used for a definitive diagnosis.
CN: Physiological integrity; CNS: Reduction of risk potential; CL: Understand

113. 1. A thrombolytic medication is given IV to break apart or dissolve blood clots. It is not given orally, does not prevent future clots from forming, and has no effect on the bronchial tubes.
CN: Physiological integrity; CNS: Pharmacological and parenteral therapies; CL: Apply

114. A client who was hospitalized for pulmonary embolism is being discharged on warfarin therapy. Which statement by the nurse about warfarin therapy is appropriate?
1. "Warfarin therapy inhibits the formation of blood clots."
2. "It is given to continue to reduce the size of the pulmonary embolism."
3. "It will reduce blood pressure and prevent venous stasis."
4. "Coagulation studies to monitor bleeding times will be necessary every 6 months."

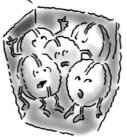

Warfarin is an anti-coagulant—that means we do what?

114. 1. Warfarin inhibits clot formation by interfering with clotting factors that are dependent on vitamin K. Warfarin does not dissolve clots and will not reduce the size of the pulmonary embolus. It does not reduce blood pressure and will not prevent venous stasis. Coagulation studies would be performed every 2 to 4 weeks while the client is receiving warfarin.
CN: Physiological integrity; CNS: Pharmacological and parenteral therapies; CL: Apply

115. A client suspected of having a pulmonary embolus is scheduled for a lung scan. What is the **most** important action for the nurse prior to the procedure?
1. Explain the procedure to the client.
2. Check all allergies of the client.
3. Watch for radioactive gas leaks.
4. Obtain the client's vital signs.

115. 2. The priority action for the nurse is checking to see if the client has any allergies, as lung scans are contraindicated in clients that have a hypersensitivity to the radiopharmaceutical dye. After that it is important to also explain the procedure, obtain the vital signs, and during the procedure watch for any gas leaks.
CN: Safe, effective care environment; CNS: Safety and infection control; CL: Apply

116. A client who has chronic bronchitis asks the nurse to identify things that will help to promote better oxygenation. Which lifestyle factor(s) will the nurse identify as affecting the client's oxygenation? Select all that apply.
1. Nutrition
2. Physical exercise
3. Ethnicity
4. Genetics
5. Anxiety

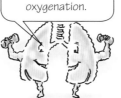

Exercise strengthens the lungs and improves oxygenation.

116. 1, 2, 5. Lifestyle factors that affect oxygenation are nutrition, physical exercise, smoking, substance abuse, and anxiety. Other factors may affect a client's oxygenation as well. Ethnicity and genetics are not lifestyle factors.
CN: Physiological integrity; CNS: Reduction of risk potential; CL: Apply

117. What is the **priority** nursing intervention when caring for a client with a pulmonary embolism?
1. Assessing oxygenation status
2. Monitoring the oxygen delivery device
3. Monitoring for other sources of clots
4. Determining if the client needs a ventilation-perfusion scan

117. 1. Nursing management of a client with a pulmonary embolism focuses on assessing oxygenation status and ensuring treatment is adequate. If the client's status begins to deteriorate, it is the nurse's responsibility to contact the health care provider and attempt to improve oxygenation. Monitoring for other clot sources, determining if a test is appropriate for the client, and ensuring the oxygen delivery device is working properly are other nursing responsibilities, but they are not the focus of care.
CN: Safe, effective care environment; CNS: Management of care; CL: Apply

118. A client with a pulmonary embolism is having a vena cava filter inserted. What is the **best** explanation by the nurse for the filter?
1. The filter prevents further clot formation
2. The filter collects clots so they do not go to the lungs
3. The filter breaks up clots into insignificantly small pieces
4. The filter contains anticoagulants that are slowly released, dissolving any clots

118. 3. The umbrella-like filter is placed in a client at high risk for the formation of more clots that could potentially become pulmonary emboli. The filter breaks the clots into small pieces that will not significantly occlude the pulmonary vasculature. The filter does not release anticoagulants and does not prevent further clot formation. The filter does not collect the clots; if it did, it would have to be emptied periodically, causing the client to require surgery in the future.
CN: Physiological integrity; CNS: Physiological adaptation; CL: Apply

119. A client with a pulmonary embolism is scheduled for an embolectomy. The client states, "I do not think I can have this surgery." Which response by the nurse is **most** appropriate?
1. "Do you know that not having this procedure could lead to death?"
2. "Surgery can be scary. Have you told your health care provider?"
3. "I will let the operating room know to cancel your surgery."
4. "Can you share with me what you are feeling at this time?"

120. A client diagnosed with a pulmonary embolism is having chest pain and apprehension. Which nursing intervention is appropriate for this client?
1. Administering analgesics
2. Using guided imagery
3. Positioning the client on the left side
4. Providing emotional support

121. A client placed on pulse oximetry monitoring asks the nurse to explain what that is. What is the **best** explanation by the nurse?
1. It is the amount of carbon dioxide in the blood
2. It is the amount of oxygen in the blood
3. It is the percentage of hemoglobin carrying oxygen
4. It is the respiratory rate

122. When providing education for the client about the importance of blood levels in relation to breathing, what is the nurse's **best** explanation?
1. "The level of hemoglobin has no effect on oxygenation."
2. "The more hemoglobin you have the less oxygen in your body."
3. "Low hemoglobin levels cause reduced oxygen-carrying capacity."
4. "Low hemoglobin levels cause increased oxygen-carrying capacity."

123. A client with atelectasis is prescribed oxygen therapy. What will the nurse expect the health care provider to prescribe for this client?
1. Ventilation with continuous positive airway pressure (CPAP)
2. Ventilation with a nasal cannula
3. Ventilation with positive end-expiratory pressure (PEEP)
4. Ventilation with a facemask only

119. 4. The nurse would discuss the client's feelings to determine why the client believes surgery cannot be performed. This discussion will guide the nurse's additional actions. The nurse should not make threatening comments, tell the client to speak with the health care provider, or immediately cancel the procedure.
CN: Psychosocial integrity; CNS: None; CL: Apply

120. 1. After the pulmonary embolism has been diagnosed and the amount of hypoxia determined, chest pain and the accompanying apprehension can be treated with analgesics. The nurse must monitor respiratory status frequently. Guided imagery and providing emotional support can be used as alternatives. Positioning the client on the left side when a pulmonary embolism is suspected may prevent a clot that has extended through the capillaries and into the pulmonary veins from breaking off and traveling through the heart into the arterial circulation, leading to a massive stroke.
CN: Physiological integrity; CNS: Physiological adaptation; CL: Apply

121. 3. Pulse oximetry determines the percentage of hemoglobin carrying oxygen. This does not ensure that the oxygen being carried through the bloodstream is actually being taken up by the tissue. Pulse oximetry does not provide information about the amount of oxygen or carbon dioxide in the blood or the client's respiratory rate.
CN: Physiological integrity; CNS: Physiological adaptation; CL: Understand

122. 3. The level of hemoglobin in one's body does have an effect on oxygenation. Hemoglobin carries oxygen to all tissues in the body. If the hemoglobin level is low, the amount of oxygen-carrying capacity is also low. More hemoglobin would increase oxygen-carrying capacity and thus increase the total amount of oxygen available in the blood.
CN: Physiological integrity; CNS: Physiological adaptation; CL: Apply

123. 3. PEEP delivers positive pressure to the lung at the end of expiration. This helps open collapsed alveoli and helps them stay open so gas exchange can occur in these newly opened alveoli, improving oxygenation. CPAP, or continuous positive airway pressure, is a treatment that uses mild air pressure to keep the airways open. CPAP typically is used by people who have breathing problems such as sleep apnea. A facemask or nasal cannula would not be helpful in this situation.
CN: Physiological integrity; CNS: Physiological adaptation; CL: Apply

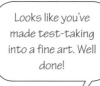
Looks like you've made test-taking into a fine art. Well done!

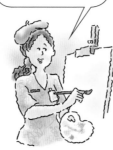

124. A client who is having difficulty breathing is told by the health care provider that oxygen will be prescribed due to collapsed alveoli. Which statement made by the nurse **best** explains to the client how opening up collapsed alveoli improves oxygenation?
  1. "Alveoli need oxygen to live."
  2. "Alveoli have no effect on oxygenation."
  3. "Collapsed alveoli increase oxygen demand."
  4. "Gaseous exchange occurs in the alveolar membrane."

125. The nurse is caring for a client prescribed continuous positive airway pressure (CPAP). The client asks the nurse, "Will I have to wear an oxygen mask?" Which response by the nurse is **best**?
  1. "Yes, a mask is what provides you with 100% oxygen."
  2. "No, a mask is not required with CPAP devices."
  3. "Yes, a mask provides pressurized oxygen so you can breathe more easily."
  4. "It depends on the type of machine you decide to purchase for home use."

126. The nurse is caring for a client with pneumonia. The health care provider prescribes 600 mg of ceftriaxone oral suspension to be given once per day. The medication label states ceftriaxone 125 mg/5 mL. How many milliliters of medication will the nurse administer to the client? Record your answer using a whole number.

_____mL

127. The nurse is caring for a client scheduled for a bronchoscopy. Which intervention(s) will the nurse perform to prepare the client for this procedure? Select all that apply.
  1. Explain the procedure.
  2. Withhold food and fluids for 2 hours before the test.
  3. Provide a clear liquid diet for 6 to 12 hours before the test.
  4. Confirm a signed informed consent form has been obtained.
  5. Ask the client to remove dentures.
  6. Administer a sedative as prescribed.

128. The nurse is auscultating a client's lungs. Identify the area on the client's vertebrae, representing the base of the lungs, where the nurse expects the breath sounds to stop at the end of expiration.

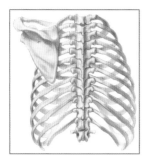

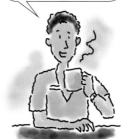

Heads up! It's one of those math questions.

Nicely done. Now put your feet up and have a cup of Joe.

124. 4. Gaseous exchange occurs in the alveolar membrane, so if the alveoli collapse, no exchange occurs. Collapsed alveoli receive oxygen, as well as other nutrients, from the bloodstream. Collapsed alveoli have no effect on oxygen demand, although by decreasing the surface area available for gas exchange, they decrease oxygenation of the blood.
CN: Physiological integrity; CNS: Physiological adaptation; CL: Apply

125. 3. The client will have to use a mask with a CPAP. The mask provides pressurized oxygen continuously through both inspiration and expiration. By providing a client with pressurized oxygen, the client has less resistance to overcome in taking in the next breath, making it easier to breathe. The mask can be set to deliver any amount of oxygen needed.
CN: Physiological integrity; CNS: Physiological adaptation; CL: Apply

126. 24.
To calculate drug dosages, use the formula:
  Dose on hand / quantity on hand = Dose desired / X
In this case,
$$125\,mg/5\,mL = 600\,mg/X.$$
Therefore, X = 24 mL.
CN: Physiological integrity; CNS: Pharmacological and parenteral therapies; CL: Analyze

127. 1, 4, 5, 6. All procedures must be explained to the client to obtain informed consent and to reduce anxiety. A signed informed consent form is required for all invasive procedures. Dentures need to be removed for bronchoscopy because they may become dislodged during the procedure. A sedative, such as lorazepam, midazolam, or diazepam, is given to relax the client. Food and fluids are restricted for 6 to 12 hours before the test to avoid the risk of aspiration during the procedure.
CN: Physiological integrity; CNS: Reduction of risk potential; CL: Apply

128. Based on posterior land marks, the lungs extend from the cervical area to the level of the tenth thoracic vertebrae (T10) at the end of expiration.

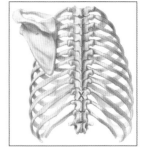

CN: Health promotion and maintenance; CNS: None; CL: Apply

Chapter 6

Neurosensory Disorders

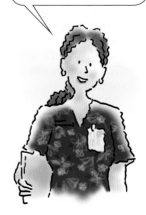

Stroke, subdural hematoma, laminectomy—they're all here in this comprehensive chapter on neurosensory disorders in adults. I've got a sixth sense you're going to do great!

Neurosensory refresher

Acute head injury

Trauma to the brain, skull, or scalp due to external mechanical force, causing brain damage including concussions, contusions, hematomas (subdural and epidural)

Key signs and symptoms

- Altered mental status using Glasgow coma scale
- Headache, dizziness, nausea, vomiting, transient amnesia
- Acute or sudden onset unequal pupil size, loss of pupillary reaction (late sign), irregular respirations, bradycardia, systolic hypertension (ominous sign)
- Babinski reflex, decorticate, decerebrate posturing

Key test results

- Computed tomography (CT) scan shows hemorrhage, cerebral edema, or shift of midline structures
- Magnetic resonance imaging (MRI) shows hemorrhage, cerebral edema, or shift of midline structures
- Positron emission tomography (PET) shows blood flow, tissue position and brain metabolism
- Cerebral angiography shows cerebral circulation
- Electroencephalography (EEG) records brain activity generated by the brain

Key treatments

- Cervical collar (until neck injury is ruled out)
- Anticonvulsant: phenytoin
- Barbiturate: pentobarbital if unable to control intracranial pressure (ICP) with diuresis
- Diuretics: mannitol, furosemide to combat cerebral edema
- Vasopressors: dopamine or phenylephrine to maintain cerebral perfusion pressure above 60 mm Hg (if blood pressure is low and ICP is elevated)
- Glucocorticoid: dexamethasone to reduce cerebral edema

- Histamine-2 (H_2) receptor antagonists: cimetidine, ranitidine, famotidine, nizatidine
- Mucosal barrier fortifier: sucralfate
- Posterior pituitary hormone: vasopressin, if client develops diabetes insipidus

Key interventions

- Obtain and maintain airway with decrease level of consciousness (LOC).
- Airway is priority with decreased LOC.
- Monitor neurologic and respiratory status (assess for clear drainage from the nose or ears indicates possible basilar skull fracture).
- Decrease stimuli to reduce intracranial pressure with quiet room, head in neutral alignment, head of bed up 30 degrees or as tolerated, reduce pain, avoid constrictive clothing, avoid straining with bowel movements, sneeze or cough with mouth open, maintain cool temperature.
- Monitor and record vital signs, intake and output, urine specific gravity, laboratory studies, and pulse oximetry values.
- Check for signs of diabetes insipidus (low urine specific gravity, high urine output).
- Cluster nursing activities to allow for frequent rest periods.

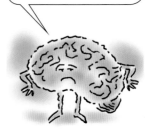

Ever since that car wreck, I've felt a little "altered."

Amyotrophic lateral sclerosis

Progressive, degenerative disorder of the myelin sheaths that affects the spinal cord

Key signs and symptoms

- Awkwardness of fine finger movements
- Muscle atrophy
- Dysphagia
- Fatigue
- Progressive disability of upper and lower extremities
- Diaphragmatic paralysis (late stage)
- No sensory loss, remains alert
- Fasciculations (twitching)
- Pseudobulbar affect (PBA) is uncontrollable bouts of laughing or crying

Key test results

- Pulmonary function testing (PFT)
- Creatine kinase level is elevated

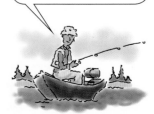

ALS is a degenerative disorder that affects motor neurons. Can you remember its symptoms?

- MRI
- Electromyography (EMG) shows impaired impulse conduction in the muscles

Key treatments
- Continuous positive airway pressure (CPAP)
- Symptomatic relief
- PBA treatment: dextromethorphan hydro-bromide and quinidine sulfate
- Neuroprotective agent: riluzole

Key interventions
- Maintain independence as long as possible.
- Prevent skin breakdown.
- Provide soft liquid diet, consider gastrostomy feeding.
- Respiratory assistance: continuous positive airway pressure (CPAP).
- Monitor neurologic and respiratory status.
- Evaluate swallow and gag reflexes.
- Monitor and record vital signs and intake and output.
- Devise an alternate method of communication when necessary.
- Support physical and emotional needs toward peaceful death.
- Assist with activities of daily living (ADLs) as long as possible.
- Suction the oropharynx as necessary.

Aphasia
Impaired ability to understand or use common words or impairment of the ability to speak, write, and/or read. Receptive (sensory) type exhibit difficulty understanding spoken or written word (temporal area: Wernicke's). Expressive (motor) type exhibit difficulty speaking or writing (frontal lobe: Broca's area).

Key signs and symptoms
Receptive
- Anomia (difficulty finding words)
- Difficulty with names of objects
- Grammatical errors
- Making up words
- Agraphia (difficulty writing)
- Alexia (difficulty recognizing words by sight)

Expressive
- Inability to speak or write

Key treatments
- Speech therapy
- Treatment of underlying cause

Key interventions
- Assess client's comprehension, understanding, writing.
- Talk slowly with normal tone and volume.

- Use alternative ways to communicate.
- Do not force client to repeat words, allow ample time to respond.
- Maintain one-way communication at all times.

Bell's palsy
Disorder of facial nerve (cranial nerve VII) causing paralysis of one side of face

Key signs and symptoms
- Inability to close eye completely on the affected side
- Decreased lacrimation (tearing)
- Pain around jaw or ear
- Unilateral facial weakness

Key test results
- EMG helps predict level of expected recovery by distinguishing temporary conduction defects from a pathologic interruption of nerve fibers

Key treatments
- Moist heat
- Corticosteroid: prednisone to reduce facial nerve edema and improve nerve conduction and blood flow
- Artificial tears to protect the cornea from injury

Key interventions
- During treatment with prednisone, watch for adverse reactions, especially gastrointestinal distress and fluid retention.
- Apply moist heat to affected side of face, taking care not to burn the skin.
- Massage client's face with a gentle upward motion two or three times daily for 5 to 10 minutes, or have client massage face oneself.
- When ready for active facial exercises, teach client to grimace in front of mirror.
- Arrange for privacy at mealtimes.
- Offer psychological support; give reassurance that recovery is likely within 1 to 8 weeks.

Brain abscess
Accumulation of infectious material within the tissue of the brain

Key signs and symptoms
- Headache, usually worse in the morning
- Chills
- Fever
- Focal deficits: weakness, decreased vision
- Symptoms of increased intracranial pressure (ICP)
- Drowsiness

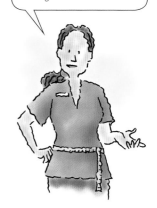

The good news about Bell's palsy is that it typically lasts for no longer than 8 weeks.

Stand back while I fight off this infection!

Key test results

- Enhanced CT scan reveals abscess site
- EEG to localize site of lesion
- CT-guided stereotactic biopsy may be performed to drain and culture the abscess
- Blood cultures if from another source

Key treatments

- Control increase of ICP
- Glucocorticoid: dexamethasone to reduce cerebral edema
- Penicillinase-resistant antibiotics: nafcillin, methicillin
- Surgical aspiration or drainage of the abscess
- Blood glucose and potassium (if steroids are administered)

Key interventions

- Frequently monitor neurologic status using GCS.
- Monitor and record vital signs at least once every hour.
- Monitor fluid intake and output carefully.
- After surgery, monitor neurologic status; monitor vital signs and intake and output.
- Watch for signs of meningitis (nuchal rigidity, headaches, chills, sweats).
- Change the dressing when damp; never allow bandages to remain damp.
- Position the client on the operative side (hemiplegia, hemiparesis likely).
- Measure drainage from a Jackson-Pratt drain or other type of drain as instructed by surgeon.

Brain tumor

Benign or malignant tumor within the cranial cavity growing as a mass or invading the tissue

Key signs or symptoms

- Various, depending on location of tumor
- Increased ICP (headache, vomiting, visual disturbances, seizures)

Key test results

- CT scan shows location and size of tumor
- Stereotactic CT shows precise location and can be used for treatment planning and prognosis
- MRI shows location and size of tumor.
- PET used to determine metabolism of the tumor and for treatment planning

Key treatments

- Craniotomy
- Radiation therapy
- Chemotherapy (with metastasis)

- Anticonvulsant: phenytoin to treat or prevent seizures
- Glucocorticoid: dexamethasone to reduce inflammation and edema around the tumor/lesion
- Osmotic diuretic: mannitol to decrease fluid volume in the brain, reducing ICP
- Histamine-2 (H_2) receptor antagonists: cimetidine, ranitidine, famotidine, nizatidine
- Mucosal barrier fortifier: sucralfate

Key interventions

- Monitor neurologic and respiratory status using GCS.
- Evaluate pain (headache characteristics should be assessed).
- Observe for signs and symptoms of increased ICP and aggressively treat.
- Monitor for signs and symptoms of syndrome of inappropriate antidiuretic hormone (SIADH; edema, weight gain, positive fluid balance, high urine specific gravity).
- Encourage client to express feelings about changes in body image and fear of dying.

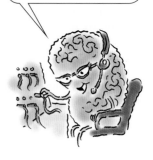

It is important to monitor neurologic status and function to ensure that all "connections" are up and running.

Cataract

Progressive opacity or cloudiness of the normally transparent lens (traumatic, congenital, or senile)

Key signs and symptoms

- Painless blurred or diminished vision
- Poor night vision
- Astigmatism
- Double vision (diplopia)
- Yellow, gray, or white lens

Key test results

- Ophthalmoscopy or slit-lamp examination confirms diagnosis by revealing a dark area in the normally homogeneous red reflex
- Visual acuity is not an accurate measure of impairment

Key treatments

- Extracapsular cataract extraction
- Intracapsular lens implant

Key interventions

- Avoid lifting, driving, sports activities until health care provider allows.
- Teach signs and symptoms of retinal detachment (floaters, flashing lights, decreased vision, pain).
- Wear eyeglasses or eye shield as prescribed; do not lay on affected side.
- Inform client that one eye at a time will be repaired.

- Teach administration of prescribed antibiotic, anti-inflammatory, corticosteroid eye drops.
- Wear sunglasses.

Cerebral aneurysm

Protrusion or sac on a cerebral blood vessel due to weakness of the vessel wall (berry, fusiform or dissection aneurysm)

Key signs or symptoms
- Sudden headache (commonly described by the client as the worst ever experienced)
- Nausea and vomiting
- Sudden changed in level of consciousness
- Seizures

Key test results
- Cerebral angiogram (CTA) identifies the aneurysm
- MRI to show the type, size, location, and presence of blood in the ventricles
- CT scan may show a shift of intracranial midline structures and blood in the subarachnoid space

Key treatments
- Aneurysm clipping
- Anticonvulsant: phenytoin
- Calcium channel blocker: nimodipine preferred to prevent cerebral vasospasm
- Glucocorticoid: dexamethasone
- Histamine-2 (H_2) receptor antagonists: cimetidine, ranitidine, famotidine, nizatidine
- Stool softener: docusate sodium

Key interventions
- Monitor neurologic status for increased ICP using GCS.
- Maintain crystalloid solutions for cerebral perfusion pressure (CPP) to prevent cerebral hypoxia.
- Monitor for cerebral vasospasm (worsening headache, decreased level of consciousness, or new neurological deficit).
- Take vital signs every 1 to 2 hours initially and then every 4 hours when the client becomes stable.
- Allow rest period between nursing activities.

Conjunctivitis

Infection of the delicate membrane lining of the eyelid and the outer surface of the eye that can result from infection, irritation, or systemic disease (can be viral, bacterial, allergic, or caused by irritants)

Key signs and symptoms
- Excessive tearing
- Itching, burning
- Thick yellow or green mucopurulent discharge (over the eyelashes after sleep)
- Blurred vision
- Redness and swelling of the conjunctiva or inner eyelid

Key test results
- Culture and sensitivity tests:
  - identify causative bacterial organism
  - indicate appropriate antibiotic therapy.

Key treatments
- Antiviral agents: oral acyclovir (if herpes simplex is cause)
- Corticosteroids: dexamethasone, fluorometholone (if cause is nonviral)
- Mast cell stabilizer: cromolyn for allergic conjunctivitis
- Topical antibiotics: according to the sensitivity of the infective organism (if bacterial)

Key interventions
- Teach proper handwashing technique.
- Avoid close contact with other people.
- Stress risk of spreading infection to family members by sharing washcloths, towels, and pillows (viral and bacterial are highly contagious).
- Warn against rubbing the infected eye (spreads infection to the other eye and to other persons).
- Apply warm compresses and therapeutic ointment or drops; do not irrigate the eye.
- Instruct the client to wash hands before using medication.
- Instruct client to use clean washcloths or towels frequently.
- Teach client to instill eye drops and ointments correctly, without touching the bottle tip to eye or lashes.

Corneal abrasion

Cut or scratch on the outer, clear layer of the eye

Key signs and symptoms
- Burning
- Pain worse when blinking; gritty or foreign body sensation
- Increased tearing
- Redness
- Sensitivity to light
- Blurred or loss of vision
- Headache

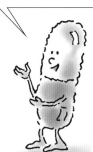

What meds are best for treating conjunctivitis?

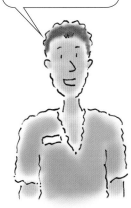

What key interventions should you undertake to assist a client with cerebral aneurysm?

Key test results

- Staining the cornea with fluorescein stain confirms diagnosis
  - injured area appears green when examined with a flashlight or slit lamp

Key treatments

- Cycloplegic agent: tropicamide
- Irrigation with saline solution
- Pressure patch (a tightly applied eye patch)
- Removal of a deeply embedded foreign body with a foreign body spud, using a topical anesthetic

Key interventions

- Assist with examination of the eye.
- Check visual acuity before beginning treatment.
- If foreign body is visible, carefully irrigate eye with normal saline solution.
- Tell the client with an eye patch to leave patch in place for 6 to 8 hours.
- May be treated with a bandage contact lens (special lens to provide pain relief and speed healing).
- Stress the importance of instilling prescribed antibiotic eye drops.

Encephalitis

Inflammation of the brain caused by an infection or allergic reaction. Viral encephalitis most often caused by herpes virus in children, by cytomegalovirus (CMV) in immunocompromised, West Nile, or postbacterial infection of the respiratory or gastrointestinal tract.

West Nile encephalitis

Inflammation of the brain caused by a mosquito-borne virus

Key signs and symptoms

- Meningeal signs (nuchal rigidity, photophobia, seizures, motor deficits, personality changes)
- Sudden onset of fever
- Severe headache
- Brain stem involvement (nystagmus, extraocular nerve palsies, hearing loss, dysphagia, respiratory dysfunction)
- Pituitary involvement (diabetes insipidus, hypothermia, SIADH)
- Vomiting

West Nile encephalitis

- Fever
- Headache
- Disorientation

Key test results

- Electroencephalogram (EEG)
- MRI

- Serology blood testing
- Cerebrospinal fluid (CSF) analysis identifies the virus

West Nile encephalitis

- Client history reveals recent mosquito bites

Key treatments

- Antiviral agents (herpes virus, CMV)
- Antibiotic
- Endotracheal (ET) intubation and mechanical ventilation (as needed)
- Nasogastric (NG) tube feedings or total parenteral nutrition (if unable to use the GI tract)
- Anticonvulsants: phenytoin, phenobarbital
- Analgesics and antipyretics: aspirin, acetaminophen to relieve headache and reduce fever
- Diuretics: furosemide, mannitol to reduce cerebral swelling
- Corticosteroid: dexamethasone to reduce cerebral inflammation and edema

West Nile encephalitis

- Symptom control (e.g., IV fluids, respiratory support)
- Antipyretic: acetaminophen

Key interventions

- Monitor neurologic status for evidence of increased ICP.
- Observe client's mental status and cognitive abilities for subtle changes in behavior or personality.
- Keep accurate intake and output records.
- Maintain seizure precautions.
- Maintain standard or viral specific isolation precautions.
- Maintain a quiet environment; dark room, avoid stimulation and agitation.

West Nile encephalitis

- Monitor respiratory status.
- Administer supplemental oxygen, as prescribed.
- Monitor neurologic status.
- Administer medications, as prescribed.
- Monitor pulse oximetry values.

Glaucoma

Group of eye disorders that causes an increase in intraocular pressure. Can damage the optic nerve if untreated. Wide angle (bilateral) or narrow angle (obstruction of outflow)

Key signs and symptoms

Normal tension glaucoma (wide angle)

- Elevated intraocular pressure (IOP)
- Optic nerve damage
- Visual field deficits

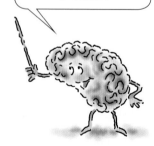

What's the condition called when I get inflamed? Can you remember?

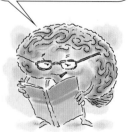

Blurred vision can be an indicator of various disorders.

Ocular hypertension (wide angle)
- Elevated IOP
- Headache or ocular pain

Chronic open-angle glaucoma (narrow angle)
- Initially asymptomatic
- Progressive visual field loss
- Ocular pain and headache

Acute angle-closure glaucoma (narrow angle)
- Rapidly progressive (emergency)
- Acute ocular pain
- Blurred vision
- Dilated pupil (vertically oval, fixed, unreactive)
- Halo vision, difficulty focusing, loss of peripheral vision
- Nausea, vomiting, bradycardia (pain associated)

Key test results
- Ophthalmoscopy shows atrophy and cupping of optic nerve head
- Tonometry shows increased intraocular pressure

Key treatments
Chronic open-angle glaucoma (narrow angle)
- Alpha$_2$-agonist: brimonidine to decrease aqueous humor production
- Beta-blocker: timolol to decrease aqueous humor production

Acute angle-closure glaucoma (narrow angle)
- Cholinergics (miotics): pilocarpine to increase outflow
- Laser iridectomy or surgical iridectomy (if pressure does not decrease with drug therapy)

Key interventions
- Monitor eye pain.
- Teach self-care (careful installation of eye drops as ordered).
- Administer medication as prescribed (monitor for adverse reactions).
- Provide referral for low vision and rehabilitation services.
- Maintain safety for loss of peripheral vision.
- Provide emotional support for lifelong disease (that may lead to blindness).

Guillain-Barré syndrome

Progressive autoimmune response causing inflammation and demyelination of the peripheral nervous system in an ascending paralysis, descending recovery process

Key signs or symptoms
- Symmetrical muscle weakness (ascending from the legs to the arms)
- Begins with toes and feet numbness
- Can impair diaphragm as it progresses
- Self-limiting in most cases

Key test results
- History of preceding febrile illness (usually a respiratory tract infection) or allergic rhinitis and typical clinical features
- Lumbar puncture with CSF protein level begins to rise, peaking in 4 to 6 weeks
- CSF white blood cell count remains normal (in severe disease, CSF pressure may rise above normal)
- Electromyogram (EMG) to measure nerve activity in the muscles
- Nerve conduction study (NCS) to measure the speed of nerve conduction

Key treatments
- Pain control
- Anticoagulants: heparin, warfarin to prevent clots when immobile
- Corticosteroid: prednisone
- ET intubation or tracheotomy, possibly mechanical ventilation
- IV fluid therapy
- NG tube feedings or parenteral nutrition (if unable to use GI tract)
- Plasmapheresis to remove antibodies may cause attack on immune system
- Intravenous immunoglobulin to block damaging antibodies

Key interventions
- Watch for ascending sensory loss, which precedes motor loss.
- Monitor vital signs and level of consciousness.
- Monitor and treat respiratory dysfunction.
- Maintain respiratory support (ventilator or CPAP) if needed.
- Reposition the client at least every 2 hours with ROM (active or passive).
- Provide aggressive physical therapy (PT) to prevent contractures and support muscle strength.
- Use adaptive devices for mobility and self-care as possible.
- Prevent aspiration by diet modifications (soft, thicken liquids) or NPO and NG tube for feeding as necessary.
- Monitor for signs and symptoms of thrombophlebitis; apply antiembolism stockings and sequential compression devices; give prophylactic anticoagulants as ordered.

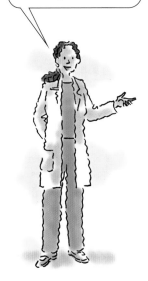

Which condition involves a progressive, autoimmune response causing inflammation and demyelination of the peripheral nervous system?

- Encourage adequate fluid intake (2,000 mL/day), unless contraindicated.
- Maintain supportive environment with family, friends, and groups.

Huntington disease

Rare, progressive, fatal, hereditary disorder that causes degeneration of basal ganglia and excess production of dopamine, leading to excessive involuntary movements and mental deterioration

Key signs and symptoms

- Personality changes, mood swings, and depression (can be mild at first but eventually disruptive
- Impaired judgment and forgetfulness
- Unsteady gait and choreiform movements (abnormal and excessive involuntary movements)
- Slurred speech, difficulty swallowing, and weight loss
- Gradual loss of musculoskeletal control (eventually leading to total dependence)

Key test results

- Genetic testing and family planning for anyone that carries the gene prior to pregnancy
- Neurological examination (tone, reflexes, coordination, balance)
- CT or MRI to show detailed images of the brain and structures
- PET detects the disease
- Deoxyribonucleic acid analysis detects the disease

Key treatments

- Monoamine depletors: tetrabenazine to decrease chorea movements
- Antidepressant: imipramine to alleviate depression
- Antipsychotics: chlorpromazine, haloperidol to help control chorea movements but may worsen dystonia and muscle rigidity
- Mood stabilizers: valproate, carbamazepine to help maintain mood with bipolar disorders
- Supportive, protective treatment aimed at relieving symptoms (Huntington disease has no known cure)

Key interventions

- Provide physical support by attending to client's basic needs (e.g., hygiene, skin care, bowel and bladder care, nutrition).
- Provide physical therapy (PT), speech therapy (ST), occupational therapy (OT), and psychotherapy to manage expectations during the progression of the disease and assess for risks of self-harm as suicide rates are high with this disease.
- Pad side rails of the bed but avoid restraints.
- Provide nutritional support as the disease progresses that may include NG tube or gastrostomy with feedings
- Offer support groups and coping strategies for end-of-life planning and care.

Ménière disease

Disorder of the inner ear, resulting in excess production of endolymphatic fluid in the semicircular canals. Can be related to blockage, immune response, allergies, infection, head trauma, or migraines

Key signs and symptoms

- Sensorineural hearing loss
- Severe vertigo that occurs without warning and lasts minutes to hours
- Nausea and vomiting related to vertigo
- Tinnitus
- Pressure in the affected ear(s)

Key test results

- Symptomatic: vertigo (two episodes lasting at least 20 minutes but not more than 24 hours)
- Videonystagmography (VNG) to assess eye movement when moving your head
- Vestibular evoked myogenic potential (VEMP) testing to show symptoms
- Audiometric studies indicate:
  ○ sensorineural hearing loss
  ○ loss of discrimination and recruitment.

Key treatments

- Restriction of sodium intake to less than 2 g/day
- Antibiotic: gentamicin injections into the ear to help control balance
- Steroids: dexamethasone injections into the ear to help control vertigo
- Anticholinergic: atropine (may stop an attack in 20 to 30 minutes)
- Antihistamine: meclizine, diphenhydramine to treat motion sickness and vertigo
- Meniett device that applies pressure to the middle ear to improve vertigo

Key interventions

- Advise client against reading and exposure to glaring lights during an attack.
- Stress safety measures.
- Instruct client not to get out of bed or walk without assistance during an attack.
- Instruct client to avoid sudden position changes.

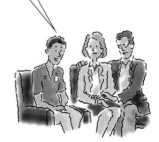

Clients diagnosed with Huntington disease may need extra care and support due to the degenerative nature of this condition.

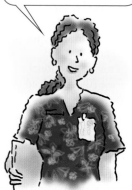

What safety measures are needed for a client with Ménière's disease and why?

- Instruct client to avoid tasks that vertigo makes hazardous.
- Before surgery, if client is vomiting, record fluid intake and output and characteristics of vomitus.
- Administer antiemetics as necessary.
- Give small amounts of fluid frequently.
- Tell client to expect dizziness and nausea for 1 or 2 days after surgery.

Meningitis

Inflammation of the meninges covering the brain and spinal cord that causes swelling resulting in symptoms. Can be bacterial (pneumococcus, meningococcus, *Haemophilus*, *Listeria*), viral (enteroviruses, usually mild), fungal (*Cryptococcus* if AIDS related, *Mycobacterium tuberculosis*) or from drug, chemical, or allergy reactions or inflammatory diseases (sarcoidosis)

Key signs and symptoms
- Anorexia
- Skin rash with meningococcal meningitis
- Chills
- Sudden high onset fever
- Headache
- Malaise
- Photophobia
- Positive Brudzinski sign (client flexes hips or knees when the nurse places the hands behind client's neck and flexes it forward)—a sign of meningeal inflammation and irritation
- Positive Kernig sign (pain or resistance when the client's leg is flexed at the hip or knee while the client is in a supine position)
- Stiff neck and back
- Vomiting

Key test results
- Blood cultures to identify the organism for specific treatment with appropriate medications
- CT or MRI to identify source of infection (sinusitis or chest) and to show inflammation
- Lumbar puncture shows:
  - elevated CSF pressure
  - cloudy or milky white CSF
  - high protein level
  - positive Gram stain and culture that usually identifies the infecting organism (unless it is a virus)
  - depressed CSF glucose concentration.

Key treatments
- Bed rest
- Hypothermia

- IV fluid administration
- Oxygen therapy, possibly with ET intubation and mechanical ventilation
- Antibiotics: penicillin G, ampicillin, or nafcillin; if allergic to penicillin, then tetracycline or chloramphenicol
- Diuretic: mannitol
- Anticonvulsants: phenytoin, phenobarbital
- Analgesics or antipyretics: acetaminophen, aspirin

Key interventions
- Monitor neurologic function often.
- Monitor and maintain ICP by reducing stressors (light, sound, position, pain, pressure, position; provide comfort, prevent shivering, no straining)
- Assess for changes in condition often.
- Monitor fluid balance; maintain adequate fluid intake.
- Relieve headache with a nonopioid analgesic.

Multiple sclerosis

Chronic, progressive, intermittent degenerative disorder that involves destruction of myelin sheath of the neurons in the brain and spinal cord

Key signs and symptoms
- Nystagmus, diplopia, blurred vision, optic neuritis
- Weakness, paresthesia, impaired sensation, paralysis
- Fatigue, dizziness, slurred speech
- Bowel and bladder function problems
- Lhermitte sign: electronic shock sensations that occur with some neck movements, particularly bending forward

Key test results
- CT scan eliminates other diagnoses such as brain or spinal cord tumors
- MRI may reveal plaques associated with multiple sclerosis
- Evoked potential tests to measure nervous system responses to stimuli

Key treatments
- Plasmapheresis to remove antibodies
- Cholinergic: bethanechol
- Glucocorticoids: prednisone, dexamethasone, corticotropin (ACTH)
- Immunosuppressants: interferon beta-1b, cyclophosphamide, methotrexate, glatiramer acetate
- Skeletal muscle relaxants: dantrolene, baclofen

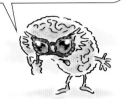

Sunglasses can help clients avoid bright lights that may exacerbate some disorders of the eye.

Key interventions

- Monitor for changes in motor coordination, paralysis, or muscle weakness.
- Encourage client to express feelings about changes in body image.
- Establish a bowel and bladder program.
- Maintain activity as tolerated (alternating rest and activity).

Myasthenia gravis

Chronic autoimmune neuromuscular disease characterized by deficiency of acetylcholine at the myoneural junction, causing extreme skeletal muscle weakness

Key signs and symptoms

- Dysphagia, drooling
- Ptosis or drooping of eyelids (early sign)
- Changes in facial expression
- Impaired speech (dysarthria)
- Muscle weakness and fatigue (typically, muscles are strongest in the morning but weaken throughout the day, especially after exercise)

Key test results

- Physical exam shows symptoms
- Blood test shows MuSK antibody (in half the cases)
- EMG shows impaired impulse conduction in the muscles
- Edrophonium test relieves symptoms after medication administration: positive indication of the disease
- CT or MRI to show thymoma

Key treatments

- Anticholinesterase inhibitors: pyridostigmine, neostigmine, ambenonium
- Immunosuppressants: azathioprine, cyclophosphamide
- Thymectomy
- Plasmapheresis to remove antibodies
- Intravenous immunoglobulin to bind to the antibodies and remove them from circulation

Key interventions

- Monitor neurologic and respiratory status.
- Prevent myasthenic crisis triggered by stressors requiring additional respiratory and muscular support.
- Prevent cholinergic crisis from too high a dose of medications or after general anesthesia
  - Flaccid paralysis, respiratory failure, increased sweating and salivation
  - Treat with antimuscarinic: atropine (antidote).
- Evaluate swallow and gag reflexes.
- Watch client for choking while eating.

Otosclerosis

Disease of the middle ear that involves progressive hardening of the ossicles

Key signs and symptoms

- Progressive hearing loss (low pitch sounds initially)
- Muffled speech tones and sounds
- Tinnitus
- Balance problems
- Dizziness

Key test results

- Audiogram to confirm hearing loss
- Tympanogram to measure sound conduction
- CT to visualize structures

Key treatments

- General screen tests
- Stapedectomy and insertion of a prosthesis to restore partial or total hearing

Key interventions

- Remove earwax blockage.
- Provide hearing aids.
- Consider cochlear implants.
- Develop alternative means of communication.
- Teach communication techniques (face the person one is speaking to, quiet setting, lower background noise, speak clearly and slowly).

Parkinson disease

Chronic, progressive, neurologic disease that involves a deficiency of dopamine production due to degeneration of substantia nigra

Key signs and symptoms

- "Pill-rolling" tremors, tremors at rest
- Masklike facial expression
- Speech and writing changes
- Shuffling gait, stiff joints, bradykinesia, "cogwheel" rigidity, stooped posture

Key test results

- EEG reveals minimal slowing of brain activity.
- No specific test to diagnose. Confirmation is typically postmortem. May have multiple tests to rule out other disorders.

Key treatments

- Antidepressant: amitriptyline
- Anticholinergic drugs: levodopa, levodopa-carbidopa, benztropine
- MAO-B inhibitors: selegiline, rasagiline, safinamide

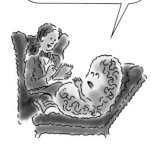

Charmed, I'm sure, but what's that ringing in my ears?

I haven't been feeling quite right lately.

- COMT inhibitors: tolcapone, entacapone
- Dopamine agonist: pramipexole, ropinirole

Key interventions

- Provide proper nutrition: diet high in fiber to prevent constipation.
- Provide PT, OT, ST.
- Monitor neurologic and respiratory status.
- Reinforce gait training for safety and balance control.
- Provide alternative therapies (massage, yoga, meditation, pet therapy).
- Suggest coping and support groups (respite care for family).
- Reinforce independence in care.

Retinal detachment

Emergent situation where the thin layer of tissue separates from the retina, depriving the eye of oxygen and nutrients

Key signs and symptoms

- Painless change in vision (floaters and flashes of light)
- Blurred vision
- Painless vision loss described as a "veil," "curtain," or "cobweb" that eliminates part of peripheral visual field (with progression of detachment)

Key test results

- Indirect ophthalmoscopy shows retinal tear or detachment
- Slit-lamp examination shows retinal tear or detachment
- Ultrasound with bleeding into the eyeball

Key treatments

- Scleral buckling to reattach the retina by sewing it into place
- Pneumatic retinopexy to inject air bubble into the eye to hold the retina into place and allow to adhere to the eye wall
- Photocoagulation to seal the retinal tear
- Cryopexy to freeze a scar into place holding the retina to the eye wall
- Vitrectomy to remove the vitreous fluid and tissue to flatten the retina (combined with scleral buckling)

Key interventions

- Postoperatively, instruct client to lie on back or on unoperated side.
- Discourage straining during defecation; bending down; and hard coughing, sneezing, or vomiting.
- Administer eye drops as prescribed.
- Leave eye shield in place as prescribed.

Spinal cord injury

Damage to spinal cord, vertebral column, supporting tissue or disks due to traumatic or nontraumatic causes that may lead to loss of motor function, sensory function, reflexes, and control of elimination

Key signs and symptoms

- Related to the level of injury (motor, sensory, or both)
- Can be total or complete transection of the cord
- Can have loss of bowel and bladder control
- Can have flaccid paralysis below the level of the injury
- Can have paresthesia below the level of the injury
- Can be ipsilateral, bilateral, or unilateral depending on the section of cord damaged
- Can have loss of pain and temperature sensation
- Can maintain light touch and vibration sensation

Key test results

- CT scan shows spinal cord edema, vertebral fracture, and spinal cord compression
- MRI shows spinal cord edema, vertebral fracture, and spinal cord compression

Key treatments

- Flat position, with neck immobilized in a cervical collar
- Maintenance of vertebral alignment through Crutchfield tongs, Gardner-Wells tongs, or Halo vest
- Surgery for stabilization of the upper spine, such as insertion of Harrington rods
- Antianxiety agent: lorazepam
- Glucocorticoid: methylprednisolone given as infusion immediately following injury (may improve neurologic recovery when administered within 8 hours of injury)
- Histamine-2 (H_2) receptor antagonists: cimetidine, ranitidine, famotidine, nizatidine
- Laxative: bisacodyl
- Mucosal barrier fortifier: sucralfate
- Muscle relaxant: dantrolene

Key interventions

- Monitor neurologic and respiratory status.
- Observe for signs and symptoms of spinal shock.
- Provide ventilator support for cervical (C4–C5) injuries if needed.
- Check for autonomic dysreflexia (sudden, extreme rise in blood pressure).
- Provide skin care.

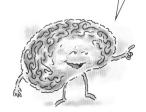

Healthy brain function is a beautiful thing.

Cerebrovascular accident (stroke)

Destruction of brain cells due to a decrease in cerebral blood flow and oxygen. Two major types: ischemic stroke and hemorrhagic stroke.

Key signs and symptoms

- Garbled or impaired speech
- Inability to move, or difficulty moving, limbs on one side of the body
- Hemianopsia (loss of half of visual field)
- Headache
- Mental impairment
- Seizures
- Coma
- Vomiting

Key test results

- CT scan reveals intracranial bleeding, infarct (shows up 24 hours after the initial symptoms), or shift of midline structures
- Digital subtraction angiography reveals occlusion or narrowing of vessels
- MRI shows intracranial bleeding, infarct, or shift of midline structures

Key treatments

- Anticoagulants: heparin, warfarin, dabigatran, apixaban, rivaroxaban, edoxaban
- Anticonvulsant: phenytoin
- Glucocorticoid: dexamethasone
- Thrombolytic therapy: tissue plasminogen activator given within first 3 hours of an ischemic stroke to:
  ○ restore circulation to the affected brain tissue
  ○ limit extent of brain injury upon review of CT scan (head).
- Antiplatelet aggregation agent: ticlopidine, clopidogrel

Key interventions

- Monitor for increased ICP and treat with mannitol as prescribed.
- Assess for cerebral perfusion (change in level of consciousness, headache, change in respirations, pupillary changes).
- Take vital signs every 1 to 2 hours initially and then every 4 hours when client becomes stable.
- Elevate the head of the bed 30 degrees or as tolerated.
- Conduct a neurologic assessment every 1 to 2 hours initially and then every 4 hours when client becomes stable using GCS and NIH stroke assessment tools.

Trigeminal neuralgia

Disorder of trigeminal nerve (cranial nerve V) that causes severe stabbing pain on one side of the face

Key signs or symptoms

- Searing pain in the facial area

Key test results

- Observation during examination shows client favoring (splinting) affected area
- To ward off painful attack, client often holds face immobile when talking
- Client may leave affected side of face unwashed and unshaven

Key treatments

- Anticonvulsants: carbamazepine or phenytoin
- Avoid trigging the nerve on effected side (washing face, brushing teeth, eating, drinking)
- Eye protection/covers to affected side
- Anticonvulsant: Carbamazepine or gabapentin to reduce the nerve transmission reducing the pain
- Surgical decompression of the nerve
- Radiofrequency thermal coagulation
- Percutaneous balloon compression

Key interventions

- Observe and record characteristics of each attack, including client's protective mechanisms.
- Provide adequate nutrition in small, frequent meals at room temperature.
- Advise client to place food in unaffected side of mouth when chewing.
- Advise client to brush teeth and rinse mouth often.
- Advise client to see dentist twice per year to detect cavities.
- After surgical decompression of the root or partial nerve dissection, check neurologic and vital signs often.
- Watch for adverse reactions to prescribed medications.

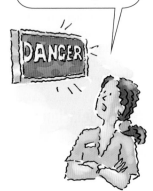

Strokes are life-threatening, and sudden symptoms of garbled or impaired speech, inability to move a limb, or loss of half the visual field should be taken seriously.

Neurosensory questions, answers, and rationales

1. A client is admitted with homonymous hemianopsia. Which intervention(s) will the nurse implement? Select all that apply.
1. Check gag reflex before allowing the client to eat.
2. Approach client each time on the unaffected side.
3. Allow enough time for the client to answer the questions.
4. Test bath water with the use of thermometer each time.
5. Gradually teach client to compensate by scanning.

1. **2, 5.** Homonymous hemianopsia is the loss of half of each visual field. This is usually seen in clients with cerebrovascular accident or stroke. The nurse should approach the client on the unaffected side and teach the client to compensate by scanning or turning the head to see things on the affected side. The other interventions are not related to homonymous hemianopsia.
CN: Safe, effective care environment; CNS: Safety and infection control; CL: Apply

2. A client is admitted with thrombotic cerebral vascular accident (CVA). The nurse understands which condition can be a contributing factor?
1. Atrial fibrillation (AF)
2. Premature ventricular contractions (PVC)
3. Deep vein thrombosis (DVT)
4. Myocardial infarction (MI)

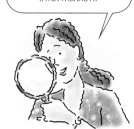

Look carefully in question #2 for the "vital" piece of information.

2. **1.** CVA is associated with cardiac arrhythmias, usually atrial fibrillation. Atrial fibrillation occurs with the irregular and rapid discharge from multiple ectopic atrial foci that cause quivering of the atria without atrial systole. This asynchronous atrial contraction predisposes to mural thrombi, which may embolize, leading to a stroke. PVCs, past MI, or DVT do not lead to arterial embolization.
CN: Physiological integrity; CNS: Physiological adaptation; CL: Understand

3. The health care provider prescribed t-PA, a thrombolytic agent, at 0.9 mg/kg over 1 hour for a client weighing 125 lb (56.7 kg). How many milligrams will the nurse give in each dose? Record your answer using a whole number.

_____ mg

3. **51**

$$\textit{full dosage ordered} \times \textit{weight} = \textit{amount by dose}$$

$$0.9\ mg/kg \times 56.7\ kg = 51.03\ mg$$

CN: Physiological integrity; CNS: Pharmacological and parenteral therapies; CL: Apply

4. A client is receiving dabigatran. Which information will the nurse include while providing client teaching?
1. Avoid people with upper respiratory infections.
2. Discontinue the medication before surgery.
3. Check daily for signs of calf pain or tenderness.
4. Take the medication with urokinase.

4. **2.** Dabigatran is an anticoagulant used to reduce the risk of having stroke, atrial fibrillation, and pulmonary embolism. It should be discontinued at least 48 hours prior to elective surgery or invasive procedures because it would cause bleeding. The client does not need to monitor daily for symptoms of deep vein thrombosis while taking anticoagulants. Giving dabigatran with antiplatelet agents, heparin, aspirin, NSAIDs, and fibrinolytic agents such as urokinase is not appropriate because this would cause further bleeding.
CN: Physiological integrity; CNS: Pharmacological and parenteral therapies; CL: Apply

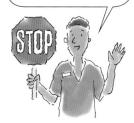

Read question #5 slowly. You are looking for the *priority*.

5. The nurse is caring for a client in the acute phase of an ischemic stroke. Which nursing intervention is **priority**?
1. Thicken all dietary liquids.
2. Recline the client to less than 30 degrees.
3. Place the client in the supine position.
4. Have tracheal suction available.

5. **4.** Because of a potential loss of gag reflex and potential altered level of consciousness, the client should be kept in Fowler's or a semi-prone position with tracheal suction available at all times. Unless heart failure is present, restricting fluids is not indicated. Thickening dietary liquids is not done until the gag reflex returns or the stroke has evolved and the deficit can be assessed.
CN: Physiological integrity; CNS: Reduction of risk potential; CL: Apply

CN: Client needs category   CNS: Client needs subcategory   CL: Cognitive level

6. A client is receiving clopidogrel bisulfate. The nurse will closely monitor the client for which potential complication(s) while on this medication? Select all that apply.
  1. Sepsis
  2. Melena
  3. Ecchymosis
  4. Drowsiness
  5. Hematuria
  6. Petechiae

6. 2, 3, 5, 6. Clopidogrel bisulfate is an antiplatelet agent. The client should be monitored for signs of bleeding like ecchymosis, melena, hematuria, and petechiae while on this medication. The other manifestations are not related to bleeding.
CN: Physiological integrity; CNS: Pharmacological and parenteral therapies; CL: Apply

7. A client is admitted with new onset ptosis, progressive muscle weakness, and blurred vision. Which nursing intervention is **priority**?
  1. Observe for bleeding.
  2. Promote mobility.
  3. Monitor breathing.
  4. Prevent dehydration.

7. 3. Myasthenia gravis is a neuromuscular disorder that causes extreme muscle weakness, ptosis (early onset), and blurred vision due to the deficiency of acetylcholine at the myoneural junction. The nurse should monitor the respiratory status frequently because the respiratory muscles may also be involved. Bleeding is not a common complication of myasthenia gravis. The nurse will need to determine the client's muscle involvement before determining if mobility is appropriate at this time. Dehydration is not an immediate complication. This may be a concern as muscle weakness progresses.
CN: Safe, effective care environment; CNS: Management of care; CL: Analyze

8. The nurse is caring for a client diagnosed with a thrombotic right brain stroke with swelling of the left arm. The nurse will monitor the client's affected extremity for which complication?
  1. Elbow contracture
  2. Loss of muscle contraction
  3. Deep vein thrombosis (DVT)
  4. Hypoalbuminemia

8. 2. In clients with hemiplegia or hemiparesis, loss of muscle contraction decreases venous return and may cause swelling of the affected extremity. Stroke is not linked to protein loss. DVT may develop in clients with a stroke but is more likely in the lower extremities. Contractures, or bony calcifications, may occur with stroke but do not appear with swelling.
CN: Physiological integrity; CNS: Physiological adaptation; CL: Apply

9. A client is diagnosed with a brain stem infarction. During assessment, the nurse will monitor the client for which conditions?
  1. Aphasia and motor deficits
  2. Bradypnea and change in pulse
  3. Contralateral hemiplegia and tachycardia
  4. Numbness of the face and arms

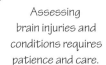

Assessing brain injuries and conditions requires patience and care.

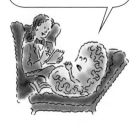

9. 2. The brain stem contains the medulla and the vital cardiac, vasomotor, and respiratory centers. A brain stem infarction leads to vital sign changes such as bradypnea. Numbness, tingling in the face, contralateral hemiplegia, and aphasia may occur with a stroke.
CN: Physiological integrity; CNS: Physiological adaptation; CL: Apply

10. A client diagnosed with a stroke involving Wernicke's area is being admitted to the unit. Which action by the nurse is **most** appropriate?
  1. Listen and watch carefully while the client is speaking.
  2. Allow enough time for the client to answer questions.
  3. Check the client's gag reflex during admission.
  4. Give the client simple and slow instructions.

10. 4. Wernicke's area is located on the left side of the temporal region and is likely the cause of receptive aphasia. Receptive aphasia means that the client is having difficulty understanding spoken and written language. Giving simple and slow directions would help the client understand the message. Listening and watching carefully while the client is speaking, and giving enough time to answer questions, are appropriate nursing interventions for a client with expressive aphasia. Checking the gag reflex is necessary for a client with dysphagia or difficulty in swallowing.
CN: Physiological integrity; CNS: Basic care and comfort; CL: Apply

11. The nurse is caring for a client postoperatively following a intracapsular lens implant. Which finding will the nurse teach the client to report **immediately** to the health care provider?
1. Blurred vision
2. Eye pain
3. Yellow glare
4. Occasional itching

12. The nurse notes clear fluid draining from the nose of a client who sustained a severe head injury. The nurse notifies the health care provider about a suspicion of which condition?
1. Basilar skull fracture
2. Cerebral concussion
3. Cerebral palsy exacerbation
4. Acute sinus infection

13. A 17-year-old client is admitted after suffering blunt trauma to the head. When offered acetaminophen, the client asks for a stronger pain medication. Which response by the nurse is **most** appropriate?
1. "You have a mild concussion; acetaminophen is the best choice right now."
2. "Opioids are avoided after a head injury because they may hide a worsening condition."
3. "Aspirin is avoided because of the danger of Reye syndrome in children or young adults."
4. "Stronger medications may lead to vomiting, which increases intracranial pressure (ICP)."

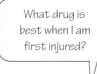

What drug is best when I am first injured?

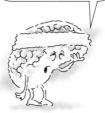

14. A client admitted to the hospital with a subarachnoid hemorrhage (SAH) reports severe headache, nuchal rigidity, and projectile vomiting. The health care provider prescribes a lumbar puncture (LP). Which action will the nurse complete **next**?
1. Have the client sign the written consent.
2. Clarify the prescription with the health care provider.
3. Obtain the equipment needed to perform a LP.
4. Anticipate admission to the intensive care unit (ICU).

15. When evaluating an arterial blood gas (ABG) from a client with a subdural hematoma, the nurse notes the client is in respiratory acidosis with hypoxia. Which nursing intervention is appropriate?
1. Increase the client's respiratory rate.
2. Give 100% oxygen via nasal cannula.
3. Administer a sedative to the client.
4. Lower the client's head of the bed.

11. 2. Pain should not be present after cataract surgery. Pain may be an indication of hyphema or clouding in the anterior chamber, and of infection. The client should be informed that blurred vision, a yellow glare, and intermittent itching may be present following the procedure.
CN: Safe, effective care environment; CNS: Management of care; CL: Apply

12. 1. Clear fluid draining from the ear or nose of a client may mean a cerebrospinal fluid leak, which is common in basilar skull fractures. Concussion is associated with a brief loss of consciousness; sinus infection is associated with facial pain and pressure with or without nasal drainage; and cerebral palsy is associated with nonprogressive paralysis present since birth.
CN: Safe, effective care environment; CNS: Management of care; CL: Apply

13. 2. Opioids may mask changes in the level of consciousness (LOC) that indicate increased ICP and should not be given. Saying acetaminophen is strong enough ignores the client's question and therefore is not appropriate. Aspirin is contraindicated in conditions that may cause bleeding, such as trauma, and for children or young adults with viral illnesses because of the danger of Reye syndrome. However, this response does not address the client's concern. Stronger medications may not necessarily lead to vomiting but will sedate the client, thereby masking changes in the LOC.
CN: Physiological integrity; CNS: Reduction of risk potential; CL: Apply

14. 2. Severe headache, nuchal rigidity, and projectile vomiting are signs of ICP. Sudden removal of cerebrospinal fluid results in pressures in the lumbar area lower than the brain and favors herniation of the brain; therefore, LP is contraindicated with increased ICP. Clarifying the procedure is priority. Because it is undetermined if a LP is appropriate for this client, obtaining consent and equipment are not needed at this time. Admission to ICU may be required but is not a priority.
CN: Safe, effective care environment; CNS: Management of care; CL: Apply

15. 1. ABGs in respiratory acidosis are pH less than 7.35 and a $PaCO_2$ more than 45 mm Hg. Hypoxia is an indication of oxygen at the tissue level and is evaluated by SpO_2 readings. The goal is to get the client to blow off more carbon dioxide (CO_2) by increasing the respiratory rate. Decreasing the respiratory rate will increase the CO_2, and 100% oxygen is not given by nasal cannula.
CN: Physiological integrity; CNS: Physiological adaptation; CL: Apply

16. A client with an open head trauma develops a urine output of 300 mL/hour, dry skin, and dry mucous membranes. Which nursing intervention is **most** appropriate?
  1. Check urine specific gravity.
  2. Anticipate treatment for renal failure.
  3. Restrict sodium intake.
  4. Increase IV fluid rate.

16. 1. Urine output of 300 mL/hour may indicate diabetes insipidus, which is failure of the pituitary to produce antidiuretic hormone. This may occur with increased intracranial pressure and head trauma; the nurse evaluates for low urine specific gravity, increased serum osmolarity, and dehydration. There is no evidence that the client is experiencing renal failure. Restricting sodium is not a priority. Increasing the IV rate may be done after the specific gravity has been evaluated.
CN: Safe, effective care environment; CNS: Management of care; CL: Apply

17. The nurse is assigned to care for four clients. Which client will the nurse see **first**?
  1. A client with meningitis experiencing nuchal rigidity
  2. A client diagnosed with a cerebrovascular accident with hemianopsia
  3. A client with myasthenia gravis reporting flu-like symptoms
  4. A client with trigeminal neuralgia with stabbing pain on the face

I just hate brain freeze, don't you!

17. 3. A client with myasthenia gravis with flulike symptoms should be checked first because infection may cause myasthenic crisis. The client may have an abrupt onset of extreme muscle weakness with inability to swallow, speak, and maintain respiration. Airway is the priority for this client. A client with meningitis is expected to have stiff neck or nuchal rigidity. Hemianopsia, or loss of half of visual field, is usually seen in clients with stroke. A client with trigeminal neuralgia will usually report stabbing pain on one side of the face during an acute episode.
CN: Safe, effective care environment; CNS: Management of care; CL: Analyze

18. A client is admitted with a brain tumor. Which vital signs will the nurse expect the client to exhibit?
  1. Temperature, 98° F (36.7° C); pulse, 108; respirations, 14; blood pressure, 120/82 mm Hg
  2. Temperature, 97° F (36.1° C); pulse, 60; respirations, 23; blood pressure, 158/94 mm Hg
  3. Temperature, 99° F (37.2° C); pulse, 52; respirations, 12; blood pressure, 176/86 mm Hg
  4. Temperature, 96° F (35.6° C); pulse, 82; respirations, 16; blood pressure, 149/82 mm Hg

18. 3. A client with brain tumor will experience an increase in intracranial pressure (ICP). One of the assessment findings in increased ICP is Cushing's triad, which includes hypertension, bradycardia, and widening pulse pressure.
CN: Physiological integrity; CNS: Physiological adaptation; CL: Apply

19. The nurse is administering mannitol to a client in the intensive care unit. Which finding indicates to the nurse the client is responding appropriately to the medication?
  1. Urine output of 450 mL in 4 hours
  2. Pupils are 8 mm and nonreactive
  3. Systolic blood pressure of 150 mm Hg
  4. Serum creatinine of 2.5 mg/dL (221 μmol/L)

19. 1. Mannitol promotes osmotic diuresis by increasing the pressure gradient in the renal tubules. The normal urine output is 30 to 50 mL/hour. A urine output of 450 mL in 4 hours indicates the client has an increase in urine output; therefore, is a sign of effectiveness of the medication. The normal serum creatinine is 0.6 to 1.2 mg/dL (53 to 106 μmol/L). Serum creatinine of 2.5 mg/dL (221 μmol/L) is not a sign of effectiveness of the medication because the result is elevated. The systolic blood pressure should go down because of diuresis. Fixed and dilated pupils are symptoms of increased ICP or cranial nerve damage.
CN: Physiological integrity; CNS: Pharmacological and parenteral therapies; CL: Analyze

20. Which nursing intervention is **most** appropriate to prevent foot drop and contractures in a client recovering from a subdural hematoma?
1. Wearing high-top sneakers
2. Starting low-dose heparin therapy
3. Referring the client to physical therapy
4. Applying sequential compression devices

20. 1. High-top sneakers are used to prevent foot drop and contractures in neurologic clients. Low-dose heparin therapy and sequential compression boots will prevent deep vein thrombosis. A consultation with physical therapy is important to prevent foot drop and should be initiated by the nurse.
CN: Physiological integrity; CNS: Basic care and comfort; CL: Apply

21. A client is diagnosed with right subarachnoid hemorrhage. It is important for the nurse to place the client in which position following assessment?
1. Elevate the head of bed.
2. Turn the client onto the right side.
3. Put the client in modified Trendelenburg.
4. Place the client supine.

21. 1. Elevating the head of the bed enhances cerebral venous return and thereby decreases intracranial pressure (ICP). The other positions would not decrease ICP.
CN: Physiological integrity; CNS: Reduction of risk potential; CL: Apply

22. The nurse teaches a client with Parkinson disease to avoid which food(s) while taking selegiline? Select all that apply.
1. Salami
2. Eggs
3. Aged cheese
4. Soy sauce
5. Milk
6. Sauerkraut

22. 1, 3, 4, 6. Selegiline is a monoamine oxidase B (MAO-B) inhibitor used in clients with Parkinson disease. The nurse should tell the client to avoid foods with high tyramine content while on this medication because it would cause hypertensive crisis. Salami, aged cheese, soy sauce, and sauerkraut are foods with high tyramine content and should be avoided. Milk and eggs can be safely given to the client while on selegiline.
CN: Physiological integrity; CNS: Pharmacological and parenteral therapies; CL: Apply

23. A client with a history of petite mal seizures reports a visual aura. Which nursing action is **priority**?
1. Ask the client to describe the aura in detail.
2. Place the client near the nurses' station.
3. Immediately notify the health care provider.
4. Pad side rails and lower the height of the bed.

23. 4. A visual aura is a warning sign of an impending seizure. The nurse should immediately institute seizure precautions such as padding the side rails and lowering the bed. Completing a more detailed assessment is important as well as notifying the health care provider and placing the client near the nurses' station, but these are not priority over client safety.
CN: Safe, effective care environment; CNS: Safety and infection control; CL: Analyze

24. A client had a lumbar laminectomy. Which nursing action is **best** postoperatively?
1. Encourage the client to be out of bed the first postoperative day.
2. Ensure the client wears a supportive brace at all times.
3. Limit movement in bed and reposition only when necessary.
4. Place a soft microfoam mattress with extra support on the client's bed.

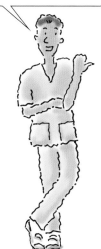

Looks like personal protective equipment is needed. What should you do?

24. 1. In most cases, clients should be out of bed the first postoperative day. Frequent repositioning, use of a chair-like brace for the lower back when out of bed, and a firm mattress will help minimize complications.
CN: Physiological integrity; CNS: Reduction of risk potential; CL: Apply

25. A client is admitted with a stiff neck, photophobia, fever, and malaise after a viral infection. The nurse will implement which precaution(s) when caring for this client? Select all that apply.
1. Wear gloves.
2. Wear a gown.
3. Wear a mask.
4. Wear goggles.
5. Wash hands.

25. 3, 5. A client with meningitis is placed on airborne precaution. The nurse should wear a mask or respirator when taking care of this client. The nurse should always wash hands before and after client care. Gloves and gown are both used for contact precaution. Goggles are used when there is any chance of splashing.
CN: Safe, effective care environment; CNS: Safety and infection control; CL: Apply

CN: Client needs category   CNS: Client needs subcategory   CL: Cognitive level

26. A client admitted with amyotrophic lateral sclerosis (ALS) is prescribed riluzole. The nurse will **immediately** notify the health care provider if which finding(s) is noted? Select all that apply.
1. History of hepatitis B
2. Client stumbles while walking
3. History of constipation
4. Blood pressure 130/86 mm Hg
5. The client is 6 weeks' pregnant

26. 1, 5. Amyotrophic lateral sclerosis (ALS), or Lou Gehrig's disease, is a progressive motor neuron disease that causes muscle wasting or atrophy. Riluzole is prescribed to delay disease progression and prolong life expectancy. Riluzole should not be prescribed to a client with liver disease, such as hepatitis B, because it can worsen liver disease. It also should not be taken while pregnant unless the benefit exceeds the risk (category C). Stumbling and constipation are common early symptoms of ALS. A blood pressure within normal range is appropriate for receiving riluzole.
CN: Safe, effective care environment; CNS: Management of care; CL: Apply

27. The nurse is preparing a client for a myelography. Which intervention will the nurse perform before the test?
1. Determine if the client is allergic to iodine.
2. Mark distal pulses on the foot in ink.
3. Check and document pain along the sciatic nerve.
4. Tell the client to cough or pant to clear the dye.

27. 1. A radiopaque dye, commonly iodine-based, is instilled into the spinal canal to outline structures during myelography; therefore, asking about iodine allergy is needed. Pain may be expected along the sciatic nerve with herniated nucleus pulposus. During cardiac catheterization, a client coughs or pants to clear the dye; before cardiac catheterization or arteriogram, the nurse marks pedal pulses in ink.
CN: Physiological integrity; CNS: Reduction of risk potential; CL: Apply

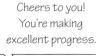

Cheers to you! You're making excellent progress.

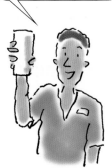

28. When assisting the client to eat during the rehabilitation phase of an ischemic stroke, the nurse will include which educational information during teaching? **Select all that apply.**
1. "Look up at the ceiling when you swallow."
2. "Tuck your chin in when you swallow."
3. "Turn your head to your weaker side when swallowing."
4. "After swallowing food, wait a few seconds then swallow again."
5. "Swallow softly between each bite of food."

28. 2, 3, 4. Tucking the chin in reduces the size of the airway opening, which helps prevent aspiration, and a double swallow helps clear the pharynx between bites of food. Having the client turn the head toward the weaker side makes swallowing easier. Waiting a few seconds before swallowing again allows time for the esophagus to clear. Swallowing forcefully reduces the amount of residual food in the client's pharynx.
CN: Physiological integrity; CNS: Basic care and comfort; CL: Apply

29. After receiving report, the nurse will see which client **first**?
1. A 17-year-old client 24 hours postappendectomy.
2. A 33-year-old client with a recent diagnosis of Guillain-Barré syndrome.
3. A 50-year-old client 3 days post–myocardial infarction (MI).
4. A 42-year-old client with diverticulitis exacerbation.

29. 2. Guillain-Barré syndrome is characterized by ascending paralysis and potential respiratory failure. The order of client assessment should follow client priorities, with disorders of airway, breathing, and then circulation. There is no information to suggest the post-MI client has an arrhythmia or other complication. There is no evidence to suggest hemorrhage or perforation for the remaining clients as a priority of care.
CN: Safe, effective care environment; CNS: Management of care; CL: Analyze

30. What will the nurse include in the plan of care when treating a client with Bell's palsy?
1. Protect the client's skin integrity.
2. Provide routine bilateral eye care.
3. Prevent complications of immobility.
4. Maintain normal bowel elimination.

30. 2. Bell's palsy is the disorder of cranial nerve VII (facial nerve) that causes weakness or paralysis of one side of the face. The client will also have difficulty closing the eye of the affected side. The nurse should provide eye care by using eye drops and an eye patch to prevent corneal dryness and to protect the eye from irritation. The other options are not appropriate.
CN: Physiological integrity; CNS: Basic care and comfort; CL: Apply

31. The nurse is discharging a 25-year-old client diagnosed with myasthenia gravis. When providing education on cyclophosphamide, which statement will the nurse include in the teaching?
1. "You need to limit your daily fluid intake to 1 liter."
2. "You may notice wounds take longer to heal while on cyclophosphamide."
3. "This medication may affect your ability to have children in the future."
4. "If you develop a fever, notify the health care provider immediately."

31. 4. Cyclophosphamide is given to clients with myasthenia gravis, an autoimmune disorder, to decrease the immune system to limit autoantibody production. These autoantibodies cause the destruction of acetylcholine receptors, which leads to muscle weakness. Clients with a fever, or any signs of an illness, should notify their health care provider immediately. Their dosage may need to be adjusted or the medication may need to be held to allow healing. Clients taking cyclophosphamide should consume ample fluids daily to prevent renal complications such as hemorrhagic cystitis. Wound healing may be delayed due to immunosuppression. Cyclophosphamide may affect fertility in both men and women.
CN: Physiological integrity; CNS: Pharmacological and parenteral therapies; CL: Apply

32. When preparing a client for an electroencephalogram (EEG), which nursing action(s) is appropriate? Select all that apply.
1. Determine if the client is allergic to iodine or shellfish.
2. Tell the client to shampoo hair before the procedure.
3. Tell the client to avoid caffeine 12 hours prior to the test.
4. Instruct the client not to eat or drink anything after midnight.
5. Inform the client that the procedure is painful.

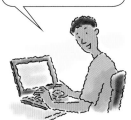

In question #32, remember to select all that apply.

32. 2, 3. EEG is a test that measures the electrical activity of the brain. The nurse should advise the client to shampoo hair and avoid using hair products before the procedure because electrodes will be placed on the client's scalp. Caffeine should also be avoided 12 hours prior to the test. A dye or contrast medium is not injected during EEG; therefore, asking the client about allergy to iodine or shellfish is not necessary. The client should avoid fasting because hypoglycemia will alter the result of the test. EEG is a painless procedure.
CN: Physiological integrity; CNS: Reduction of risk potential; CL: Apply

33. One hour after receiving pyridostigmine, a client reports difficulty swallowing and excessive respiratory secretions. The nurse notifies the health care provider and prepares to administer which medication?
1. Pyridostigmine
2. Atropine
3. Edrophonium
4. Acyclovir

33. 2. These symptoms suggest cholinergic crisis or excessive acetylcholinesterase medication, typically appearing 45 to 60 minutes after the last dose of acetylcholinesterase inhibitor. Atropine, an anticholinergic drug, is used to antagonize acetylcholinesterase inhibitors. The other drugs are acetylcholinesterase inhibitors. Edrophonium is used to diagnose myasthenia gravis, and pyridostigmine is used to treat the condition and would worsen the symptoms. Acyclovir is an antiviral and would not be used to treat the client's symptoms.
CN: Physiological integrity; CNS: Pharmacological and parenteral therapies; CL: Analyze

34. A client diagnosed with a brain abscess is prescribed nafcillin. Which finding(s) noted in the client's history will cause the nurse to question this prescription? Select all that apply.
1. History of asthma
2. Allergy to penicillin
3. Blood urea nitrogen (BUN) 15 mg/dL (5.4 mmol/L)
4. Alanine aminotransferase (ALT) 30 u/L (0.5 μkat/L)
5. Urine output 865 mL over the past 24 hours

34. 2. Nafcillin is a penicillin antibiotic given to treat bacterial infections. Clients with previous hypersensitivity reactions to penicillins or cephalosporins should not receive nafcillin due to the high risk of an anaphylactic reaction. Clients with a history of asthma should be monitored closely for a reaction, but can receive nafcillin. The BUN and ALT levels and urine output are all within normal range; therefore, the client can receive nafcillin. Clients with liver or renal impairment may not be candidates for nafcillin therapy.
CN: Physiological integrity; CNS: Pharmacological and parenteral therapies; CL: Apply

35. The nurse is assessing a client with increased intraocular pressure (IOP). The nurse will expect which finding(s)? Select all that apply.
1. Severe eye pain
2. Halos around lights
3. Loss of central vision
4. Soft globe on palpation
5. Decreased accommodation

35. 1, 2, 5. Glaucoma is largely asymptomatic. Symptoms can include: severe eye and head pain, loss of peripheral vision or blind spots, reddened sclera, firm globe, decreased accommodation, halos around lights, and occasional eye pain. Loss of central vision is seen in clients with macular degeneration.
CN: Physiological integrity; CNS: Physiological adaptation;
CL: Apply

36. The nurse is educating a client with an acute head injury on famotidine capsules. Which statement made by the client indicates the education is understood?
1. "I will be sure to take this medication with food."
2. "I will take famotidine once every day."
3. "I can take famotidine even though I am allergic to ranitidine."
4. "It is okay to chew or crush this medication."

36. 2. Famotidine is a histamine-2 (H2)-receptor antagonist, which decreases acid produced by the stomach. Famotidine can be taken with or without food once a day. Clients allergic to another H2-receptor antagonist should not take famotidine due to the high probability of hypersensitivity. Capsules should not be crushed or chewed. If the client cannot swallow the pill, a chewable tablet may be prescribed.
CN: Physiological integrity; CNS: Pharmacological and parenteral therapies; CL: Apply

37. The nurse is caring for a client with a cerebral injury who is showing signs of receptive aphasia and unilateral deafness. Which part of the brain does the nurse suspect has been affected?
1. Frontal lobe
2. Parietal lobe
3. Occipital lobe
4. Temporal lobe

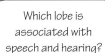

Which lobe is associated with speech and hearing?

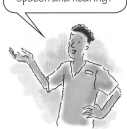

37. 4. The portion of the cerebrum that controls speech and hearing is the temporal lobe. Injury to the frontal lobe causes personality changes, difficulty speaking, and disturbances in memory, reasoning, and concentration. Injury to the parietal lobe causes sensory alterations and problems with spatial relationships. Damage to the occipital lobe causes vision disturbances.
CN: Physiological integrity; CNS: Physiological adaptation;
CL: Understand

38. The nurse is caring for a client with an essential tremor and pending diagnosis of Parkinson disease. For which complication will the nurse observe this client?
1. Bilateral exophthalmos
2. Diminished distal extremity sensation
3. Excessive involuntary movements
4. Bradykinesia and shuffling gate

38. 4. Parkinson disease is characterized by the slowing of voluntary muscle movement (bradykinesia), muscular rigidity, shuffling gate, and resting tremor. Dopamine is deficient in this disorder. Diminished distal extremity sensation does not occur in Parkinson disease. Bulging eyeballs (exophthalmos) occurs in Graves' disease. Excessive involuntary movement is a sign of Huntington disease.
CN: Physiological integrity; CNS: Physiological adaptation;
CL: Apply

39. The nurse is caring for a client prescribed neostigmine. The nurse will be **most** concerned if which symptom(s) is noted? Select all that apply.
1. Dry mouth
2. Abdominal cramps
3. Increased sweating
4. Sudden tachycardia
5. Increased urination

39. 1, 4. Neostigmine is an anticholinesterase drug used to improve muscle strength in clients with myasthenia gravis. It blocks the action of cholinesterase and increases the level of acetylcholine at the neuromuscular junction. This drug causes excessive salivation, not dry mouth. The client may also experience bradycardia, not tachycardia. Therefore, the nurse would be most concerned about any unexpected symptoms. Abdominal cramps, increased sweating, and increased urination are all side effects of neostigmine.
CN: Safe, effective care environment; CNS: Management of care;
CL: Apply

CN: Client needs category   CNS: Client needs subcategory   CL: Cognitive level

40. The nurse understands which client is **most** at risk for secondary Parkinson disease caused by pharmacotherapy?
1. A 30-year-old client with schizophrenia taking chlorpromazine
2. A 50-year-old client taking nitroglycerin tablets for angina
3. A 60-year-old client taking prednisone for chronic obstructive pulmonary disease
4. A 75-year-old client using naproxen for rheumatoid arthritis

40. 1. Phenothiazines, such as chlorpromazine, deplete dopamine, which may lead to tremor and rigidity (extrapyramidal effects). The other clients are not at a greater risk for developing Parkinson disease caused by pharmacotherapy.
CN: Physiological integrity; CNS: Pharmacological and parenteral therapies; CL: Analyze

41. The nurse is assigned to care for a client with Parkinson disease who practices orthodox Judaism. Which dietary instruction(s) will the nurse consider when developing the client's plan of care? Select all that apply.
1. Any combination of meat and milk is forbidden.
2. Strictly adhere to lacto-ovo-vegetarian diet.
3. Only fish that have scales and fins can be offered.
4. Meat products not ritually slaughtered are forbidden.
5. Fasting is observed during the month of Ramadan.

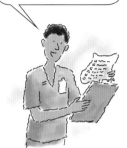

With orthodox Jewish clients, keep it kosher.

41. 1, 3, 4. Jewish dietary kosher laws include eating only fish that have scales and fins, prohibiting eating meat products not ritually slaughtered, and avoiding eating meat with milk products. Seventh Day Adventists and Buddhists may follow a lacto-ovo-vegetarian diet. Muslims may fast during the month of Ramadan.
CN: Psychosocial integrity; CNS: None; CL: Apply

42. To evaluate the effectiveness of levodopa–carbidopa in a client with Parkinson disease, the nurse will observe for which outcome?
1. Improved visual acuity
2. Increased dyskinesia
3. Reduced short-term memory
4. Lessened rigidity and tremor

42. 4. Levodopa–carbidopa increases the amount of dopamine in the central nervous system, allowing for smooth, purposeful movements. The drug does not affect visual acuity and should improve dyskinesia and short-term memory.
CN: Physiological integrity; CNS: Pharmacological and parenteral therapies; CL: Apply

43. After starting therapy with sucralfate, a client reports a dry mouth. Which nursing intervention is **best** to relieve the client's dry mouth?
1. Offer the client ice chips and frequent sips of water.
2. Withhold the drug and notify the health care provider.
3. Change the client's diet to clear liquid until symptoms subside.
4. Encourage the client to brush teeth after each meal.

43. 1. Sucralfate is an anti-ulcer medication that may cause constipation, dry mouth, upset stomach, and nausea. Ice chips and frequent sips of water will help relieve the client's dry mouth. There is no need to withhold the drug unless these symptoms persist or worsen. A clear liquid diet does not provide adequate nutrition and will not provide relief from dry mouth. Frequent oral hygiene may be helpful, but would not provide as much relief as ice and water.
CN: Physiological integrity; CNS: Pharmacological and parenteral therapies; CL: Apply

44. The nurse is administering acyclovir to a client with encephalitis. Which laboratory test(s) will the nurse monitor while the client is taking acyclovir? Select all that apply.
1. Amylase
2. Creatinine
3. Lipase
4. Blood urea nitrogen (BUN)
5. Aspartate aminotransferase (AST)
6. Alanine aminotransferase (ALT)

44. 2, 4, 5, 6. Acyclovir is antiviral medication. The nurse should monitor the BUN and creatinine because this drug is nephrotoxic. AST and ALT should also be monitored because acyclovir is hepatotoxic. The other tests are not indicated.
CN: Physiological integrity; CNS: Pharmacological and parenteral therapies; CL: Apply

CN: Client needs category   CNS: Client needs subcategory   CL: Cognitive level

45. A client is receiving levodopa–carbidopa. Which information will the nurse include while providing client teaching? Select all that apply.
1. Avoid sudden changes in position.
2. Always take with grapefruit.
3. Avoid eating high-protein foods.
4. Encourage use of central nervous system depressants.
5. Avoid large doses of pyridoxine.

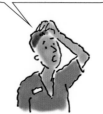

What is levodopa–carbidopa used to treat?

45. 1, 3, 5. Levodopa–carbidopa is used to treat symptoms of Parkinson disease. The client should avoid sudden changes in position because the medication will cause orthostatic hypotension. High-protein diet and large doses of pyridoxine (vitamin B_6) should be avoided, because they will reduce the effectiveness of the levodopa–carbidopa. Because the medication will cause drowsiness, central nervous system depressants should also be avoided. Grapefruit should be avoided because it will decrease the breakdown of the medication by the liver and cause increased drug level in the blood.

CN: Physiological integrity; CNS: Pharmacological and parenteral therapies; CL: Apply

46. An adult client is admitted with myasthenia gravis. While reviewing the client's chart, the nurse noticed the medication administration record, noted below. Based on the findings, what will the nurse do **next**?

Progress notes	
	Medications
	Furosemide 20 mg PO bid
	Neostigmine 15 mg PO every 4 hours
	Potassium chloride 20 mEq PO once a day
	Morphine sulfate 10 mg IM every 4 hours
	Docusate sodium 100 mg PO once a day

1. Administer neostigmine and morphine together.
2. Administer the morphine sulfate and hold the neostigmine.
3. Check the platelet count before administering neostigmine.
4. Call the health care provider and question the morphine sulfate prescription.

46. 4. Myasthenia gravis is a neuromuscular disease characterized by deficiency of acetylcholine at the myoneural junction, causing extreme voluntary muscle weakness. Clients with myasthenia gravis are usually given an anticholinesterase drug like neostigmine to improve muscle strength. Anticholinesterase drugs may potentiate the effect of morphine. The nurse should inform the health care provider and question the medication because narcotic analgesic such as morphine may cause respiratory depression.

CN: Safe, effective care environment; CNS: Management of care; CL: Apply

47. A client with a history of seizures is receiving gabapentin. For which side effect(s) will the nurse monitor this client? Select all that apply.
1. Drowsiness
2. Transient dizziness
3. Increased salivation
4. Weight loss
5. Noticeable tremors

47. 1, 2, 5. Gabapentin is a medication used for seizures and neuropathic pain. The nurse should monitor for the side effects of this drug, which include drowsiness, dizziness, and tremors. Gabapentin also causes weight gain and dry mouth.

CN: Physiological integrity; CNS: Pharmacological and parenteral therapies; CL: Apply

48. Which intervention will the nurse emphasize when providing education for a client with multiple sclerosis (MS) to avoid exacerbation of the disease?
1. Patch the affected eye.
2. Get adequate rest each night.
3. Take hot baths for relaxation.
4. Drink 2,000 mL of fluid daily.

48. 2. MS is exacerbated by exposure to stress, fatigue, and heat. Clients should balance activity with rest. Patching the affected eye may result in improvement in vision and balance but will not prevent exacerbation of the disease. Adequate hydration will help prevent urinary tract infections secondary to a neurogenic bladder.

CN: Physiological integrity; CNS: Reduction of risk potential; CL: Apply

CN: Client needs category   CNS: Client needs subcategory   CL: Cognitive level

49. A client is admitted with complications related to myasthenia gravis. Which medication(s) will the nurse question administering to this client? Select all that apply.
1. Lithium
2. Ciprofloxacin
3. Pyridostigmine
4. Propranolol
5. Ambenonium

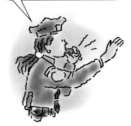

Caution! Some drugs can cause further muscle weakness in clients with myasthenia gravis.

49. 1, 2, 4. The client with myasthenia gravis should avoid taking ciprofloxacin, propranolol, and lithium because these drugs will further cause muscle weakness. Pyridostigmine and ambenonium are anticholinesterase agents used in clients with myasthenia gravis.
CN: Physiological integrity; CNS: Pharmacological and parenteral therapies; CL: Analyze

50. When reviewing the cerebrospinal fluid (CSF) laboratory results of a client diagnosed with multiple sclerosis (MS), what does the nurse expect to find?
1. Presence of blood in the CSF
2. Elevated white blood cell count
3. Increased glucose level
4. Increased protein levels

50. 4. Elevated gamma globulin fraction in CSF without the presence of blood occurs in MS. Blood may be found with trauma or subarachnoid hemorrhage. Increased glucose concentration is a nonspecific finding indicating infection or subarachnoid hemorrhage. Elevated WBCs or pus indicate infection.
CN: Physiological integrity; CNS: Physiological adaptation; CL: Apply

51. During the assessment of a client with suspected meningitis, which nursing finding(s) indicates support of the diagnosis? Select all that apply.
1. Turner sign
2. Brudzinski sign
3. Murphy sign
4. Kernig sign
5. Cullen sign
6. Battle sign

51. 2, 4. A client with meningitis will experience signs of meningeal irritation, which include nuchal rigidity (stiff neck), Brudzinski sign, and Kernig sign. Brudzinski sign is flexion at the hip and knee in response to forward flexion of the neck. Kernig sign is severe stiffness and pain in the hamstring muscle when attempting to extend the leg when the hip is flexed. Turner sign and Cullen sign are both signs of retroperitoneal bleeding seen in clients with acute pancreatitis. Murphy sign is used to assess for gallbladder inflammation. Battle sign is the ecchymosis behind the ear, which is a sign of head injury.
CN: Physiological integrity; CNS: Physiological adaptation; CL: Apply

52. Which nursing intervention is **priority** for the client experiencing a tonic–clonic seizure?
1. Maintain a patent airway.
2. Time the duration of the seizure.
3. Note the origin of seizure activity.
4. Insert tongue blade inside the mouth.

You're so brainy! I can't believe how well you're doing.

52. 1. The priority during and after a seizure is to maintain a patent airway. Noting the origin of the seizure activity and the duration of the seizure are important, but they do not take priority over maintenance of a patent airway. Nothing should be placed in the client's mouth during a seizure because teeth may be dislodged or the tongue pushed back, further obstructing the airway.
CN: Safe, effective care environment; CNS: Management of care; CL: Apply

53. A client is receiving dabigatran. Which medication instruction(s) will the nurse include during client teaching? Select all that apply.
1. Avoid eating green, leafy vegetables.
2. Do not chew, break, or open capsules.
3. Immediately report signs of bleeding.
4. Take medication with a full glass of water.
5. Monitor prothrombin time (PT) regularly.

53. 2, 3, 4. Dabigatran is a direct thrombin inhibitor that reduces the risk of cerebrovascular accident, atrial fibrillation, deep vein thrombosis, and pulmonary embolism. Unlike warfarin, there is no need to avoid foods high in vitamin K and it is not necessary to monitor the PT/international normalized ratio (INR) while on this medication. Client should not chew, break, or open capsules while taking this drug. The medication should also be taken with full glass of water. Signs of bleeding should be immediately reported because of its anticoagulant effect.
CN: Physiological integrity; CNS: Pharmacological and parenteral therapies; CL: Apply

CN: Client needs category   CNS: Client needs subcategory   CL: Cognitive level

54. The nurse is caring for a client prescribed phenytoin 750 mg IV now followed by 100 mg PO three times per day. The client asks the nurse, "Why do I have to take some of the medication through an IV?" Which nursing response is appropriate?
1. "The IV dose is to ensure that the drug reaches the cerebrospinal fluid."
2. "Getting both IV and oral phenytoin will omit the need for surgery."
3. "The IV form will help to reduce secretions in case another seizure occurs."
4. "The stronger IV dose will help you reach a therapeutic level quickly."

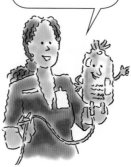

Here's your loading dose. He helps speed up your treatment.

54. 4. A loading dose of phenytoin and other drugs is given to reach therapeutic levels more quickly; maintenance dosing follows. A loading dose of phenytoin can be oral or parenteral. Surgical excision of an epileptic focus is considered when seizures are not controlled with anticonvulsant therapy. Phenytoin does not reduce secretions.

CN: Physiological integrity; CNS: Pharmacological and parenteral therapies; CL: Apply

55. Which finding(s) in a client with a seizure disorder prescribed phenytoin **most** concerns the nurse? Select all that apply.
1. Red rash on the torso
2. Behavior changes
3. Client is breastfeeding
4. History of depression
5. Drowsiness

55. 1, 2, 3, 4. Phenytoin is an anti-epileptic drug used to control seizures. A skin rash of any kind, fever, severe weakness, jaundice, or blood dyscrasias can indicate a severe reaction to phenytoin and should be reported to the health care provider immediately. Clients taking phenytoin are at increased risk of suicide; therefore, behavior changes and a history of depression would concern the nurse. Clients taking phenytoin should not breastfeed because it will pass into the milk and is not safe for infants. Side effects of phenytoin include drowsiness, confusion, and slurred speech.

CN: Safe, effective care environment; CNS: Management of care; CL: Analyze

56. A client has a phenytoin level of 32 mg/dL (127 μmol/L). For which symptoms will the nurse monitor the client, based on this level?
1. Ataxia and confusion
2. Hyponatremia and confusion
3. Tonic–clonic seizure and ataxia
4. Urinary incontinence and hematuria

56. 1. A therapeutic phenytoin level is 10 to 20 mg/dL (39.7 to 79.4 μmol/L). A level of 32 mg/dL (127 μmol/L) indicates phenytoin toxicity. Symptoms of toxicity include confusion and ataxia. Phenytoin does not cause hyponatremia, hematuria seizure, or urinary incontinence. Incontinence may occur during or after a seizure.

CN: Physiological integrity; CNS: Pharmacological and parenteral therapies; CL: Apply

57. Which precaution will the nurse take when giving phenytoin to a client with a nasogastric (NG) tube for feeding?
1. Check the phenytoin level after giving the drug.
2. Place the client supine before administering phenytoin.
3. Give phenytoin 1 hour before or 2 hours after NG tube feedings.
4. Place the end of the tube in water to verify proper NG tube placement.

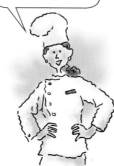

Be sure to take precautions with nasogastric tube feedings.

57. 3. Nutritional supplements and milk interfere with the absorption of phenytoin, decreasing its effectiveness. The nurse verifies NG tube placement by checking for stomach contents before giving drugs and feedings. The head of the bed is elevated when giving all drugs or solutions. Phenytoin levels are checked before giving the drug, and the drug is withheld for elevated levels to avoid compounding toxicity.

CN: Physiological integrity; CNS: Pharmacological and parenteral therapies; CL: Apply

58. The nurse is providing education to a client taking phenytoin. The client asks, "Can I still drink beer with dinner?" What is the **best** response by the nurse?

1. "The research is not clear regarding alcohol with phenytoin, so ask your health care provider."
2. "It is very dangerous for you to drink alcohol, because it will raise your seizure threshold."
3. "You can drink alcohol, but you need to understand it will impair judgment and coordination."
4. "You should avoid alcohol because it will decrease the effectiveness of your phenytoin."

58. 4. The greatest concern is that alcohol will lower phenytoin levels. Telling the client to ask another health care provider is not appropriate. Phenytoin will lower the client's seizure threshold. Alcohol should not be consumed due to it decreasing the drug's effectiveness.
CN: Physiological integrity; CNS: Pharmacological and parenteral therapies; CL: Apply

59. The nurse is obtaining vital signs for a client with an unstable seizure disorder. Which method will the nurse use to obtain the **most** accurate measurements?

1. Assess for a pulse deficit.
2. Review for pulsus paradoxus.
3. Perform an axillary temperature.
4. Check the blood pressure for an auscultatory gap.

59. 3. To reduce the risk of injury, the nurse should take an axillary temperature, or the nurse should use a metal thermometer when taking an oral temperature to prevent injury if a seizure occurs. An auscultatory gap occurs in hypertension. Pulse deficit occurs in an arrhythmia. Pulsus paradoxus may occur with cardiac tamponade.
CN: Physiological integrity; CNS: Reduction of risk potential; CL: Apply

60. The emergency room nurse is assigned a client who is suspected to have a brain injury after falling out of a tree. When the nurse enters the client's room, the nurse notes the client is lying rigidly on the stretcher, with the arms bent toward the chest, clenched fists, extension and internal rotation of the legs, and plantar flexion of the feet. The client does not respond to verbal stimuli. Which action will the nurse take **next**?

1. Assess the client's vital signs.
2. Monitor the client's pupils.
3. Perform sternal rub.
4. Notify the health care provider.

60. 4. The nurse would first notify the health care provider. The client is exhibiting signs of decorticate posturing, which is seen in clients with damage in the corticospinal tract. This is an emergency situation and generally requires intubation and admission to the intensive care unit. The nurse would assess the client's vital signs after notifying the health care provider as intubation is priority for this client. It is not appropriate to monitor the client's pupils or perform sternal rub at this time.
CN: Safe and effective care environment; CNS: Management of care; CL: Analyze

61. A client is admitted to the emergency department following a head-on motor vehicle collision. Which nursing intervention will the registered nurse do **first**?

1. Perform full range of motion (ROM).
2. Call for an immediate chest x-ray.
3. Immobilize the client's head and neck.
4. Open airway using head tilt/chin lift maneuver.

In question #61, focus on what should be done **first**.

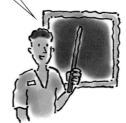

61. 3. All clients with a head injury are treated as if a cervical spine injury is present until x-rays confirm their absence. Performing ROM would be contraindicated at this time. There is no indication the client needs a chest x-ray. The airway does not need to be opened because the client appears alert and not in respiratory distress. In addition, the head tilt/chin lift maneuver would not be used until cervical spine injury is ruled out.
CN: Physiological integrity; CNS: Reduction of risk potential; CL: Apply

62. A client with a diving injury is admitted to the emergency department. What assessment finding does the nurse expect?
1. Aphasia
2. Hemiparesis
3. Paraplegia
4. Quadriplegia

63. A client has a spinal cord transection at the level of the nipple line. The nurse will expect the client to have which symptom?
1. Paraplegia
2. Quadriplegia
3. Autonomic dysreflexia
4. Hemiplegia

64. A client is admitted with a burst fracture at the level of T12 and reports loss of movement of the lower extremities. Which medication will the nurse anticipate administering to this client?
1. Acetazolamide
2. Furosemide
3. Methylprednisolone
4. Sodium bicarbonate

65. A client is admitted to the progressive care unit with an acute injury to the cervical spine from a motorcycle collision. Which nursing action is **priority**?
1. Assessing for bladder distention
2. Monitoring neurologic deficit
3. Checking pulse oximetry readings
4. Referral for rehabilitation evaluation

66. The nurse is caring for a client with C8 quadriplegia 8 hours after the injury. During assessment the nurse notes: blood pressure, 80/44 mm Hg; pulse, 48 beats/minute; and respiratory rate, 18 breaths/minute. The nurse suspects which condition?
1. Neurogenic shock
2. Autonomic dysreflexia
3. Hemorrhagic shock
4. Pulmonary embolism

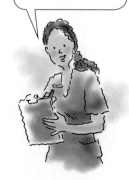
Wow—those are low numbers. Which condition is most likely to produce them?

62. 4. Quadriplegia occurs as a result of cervical spine injuries. Paraplegia occurs as a result of injury to the thoracic cord and below. Hemiparesis describes weakness of one side of the body. Aphasia refers to difficulty expressing or understanding spoken words.
CN: Physiological integrity; CNS: Physiological adaptation; CL: Apply

63. 1. Spinal cord injuries at the T4 level affect all motor and sensory nerves below the level of injury and result in dysfunction of legs, bowel, and bladder. Paraplegic injuries involve the thoracic, lumbar, or sacral region of the spinal cord. Quadriplegic injuries result from damage to the cervical region of the spine. Autonomic dysreflexia occurs because of a massive sympathetic discharge of stimuli from the autonomic nervous system.
CN: Physiological integrity; CNS: Physiological adaptation; CL: Apply

64. 3. High doses of methylprednisolone are used within 24 hours of spinal cord injury to reduce cord swelling and limit neurologic deficits. The other drugs are not indicated in this circumstance.
CN: Physiological integrity; CNS: Pharmacological and parenteral therapies; CL: Apply

65. 3. After a spinal cord injury, ascending cord edema may cause a higher level of injury. The diaphragm is innervated at the level of C4, so assessment of adequate oxygenation and ventilation through pulse oximetry readings is necessary. Although the other options would be necessary at a later time, observation for respiratory failure is the priority.
CN: Safe, effective care environment; CNS: Management of care; CL: Analyze

66. 1. Symptoms of neurogenic shock include hypotension, bradycardia, and warm, dry skin due to loss of adrenergic stimulation below the level of the lesion. Hypertension, bradycardia, flushing, and sweating of the skin are seen with autonomic dysreflexia. Hemorrhagic shock presents with anxiety, tachycardia, and hypotension; this would not be suspected without an injury. Pulmonary embolism presents with chest pain, hypotension, hypoxemia, tachycardia, and hemoptysis; this may be a later complication of spinal cord injury due to immobility.
CN: Physiological integrity; CNS: Reduction of risk potential; CL: Analyze

67. A client with quadriplegia is apprehensive and flushed, and has a blood pressure of 210/100 mm Hg and heart rate of 50 beats/minute. Which intervention will the nurse complete **first**?
1. Place the client in the supine position.
2. Check patency of the indwelling urinary catheter.
3. Give one sublingual nitroglycerin tablet.
4. Raise the head of the bed to 90 degrees.

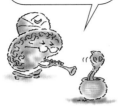

Sometimes simple interventions can calm a client's anxieties and fears.

67. 4. Anxiety, flushing above the level of the lesion, piloerection, hypertension, and bradycardia are symptoms of autonomic dysreflexia, typically caused by such noxious stimuli as a full bladder, fecal impaction, or pressure injury. The client is immediately placed in a sitting position to lower blood pressure. Placing the client flat will cause the blood pressure to increase. Nitroglycerin is given to relieve chest pain and reduce preload; it is not used for hypertension or dysreflexia. The indwelling urinary catheter should be checked immediately after the head of the bed is raised.
CN: Safe, effective care environment; CNS: Management of care; CL: Analyze

68. Which nursing response is **most** appropriate for the client newly diagnosed with paraplegia who becomes verbally aggressive while transferring to a wheelchair?
1. "You know I want to help you; I have offered several times."
2. "I will pick these things up for you and come back later."
3. "You seem angry today. How do you feel about your transfer to rehab?"
4. "If you will cooperate, you will be able to get into the wheelchair."

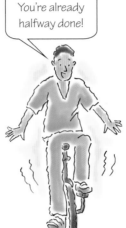

Impressive. You're already halfway done!

68. 3. The nurse should always focus on the feelings underlying a particular action. The nurse saying that he or she offered to help or telling the client to cooperate is confrontational. Offering to pick up the client's belongings does not deal with the situation and assumes the client cannot do it alone.
CN: Psychosocial integrity; CNS: None; CL: Apply

69. A client with a cervical spine injury is placed in a Minerva body vest. The client is uncomfortable and would like to try a different device. Which information will the nurse explain to the client?
1. The vest protects the neck against excessive motion.
2. The vest will provide significant immobilization, including lateral flexion.
3. The vest will provide for immobilization of the mid-cervical segments.
4. There are other soft-type collars that can be used.

69. 2. The Minerva vest will provide significant immobilization, including lateral flexion. Most soft collars do not limit cervical motion but act as a reminder against excessive motion. More rigid devices such as the Philadelphia collar provide reasonable immobilization of the mid-cervical segments for flexion and extension but not for lateral flexion.
CN: Physiological integrity; CNS: Physiological adaptation; CL: Apply

70. When discharging a client with a halo vest from the hospital, which statement will the nurse provide to the client and family?
1. "You really need to be extra careful while you are driving a car."
2. "Keep the wrench that opens the vest attached to the client at all times."
3. "Clean the pin sites every other day especially when there is drainage."
4. "Perform range of motion (ROM) exercises to the neck and shoulders four times daily."

70. 2. The wrench must be attached at all times to remove the vest in case the client needs cardiopulmonary resuscitation. The vest is designed to improve mobility; the client may use a wheelchair but cannot drive as movement is limited. The pins are cleaned daily. The purpose of the vest is to immobilize the neck; ROM exercises to the neck are prohibited but should be performed to other areas.
CN: Physiological integrity; CNS: Reduction of risk potential; CL: Apply

CN: Client needs category   CNS: Client needs subcategory   CL: Cognitive level

71. When caring for a client with trigeminal neuralgia, the client tells the nurse, "I have severe stabbing pain on my effected side." Which action will the nurse perform **first**?
1. Ask the client to take slow deep breaths.
2. Medicate the client as prescribed.
3. Notify the health care provider.
4. Assess for pain using a numerical scale.

72. Which early intervention describes an appropriate bladder program for a client in rehabilitation for spinal cord injury?
1. Insert an indwelling urinary catheter.
2. Schedule intermittent catheterization every 2 to 4 hours.
3. Perform a straight catheterization every 8 hours while awake.
4. Perform Credé maneuver to the lower abdomen before the client voids.

73. The nurse is caring for a client who underwent a stapedectomy. The nurse knows which position will have the **greatest** benefit for this client?
1. Lying in the prone position
2. Lying on the unaffected side
3. Sitting semi- to high-Fowler's
4. Being in modified Trendelenburg

74. A client with breast cancer reports back pain and difficulty in moving the legs. Which nursing intervention is **most** appropriate?
1. Notify the client's health care provider.
2. Prop the client on the side with a foam wedge.
3. Request a physical therapy consultation.
4. Administer 1,000 mg acetaminophen orally.

75. A client is admitted to the hospital with a diagnosis of transient ischemic attack (TIA) secondary to atrial fibrillation. Which medication will the nurse administer to prevent further neurologic deficit?
1. Digoxin
2. Diltiazem
3. Heparin
4. Quinidine gluconate

76. A client is admitted with Ménière disease. Which condiment(s) will the nurse educate the client to avoid? Select all that apply.
1. Soy sauce
2. Pepper
3. Vinegar
4. Olive oil
5. Ketchup

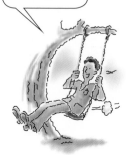

Looks like you are in the swing of things.

71. 4. A pain assessment should be completed prior to medicating a client. The health care provider does not need to be notified as this is an expected finding. Diversion techniques are not priority at this time.
CN: Safe, effective care environment; CNS: Management of care; CL: Analyze

72. 2. Intermittent catheterization should begin every 2 to 4 hours early in treatment. When residual volume is less than 400 mL, the schedule may advance to every 4 to 6 hours. Indwelling catheters may predispose the client to infection and are removed as soon as possible. Credé maneuver is applied after voiding to enhance bladder emptying.
CN: Physiological integrity; CNS: Basic care and comfort; CL: Apply

73. 2. The client should be positioned on the unaffected side with the operative ear up. Semi- or high-Fowler's position does not facilitate drainage or hearing. Modified Trendelenburg is contraindicated as the client should not be flat with legs up.
CN: Physiological integrity; CNS: Physiological adaptation; CL: Apply

74. 1. Symptoms of back pain and neurologic deficits may indicate metastasis; therefore, the health care provider should be notified. Repositioning the client, physical therapy, or acetaminophen may help the pain but may delay evaluation and treatment.
CN: Health promotion and maintenance; CNS: None; CL: Analyze

75. 3. Atrial fibrillation may lead to the formation of mural thrombi, which may embolize to the brain. Heparin will prevent further clot formation and clot enlargement. The other drugs are used in the treatment and control of atrial fibrillation but will not affect clot formation.
CN: Physiological integrity; CNS: Pharmacological and parenteral therapies; CL: Apply

76. 1, 5. Ménière disease is a disorder of the inner ear in which there is an excess production of endolymphatic fluid in the semicircular canals. The client's diet should be low in sodium. Both soy sauce and ketchup are high in sodium and should be avoided.
CN: Health promotion and maintenance; CNS: None; CL: Apply

77. The nurse is caring for a client with Ménière disease. Which symptom(s) will the nurse report to the health care provider? Select all that apply.
1. Dizziness
2. Vertigo
3. Epistaxis
4. Facial pain
5. Ptosis
6. Tinnitus

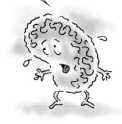

Do you hear that ringing sound?

77. 3, 4, 5. The nurse would report unexpected findings. Epistaxis, facial pain, and ptosis are not expected findings in clients with Ménière disease. Facial pain may occur with trigeminal neuralgia. Ptosis occurs with a variety of conditions, including myasthenia gravis. Epistaxis may occur with a variety of blood dyscrasias or local lesions. Tinnitus, dizziness, and vertigo occur in Ménière disease.
CN: Safe, effective care environment; CNS: Management of care; CL: Apply

78. Which nursing intervention is **priority** when caring for a client with a foreign body protruding from the eye following head trauma?
1. Irrigating the eye with sterile saline
2. Assessing visual acuity with a Snellen chart
3. Removing the object with sterile forceps
4. Temporarily patching both eyes

78. 4. One or both eyes may be patched to prevent pain with extraocular movement or accommodation. Assessment of visual acuity is not a priority, although it may be done after treatment. Chemicals or small foreign bodies may be irrigated. Protruding objects are not removed by the nurse because the vitreous body may rupture.
CN: Safe, effective care environment; CNS: Management of care; CL: Apply

79. The health care provider prescribed a nasogastric tube to be inserted on a client with dysphagia. Place the following nursing actions in chronological order of how the nurse will perform the procedure. Use each option once.

1. Instruct client to hyperextend the head.

2. Advance tube 1 to 2 in (2.5 to 5 cm) with each swallow.

3. Instruct client to flex head forward.

4. Position client in high Fowler's.

5. Measure distance to insert tube.

6. Pass lubricated tube along floor of nasal passage.

79. Ordered Response:

4. Position client in high Fowler's.

5. Measure distance to insert tube.

1. Instruct client to hyperextend the head.

6. Pass lubricated tube along floor of nasal passage.

3. Instruct client to flex head forward.

2. Advance tube 1 to 2 in (2.5 to 5 cm) with each swallow.

CN: Physiological integrity; CNS: Reduction of risk potential; CL: Apply

80. A health care provider instills a topical anesthetic in the affected eye of a client with severe eye pain. The client asks the nurse, "Will I get a prescription for those drops?" Which nursing response is **most** appropriate?
1. "Overuse of these drops can lead to an increased risk of eye infections."
2. "No; damage could occur to the cornea because of lack of sensation."
3. "These drops cannot be taken at home because they cause dependence and rebound pain."
4. "You will have to ask the health care provider if you will be given a prescription."

80. 2. Corneal damage may occur with the prolonged use of topical anesthetics. Infections, dependence and rebound pain do not occur from topical anesthetics. Telling the client to ask the health care provider is not therapeutic and does not address the client's question.
CN: Physiological integrity; CNS: Reduction of risk potential; CL: Apply

81. During the assessment of an older adult client, the nurse notes the client has decreased hearing bilaterally. Which method will the nurse use **first** when communicating with this client?
1. Speak loudly when talking to the client.
2. Lower voice pitch while facing the client.
3. Ask the family to locate the hearing aids.
4. Write down all words spoken to the client.

81. 2. Hearing loss in the older adult typically involves the upper ranges; lowering the pitch of the voice and facing the client is essential for the client to use other means of understanding, such as lip reading, mood, and so on. Shouting is typically in the upper ranges and could cause the client to become anxious. Alternate means of communication, such as writing, may be used if speaking in a lower range is not sufficient.

CN: Physiological integrity; CNS: Basic care and comfort; CL: Apply

82. A client is scheduled for magnetic resonance imaging (MRI) of the head. The nurse knows which assessment finding(s) is **priority** before the procedure? Select all that apply.
1. History of claustrophobia
2. Presence of metal fillings, prostheses, or pacemaker
3. Food or drink intake within the past 8 hours
4. Presence of carotid artery disease
5. Voiding before the procedure

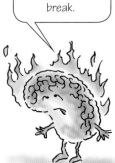

If your brain feels like it's on fire, you might want to take a break.

82. 1, 2. Strong magnetic waves may dislodge metal in the client's body, causing tissue injury. Although the client may be told to restrict food for 8 hours, particularly if contrast is used, metal is an absolute contraindication for this procedure. The client with history of claustrophobia should be evaluated because the client will be confined in a small, enclosed, tube-shaped machine during MRI. Voiding beforehand would make the client more comfortable and better able to remain still during the procedure, but it is not essential for the test. Having carotid artery disease is not a contraindication to having an MRI.

CN: Safe, effective care environment; CNS: Safety and infection control; CL: Analyze

83. After cataract surgery, the nurse will provide which discharge education to the client? Select all that apply.
1. Avoid bending over at the waist.
2. Reduce sodium intake to reduce intraocular pressure.
3. If you notice flashing lights, sit and rest for 15 minutes.
4. Eye makeup can be applied beginning tomorrow.
5. Call your health care provider if you have vision loss.
6. When sleeping, lie on the unaffected side.

83. 1, 5, 6. Bending over may increase intraocular pressure and strain the sutures. Vision loss or seeing flashing lights may signal complications, such as retinal detachment or increased intraocular pressure, and should be reported. Intraocular pressure is reduced when sleeping on the nonsurgical side. Reducing sodium intake does not decrease intraocular pressure. Applying eye makeup may introduce infection and cause irritation.

CN: Physiological integrity; CNS: Reduction of risk potential; CL: Apply

84. When administering cromolyn ophthalmic drops to an adult client, which nursing action is appropriate?
1. Place the client supine and hold the eye open.
2. Tilt the client's head back and pull the lower conjunctival sack down.
3. Place the tip of the dropper to the corner of the client's eye.
4. Have the client blink repeatedly immediately following administration.

84. 2. To administer ophthalmic drops, the nurse should slightly tilt the client's head back and pull the lower conjunctival sack downward to create a small pocket. The nurse would then administer the prescribed number of drops into the pocket and have the client close the eyes for 2 to 3 minutes, without blinking or squinting. Touching the tip to the client's eye will contaminate the dropper and could lead to infection.

CN: Physiological integrity; CNS: Pharmacological and parenteral therapies; CL: Apply

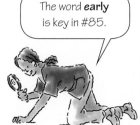

The word **early** is key in #85.

85. The nurse recognizes which finding as an early sign of increased intracranial pressure (ICP)?
1. New onset bradycardia
2. Restlessness and confusion
3. Widened pulse pressure
4. Large amounts of very dilute urine

85. 2. The earliest symptom of increased ICP is a change in mental status. Bradycardia, widened pulse pressure, and bradypnea occur later. The client may void large amounts of very dilute urine if there is damage to the posterior pituitary.

CN: Physiological integrity; CNS: Physiological adaptation; CL: Apply

86. A client admitted to the emergency department for head trauma following a skiing accident is diagnosed with an epidural hematoma. What is the **priority** nursing action?
1. Prepare the client for emergency surgery.
2. Monitor the client closely for 24 hours.
3. Apply direct pressure to the scalp.
4. Obtain vital signs every hour.

86. 1. Epidural hematoma or extradural hematoma is usually caused by laceration of the middle meningeal artery. This condition is emergent and requires immediate evacuation of the hematoma. Monitoring the client for 24 hours is not an appropriate action because the client will require emergency surgery to evacuate the hematoma. Applying direct pressure to the scalp is an ineffective treatment because the artery that is ruptured is not a surface vessel. Vital signs will be obtained at least every 15 minutes prior to surgery.
CN: Safe, effective care environment; CNS: Management of care; CL: Apply

87. The nurse notes clear fluid draining from the right ear and nose of a client after a blunt trauma to the head. Which nursing intervention is **priority**?
1. Position the client in the supine position.
2. Check the fluid for glucose with a dipstick.
3. Suction the nose to maintain airway patency.
4. Insert nasal and ear packing with sterile gauze.

87. 2. Clear liquid from the nose (rhinorrhea) or ear (otorrhea) can be determined to be cerebral spinal fluid or mucus by the presence of glucose. Glucose would be present in cerebral spinal fluid. Placing the client flat in bed may increase intracranial pressure and promote pulmonary aspiration. Nothing is inserted into the ears or nose of a client with a skull fracture because of the risk of infection. The nose would not be suctioned because of the risk of suctioning brain tissue through the sinuses.
CN: Safe, effective care environment; CNS: Management of care; CL: Apply

88. The nurse notes lucid intervals in a client following a closed head injury. How will the nurse document this finding?
1. Experiences neurological aura intermittently
2. Speech is garbled, and unclear sounds are made
3. Awake, alert to person and time but cannot recall recent events
4. Oriented to person, place, and time but then becomes somnolent

88. 4. A lucid interval is described as a brief period of unconsciousness at the time of the trauma followed by alertness; after several hours, the client deteriorates neurologically. Garbled speech is known as dysarthria. An interval in which the client is alert but cannot recall recent events is known as amnesia. Warning symptoms or auras typically occur before seizures.
CN: Health promotion and maintenance; CNS: None; CL: Understand

89. The nurse will assess which client on the rehabilitation unit **most** closely for the development of autonomic dysreflexia?
1. A client with a traumatic brain injury
2. A client with a herniated nucleus pulposus
3. A client with a high cervical spine injury
4. A client with a frontal ischemic stroke

89. 3. Autonomic dysreflexia refers to uninhibited sympathetic outflow in clients with spinal cord injuries above the level of T10. The other clients are not prone to dysreflexia.
CN: Safe, effective care environment; CNS: Management of care; CL: Analyze

90. The nurse is educating the family of a client being discharged on tracheostomy suctioning. The nurse will include which information in the teaching?
1. Suction for no more than 20 seconds when withdrawing the catheter.
2. Regulate the suction machine to intermittent suction at 200 cm.
3. Apply suction to the catheter when inserting until meeting resistance.
4. Pass the suction catheter into the opening of the tracheostomy 1 to 1.5 in (2.5 to 3.75 cm).

When possible, recruit family members to help provide basic comfort and care measures for the client.

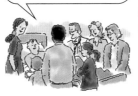

90. 1. Suction should be applied no more than 20 seconds at a time. When suctioning the trachea, the catheter is inserted 4 to 6 in (10 to 15 cm) or until resistance is felt. Suction should be applied only during withdrawal of the catheter. Suction is regulated to 80 to 120 cm.
CN: Safe, effective care environment; CNS: Safety and infection control; CL: Apply

CN: Client needs category   CNS: Client needs subcategory   CL: Cognitive level

91. The family of a client diagnosed with hemorrhagic stroke asks the nurse, "What can cause this?" The nurse will include which risk factor(s) in the response? Select all that apply.

1. Coronary artery disease
2. Juvenile onset diabetes
3. Uncontrolled hypertension
4. Recent viral infection
5. Cerebral aneurysm

92. The nurse is assisting a client during lumbar puncture. Which position will the nurse place the client in for this procedure?

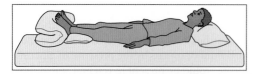
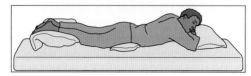
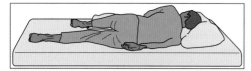
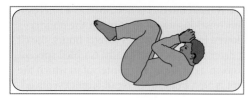

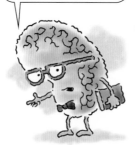

Hemorrhagic strokes are caused by bleeding from a ruptured blood vessel in the brain. What risk factors would contribute to this condition?

91. 3, 5. Uncontrolled hypertension and cerebral aneurysm are major causes of hemorrhagic stroke. The other options are not directly linked to this condition.

CN: Physiological integrity; CNS: Reduction of risk potential; CL: Apply

92. 4. During lumbar puncture, the client will be placed on a lateral (side-lying) position to widen the intervertebral spaces for easy insertion of the spinal needle.

CN: Physiological integrity; CNS: Reduction of risk potential; CL: Apply

93. Which assessment finding indicates to the nurse spinal shock is resolving in a client with C7 quadriplegia?

1. No pain sensation in the chest
2. Noted reflexes
3. Spontaneous respirations
4. Urinary continence

93. 2. Spasticity, the return of reflexes, is a sign of resolving shock. Spinal or neurogenic shock is characterized by hypotension, bradycardia, dry skin, flaccid paralysis, or the absence of reflexes below the level of injury. Slight muscle contraction at the bulbocavernosus reflex occurs but not enough for urinary continence. Spinal shock descends from the injury, and respiratory difficulties occur at C4 and above. The absence of pain sensation in the chest does not apply to spinal shock.

CN: Physiological integrity; CNS: Physiological adaptation; CL: Apply

94. When discharging a client from the hospital after a cervical laminectomy, the nurse recognizes further education is necessary when the client makes which statement?

1. "I will sleep on a firm mattress using only one pillow."
2. "I will not drive for 2 to 4 weeks until I see the health care provider."
3. "When I pick things up, I will always bend my knees."
4. "I cannot wait to toss my granddaughter up in the air."

94. 4. Lifting more than 10 lb (4.5 kg) for several weeks after surgery is contraindicated. The other responses are appropriate.

CN: Physiological integrity; CNS: Reduction of risk potential; CL: Apply

CN: Client needs category   CNS: Client needs subcategory   CL: Cognitive level

95. The nurse is collecting data on a client with herniated nucleus pulposus (HNP) of L4–L5. Which finding(s) will the nurse anticipate? Select all that apply.
1. Urinary incontinence
2. Increased muscle weakness
3. Paresthesia
4. Constant low back pain
5. Pain radiating across the buttocks
6. Positive Kernig's sign

96. The nurse is discharging a client with autonomic dysreflexia. The nurse teaches the client to carefully monitor for which potential complication?
1. Moderate tension headache
2. Low back strain when lifting
3. Decreased temperature sensation
4. Fecal impaction or distended bladder

97. The nurse is providing dietary instructions to a client with Parkinson disease. Which findings are **most** important for the nurse to address?
1. Leaking of urine and dementia
2. Tremors and a distorted sense of smell
3. Confusion in the afternoon and drooling
4. Dysphagia and increased difficulty standing

98. When treating a client after a spinal cord injury for spastic leg syndrome, the nurse will prepare to administer which medication?
1. Hydralazine
2. Baclofen
3. Lidocaine
4. Methylprednisolone

99. The nurse is performing a neurological assessment on the client's cranial nerves (CN). Which technique will the nurse use to assess the function of the facial nerve (CN VII)?
1. Have the client tightly clench the teeth.
2. Place a tongue applicator against the pharynx.
3. Ask the client to frown, smile, and raise the eyebrows.
4. Give the client a straw to suck on and swallow.

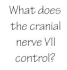

What does the cranial nerve VII control?

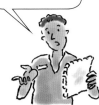

100. The nurse is assessing a client in the emergency department and notes: blood pressure, 82/40 mm Hg; pulse, 34 beats/minute; dry skin; and flaccid paralysis of the lower extremities. Which condition will the nurse suspect?
1. Neurogenic shock
2. Septic shock
3. Autonomic dysreflexia
4. Absolute hypervolemia

95. 1, 2, 3. Progressive neurologic deficits at L4–L5 including worsening muscle weakness, paresthesia, and loss of bowel and bladder control are symptoms of spinal cord compression. The other symptoms usually occur in clients with HNP without spinal cord compression.
CN: Physiological integrity; CNS: Physiological adaptation; CL: Apply

96. 4. Noxious stimuli, such as a full bladder, fecal impaction, or a pressure injury, may cause autonomic dysreflexia. Autonomic dysreflexia is most commonly seen with injuries at T10 or higher. A headache is a symptom, not a cause, of autonomic dysreflexia. The client will not be able to lift as the level of injury is at T10.
CN: Physiological integrity; CNS: Physiological adaptation; CL: Apply

97. 4. All of the findings are expected with Parkinson disease. However, the nurse would be most concerned with dysphagia due to the risk of choking and aspiration, and increased difficulty standing due to the risk for falling.
CN: Safe, effective care environment; CNS: Management of care; CL: Analyze

98. 2. Baclofen is a skeletal muscle relaxant used to decrease spasms. Methylprednisolone, an anti-inflammatory drug, is used to decrease spinal cord edema. Hydralazine is an antihypertensive and afterload-reducing agent. Lidocaine is an antiarrhythmic and a local anesthetic agent.
CN: Physiological integrity; CNS: Pharmacological and parenteral therapies; CL: Apply

99. 3. To check the motor function of CN VII, the nurse should ask the client to frown, smile, and raise the eyebrows. If these facial expressions are symmetrical, motor function is intact. Jaw clenching is a test for CN V function. Testing the gag reflex by placing an applicator against the pharynx, and checking swallowing ability, are ways to evaluate CN IX function. Testing the gag reflex also helps evaluate CN X function.
CN: Health promotion and maintenance; CNS: None; CL: Understand

100. 1. Loss of sympathetic control and unopposed vagal stimulation below the level of the injury typically cause hypotension, bradycardia, pallor, flaccid paralysis, and warm, dry skin in the client in neurogenic shock. Hypervolemia is indicated by a bounding and rapid pulse and edema. Autonomic dysreflexia occurs after neurogenic shock abates. Signs of sepsis would include elevated temperature, increased heart rate, and increased respiratory rate.
CN: Physiological integrity; CNS: Physiological adaptation; CL: Apply

101. A client with quadriplegia is flushed, anxious, and reports a pounding headache. During assessment, the nurse will anticipate which additional finding?
1. Decreased urinary output and bradycardia
2. Hypertension and bradycardia
3. Acute respiratory failure and fatigue
4. Tachycardia and dilated pupils

102. A client has suffered a high cervical cord injury after a fall. Which nursing intervention is **priority** during the acute phase of treatment?
1. Monitor urine output.
2. Discuss assistive devices for eating.
3. Assess for extremity paralysis.
4. Provide mechanical ventilator support.

103. When providing care for a client with a thoracic cord transection, which nursing intervention is **priority**?
1. Forcing fluids
2. Supporting breathing
3. Maintaining skin integrity
4. Obtaining adaptive devices

104. The nurse is caring for a client diagnosed with a transient ischemic attack (TIA). The family asks how this stroke is different than the transient ischemic attack the client had in the past. Which response by the nurse is **best**?
1. "A TIA typically resolves in 24 hours."
2. "Many times TIA is hemorrhagic in origin."
3. "A TIA causes paralysis in both sides of the body."
4. "A TIA often leads to a myocardial infarction (MI)."

105. During care of a client with a right-sided cerebral vascular accident (CVA), the nurse will use which intervention to help prevent contractures of the left shoulder?
1. Splinting the wrist on both sides for support
2. Using an air splint on the cervical spine to align
3. Putting the affected arm in a sling to keep in position
4. Performing range-of-motion (ROM) exercises for mobility

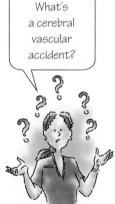

What's a cerebral vascular accident?

101. 2. Hypertension, bradycardia, anxiety, blurred vision, and flushing above the lesion occur with autonomic dysreflexia due to uninhibited sympathetic nervous system discharge. The other findings are not associated.
CN: Physiological integrity; CNS: Physiological adaptation; CL: Analyze

102. 4. The diaphragm is stimulated by nerves at the level of C4. Initially, this client may need mechanical ventilation because of cord edema, which would be priority. This may resolve in time. The nurse will assess for paralysis, discuss the potential use of assistive devices, and monitor urine output. However, these are not priority over airway management.
CN: Safe, effective care environment; CNS: Management of care; CL: Analyze

103. 2. Clients with quadriplegia have paralysis or weakness of the diaphragm, abdominal, or intercostal muscles. Maintenance of airway and breathing take top priority. Although forcing fluids, maintaining skin integrity, and obtaining adaptive devices for more independence are all important interventions, preventing atelectasis has more priority.
CN: Safe, effective care environment; CNS: Management of care; CL: Analyze

104. 1. Symptoms of a TIA result from a transient lack of oxygen to the brain and usually resolve within 24 hours. Hemorrhage into the brain has the worst neurologic outcome and is not associated with TIA. Permanent motor deficits do not result from TIA. Unstable angina, not a TIA, may predispose the client to a future MI.
CN: Physiological integrity; CNS: Physiological adaptation; CL: Understand

105. 3. Because of the weight of the flaccid extremity, the shoulder may disarticulate. A sling will support the extremity. The other options will not support the shoulder.
CN: Physiological integrity; CNS: Basic care and comfort; CL: Apply

106. The nurse is caring for a client with a history of a traumatic lumbar spinal cord injury who is experiencing constipation. Which prescription will the nurse question?
1. Administer bisacodyl 10 mg rectally daily.
2. Increase daily intake of fiber.
3. Encourage increased oral fluid intake.
4. Increase passive range of motion exercises.

106. 4. Increasing passive range of motion exercise will not affect the client's constipation. Bisacodyl is a laxative used to treat constipation. Increasing fiber and fluids can also assist with bowel movements.
CN: Physiological integrity; CNS: Basic care and comfort; CL: Apply

107. When assessing a client's pupillary responses, which method will the nurse use to evaluate pupil accommodation?
1. Check for peripheral vision using a blinking light.
2. Touch each cornea lightly with a wisp of cotton watching for a blink.
3. Have the client follow an object upward, downward, obliquely, and horizontally.
4. Observe for pupil constriction and convergence while focusing on an oncoming object.

107. 4. Accommodation refers to convergence and constriction of the pupil while focusing on a nearing object. Touching the cornea lightly with a wisp of cotton describes evaluation of the corneal reflex. Having the client follow an object upward, downward, obliquely, and horizontally refers to cardinal fields of gaze. Checking for peripheral vision refers to visual fields.
CN: Health promotion and maintenance; CNS: None; CL: Understand

108. The health care provider diagnosed a client with nyctalopia. The nurse understands which nutrient will **most** benefit the client?
1. Vitamin A
2. Vitamin B₆
3. Vitamin C
4. Vitamin K

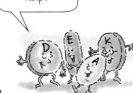

Which one of us should help?

108. 1. Night blindness (nyctalopia) may be caused from a vitamin A deficiency or dysfunctional rod receptors. None of the other deficiencies leads to nyctalopia.
CN: Physiological integrity; CNS: Basic care and comfort; CL: Apply

109. When discharging a client with a neurogenic bladder, the nurse will gather which equipment to use when providing educating?
1. Intermittent catheterization kit
2. Suprapubic catheter bag
3. Transurethral conduit drain
4. Ureterostomy pouch

109. 1. Intermittent catheterization, starting with 2-hour intervals and increasing to 4- to 6-hour intervals, is used to manage neurogenic bladder. A suprapubic catheter is a surgically implanted catheter above the pubis in the abdomen. An ileostomy or ureterostomy is not necessary. Transurethral prostatectomy is indicated for obstruction to urinary outflow by benign prostatic hyperplasia or for the treatment of cancer and does not require a drain.
CN: Safe, effective care environment; CNS: Safety and infection control; CL: Apply

110. When using a Snellen alphabet chart, the nurse records the client's vision as 20/40. What does this evaluation determine for the client?
1. The client can read 40% of the lines and 20% of the letters.
2. The client can see at 20 feet what the person with normal vision sees at 40 feet.
3. The client can see at 40 feet what the person with normal vision sees at 20 feet.
4. The client has a 20% decrease in acuity in one eye and a 40% decrease in the other eye.

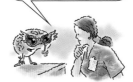

Sometimes neurosensory disorders can be difficult to identify.

110. 2. The numerator refers to the client's vision while comparing the normal vision in the denominator. Alterations in near vision may be due to loss of accommodation caused by the aging process (presbyopia) or farsightedness.
CN: Physiological integrity; CNS: Physiological adaptation; CL: Understand

111. Which herb will the nurse educate a client to avoid while taking rivaroxaban?
1. Bilberry
2. Goldenseal
3. Kava
4. Valerian

111. 2. Rivaroxaban is an anticoagulant that reduces the risk of cerebrovascular accident, atrial fibrillation, deep vein thrombosis, and pulmonary embolism. Goldenseal has an anticoagulant effect and could predispose the client to bleeding when given with rivaroxaban. Bilberry is used for improving eyesight. Kava and valerian are both used to decrease anxiety, stress, restlessness, and insomnia.
CN: Physiological integrity; CNS: Pharmacological and parenteral therapies; CL: Apply

112. After instilling atropine drops in both eyes of a client undergoing an ophthalmic examination, the nurse will educate the client on which safety issue?
1. Be careful because the blink reflex is paralyzed.
2. Avoid wearing regular glasses when driving.
3. It is normal to expect that the pupils may be unusually small.
4. Wear dark glasses in bright light because the pupils are dilated.

112. 4. Atropine, an anticholinergic drug, has mydriatic effects causing pupil dilation. This allows more light onto the retina and causes photophobia and blurred vision. Atropine does not paralyze the blink reflex or cause miosis (pupil constriction). Driving may be contraindicated because of blurred vision.
CN: Physiological integrity; CNS: Pharmacological and parenteral therapies; CL: Apply

113. The nurse is discussing risk factors for stroke and cerebrovascular accident (CVA) with an older adult client. Which risk factor(s) are **priority** for the nurse to include in the teaching? Select all that apply.
1. Hypertension
2. Diabetes mellitus
3. Oral contraceptive use
4. Atherosclerosis
5. Obesity

113. 1, 2, 4, 5. Atherosclerosis, hypertension, diabetes mellitus, and obesity are risk factors for the development of a stroke or CVA. The use of oral contraceptives can be a risk factor, but the client is an older adult, so this is not a priority.
CN: Health promotion and maintenance; CNS: None; CL: Apply

114. A client is scheduled for cataract surgery of the right eye. Which nursing action will be included in preparing a client for the surgical procedure?
1. Clip the client's eyelashes.
2. Put a patch on the affected eye.
3. Keep the client NPO.
4. Obtain informed consent.

114. 3. Maintaining nothing-by-mouth (NPO) status for at least 8 hours before surgical procedures prevents vomiting and aspiration. The health care provider is responsible for obtaining informed consent; the nurse validates that the consent is obtained. There is no need to patch an eye before most surgeries or to clip the eyelashes unless specifically prescribed by the health care provider.
CN: Physiological integrity; CNS: Reduction of risk potential; CL: Apply

115. When teaching a group of clients in a senior center, the nurse describes open angle glaucoma using which information?
1. The visual changes are easily corrected with eyeglasses.
2. The condition can be painless with loss of peripheral vision.
3. The disorder will not lead to complete loss of vision.
4. Narcotic medications are prescribed if pressures become uncomfortable.

If glaucoma is suspected, be sure to check to check the client's peripheral vision.

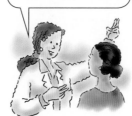

115. 2. Open-angle glaucoma causes a painless increase in intraocular pressure with loss of peripheral vision. A variety of miotics and agents to decrease intraocular pressure (and occasionally surgery) are used to treat glaucoma. The other options are not correct.
CN: Health promotion and maintenance; CNS: None; CL: Understand

116. The nurse is discharging a client following an intracapsular lens implant of the left eye. Which statement by the client is **most** concerning to the nurse?
1. "I will avoid eating until I notice the nausea subside."
2. "I will place a soft pillow under my left eye when I lay down."
3. "I will avoid bending over to put on my socks and shoes."
4. "I will wear the eye shield to protect the operative eye."

116. 2. Laying down should be with the operative side up, not on the affected side. Preventing nausea and subsequent vomiting will prevent increased intraocular pressure, as will avoiding bending or placing the head in a dependent position. The client will be wearing an eye shield to protect the affected eye.
CN: Safe, effective care environment; CNS: Management of care; CL: Apply

117. The nurse is caring for a client with chronic open-angle glaucoma. Which medication(s) will the nurse expect the client to be prescribed?
1. Brimonidine
2. Timolol
3. Furosemide
4. Urokinase
5. Atropine

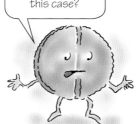

Which medications are the right ones in this case?

117. 1, 2. Brimonidine, an alpha₂-agonist, and timolol, a beta-blocker, are used to decrease intraocular pressure by decreasing aqueous humor production in clients with chronic open-angle glaucoma. Urokinase is a thrombolytic agent, and furosemide is a loop diuretic; these are not used in the treatment of glaucoma. Atropine dilates the pupil and decreases outflow of aqueous humor, causing a further increase in intraocular pressure.
CN: Physiological integrity; CNS: Pharmacological and parenteral therapies; CL: Apply

118. During assessment of a client admitted with signs of retinal detachment, the nurse will anticipate which finding(s)? Select all that apply.
1. Flashing lights
2. Homonymous hemianopia
3. Loss of central vision
4. Drooping of the eyelids
5. Visualization of floaters
6. Seeing shadows

118. 1, 5, 6. Signs and symptoms of retinal detachment include abrupt flashing lights, floaters, and a sudden shadow or curtain in the vision. Occasionally, vision loss is gradual. Homonymous hemianopia is the loss of half of the visual field; it is seen in clients with cerebrovascular accident or stroke. Loss of central vision is for macular degeneration. Ptosis or drooping of the eyelid is an early sign of myasthenia gravis.
CN: Physiological integrity; CNS: Physiological adaptation; CL: Apply

119. The nurse is providing education to a client receiving pilocarpine eye drops. Which statement made by the client indicates to the nurse the client needs additional teaching?
1. "The medication may make it hard for me to see at night."
2. "I cannot wear my contact lenses while taking this medication."
3. "The medication may cause me to have blurred vision."
4. "I may notice mild burning when I administer the drops."

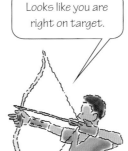

Looks like you are right on target.

119. 2. Pilocarpine is a miotic drug that causes constriction of the pupils. It is given to a client with glaucoma to decrease the intraocular pressure. The client can wear contact lenses; however, they should be removed prior to instillation and left out for 10 minutes after instillation. Pilocarpine can make it difficult for the client to see well at night or in low light; cause blurred vision; and cause mild burning, stinging, or discomfort of the eyes.
CN: Physiological integrity; CNS: Pharmacological and parenteral therapies; CL: Apply

120. The nurse is assessing a client 6 weeks after an emergent enucleation of the right eye. Which nursing intervention is appropriate for this client?
1. Instill pilocarpine to the left eye as prescribed.
2. Assess the client's ability to properly clean the prosthesis.
3. Determine reactivity of the pupils to light and accommodation.
4. Teach the client to avoid straining with bowel movements.

120. 2. Enucleation of the eye refers to surgical removal of the entire eye; therefore, the client needs instructions about the prosthesis. There are no activity restrictions or need for eye drops; however, prophylactic antibiotics may be used in the immediate postoperative period.
CN: Physiological integrity; CNS: Physiological adaptation; CL: Apply

CN: Client needs category CNS: Client needs subcategory CL: Cognitive level

121. Which is the **priority** nursing action prior to administering a gentamicin otic medication to a client?
1. Check and verify the client's name.
2. Warm the solution to prevent dizziness.
3. Hold an emesis basin under the client's ear.
4. Place the client in the semi-Fowler's position.

121. 1. When giving medications, a nurse follows the rights of medication administration: right client, right drug, right dose, right route, and right time, right documentation, right assessment, right to refuse, right evaluation, and right client education or information. The nurse would put the client in the lateral position, not semi-Fowler's position, for 5 minutes to prevent the drops from draining out. The drops may be warmed to prevent pain or dizziness, but this is not the first action. An emesis basin would be used for irrigation of the ear.
CN: Physiological integrity; CNS: Pharmacological and parenteral therapies; CL: Apply

122. The nurse is caring for a client newly diagnosed with Ménière's disease. Which prescription will the nurse question?
1. Administer meclizine
2. Strict bedrest
3. Diphenhydramine 25 mg TID PRN motion sickness
4. Limit daily sodium intake to 2 g

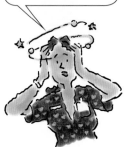

Ugghh. I think I got up too quickly. Everything is spinning.

122. 2. A client with Ménière's disease may experience dizziness, vertigo, ear pressure, hearing loss, and tinnitus. The client should not be placed on strict bedrest; however, the client should be assisted with ambulation until symptoms are controlled. Meclizine and diphenhydramine are used to decrease motion sickness and vertigo in clients with Ménière's disease. High sodium diets, smoking, infections, and caffeine may worsen symptoms.
CN: Physiological integrity; CNS: Reduction of risk potential; CL: Apply

123. A client is receiving phenytoin. Which response by a client **best** indicates to the nurse the client has an understanding of the adverse effects of the medication?
1. "I should take the medication without food."
2. "I can stop this medication if seizures stop."
3. "I need to see the dentist every 6 months."
4. "I should report drowsiness immediately."

123. 3. Phenytoin can cause hypertrophy of the gums and gingivitis; therefore, regular dental checkups are essential. Phenytoin needs to be taken with food or after meals to decrease adverse gastrointestinal reactions and should never be discontinued unless prescribed by the health care provider. Some drowsiness is expected initially; however, this usually decreases with continued use.
CN: Physiological therapy; CNS: Pharmacological and parenteral therapies; CL: Apply

124. After an assessment of a client's cranial nerves, the nurse documents the client's extraocular eye movements to be within normal limits. Which cranial nerve(s) will the nurse document as normal? Select all that apply.
1. Optic nerve (II)
2. Oculomotor nerve (III)
3. Trochlear nerve (IV)
4. Trigeminal nerve (V)
5. Abducens nerve (VI)

124. 2, 3, 5. Cranial nerve (CN) III (oculomotor), CN IV (trochlear), and CN VI (abducens) are all responsible for the movement of the eye. CN II is the optic nerve, which controls vision. CN V is the trigeminal nerve, which innervates the muscles of chewing.
CN: Health promotion and maintenance; CNS: None; CL: Apply

125. A client is taking carbamazepine. The nurse will monitor the client for which potential complication(s)? Select all that apply.
1. Respiratory distress
2. Diplopia
3. Ataxia
4. Dry skin
5. Leukocytosis

125. 2, 3. Carbamazepine is likely to cause diplopia, dizziness, ataxia, and a rash. Carbamazepine causes agranulocytosis because of the reduction in leukocytes. Respiratory distress and dry skin are not complications.
CN: Physiological integrity; CNS: Pharmacological and parenteral therapies; CL: Apply

CN: Client needs category   CNS: Client needs subcategory   CL: Cognitive level

126. The nurse is observing a client with cerebral edema for evidence of increasing intracranial pressure. The client's current blood pressure is 170/80 mm Hg. What will the nurse document as the client's pulse pressure? Record your answer using a whole number.

_____

127. After a client suffered a blunt trauma to the head, the nurse will include which statement when teaching the client's caregiver?
1. "Monitor for keyhole pupils over the next day and report to the health care provider."
2. "Expect profuse vomiting for the next few hours and keep the client NPO."
3. "Wake the client every hour and check orientation to person, time, and place."
4. "Notify the health care provider immediately if the client experiences a headache."

128. Which manifestation will the nurse expect to observe in a client with thalamic syndrome?
1. Aching sensation over one-half of the body
2. Grand mal seizure activity
3. Problems with initiating body movement
4. Chronic memory lapses

129. The nurse is making assignments for the day. Which task will the nurse appropriately delegate to the assistive personnel (AP)?
1. Performing assessment on a client with encephalitis
2. Feeding a client with stroke reporting dysphagia
3. Measuring the intake of a client with multiple sclerosis
4. Turning a client with fracture of cervical spine

130. A client is admitted after falling and hitting the back of the head on a curb. Which nursing action is appropriate for this client?
1. Test water temperature before bathing or showering.
2. Assist client while walking due to loss of balance.
3. Monitor the client for visual disturbances.
4. Evaluate the client's hearing condition.

Yahoo! You're almost done. Keep going.

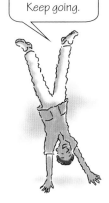

126. 90.
Pulse pressure is the difference between the systolic blood pressure and the diastolic blood pressure. For this client:

$$170 \; mm \; Hg - 80 \; mm \; Hg = 90 \; mm \; Hg$$

CN: Physiological integrity; CNS: Reduction of risk potential; CL: Apply

127. 3. Changes in level of consciousness (LOC) may indicate expanding lesions such as subdural hematoma; orientation and LOC are assessed frequently for 24 hours. Profuse or projectile vomiting is a symptom of increased intracranial pressure and should be reported immediately. A slight headache may last for several days after concussion; severe or worsening headaches should be reported. A keyhole pupil is found after iridectomy.

CN: Physiological integrity; CNS: Physiological adaptation; CL: Apply

128. 1. Damage to the thalamus may result in thalamic syndrome, which is characterized by pain, burning, or an aching sensation over one-half of the body. It is often accompanied by mood swings. Problems initiating movement are associated with the basal ganglia and memory problems with the hippocampus. Seizures are not specific to thalamic injury.

CN: Physiological integrity; CNS: Physiological adaptation; CL: Apply

129. 3. The AP can be assigned to perform a routine task such as measuring the intake of a client with multiple sclerosis. However, AP cannot be assigned to a client who is not stable. A client with a stroke may have dysphagia or difficulty swallowing. This client should not be assigned to a AP because of risk of aspiration. A client with fracture of the cervical spine should not be assigned to AP because the client is also unstable. Performing assessment is not within the scope of practice of AP.

CN: Safe, effective care environment; CNS: Management of care; CL: Apply

130. 3. The nurse should monitor client for visual disturbances since occipital lobe regulates vision. The parietal lobe primarily regulates sensory function. The cerebellum controls balance. The temporal lobe is involved in hearing.

CN: Physiological integrity; CNS: Basic care and comfort; CL: Apply

131. The nurse is caring for a client diagnosed with Huntington disease. Which prescription(s) will the nurse question? Select all that apply.
1. Tetrabenazine
2. Imipramine
3. Chlorpromazine
4. Pramipexole
5. Entacapone

131. 4, 5. Huntington disease (HD) is an inherited, progressive disease where the nerve cells in the basal ganglia region of the brain break down over time. Symptoms of HD include uncontrollable movements, memory loss, confusion, difficulty speaking, depression, and impaired cognitive function. Pramipexole (dopamine agonist) and entacapone (catechol-O-methyltransferase [COMT] inhibitor) are both used to treat Parkinson disease. Tetrabenazine and chlorpromazine are used to decrease chorea movements in clients with HD. Imipramine is used to treat depression in clients with HD.
CN: Physiological integrity; CNS: Physiological adaptation; CL: Apply

132. The nurse is preparing a client who suffered a cerebral hemorrhage from a cerebral aneurysm for an electroencephalogram (EEG). Which finding will the nurse report to the health care provider?
1. The client has a pacemaker.
2. The client is allergic to iodine.
3. The client cannot be taken off oxygen.
4. The client is prescribed nimodipine.

132. 3. An EEG measures the electrical activity of the brain. The only potential contraindication to undergoing an EEG is if the client requires a high concentration of oxygen. This is because of the risk of fire if the electrical current from the EEG machine ignites the oxygen. An EEG is noninvasive; therefore, there are no other contraindications or risks associated with proper use. Nimodipine is a calcium channel blocker given to prevent brain damage by improving blood flow in the brain.
CN: Safe, effective care environment; CNS: Management of care; CL: Apply

133. The nurse is caring for a client with multiple sclerosis (MS). Which complication(s) will the nurse expect the client to experience? Select all that apply.
1. Visual disturbances
2. Coagulation abnormalities
3. Impaired motor function
4. Immunity compromise
5. Decreased sensation

133. 1, 3, 5. Multiple sclerosis, a neuromuscular disorder, may cause visual disturbances, impaired sensation, and impaired motor function. MS does not cause coagulation abnormalities or immunity problems.
CN: Physiological integrity; CNS: Reduction of risk potential; CL: Apply

134. The nurse is teaching a client with trigeminal neuralgia on how to minimize pain episodes. Which comment(s) by the client indicates correct understanding of the nurse's education? Select all that apply.
1. "I will eat food that is very hot or cold."
2. "I will chew food on the unaffected side."
3. "I can wash my face with icy water."
4. "I will drink fluids at room temperature."
5. "I will perform mouth care after meals."

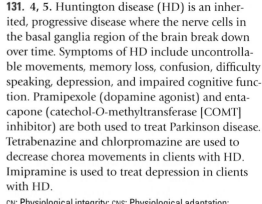

With trigeminal neuralgia, remember to chew on the good side.

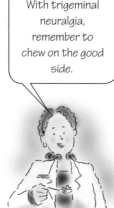

crackle crackle

134. 2, 4, 5. The facial pain of trigeminal neuralgia is triggered by mechanical or thermal stimuli. Chewing food on the unaffected side and rinsing the mouth rather than brushing the teeth reduce mechanical stimulation. Drinking fluids at room temperature reduces thermal stimulation. Eating hot or cold food and washing the face with cold water are likely to trigger pain.
CN: Health promotion and maintenance; CNS: None; CL: Apply

135. The nurse is caring for a client experiencing problems with balance and fine gross motor function. Identify the area of the client's brain the nurse will document as effected.

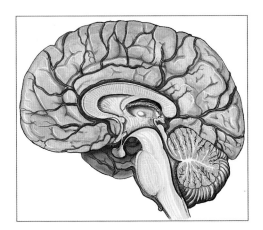

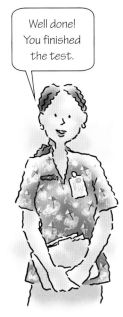

Well done! You finished the test.

135. The cerebellum is the portion of the brain that controls balance and fine and gross motor function.

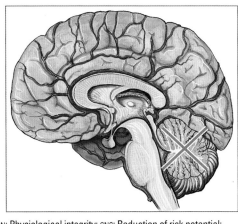

CN: Physiological integrity; CNS: Reduction of risk potential; CL: Apply

Chapter 7

Musculoskeletal Disorders

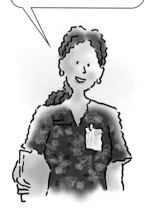

Here's a test that covers nursing care for clients with a disorder of the musculoskeletal system. So get moving and break a leg. Oh—I mean good luck!

Musculoskeletal refresher

Arm and leg fractures

Complete or incomplete break in a bone resulting from the application of excessive force

Key signs and symptoms
- Loss of limb function, altered mobility
- Swelling, pallor, ecchymosis of surrounding subcutaneous tissue
- Pain
- Absent or decreased pulses distal to the fracture
- Deformity

Key test results
- Anterior, posterior, and lateral x-rays of the suspected fracture as well as x-rays of the joints above and below it confirms diagnosis

Key treatments
- Closed reduction procedure to restore displaced bone segments to their normal position
- Immobilization with a splint, cast, or traction
- Open reduction and internal fixation (ORIF) is a surgical procedure to reduce and immobilize the fracture with rods, plates, pins, or screws when closed reduction is impossible, usually followed by application of a cast
- Analgesics: morphine, ibuprofen, acetaminophen, oxycodone, hydrocodone

Key interventions
- Monitor vital signs and be especially alert for rapid pulse, decreased blood pressure, pallor, and cool, clammy skin.
- Maintain IV fluids as prescribed.
- Provide analgesics: acetaminophen, hydrocodone, morphine sulfate, oxycodone.
- Reposition the immobilized client often.
- Assist with active range-of-motion (ROM) exercises to the unaffected extremities.
- Encourage deep breathing and coughing.
- Ensure that immobilized client receives adequate fluid intake.

- Watch for signs of renal calculi, such as flank pain, nausea, and vomiting.
- Provide cast care.
- Encourage the client to start moving about as soon as possible.
- Assist with walking, keeping in mind that a client who has been bedridden for some time may be dizzy at first.
- Demonstrate proper crutch use.

Carpal tunnel syndrome

Pressure on the median nerve as it passes under the transverse carpal ligament in the wrist

Key signs and symptoms
- Numbness, burning, or tingling in the hand and arm
- Pain in arm and hand
- Weakness in arm and hand

Key test results
- Blood pressure cuff on the forearm inflated above systolic pressure for 1 to 2 minutes evokes pain and paresthesia along the median nerve
- Tinel's test by tapping on the inside of the client's wrist over the median nerve to assess for numbness or tingling in the fingers
- Electromyography detects median nerve motor conduction delay of more than 5 milliseconds

Key treatments
- Resting the hands by splinting the wrist in neutral position for 1 to 2 weeks
- Possibly changing occupations (if definite link has been established between client's occupation and development of carpal tunnel syndrome)
- Corticosteroid injections: betamethasone, hydrocortisone
- Nonsteroidal anti-inflammatory drugs (NSAIDs): indomethacin, ibuprofen, naproxen
- A carpal tunnel release may be needed if nonsurgical techniques are not effective

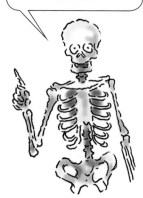

No bones about it—you're going to break these questions down like a compound fracture.

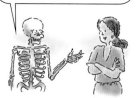

What could be causing this pain in my arms and hands?

Key interventions
- Administer NSAIDs as needed: ibuprofen, indomethacin, naproxen.
- Administer corticosteroids: betamethasone, hydrocortisone.
- Assist with eating and bathing if client's dominant hand has been impaired.
- Monitor vital signs and regularly check color, sensation, and motion of affected hand, if surgery is performed.

Compartment syndrome
Serious condition that involves increased pressure in a muscle compartment, compromising circulation

Key signs and symptoms
- Severe pain that is more intense than expected for the injury and is unrelieved by analgesics
- Loss of distal pulse
- Tense, swollen muscle
- Pale, cool extremity
- Paresthesia

Key test results
- Intracompartmental pressure is elevated, as indicated by a blood pressure sphygmomanometer

Key treatments
- Fasciotomy
- Positioning the affected extremity lower than the heart
- Removal of dressings or constrictive coverings from the area

Key interventions
- Monitor the affected extremity.
- Perform frequent neurovascular checks.
- Perform dressing changes after fasciotomy, and reinforce dressings frequently (expect a large amount of bloody drainage).

Gout
Disease in which defective metabolism of uric acid causes arthritis

Key signs or symptoms
- Inflamed, painful joints

Key test results
- Blood studies indicate:
  - elevated serum uric acid level
  - urine uric acid level usually higher in secondary gout than in primary gout.

Key treatments
- Antigout drugs: colchicine, allopurinol, febuxostat
- Uricosuric drugs: probenecid, sulfinpyrazone, lesinurad
- Corticosteroids: betamethasone, hydrocortisone
- NSAIDs: ibuprofen, naproxen, indomethacin, celecoxib

Key interventions
- Encourage bed rest, and use a bed cradle to reduce discomfort.
- Apply hot or cold packs to inflamed joints.
- Administer analgesics, anti-inflammatory medications, and other drugs as needed.
- Limit intake of foods high in purines, alcoholic beverages, and drinks sweetened with fructose.
- Urge client to drink plenty of fluids (up to 2 L/day).
- Record intake and output accurately.
- Alkalinize urine with sodium bicarbonate as needed.
- Ensure client understands importance of having serum uric acid levels checked periodically.

Herniated nucleus pulposus
Disk is displaced from its normal position in between the vertebral bodies of spine

Key signs and symptoms
In lumbosacral area
- Acute pain in lower back that radiates across the buttock and down the leg
- Pain on ambulation
- Weakness, numbness, and tingling of foot and leg

In cervical area
- Neck pain that radiates down arm to the hand
- Neck stiffness
- Weakness of the affected upper extremities
- Weakness, numbness, and tingling of hand

Key test results
- Myelogram shows compression of the spinal cord
- X-ray shows narrowing of disk space
- Magnetic resonance imaging identifies the herniated disk

Key treatments
- Corticosteroid: cortisone

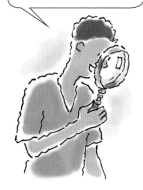
What signs should you look for in compartment syndrome?

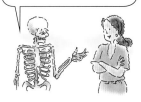
So, my gout has really been flaring up lately. What should I do about it?

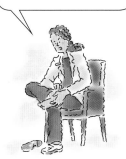
Arrgghh! My gout is acting up. I guess I need to drink more water.

- NSAIDs: indomethacin, ibuprofen, sulindac, piroxicam, flurbiprofen, diclofenac sodium, naproxen, diflunisal

Key interventions

- Monitor neurovascular status.
- Turn the client every 2 hours using the log-rolling technique.

Hip fracture

Fracture of the femoral neck

Key signs and symptoms

- Shorter appearance and outward rotation of affected leg, resulting in limited or abnormal ROM
- Edema and discoloration of surrounding tissue

Key test results

- Computed tomography scan pinpoints abnormalities (for complicated fractures)
- X-ray reveals a break in the continuity of the bone

Key treatments

- Surgical immobilization or joint replacement
- Abductor splint or trochanter roll between legs to prevent loss of alignment (postoperatively)
- Anticoagulant: warfarin (postoperatively)

Key interventions

- Monitor neurovascular and respiratory status.
- Priority: check for compromised circulation, hemorrhage, and neurologic impairment in the affected extremity and pneumonia in the bedridden client.
- Provide active and passive ROM and isometric exercises for unaffected limbs.
- Provide a trapeze.
- Maintain traction before surgery at all times, if using conservative treatment.

Osteoarthritis

Type of arthritis caused by inflammation, breakdown, and eventual loss of cartilage in the joints

Key signs and symptoms

- Crepitation
- Joint stiffness
- Pain relieved by resting the joints

Key test results

- Arthroscopy reveals bone spurs and narrowing of joint space
- X-rays show joint deformity, narrowing of joint space, and bone spurs

Key treatments

- Exercise
- Application of warm, moist heat
- NSAIDs: indomethacin, ibuprofen, naproxen, diflunisal, celecoxib

Key interventions

- Evaluate musculoskeletal status.
- Observe for increased bleeding or bruising tendency.

Osteomyelitis

Bone infection caused by bacteria or other germs

Key signs and symptoms

- Pain
- Tenderness
- Swelling

Key test results

- Blood cultures identify causative organism
- Erythrocyte sedimentation rate and C-reactive protein (CRP) are elevated (CRP appears to be a better diagnostic tool)

Key treatments

- Immobilization of affected bone by plaster cast, traction, or bed rest
- Antibiotics: large doses of IV antibiotics after blood cultures are taken, usually:
  - penicillinase-resistant penicillin (nafcillin and oxacillin)
  - cephalosporin (cefazolin)

Key interventions

- Use strict aseptic technique when changing dressings and irrigating wounds.
- Check vital signs and wound appearance daily; monitor for new pain.
- Check circulation and drainage; if wet spot appears on cast, circle it with a pen and note the date and time of appearance (on the cast); be aware of how much drainage is expected; check the circled spot at least every 4 hours; watch for any enlargement.

Osteoporosis

Softening of the bones that gradually increases and makes them more fragile

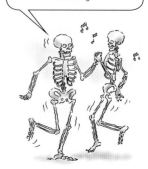

Shake those bones! Exercise helps keep bones and joints healthy.

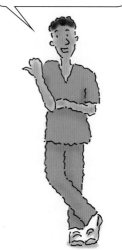

"Crepitation." That word gives me the creeps.

Key signs and symptoms
- Deformity
- Kyphosis
- Pain

Key test results
- X-rays show typical degeneration in the lower thoracic and lumbar vertebrae
- Vertebral bodies may appear flattened and may look denser than normal
- Loss of bone mineral becomes evident in later stages
- Dual-energy x-ray absorptiometry (DXA) shows bone mineral density at the spine and hip

Key treatments
- Physical therapy consisting of weight-bearing exercise and activity

- Hormonal agents: conjugated estrogen, calcitonin, teriparatide, calcitonin
- Vitamin D supplements
- Antiosteoporotics: alendronate, risedronate, raloxifene, ibandronate
- Calcium supplements

Key interventions
- Check the client's skin daily for redness, warmth, and new sites of pain.
- Encourage activity; help client walk several times daily.
- Perform passive ROM exercises, or encourage the client to perform active exercises.
- Encourage regular attendance at physical therapy sessions.
- Provide a balanced diet high in vitamin D, calcium, and protein.
- Administer analgesics and apply heat.

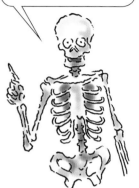

Make sure you're getting enough calcium and vitamin D, my friend. I need to stay strong and healthy for years to come.

thePoint® You can download tables of drug information to help you prepare for the NCLEX®! View Generic Drug Names, Drug Classifications, Drug Actions, and Nursing Implications for the drugs discussed in this refresher at **http://thePoint.lww.com.**

Musculoskeletal questions, answers, and rationales

1. The emergency room nurse is caring for a client with a history of osteoporosis who sustained right wrist and hip fractures after a fall. Which nursing intervention is **priority**?
1. Administer opioid analgesics.
2. Assist with activities of daily living.
3. Give the client water as requested.
4. Assess the client's living arrangements.

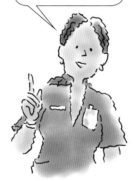

Remember, the **priority** is the intervention to take first.

2. An older adult client reports pain in the lower back and is diagnosed with osteoporosis. Which education is **priority** for the nurse to provide?
1. Pain control options
2. Safety precautions to avoid fractures
3. Effect of the disease process on the bones
4. Supplement usage

3. The nurse is providing education for a client on preventing complications of primary osteoporosis. Which statement made by the client indicates a proper understanding of the education provided?
1. "I will refrain from drinking any alcoholic beverages."
2. "I will be sure to take my calcium supplements each day."
3. "I must eat three balanced meals each day and have a light snack."
4. "I cannot stop complications because I have rheumatoid arthritis, too."

1. 1. Relieving pain and making the client more comfortable should have priority. Water should not be administered unless cleared by the health care provider in case the client requires surgery. Obtaining data regarding living arrangements and assisting with activities of daily living are important after the fractures are stabilized or repaired. CN: Safe, effective care environment; CNS: Safety and infection control; CL: Analyze

2. 2. The primary complication of osteoporosis is fractures, so education on safety precautions to avoid them would be priority. Pain may occur, but fractures can be life-threatening. Education on the disease process and supplement usage would not help prevent complications. CN: Safe, effective care environment; CNS: Management of care; CL: Analyze

3. 2. Hormonal imbalance, faulty metabolism, and poor dietary intake of calcium cause primary osteoporosis. Therefore, taking calcium supplements each day is of primary importance for clients with primary osteoporosis. Malnutrition, alcoholism, osteogenesis imperfecta, rheumatoid arthritis, liver disease, scurvy, lactose intolerance, hyperthyroidism, and trauma cause secondary osteoporosis. So, eating balanced meals and refraining from alcohol would not prevent complications in primary osteoporosis, and a client with primary osteoporosis would not necessarily have rheumatoid arthritis. CN: Physiological integrity; CNS: Physiological adaptation; CL: Apply

CN: Client needs category   CNS: Client needs subcategory   CL: Cognitive level

4. The nurse is caring for a 50-year-old client who recently had a hysterectomy with salpingo-oophorectomy. Which response by the client indicates the nurse's education has been effective?
1. "My risk for osteoporosis is low because I still have my thyroid gland."
2. "I am fine because osteoporosis only affects women over 65 years of age."
3. "I am still producing hormones, so I do not have to worry about osteoporosis."
4. "Since my surgery, I now need to take precautions to protect against osteoporosis."

5. The nurse is providing nutritional information to a client with a diagnosis of gout. The nurse will recommend the client avoid which food(s)? Select all that apply.
1. Blackberries
2. Tofu
3. Liver
4. Tomatoes
5. Bacon
6. Anchovies

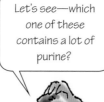

6. A client who is hospitalized is at risk for developing osteoporosis. Which intervention focused on primary prevention will the nurse include when caring for the client?
1. Placing personal items within reach of the client
2. Placing the client in a room with bars in the bathroom
3. Maintaining optimal calcium and vitamin D intake
4. Contacting case management to get the client a professional alert system

7. The nurse is caring for a client with an acute attack of gout. Which action will the nurse take **first**?
1. Force fluids.
2. Provide relaxation techniques.
3. Encourage bed rest.
4. Administer analgesics.

8. The nurse is caring for a male client diagnosed with acute gout. Which finding will the nurse highlight for the primary health care provider to review?
1. Client reports pain for the past 48 hours.
2. Client reports multiple joints are involved.
3. Oral temperature is 99°F (37.2°C).
4. Uric acid level 4.6 mg/dL (273.63 μmol/L).

4. 4. A hysterectomy with salpingo-oophorectomy places the client in surgically induced menopause; with her ovaries removed, she is no longer producing the necessary hormones. Therefore, she must now take precautions to protect against osteoporosis. This client's thyroid gland will not protect her from menopause. Although age is a risk factor for osteoporosis, women younger than 65 years can be affected by this disease, and menopause at any age puts women at risk for osteoporosis because of the associated hormonal imbalance.
CN: Physiological integrity; CNS: Physiological adaptation; CL: Apply

5. 3, 5, 6. A client with gout should reduce intake of purine-rich foods, such as liver; bacon; select seafood, fish, and shellfish; and alcohol. Blackberries, tofu, and tomatoes are not rich in purine.
CN: Physiological integrity; CNS: Basic care and comfort; CL: Apply

6. 3. Primary prevention of osteoporosis includes maintaining optimal calcium and vitamin D intake. Using a professional alert system in the home, installing bars in bathrooms to prevent falls, and placing items within reach of the client are all secondary and tertiary prevention methods.
CN: Health promotion and maintenance; CNS: None; CL: Apply

7. 4. Administering analgesics to relieve the pain of gout should be the priority. The other actions are appropriate measures to institute but are not the priority.
CN: Safe, effective care environment; CNS: Management of care; CL: Analyze

8. 2. The nurse would highlight multiple joint involvement as this is seen with chronic, not acute gout. Acute gout is a painful attack (joint inflammation) following trauma or activity that increases uric acid levels, such as alcohol consumption. Symptoms generally ease after 7 to 10 days. Inflammation may lead to a slight elevation in temperature. The normal uric acid level range for males is 3.4 to 7 mg/dL (202.25 to 416.39 μmol/L).
CN: Safe, effective care environment; CNS: Management of care; CL: Apply

9. The nurse is ordering breakfast for a client with gout. Which is the **best** meal for the nurse to order the client?
1. Egg omelet with cheese and anchovies, along with milk
2. Bacon and liver mush biscuit with orange juice
3. Eggs with turkey bacon, and chocolate milk
4. Jelly biscuit, scrambled eggs, and water

9. **4.** A client with gout should limit purine consumption. Anchovies, bacon, turkey, organ meats, and fish are high in purines and thus should be avoided in clients with gout.
CN: Physiological integrity; CNS: Basic care and comfort; CL: Apply

10. A client is recovering from a gout attack. Which rationale will the nurse provide the client regarding the need to lose weight?
1. Weight loss will decrease purine levels without a change in diet.
2. Weight loss will decrease inflammation in the joints.
3. Weight loss will increase life expectancy by decreasing uric acid levels.
4. Weight loss will decrease uric acid levels and decrease stress on the joints.

10. **4.** Weight loss will decrease uric acid levels and decrease stress on the joints. Weight loss will not decrease purine levels, increase life expectancy, or decrease inflammation in the joints.
CN: Health promotion and maintenance; CNS: None; CL: Apply

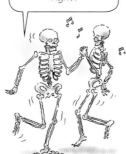

Well, rattle my bones—I think you got that one right!

11. The nurse is caring for a client reporting sudden-onset right foot pain, especially in the great toe. While reviewing the client's laboratory results, the nurse notes a uric acid level of 9.8 mg/dL (582.95 μmol/L). Which primary health care provider prescription will the nurse question?
1. Give acetaminophen 500 mg every 6 hours PRN pain.
2. Limit dietary intake of purines.
3. Apply ice to the affected foot and elevate.
4. Give prednisone 30 mg daily.

11. **1.** The findings indicate an acute gout attack. The nurse would question a prescription for acetaminophen. Nonsteroidal anti-inflammatory drugs (NSAIDs) are the drug of choice to quickly relieve inflammation and pain for an acute gout attack. It is best to take an NSAID within the first 24 hours after symptom onset. Avoiding purines, applying ice and elevating the affected joint, and corticosteroids are common treatments for gout.
CN: Safe, effective care environment; CNS: Management of care; CL: Analyze

12. Which statement by a client diagnosed with gout indicates to the nurse the client understands the proper rationale for increasing fluid intake, as directed in discharge instructions?
1. "Increasing fluids will help provide a cushion for my bones."
2. "I will increase my fluids so the inflammation will be reduced."
3. "Increasing fluid intake will increase the calcium my body absorbs."
4. "Increasing fluid intake will cause my body to excrete more uric acid."

12. **4.** Fluids promote the excretion of uric acid. Fluids do not decrease inflammation, increase calcium absorption, or provide a cushion for bones.
CN: Physiological integrity; CNS: Physiological adaptation; CL: Apply

13. A client recently diagnosed with gout asks the nurse to explain the needs to take colchicine. Which nursing response is **most** appropriate?
1. "Colchicine decreases inflammation."
2. "Colchicine increases estrogen levels in the bloodstream."
3. "Colchicine decreases the risk of infection."
4. "Colchicine decreases bone demineralization."

13. **1.** The action of colchicine is to decrease inflammation by reducing the migration of leukocytes to synovial fluid. Colchicine does not decrease the risk of infection, increase estrogen levels, or decrease bone demineralization.
CN: Physiological integrity; CNS: Pharmacological and parenteral therapies; CL: Apply

14. The nurse is assessing a client with osteoarthritis. Which finding(s) **most** concerns the nurse? Select all that apply.
1. Joint pain after exercise
2. Symmetrical swelling of hand joints
3. Joint stiffness
4. Fever
5. Crepitation

14. 2, 4. Symmetrical swelling of hand joints and fever are consistent with rheumatoid arthritis, not osteoarthritis. Unexpected findings such as these would be most concerning. The expected symptoms of osteoarthritis are joint pain after exercise or weight bearing (usually relieved by rest), joint stiffness, and crepitation.
CN: Safe, effective care environment; CNS: Management of care; CL: Apply

15. Which instruction will the nurse provide for a client diagnosed with osteoarthritis taking nonsteroidal anti-inflammatory drugs (NSAIDs)?
1. Bleeding is not a problem with NSAIDs.
2. Take NSAIDs with food to avoid an upset stomach.
3. Take NSAIDs with acidic juice to increase absorption.
4. Do not take NSAIDs at bedtime because they may cause insomnia.

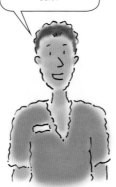

Great! I'm always looking for an excuse to eat.

15. 2. NSAIDs should be taken with food to avoid an upset stomach. NSAIDs should not be taken with acidic juice because the combination of the two can irritate the gastrointestinal mucosa and lead to gastrointestinal bleeding. NSAIDs can cause drowsiness (not insomnia) and complications from bleeding.
CN: Physiological integrity; CNS: Pharmacological and parenteral therapies; CL: Apply

16. Which statement will the nurse include when educating a client newly diagnosed with osteoarthritis?
1. "Osteoarthritis is rarely debilitating."
2. "There is no treatment for osteoarthritis."
3. "Osteoarthritis affects people older than 60 years."
4. "Osteoarthritis is the most common form of arthritis."

16. 4. Osteoarthritis is the most common form of arthritis. It can affect people of any age, although it is most common in older adults, and can be extremely debilitating. Treatments, such as NSAIDs, are available for osteoarthritis.
CN: Physiological integrity; CNS: Physiological adaptation; CL: Apply

17. A client diagnosed with primary osteoarthritis asks the nurse, "What caused this disease?" Which rationale(s) is appropriate for the nurse to include in the response? Select all that apply.
1. Joint overuse
2. Obesity
3. Congenital abnormality
4. Aging process
5. Diabetes mellitus

17. 1, 2, 4. Primary osteoarthritis may be caused by the overuse of joints, aging, or obesity. Congenital abnormalities and diabetes mellitus can cause secondary osteoarthritis.
CN: Physiological integrity; CNS: Physiological adaptation; CL: Apply

18. The nurse knows a client with osteoarthritis of the knee understands the discharge instructions when the client makes which statement?
1. "I will take my ibuprofen on an empty stomach."
2. "I will try taking a warm shower in the morning."
3. "I will wear my knee splint every night."
4. "I will jog at least a mile every evening."

18. 2. A client with osteoarthritis has joint stiffness that may be partially relieved with a warm shower on arising in the morning. Ibuprofen should be taken with food, as should all nonsteroidal anti-inflammatory drugs. Splints are usually used by clients with rheumatoid arthritis. Because osteoarthritis continually stresses the joint, exercise that puts less strain on the joint, such as swimming, would be a better choice.
CN: Physiological integrity; CNS: Basic care and comfort; CL: Apply

19. A client is taking aspirin for osteoarthritis. The nurse will carefully monitor the client for which complication?
1. Hearing loss
2. Increasing joint pain
3. Decreased calcium levels
4. Increased bone demineralization

19. 1. Many older adults already have diminished hearing, and salicylate use can lead to further or total hearing loss. Salicylates, such as aspirin, do not increase bone demineralization, decrease calcium absorption, or increase pain in joints.
CN: Physiological integrity; CNS: Pharmacological and parenteral therapies; CL: Analyze

CN: Client needs category   CNS: Client needs subcategory   CL: Cognitive level

20. The nurse is caring for a client diagnosed with osteoarthritis who has been prescribed bed rest. Which nursing intervention(s) is appropriate for this client? Select all that apply.
1. Limit oral fluid intake.
2. Providing passive range of motion.
3. Decrease stimulation.
4. Encourage the client to lie still in the bed.
5. Turn the client every 2 hours.
6. Teach coughing and deep breathing.

21. The nurse will recommend a client with osteoarthritis use which type(s) of clothing at home to assist in performing activities of daily living? Select all that apply.
1. Zippered clothing
2. Rubber grippers
3. Velcro clothing
4. Slip-on shoes
5. Tied shoes

22. The nurse is caring for a client prescribed indomethacin for osteoarthritis. Which finding will the nurse report to the primary health care provider?
1. The client is currently 34 years of age.
2. The client has a history of a stomach ulcers.
3. The client's grandfather had a myocardial infarction (MI).
4. The client gained 10 lb (4.5 kg) over the past 6 months.

23. An older adult client is seen in the clinic with reports of right hip pain that worsens after activity, decreased range of motion (ROM) of the right hip, and difficulty getting up after sitting for long periods. The nurse hears crepitus in the right hip upon movement and prepares to provide care for which condition?
1. Gout
2. Osteoarthritis
3. Rheumatoid arthritis
4. Hip fracture

24. Which education provided by the nurse will help prevent injury in a client diagnosed with osteoarthritis? Select all that apply.
1. Stay on bed rest.
2. Avoid physical activity.
3. Avoid repetitive tasks.
4. Warm up before exercise.
5. Apply ice to the joints.

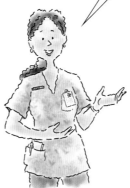

The answer to question #20 is a real turn-on.

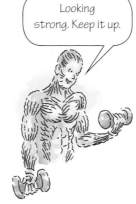

Looking strong. Keep it up.

20. 5, 6. A bedridden client needs to be turned every 2 hours, have adequate nutrition, and cough and deep breathe. Providing adequate pain medication, active *and* passive range of motion, and oral hydration are also appropriate nursing measures. The nurse should not encourage the client to lie still in bed (to prevent contractures), decrease stimulation, or limit fluid intake.
CN: Physiological integrity; CNS: Basic care and comfort; CL: Apply

21. 2, 3, 4. Velcro clothing, slip-on shoes, and rubber grippers make it easier for the client to dress and grip objects. Zippers and tied shoes may be difficult for the client to use.
CN: Physiological integrity; CNS: Basic care and comfort; CL: Apply

22. 2. Indomethacin is a NSAID used to treat osteoarthritis. For clients with a history of stomach ulcers or bleeding, the nurse should notify the health care provider before the client begins the prescription for indomethacin, as this drug may cause fatal gastrointestinal (GI) bleeding. The risk of GI bleeding is higher in older adult clients. Clients with a history of heart disease, MI, or stroke should also have a consult with their health care provider before treatment. A distant family history of heart disease and prior weight gain are not concerning.
CN: Safe, effective care environment; CNS: Management of care; CL: Analyze

23. 2. Osteoarthritis of the hip is associated with joint pain that worsens with activity, diminished ROM, joint crepitus, and difficulty arising after long periods of rest. Gout is associated with intermittent periods of joint pain that resolve. Rheumatoid arthritis is a systemic disease that affects multiple joints. Clients with hip fractures have severe pain in the hip or groin and are unable to bear weight, and the leg may be externally rotated.
CN: Physiological integrity; CNS: Physiological adaptation; CL: Analyze

24. 3, 4. Primary prevention of injury from osteoarthritis includes warming up and avoiding repetitive tasks. Physical activity is important to remain fit and healthy and to maintain joint function. Bed rest would contribute to many other systemic complications. Applying ice would help reduce inflammation and dull the pain sensation; however, this would not help prevent injury.
CN: Health promotion and maintenance; CNS: None; CL: Apply

25. Which statement by the client indicates to the nurse that additional education regarding celecoxib is needed?
1. "I can open the capsule and sprinkle the medicine in applesauce."
2. "I can take this medication with or without food."
3. "I will report any rectal bleeding immediately."
4. "I can take this even though I am allergic to sulfonamides."

26. A client with osteoarthritis is refusing to perform independent daily care. Which nursing approach is **most** appropriate to use with this client?
1. Have the assistive personnel (AP) perform the care for the client.
2. Explain that complete independence should be maintained.
3. Encourage the client to perform as much care as pain allows.
4. Inform the client after care is completed, pain medication will be administered.

27. The nurse is gathering data from a client newly diagnosed with osteoarthritis and asks the client to describe the pain. What description **most** concerns the nurse?
1. Grating
2. Dull ache
3. Deep, aching pain
4. Deep aching, relieved with rest

28. A client is prescribed a cane to use for assistance with walking. The nurse is teaching the client how to use the cane. Which instruction will the nurse include in the teaching? Select all that apply.
1. Hold the cane in the hand on your unaffected side.
2. Move the cane and affected leg forward simultaneously.
3. Lean your weight on the cane as needed.
4. Do not use the cane when walking up or down stairs.
5. Take the first step with the unaffected leg.

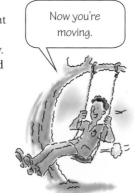

Now you're moving.

29. The nurse is providing discharge instructions to a client diagnosed with osteoarthritis. Which discharge instruction about home activity will the nurse include in the teaching?
1. Learn to pace activity.
2. Remain as sedentary as possible.
3. Return to a normal level of activity.
4. Include vigorous exercise in daily routine.

25. 4. Celecoxib is a nonsteroidal anti-inflammatory drug (NSAID) used to treat osteoarthritis. A client allergic to sulfa drugs, aspirin, or NSAIDs should not take celecoxib. Celecoxib can be sprinkled on food if the client cannot swallow the capsule. It can also be taken with or without food. Any signs of gastrointestinal bleeding should be reported immediately, as bleeding may be fatal.
CN: Physiological integrity; CNS: Pharmacological and parenteral therapies; CL: Apply

26. 3. A client with osteoarthritis should be encouraged to perform as much of the client's own care as possible. The nurse's goal should be to allow the client to maintain her self-care abilities with help as needed. It is never appropriate to use pain medication as a bargaining tool.
CN: Psychosocial integrity; CNS: None; CL: Apply

27. 1. This indicates the client is actually in the late stages of osteoarthritis. As the disease progresses, the cartilage covering the ends of bones is destroyed and bones rub against each other. Osteophytes, or bone spurs, may also form on the ends of bones. A dull ache and deep, aching pain that may be relieved with rest is usually seen in the earlier stages of osteoarthritis.
CN: Safe, effective care environment; CNS: Management of care; CL: Apply

28. 1, 2, 3. A cane should be used on the unaffected side. The client should move the affected leg and cane forward together and can lean weight through the arm holding the cane as needed. A cane can be used when walking on stairs. The client should take the first step with the affected leg and cane.
CN: Safe, effective care environment; CNS: Safety and infection control; CL: Apply

29. 1. A client with osteoarthritis should pace activities to avoid overexertion. Overexertion can increase degeneration and cause pain. The client should not become sedentary, as this would lead to a higher risk of pneumonia and contractures. The client should not return to a normal level of activity (as before developing osteoarthritis) or engage in vigorous exercise on a daily basis, as these would likely lead to overexertion.
CN: Physiological integrity; CNS: Physiological adaptation; CL: Apply

30. The nurse is educating a client newly prescribed ibuprofen for osteoarthritis. Which statement by the client indicates the nurse's education has been effective?
1. "If I am not free from pain in a week, I will come back to the clinic."
2. "It can take 2 to 3 weeks for me to feel the full effects of the medicine."
3. "I will increase from one pill to two pills a day if I am not better in a week."
4. "If I do not experience pain relief in a few days, I will stop taking the medication."

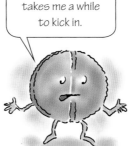

Patience. Sometimes it takes me a while to kick in.

31. A client reports low back pain that radiates down the right leg, with numbness and weakness of the right leg. The nurse will plan to provide the client interventions for which disorder?
1. Herniated nucleus pulposus (HNP)
2. Muscular dystrophy
3. Parkinson's disease
4. Osteoarthritis

32. A client is diagnosed with a herniated nucleus pulposus (HNP) and prescribed flurbiprofen. Which statement will the nurse include when educating the client?
1. "Stop taking flurbiprofen if you experience indigestion."
2. "Call your health care provider before taking any cold medicines."
3. "You will need to have your hematocrit monitored monthly."
4. "Flurbiprofen decreases your chance of having a stroke."

33. A client is being treated conservatively for a herniated nucleus pulposus (HNP). Which intervention(s) will the nurse include in the client's plan of care? Select all that apply.
1. Pain medication
2. Bone fusion
3. Heat application
4. Physiotherapy
5. Surgery

34. A client is admitted for closed spine surgery to repair a herniated disk. Which instruction will the nurse include in the client's preoperative education?
1. "This procedure is riskier than open spine surgery."
2. "Intense physical therapy is needed after the procedure."
3. "An endoscope is used to perform the surgery."
4. "Recovery time is longer than with open spine surgery."

30. 2. Anti-inflammatory drugs, such as ibuprofen, may take 3 weeks for full benefits to be achieved. If the client can tolerate the pain, the dose should not change and other pain reduction measures should be attempted, such as rest, massage, heat, or cold. Clients should never adjust their dosage or discontinue a medication without consulting the health care provider.
CN: Physiological integrity; CNS: Pharmacological and parenteral therapies; CL: Apply

31. 1. Compression of nerves by the HNP causes back pain that radiates into the leg, with numbness and weakness of the leg. Muscular dystrophy causes wasting of skeletal muscles. Parkinson's disease is characterized by progressive muscle rigidity and tremors. Osteoarthritis causes deep, aching joint pain.
CN: Physiological integrity; CNS: Physiological adaptation; CL: Analyze

32. 2. Flurbiprofen is a nonsteroidal anti-inflammatory drug (NSAID) used to treat HNP. The nurse would tell the client to notify the health care provider before taking cold medications to determine safety. Many cold medications contain aspirin, and should not be taken with flurbiprofen due to the increased risk of gastrointestinal bleeding. Indigestion is a common side effect of flurbiprofen. There is no need to have laboratory work monitored monthly. The drug increases a client's chance of having a stroke or myocardial infarction when used long term or in high doses.
CN: Physiological integrity; CNS: Pharmacological and parenteral therapies; CL: Apply

33. 1, 3, 4. Conservative treatment of an HNP may include heat application, pain medication, and physiotherapy. Aggressive treatment may include surgery, such as a bone fusion.
CN: Physiological integrity; CNS: Reduction of risk potential; CL: Apply

34. 3. Closed spine surgery uses endoscopy to fix a herniated disk. It is less risky than open surgery and has a shorter recovery time; it is commonly done as a same-day surgical procedure. Physical therapy may be less intensive or not needed at all.
CN: Physiological integrity; CNS: Reduction of risk potential; CL: Apply

CN: Client needs category   CNS: Client needs subcategory   CL: Cognitive level

35. A client asks the nurse, "Why do I need to apply a cold pack to my sprained ankle?" Which response by the nurse is **most** appropriate?
1. "The ice decreases pain and increases circulation."
2. "The ice numbs the nerves and dilates the blood vessels."
3. "The ice promotes circulation and reduces muscle spasm."
4. "The ice constricts local blood vessels and decreases swelling."

36. A client is being seen in the emergency department for severe lower back pain, weakness, and atrophy of the leg muscles. The nurse anticipates preparing the client for which diagnostic test(s)? Select all that apply.
1. Magnetic resonance imaging (MRI)
2. Computerized tomography (CT) scan
3. Lumbar puncture
4. Myelography
5. Chest x-ray

37. The nurse is caring for a client who has experienced a vertebral herniation. Which areas will the nurse assess **first**?
1. L1–L2, L4–L5 vertebrae
2. L1–L2, L5–S1 vertebrae
3. L4–L5, L5–S1 vertebrae
4. L5–S1, S2–S3 vertebrae

38. Which response(s) by the client indicates the nurse's education regarding back safety has been effective? Select all that apply.
1. "I will carry objects at arm's length from my body."
2. "I will sleep on my back at night."
3. "I will carry objects close to my body."
4. "I will lift items by bending over at my waist."
5. "I will maintain a healthy weight."

39. A client has been prescribed cyclobenzaprine. After the nurse has instructed the client about taking the medication, which client statement(s) indicates further education is needed? Select all that apply.
1. "I will stand up slowly while I am taking cyclobenzaprine."
2. "If I miss a dose of the medicine, I will take an extra pill at the next dose."
3. "I will call my health care provider before taking over-the-counter medications."
4. "I will avoid activities that require alertness while taking the medication."
5. "If I experience a dry mouth or heartburn, I will call my health care provider."

Feeling sleepy? Grab a cup of coffee.

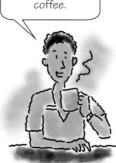

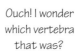

Ouch! I wonder which vertebra that was?

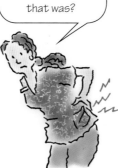

35. 4. Application of a cold pack causes the blood vessels to constrict, which reduces the leakage of fluid into the tissues and prevents swelling. It may have an effect on muscle spasms. Cold therapy may reduce pain by numbing the nerves and tissues. Cold therapy does not promote circulation or dilate the blood vessels.
CN: Physiological integrity; CNS: Basic care and comfort; CL: Apply

36. 1, 2, 4. The nurse should suspect that the client has a herniated nucleus pulposus (HNP). Tests used to diagnose a HNP include myelography, MRI, and CT scan. Lumbar puncture and chest x-ray are not conclusive tests for a herniated disk.
CN: Physiological integrity; CNS: Physiological adaptation; CL: Analyze

37. 3. The nurse will assess the L4–L5 and L5–S1 vertebrae first because this is the area in which most herniations occur.
CN: Health promotion and maintenance; CNS: None; CL: Apply

38. 3, 5. Keeping objects close to the body's center of gravity by carrying them close to the body lessens strain on the back. Maintaining a healthy weight decreases the incidence of back pain. Carrying objects away from the body, sleeping on the back, and bending over at the waist to lift objects all increase back strain.
CN: Health promotion and maintenance; CNS: None; CL: Apply

39. 2, 5. It is not appropriate to take more than the prescribed dosage, as serious adverse effects can occur. A dry mouth and pyrosis are common side effects of cyclobenzaprine and thus do not need to be reported to the health care provider. Changing position slowly helps avoid dizziness while on the medication. Over-the-counter medications may intensify adverse effects; therefore, the client should check with the health care provider before taking them. Skeletal muscle relaxants such as cyclobenzaprine can cause drowsiness.
CN: Physiological integrity; CNS: Pharmacological and parenteral therapies; CL: Apply

40. The nurse is caring for a client with a cast on the right forearm. Which finding(s) indicate to the nurse the client is experiencing compartment syndrome? Select all that apply.
1. Cool, pale fingers
2. Inability to move the fingers
3. Numbness in the fingers
4. Persistent, intense pain
5. Decreased oxygen saturation level

40. 1, 2, 3, 4. With compartment syndrome, the nurse should expect to find pain, pallor, paresthesia, pulselessness, and paralysis. A decrease in the client's oxygen saturation level does not indicate compartment syndrome.
CN: Safe, effective care environment; CNS: Management of care; CL: Analyze

41. The nurse is caring for a client experiencing hemorrhage from compartment syndrome. Which symptom(s) will the nurse expect to find? Select all that apply.
1. Edema
2. Increased venous pressure
3. Increased venous circulation
4. Increased arterial circulation
5. Tachycardia

How do all of these symptoms fit together?

41. 1, 2, 5. The hemorrhage in compartment syndrome causes edema, increased venous pressure, tachycardia, and decreased venous and arterial circulation.
CN: Physiological integrity; CNS: Physiological adaptation; CL: Apply

42. A client who was casted for a fracture of the right ulna reports severe pain, numbness, and tingling of the right arm. What will the nurse do **next**?
1. Administer acetaminophen as prescribed.
2. Lower the arm below the level of the heart.
3. Notify the health care provider.
4. Apply a heating pad to the area.

42. 3. Severe pain, numbness, and tingling are symptoms of impaired circulation due to compartment syndrome, which is a medical emergency. Do not give analgesics until the client has been assessed and treated. Lowering the arm below the level of the heart and applying heat would decrease venous outflow and impair the circulation even more.
CN: Safe, effective care environment; CNS: Management of care; CL: Analyze

43. A client has developed compartment syndrome from full-thickness burns on both arms. The nurse will prepare the client for which treatment?
1. Amputation
2. Fasciotomy
3. Casting
4. Observation

43. 2. Treatment of compartment syndrome includes a fasciotomy. A fasciotomy involves cutting the fascia over the affected area to permit muscle expansion. Casting, observation, and amputation are not treatments for compartment syndrome.
CN: Physiological integrity; CNS: Physiological adaptation; CL: Apply

44. A client presented to the emergency department with a foot fracture and the health care provider placed the foot in a medical boot. Which information will the nurse include when discharging the client?
1. Apply ice to the foot for 45-minute intervals.
2. Take narcotic medication as prescribed.
3. Do not bear weight on the affected extremity.
4. The brace can be worn in the shower.

44. 2. The client should be told to take narcotics only as prescribed to limit abuse and dependence. The purpose of the medical boot is to act as a splint, prevent direct contact, and maintain immobility. Ice should be applied for 15 to 20 minutes at a time. Boots allow weight bearing and should be removed before showering or bathing.
CN: Physiological integrity; CNS: Reduction of risk potential; CL: Apply

45. A client arrives in the emergency department reporting he fell down the stairs and thinks he broke his leg. Which finding(s) indicates to the nurse the client might be correct in the belief that he broke his leg? Select all that apply.
1. Tingling
2. No pedal pulse
3. Coolness
4. Redness
5. Warmth
6. Pain at the site of injury

45. 4, 5, 6. Signs of a fracture may include redness, warmth, and intense pain at the fracture site. Coolness, tingling, and loss of pulses are signs of arterial insufficiency.
CN: Physiological integrity; CNS: Physiological adaptation; CL: Apply

CN: Client needs category   CNS: Client needs subcategory   CL: Cognitive level

46. After treatment of compartment syndrome, a client reports experiencing paresthesia. Which findings will the nurse monitor for?
  1. Fever and chills
  2. Changes in range of motion (ROM)
  3. Pain and blanching
  4. Numbness and tingling

47. The nurse is teaching a client with a recent leg fracture and cast. Which statement(s) by the client indicates to the nurse further education is needed? Select all that apply.
  1. "I need to report any numbness or tingling in my leg at once."
  2. "It is normal to have some numbness or tingling following a fracture."
  3. "It is normal to have severe pain even after the cast is on."
  4. "I need to keep my leg elevated as much as possible."
  5. "The color and temperature of my toes will be checked frequently."
  6. "It is normal to have swelling and for the cast to feel really tight."

48. The nurse is caring for a client taking warfarin admitted for a possible right hip fracture. Which primary health care provider prescription will the nurse question?
  1. Administer morphine sulfate IM for pain.
  2. Insert an indwelling urinary catheter.
  3. Place the client in Buck's traction.
  4. Prepare the client for a portable x-ray.

49. A client has a long leg cast applied for a tibia fracture. Which statement made by the client indicates to the nurse that compartment syndrome may be developing?
  1. "I have some discomfort when I move my foot around."
  2. "My toenails are pink on both feet."
  3. "My leg really itches under this cast."
  4. "I am having a decrease in sensation in my toes."

50. The nurse is assessing a client who is at risk for impaired neurovascular function from a cast application. Which data are important for the nurse to gather from this client?
  1. Orientation, movement, pulses, warmth
  2. Capillary refill, movement, pulses, warmth
  3. Orientation, pupillary response, temperature, pulses
  4. Respiratory pattern, orientation, pulses, temperature

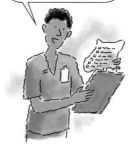

Sometimes I get paresthesia when I sleep on my arm.

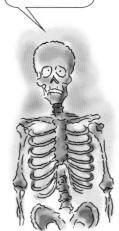

Hip fractures are definitely not "hip."

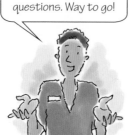

You've already finished 50 questions. Way to go!

46. 4. Paresthesia is described as numbness and tingling. It does not include pain or blanching, and is not associated with fever and chills or change in ROM.
CN: Physiological integrity; CNS: Physiological adaptation; CL: Apply

47. 2, 3, 6. Paresthesia (numbness or tingling) is the earliest sign of compartment syndrome while severe pain is a later sign; both should be reported at once. Elevating the leg would help prevent venous stasis, edema, and impaired circulation. Circulation and limb sensation need to be monitored frequently by checking the color and temperature of the toes. Swelling and tightness of the cast are not normal and should be reported.
CN: Physiological integrity; CNS: Physiological adaptation; CL: Analyze

48. 1. The nurse would question administering the client taking warfarin an intramuscular injection due to the increased risk of bleeding. A urinary catheter will limit the client having to move before surgery. Traction is used to restore alignment and decrease pain. An x-ray will assist in diagnosing the hip fracture.
CN: Safe, effective care environment; CNS: Management of care; CL: Analyze

49. 4. Compartment syndrome can occur from internal (due to bleeding) and external (due to the cast or dressing) pressure and can cause a feeling similar to the foot "falling asleep" (related to a lack of sensation). Blood flow is impaired in compartment syndrome. Normally, the toenails should be pink and capillary refill less than 3 seconds. It is normal to have some discomfort with movement and for the leg to itch underneath the cast; the nurse should reinforce that no objects should be placed under the cast to scratch the skin. This can damage skin integrity and predispose the client to infection.
CN: Physiological integrity; CNS: Physiological adaptation; CL: Apply

50. 2. A thorough neurovascular assessment should include checking capillary refill, movement, pulses, and warmth. Neurovascular assessment involves nerve and blood supply to an area. Respiratory pattern, orientation, temperature, and pupillary response are not part of a neurovascular examination.
CN: Physiological integrity; CNS: Reduction of risk potential; CL: Apply

CN: Client needs category   CNS: Client needs subcategory   CL: Cognitive level

51. The nurse has provided instruction for a client to accurately measure the circumference of both calves each morning and to report any increase in circumference. Which client statement indicates the nurse's education has been effective?
1. "I will use a measuring tape to check circumference."
2. "I only have to call if one leg is significantly larger than the other."
3. "I can measure my calves either near the knee or closer to the ankle."
4. "I will use the standardized chart for limb circumference."

52. The nurse is unable to detect a dorsalis pedal pulse on the left foot. What is the **priority** action by the nurse?
1. Recheck the pulse in 1 hour.
2. Notify the health care provider.
3. Verify the finding with a handheld Doppler.
4. Check for a pulse in the right foot.

53. A client calls the clinic and informs the nurse there is a foul odor coming from the cast. What is the **best** action by the nurse?
1. Tell the client to come to the clinic immediately.
2. Educate on proper cast care and hygiene measures.
3. Inform the client that odor is normal.
4. Advise the client to check temperature each morning.

54. The client calls the clinic nurse and states, "My cast feels very rough around the edges and is scratching my skin." Which nursing response is **best**?
1. "Apply moleskin or pink tape around the edges."
2. "Elevate the limb above the level of the heart."
3. "Break off the rough area and file it down."
4. "Cover the cast with a gauze wrap."

55. The nurse is providing education on cast care for a client with a cast on the arm. How will the nurse instruct the client to place the casted limb, if swelling occurs?
1. Close to the body
2. On the side while in a side-lying position
3. Behind the client's back
4. Above the level of the heart

51. 1. The correct method for measuring calf circumference is to use a measuring tape, place the tape at the level where the calf circumference is largest, and measure at this same place each time. The client was instructed to report any increase in circumference. A significant increase in calf circumference size might be unilateral or bilateral. There is no standardized chart for limb circumference.
CN: Health promotion and maintenance; CNS: None; CL: Apply

52. 3. If pulses are not palpable, verify the observation with Doppler ultrasonography. If pulses cannot be found with a handheld Doppler, immediately notify the health care provider. There is no reason for the nurse to assess the right pedal pulse at this time, and the nurse should not recheck the pulse in 1 hour.
CN: Safe, effective care environment; CNS: Management of care; CL: Analyze

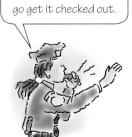
Foul odor coming from the cast? Stop what you're doing and go get it checked out.

53. 1. A foul odor from a cast may be a sign of infection. The nurse needs to monitor the client for fever, malaise, and possibly an elevation in white blood cells. Odor from a cast is never normal. Although education on proper cast care and hygiene measures and checking the temperature may be appropriate, the priority action is to have the client come to the clinic for assessment.
CN: Physiological integrity; CNS: Reduction of risk potential; CL: Analyze

54. 1. To reduce the roughness of the cast, apply moleskin or pink tape around the rough edges. Elevating the limb would prevent swelling but would not alleviate scratching. The client should never break a rough area off the cast. There is not a reason to cover the cast.
CN: Physiological integrity; CNS: Basic care and comfort; CL: Apply

What can I say? I'm a glutton for punishment.

55. 4. To reduce swelling, the client should place the limb with the cast above the level of the heart. Placing it below or at the level of the heart will not reduce swelling. To elevate a cast, the limb may need to be extended from the body. The client need not be in the side-lying position nor place the arm with the cast behind the back.
CN: Physiological integrity; CNS: Physiological adaptation; CL: Apply

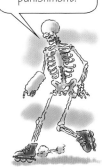

56. A client who being discharged with an arm cast wants to shower at home. The nurse will include which rationale for keeping the cast dry?
1. A wet cast can cause a foul odor.
2. A wet cast will weaken or decompose.
3. A wet cast is heavy and difficult to maneuver.
4. A wet cast is more likely to cause infection.

56. 2. A wet cast will weaken or decompose. A foul odor is a sign of infection. It is never appropriate to get a cast wet.
CN: Physiological integrity; CNS: Reduction of risk potential;
CL: Apply

57. A client with a fractured femur is in Russell's traction and asks the nurse to help with back care. Which nursing action is **most** appropriate?
1. Tell the client back care cannot be performed while in traction.
2. Remove the weight to give the client slack to move.
3. Support the weight to provide correct tension.
4. Tell the client to use the trapeze to lift the back off the bed.

57. 4. The traction must not be disturbed to maintain correct alignment. Therefore, the client should use the trapeze to lift the back off of the bed. The client can have back care as long as the trapeze is used and the alignment is not disturbed. The weight should not be moved without a health care provider's prescription; it should hang freely without touching anything.
CN: Physiological integrity; CNS: Reduction of risk potential;
CL: Apply

58. A client is involved in a motor vehicle accident (MVA) and is being transferred to a trauma center. The nurse will **first** assess the client for which fracture(s)? Select all that apply.
1. Brachial fracture
2. Clavicle fracture
3. Fibula fracture
4. Humerus fracture
5. Occipital fracture

58. 2, 4. Classic fractures that occur with trauma are those of the humerus and clavicle. There are no brachial bones. Occipital and fibula bones are not usually involved in a traumatic injury.
CN: Physiological integrity; CNS: Physiological adaptation;
CL: Apply

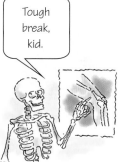

Tough break, kid.

59. A client comes to the emergency department reporting dull, deep bone pain unrelated to movement. Which action will the nurse complete **first**?
1. Assess the client's oxygen saturation level.
2. Prepare the client to receive a cast.
3. Notify the primary health care provider.
4. Ask when the pain started.

59. 4. It is priority to assess when the pain started and what caused the injury. Other actions listed are not priority, as respiratory distress is not suspected and the nurse does not know whether a fracture is present. The health care provider should be notified if needed, but after assessing the client.
CN: Safe, effective care environment; CNS: Management of care;
CL: Analyze

60. A client asks the nurse, "Why am I being placed in traction prior to surgery?" Which response by the nurse is **most** appropriate?
1. "Traction will help prevent your skin from breaking down."
2. "Traction helps with repositioning while in bed."
3. "Traction allows for more activity with decreased pain."
4. "Traction helps to prevent trauma and overcome muscle spasms."

60. 4. Traction prevents trauma and overcomes muscle spasms. Traction does not help in preventing skin breakdown, repositioning the client, or allowing the client to be active.
CN: Physiological integrity; CNS: Basic care and comfort; CL: Apply

61. A client who is in traction for a right leg skeletal fracture reports severe right leg pain. Which action will the nurse take **first**?
1. Call the health care provider.
2. Check the client's alignment in bed.
3. Remove the weights from the fracture.
4. Administer morphine sulfate.

61. 2. A client who reports severe leg pain may need realignment to ease some pressure on the fracture site. If this is ineffective, then the health care provider would be notified. The weights prescribed may be too heavy, but the nurse cannot remove them without a health care provider's prescription. Administering pain medication is not priority.
CN: Safe, effective care environment; CNS: Management of care;
CL: Analyze

CN: Client needs category   CNS: Client needs subcategory   CL: Cognitive level

62. The nurse is examining an older adult client with a fracture. Identify the location of the **most** common fracture in older adults to cause death within 1 year of sustaining the fracture.

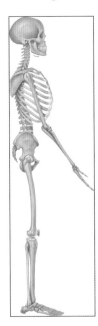

63. The nurse is caring for an older adult client with Paget's disease. The client reports decreased mobility and pain of the left arm after falling in the bathroom. The nurse notes swelling of the left forearm and fingers. Which action will the nurse complete **next**?
1. Put an ice pack on the arm.
2. Apply a splint to the arm.
3. Obtain the client's vital signs.
4. Prepare the client for an x-ray.

64. A healthy 8-year-old client is reporting severe pain in the right upper arm. Which x-ray finding **most** concerns the nurse?
1. A longitudinal fracture
2. An oblique fracture
3. A spiral fracture
4. A transverse fracture

65. A client undergoes an open reduction internal fixation for a femur fracture. Which action by the nurse caring for the client is **priority** immediately following surgery?
1. Assess urine output.
2. Monitor vital signs.
3. Give pain medication.
4. Change the surgical dressing.

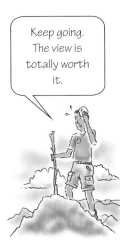

Keep going. The view is totally worth it.

62. Hip fracture is the most common injury in the older adult population and has a high rate of mortality due to complications of surgery and prolonged immobility.

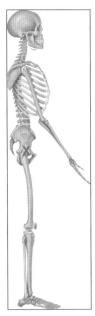

CN: Physiological integrity; CNS: Reduction of risk potential; CL: Understand

63. 2. The nurse would first splint the affected arm to prevent further injury. The nurse would suspect the client has a transverse fracture, which commonly occurs with Paget's disease. The nurse would then notify the health care provider. Ice may be applied to decrease swelling and limit pain. Vital signs would be obtained because the client experienced a fall. The nurse would anticipate preparing the client for an x-ray to confirm a fracture.
CN: Safe, effective care environment; CNS: Management of care; CL: Analyze

64. 3. Spiral fractures are commonly seen in the upper extremities and are related to physical abuse. Oblique and longitudinal fractures generally occur with trauma. A transverse fracture commonly occurs with such bone diseases as osteomalacia and Paget's disease.
CN: Safe, effective care environment; CNS: Management of care; CL: Analyze

65. 2. It is priority for the nurse to assess the client's vital signs to monitor for postoperative complications. The nurse should monitor urine output over the next several hours, not immediately. Pain medication should be administered based on the client's pain level and need. The nurse should not change the surgical dressing; this is generally done by the surgeon.
CN: Safe, effective care environment; CNS: Management of care; CL: Analyze

CN: Client needs category   CNS: Client needs subcategory   CL: Cognitive level

66. A client just had a plaster cast applied to the right forearm following reduction of a closed radius fracture. Which nursing action is **most** important?

1. Determine whether the cast is completely dry.
2. Assess sensation and movement of the fingers.
3. See whether the client is having any pain.
4. Decide whether the cast needs petaling.

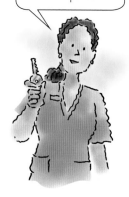

*The key words in question #66 are "**most** important."*

66. 2. Neurovascular checks are most important because they are used to determine whether any impairment exists after cast application and reduction of the fracture. Checking to see whether the cast is completely dry is not the nurse's priority. Checking to see whether the client has pain is important but not the priority. Petaling to smooth the cast edge is done when the cast is completely dry.

CN: Physiological integrity; CNS: Reduction of risk potential; CL: Analyze

67. A client is diagnosed with a femur fracture. The nurse will monitor this client for which potential complication(s)? Select all that apply.

1. Hemorrhage
2. Fat embolism
3. Compartment syndrome
4. Infection
5. Malalignment

67. 1, 2, 3, 4. Hemorrhage (from torn or punctured vessels), fat embolism, compartment syndrome, and infection are potential complications from a femur fracture. Malalignment is a potential complication following surgery, but not from the femur fracture itself.

CN: Physiological integrity; CNS: Physiological adaptation; CL: Apply

68. A client is diagnosed with a fat embolus. Which finding(s) will the nurse expect to find when assessing this client? Select all that apply.

1. Paresthesia
2. Tachypnea
3. Tachycardia
4. Shortness of breath
5. Petechial rash

68. 2, 3, 4, 5. Signs and symptoms of fat emboli include tachypnea, tachycardia, shortness of breath, and a petechial rash on the chest and neck. The fat molecules enter the venous circulation and travel to the lung, obstructing pulmonary circulation. Paresthesia is not a usual symptom.

CN: Health promotion and maintenance; CNS: None; CL: Apply

69. The community health nurse found an older adult client lying in the snow, unable to move the right leg due to a fracture. What is the nurse's **priority**?

1. Realign the fracture.
2. Take the client indoors.
3. Immobilize the fracture.
4. Elevate the leg.

69. 3. Initial treatment of obvious and suspected fractures includes immobilizing and splinting the limb to prevent further injury. Any attempt to realign the fracture at the site may cause further injury and complications. The client may be taken indoors and the leg elevated only after immobilization.

CN: Safe, effective care environment; CNS: Management of care; CL: Apply

70. A high-protein diet is prescribed for a client recovering from a fracture. Which meal will the nurse order the client?

1. Baked shrimp, garlic bread, beans, vanilla Greek yogurt, and milk
2. Macaroni and cheese, steamed carrots, fresh fruit cup, and soy milk
3. Fried chicken, spinach salad with goat cheese, orange, and tea
4. Vegetable sub sandwich, boiled egg, chocolate cake, and juice

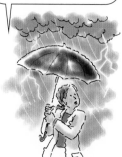

Feeling overwhelmed? Take a deep breath and keep on going. You'll ride out the storm.

70. 1. High-protein intake promotes cell growth and bone union. Foods high in protein include meat, milk, cheese, yogurt, beans, eggs, and soy.

CN: Physiological integrity; CNS: Basic care and comfort; CL: Apply

71. The nurse is providing education for a client on 3-point gait using crutches. The client demonstrates a proper understanding when placing weight on what part of the body?

1. Feet
2. Axillary areas
3. Palms of the hands
4. Palms and axillary areas

71. 3. To avoid damage to the brachial plexus nerves in the axilla, the palms of the hands should bear the client's weight. Minimal weight should be placed on the affected leg.

CN: Physiological integrity; CNS: Basic care and comfort; CL: Understand

CN: Client needs category   CNS: Client needs subcategory   CL: Cognitive level

72. The nurse is caring for a client experiencing a flare-up of acute gout. Identify the location of the **most** common site of acute gout.

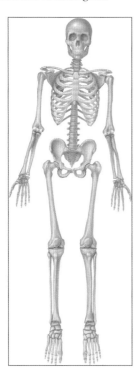

73. The nurse is caring for a client prescribed nafcillin for osteomyelitis. Which finding will the nurse highlight for the primary health care provider to review?
1. The client's sodium level of 156 mEq/L (156 mmol/L).
2. The client is allergic to levofloxacin.
3. The client's heart rate is 75 beats/minute.
4. The client's 24-hour urine output was 980 mL.

74. The registered nurse (RN) is instructing an assistive personnel (AP) on the proper care of a client in Buck's traction following a left fibula fracture. Which observation by the RN indicates the education was effective?
1. The AP allows the weights to hang freely over the end of the bed.
2. The AP lifts the weights when assisting the client to move up in bed.
3. The AP keeps the leg in traction externally rotated.
4. The AP instructs the client to perform ankle rotation exercises.

72. Pain and inflammation of a gout attack usually occur in one or more small joints of the great toe; the metatarsophalangeal joint of the great toe is most common.

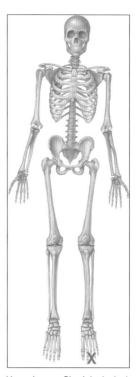

CN: Physiological integrity; CNS: Physiological adaptation; CL: Understand

73. **1.** The nurse would highlight the client's sodium level. The normal range for sodium is 135 to 145 mEq/L (135 to 145 mmol/L). The client who is allergic to levofloxacin, a fluoroquinolone, can take nafcillin but should be monitored closely. Clients allergic to penicillins should not be prescribed nafcillin. The client's heart rate and urine output are in normal range.
CN: Physiological integrity; CNS: Pharmacological and parenteral therapies; CL: Apply

74. **1.** In Buck's traction, the weights should hang freely without touching the bed or floor. Lifting the weights would break the traction. The client should be moved up in bed, allowing the weights to move freely along with the client. The leg should be kept in straight alignment. Performing ankle rotation exercises could cause the leg to go out of alignment.
CN: Physiological integrity; CNS: Basic care and comfort; CL: Apply

75. The nurse is providing nutritional counseling to a client following application of a plaster cast for a fracture. Which statement by the client indicates additional education is needed?
1. "I will eat foods fortified with vitamin D or spend time outside daily."
2. "I will consume at least 1,000 mg of calcium per day."
3. "I will include citrus fruits and green vegetables in my diet."
4. "I will increase fiber and decease protein in my diet."

76. The registered nurse (RN) is instructing an assistive personnel (AP) on how to properly position a client who underwent a total hip replacement. The RN knows the AP understood the education if the client's hip is observed to be in which position following a bed bath?
1. Straight with the knee flexed
2. In an abducted position
3. In an adducted position
4. Externally rotated

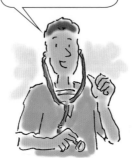

My next door neighbor says he was *abducted* by aliens.

77. A client underwent a bipolar hip replacement after a fracture. Which nursing intervention(s) will help prevent deep vein thrombosis (DVT) after surgery? Select all that apply.
1. Promotion of bed rest
2. Placing an egg crate mattress on the bed
3. Vigorous pulmonary care
4. Administration of subcutaneous heparin
5. Application of pneumatic compression boots

78. The nurse is caring for a postoperative client. Identify the location of the **most** likely site of deep vein thrombosis (DVT) for this client.

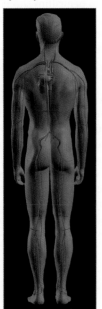

75. 4. The client should increase the protein in the diet to aid in bone repair and regrowth. Vitamin D allows the body to use vitamin C, which assists the body in making collagen to repair the bone. Vitamin C is found in citrus fruits, green vegetables, potatoes, peppers, and berries. The average adult needs 1,000 to 1,200 mg of calcium per day.
CN: Physiological integrity; CNS: Physiological adaptation; CL: Apply

76. 2. An abducted position keeps the new joint from becoming displaced out of the socket. The client can keep his or her hip straight with the knee flexed as long as an abductor pillow is kept in place. Keeping the hip adducted or externally rotated could dislocate the hip joint.
CN: Physiological integrity; CNS: Basic care and comfort; CL: Apply

77. 4, 5. To prevent DVTs after hip surgery, subcutaneous heparin and pneumatic compression boots are used. Egg crate mattresses and pulmonary care do not prevent DVT. Bed rest can *cause* DVT.
CN: Physiological integrity; CNS: Reduction of risk potential; CL: Apply

78. A DVT is a blood clot that forms in a vein deep in the body. Most deep vein blood clots occur in the lower leg.

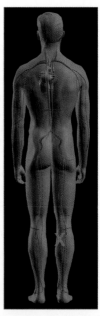

CN: Physiological integrity; CNS: Physiological adaptation; CL: Understand

79. A client who had a recent total hip replacement is being seen by the home care nurse. When the nurse arrives, there are a large number of small carpets scattered throughout the client's home. Which action by the nurse is appropriate?
1. Ask the client why there are so many scattered carpets throughout the home.
2. Explain the hazard that small carpets pose for a person with musculoskeletal impairment.
3. Collect the small carpets and place them together near the main door of the home.
4. Nothing; there is nothing wrong with having small carpets scattered throughout the home.

80. A client is in traction for a fracture. Which nursing intervention is appropriate for this client?
1. Assessing the client's pin sites every shift
2. Adding and removing weights as the client desires
3. Making sure the knots in the rope catch on the pulley
4. Giving range of motion (ROM) to all joints every shift

81. The nurse reads the progress note in the chart exhibited below for a client who had surgical repair of a right hip fracture. The nurse suspects the client is experiencing which condition?

Progress notes	
4/30	The client reports new left calf pain
1400	(4/5 on the pain scale) that worsens with
	touch of the left foot. +4 nonpitting edema
	from the left foot to the knee is noted.
	Prominent superficial veins are noted on the
	left leg. Dr. Smith has been notified.
	—M. Lopez, RN

1. Deep vein thrombosis (DVT)
2. Fat embolus
3. Infection
4. Pulmonary embolism

82. The health care provider has just removed the cast from a client's lower leg. During the removal, a small superficial abrasion occurred over the ankle. Which statement by the client indicates to the nurse the need for additional education?
1. "I must use a moisturizing lotion on the dry areas."
2. "The dry, peeling skin will go away in a few days."
3. "I can wash the abrasion on my ankle with soap and water."
4. "I will wait until the abrasion is healed before I go swimming."

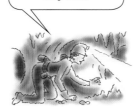
Always be on the lookout for safety hazards your client may face.

79. 2. The nurse should review the hazards of having small carpets on the floors so that the client can take the appropriate action and reduce her likelihood of injury by removing the carpets. Questioning the client about the small scattered carpets would only begin to help the client understand the role she plays in causing home injuries, especially for a person with an alteration in musculoskeletal status, and might come across as accusatory. Collecting the small carpets and doing nothing are not appropriate actions for the nurse.
CN: Safe, effective care environment; CNS: Safety and infection control; CL: Apply

80. 1. Nursing care for a client in traction may include assessing pin sites every shift (and as needed) and making sure the knots in the rope do not catch on the pulley. The nurse should add and remove weights only as the health care provider prescribes, and every shift the nurse should give ROM to all joints *except* those immediately proximal and distal to the fracture.
CN: Physiological integrity; CNS: Basic care and comfort; CL: Apply

81. 1. Unilateral leg pain and edema with calf pain might be symptoms of DVT. Tachycardia, chest pain, and shortness of breath may be symptoms of a pulmonary embolism. It is unlikely an infection would occur on the opposite side of the fracture without cause. Fat emboli are associated with the symptoms of restlessness, tachypnea, and tachycardia and are more common in long-bone injuries than in hip injuries.
CN: Physiological integrity; CNS: Reduction of risk potential; CL: Apply

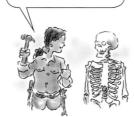
Progress notes are an important tool of the trade in nursing.

82. 1. The dry, peeling skin will heal in a few days with normal cleaning; therefore, lotions are unnecessary. Vigorous scrubbing is not necessary. Washing the abrasion and delaying swimming until healing are correct procedures to follow after removal of a cast.
CN: Physiological integrity; CNS: Reduction of risk potential; CL: Apply

CN: Client needs category   CNS: Client needs subcategory   CL: Cognitive level

83. A client who fell has a fractured right ankle and is being fitted with a cast. After assisting with the cast application, which instruction will the nurse provide to the client?
1. Go home and stay in bed for a few days.
2. Expect some swelling and blueness of the toes.
3. Keep the cast covered with plastic until it feels dry.
4. Move the toes on the right foot for several minutes every hour.

83. 4. Moving the toes is encouraged to facilitate circulation and prevent swelling. By moving the toes, the client becomes aware of any numbness or swelling and can take appropriate action, such as elevating the extremity and reporting the findings to the health care provider. Usually, clients are instructed to remain in bed for only 24 hours while the cast dries. Prolonged immobility creates problems for the client. While the cast is still damp, the ankle should be elevated on a pillow that is protected with plastic; the cast itself should be left open to the air. Swelling and a bluish color of the toes are not expected; they indicate compromised circulation and should be reported immediately.
CN: Physiological integrity; CNS: Reduction of risk potential; CL: Apply

84. The nurse is caring for a female client prescribed oral ibandronate sodium for osteoporosis. Which finding concerns the nurse?
1. The client became postmenopausal 2 years ago.
2. The client has a history of severe gastroesophageal reflux.
3. The client's calcium level is 9.8 mEq/L (2.45 mmol/L).
4. The client states she does not like the taste of fruit juice.

84. 2. Ibandronate sodium is a bisphosphate prescribed to slow bone loss and decrease the risk for bone fractures in women with osteoporosis after menopause. Esophageal damage can occur, and the drug should be used very cautiously in clients with preexisting esophageal damage. The client must remain upright and not take vitamins, calcium, or antacids for 60 minutes after taking ibandronate sodium to prevent serious esophageal damage. This medication can cause hypocalcemia and should not be taken by clients with existing hypocalcemia. A calcium level of 9.8 mEq/L (2.45 mmol/L) is within the normal range of 8.5 to 10.5 mEq/L (2.13 to 2.63 mmol/L). This medication should be taken with water only, so the client not preferring fruit juice is not a complication.
CN: Physiological integrity; CNS: Pharmacological and parenteral therapies; CL: Apply

85. Which statement by a client who recently had a cast applied indicates the nurse's education has been effective?
1. "The cast will need to be removed if I feel any heat."
2. "Heat is a normal sensation as a cast dries."
3. "The heat I feel is most likely caused by an infection."
4. "I will call my health care provider if I feel any heat."

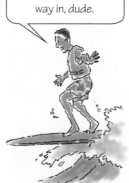

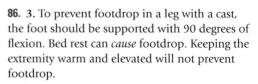

Looking good. Ride that wave all the way in, dude.

85. 2. Normally, as the cast dries, a client may report heat from the cast. The nurse should reassure the client. The cast will not need to be removed and the health care provider does not need to be notified. Heat from the cast is not a sign of infection.
CN: Physiological integrity; CNS: Reduction of risk potential; CL: Apply

86. The nurse is providing care for a client with a leg cast. To help prevent footdrop, which action by the nurse is **most** appropriate?
1. Encouraging bed rest
2. Placing the foot on several pillows
3. Supporting the foot with 90 degrees of flexion
4. Placing a stocking on the foot to provide warmth

86. 3. To prevent footdrop in a leg with a cast, the foot should be supported with 90 degrees of flexion. Bed rest can *cause* footdrop. Keeping the extremity warm and elevated will not prevent footdrop.
CN: Health promotion and maintenance; CNS: None; CL: Apply

87. A client is diagnosed with gout. Which food(s) will the nurse instruct the client to avoid? Select all that apply.
1. Green leafy vegetables
2. Liver
3. Cod
4. Chocolate
5. Sardines
6. Eggs

88. The nurse is caring for a client who developed osteomyelitis 2 weeks after a fishhook was removed from the foot. Which rationale **best** explains the need for long-term antibiotic therapy?
1. Bone has poor circulation.
2. Tissue trauma requires antibiotics.
3. Feet are normally difficult to treat.
4. Fishhook injuries are highly contaminated.

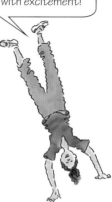

You're almost done. I'm giddy with excitement!

89. Which information is **priority** for the nurse to include in the discharge plan for a client leaving the hospital in a leg cast?
1. Cast care procedures and devices to relieve itching
2. Skin care, mouth care, and cast removal procedures
3. Cast care, neurovascular checks, and hygiene measures
4. Cast removal procedures, neurovascular checks, and devices to relieve itching

90. A client has just returned from the postanesthesia care unit after undergoing internal fixation of a left femoral neck fracture. The nurse notes the client positioned on the right side with the left knee bent. Which action will the nurse perform **first**?
1. Complete an initial head-to-toe assessment.
2. Reposition the client supine with two pillows between the legs.
3. Review the primary health care provider's postoperative prescriptions.
4. Determine the client's pain level and provide medication if needed.

87. 2, 3, 5. The client with gout should avoid foods that are high in purines, such as liver, cod, and sardines. Other foods that should be avoided include anchovies, kidneys, sweetbreads, lentils, and alcoholic beverages, especially beer and wine. Green leafy vegetables, chocolate, and eggs are not high in purines, and therefore are not restricted in the diet of a client with gout.
CN: Physiological integrity; CNS: Basic care and comfort; CL: Apply

88. 1. Bone has poor circulation, making it difficult to treat an infection in the bone. This requires long-term use of IV antibiotics to make sure the infection is cleared. Tissue trauma does not always require antibiotics, at least not long term. Fishhooks may not be any more contaminated than another instrument that causes an injury. Feet are not more difficult to treat than other parts of the body unless the client has a circulatory problem or diabetes.
CN: Physiological integrity; CNS: Pharmacological and parenteral therapies; CL: Apply

89. 3. The discharge plan for a client with a leg cast should include proper cast care procedures, such as observing the skin nearest the cast edges for signs of pressure ulcers, keeping the cast dry and intact, and avoiding the use of insertable devices (such as wire hangers or sticks) to relieve itching. Frequent neurovascular checks should also be included, as they can reveal evidence of pressure or impaired circulation to the leg under the cast. They include checking the toes frequently for discoloration, swelling, or lack of movement or sensation. Hygiene measures should also be included, such as resuming normal elimination patterns and the importance of cleanliness after elimination, as well as the need to maintain skin integrity by taking sponge baths and caring for dry skin. Devices should never be inserted between the cast and the skin. Although mouth care and cast removal are important issues, they are not priority discharge instructions in this case.
CN: Safe, effective care environment; CNS: Management of care; CL: Apply

90. 2. The operative leg must be kept abducted to prevent dislocation of the hip. Placing the client side-lying with knee bent does not promote abduction. The nurse will complete an assessment, review prescriptions, and assess pain; however, these are not a higher priority than client safety.
CN: Safe, effective care environment; CNS: Safety and infection control; CL: Analyze

CN: Client needs category   CNS: Client needs subcategory   CL: Cognitive level

91. The health care provider prescribes heparin 8,000 units to be administered subcutaneously to a client following a total hip replacement. The label on the heparin vial reads: heparin 10,000 units/mL. How many milliliters of heparin will the nurse administer to the client? Record your answer using one decimal place.

_____ mL

92. The nurse is providing preoperative education for a client having a total hip arthroplasty and explaining which actions to avoid postoperatively. Which statement(s) made by the client indicates the need for additional teaching? Select all that apply.
1. "I will keep my legs apart while lying in bed."
2. "I will periodically tighten my leg muscles."
3. "I will rotate my feet internally."
4. "I will bend from my waist to pick items up from the floor."
5. "I will sleep in a side-lying position on the unaffected side."

93. A client had knee replacement surgery 2 weeks ago and has been on warfarin therapy. The client's most recent international normalized ratio (INR) was 5.6. Which intervention will the nurse do **next**?
1. Administer vitamin K as prescribed.
2. Assess the client's surgical site.
3. Schedule the client for repeat laboratory testing.
4. Decrease the client's warfarin dosage.

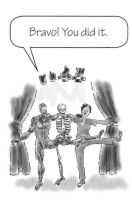

Bravo! You did it.

91. 0.8.
This formula is used to calculate drug dosages:

$$Dose\ on\ hand = \frac{Dose\ desired}{X}$$

In this example, the equation is as follows:

$$10,000\ units/mL = \frac{8,000\ units}{X}$$

$$X = 0.8\ mL$$

CN: Physiological integrity; CNS: Pharmacological and parenteral therapies; CL: Apply

92. 3, 4. After hip replacement surgery, the client should avoid internally rotating the feet and bending more than 90 degrees. These activities can compromise the hip joint. The client should lie with the legs abducted. Leg-strengthening exercises, such as periodically tightening the leg muscles, are recommended to maintain muscle strength and reduce the risk of thrombus formation. A side-lying position is acceptable; however, some health care providers restrict lying on the operative side.

CN: Physiological integrity; CNS: Reduction of risk potential; CL: Apply

93. 1. The client's INR is elevated, meaning that clotting time is too high and, therefore, the dosage of warfarin is likely too high. The client needs an antidote to warfarin to reduce clotting time and INR. The antidote for warfarin is vitamin K and would be administered as prescribed. The nurse would assess the surgical site, but this is not priority over safety. The primary health care provider will determine if additional testing or a change in dosage is needed.

CN: Physiological integrity; CNS: Pharmacological and parenteral therapies; CL: Apply

CN: Client needs category   CNS: Client needs subcategory   CL: Cognitive level

Chapter 8

Gastrointestinal Disorders

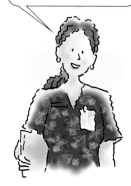

From hiatal hernia to diverticulitis to pancreatitis, this chapter covers all the GI disorders you could ask for, in one handy package. Are you ready to attack this chapter? Remember—no guts, no glory!

Gastrointestinal refresher

Appendicitis

Inflammation of the appendix resulting from blockage of the organ, which causes infection, inflammation, and pus accumulation

Key signs and symptoms
- Anorexia, nausea, and vomiting
- Abdominal pain that localizes in the right lower abdomen (McBurney's point) or in the periumbilical area
- Sudden cessation of pain indicates rupture

Key test results
- Hematology shows moderately elevated white blood cell count

Key treatments
- Appendectomy

Key interventions
- Monitor vital signs, GI status, and pain.
- Maintain nothing-by-mouth (NPO) status until bowel sounds return postoperatively; advance diet as tolerated.
- Monitor for signs of peritonitis (rigid abdomen and guarding).

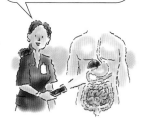

Uh oh. Looks like we have an inflamed appendix here. There's only one treatment.

Cancer of the gastrointestinal system

Colorectal
Abnormal growth (adenoma) occurring in the inner lining of the colon or rectum

Esophageal
Growth of cancer in the cells that line the inside of the esophagus

Gastric
Growth of cancer cells in the mucus-producing cells of the gastric lining

Pancreatic
Growth of cancer cells in the pancreas

Key signs and symptoms

Colorectal
- Change of bowel habits, abdominal pain, bloody stools, and rectal bleeding

Esophageal
- Nagging cough, dysphagia, hoarseness, and sub-sternal pain

Gastric
- Anorexia, epigastric fullness, and pain after eating not relieved by antacids
- Unexplained nausea, indigestion, or heartburn

Pancreatic
- Asymptomatic until late stages; may have jaundice and upper abdominal pain that radiates to the back

Key test results

Colorectal
- Colonoscopy identifies and locates a mass
- Digital rectal examination reveals a mass
- Fecal occult blood positive (screen for fecal occult blood starting at age 50)

Esophageal
- Endoscopic examination of the esophagus, biopsies, and cytological test confirm esophageal tumors; computed tomography (CT) and positron emission tomography (PET) scans for tumor staging

Gastric
- Gastric analysis shows positive cancer cells and achlorhydria
- Gastric biopsy reveals cancer cells

Pancreatic
- Ultrasound, CT scan, and magnetic resonance imaging (MRI)

Key treatments
- Surgery to remove the tumor or resect the bowel depending on tumor location
- Radical surgery to excise the tumor and resect the esophagus or both the stomach and esophagus (gastroduodenostomy, gastrojejunostomy, partial gastric resection, total gastrectomy)
- Radiation to reduce tumor size
- Chemotherapy: 5-fluorouracil common use for each type along with doxorubicin for colorectal; cisplatin for esophageal; carmustine for gastric
- Palliative or hospice care referrals

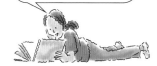

Wow. I never realized how many different types of GI cancer there are, all with different symptoms.

- Support groups and organizations for emotional health

Key interventions

- Surgery
  - Preoperative:
    - answer client's questions
    - explain what to expect after surgery (gastrostomy tubes, closed chest drainage, and NG suctioning)
    - witness the consent
    - prep the skin and surgical region/area
    - maintain IV site access
    - monitor labs
    - administer pre-op meds.
- Radiation therapy:
  - leave skin markings intact
  - avoid creams, lotions, deodorants, and perfumes
  - use lukewarm water to clean skin and assess skin for redness and cracking
  - teach client to wear loose-fitting clothes.
- Chemotherapy:
  - assess breath sounds, vital signs, cardio-vascular system, and renal, skin, hair, and lab results
  - monitor for signs of infection (fever, sore throat, elevated WBC)
  - assess for stomatitis (erythema, ulcers, and bleeding)
  - rinse the mouth with saline or chlorhexidine
  - avoid toothbrushes, lemon-glycerin swabs, dental floss, and hot or spicy foods
  - use topical anesthetics and antifungals (nystatin swish and swallow)
  - encourage deep breathing and meticulous hygiene
  - inspect IV site for infection
  - place in private room if possible and do not allow fresh salads, fruit, or flowers in room
  - perform meticulous hand hygiene and avoid contact with staff or visitors who have cold or flu-like symptoms.
- Encourage participation in self-care and decision-making.
- Provide referrals to support groups and organizations.
- Maintain comfort and allow verbalization of feelings.
- Provide supportive care for the client and family.
- Encourage verbalization of feelings.
- Promote adequate nutrition, and evaluate the client's nutritional and hydration status.

Esophageal and gastric cancer
- Place the client in Fowler's position for meals and allow plenty of time to eat.

- Provide high-calorie, high-protein, pureed diet as needed.
- Place client with esophageal anastomosis supine.
- Gastrostomy tube:
  - administer feeding slowly
  - use gravity to adjust flow rate
  - offer something to chew before each feeding
  - provide mouth care.
- Esophageal and gastric surgery:
  - monitor for signs and symptoms of dumping syndrome (can occur after removal of parts of the stomach or esophagus [diaphoresis, hypotension, tachycardia, and diarrhea])
  - teach client how to prevent dumping syndrome (restrict fluids 1 hour before meals or 1 hour after meals)
  - instruct client to eat sitting up in semi-Fowler's
  - instruct client to lie down 20 minutes after eating
  - instruct client to eat small, frequent meals
  - encourage a low-carbohydrate and low-fiber diet
  - take antispasmodics as prescribed.

Colorectal cancer
- Provide ostomy care as indicated

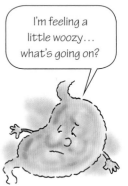

I'm feeling a little woozy... what's going on?

Cholecystitis

Inflammation of the gallbladder resulting from infection and by blockage of the common bowel duct by stones, problems with the duct, or tumors

Key signs and symptoms

- Episodic colicky pain in epigastric area, which radiates to the back and shoulder
- Indigestion or chest pain after eating fatty or fried foods
- Nausea, vomiting, and flatulence

Key test results

- Blood chemistry reveals increased alkaline phosphatase, bilirubin, direct bilirubin transaminase, amylase, lipase, aspartate aminotransferase (AST), and lactate dehydrogenase (LD) levels
- Cholangiogram shows stones in the biliary tree

Key treatments

- Cholecystostomy—opening the gallbladder and removing the stones
- Extracorporeal shock wave therapy (ESWL)—shock wave therapy to destroy the stones

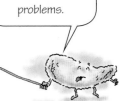

Remember, my stones could feel like stomach problems.

- Cholecystectomy—removal of the gallbladder laparoscopically or by open abdominal incision
- Choledochostomy—opening the common bowel duct and removal of the stones with insertion of a drainage tube (T-tube) to a drainage device
- Analgesic: morphine, hydromorphone, ketorolac
- Antibiotics: piperacillin/tazobactam, ceftriaxone
- Antiemetics: ondansetron, metoclopramide

Key interventions
- Assess abdominal status, color of stools, and pain.
- Administer analgesics and antibiotics as prescribed.
- Monitor fluid and electrolyte balance.
- Provide postoperative care; if open cholecystectomy, monitor and record T-tube drainage-report >1,000 mL/day.
- Maintain the position, patency, and low suction of the nasogastric (NG) tube.

Cirrhosis

Irreversible scarring of the liver that disrupts structure and functioning; causes include hepatitis, chronic alcohol abuse, biliary disease, or severe right-sided heart failure

Key signs and symptoms
- Abdominal pain (possibly because of an enlarged liver)
- Anorexia
- Ascites (which can cause dyspnea)
- Fatigue
- Jaundice
- Nausea and or vomiting
- Dark urine and clay-colored stools
- Pruritus and easy bruising or bleeding

Key test results
- Liver biopsy—definitive test for cirrhosis; detects destruction and fibrosis of hepatic tissue
- Computed tomography (CT) scan with IV contrast reveals enlarged liver, identifies liver masses, and visualizes hepatic blood flow and obstruction, if present

Key treatments
- IV therapy using colloid volume expanders or crystalloids
- Diuretics: furosemide, spironolactone for edema
- Lactulose to reduce ammonia levels
- Vitamin K: phytonadione for bleeding tendencies due to hypoprothrombinemia

- Vasopressin and sclerotherapy for esophageal varices
- Gastric intubation and esophageal balloon tamponade for bleeding esophageal varices (Sengstaken-Blakemore-4 lumen tube and Minnesota-3 lumen tube)
- Blood transfusions to replace loss and shunt insertion to relieve portal hypertension

Key interventions
- Monitor cardiac status.
- Monitor respiratory status.
- Monitor level of consciousness (observe for behavioral or personality changes, increased confusion, stupor, lethargy, hallucinations, and neuromuscular dysfunction).
- Measure intake and output (I&O).
- Maintain fluid restriction (if indicated).
- Weigh daily.
- Measure abdominal girth.
- Check prescriptions regarding T-tube clamping before and after meals.
- Provide appropriate nutrition:
  - early stages: high protein and carbohydrates
  - advanced stages: high calorie, low protein, low fat, low sodium.
- Provide skin care, avoid strong soaps.
- Position frequently for comfort.
- Provide pain medication as needed and promote rest.
- Monitor for bleeding (check skin, gums, stool, and emesis) and monitor Na+, K+, ammonia level, platelets, PT/INR, CBC, WBC, and bilirubin.
- Carefully evaluate before, during, and after paracentesis.
- Administer diuretics and other medications as prescribed.

Crohn's disease

Inflammation of the large or small intestine with ulcers that have a "cobblestone" appearance, separated by normal tissue; can affect areas from the mouth to the anus

Key signs and symptoms
- Abdominal pain (right lower quadrant) aggravated by eating
- Chronic diarrhea, mucus, pus and fat (steatorrhea) in stools
- Weight loss (emaciation can occur)

Key test results
- Upper GI series shows classic string sign: segments of stricture separated by normal bowel

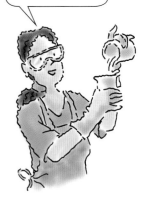
It is best to use precision when measuring fluids.

Key treatments

- Hemicolectomy or ileostomy in clients with extensive disease of the large intestine and rectum
- Antibiotics: sulfasalazine, metronidazole
- Anticholinergics: propantheline, dicyclomine hydrochloride
- Antidiarrheal: diphenoxylate hydrochloride-atropine sulfate
- Corticosteroid: prednisone
- Immunosuppressants: mercaptopurine, azathioprine

Key interventions

- Monitor GI status (note excessive abdominal distention).
- Monitor fluid balance.
- Encourage rest.
- Encourage client to minimize stress.
- Promote verbalization of feelings.
- Encourage maintenance of high-calorie, high-protein, low-fiber, low-fat and dairy-free diet.
- Encourage client to avoid caffeine, alcohol, and smoking.
- TPN for those on bowel rest is indicated in some cases.
- Administer medications as prescribed.
- Encourage client to avoid foods and other things that produce flare-ups.

Dental caries

Erosive process of the teeth caused by the action of bacteria, medications, or other substances or fermentables when acid if formed

Key signs and symptoms

- Halitosis, tooth discoloration, bleeding gums, pain, and tooth erosion

Key test results

- X-ray of teeth and gums reveals tooth destruction

Key treatments

- Extraction, filling, or deep scaling with antibiotic treatment
- Prevention: Dental hygiene and mouth care, especially for at-risk clients (those who are intubated, NPO, in septic shock, and multisystem organ failure)
- Fluoridation of water sources or supplementation with fluoride rinses

Key interventions

- Teach prevention measures:
  - brush after eating
  - floss regularly
  - consume a diet high in fresh fruits and vegetables, nuts, cheese, and plain yogurt.

- If water is not fluoridated (well-water), obtain fluoride from another source.
- Encourage client to see a dentist regularly.
- Provide meticulous mouth care for clients who are:
  - receiving gastric suctioning
  - receiving enteral or parenteral feedings
  - on ventilators
  - NPO and are not able to perform self-care.

Diverticular disease

Sacs or pouch-like projections in the wall of the intestine that can become infected, inflamed, or obstructed

Diverticulosis
- Pouch-like projections (sacs) along the wall of the intestine

Diverticulitis
- Inflammation of the one or more diverticula (sacs)

Key signs and symptoms

- Change in bowel habits (alternating diarrhea and constipation) and decreased bowel sounds
- Left lower quadrant pain or mid-abdominal pain (colicky or cramping pain that radiates to the back)
- Fever and increased WBCs

Key test results

- Sigmoidoscopy shows a thickened wall in the diverticula

Key treatments

- Colon resection or temporary colostomy (for hemorrhage, abscess, perforation, peritonitis, obstruction, or fistula that accompanies diverticulitis)
- Liquid diet for mild diverticulitis or diverticulosis before pain subsides
- High-fiber, low-fat diet for mild diverticulitis or diverticulosis after pain subsides
- Analgesic: morphine
- Antibiotics: metronidazole, ciprofloxacin, sulfamethoxazole, and trimethoprim for mild diverticulitis
- Anticholinergic: oxyphencyclimine or propantheline

Key interventions

- Monitor the following for complications:
  - abdominal distention
  - bowel sounds
  - bowel elimination patterns.
- NPO to rest bowel then clear liquids; increase fluid intake to 3 L/day.

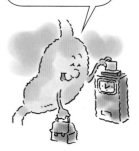

Healthy digestion is all in a day's work.

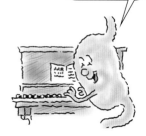

Diagnosis can be aided by assessment of bowel sounds.

- Prepare the client for surgery, if indicated (administer cleansing enemas, osmotic purgative, oral and parenteral antibiotics).
- Postoperative care: see post-op care.

Gastritis

Inflammation or irritation of the lining of the stomach caused by stress, medications, alcohol consumption, or *Helicobacter pylori* bacteria

Key signs and symptoms
- Abdominal cramping and bloating
- Epigastric discomfort (burning between meals or at night)
- Hematemesis
- Indigestion

Key test results
- Upper GI endoscopy with biopsy confirms the diagnosis when performed within 24 hours of bleeding

Key treatments
- Histamine-2 (H_2) receptor antagonists: cimetidine, ranitidine, famotidine, nizatidine
- Proton pump inhibitors: omeprazole
- IV fluid therapy and NG lavage to control bleeding if present

Key interventions
- Administer antiemetic and IV fluids as prescribed.
- Monitor I&O and electrolytes.
- NPO and progress to a bland diet.
- Monitor the client for recurrent symptoms as food is reintroduced.
- Offer small, frequent meals and eliminate foods that cause gastric upset.
- Administer antacids and other prescribed medications.
- Provide emotional support to the client and collaborate for referral for alcohol abuse if verified.
- If surgery is necessary, prepare client preoperatively and provide appropriate postoperative care.
- Teach client to avoid medications that may aggravate GI lining (NSAIDs).

Gastroenteritis

Inflammation of the stomach and intestines caused by an irritant, bacteria, parasite, or virus that produces vomiting and diarrhea

Key signs and symptoms
- Abdominal discomfort
- Diarrhea
- Nausea and vomiting

Key test results
- Stool culture identifies the causative bacteria, parasites, or amoebae

Key treatments
- IV fluid and electrolyte replacement
- Antidiarrheals: diphenoxylate hydrochloride-atropine sulfate, loperamide

Key interventions
- Collect stool specimens as prescribed.
- Administer medications.
- Correlate dosages, routes, and times appropriately with the client's meals and activities.
- Give antiemetics 30 to 60 minutes before meals.
- If client is unable to tolerate food, replace lost fluids and electrolytes with clear liquids and sports drinks.
- Record strict I&O.
- Monitor for signs of dehydration (dry skin and mucous membranes, fever, and sunken eyes).
- Provide perineal care and wash hands thoroughly after providing care.

Gastroesophageal reflux disease

Backup of stomach contents through the lower esophageal sphincter (LES) that does not close properly

Key signs and symptoms
- Dysphagia, dyspepsia, belching, and regurgitation of food
- Heartburn (burning sensation in the upper abdomen)

Key test results
- Barium swallow fluoroscopy indicates reflux
- Esophagoscopy shows reflux
- Endoscopy allows visualization and confirmation of pathologic changes in the mucosa

Key treatments
- Positional therapy to help relieve symptoms by decreasing intra-abdominal pressure:
- Histamine blockers: famotidine, ranitidine, cimetidine
- Proton pump inhibitors: omeprazole, esomeprazole, or pantoprazole may be given IV

Key interventions
- Dietary planning:
  - take into account client's food preferences

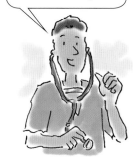

Gastroenteritis, eh? What lab test will help us figure out what's causing it?

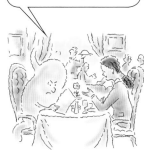

No caffeine, no chocolate, no alcohol, no fatty foods—GERD takes all the fun out of eating.

- limit or eliminate chocolate, caffeine, alcohol, carbonated beverages, and spicy, fatty, or acidic foods (decrease LES pressure)
- encourage four to six small meals per day.
- Encourage client to wear loose clothing.
- Elevate the head of the bed 6″ to 12″ (15 to 30 cm)—reverse Trendelenburg position, and encourage client to sleep on right side
- Encourage smoking cessation, alcohol cessation, and weight reduction programs.

Hepatitis

Inflammation of the liver caused by infectious organisms, toxins, or chemicals that invaded the organ.

Hepatitis A
- Fecal-oral/person-person

Hepatitis B
- Blood and body fluids

Hepatitis C
- Blood-borne and illicit IV drug sharing

Key signs and symptoms

Pre-icteric phase (usually 1 to 5 days)
- Clay-colored stools
- Fatigue
- Right upper quadrant pain
- Dark urine

Icteric phase (~1 to 2 weeks)
- Jaundice and yellow sclera
- Pruritus
- Weight loss

Post-icteric or recovery phase (~2 to 12 weeks or longer in clients with hepatitis B, C, or E)
- Decreased hepatomegaly
- Decreased jaundice
- Fatigue

Key test results

- Blood chemistry shows increased:
  - alanine aminotransferase (ALT)
  - aspartate aminotransferase (AST)
  - alkaline phosphatase (ALP)
  - lactate dehydrogenase (LD)
  - bilirubin
  - erythrocyte sedimentation rate (ESR)
- Serologic tests identify hepatitis A virus, hepatitis B virus, hepatitis C virus, and delta antigen, if present

Key treatments

- Vitamins and minerals: vitamin K, vitamin C (ascorbic acid), vitamin B-complex (mega-B)
- Antivirals: lamivudine, interferon, peginterferon-alfa 2b

Key interventions

- Monitor GI status.
- Provide symptomatic care.
- Watch for bleeding and fulminant hepatitis.
- Provide for rest and maintain high-carbohydrate, high-protein, and low-fat diet.
- Avoid hepatotoxic OTC/prescription medications (acetaminophen and sedatives).
- Maintain standard and appropriate transmission-based precautions.

Hiatal hernia

Protrusion of a portion of the stomach through the esophageal hiatus of the diaphragm

Key signs and symptoms

- Regurgitation
- Persistent heartburn and dysphagia
- Sternal pain and breathlessness after eating

Key test results

- Barium swallow with fluoroscopy reveals protrusion of the hernia
- Chest x-ray shows protrusion of abdominal organs into the thorax
- Esophagoscopy shows incompetent cardiac sphincter

Key treatments

- Bland diet; small, frequent meals with decreased intake of caffeine and spicy foods
- Anticholinergic: propantheline
- Histamine-2 (H_2) receptor antagonists: cimetidine, ranitidine, famotidine
- Proton pump-inhibitors: omeprazole
- Surgery to tighten cardiac sphincter

Key interventions

- Obtain diet history.
- Encourage small, frequent meals.
- Have client sit up 1 to 2 hours after meals, and avoid eating 3 hours prior to bedtime.
- Reinforce need to avoid tight clothing, straining, and flexion at the waist.
- Encourage weight reduction for clients with BMI > 25.
- Monitor for respiratory issues:
  - aggravation of asthma
  - onset of pulmonary edema
  - chronic cough (this is reason to delay surgery).
- Monitor for GI complications, such as esophageal ulcers or bleeding.
- Provide pre-op and post-op care for abdominal surgery.
- Remind client of no heavy lifting for 6 weeks after surgery.

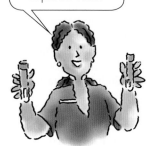

A blood test can really help diagnose the correct hepatitis virus.

Intestinal obstruction

Partial or complete blockage of the lumen in the small or large intestine; small bowel obstruction (SBO) is the most common and serious

Key signs and symptoms
- Abdominal distention with cramping pain
- Vomiting with SBO
- Unable to pass gas or stool for >8 hours; leakage of loose stool if there is blockage of large intestine (sign of impaction)
- Bowel sounds:
  - hyperactive above the obstruction
  - hypoactive below the obstruction

Key test results
- Abdominal x-ray shows increased amount of gas in bowel
- Endoscopy and CT scan reveals a mass or obstruction and the location
- Barium enema: shows the flow of barium stops at area of obstruction

Key treatments
- Bowel resection with or without anastomosis
- GI decompression using NG, Miller-Abbott, or Cantor tube
- Fluid and electrolyte replacement

Key interventions
- Maintain NPO.
- Assess bowel sounds.
- Measure and record abdominal girth.
- Monitor IV fluids and measure I&O.
- Monitor for fluid and electrolyte deficits and imbalances.
- Maintain the position, patency, and low intermittent suction of NG tubes.
- Provide pre-op and post-op care if indicated.

Irritable bowel syndrome

Chronic condition with recurrent diarrhea, constipation, and abdominal pain with bloating

Key signs and symptoms
- Erratic bowel patterns and bloating
- Abdominal pain (relieved by defecation)
- Constipation, diarrhea, or both
- Passage of mucus in stool

Key test results
- Sigmoidoscopy may disclose spastic contraction of the colon

Key treatments
- Dietary management
- Stress management
- Antispasmodic: propantheline
- Antidiarrheal: diphenoxylate hydrochloride-atropine sulfate

Key interventions
- Teach client to:
  - eat slowly
  - eat at regular times
  - chew food thoroughly
  - drink adequate fluids.
- Encourage the client to:
  - eat 15 to 20 g of fiber daily
  - maintain a food diary to identify triggers
  - avoid food intolerances.
- Encourage regular exercise (walking and yoga).
- Assist client to deal with stress and warn against dependence on sedatives or antispasmodics.

Pancreatitis

Acute
Inflammation of the pancreas by auto-digestion due to diminished functioning (life threatening)

Chronic
Progressive disease of the pancreas that is associated with remissions and exacerbations

Key signs and symptoms
- Abrupt onset of pain in the epigastric area that radiates to the shoulder, substernal area, back, and flank (intensifies after meals or lying down)
- Abdominal tenderness, nausea, vomiting, and fatty stools (steatorrhea)
- Positive Turner's sign and Cullen's sign

Key test results
- Elevated amylase, lipase, liver enzymes, lactate dehydrogenase (LD), glucose, aspartate aminotransferase (AST), and lipid levels; decreased calcium and potassium levels
- CT scan and ultrasonography reveal cysts, bile duct inflammation, and dilation

Key treatments
- IV fluids, antibiotic therapy, and TPN
- Anticholinergics; Histmaine-2 (H_2) receptor antagonists or proton pump inhibitors
- Opioid analgesic: morphine, hydromorphone; meperidine contraindicated
- Blood sugar control: insulin and pancreatic enzymes

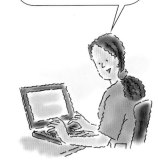

Which tests are used to determine the cause of an intestinal obstruction?

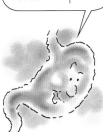

You'd be irritable, too, if you had recurrent diarrhea, constipation, and abdominal pain.

- Potassium supplement: IV potassium chloride
- Surgery:
  - endoscopic retrograde cholangiopancreatography (ERCP) to create an opening in the sphincter of Oddi
  - cholecystectomy
  - pancreaticojejunostomy (Roux-en-Y) to reroute pancreatic enzymes to the jejunum

Key interventions

- Maintain NPO; after 24 to 48 hours start jejunal feedings; when food is tolerated advance to small, frequent meals (moderate to high carbohydrate, high-protein, and low-fat meals).
- Maintain patency of NG tube.
- Monitor abdominal, cardiac, and respiratory status (watch for respiratory failure and tachycardia—signs of hypocalcemia and hypomagnesemia).
- Maintain IV fluids and monitor I&O.
- Monitor blood glucose, laboratory results.
- Position for comfort (knee chest, sitting up, leaning forward).
- Administer pain medications.
- Reassure client and explain procedures to reduce anxiety.

Peptic ulcer disease

Ulceration of the stomach or duodenal lining that is caused by destruction of the mucosal tissue

Key signs and symptoms

- Anorexia
- Hematemesis
- Left epigastric pain 1 to 2 hours after eating
- Relief of pain after administration of antacids

Key test results

- Urea breath test to detect presence of *Helicobacter pylori*
- Barium swallow shows ulceration of the gastric mucosa
- Upper GI endoscopy shows the location of the ulcer

Key treatments

- If GI hemorrhage: gastric surgery that may include gastroduodenostomy, gastrojejunostomy, partial gastric resection, and total gastrectomy
- Saline lavage by NG tube until return is clear (if bleeding is present)
- Antibiotic if *Helicobacter pylori* is present
- Histamine-2 (H_2) receptor antagonists: cimetidine, ranitidine, nizatidine, famotidine
- Mucosal barrier fortifier: sucralfate

Key interventions

- Teach client to eat small, frequent meals three times a day (not necessary if on histamine-2 [H_2] receptor antagonist).
- Teach client to avoid caffeine, alcohol, spicy foods, milk, and cream.
- Teach client to reduce stress and take medications as prescribed.
- Post-op care for gastric resection, total or partial gastrectomy with esophageal anastomosis:
  - administer B_{12} supplementation via parenteral route
  - maintain NG tube
  - auscultate bowel sounds and when able to eat again teach preventive measures for "dumping syndrome" (rapid passage of food to stomach, causing diaphoresis, tachycardia, diarrhea, and hypotension) usually 15 minutes after eating
  - restrict fluids with meals
  - avoid stress after eating
  - eat smaller, frequent meals
  - lie down 20 minutes after eating.

Peritonitis

Inflammation of the peritoneal membrane that covers the abdominal organs

Key signs and symptoms

- Abdominal rigidity and muscle guarding
- Constant, intense abdominal pain
- Decreased or absent bowel sounds
- Shock (weak rapid pulse, pallor, diaphoresis) and elevated temperature

Key test results

- Abdominal x-ray shows free air in the abdomen under the diaphragm

Key treatments

- IV fluids and antibiotics
- Gastric decompression: NG tube to low intermittent suction
- Surgical intervention when the client's condition has stabilized (to treat the cause [e.g., if client has a perforated appendix, then an appendectomy is indicated]; drains would also be placed for drainage of infected material)

Key interventions

- Monitor abdominal, cardiovascular, and respiratory status.
- Watch for fluid and electrolyte imbalance.
- Monitor and record vital signs, intake and output, laboratory studies, daily weight, and urine specific gravity.

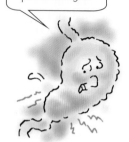

Stress is a real pain in the gut!

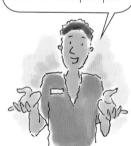

What's that bacterium that causes ulcers? Helicopter pie?

- Administer IV fluids and antibiotics.
- Maintain NPO and NG tube to low-intermittent suction.
- Provide postoperative care as indicated.
- Monitor for salivary, oral, and pharyngeal disorders.

Oral candidiasis (thrush), parotitis, sialadenitis, sialolithiasis, stomatitis, esophageal cancer

Disorders that affect lubrication, protection from harmful bacteria, and digestion

Key signs and symptoms

- Pain, inflammation, and redness
- Cheesy white plaque on the tongue (oral candidiasis)
- Persistent, painless lesion the does not heal (cancer)
- Xerostomia (dry mouth), sticky and stringy saliva, change in taste

Key test results

- Biopsy of cells of the lips to rule out Sjögren's syndrome (autoimmune disease in which the WBCs attack the moisture-producing glands)
- Oral examination, tissue scraping, and brushing

Key treatments

- Preventative: regular dental and oral screenings
- Pilocarpine or cevimeline to stimulate saliva production
- Mycostatin to treat candidiasis

Key interventions

- Monitor nutritional status and chewing and swallowing ability, and ensure adequate food intake.
- Provide support to client and family and encourage verbalization of feelings (cancer).
- Provide mouth care and teach regular and thorough oral hygiene.
- Administer pain medication and monitor for infection.
- Encourage a positive self-image.
- Maintain methods of alternative communication when needed.

Ulcerative colitis

Inflammation of the colon characterized by eroded areas of the mucous membrane and underlying tissue

Key signs and symptoms

- Abdominal cramping and fecal incontinence
- Bloody, purulent, mucoid, watery stools (10 to 20 per day)
- Hyperactive bowel sounds
- Weight loss (unintentional)

Key test results

- Barium enema shows ulcerations
- Sigmoidoscopy shows ulceration and hyperemia

Key treatments

- Colectomy or pouch ileostomy
- Total parenteral nutrition (TPN) if necessary to rest the GI tract
- Antibiotic: sulfasalazine
- Anticholinergics: propantheline, dicyclomine hydrochloride
- Antidiarrheals: diphenoxylate hydrochloride-atropine sulfate, loperamide
- Antiemetic: prochlorperazine
- Corticosteroid: hydrocortisone
- Immunosuppressants: azathioprine, cyclophosphamide

Key interventions

- Monitor GI and cardiovascular status (irregular pulse) and for edema.
- Monitor I&O (especially number, amount, and character of stools) and for fluid and electrolyte imbalance.
- Maintain IV fluids, TPN, or enteral feedings for nutritional support.
- Maintain the position, patency, and low suction of NG tube.
- Provide skin care and perineal care, and observe for vitamin and mineral deficiency.
- Postoperative: provide ostomy care if indicated.

Postoperative care for abdominal surgery

- Postoperative care interventions: assess neuro, heart, lungs, GI-focused assessment (assess abdomen: bowel sounds, passage of flatus or stool, distention, bruising, tone, etc.), pain, and renal systems.
- Monitor vital signs and I&O.
- Maintain NG tube patency, do not reposition the NG tube:
  - irrigate NG tube gently if prescribed
  - lubricate nares with water-soluble lubricant
  - perform meticulous mouth care
  - monitor NG output.

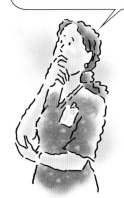

Which interventions are needed for a client with ulcerative colitis?

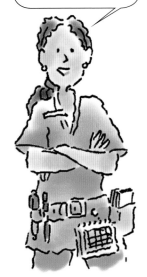

Make sure you have all the tools you need before assessing your client.

- Maintain IV fluids and TPN if prescribed.
- Administer pain medications as prescribed.
- Teach client proper use of patient-controlled anesthesia (PCA) pump.
- Monitor dressings and drains (note the size of any drainage or blood on dressings).
- Monitor ostomy drainage and perform ostomy care as needed.
- Apply sequential compression device (SCD) while on bedrest.
- Turn and reposition client for comfort.
- Encourage deep breathing, coughing, and use of incentive spirometer.
- Get client out of bed as soon as prescribed.
- Teach client to splint the incision and to change positions slowly.
- Monitor lab results (CBC with differential, chemistry or metabolic panel, coagulation panel if liver involvement or on anticoagulants, liver panel if indicated).

- Monitor for signs and symptoms of:
  - atelectasis (dyspnea, cyanosis)
  - bleeding/hemorrhage (decreased blood pressure; increased pulse rate; cool, clammy skin)
  - peritonitis (rigid abdomen and guarding)
  - fluid and electrolyte disturbances
  - infection
  - paralytic ileus (absence of bowel sounds, inability to pass gas or stool, and abdominal distention)
  - dehiscence (unexpected opening of surgical incision caused by infection or improper wound healing)
  - wound evisceration (care for organ protrusion through the wound: use moist, sterile saline gauze to cover the organs/wound and notify the primary health care provider immediately; if client is at home instruct to cover with wax paper and call 911).

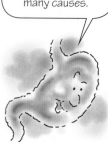

Stomach irritation can have many causes.

thePoint® You can download tables of drug information to help you prepare for the NCLEX®! View Generic Drug Names, Drug Classifications, Drug Actions, and Nursing Implications for the drugs discussed in this refresher at **http://thePoint.lww.com**

Gastrointestinal questions, answers, and rationales

1. The nurse administers lactulose to a client with cirrhosis. Which assessment finding indicates to the nurse the medication is effective?
   1. Four or more loose stools in 24 hours
   2. Serum sodium level of 135 mEq/L (135 mmol/L)
   3. Improvement in mental status
   4. Reduction in abdominal ascites

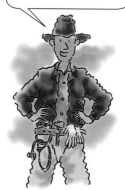

Ready to wrangle up some multiple choice answers? Let's roll.

1. **3.** Lactulose, used to treat portal-systemic encephalopathy in clients with cirrhosis, works by acidifying colonic contents and trapping ammonia in the colon. The laxative action of lactulose assists in expelling the ammonia from the colon. This leads to a reduction in serum ammonia levels and improvements in mental and cardiac status. Lactulose causes diarrhea as a side effect and is expected—but it is not the intended effect of the medication. Adverse effects of lactulose are increased serum sodium and decreased serum potassium levels. Abdominal ascites is not affected by this medication.
CN: Physiologic integrity; CNS: Pharmacological and parenteral therapies; CL: Apply

2. The nurse interviews a client presenting to the clinic with reports of nausea, dark urine, weight loss, and fatigue for the past 2 weeks. Which additional information will the nurse gather from this client related to the presenting symptoms?
   1. Presence of anorexia
   2. 24-hour dietary history
   3. Number and color of stools
   4. Use of over-the-counter medications

2. **3.** Weight loss, nausea, fatigue, and dark urine lasting 2 weeks or more are signs of hepatitis. The nurse should question the client about the presence of clay-colored stools. This additional symptom would prompt the nurse to look at the eyes for the presence of a yellow sclera (jaundice). A 24-hour diet history is not appropriate in a case in which the nausea has been ongoing for 2 weeks but is useful in cases in which nausea and vomiting have just started. A client who has nausea does not eat as much as he or she normally would if not nauseated. Asking about loss of appetite does not add to what the nurse already knows in the presenting report. Use of over-the-counter medications is not related to the client's presenting symptoms.
CN: Physiological integrity; CNS: Physiological adaptation; CL: Analyze

CN: Client needs category   CNS: Client needs subcategory   CL: Cognitive level

3. The nurse provides home care instructions to a client with a diagnosis of hiatal hernia. Which statement made by the client indicates a proper understanding of the instructions?
1. "I will drink carbonated cola beverages with my meals."
2. "I will be sure to lie down immediately after eating."
3. "I should eat three large, high-carbohydrate meals each day."
4. "I will sleep with my head elevated about 3 to 4 inches."

4. The nurse will expect to prepare a client for which test to aid in diagnosing a hiatal hernia?
1. Colonoscopy
2. Lower gastrointestinal (GI) series
3. Barium swallow
4. Abdominal x-ray series

5. Which nursing intervention is **priority** when providing care for a client following an appendectomy for an appendix that spontaneously ruptured?
1. Monitoring for pain
2. Encouraging oral intake of fluids
3. Providing discharge education
4. Monitoring for peritonitis

6. Which intervention will the nurse expect to perform while caring for a client with acute pancreatitis?
1. Institute transmission-based precautions.
2. Administer sedatives to control anxiety.
3. Withhold oral intake as prescribed.
4. Encourage the client to ambulate.

7. A client is brought to the emergency room with suspected cholecystitis. Which finding(s) is characteristic of this diagnosis? Select all that apply.
1. Epigastric pain radiating to the back
2. Indigestion after eating fatty foods
3. Blood-tinged emesis
4. Abdominal distention
5. Itching and dry skin

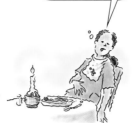

Ugh. I need to work on my portion control.

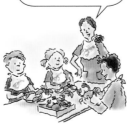

No, Brian. Eating it with the shell on will give you serious GI issues.

3. **4.** With a hiatal hernia, sleeping with the head of the bed elevated 30 degrees (about 3 to 4 inches [7.5 to 10 cm]) prevents stomach acids from refluxing into the esophagus. Carbonated beverages would create gas and belching (eructation), causing an increase in intra-abdominal pressure, which would irritate the herniated area. Lying down immediately after eating leads to the reflux of stomach acids, causing irritation. Clients with hiatal hernia should eat small meals.
CN: Physiological integrity; CNS: Reduction of risk potential; CL: Apply

4. **3.** A barium swallow with fluoroscopy shows the position of the stomach in relation to the diaphragm, which is pertinent in diagnosing a hiatal hernia. A colonoscopy and a lower GI series show disorders of the intestine. An abdominal x-ray series would show structural defects but not necessarily a hiatal hernia, unless it is sliding or rolling at the time of the x-ray.
CN: Physiological integrity; CNS: Reduction of risk potential; CL: Understand

5. **4.** The priority of care is to monitor for peritonitis, or inflammation of the peritoneal cavity. Peritonitis is caused by appendix rupture and invasion of bacteria, which could be lethal. Postoperative pain management is not a priority because this is not life-threatening. The nurse should encourage oral intake; however, it is not a priority. Discharge education is important, but management should focus on minimizing complications and recognizing when they may be occurring for rapid intervention.
CN: Safe, effective care environment; CNS: Management of care; CL: Apply

6. **3.** Clients admitted with pancreatitis are acutely ill and should be NPO on admission. Maintain NPO status as prescribed by the health care provider. Transmission-based precautions are not indicated because this is not an infectious process spread by contact with body fluids or by airborne or direct contact modes of transmission. Administer morphine or hydromorphone for pain relief, not sedatives. During acute pancreatitis, the client is on bed rest and not encouraged to ambulate.
CN: Physiological integrity; CNS: Physiological adaptation; CL: Apply

7. **1, 2.** Cholecystitis has characteristic symptoms of epigastric pain radiating to the back and indigestion after eating fatty foods. Hematemesis, or blood in the vomit, may be a symptom of cirrhosis, gastritis, or peptic ulcer disease but is not associated with cholecystitis. Itching, dry skin is associated with pancreatic cancer. Abdominal bloating is associated with irritable bowel syndrome.
CN: Physiological integrity; CNS: Physiological adaptation; CL: Apply

8. A client with acute pancreatitis is admitted to the hospital. Which health care provider prescription will the nurse question?
   1. Start a normal saline (0.9% NaCl) IV to run at 100 mL/hour.
   2. Give meperidine 4 mg IM every 6 hours PRN pain.
   3. Monitor blood glucose levels every 6 hours.
   4. Connect NG tube to low intermittent suction.

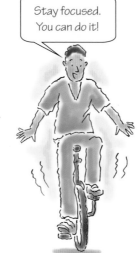

9. Which finding(s) will the nurse expect when assessing a client admitted with suspected appendicitis? Select all that apply.
   1. Loss of appetite
   2. Nausea and vomiting
   3. Sudden cessation of pain
   4. Yellow pigment to the skin
   5. Right lower quadrant pain
   6. Abdominal rigidity and tenderness

10. The nurse will place a client with appendicitis in which position to help relieve pain?

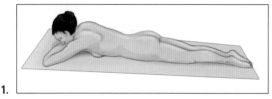
1.

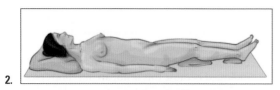
2.

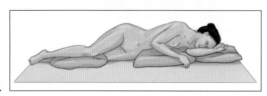
3.

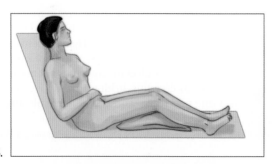
4.

8. **2.** The use of meperidine in the treatment of clients with pancreatitis and other biliary disorders is contraindicated because it causes spasm of the sphincter of Oddi. Morphine is one of the medications of choice used to treat pain associated with biliary disorders. IV fluids are given to prevent fluid volume deficit. Blood glucose monitoring is indicated because the pancreas is responsible for the release of insulin that is needed for glucose metabolism; when inflamed the organ does not function normally. Connecting the NG tube to low intermittent suction is indicated for very ill clients or for those with vomiting that is intractable.
CN: Safe, effective care environment; CNS: Management of care; CL: Apply

9. **1, 2, 5.** The pain begins in the periumbilical region and then shifts to the right lower quadrant (McBurney's point) and becomes steady. The pain may range from moderate to severe. Other signs and symptoms include anorexia, nausea, and vomiting. Sudden cessation of the pain indicates rupture of the appendix and requires surgery. Yellow-pigmented skin (jaundice) is a sign of hepatitis or liver failure/cirrhosis. Abdominal rigidity and tenderness are signs of peritonitis.
CN: Physiological integrity; CNS: Physiological adaptation; CL: Apply

10. **4.** The nurse should place the client in the Fowler's position with a pillow at the knees. Lying still with the legs drawn up toward the chest helps relieve tension on the abdominal muscles, which helps to reduce the amount of discomfort felt. Lying flat or sitting may increase the amount of pain experienced.
CN: Physiological integrity; CNS: Basic care and comfort; CL: Apply

CN: Client needs category   CNS: Client needs subcategory   CL: Cognitive level

11. Which nursing intervention is **priority** during the immediate postoperative care of a client who has undergone gastric surgery?
1. Monitor gastric pH.
2. Assess bowel sounds.
3. Provide nutritional support.
4. Monitor for hemorrhage.

11. 4. Hemorrhage is a postoperative complication detected by monitoring vital signs, abdominal dressings, and nasogastric tube drainage for bleeding. Monitor the postoperative client closely for signs and symptoms of hemorrhage, such as bright red blood in the nasogastric tube suction, tachycardia, or a drop in blood pressure. Monitoring gastric pH helps to evaluate the need for histamine-2 receptor antagonists but is not a priority. Bowel sounds may not return for up to 72 hours postoperatively. Providing nutritional support is not an immediate priority.
CN: Physiological integrity; CNS: Reduction of risk potential; CL: Apply

12. The nurse receives shift report on a client who underwent a bowel resection 2 days ago and reports sudden onset of pain unrelieved by medications. The client's abdomen is rigid and bowel sounds are absent. Which action will the nurse take **next**?
1. Administer an increased dosage of pain medication.
2. Perform an in-depth abdominal assessment.
3. Obtain a complete set of vital signs.
4. Notify the client's primary health care provider.

12. 3. The client is exhibiting signs of peritonitis. The nurse needs a set of vital signs to make sure the client is not going into shock from hidden bleeding before calling the health care provider. An in-depth abdominal assessment is not necessary based on the client's current status. Once the vital signs are gathered, then the health care provider should be notified. The client is already receiving pain medication, and it is not relieving the pain. The nurse would assess for complications before increasing the medication dosage.
CN: Safe, effective care environment; CNS: Management of care; CL: Analyze

13. Which intervention(s) will the nurse perform when caring for a client with acute gastritis? Select all that apply.
1. Maintain bed rest.
2. Prepare for gastric resection.
3. Monitor laboratory values.
4. Administer parenteral nutrition.
5. Assess for changes in abdominal status.
6. Administer antispasmodics as prescribed.

13. 3, 5. The nurse will monitor lab values for changes in hematocrit, hemoglobin, and electrolytes. The nurse will also assess for changes in abdominal status, which includes increased tenderness, distention, pain, bowel sounds, etc. Gastric resection is an option only when serious erosion has occurred. Antispasmodics are for irritable bowel syndrome. Bed rest is not necessary unless the client is unstable, and neither is parenteral nutrition.
CN: Safe, effective care environment; CNS: Management of care; CL: Apply

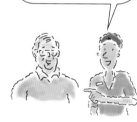
Remember to carefully review your client's medications, as they can contribute to some gastrointestinal disorders.

14. When talking with a client, which finding leads the nurse to suspect the client is at risk for developing chronic gastritis?
1. The client consumes an occasional glass of wine with dinner
2. The client is finishing a 7-day course of amoxicillin for an infection
3. The client is 28 years old with a history of gallbladder disease
4. The client is taking naproxen three times a day for a sports injury

14. 4. Overuse of nonsteroidal anti-inflammatory drugs (such as naproxen), alcohol overuse, and bacterial colonization with *Helicobacter pylori* in the gastrointestinal tract can lead to chronic atrophic gastritis. Conditions that allow reflux of bile acids into the stomach can also cause gastritis. Chronic gastritis can occur at any age but is more common in older adults; antibiotics, occasional alcohol consumption, and gallbladder disease are not causes of gastritis.
CN: Physiological integrity; CNS: Physiological adaptation; CL: Analyze

15. The nurse admits a client with Crohn's disease who is experiencing an exacerbation. Which intervention is the nurse's **priority**?
1. Maintaining current weight
2. Encouraging ambulation
3. Promoting bowel rest
4. Providing mouth care

15. 3. Promoting bowel rest is the priority during an acute exacerbation. This is accomplished by decreasing activity and initially putting the client on nothing-by-mouth (NPO) status. Weight loss may occur and providing mouth care may be indicated, but the priority is bowel rest.
CN: Safe, effective care environment; CNS: Management of care; CL: Analyze

16. Which instruction is **most** appropriate for the nurse to give a client reporting cramping abdominal pain, vomiting, and the inability to pass gas and stool 5 days after undergoing open abdominal surgery to remove an intestinal mass?
1. "Add additional fiber and fluids to your diet."
2. "Eat dried prunes to help you have a bowel movement."
3. "Sip on clear liquids until the vomiting subsides."
4. "Go to the emergency department for evaluation."

16. 4. The client is exhibiting symptoms of an intestinal obstruction. The nurse should advise the client to go to the emergency department for evaluation of the symptoms, especially when this occurs after open abdominal surgery (inflammation of the colon and scar tissue development are causes of intestinal obstruction). Signs and symptoms of an intestinal obstruction include abdominal distention, nausea, vomiting, diarrhea, crampy abdominal pain, and inability to pass gas and stool. Consuming foods that are high in indigestible fiber (such as bran cereal, lettuce, apricots, raisins, dried prunes, brown rice, and fresh peeled apples) promotes regular bowel movements and the passage of gas. The client in this case is vomiting; therefore, offering this advice, as well as the advice to sip on clear liquids, is not appropriate.
CN: Physiological integrity; CNS: Reduction of risk potential; CL: Apply

17. The nurse is providing discharge education for a client treated for acute diverticulitis. Which statement by the client indicates the client understands the discharge instructions?
1. "I will reduce my fluid intake."
2. "I will decrease the fiber in my diet."
3. "I will take all of my antibiotics."
4. "I will exercise to increase my intra-abdominal pressure."

17. 3. Antibiotics are used to reduce inflammation. The client with acute diverticulitis typically is not allowed anything orally until the acute episode subsides. Parenteral fluids are given until the client feels better; then it is recommended the client drink eight 8-ounce (237 mL) glasses of water per day and gradually increase fiber in the diet to improve intestinal motility. During the acute phase, activities that increase intra-abdominal pressure should be avoided to decrease pain and the chance of intestinal obstruction.
CN: Physiological integrity; CNS: Reduction of risk potential; CL: Apply

18. The nurse provides education to a teenage client and parents about Crohn's disease and the dietary changes needed. Which statement made by the parents indicates an accurate understanding of the child's dietary needs?
1. "We will need to include plenty of calories in our child's diet."
2. "We will need to make certain our child's food is gluten-free."
3. "We will only give our child foods that are low in sodium."
4. "We will be sure to provide foods high in fiber for our child."

18. 1. Crohn's disease is an inflammatory bowel disease that causes diarrhea with subsequent weight loss and malnutrition. A high-calorie, nutritious diet helps replenish nutrients that are lost through the affected bowel. A gluten-free diet is appropriate for a client with celiac disease, not Crohn's disease. A client with Crohn's disease does not need to restrict dietary sodium but should avoid high-fiber foods during a flare-up of the disease, because these foods can contribute to bowel irritation.
CN: Physiological integrity; CNS: Basic care and comfort; CL: Apply

19. A client with irritable bowel syndrome (IBS) is reporting pain. The nurse will expect to administer which medication to help alleviate the underlying cause of the client's pain?
1. Acetaminophen
2. Morphine sulfate
3. Prednisone
4. Docusate sodium

19. 3. The pain of IBS is caused by inflammation, which steroids can reduce. Acetaminophen has little effect on the pain, and opiates will not treat its underlying cause. Stool softeners are not necessary.
CN: Physiological integrity; CNS: Pharmacological and parenteral therapies; CL: Apply

CN: Client needs category   CNS: Client needs subcategory   CL: Cognitive level

20. The nurse provides discharge education to a client with Crohn's disease. Which long-term symptom management instruction will the nurse include in the teaching?
   1. "Increase your intake of fiber and take a probiotic daily."
   2. "Join a support group and exercise three times a day."
   3. "Take your multivitamin and corticosteroid for a year."
   4. "Keep a food diary and eat small, frequent meals."

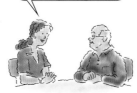

Take time to carefully explain any needed dietary changes to clients.

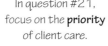

In question #21, focus on the **priority** of client care.

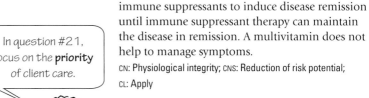

21. The nurse is caring for a client during the initial days following ostomy surgery for ulcerative colitis. Which area of care is the nurse's **priority**?
   1. Body image
   2. Ostomy care
   3. Sexual concerns
   4. Skin care

22. The nurse is caring for a client who has undergone an open surgical procedure for hiatal hernia repair. Which nursing intervention is **priority**?
   1. Turn and reposition the client.
   2. Encourage incentive spirometer use.
   3. Palpate the bladder for distention.
   4. Administer pain medications.

23. A client with gastric cancer is scheduled for a gastric resection. Preoperative, which nursing intervention is **priority** for this client?
   1. Discharge planning
   2. Correction of nutritional deficits
   3. Prevention of deep vein thrombosis
   4. Instruction regarding radiation treatment

24. The nurse is reviewing laboratory results for a client with peritonitis. Which result will the nurse expect to observe?
   1. Partial thromboplastin time (PTT) longer than 100 seconds
   2. Hemoglobin level below 10 g/dL (100 g/L)
   3. Potassium level above 5.5 mEq/L (5.5 mmol/L)
   4. White blood cell (WBC) count above 15,000/µL (15×10^9/L)

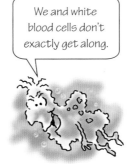

We and white blood cells don't exactly get along.

20. 4. Keeping a food diary to determine foods that produce or aggravate symptoms and eating small, frequent meals help to manage symptom flare-ups long term. Managing stress with exercise can increase the time between flare-ups; however, joining a support group may not help to manage symptoms. Increased fiber, fatty foods, dairy products, alcohol, smoking, and caffeine can aggravate symptoms. Probiotics have not shown any benefit with the management of Crohn's disease symptoms. Steroids are not for long-term use. Short-term (3 to 4 months) steroid therapy is used with immune suppressants to induce disease remission until immune suppressant therapy can maintain the disease in remission. A multivitamin does not help to manage symptoms.
CN: Physiological integrity; CNS: Reduction of risk potential; CL: Apply

21. 2. Although all of these are concerns the nurse should address, it is crucial the client is able to safely manage the ostomy before discharge.
CN: Safe, effective care environment; CNS: Management of care; CL: Analyze

22. 2. Although all of these are concerns the nurse should address, it is crucial the client use the incentive spirometer to maintain lung expansion and prevent atelectasis.
CN: Safe, effective care environment; CNS: Management of care; CL: Analyze

23. 2. Clients with gastric cancer commonly have nutritional deficits and may be cachectic. Discharge planning before surgery is important, but correcting the nutritional deficit is the priority. Prevention of deep vein thrombosis also is not the priority before surgery, though it assumes greater importance after surgery. At present, radiation therapy has not been proven effective for gastric cancer, and teaching about it preoperatively would not be appropriate.
CN: Physiological integrity; CNS: Reduction of risk potential; CL: Apply

24. 4. Because of infection, the client's WBC count would be elevated. A PTT longer than 100 seconds may suggest disseminated intravascular coagulation, a serious complication of septic shock. A hemoglobin level below 10 mg/dL (100 g/L) may occur from hemorrhage. A potassium level above 5.5 mEq/L (5.5 mmol/L) may suggest renal failure.
CN: Physiological integrity; CNS: Reduction of risk potential; CL: Apply

25. A client had a gastroscopy while under local anesthesia. Before resuming the client's oral fluid intake, which action will the nurse take **first**?
1. Listen for bowel sounds.
2. Determine whether the client can talk.
3. Check for a gag reflex.
4. Determine the client's mental status.

26. A recently admitted client suspected of having peritonitis is requesting a glass of water to drink. What is the **best** response by the nurse?
1. "I can give you small amounts of water frequently."
2. "You are getting your fluids intravenously."
3. "I will check with your health care provider."
4. "It would not be safe to give you anything to drink."

27. The nurse is caring for a client with acute pancreatitis. The nurse knows it is **most** important to monitor the client closely for which complication?
1. Increased appetite
2. Vomiting
3. Hypoglycemia
4. Pain

28. The nurse is completing the intake record for a client with chronic pancreatitis. The client has the intake during the previous 8 hours listed below.
Intake:
4 oz apple juice
½ cup fruit-flavored gelatin
6 oz water
500 mL 0.45% sodium chloride IV
How many milliliters will the nurse record as the client's intake? Record your answer using a whole number.

——————————— mL

29. Several children at a day care center have been infected with the hepatitis A virus. Which instruction will the nurse include when educating the day care staff?
1. Hand washing after diaper changes
2. Isolation of the sick children
3. Using masks during contact with children
4. Sterilization of all eating utensils

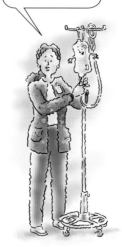

For clients with peritonitis, IV fluids are important for hydration.

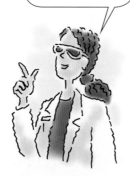

Your future's so bright, you have to wear shades.

25. 3. After a gastroscopy, the nurse should check for the presence of a gag reflex before giving oral fluids. This step is essential to prevent aspiration. The presence of bowel sounds, the ability to speak, and mental status within normal limits would not ensure the presence of a gag reflex.
CN: Physiological integrity; CNS: Reduction of risk potential; CL: Apply

26. 4. The client with peritonitis commonly is not allowed anything orally until the source of the peritonitis is confirmed and treated. IV fluids are given to maintain hydration and hemodynamic stability and to replace electrolytes; however, saying, "You are getting your fluids intravenously" does not explain to the client why oral fluids are not permitted. Checking with the health care provider is not necessary.
CN: Physiological integrity; CNS: Physiological adaptation; CL: Apply

27. 2. Acute pancreatitis is commonly associated with fluid isolation and accumulation in the bowel secondary to ileus or peripancreatic edema. Fluid and electrolyte loss from vomiting is the primary concern. A client with acute pancreatitis may have increased pain on eating and is unlikely to demonstrate an increased appetite. A client with acute pancreatitis is at risk for hyperglycemia, not hypoglycemia. Although pain is an important concern, it is less significant than vomiting.
CN: Physiological integrity; CNS: Physiological adaptation; CL: Apply

28. 920.
Fluid intake for this client includes 4 oz (120 mL) apple juice, 1/2 cup (120 mL) fruit-flavored gelatin, 6 oz (180 mL) water, and 500 mL 0.45% sodium chloride IV for a total of 920 mL.
CN: Physiological integrity; CNS: Basic care and comfort; CL: Apply

29. 1. Children in day care centers are at risk of hepatitis A infection, which is transmitted via the fecal-oral route due to poor hand hygiene practices and poor sanitation. Isolation of sick children, use of masks during contact, and sterilization of all eating utensils would not be useful in breaking the chain of infection.
CN: Safe, effective care environment; CNS: Safety and infection control; CL: Apply

30. The nurse is caring for a client diagnosed with hepatitis A. Which client statement indicates the nurse's education about hepatitis A was effective?
1. "I will wear a mask all of the time."
2. "I should keep my door closed."
3. "I should wash my hands frequently."
4. "I will save part of my sandwich for my wife."

31. A client with a liver disorder is having an invasive procedure. It is **priority** for the nurse to review which of the client's laboratory tests?
1. Coagulation studies
2. Liver enzyme levels
3. Serum chemistries
4. White blood cell count

32. The nurse is providing discharge instructions to a client with chronic cholecystitis. Which response by the client indicates the education has been effective?
1. "I need to rest more during the day."
2. "I should avoid taking antacids for heartburn."
3. "I should increase the fat intake in my diet."
4. "I will take my anticholinergic medications as prescribed."

33. After a laparoscopic cholecystectomy, a client reports abdominal pain. The nurse prepares to administer morphine sulfate 2 mg. The label on the morphine vial reads 10 mg/mL. How many milliliters will the nurse administer to the client? Record your answer using one decimal place.

_____ mL

34. The nurse obtains data from a client admitted with a diagnosis of cirrhosis and ascites. The client is lethargic and confused. Which action will the nurse take?
1. Elevate the head of the bed.
2. Notify the health care provider.
3. Reorient to time, place, and circumstance.
4. Apply 2 L of oxygen via nasal cannula.

30. 3. Hepatitis A is transmitted through the fecal-oral route, so frequent hand washing, especially after elimination, helps prevent transmission. It is not necessary to wear a mask or keep the door closed. Sharing food allows for viral transmission.
CN: Safe, effective care environment; CNS: Safety and infection control; CL: Apply

31. 1. The liver produces coagulation factors. If the liver is affected negatively, production of these factors may be altered, placing the client at risk for hemorrhage. The other laboratory tests should be monitored as well, but the results may not necessarily relate to the safety of the procedure.
CN: Physiological integrity; CNS: Reduction of risk potential; CL: Analyze

32. 4. Conservative therapy for chronic cholecystitis includes weight reduction by increasing physical activity, a low-fat diet, antacid use to treat dyspepsia, and anticholinergic use to relax smooth muscles and reduce ductal tone and spasm, thereby reducing pain.
CN: Physiological integrity; CNS: Pharmacological and parenteral therapies; CL: Apply

33. 0.2.
This formula is used to calculate drug dosages:

$$\frac{Dose\ on\ hand}{Quantity\ on\ hand} = \frac{Dose\ desired}{X}$$

In this example, the formula for calculating the amount of morphine is as follows:

$$\frac{10\ mg}{mL} = \frac{2\ mg}{X}$$

$$X = 0.2\ mL$$

CN: Physiological integrity; CNS: Pharmacological and parenteral therapies; CL: Apply

34. 2. Notify the health care provider for changes in the level of consciousness (observe for behavioral or personality changes, increased confusion, stupor, lethargy, hallucinations, and neuromuscular dysfunction), which indicate hepatic encephalopathy due to increased ammonia levels. Ammonia is a byproduct of the metabolism of nitrogen-containing compounds and is neurotoxic. Elevating the head of the bed would not improve confusion and lethargy and may be appropriate if the client was semiconscious. Reorientation would not improve the confusion, and although O_2 may also be needed, it would not fix the problem (elevated ammonia and possible swollen brain).
CN: Physiological integrity; CNS: Physiologic adaptation; CL: Analyze

35. Which instruction will the nurse give to a client with pancreatitis during discharge education?
1. Consume high-fat meals.
2. Consume low-calorie meals.
3. Limit daily intake of alcohol.
4. Avoid beverages that contain caffeine.

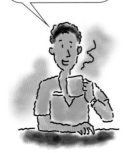

Don't panic. You're doing fine. Try some herbal tea.

36. A client undergoes a barium swallow fluoroscopy that confirms gastroesophageal reflux disease (GERD). Based on this diagnosis, the nurse will instruct the client to take which action(s)? Select all that apply.
1. Follow a high-fat, low-fiber diet.
2. Avoid caffeine and carbonated beverages.
3. Sleep with the head of the bed flat.
4. Stop smoking.
5. Take antacids 1 hour after meals and at bedtime.
6. Limit alcohol consumption to one drink per day.

37. A client with osteoarthritis is admitted to the hospital with peptic ulcer disease. Which finding(s) will the nurse expect to assess in this client? Select all that apply.
1. Localized, colicky periumbilical pain
2. History of nonsteroidal anti-inflammatory drug (NSAID) use
3. Epigastric pain relieved by antacids
4. Tachycardia
5. Nausea
6. Weight loss
7. Low-grade fever

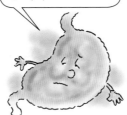

I'm feeling a little nausea and stomach pain. Could you pop an antacid?

38. A client is prescribed 1 g of neomycin sulfate orally every hour times 4 doses followed by 1 g orally every 4 hours for the remaining balance of the 24 days. Neomycin sulfate tablets are available in 500 mg per tablet. How many tablets will the nurse administer the client for each dose? Record your answer using a whole number.

_____ tablets

39. A client with cirrhosis is prescribed lactulose 2 tablespoons orally every day, to start if indicated by the client's lab results or signs and symptoms. Which finding indicates to the nurse a need to administer the medication?
1. Increasing confusion
2. Potassium level 5.6 mEq/dL (5.6 mmol/L)
3. Blood pressure 158/94 mm Hg
4. Increase in ascites

35. 4. Caffeine must be avoided because it is a stimulant, which would further irritate the pancreas. A client with pancreatitis must avoid all alcohol because chronic alcohol use is one of the causes of pancreatitis. The diet should be low in fat and high in calories, especially from carbohydrates.
CN: Physiological integrity; CNS: Reduction of risk potential; CL: Apply

36. 2, 4, 5. The nurse should instruct the client with GERD to follow a low-fat, high-fiber diet. Caffeine, carbonated beverages, alcohol, and smoking should be avoided because they aggravate GERD. In addition, the client should take antacids as prescribed (typically 1 hour after meals and at bedtime). Lying down with the head of the bed elevated, not flat, reduces intra-abdominal pressure, thereby reducing the symptoms of GERD.
CN: Health promotion and maintenance; CNS: None; CL: Apply

37. 2, 3, 5, 6. Peptic ulcer disease is characterized by nausea, hematemesis, melena, weight loss, and left-sided epigastric pain—occurring 1 to 2 hours after eating—that is relieved with antacids. NSAID use is also associated with peptic ulcer disease. Appendicitis begins with generalized or localized colicky periumbilical or epigastric pain, followed by anorexia, nausea, a few episodes of vomiting, low-grade fever, and tachycardia.
CN: Physiological integrity; CNS: Physiological adaptation; CL: Apply

38. 2.
First, convert from g to mg.
1 g to mg: 1,000 mg = 1 g, therefore the prescription is for 1,000 mg of neomycin.
Then use this formula for calculating the number of tablets to administer:

$$\frac{Desired\ dose}{Form\ on\ hand} = Dose$$

$$\frac{1,000\ mg}{500\ mg} = 2\ tablets$$

CN: Physiological integrity; CNS: Pharmacological and parenteral therapies; CL: Apply

39. 1. Lactulose is given when the client's ammonia level is elevated. The only sign of elevation in the ammonia levels is increasing confusion, which can indicate hepatic encephalopathy. Elevation in blood pressure and potassium level is not an indicator of elevated ammonia, nor is an increase in ascites.
CN: Physiological integrity; CNS: Pharmacological and parenteral therapies; CL: Analyze

CN: Client needs category   CNS: Client needs subcategory   CL: Cognitive level

40. The nurse is assigned to care for a client with peptic ulcer disease. Which finding will the nurse report **immediately** to the primary health care provider?
1. Black, tarry stools
2. Abdominal pain
3. Loss of appetite
4. Tachycardia

41. While caring for a client with cirrhosis, the nurse reviews the laboratory data in the client's chart. Which data will the nurse report **immediately** to the primary health care provider?
1. White blood cells (WBC) 12,8000 mm³ (12.8×10^9/L)
2. Red blood cells (RBC) 5.3 mm³ (5.03×10^{12}/L)
3. Prothrombin time (PT) 18 seconds
4. Total bilirubin 0.6 mg/dL (10.26 μmol/L)

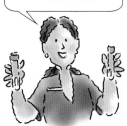

Do you choose the results of test tube A or test tube B?

42. When counseling a client in the ways to prevent cholecystitis, which guideline is appropriate for the nurse to include?
1. Eat low-protein foods.
2. Eat high-fat, high-cholesterol foods.
3. Limit exercise to 10 minutes per day.
4. Keep weight proportional to height.

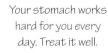

Your stomach works hard for you every day. Treat it well.

43. A client is brought to the emergency room with severe nausea, vomiting, and diarrhea for 36 hours. The client is admitted for gastroenteritis. Which action will the nurse take **first**?
1. Initiate NPO status for the client.
2. Encourage sips of an electrolyte-replacement drink.
3. Administer promethazine 25 mg orally.
4. Insert an IV and give fluids as prescribed.

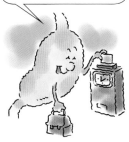

44. The nurse is caring for a client immediately after a liver biopsy. Which finding indicates to the nurse the client is experiencing a post-procedure complication?
1. Abdominal cramping
2. Weak, rapid pulse
3. Onset of vomiting
4. Temperature of 100.1°F (37.8°C)

40. 4. Pulse rate is a cardiovascular system assessment and tachycardia is an indicator of hidden bleeding, as well as a compensatory mechanism when a client is in the early stage of shock. Loss of appetite can occur from a number of factors and is not something to be alarmed about. Abdominal pain and black, tarry stools are expected with peptic ulcer disease. As blood from the gastrointestinal tract passes through the intestines, bacterial action causes it to become black and tarry colored.
CN: Safe, effective care environment; CNS: Management of care; CL: Apply

41. 3. Clotting factors may not be produced normally when a client has cirrhosis, increasing the potential for bleeding. PT measures the time required for a fibrin clot to form and is normally 11 to 13.5 seconds. The WBC count can be elevated in acute cirrhosis but is not always altered. The total bilirubin level would be elevated in cirrhosis of the liver. The elevation in bilirubin levels is what causes jaundice. The RBC count is not abnormal.
CN: Physiological integrity; CNS: Reduction of risk potential; CL: Analyze

42. 4. Obesity is a known cause of gallstones, and maintaining a recommended weight helps to protect against cholecystitis. Excessive dietary intake of cholesterol is associated with the development of gallstones in many people. Dietary protein is not implicated in cholecystitis. Liquid protein and low-calorie diets (with rapid weight loss of more than 5 lb [2.3 kg] per week) are implicated as the cause of some cases of cholecystitis. Regular exercise (30 minutes/three times per week) may help to reduce weight and improve fat metabolism.
CN: Health promotion and maintenance; CNS: None; CL: Apply

43. 4. First, the nurse would start an IV and administer fluids to restore the client's fluid imbalance. An antiemetic, such as promethazine, can be given to control nausea and vomiting The nurse would make the client NPO until 2 to 3 hours after the nausea and vomiting subsided. Sips of an electrolyte-replacement drink can be offered after the antiemetic to increase the chances of the client keeping the fluids down.
CN: Safe, effective care environment; CNS: Management of care; CL: Apply

44. 2. The liver is so vascular that taking a biopsy could cause the client to hemorrhage. Hemorrhage may be hidden, frank, or slow; therefore, monitor the dressing for visible bleeding and monitor the client's vital signs (changes in pulse rate, quality, and rhythm and a drop in blood pressure). The client may experience some discomfort but typically not cramping. Nausea and vomiting may be present and infection may occur, but not immediately after the procedure.
CN: Physiological integrity; CNS: Reduction of risk potential; CL: Apply

CN: Client needs category   CNS: Client needs subcategory   CL: Cognitive level

45. A client has just been given a prescription for diphenoxylate hydrochloride-atropine sulfate. Which information will the nurse provide about the use of this medication?
1. Drooling is a side effect of this medication
2. Irritability is an adverse effect of the medication
3. This medication can be habit-forming
4. Finish all of the medicine as prescribed

46. Oral lactulose is prescribed for a client with a hepatic disorder, and the nurse provides instructions to the client regarding this medication. Which statement by the client indicates a correct understanding of the instructions?
1. "Increasing my fluid intake will make the medication work better."
2. "I should remain close to the restroom when I take the medication."
3. "I need to include more high-fiber foods in my diet."
4. "I should call my health care provider immediately if I start having nausea."

47. The nurse is caring for a client who just underwent bowel resection and has a nasogastric (NG) tube connected to low intermittent suction. Which nursing intervention will the nurse include in the plan of care?
1. Flush the NG with saline once per shift.
2. Offer ice chips to moisturize the mouth.
3. Secure the suction tubing to the bed rail.
4. Provide meticulous mouth care as needed.

48. The nurse assesses a client with ascites from liver cirrhosis who is taking spironolactone. Which finding indicates to the nurse the client is responding well to the medication?
1. Decrease in abdominal circumference
2. Increase in urine output to 50 mL/hour
3. Serum potassium level of 5.8 mEq/L (5.8 mmol/L)
4. Improvement in breathing pattern

45. 3. Diphenoxylate hydrochloride-atropine sulfate is an antidiarrheal. The client should not exceed the recommended dose of this medication because it may be habit-forming. Because this medication is an antidiarrheal, it should not be taken until it is finished. Side effects of the medication include dry mouth and drowsiness, not drooling or irritability.
CN: Physiological integrity; CNS: Pharmacological and parenteral therapies; CL: Apply

46. 2. Lactulose retains ammonia in the colon and promotes increased peristalsis and bowel evacuation, expelling ammonia from the colon. Therefore, the client should remain close to the restroom when taking the medication. It should be taken with water or juice to aid in softening the stool. An increased fluid intake and a high-fiber diet would promote defecation but is unrelated to the medication and why it is being given to this client. Nausea is a side effect and the client should be instructed to drink cola and eat unsalted crackers or dry toast. It is not necessary to notify the health care provider should nausea occur.
CN: Physiological integrity; CNS: Pharmacological and parenteral therapies; CL: Apply

47. 4. Provide mouth care for clients who are receiving enteral or parenteral feedings or NPO and are not able to perform for themselves. The NG tube should not be flushed once per shift; the health care provider's prescription would determine the frequency of flushing if prescribed. A client who is on gastric suctioning should be NPO. Avoid securing the suction tubing to the bed rail; doing so may cause the NG tube to become dislodged if the bedrail is let down, which can inadvertently dislodge the NG tube.
CN: Physiological integrity; CNS: Basic care and comfort; CL: Apply

48. 1. In clients with ascites, spironolactone is used to reduce ascites and portal hypertension that causes the ascites. The medication helps to reduce the accumulation of fluid in the abdominal region and other regions of the body, which would be indicated by a decrease in abdominal circumference. Spironolactone is a potassium-sparing diuretic, which can cause potassium levels to rise dramatically in clients, so this should be monitored. Elevation of serum potassium levels above the normal range should be reported. Increased urine output is an expected finding but does not indicate how well the client's ascites is responding to the medication. Breathing pattern is also not an indicator of the client's response to spironolactone.
CN: Physiological integrity; CNS: Pharmacological and parenteral therapies; CL: Analyze

49. A client who takes famotidine for gastritis asks the home care nurse which medication is **best** to take for a headache. Which over-the-counter medication will the nurse suggest for this client?
1. Acetylsalicylic acid
2. Acetaminophen
3. Ibuprofen
4. Naproxen

50. The nurse prepares to administer morning medications to a client with hepatitis. The client's medications are listed below. Which medication will the nurse withhold?
1. Lamivudine 150 mg orally twice daily
2. Acetaminophen 650 mg orally every day
3. Vitamin B_{12} one capsule twice daily
4. Phytonadione 5 mg IM once daily

51. Which manifestations reported by a client will lead the nurse to suspect Crohn's disease affecting the small intestine?
1. Nausea accompanied by vomiting
2. Weight gain and fluid retention
3. Diarrhea alternating with constipation
4. Stools that have an oily consistency

52. The nurse assesses a client with colon cancer. Which finding(s) will the nurse report **immediately** to the health care provider? Select all that apply.
1. Change in bowel habits
2. A palpable abdominal mass
3. Fecal smears in client's underwear
4. Reports of rectal bleeding
5. Diarrhea and constipation
6. Abdominal swelling and tenderness

53. Which intervention will the nurse provide for a client admitted with a perforated gastric ulcer?
1. Administration of antacids
2. Fluid and electrolyte replacement
3. Removal of nasogastric (NG) tube
4. Histamine-2 (H_2) receptor antagonist administration

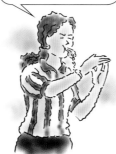

Which medication is hardest on the liver?

Time out! Take a careful look at all the options in question #52 and then select all that apply.

49. 2. The client is taking famotidine, a histamine-2 receptor antagonist. This implies the client has a disorder characterized by gastrointestinal (GI) irritation. The only medication among the answer choices that is not irritating to the GI tract is acetaminophen. The other medications could aggravate an already-existing GI problem.
CN: Physiological integrity; CNS: Pharmacological and parenteral therapies; CL: Analyze

50. 2. Acetaminophen is contraindicated in clients with liver disorders. The medication should be withheld, and the health care provider should be contacted regarding this medication. Lamivudine is an antiviral used to treat hepatitis B; B_{12} is a vitamin supplement used to treat anemia associated with hepatitis; and phytonadione, a form of vitamin K, is used to prevent bleeding when the liver is not functioning properly and does not produce adequate amounts of clotting factors to support clotting.
CN: Physiological integrity; CNS: Pharmacological and parenteral therapies; CL: Analyze

51. 4. Excessive amounts of fat in the feces due to malabsorption can occur with Crohn's disease. Weight loss (not weight gain) due to malabsorption is common. Nausea, vomiting, diarrhea, and constipation are symptoms of many different GI disorders. Fluid loss (not fluid retention) occurs with Crohn's disease due to diarrhea.
CN: Health promotion and maintenance; CNS: None; CL: Understand

52. 2, 3, 6. A mass is not usually palpable in the abdomen unless this is an advanced case. The fecal smearing is a sign of incontinence caused by loss of sphincter control/tone or diarrhea. Abdominal swelling would not be expected with colon cancer and thus may be a sign of another gastrointestinal (GI) problem. The key signs and symptoms of colon cancer are: change in bowel habits and shape of stools; abdominal pain (bloating, gas, cramps), diarrhea, and constipation; bloody stools or rectal bleeding; and weight loss from GI irritation.
CN: Physiological integrity; CNS: Physiological adaptation; CL: Apply

53. 2. The client should be treated with fluid and electrolyte replacement, blood products, and antibiotics. NG tube suctioning may also be performed to prevent further spillage of stomach contents into the peritoneal cavity. Antacids and H_2 receptor antagonists are not helpful in this situation.
CN: Physiological integrity; CNS: Physiological adaptation; CL: Apply

CN: Client needs category   CNS: Client needs subcategory   CL: Cognitive level

54. When providing discharge education for a client with ulcerative colitis, the nurse emphasizes the importance of regular examinations. Which statement by the client indicates a proper understanding of the instructions?
  1. "People who have ulcerative colitis tend to have more problems with their teeth than those with other GI problems."
  2. "I should report any rectal bleeding to my health care provider because this could indicate I have developed an ulcer."
  3. "My health care provider needs to see me frequently because my chance of developing appendicitis is higher."
  4. "I will need to have routine screenings because having ulcerative colitis places me at risk for colon cancer."

54. 4. Clients with chronic ulcerative colitis, granulomas, and familial polyposis have an increased risk of developing colon cancer. Clients with ulcerative colitis do not have an increased risk of developing the other disorders.
CN: Health promotion and maintenance; CNS: None; CL: Apply

55. The nurse is caring for a client with chronic pancreatitis. Which response by the client indicates discharge education has been effective?
  1. "I will eat a low-carbohydrate diet."
  2. "I can have an occasional glass of wine."
  3. "I will take pancreatic enzymes with each meal."
  4. "I will take pancreatic enzymes before breakfast and at bedtime."

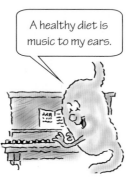

A healthy diet is music to my ears.

55. 3. Oral pancreatic enzymes are taken with each meal to aid digestion and control steatorrhea. The client should adhere to a low-fat (not low-carbohydrate) diet. The client should eliminate alcohol from the diet completely, as it would continue to cause pancreatic damage.
CN: Physiological integrity; CNS: Physiological adaptation; CL: Apply

56. The nurse is caring for a client with alcohol-related acute pancreatitis. Which intervention is **most** appropriate to reduce the exacerbation of pain?
  1. Lying supine
  2. Taking aspirin
  3. Eating low-fat foods
  4. Abstaining from alcohol

56. 4. Abstaining from alcohol is imperative to reduce injury to the pancreas; in fact, it may be enough to completely control pain. Lying supine usually aggravates the pain because it stretches the abdominal muscles. Taking aspirin can cause bleeding in hemorrhagic pancreatitis. During an attack of acute pancreatitis, the client usually is not allowed to ingest anything orally.
CN: Physiological integrity; CNS: Reduction of risk potential; CL: Apply

57. Which nursing intervention is **priority** when caring for a client with esophageal varices?
  1. Recognizing hemorrhage
  2. Controlling blood pressure
  3. Encouraging nutritional intake
  4. Provide education about varices

57. 1. Recognizing the rupture of esophageal varices, or hemorrhage, is the focus of nursing care because the client could succumb to this quickly. Controlling blood pressure is also important because it helps reduce the risk of variceal rupture. It is also important to educate the client on what varices are and what foods the client should avoid, such as spicy foods.
CN: Safe, effective care environment; CNS: Management of care; CL: Apply

58. A client diagnosed with peptic ulcer disease is prescribed ranitidine. The client asks the nurse, "What is the action of ranitidine?" Which response by the nurse is appropriate?
  1. "It neutralizes stomach acid."
  2. "It reduces acid secretions."
  3. "It stimulates gastrin release."
  4. "It protects the mucosal barrier."

58. 2. Ranitidine is a histamine-2 receptor antagonist, which reduces acid secretion by inhibiting gastrin secretion. Antacids neutralize acid, and mucosal barrier fortifiers protect the mucosal barrier.
CN: Physiological integrity; CNS: Pharmacological and parenteral therapies; CL: Understand

CN: Client needs category   CNS: Client needs subcategory   CL: Cognitive level

59. The nurse is preparing to obtain a stool sample from a client admitted with suspected hepatitis. Which precaution(s) will the nurse take when caring for this client? Select all that apply.

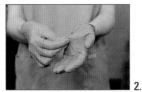
1.

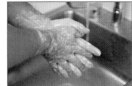
2.

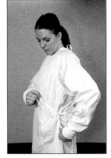
3.

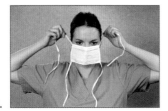
4.

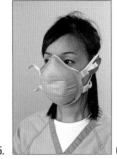
5.

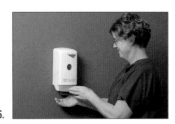
6.

59. **1, 2, 3, 6.** Hepatitis transmission occurs via the fecal-oral route, exposure to infected blood feces and urine, and through the ingestion of contaminated food or liquids. To collect a specimen when the type of hepatitis in unknown, the nurse should take these precautions: wear gloves and a gown, perform meticulous hand washing, and use an alcohol-based hand sanitizer to reduce the possibility of spreading infection. A mask and goggles are not needed unless there is the possibility of splashing (e.g., when performing gastric lavage; flushing G-tubes or catheters; suctioning; and when working with clients who are vomiting, have explosive diarrhea, or are vomiting/coughing up blood).
CN: Safe, effective care environment; CNS: Safety and infection control; CL: Apply

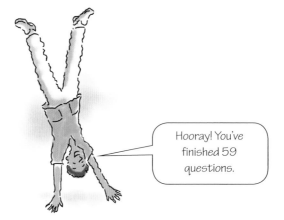

Hooray! You've finished 59 questions.

60. The nurse is reviewing data in a client's chart suspected to have cholecystitis. Which test result will help confirm a diagnosis of cholecystitis?
1. Results of a colonoscopy
2. Results of an abdominal ultrasound
3. Results of barium swallow
4. Results of endoscopy

60. **2.** An abdominal ultrasound can show whether the gallbladder is enlarged, gallstones are present, the gallbladder wall is thickened, or distention of the gallbladder lumen is present. A colonoscopy looks at the inner surface of the colon. A barium swallow looks at the stomach and the duodenum. Endoscopy looks at the esophagus, stomach, and duodenum.
CN: Health promotion and maintenance; CNS: None; CL: Understand

61. The nurse is planning care for a client following a gastric resection. Which item is the nurse's **priority**?
1. Body image
2. Nutritional needs
3. Skin care
4. Spiritual needs

61. **2.** After gastric resection, a client may require total parenteral nutrition or jejunostomy tube feedings to maintain adequate nutritional status. Body image is not much of a problem for this client because clothing can cover the incision site. Wound care of the incision site is necessary to prevent infection; otherwise, the skin should not be affected. Spiritual needs may be a concern, depending on the client, and should be addressed as the client demonstrates readiness to share concerns.
CN: Physiological integrity; CNS: Reduction of risk potential; CL: Apply

62. The nurse assesses a client at the clinic for follow-up after being treated in the hospital for pancreatitis. When assessing the client, which finding will the nurse **immediately** report to the health care provider?
1. Dry, itchy, and scaly skin
2. Abdomen bloated but non-tender
3. Greenish-yellow bruise over the IV site
4. Shortness of breath with minimal exertion

62. **4.** In pancreatitis, the nurse should watch for signs and symptoms of worsening of the condition: shortness of breath with minimal exertion; respiratory failure and tachycardia (signs of hypocalcemia and hypomagnesemia); and acute changes in abdominal symptoms/size. The other findings are expected and are not a reason to be alarmed.
CN: Safe, effective care environment; CNS: Management of care; CL: Apply

63. The nurse is educating a 52-year-old client on cancer screening. The nurse emphasizes the client needs which diagnostic test annually after age 50 years to screen for colon cancer?
1. Abdominal computed tomography (CT) scan
2. Abdominal x-ray
3. Colonoscopy
4. Fecal occult blood test

63. **4.** Annual screenings for colon cancer using fecal occult blood tests beginning at age 50 years are recommended. Surface blood vessels of polyps and cancers are fragile and often bleed with the passage of stools, so a fecal occult blood test should be performed annually. CT scan and abdominal x-ray can help establish tumor size and metastasis. A colonoscopy can help locate a tumor as well as polyps and can be used for screening every 10 years.
CN: Health promotion and maintenance; CNS: None; CL: Apply

64. A client with colon cancer asks the nurse, "Why am I getting radiation therapy before surgery?" Which response by the nurse is **most** appropriate?
1. "It helps reduce the size of the tumor."
2. "It eliminates the malignant cells."
3. "The chances of curing the cancer are improved."
4. "The therapy helps to heal the bowel after surgery."

64. **1.** Radiation therapy is used to treat colon cancer before surgery to reduce the size of the tumor, making it easier to resect. Radiation therapy cannot eliminate the malignant cells (though it helps to define tumor margins), is not curative, and could slow postoperative healing.
CN: Physiological integrity; CNS: Physiological adaptation; CL: Apply

65. Which symptom reported by a client leads the nurse to suspect gastric cancer?
1. Abdominal cramping
2. Constant hunger
3. Feeling of fullness
4. Weight gain

65. **3.** The client with gastric cancer may report a feeling of fullness in the stomach but not enough to seek medical care. Abdominal cramping is not associated with gastric cancer. Anorexia and weight loss (not increased hunger or weight gain) are common symptoms of gastric cancer.
CN: Physiological integrity; CNS: Physiological adaptation; CL: Apply

66. A client is suspected of having gastric cancer. The nurse will expect to prepare the client for which diagnostic test?
1. Barium enema
2. Colonoscopy
3. Gastroscopy
4. Serum chemistry levels

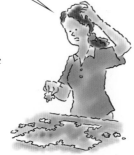

Puzzled by a question? Try to eliminate as many wrong answers as you can before answering.

66. **3.** A gastroscopy allows direct visualization of the tumor. A barium enema or colonoscopy would help to diagnose colon cancer. Serum chemistry levels do not contribute data useful to the assessment of gastric cancer.
CN: Health promotion and maintenance; CNS: None; CL: Understand

67. A client is prescribed carmustine. Which nursing intervention is appropriate when caring for this client?
1. Allow the client to hold the medication in the hand.
2. Give an antiemetic before giving carmustine.
3. Monitor the client's electrolyte levels daily.
4. Apply a heart monitor to assess cardiac function.

67. **2.** The nurse would give an antiemetic before administering carmustine to reduce nausea. The medication should not touch skin because it may stain the skin brown. The nurse should monitor the client's liver, renal, and pulmonary function tests. Electrolytes should be monitored when taking cisplatin. Cardiac function should be monitored when taking doxorubicin.
CN: Physiological integrity; CNS: Pharmacological and parenteral therapies; Apply

68. A client recently diagnosed with colon cancer tells the nurse, "I am having trouble sleeping because of thoughts of how life will change after surgery." Which action will the nurse take in this situation?
1. Request a chaplain to come and talk to the client.
2. Refer the client to a cancer support group.
3. Discuss the client's remarks with the charge nurse.
4. Encourage the client to discuss personal feelings.

69. To reduce occurrence of dumping syndrome, which action will the nurse instruct a client to take?
1. Sip fluids while eating meals.
2. Consume three meals daily.
3. Rest after meals for 20 to 30 minutes.
4. Eat high-carbohydrate, low-fat foods.

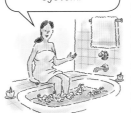

A bath is a great way to engage your parasympathetic (rest-and-digest) system.

70. Which finding(s) in a client with Crohn's disease indicates early signs of dehydration? Select all that apply.
1. Poor skin turgor
2. Decreased creatinine
3. Low specific gravity
4. Elevated blood pressure
5. Increased heart rate
6. Bradypnea

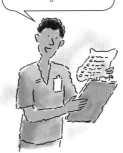

Dehydration is serious business. Remember to stay well hydrated.

71. The nurse is caring for an adult client prescribed phytonadione. Which nursing action is **priority**?
1. Monitor the client's sclera for signs of jaundice.
2. Assess the client's electrolyte levels closely.
3. Educate the client on dietary restrictions.
4. Get liver function tests before giving the first dose.

72. A client who underwent a colon resection 1 week ago calls the nurse and says, "My incision is wide open on one side and something is poking out of it." Which instruction is **priority** for the nurse to give this client?
1. "Drive to the nearest emergency department to be evaluated by a health care provider."
2. "Wrap an ace bandage around your abdomen and monitor for bleeding."
3. "Place wax paper over the wound and call an ambulance immediately."
4. "Apply petroleum jelly gauze over the wound and come to the office."

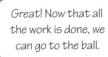

Great! Now that all the work is done, we can go to the ball.

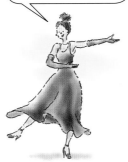

68. 4. The client is having trouble sleeping because of concerns about life changes. The client may be experiencing anxiety and powerlessness. Encouraging the client to verbalize feelings helps the nurse to determine how to assist the client and may reduce the client's anxiety. The other options do not directly address the client's comments and concerns.
CN: Psychosocial integrity; CNS: None; CL: Apply

69. 3. To reduce occurrences of dumping syndrome, clients should be taught to lie down for 20 to 30 minutes after eating; take fluids between meals only; eat smaller amounts more frequently in a semi-recumbent position; follow a low-carbohydrate diet, with high-protein and moderate-fat foods; and avoid sweets.
CN: Physiological integrity; CNS: Reduction of risk potential; CL: Apply

70. 1, 5. Signs and symptoms of dehydration include poor skin turgor, increased heart rate, concentrated urine, and decreased blood pressure. Other signs are dry skin and mouth, sunken eyes, and lethargy. Decreased creatinine level and bradypnea are not early signs of dehydration.
CN: Physiological integrity; CNS: Physiological adaptation; CL: Apply

71. 4. The nurse would obtain liver function tests, platelet count, prothrombin time (PT), and international normalized ratio (INR) before starting therapy to have a baseline. The nurse would monitor newborn clients for jaundice. There is not a need to assess electrolyte levels. There are no dietary restrictions for phytonadione.
CN: Physiological integrity; CNS: Pharmacological and parenteral therapies; CL: Apply

72. 3. The client is experiencing wound evisceration (occurs 5 to 7 days after surgery). The nurse should instruct the client to cover the wound with wax paper to maintain moisture of the internal organs and call 911 for ambulance transport to the hospital. Petroleum products, an elastic bandage, and driving to the hospital are contraindicated in the care of this client.
CN: Physiological integrity; CNS: Physiological adaptation; CL: Apply

Chapter 9

Endocrine Disorders

Endocrine refresher

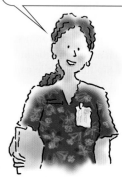

Time to get all hormonal ... this chapter covers diabetes and other endocrine disorders, typically a difficult area for nursing students. Don't worry though—I'll help you through all the tough spots.

Acromegaly and gigantism (hyperpituitarism)

Acromegaly
Over-secretion of growth hormone (GH) by the pituitary gland in adulthood (after closure of the epiphyseal plates)

Gigantism
Over-secretion of growth hormone (GH) prior to puberty (before closure of the epiphyseal plates)

Key signs and symptoms

Acromegaly
- Enlarged supraorbital ridge
- Thickened ears and nose
- Thickening of the tongue

Gigantism
- Excessive growth in all parts of the body

Key test results
- Plasma human growth hormone (HGH) levels measured by radioimmunoassay typically are elevated. However, because HGH secretion is pulsatile, the results of random sampling may be misleading. IGF-1 (somatomedin-C) levels offer a better screening alternative.

Key treatments
- Surgery to remove the affecting tumor (transsphenoidal hypophysectomy)
- Thyroid hormone replacement therapy after surgery: levothyroxine
- Inhibitor of HGH release: bromocriptine, pegvisomant
- Somatotropic hormone: octreotide

Key interventions
- Provide the client with emotional support.
- Perform or assist with range-of-motion (ROM) exercises.
- This disease can also cause inexplicable mood changes; reassure the family that these mood changes result from the disease and can be modified with treatment.
- After surgery, monitor vital signs and neurologic status; be alert for any alterations in level of consciousness, pupil equality, or visual acuity as well as vomiting, falling pulse rate, and rising blood pressure.
- Check blood glucose levels.
- Measure intake and output hourly, watching for large increases.
- Encourage the client to ambulate on the first or second day after surgery.

Diabetes insipidus

Insufficient antidiuretic hormone (ADH) secreted by the pituitary gland resulting in excretion of copious volumes of urine

Key signs and symptoms
- Polydipsia (consumption of 4 to 40 L/day)
- Polyuria (greater than 5 L/day of dilute urine)

Key test results
- Urine chemistry shows urine specific gravity less than 1.005, osmolality 50 to 200 mOsm/kg (50 to 200 mmol/kg), decreased urine pH, and decreased sodium and potassium levels

Key treatments
- IV therapy: hydration (when first diagnosed, intake and output must be matched milliliter to milliliter to prevent dehydration), electrolyte replacement
- ADH replacement: desmopressin

Key interventions
- Monitor fluid balance and daily weight.
- Monitor and record vital signs, intake and output (urine output should be measured every hour when first diagnosed), urine specific gravity (check every 1 to 2 hours when first diagnosed), and laboratory studies.
- Maintain IV fluid.

Syndrome of inappropriate antidiuretic hormone secretion (SIADH)

Posterior pituitary gland disorder in which there is a continued release of ADH that results in renal reabsorption of water rather than its normal excretion

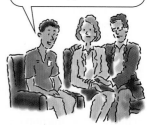

Acromegaly can affect both the client's appearance and mood, so be prepared to provide emotional support.

Key signs and symptoms

- Water retention, edema, weight gain
- Oliguria
- Headache
- Muscle cramps
- Anorexia
- With worsening of condition: nausea, vomiting, muscle twitching, and changes in level of consciousness (LOC)

Key test results

- Decreased serum sodium and osmolality
- Increased urine sodium and osmolality

Key treatments

- Eliminate underlying cause
- Osmotic diuretics (mannitol)
- Loop diuretics (furosemide)
- IV administration of a 3% hypertonic sodium chloride solution for severe hyponatremia

Key interventions

- Monitor intake and output.
- Assess LOC frequently.
- Monitor for signs and symptoms of fluid overload and hyponatremia.

Addison's disease (primary adrenal insufficiency)

Disorder that results from destruction of the adrenal cortex by disease; this results in decreased adrenal cortical function

Key signs and symptoms

- Orthostatic hypotension
- Weakness and lethargy
- Weight loss

Key test results

- Blood chemistry reveals decreased cortisol, glucose, sodium, chloride, and aldosterone levels; and increased blood urea nitrogen (BUN), potassium level, and plasma ACTH
- Hematology tests reveal elevated hematocrit and decreased hemoglobin
- Blood or capillary glucose levels reveal hypoglycemia
- Urine chemistry shows decreased 17-ketosteroids and hydroxycorticosteroids (17-OHCS)

Key treatments

- With adrenal crisis, IV hydrocortisone given promptly along with 3 to 5 L of normal saline solution
- Glucocorticoids: hydrocortisone
- Mineralocorticoid: fludrocortisone

Key interventions

- Administer appropriate medications.
- Maintain IV fluids.
- Do not allow the client to sit up or stand quickly.

Cushing's syndrome (adrenocortical hyperfunction)

Excessive secretion of hormones by the adrenal cortex

Key signs and symptoms

- History of amenorrhea
- History of mood swings
- Hypertension
- Muscle wasting
- Weight gain, especially truncal obesity, "buffalo hump," and "moonface"

Key test results

- Blood chemistry shows increased cortisol, aldosterone, sodium, corticotropin, and glucose levels, and a decreased potassium level
- Dexamethasone suppression test shows no decrease in 17-OHCS
- Magnetic resonance imaging shows pituitary or adrenal tumors

Key treatments

- Hypophysectomy or bilateral adrenalectomy
- Control excess production of cortisol: ketoconazole, mitotane, and metyrapone

Key interventions

- Perform postoperative care.
- Observe for edema.
- Limit water intake.
- Weigh the client daily.

Diabetes mellitus

Metabolic disorder of the pancreas that affects carbohydrate, fat, and protein metabolism

- Type 1 is characterized by no insulin production by the pancreas; onset most likely to occur in childhood and adolescence
- Type 2 is characterized by insulin resistance or insufficient insulin production; more common in aging adults

Key signs and symptoms

- Polydipsia
- Polyphagia
- Polyuria
- Weight loss (with type 1)

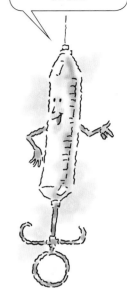

Diuretics are the "appropriate" treatment for SIADH.

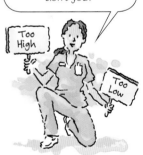

Cushing's syndrome is characterized by adrenocortical hyperfunction. You remember what "hyper" means, don't you?

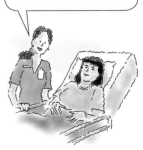

When assessing for diabetes mellitus, remember the three "polys": -dipsia, -phagia, and -uria.

Key test results

- Fasting blood glucose level is increased (greater than or equal to 126 mg/dL [6.99 mmol/L])
- Glycosylated hemoglobin assay is increased to 7 (0.07) or above
- 2-hour postprandial blood glucose level shows hyperglycemia (greater than 200 mg/dL [11.10 mmol/L])

Key treatments

- Antidiabetic agents: insulin or oral agents, such as glimepiride, glyburide, glipizide, metformin

Key interventions

- Monitor acid-base and fluid balance.
- Monitor for signs of hypoglycemia (altered mental status, dizziness, weakness, pallor, tachycardia, diaphoresis, seizures, and coma), ketoacidosis (acetone breath, dehydration, weak or rapid pulse, Kussmaul's respirations), and hyperosmolar coma (polyuria, thirst, neurologic abnormalities, stupor).
- Be prepared to treat hypoglycemia; immediately give carbohydrates in the form of skim milk, fruit juice, hard candy, or honey. If the client is unconscious, maintain safety until glucagon or dextrose is administered IV.
- Be prepared to maintain IV fluid; administer insulin and, usually, potassium replacement for ketoacidosis or hyperosmolar coma.
- Monitor wound healing.
- Maintain the client's diet.
- Provide meticulous skin and foot care; clients with diabetes are at increased risk for infection from impaired leukocyte activity.
- Foster independence.

Goiter

Enlarged thyroid gland; endemic goiter is caused by dietary deficiency of iodine or the inability of the thyroid gland to utilize iodine

Key signs and symptoms

- Single or multinodular, firm, irregular enlargement of the thyroid gland
- Dizziness or syncope when the client raises the arms above the head (Pemberton's sign)
- Dysphagia

Key test results

- Laboratory tests reveal high or normal thyroid-stimulating hormone (TSH), low serum thyroxine (T4) concentrations, and increased iodine-131 uptake

Key treatments

- Subtotal thyroidectomy
- Thyroid hormone replacement: levothyroxine

Key interventions

- Measure the client's neck circumference. Also check for the development of hard nodules in the gland.
- Provide preoperative teaching and postoperative care if subtotal thyroidectomy is indicated.

Hyperthyroidism

Hypersecretion of thyroid hormones (T3, T4) that results in an increased metabolic rate

Key signs and symptoms

- Atrial fibrillation
- Bruit or thrill over thyroid
- Diaphoresis
- Palpitations
- Tachycardia

Key test results

- Blood chemistry shows increased triiodothyronine (T3), T4, and free thyroxine levels; also shows decreased TSH and cholesterol levels
- Radioactive iodine uptake (RAIU) is increased

Key treatments

- Radiation therapy
- Thyroidectomy
- Iodine preparations: potassium iodide (SSKI), radioactive iodine

Key interventions

- Monitor cardiovascular status.
- Avoid stimulants, such as caffeine-containing drugs and foods.
- Maintain IV fluids.
- Weigh the client daily.
- Provide postoperative care.

Hypothyroidism

Thyroid gland fails to secrete adequate amounts of thyroid hormones; this results in slowing of all metabolic processes

Key signs and symptoms

- Dry, flaky skin
- Thinning nails
- Fatigue
- Hypothermia
- Menstrual disorders
- Mental sluggishness
- Weight gain or anorexia

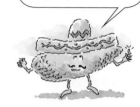

Hey, everybody— the insulin has arrived. Let's get this party started!

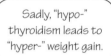

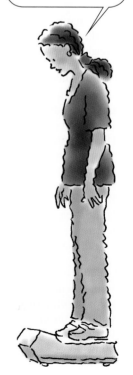

Sadly, "hypo-" thyroidism leads to "hyper-" weight gain.

Key test results

- Blood chemistry shows decreased T3, T4, free thyroxine, and sodium levels; TSH levels are increased with thyroid insufficiency and decreased with hypothalamic or pituitary insufficiency
- RAIU is decreased

Key treatments

- Thyroid hormone replacement: levothyroxine, liothyronine

Key interventions

- Avoid sedation; administer one-half to one-third the normal dose of sedatives or opioids.
- Check for constipation and edema.
- Encourage fluids.

Thyroid cancer

Growth of malignant cells in the thyroid gland

Key signs and symptoms

- Enlarged thyroid gland
- Painless, firm, irregular, and enlarged thyroid nodule or mass

Key test results

- Blood chemistry shows increased calcitonin, serotonin, and prostaglandin levels
- RAIU shows a "cold" or nonfunctioning nodule
- Thyroid biopsy shows cytology positive for cancer cells

Key treatments

- Radiation therapy
- Thyroidectomy (total or subtotal) with or without radical neck excision

Key interventions

- Monitor respiratory status for signs of airway obstruction.
- Evaluate ability to swallow.
- Provide postoperative thyroidectomy care.

Thyroiditis

Inflammation of the thyroid gland that involves release of excessive amounts of thyroid hormones; this results in thyroid dysfunction from hyperactivity to eventual hypoactivity as the stores of thyroid hormones in the gland are depleted. Hashimoto's thyroiditis (an autoimmune disorder) is the most common form.

Key signs and symptoms

- Thyroid enlargement
- Fever
- Pain
- Tenderness and reddened skin over the gland

Key test results

- Precise diagnosis depends on the type of thyroiditis:
    - With autoimmune thyroiditis, high titers of thyroglobulin and microsomal antibodies may be present in serum
    - With subacute granulomatous thyroiditis, tests may reveal elevated erythrocyte sedimentation rate, increased thyroid hormone levels, and decreased thyroidal RAIU
    - With chronic infective and noninfective thyroiditis, varied findings occur, depending on underlying infection or other disease

Key treatments

- Partial thyroidectomy to relieve tracheal or esophageal compression in Riedel thyroiditis
- Thyroid hormone replacement: levothyroxine for accompanying hypothyroidism

Key interventions

- Check vital signs and examine the client's neck for unusual swelling, enlargement, or redness.
- If the neck is swollen, measure and record the circumference daily.
- After thyroidectomy:
    - Check vital signs every 15 to 30 minutes until the client's condition stabilizes. Stay alert for signs of tetany secondary to unintentional parathyroid injury during surgery. Keep 10% calcium gluconate available for IM use if needed.
    - Check dressings frequently for excessive bleeding.
    - Keep the head of the client's bed elevated.
    - Watch for signs of airway obstruction, such as difficulty talking and increased swallowing; keep tracheotomy equipment handy.

Hyperparathyroidism

Excessive secretion of parathormone (parathyroid hormone) which results in increased urinary excretion of phosphorus and loss of calcium from the bones

Key signs and symptoms

- Fatigue and muscle weakness
- Bone pain, especially on weight bearing

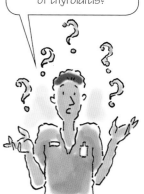

Can you remember the signs and symptoms of thyroiditis?

- Pathologic fractures
- Calcium renal calculi (stones)

Key test results

- Increased serum calcium levels
- Decreased serum phosphorus levels
- Elevated urine calcium levels in a 24-hour collection

Key treatments

Primary hyperparathyroidism
- Surgical excision of the hypertrophied glandular tissue or adenoma

Secondary hyperparathyroidism
- Correct the underlying cause (vitamin D therapy, management of renal failure, calcium restricted diet)

Key interventions

- Measure intake and output.
- Observe for development of renal calculi (flank pain, increased serum calcium, decreased urine output).
- Increase PO fluid intake.
- Frequent rest periods.
- Maintain postoperative care similar to care after thyroidectomy.

Hypoparathyroidism

Insufficient secretion of parathormone due to trauma or inadvertent removal of all (or nearly all) of the glands during thyroidectomy

Key signs and symptoms

- Tetany
- Numbness in fingers, toes, or around the lips
- Positive Chvostek's sign, Trousseau's sign
- Laryngeal spasm

Key test results

- Elevated serum phosphorus level
- Decreased serum calcium level
- Decreased urinary calcium and phosphorus levels

Key treatments

- Administration of an IV calcium salt
- Intubation and mechanical ventilation for acute respiratory distress
- Long-term treatment: oral calcium supplements, vitamin D or D2 (calcitriol), and a high calcium, low phosphorus diet

Key interventions

- Observe for tetany and assess Chvostek's and Trousseau's signs.
- Insert IV line for emergency administration of calcium.
- Observe during calcium administration for adverse effects (bradycardia, flushing, tingling in the arms and legs, metallic taste).
- Observe for respiratory distress and keep emergency equipment for intubation/tracheostomy/mechanical ventilation at the bedside.
- To prevent muscle contractions and convulsions, keep noise, movement, and other environmental triggers to a minimum.

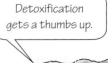

Detoxification gets a thumbs up.

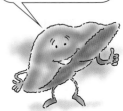

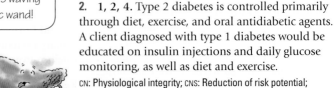

thePoint® You can download tables of drug information to help you prepare for the NCLEX®! View Generic Drug Names, Drug Classifications, Drug Actions, and Nursing Implications for the drugs discussed in this refresher at **http://thePoint.lww.com**

Endocrine questions, answers, and rationales

1. After assessing a client, which symptom(s) will lead the nurse to suspect hyperglycemia? Select all that apply.
 1. Polydipsia
 2. Polyuria
 3. Diaphoresis
 4. Tachycardia
 5. Polyphagia
 6. Irritability

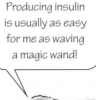

Producing insulin is usually as easy for me as waving a magic wand!

2. A client is newly diagnosed with type 2 diabetes. The nurse will educate the client on which intervention(s)? Select all that apply.
 1. Exercise
 2. Diabetic diet
 3. Insulin injections
 4. Metformin administration
 5. Daily glucose monitoring

1. **1, 2, 5.** Symptoms of hyperglycemia include polydipsia, polyuria, and polyphagia. Irritability, diaphoresis, and tachycardia are symptoms of hypoglycemia.
CN: Physiological integrity; CNS: Reduction of risk potential;
CL: Apply

2. **1, 2, 4.** Type 2 diabetes is controlled primarily through diet, exercise, and oral antidiabetic agents. A client diagnosed with type 1 diabetes would be educated on insulin injections and daily glucose monitoring, as well as diet and exercise.
CN: Physiological integrity; CNS: Reduction of risk potential;
CL: Apply

CN: Client needs category   CNS: Client needs subcategory   CL: Cognitive level

3. A client presents with diaphoresis, palpitations, jitters, and tachycardia approximately 4 hours after taking the morning dose of insulin. What is the nurse's **priority** action?
1. Check blood glucose level and administer carbohydrates as indicated.
2. Give nitroglycerin and perform an electrocardiogram (ECG).
3. Check pulse oximetry and administer oxygen therapy.
4. Restrict salt, administer diuretics, and perform paracentesis.

4. The nurse is caring for a client receiving isophane insulin suspension. Which assessment finding(s) will lead the nurse to suspect the client is experiencing hypoglycemia? Select all that apply.
1. Diaphoresis
2. Hunger
3. Increased urination
4. Excessive thirst
5. Confusion
6. Headache
7. Dizziness

5. The nurse is caring for a client who vomits 1 hour after taking the morning dose of glyburide. What is the **priority** nursing action?
1. Administer another dose of glyburide to the client.
2. Give subcutaneous insulin and monitor blood glucose.
3. Monitor blood glucose and look for signs of hypoglycemia.
4. Notify the client's primary health care provider.

6. The nurse is discussing exercise with a client newly diagnosed with type 2 diabetes mellitus. Which statement by the client indicates to the nurse additional education is needed?
1. "I need to carry candy or juice when I go jogging."
2. "I should wait to eat until after I have finished exercising."
3. "I should give my insulin in my abdomen."
4. "I should warm up before my aerobic exercise."

7. During client rounding, the primary health care provider informed the nurse a client would be prescribed a long-acting insulin for treatment. Which prescription(s) will the nurse question if prescribed by the health care provider? Select all that apply.
1. Insulin aspart
2. Insulin glargine
3. Insulin detemir
4. Isophane insulin suspension
5. Insulin lispro

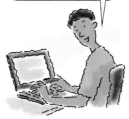
I wish someone would administer some carbohydrates to me.

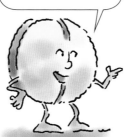
Vomiting may be a sign that I'm working a little *too* well.

3. 1. The client is experiencing symptoms of hypoglycemia. Checking the blood glucose level and administering carbohydrates would elevate blood glucose. ECG and nitroglycerin are treatments for myocardial infarction. Administering oxygen would not help correct the low blood glucose level. Restricting salt, administering diuretics, and performing paracentesis are treatments for ascites.
CN: Safe, effective care environment; CNS: Management of care; CL: Analyze

4. 1, 2, 5, 6, 7. Signs and symptoms of hypoglycemia include: diaphoresis, weakness, headache, nausea, drowsiness, nervousness, hunger, tremors, malaise, characteristic behavioral changes, confusion, and dizziness. Excessive thirst and polyuria suggest hyperglycemia rather than hypoglycemia.
CN: Physiological integrity; CNS: Physiological adaptation; CL: Apply

5. 3. When a client who has taken an oral antidiabetic agent vomits, the nurse should monitor glucose and assess frequently for signs of hypoglycemia. Most of the medication has probably been absorbed. Therefore, repeating the dose would further lower glucose levels later in the day. Giving insulin would also lower glucose levels, causing hypoglycemia. There is not a reason to notify the health care provider at this time.
CN: Physiological integrity; CNS: Pharmacological and parenteral therapies; CL: Apply

6. 2. The client should eat before exercising to prevent hypoglycemia. Carbohydrate snacking may be necessary with prolonged exercise. Insulin should be given in the abdomen before exercise because it is more rapidly absorbed. Warming up is effective in any exercise plan.
CN: Physiological integrity; CNS: Physiological adaptation; CL: Apply

7. 1, 4, 5. Insulins aspart and lispro are rapid-acting insulins. Isophane insulin suspension is an intermediate-acting insulin. Insulin glargine and insulin detemir are long-acting insulins.
CN: Physiological integrity; CNS: Pharmacological and parenteral therapies; CL: Apply

CN: Client needs category   CNS: Client needs subcategory   CL: Cognitive level

8. The nurse is educating a client on chronic complications of diabetes. The nurse will include which condition(s) in the education? Select all that apply.
   1. Dyspnea on exertion
   2. Retinopathy
   3. Neuropathy
   4. Coronary artery disease
   5. Cerebral ischemic events
   6. Pulmonary infarcts
   7. Muscle weakness

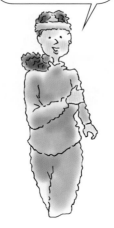

Pace yourself. The NCLEX-RN is more like a marathon than a sprint.

8. 2, 3, 4. Retinopathy, neuropathy, and coronary artery disease are all chronic complications of diabetes. Dyspnea on exertion and muscle weakness are complications of a host of other disorders. Cerebral ischemic events and pulmonary infarcts are complications of sickle cell anemia.
CN: Physiological integrity; CNS: Reduction of risk potential; CL: Apply

9. When caring for a client with a diagnosis of type 2 diabetes mellitus, the nurse will anticipate preparing the client for which diagnostic test(s)? Select all that apply.
   1. Fasting blood glucose
   2. Glycosylated hemoglobin
   3. Pancreatic CT scan
   4. Postprandial glucose
   5. Cardiac catheterization

9. 1, 2, 4. Screening for diabetes mellitus is relatively simple. Insulin resistance or insufficient insulin production is reflected in faulty glucose metabolism. Fasting blood glucose and postprandial glucose reflect current glucose levels. Glycosylated hemoglobin reflects average glucose levels over the preceding 120 days. Pancreatic CT scan does not assess diabetes mellitus. Cardiovascular complications may eventually necessitate cardiac catheterization; however, it is not a diagnostic test for diabetes mellitus.
CN: Physiological integrity; CNS: Reduction of risk potential; CL: Apply

10. A client reports weight gain and tiredness. Based on the assessment data, the nurse determines the client is experiencing which condition?

Vital Signs	
Blood pressure	120/74 mm Hg
Pulse	52 beats/minute
Respiratory rate	20 breaths/minute
Temperature	98°F (36.7°C)
Laboratory Results	
Thyroxine (T4)	3.1 µg/dL (39.9 nmol/L)
Triiodothyronine (T3)	30 ng/dL (0.46 nmol/L)

   1. Tetany
   2. Hypothyroidism
   3. Hyperthyroidism
   4. Hypokalemia

10. 2. Weight gain, lethargy, and slow pulse rate along with decreased T3 and T4 levels indicate hypothyroidism. T3 and T4 are thyroid hormones that affect growth and development as well as metabolic rate. Tetany is related to low calcium levels. Hypokalemia is a low potassium level.
CN: Physiological integrity; CNS: Physiological adaptation; CL: Analyze

11. The nurse administers a client isophane insulin at 0730. At 1230, the client reports shakiness and increasing anxiety. When nursing action is **most** appropriate?
   1. Administer intravenous glucagon.
   2. Check the client's glucose level.
   3. Have the client eat a snack.
   4. Give oral diazepam.

11. 2. Isophane insulin suspension is an intermediate-acting insulin with a peak (when hypoglycemia is most likely to occur) of 4 to 12 hours. Shakiness and anxiety are symptoms of hypoglycemia, indicating to the nurse the need to assess the client's glucose level. Further interventions, such as a snack or administering glucagon or diazepam, would be determined based on the glucose level.
CN: Safe, effective care environment; CNS: Management of care; CL: Analyze

CN: Client needs category   CNS: Client needs subcategory   CL: Cognitive level

12. Which medication(s) will the nurse expect the primary health care provider to prescribe for a client with hypothyroidism? Select all that apply.
1. Dexamethasone
2. Lactulose
3. Levothyroxine
4. Lidocaine
5. Potassium iodide

12. 3. Levothyroxine, a synthetic form of the thyroid hormone thyroxine, is the medication of choice for treating hypothyroidism. Dexamethasone is a steroid and an antithyroid medication. Lactulose is a laxative used to treat constipation. Lidocaine is used to treat ventricular dysrhythmias. Potassium iodide is an antithyroid medication used to treat hyperthyroidism.
CN: Physiological integrity; CNS: Pharmacological and parenteral therapies; CL: Apply

13. The nurse and a client have just discussed the client's recent diagnosis of hypothyroidism and its causes and effects. Which statement indicates to the nurse the client needs further instruction?
1. "Now I see—my clumsiness is caused by a hormone problem."
2. "I just eat too much. That is why I am depressed and overweight."
3. "No wonder I am constipated. I am predisposed to it no matter what I eat."
4. "I am not cold all the time because I am getting older; I have a metabolic problem."

13. 2. Hypothyroidism results from an inadequate secretion of thyroid hormones, which slows metabolic processes and can cause depression and weight gain. A client with hypothyroidism who insists that overeating has caused depression and obesity needs further instruction about the effects of the disease. The other statements reflect an accurate understanding that hypothyroidism can cause clumsiness, constipation, and a feeling of coldness.
CN: Physiological integrity; CNS: Reduction of risk potential; CL: Apply

14. The nurse will monitor which client(s) with hypothyroidism **most** carefully for myxedema coma? Select all that apply.
1. A client who was in a motor vehicle accident
2. A client undergoing an emergency appendectomy
3. A client who just lost a spouse of 30 years
4. A client taking opioids several times a day
5. A client being treated for bronchitis

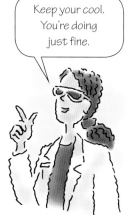

Keep your cool. You're doing just fine.

14. 1, 2, 3, 4, 5. Myxedema coma represents the most severe form of hypothyroidism. The client develops severe hypothermia and hypoglycemia and becomes comatose. Myxedema coma can be precipitated by opioids, stress (such as surgery or loss of a loved one), trauma, and infections.
CN: Physiological integrity; CNS: Reduction of risk potential; CL: Analyze

15. The nurse is caring for an older adult client being treated for hypothyroidism. For which complication will the nurse monitor the client?
1. Acute hemolytic reaction
2. Cardiac dysrhythmia
3. Retinopathy
4. Thrombocytopenia

15. 2. Precipitation of cardiac dysrhythmia is a potentially serious complication of hypothyroidism treatment, especially for older adult clients or those with underlying heart disease. Acute hemolytic reaction is a complication of blood transfusions. Retinopathy is usually a complication of diabetes. Thrombocytopenia is defined as a platelet count of less than 150,000/mm³ (150,000 × 10⁹/L) and does not result from treating hypothyroidism.
CN: Physiological integrity; CNS: Reduction of risk potential; CL: Apply

16. A client is suspected of having hypothyroidism. Which diagnostic tests is **most** appropriate for the nurse to monitor?
1. Liver function studies and sodium level
2. Hemoglobin A1c and calcium level
3. Thyroxine (T4) and thyroid-stimulating hormone (TSH) levels
4. 24-hour urine collection for cortisol and bacteria

16. 3. T4 and TSH are diagnostic tests for hypothyroidism. Liver function studies are indicated in many disorders to check for liver damage. Hemoglobin A1c measurement is used to assess hyperglycemia. Cortisol levels would be checked if adrenal insufficiency is suspected. There are no indications of sodium- or calcium-related complications.
CN: Safe, effective care environment; CNS: Management of care; CL: Apply

17. The nurse is caring for a client with hypothyroidism. Which finding(s) will the nurse report to the health care provider? Select all that apply.
1. Hair loss
2. Cold intolerance
3. Weight gain
4. Constipation
5. Nervousness

18. The nurse is caring for a client admitted with an adrenal malfunction. Which hormone level(s) will the nurse anticipate the health care provider prescribing? Select all that apply.
1. Epinephrine
2. Norepinephrine
3. Thyroxine (T4)
4. Triiodothyronine (T3)
5. Calcitonin
6. Insulin
7. Somatostatin

19. While monitoring a client with hypothyroidism, the nurse notes hypoactive bowel sounds. Which action will the nurse complete?
1. Continue to monitor the client.
2. Notify the health care provider.
3. Assess the client's heart rate.
4. Decrease the temperature of the room.

20. When preparing a client for a thyroid function test, the nurse questions the client about medications. The nurse will notify the health care provider if the client is taking which medications?
1. Acetaminophen and aspirin
2. Estrogen and amphetamines
3. Insulin and oral antidiabetic agents
4. Topical antiseptics and multivitamins

21. A client with Cushing's syndrome is admitted to the medical-surgical unit. While assessing the client, the nurse notes the client is agitated and irritable, has poor memory, reports a loss of appetite, and is disheveled. The nurse recognizes these findings are associated with which condition?
1. Depression
2. Neuropathy
3. Hypoglycemia
4. Hyperthyroidism

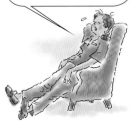
Ugh! I feel so "hypo" today. Maybe I should have my hormone levels checked out.

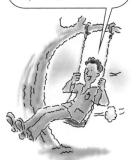
Looks like your knowledge is on the upswing. Well done!

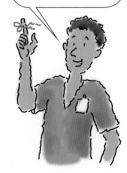
Hmm. What condition is associated with poor memory? I forget.

17. 1, 5. The nurse would report unexpected findings, such as hair loss and nervousness. Hyperthyroidism has symptoms of heat intolerance, nervousness, weight loss, and hair loss. Cold intolerance, weight gain, and constipation are symptoms of hypothyroidism secondary to a decrease in cellular metabolism.
CN: Safe, effective care environment; CNS: Management of care; CL: Apply

18. 1, 2. The medulla of the adrenal gland causes the release of epinephrine and norepinephrine. Glucocorticoids, mineralocorticoids, and androgens are released from the adrenal cortex. T4, T3, and calcitonin are secreted by the thyroid gland. The islet cells of the pancreas secrete insulin, glucagon, and somatostatin.
CN: Safe, effective care environment; CNS: Management of care; CL: Apply

19. 1. Hypothyroidism is associated with a general slowing of body systems as indicated by hypoactive bowel sounds. The nurse would continue to monitor this client. There is not a need to notify the health care provider of expected findings. The nurse would not assess the heart rate due to hypoactive bowel sounds. Clients with hypothyroidism are generally sensitive to cold environments.
CN: Physiological integrity; CNS: Physiological adaptation; CL: Apply

20. 4. Topical antiseptics and multivitamins contain iodine and can alter thyroid function test results. Estrogen and amphetamines do not contain iodine but may alter thyroid function test results. Insulin, oral antidiabetic agents, acetaminophen, and aspirin will not affect a thyroid test.
CN: Physiological integrity; CNS: Pharmacological and parenteral therapies; CL: Analyze

21. 1. Agitation, irritability, poor memory, loss of appetite, and neglect of one's appearance may signal depression, which is common in clients with Cushing's syndrome. Neuropathy affects clients with diabetes, not Cushing's syndrome. Although hypoglycemia can cause irritability, it also produces increased appetite rather than loss of appetite. Hyperthyroidism typically causes such signs as goiter, nervousness, heat intolerance, and weight loss despite increased appetite.
CN: Psychosocial integrity; CNS: None; CL: Apply

22. The nurse is providing education to a client on how to correctly self-administer 3 units of regular insulin and 4 units of NPH insulin daily. Which client statement demonstrates the education has been successful?

1. "I will check my blood sugar after breakfast and lunch, and give myself shots in my stomach as needed."
2. "After taking my insulin out of the refrigerator, I will draw up the clear insulin first to the line for 3 units, and then cloudy insulin until there is a total of 7 units in the syringe."
3. "First, I will check my blood sugar; then I will get insulin from the refrigerator and withdraw 7 units."
4. "I should inject the insulin into a different site each time and then put it back in the pantry for safekeeping."

22. **2.** By indicating the proper dosage and prescription in which the insulin should be drawn, the client reveals a higher level of knowledge and demonstrates greater readiness to manage personal care alone. The next step would be to ask the client to demonstrate how an actual injection would be given. Blood sugar should be checked before meals, and insulin should be kept refrigerated. The statement by the client to check the blood sugar, get the insulin, and withdraw 7 units suggests the client does not understand how the insulin is drawn into the syringe.

CN: Physiological integrity; CNS: Pharmacological and parenteral therapies; CL: Apply

23. A client reports muscle weakness, anorexia, and darkening of the skin. The nurse reviews laboratory data and notes decreased sodium and high potassium levels. The nurse will anticipate the client will be diagnosed with which condition?

1. Addison's disease
2. Cushing's syndrome
3. Diabetes insipidus
4. Thyrotoxic crisis

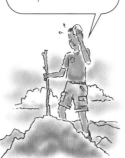

Keep on truckin'. The view from the top is worth it.

23. **1.** The clinical picture of Addison's disease includes muscle weakness, anorexia, darkening of the skin's pigmentation, low sodium level, and high potassium level. Cushing's syndrome involves obesity, "buffalo hump," "moonface," and thin extremities. Symptoms of diabetes insipidus include excretion of large volumes of dilute urine. Thyrotoxic crisis can occur with severe hyperthyroidism.

CN: Physiological integrity; CNS: Physiological adaptation; CL: Apply

24. The nurse is caring for a client following surgical ablation of the pituitary gland. For which condition **must** the nurse be alert?

1. Addison's disease
2. Cushing's syndrome
3. Diabetes insipidus
4. Hypothyroidism

24. **3.** The cause of diabetes insipidus is unknown, but it may be secondary to head trauma, brain tumors, or surgical ablation of the pituitary gland. Addison's disease is caused by a deficiency of cortical hormones, whereas Cushing's syndrome is an excess of cortical hormones. Hypothyroidism occurs when the thyroid gland secretes low levels of thyroid hormone.

CN: Safe, effective care environment; CNS: Management of care; CL: Apply

25. A client who sustained a head injury is diagnosed with diabetes insipidus. The health care provider prescribes desmopressin acetate. Which finding **most** concerns the nurse?

1. Client reports a headache, muscle cramps, and unsteady gait
2. Blood pressure is 110/70 mm Hg standing and 108/68 mm Hg lying in bed
3. Client removes bandage from superficial head wound
4. Client reports increased thirst and the nurse notes colorless urine

25. **1.** Diabetes insipidus (DI) results from a deficiency of circulating antidiuretic hormone (vasopressin). Desmopressin acetate, a synthetic vasopressin, is the medication of choice for treating diabetes insipidus. A client with hyponatremia should not take desmopressin. Headache, muscle cramps, and unsteady gait are symptoms of hyponatremia. The nurse would be concerned if the client had hypertension, not normal blood pressure. The nurse would need to determine why the client removed the bandage and reapply as necessary; however, this is not greatly concerning because it is a superficial wound. Increased thirst and colorless urine are expected with DI.

CN: Safe, effective care environment; CNS: Management of care; CL: Analyze

26. A client with diabetes insipidus has had limited fluid intake over the past 12 hours. Which complication(s) will the nurse monitor the client for? Select all that apply.
 1. Hypertension
 2. Bradycardia
 3. Glucosuria
 4. Hyperglycemia
 5. Severe dehydration
 6. Hypernatremia

26. 5, 6. A client with diabetes insipidus has high volumes of urine, even without fluid replacement. Therefore, limited fluid intake would cause severe dehydration and hypernatremia. A client undergoing a fluid deprivation test may experience tachycardia and hypotension. A client with diabetes insipidus would not have glucose in the urine. Diabetes insipidus has no effect on blood glucose; therefore, the client would not suffer from hyperglycemia.
CN: Physiological integrity; CNS: Physiological adaptation; CL: Analyze

27. When caring for a client with a diagnosis of diabetes insipidus, which nursing intervention is **priority**?
 1. Watch for signs and symptoms of septic shock.
 2. Maintain an adequate fluid intake.
 3. Check the client's weight every 3 days.
 4. Monitor urine for specific gravity greater than 1.030.

> Clients with diabetes insipidus have to pee a lot, which puts them at risk of dehydration. So, what should you encourage them to do?

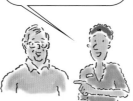

27. 2. In a client with diabetes insipidus, maintaining fluid intake is essential to prevent severe dehydration. The client is at risk for developing hypovolemic shock because of increased urine output. Weight should be measured on a daily basis to check for adequate fluid balance. Urine specific gravity should be monitored for low osmolality, generally less than 1.005, due to the body's inability to concentrate urine.
CN: Safe, effective care environment; CNS: Management of care; CL: Apply

28. A client experiences polydipsia and is voiding large amounts of water-like urine with a specific gravity of 1.003. Which health care provider prescription will the nurse question?
 1. Administer desmopressin.
 2. Provide a regular diet.
 3. Provide strict intake and output (I&O) measurement.
 4. Increase oral fluid intake.

28. 2. The nurse would suspect the client has diabetes insipidus, which is characterized by polydipsia and large amounts of water-like urine, which has a specific gravity of 1.001 to 1.005. The nurse would question providing the client a regular diet. The client should be provided with a low-sodium diet. Desmopressin is given to decrease urine production. Strict monitoring of intake and output is needed to monitor for improvement or complications. Increased oral fluid intake and possibly intravenous fluids are given to restore volume.
CN: Safe, effective care environment; CNS: Management of care; CL: Analyze

29. The nurse is caring for a client with syndrome of inappropriate antidiuretic hormone secretion (SIADH). Which finding(s) will the nurse report to the health care provider? Select all that apply.
 1. History of a head injury
 2. Water retention
 3. Excessive thirst
 4. Weight loss
 5. Oliguria

> Hooray! You've finished 30 questions.

29. 3, 4. SIADH is a disorder of excessive antidiuretic hormone secretion by the posterior pituitary gland. Causes include head trauma. It is manifested by water retention, edema, and weight gain, not weight loss. Excessive thirst is a symptom of diabetes insipidus, a disorder of insufficient ADH secretion.
CN: Physiological integrity; CNS: Physiological adaptation; CL: Apply

30. A client is diagnosed with diabetes insipidus. The nurse will develop the care plan based on the understanding that which hormone is deficient?
 1. Androgen
 2. Epinephrine
 3. Norepinephrine
 4. Vasopressin

30. 4. Clients with diabetes insipidus have a deficiency of vasopressin, the antidiuretic hormone. Androgen, epinephrine, and norepinephrine are hormones secreted by the adrenal gland and are not related to diabetes insipidus.
CN: Physiological integrity; CNS: Physiological adaptation; CL: Understand

CN: Client needs category   CNS: Client needs subcategory   CL: Cognitive level

31. A client is suspected of having diabetes insipidus. The nurse will prepare the client for which diagnostic test?
1. Capillary blood glucose test
2. Fluid deprivation test
3. Serum ketone test
4. Urine glucose test

31. 2. The fluid deprivation test involves withholding water for 4 to 18 hours and checking urine and plasma osmolality periodically for signs of diabetes insipidus. The capillary blood glucose test allows a rapid measurement of glucose in whole blood and would be used to assess for diabetes mellitus. The serum ketone test documents diabetic ketoacidosis. The urine glucose test monitors glucose levels in urine, but diabetes insipidus does not affect urine glucose levels.
CN: Physiological integrity; CNS: Reduction of risk potential; CL: Apply

32. The nurse is reviewing data in the progress notes entry of a client with adrenocortical insufficiency. The client reports difficulties in the work environment and a recent upper respiratory infection. The nurse identifies the client is **most** at risk for which condition?
1. Adrenal crisis
2. Diabetic ketoacidosis
3. Myxedema
4. Thyrotoxic crisis

32. 1. As Addison's disease progresses, the client may develop a life-threatening emergency—adrenal crisis, which is related to insufficient levels of cortisol, a hormone produced by the adrenal glands. The crisis occurs as a result of deterioration of the adrenal gland or inadequate treatment of adrenal insufficiency. Stress and infection can both necessitate a dose adjustment in corticosteroid therapy to prevent adrenal insufficiency and the development of adrenal crisis. Diabetic ketoacidosis is a form of hyperglycemia. Myxedema is a form of severe hypothyroidism. Thyrotoxic crisis is a form of severe hyperthyroidism.
CN: Physiological integrity; CNS: Physiological adaptation; CL: Analyze

33. The nurse is reviewing a client's laboratory findings, which indicate a deficiency of cortical hormones. The nurse will expect the client to be treated for which diagnosis?
1. Addison's disease
2. Cushing's syndrome
3. Diabetes
4. Diabetic ketoacidosis

33. 1. Addison's disease is caused by a deficiency of cortical hormones. Cushing's syndrome is the opposite of Addison's disease and includes excessive adrenocortical activity. Diabetes is an insulin deficiency. Diabetic ketoacidosis is severe hyperglycemia, causing acidosis.
CN: Physiological integrity; CNS: Physiological adaptation; CL: Apply

34. The nurse is caring for a client undergoing evaluation of endocrine function, and laboratory findings indicate excessive levels of adrenocortical hormones. This would correlate with which disease?
1. Cushing's syndrome
2. Diabetes
3. Hypothyroidism
4. Addison's disease

34. 1. Cushing's syndrome is indicated by excessive levels of adrenocortical hormones. Low levels of glucose and sodium, along with high levels of potassium and white blood cells, are diagnostic of Addison's disease. Diabetes causes increased blood glucose levels. Hypothyroidism results in low levels of thyroid hormone.
CN: Physiological integrity; CNS: Physiological adaptation; CL: Apply

T3 and T4 are hormones secreted by the thyroid. So, increased levels would point to what condition?

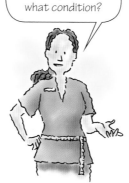

35. The nurse reviews the laboratory data of a client. The data reveal increased blood and urine levels of triiodothyronine (T3) and thyroxine (T4). The nurse will suspect the client will be treated for which complication?
1. Hyperthyroidism
2. Addison's disease
3. Cushing's syndrome
4. Hypopituitarism

35. 1. Hyperthyroidism causes high levels of T3 and T4. A definitive diagnosis of Addison's disease must reflect low levels of adrenocortical hormones. Cushing's syndrome manifests as excessive amounts of adrenocortical hormones. Lower pituitary hormone secretion levels are consistent with hypopituitarism.
CN: Physiological integrity; CNS: Physiological adaptation; CL: Apply

CN: Client needs category   CNS: Client needs subcategory   CL: Cognitive level

36. The health care provider prescribes an oral antidiabetic medication and weekly glucose monitoring for a client who is overweight, with a poor diet and stressful job, and recently diagnosed with type 2 diabetes. The client asks the nurse how this will impact life. Which nursing response is **most** appropriate?

1. "The medication will help maintain a steady glucose level, but you need to cut back on snacking."
2. "Type 2 diabetes is common and easily treated. You do not have to make dietary or lifestyle changes."
3. "I will refer you to a diabetes nurse specialist. The nurse will be able to help you develop a plan."
4. "You may want to change careers because your job requires so much of your daily energy."

37. The nurse is caring for a client with syndrome of inappropriate antidiuretic hormone secretion (SIADH). The client becomes confused and develops crackles and dyspnea. What is the **priority** action of the nurse?

1. Administer an IV fluid bolus.
2. Notify the health care provider.
3. Monitor serum sodium level.
4. Weigh the client.

38. The nurse is caring for a client admitted with a diagnosis of Addison's disease. Which nursing intervention is appropriate?

1. Provide frequent rest periods.
2. Administer diuretics.
3. Encourage a high potassium diet.
4. Maintain fluid restrictions.

39. A client had a subtotal thyroidectomy at 0730. During evening rounds, the nurse obtains data from the client, who now has nausea, a temperature of 105°F (40.6°C), tachycardia, and extreme restlessness. Which complication does the nurse suspect?

1. Diabetic ketoacidosis
2. Thyroid crisis
3. Hypoglycemia
4. Tetany

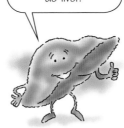

Great job answering these questions. You really know how to de-liver.

A temperature of 105°F (40.6°C) sounds like a crisis to me.

36. 3. A referral to a nurse specialist who can develop an ongoing relationship with the client, spend more time assessing personal needs, and develop a workable plan would be most appropriate. Although the medication does help to maintain steady glucose levels, this response ignores the other factors contributing to the client's poor health habits. Telling the client that there will not be lifestyle changes is inappropriate, as is suggesting the client change careers.
CN: Health promotion and maintenance; CNS: None; CL: Apply

37. 2. Confusion and respiratory distress are indicators of fluid overload, which can be a life-threatening complication of SIADH. The nurse notifies the health care provider immediately of a change in level of consciousness. The nurse would not administer a fluid bolus as this would further complicate the client's condition. Weighing the client is not a priority. Hyponatremia does not manifest with these symptoms.
CN: Safe, effective care environment; CNS: Management of care; CL: Analyze

38. 1. A client with Addison's disease is dehydrated, hypotensive, and very weak. Frequent rest periods are needed to prevent exhausting the client. Diuretics would cause further dehydration and are contraindicated in a client with Addison's disease. Potassium levels are usually elevated in Addison's disease because aldosterone secretion is decreased, resulting in decreased sodium and increased potassium. Fluid intake would be encouraged, not restricted, in a dehydrated client.
CN: Physiological integrity; CNS: Physiological adaptation; CL: Apply

39. 2. Thyroid crisis usually occurs in the first 12 hours after thyroidectomy and causes exaggerated signs of hyperthyroidism, such as high fever, tachycardia, and extreme restlessness. Diabetic ketoacidosis is more likely to produce polyuria, polydipsia, and polyphagia. Hypoglycemia typically produces weakness, tremors, profuse perspiration, and hunger. Tetany typically causes uncontrollable muscle spasms, stridor, cyanosis, and possibly asphyxia.
CN: Physiological integrity; CNS: Physiological adaptation; CL: Apply

40. The nurse will expect to see which signs and symptoms when a pediatric client overproduces adrenocortical hormone? Select all that apply.
1. Slow growth rate
2. Obesity
3. Weight loss
4. Heat intolerance
5. Changes in skin texture
6. Low body temperature
7. Polyuria
8. Dehydration

40. 1, 2. Overproduction of adrenocortical hormone results in slow growth rate and obesity. Weight loss and heat intolerance indicate thyroid hormone overproduction. Changes in skin texture and low body temperature indicate thyroid hormone underproduction. Polyuria and dehydration indicate diabetic ketoacidosis.
CN: Physiological integrity; CNS: Physiological adaptation; CL: Apply

41. Assessment of a client reveals thin extremities with an obese truncal area and a "buffalo hump" at the shoulder area with reports of weakness and disturbed sleep. The nurse will anticipate which prescription from the health care provider?
1. Administer prednisone.
2. Give ketoconazole.
3. Place client on bed rest.
4. Monitor respiratory rate.

41. 2. The nurse would suspect the client has Cushing's syndrome, which is treated with ketoconazole, mitotane, and metyrapone. Steroid usage should be reduced. There is no need to place the client on bed rest or monitor respiratory status.
CN: Physiological integrity; CNS: Physiological adaptation; CL: Apply

42. The nurse is caring for a client with Cushing's syndrome experiencing sodium and water retention. The nurse will assess the client for which disorder(s)? Select all that apply.
1. Hypoglycemia
2. Dehydration
3. Pulmonary edema
4. Hypertension
5. Heart failure

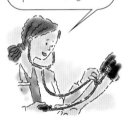

You remember what effect increased sodium has on blood pressure, right?

42. 4, 5. Increased mineralocorticoid activity in a client with Cushing's syndrome commonly contributes to hypertension and heart failure. Hypoglycemia and dehydration are uncommon in a client with Cushing's syndrome. Pulmonary edema also is not a complication of Cushing's syndrome.
CN: Physiological integrity; CNS: Physiological adaptation; CL: Apply

43. The nurse is caring for a client with high serum sodium and glucose levels, low potassium level and eosinophil count, and disappearance of lymphoid tissue. The nurse will expect this client to be diagnosed with which condition?
1. Graves' disease
2. Myxedema
3. Addison's disease
4. Cushing's syndrome

43. 4. Test results in Cushing's syndrome include high serum sodium and glucose levels, low potassium level, reduction of eosinophils, and disappearance of lymphoid tissue. Addison's disease is the opposite of Cushing's syndrome, with low serum sodium and glucose levels and a high potassium level. Graves' disease causes increased thyroid hormone levels. Myxedema results in low levels of thyroid hormones.
CN: Physiological integrity; CNS: Physiological adaptation; CL: Apply

44. A client presents with a "buffalo hump" at the shoulder area and an obese truncal area with thin extremities. The nurse will anticipate preparing the client for which test?
1. Fluid deprivation test
2. Glucose tolerance test
3. Low-dose dexamethasone suppression test
4. Thallium stress test

44. 3. A low-dose dexamethasone suppression test is used to detect changes in plasma cortisol levels in the diagnosis of Cushing's syndrome, which is characterized by a "buffalo hump" at the shoulder area and an obese truncal area with thin extremities. A fluid deprivation test is used in the diagnosis of diabetes insipidus. The glucose tolerance test is used to determine gestational diabetes in pregnant women. A thallium stress test is used to monitor heart function under stress.
CN: Physiological integrity; CNS: Physiological adaptation; CL: Analyze

45. The nurse is caring for a client with adrenocortical hyperfunction after a bilateral adrenalectomy. Which nursing intervention(s) will the nurse implement when caring for this client? Select all that apply.
1. Administer corticosteroids as prescribed.
2. Observe closely for signs and symptoms of acute adrenal crisis.
3. Maintain strict aseptic technique during dressing changes.
4. Weigh the client prior to administering corticosteroids.
5. Administer analgesics only for severe pain.

46. The nurse is caring for a client with hypoparathyroidism. During the assessment, the nurse will perform which action?
1. Monitor the client for heart failure.
2. Assess the client for seizure activity.
3. Flex the client's neck to see if hips and knees flex.
4. Tap the client's face 0.75 in (2 cm) anterior to the earlobe.

47. Which nursing intervention will be performed for a client with Cushing's syndrome?
1. Suggest clothing or bedding that feel cool and comfortable.
2. Recommend consumption of high-carbohydrate and low-protein foods.
3. Explain that physical changes are a result of excessive corticosteroids.
4. State the rationale for increasing salt and fluids during illness, stress, and heat.

48. A client was recently admitted with a diagnosis of diabetes. During assessment, the nurse notes the client has acetone breath, a weak and rapid pulse, and Kussmaul's respirations. The nurse anticipates which prescription from the health care provider?
1. Respiratory monitoring
2. Administer magnesium
3. Fluid replacement
4. Mouth care

49. The nurse is caring for a client with type 1 diabetes who does not adhere to an insulin regimen regularly. The nurse will identify that the client is at risk for developing which complication?
1. Diabetic ketoacidosis
2. Hypoglycemia
3. Pancreatitis
4. Respiratory failure

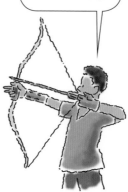

Aim for success ... it makes it a lot easier to hit it.

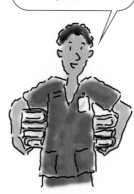

Hint: The symptoms described in question #48 point to hyperglycemia.

45. 1, 2, 3. Bilateral adrenalectomy results in acute adrenal insufficiency that is treated by corticosteroid replacement. It is critical that supplemental corticosteroids be administered in the right dose and time. The client needs to be monitored closely for signs and symptoms of adrenal crisis, which may occur if the prescribed corticosteroid dose is inadequate or the prescribed dose is not administered. Aseptic technique is critical due to immunosuppression secondary to steroid therapy. Weighing the client before a corticosteroid dose is not necessary. Pain management before it becomes severe is indicated.
CN: Physiological integrity; CNS: Reduction of risk potential; CL: Apply

46. 4. Clients with hypoparathyroidism can present with hypocalcemia and hyperphosphatemia. Heart failure and seizure activity are seen in hypophosphatemia. Spasms of the facial nerve when tapped (positive Chvostek's sign) is an indication of hypocalcemia. Flexing of the hips and knees with neck flexion (Brudzinski's sign) is indicative of meningitis.
CN: Physiological integrity; CNS: Reduction of risk potential; CL: Analyze

47. 3. Clients with Cushing's syndrome have physical changes related to excessive corticosteroids. Clients with hyperthyroidism are heat intolerant and must have comfortable, cool clothing and bedding. Clients with Cushing's syndrome should eat a high-protein, not low-protein, diet. Clients with Addison's disease must increase sodium intake and fluid intake in times of stress to prevent hypotension.
CN: Physiological integrity; CNS: Physiological adaptation; CL: Apply

48. 3. The nurse would suspect the client is experiencing diabetic ketoacidosis, caused by inadequate amounts of insulin or absence of insulin, which leads to a series of biochemical disorders. Treatment includes fluid replacement, cardiac monitoring, insulin, and potassium replacement. There is no indication for respiratory monitoring, magnesium, or mouth care.
CN: Safe, effective care environment; CNS: Management of care; CL: Apply

49. 1. A client with type 1 diabetes who fails to regularly take insulin is at risk for hyperglycemia, which could lead to diabetic ketoacidosis. Hypoglycemia would not occur because the lack of insulin would lead to increased levels of glucose in the blood. A client with chronic pancreatitis may develop diabetes (secondary to the pancreatitis), but insulin-dependent diabetes does not lead to pancreatitis. Respiratory failure is not related to insulin levels.
CN: Physiological integrity; CNS: Physiological adaptation; CL: Apply

50. A client with diabetes exhibits polyphagia, polydipsia, and oliguria and also reports headache, malaise, and some vision changes with signs of dehydration present. Which intervention is appropriate for the nurse to complete for this client?
1. Check creatinine levels.
2. Assess for ketones.
3. Send client for a renal scan.
4. Decrease environmental stimuli.

50. 2. The nurse suspects the client is experiencing diabetic ketoacidosis (DKA). The nurse would assess the client for ketones to determine the severity. Creatinine is not altered in a client with DKA. Renal scans measure renal function. Decreasing environmental stimuli would not improve the client's headache, as it is a result of dehydration.
CN: Physiological integrity; CNS: Physiological adaptation; CL: Analyze

51. The nurse is caring for a client with a history of hypothyroidism. Which clinical manifestation(s) indicates to the nurse the progression to myxedemic crisis? Select all that apply.
1. Hypothermia
2. Hypoglycemia
3. Hypotension
4. Hypoventilation
5. Irritability

51. 1, 2, 3, 4. Myxedemic crisis or coma is a life-threatening event of severe hypothyroidism. Signs are hypothermia, hypotension, hypoglycemia, and hypoventilation. Irritability is seen in *hyper*thyroidism.
CN: Physiological integrity; CNS: Reduction of risk potential; CL: Apply

52. The nurse is assessing an older adult client being screened for hypothyroidism. Which statement by the nurse demonstrates a correct understanding of the effects of aging?
1. "Thyroid disorders are rare in the older adult population."
2. "Hypothyroidism symptoms may resemble normal aging."
3. "Older adults with hypothyroidism need larger doses of thyroid replacement hormones."
4. "Older adults receiving thyroid replacement drugs have a decreased risk of adverse reactions."

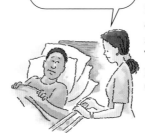

Sometimes listening to your client is the best intervention.

52. 2. Hypothyroidism is more difficult to diagnose in the aging population because many of the symptoms closely resemble normal aging and other chronic diseases. Dosages of thyroid replacement drugs are lower in older adults. Therapy is initiated more slowly and doses are increased with caution. Older adults have an increased risk of adverse reactions associated with cardiac function. Thyroid disorders are not rare in the older adult population.
CN: Health promotion and maintenance; CNS: None; CL: Analyze

53. The nurse is caring for a client who has hypothyroidism. Which health care provider prescription will the nurse question?
1. Administer levothyroxine.
2. Monitor heart rate.
3. Maintain a cool room temperature.
4. Check cholesterol levels.

53. 3. The nurse would question a cool room temperature because many clients with hypothyroidism experience cold intolerance. Levothyroxine is given to replace the thyroid hormone. Monitoring the heart will assist in monitoring for complications such as bradycardia. Cholesterol levels should be monitored for overproduction.
CN: Safe, effective care environment; CNS: Management of care; CL: Analyze

54. A client with hyperthyroidism develops a high fever, extreme tachycardia, and altered mental status. Which condition will the nurse suspect the client is developing?
1. Hepatic coma
2. Thyroid storm
3. Myxedema coma
4. Hyperosmolar hyperglycemic nonketotic syndrome (HHNS)

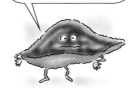

I don't know about you, but storms always get my heart rate up and alter my mental status.

54. 2. Thyroid storm is a form of severe hyperthyroidism that can be precipitated by stress, injury, or infection. Hepatic coma occurs in clients with profound liver failure. Myxedema coma is a rare disorder characterized by hypoventilation, hypotension, hypoglycemia, and hypothyroidism. HHNS occurs in clients with type 2 diabetes who are dehydrated and have severe hyperglycemia.
CN: Physiological integrity; CNS: Physiological adaptation; CL: Apply

55. When assisting with the development of a care plan for a client with hyperthyroidism, the nurse will anticipate which treatment?
1. Cholelithotomy
2. Irradiation of the thyroid
3. Oral thyroid hormones
4. Whipple procedure

55. 2. Irradiation, involving the administration of I-31I, destroys the thyroid gland, thereby treating hyperthyroidism. Cholelithotomy is used to treat gallstones. Oral thyroid hormones are the treatment for hypothyroidism. The Whipple procedure is a surgical treatment for pancreatic cancer.
CN: Physiological integrity; CNS: Pharmacological and parenteral therapies; CL: Apply

56. The nurse is assessing an older adult client diagnosed with hyperthyroidism. Which symptom(s) of hyperthyroidism will the nurse expect to find? Select all that apply.
1. Depression
2. Apathy
3. Weight loss
4. Palpitation
5. Irritability

56. 1, 2, 3. Older adult clients demonstrate depression, apathy, and weight loss, which are typical signs and symptoms of hyperthyroidism. Palpitations and irritability can be present with hyperthyroidism, but these are not typical symptoms in older adult clients.
CN: Physiological integrity; CNS: Physiological adaptation; CL: Apply

57. A client is admitted with Graves' disease. Which laboratory test will the nurse expect the primary health care provider to prescribe?
1. Serum glucose
2. Serum calcium
3. Lipid panel
4. Thyroid panel

57. 4. Graves' disease is also known as hyperthyroidism. The nurse should expect a thyroid panel to be prescribed. Graves' disease is not associated with alterations in serum levels of glucose, calcium, or lipids, so these laboratory tests would not be prescribed.
CN: Safe, effective care environment; CNS: Management of care; CL: Apply

58. The nurse is caring for a client receiving radioactive iodine (I-131) treatment for thyroid cancer. Which teaching will the nurse provide this client to reduce exposure of family members? Select all that apply.
1. "Wash hands carefully after using the bathroom."
2. "Wear clothing that covers the throat."
3. "Prepare food separately from family members."
4. "Flush the toilet several times after use."
5. "Avoid sexual contact and kissing."

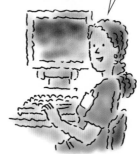

Remember to "select all that apply" in question #58.

58. 1, 4, 5. Radioactive iodine (I-131) is a form of systemic internal radiation therapy that is primarily excreted in urine, but also in saliva, sweat, and feces. I-131 has a half-life of approximately 8 days, so precautions should be followed for that period of time. Precautions include: washing hands after using the toilet, flushing the toilet at least twice after use, and avoiding kissing and sexual contact. Food does not need to be prepared separately, but separate utensils should be used. Covering the throat with clothing does not reduce exposure because effects are systemic.
CN: Safe, effective care environment; CNS: Safety and infection control; CL: Apply

59. During assessment, the nurse notes a client has flushed skin, bulging eyes, increased perspiration, and palpitations. Which action by the nurse is **most** appropriate?
1. Notify the health care provider.
2. Document the findings.
3. Assess the client's temperature.
4. Apply a cardiac monitor.

59. 1. Signs and symptoms of hyperthyroidism include nervousness, palpitations, irritability, bulging eyes, heat intolerance, weight loss, and weakness. The nurse would first notify the health care provider to begin treatment. The nurse would document the findings and assess a temperature; however, these are not priority. Applying a cardiac monitor may be prescribed because the client is having palpitations.
CN: Physiological integrity; CNS: Physiological adaptation; CL: Apply

60. Which technique is appropriate for the nurse to use when administering insulin to a client with diabetes?
1. Grasp the skin tightly.
2. Rotate injection sites.
3. Massage the site vigorously.
4. Inject into the deltoid muscle.

60. 2. The nurse should rotate insulin injection sites systematically to minimize tissue damage, promote absorption, avoid discomfort, and prevent lipodystrophy. Grasping the skin tightly can traumatize the skin; therefore, the nurse should hold it gently but firmly when giving an injection. Massaging the site vigorously is contraindicated because it hastens insulin absorption, which is not recommended. Usually, insulin is administered subcutaneously, rather than into a muscle, because muscular activity increases insulin absorption.
CN: Physiological integrity; CNS: Pharmacological and parenteral therapies; CL: Apply

61. A client in the emergency department has a brain stem contusion. Two days after admission, the client has a large amount of urine output and a serum sodium level of 155 mEq/dL (155 mmol/L). Which condition does the nurse suspect the client is developing?
1. Myxedema coma
2. Diabetes insipidus
3. Type 1 diabetes
4. Syndrome of inappropriate antidiuretic hormone (SIADH) secretion

61. 2. Two leading causes of diabetes insipidus are hypothalamic or pituitary tumors and closed-head injuries. Myxedema coma is a form of hypothyroidism. Type 1 diabetes is not caused by a brain injury. A client with SIADH secretion would have symptoms of hyponatremia; this client's sodium level was 155 mEq/dL (155 mmol/L), which is above the normal levels of 135 to 145 mEq/dL (135 to 145 mmol/L).
CN: Physiological integrity; CNS: Physiological adaptation; CL: Apply

62. A client with a history of diabetes has serum ketones and a serum glucose level above 300 mg/dL (16.65 mmol/L). Which condition does the nurse expect is the cause?
1. Diabetes insipidus
2. Diabetic ketoacidosis
3. Hypoglycemia
4. Somogyi phenomenon

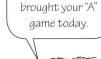

Looks like you brought your "A" game today.

62. 2. Clients with serum ketones and serum glucose levels above 300 mg/dL (16.65 mmol/L). could be diagnosed with diabetic ketoacidosis. Diabetes insipidus is an overproduction of antidiuretic hormone and does not create ketones in the blood. Hypoglycemia causes low blood glucose levels. The Somogyi phenomenon is rebound hyperglycemia following an episode of hypoglycemia.
CN: Physiological integrity; CNS: Physiological adaptation; CL: Apply

63. The nurse is caring for a client diagnosed with ketoacidosis. Which prescribed treatment(s) will the nurse anticipate administering? Select all that apply.
1. Insulin
2. Glucagon
3. Blood products
4. Glucocorticoids
5. Intravenous fluids

63. 1, 5. A client with diabetic ketoacidosis would receive insulin to lower glucose and would receive IV fluids to correct hypotension. Glucagon is given to treat hypoglycemia; diabetic ketoacidosis involves hyperglycemia. Blood products are not needed to correct diabetic ketoacidosis. Glucocorticoids are unnecessary because the adrenal glands are not involved.
CN: Physiological integrity; CNS: Pharmacological and parenteral therapies; CL: Apply

64. Which method of insulin administration will the nurse expect to be used **first** in the initial treatment of hyperglycemia in a client with diabetic ketoacidosis?
1. Subcutaneous
2. Intramuscular
3. Intravenous bolus
4. Continuous infusion

64. 3. An intravenous bolus of insulin is given initially to control the hyperglycemia, followed by a continuous infusion, titrated to control blood glucose. After the client is stabilized, subcutaneous insulin is given. Insulin is never given intramuscularly.
CN: Physiological integrity; CNS: Pharmacological and parenteral therapies; CL: Apply

65. The nurse is teaching a client diagnosed with diabetes about glycosylated hemoglobin (HbA1c) testing. Which statement by the client indicates the education has been effective?
1. "It is used to monitor the control of my disease."
2. "It is used to diagnose diabetes."
3. "It is useful in determining if I have anemia."
4. "It reflects the average blood glucose level for the previous 3 weeks."

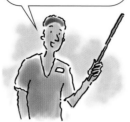

In other words, which statement by the client in question #65 is correct?

65. 1. The HbA1c test is used to gather data and to monitor progress of diabetes control. It is not used to diagnose diabetes or anemia. Red blood cells live in the body for about 3 months. When the glucose that is attached to the hemoglobin is measured, it reflects the average blood glucose level for the previous 2 to 3 months.
CN: Physiological integrity; CNS: Physiological adaptation; CL: Understand

66. Which potential complications will the nurse carefully monitor for when administering intravenous insulin to a client diagnosed with diabetic ketoacidosis?
1. Hypokalemia and hypoglycemia
2. Hypocalcemia and hyperkalemia
3. Hyperkalemia and hyperglycemia
4. Hypernatremia and hypercalcemia

66. 1. Blood glucose must be monitored because there is a chance for hypokalemia or hypoglycemia. Hypokalemia might occur because intravenous insulin forces potassium into cells, thereby lowering the plasma levels of potassium. Hypoglycemia might occur if too much insulin is administered. The client with diabetic ketoacidosis would not have hyperkalemia or hyperglycemia. Calcium and sodium levels are not affected.
CN: Physiological integrity; CNS: Pharmacological and parenteral therapies; CL: Apply

67. The nurse is caring for a client with acromegaly. The client asks the nurse to explain the difference between acromegaly and gigantism. The nurse will differentiate between the two with which statement?
1. "Acromegaly is an endocrine disorder of the pituitary gland and gigantism is a disorder of the musculoskeletal system."
2. "Acromegaly affects primarily children and young adults and gigantism affects the aging population."
3. "Both are characterized by excessive growth hormone production; acromegaly occurs after puberty and gigantism before puberty."
4. "Acromegaly and gigantism are actually terms that are used interchangeably to refer to the same condition of excessive growth hormone secretion."

I see great things in your nursing future.

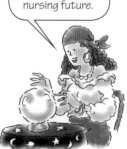

67. 3. Acromegaly and gigantism are both pituitary disorders characterized by excessive production of growth hormone (GH). Acromegaly is the excessive production of GH after the epiphyseal plates have closed (after puberty) and gigantism is excessive production of growth hormone prior to closure of the epiphyseal plates. The terms are not interchangeable.
CN: Physiological integrity; CNS: Physiological adaptation; CL: Understand

68. The nurse is caring for a client with diabetes. Which statement(s) by the client demonstrates an accurate understanding of foot care education provided by the nurse? Select all that apply.
1. "I should cut my toenails once a week."
2. "I should never go barefoot in or outside."
3. "I should wash with very hot water and dry my feet well."
4. "I should inspect the skin on my feet every week for open areas."
5. "I should apply moisturizer to my feet every day."
6. "I should wear cotton socks."

68. 2, 5, 6. The client with diabetes is prone to the development of foot problems, such as ulcers and infection, due to the combination of vascular disease and neuropathy. Daily moisturizer should be applied to prevent drying and cracking. Going barefoot subjects the feet to potential injury. Cotton socks worn with leather shoes keep the feet dry and protected from injury. A podiatrist should routinely examine the feet, and cut the nails as needed. Washing with hot water can result in burns; using lukewarm water is recommended. Visual inspection of the feet should be performed daily.
CN: Physiological integrity; CNS: Reduction of risk potential; CL: Apply

CN: Client needs category CNS: Client needs subcategory CL: Cognitive level

69. A client with diabetes who had a stroke has right-sided paralysis and incontinence. Which nursing action is **priority** when caring for the client?
   1. Apply body powder every 4 hours.
   2. Maintain bed rest when not in therapy.
   3. Insert an indwelling urinary catheter.
   4. Wash the skin with soap and water, gently pat dry.

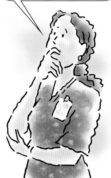

Let's see. A client with diabetes who is confined to bed and incontinent is at risk for skin breakdown and infection. Which intervention is the best way to prevent this?

70. An older adult client who has been on long-term steroid therapy now has drug-induced Cushing's syndrome. Which condition will the nurse determine closely relates to chronic steroid use?
   1. Periods of hypoglycemia
   2. Periods of euphoria
   3. Thin, easily damaged skin
   4. Weight loss

71. The nurse is assessing a client with possible hyperaldosteronism. Which nursing intervention is **priority**?
   1. Monitoring blood glucose levels
   2. Auscultating for breath sounds
   3. Monitoring arterial blood gas (ABG) levels
   4. Weighing the client weekly

72. The nurse is caring for a client with acute hypoparathyroidism. Which nursing intervention(s) is appropriate for this client? Select all that apply.
   1. Keep noise and movement to a minimum.
   2. Assess Trousseau's sign.
   3. Observe for development of renal calculi.
   4. Insert an intravenous line.
   5. Keep emergency intubation equipment at the bedside.

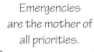

Emergencies are the mother of all priorities.

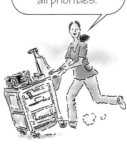

69. 4. The skin of a diabetic client should be kept dry to prevent breakdown and infection. The nurse should avoid excessive use of powders, which can cake with perspiration and cause irritation. Clients undergoing rehabilitation should be upright in a chair, except for short rest periods during the day, to promote optimal recovery. Clients with diabetes are especially prone to infections. Urinary tract infections are commonly caused by the use of indwelling catheters. Other methods should be used to encourage continence.
CN: Safe, effective care environment; CNS: Management of care; CL: Apply

70. 3. Clients taking steroids on a long-term basis lose subcutaneous fat under the skin and are especially vulnerable to skin breakdown and bruising. Such clients should take great care when performing tasks that may injure the skin, and should anticipate delayed healing when injuries occur. Clients taking long-term steroids are likely to have hyperglycemia. Prolonged steroid use can cause depression. Clients taking long-term steroids should be monitored for weight gain and edema, not weight loss.
CN: Physiological integrity; CNS: Pharmacological and parenteral therapies; CL: Apply

71. 2. Aldosterone is secreted by the adrenal cortex. One of its major functions is causing the kidneys to retain saline in the body. A client with hyperaldosteronism should be observed for signs of respiratory distress, crackles, and the use of accessory muscles. Blood glucose and ABG levels are not immediate priorities when assessing a client with hyperaldosteronism. Rapid weight gain can indicate fluid volume excess, but the client should be weighed daily, not weekly.
CN: Safe, effective care environment; CNS: Management of care; CL: Apply

72. 1, 2, 4, 5. In acute hypoparathyroidism, there are decreased serum calcium levels that put the client at risk for tetany, convulsions, and laryngeal spasms. The nurse observes for neuromuscular irritability by assessing Chvostek's and Trousseau's signs. The environment must be kept quiet and nondisruptive to prevent convulsions. Emergency intubation/mechanical ventilation equipment should be kept at the bedside in case laryngeal spasms occur and the client's respiratory status is compromised. An intravenous line needs to be in place for the emergency administration of a calcium salt. Renal calculi may develop in hyperparathyroidism, not hypoparathyroidism.
CN: Physiological integrity; CNS: Physiological adaptation; CL: Apply

73. A client with hyperparathyroidism develops renal calculi. The nurse will expect to see which electrolyte level?
1. Increased sodium level
2. Increased calcium level
3. Increased potassium level
4. Increased magnesium level

74. The nurse is caring for a client with suspected parathyroid dysfunction. Which laboratory results indicate to the nurse the client has primary hyperparathyroidism?
1. High parathyroid hormone and high calcium levels
2. High magnesium and high thyroid hormone levels
3. Low parathyroid hormone and low potassium levels
4. Low thyroid-stimulating hormone (TSH) and high phosphorus levels

75. The nurse is caring for a client with hyperparathyroidism. Which classification of drug will the nurse question prior to administration?
1. Nonsteroidal anti-inflammatory drugs (NSAIDs)
2. Salicylates
3. Potassium-wasting diuretics
4. Thiazide diuretics

76. In clients with hyperparathyroidism, which calcium level would indicate to the nurse an acute hypercalcemic crisis?
1. 2 mg/dL (0.5 mmol/L)
2. 4 mg/dL (1 mmol/L)
3. 10.5 mg/dL (2.63 mmol/L)
4. 15 mg/dL (3.75 mmol/L)

77. On reviewing a client's laboratory results, the nurse notes increased serum phosphate levels and decreased serum calcium levels. The nurse suspects the client will be diagnosed with which disorder?
1. Cushing's syndrome
2. Graves' disease
3. Hypoparathyroidism
4. Hypothyroidism

78. A client is admitted with hypoparathyroidism. When assessing the client, the nurse will expect which finding?
1. Chest pain
2. Exophthalmos
3. Shortness of breath
4. Hand twitching

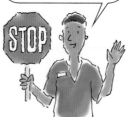

Which drug class in question #75 might actually worsen the effects of hyperparathyroidism?

73. 2. Renal calculi usually consist of calcium and phosphorus. In hyperparathyroidism, serum calcium levels are high, leading to renal calculi formation. Potassium, magnesium, and sodium do not form renal calculi, and levels of these minerals are not high in clients with hyperparathyroidism.
CN: Physiological integrity; CNS: Physiological adaptation; CL: Apply

74. 1. A diagnosis of primary hyperparathyroidism is established based on increased serum calcium levels and elevated parathyroid hormone levels. Potassium, magnesium, TSH, and thyroid hormone levels are not used to diagnose hyperparathyroidism.
CN: Physiological integrity; CNS: Physiological adaptation; CL: Apply

75. 4. Thiazide diuretics should not be used because they decrease renal excretion of calcium, thereby raising serum calcium levels even higher. There are no contraindications to NSAIDs or salicylates for clients with hyperparathyroidism. Potassium loss is not an issue for clients with hyperparathyroidism.
CN: Physiological integrity; CNS: Pharmacological and parenteral therapies; CL: Analyze

76. 4. Normal calcium levels are 8.5 to 10.5 mg/dL (2.13 to 2.63 mmol/L), so a level of 15 mg/dL (3.75 mmol/L) is dangerously high.
CN: Physiological integrity; CNS: Physiological adaptation; CL: Understand

77. 3. Symptoms of hypoparathyroidism include hyperphosphatemia and hypocalcemia. Excessive adrenocortical activity indicates Cushing's syndrome. Excessive thyroid hormone levels indicate Graves' disease (hyperthyroidism). Low thyroid hormone levels indicate hypothyroidism.
CN: Physiological integrity; CNS: Physiological adaptation; CL: Apply

78. 4. Tetany, which is manifested by muscle twitching or spasms, is the chief symptom of hypoparathyroidism. Chest pain and shortness of breath are not usually symptoms of hypoparathyroidism. Exophthalmos, or bulging eyes, is a common symptom of hyperthyroidism.
CN: Physiological integrity; CNS: Physiological adaptation; CL: Apply

79. A client is prescribed oral calcium supplements. Which additional supplement will the nurse encourage the client to consume?
1. Magnesium
2. Fennel
3. Vitamin D
4. Folic acid

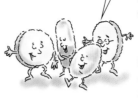

Which supplement is calcium's best buddy?

80. The nurse is caring for a client who had a subtotal thyroidectomy to treat hyperthyroidism. Which finding indicates to the nurse the client is bleeding at the incision site?
1. Hoarseness
2. Severe stridor
3. Client report of a tight dressing
4. Difficulty swallowing

81. The nurse is caring for a client with pituitary gigantism. Which prescription will the nurse question?
1. Octreotide analog injection
2. Pegvisomant injection
3. Thyroid function testing
4. Thyroid-stimulating hormone (TSH)

82. The nurse is caring for a client newly diagnosed with hyperthyroidism. Which nursing intervention is **priority** to decrease the client's anxiety?
1. Keeping the client warm
2. Encouraging the client to increase activity
3. Providing a calm, restful environment
4. Placing the client in semi-Fowler's position

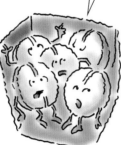

Sometimes relaxation is the best medicine.

83. After undergoing a thyroidectomy, a client develops hypocalcemia and tetany. Which medication will the nurse anticipate administering?
1. Calcium gluconate
2. Potassium chloride
3. Sodium bicarbonate
4. Sodium phosphorus

84. The nurse is providing dietary teaching to a client with an endemic goiter. The nurse identifies the education has been successful when the client selects which food(s) as good sources of iodine? Select all that apply.
1. Spinach
2. Codfish
3. Shrimp
4. Peanut butter
5. Eggs
6. Oranges

79. 3. Variable doses of vitamin D preparations enhance the absorption of calcium from the gastrointestinal tract. Magnesium, fennel, and folic acid are not involved in this process.
CN: Physiological integrity; CNS: Pharmacological and parenteral therapies; CL: Apply

80. 3. Reports of a tight dressing indicate postoperative bleeding. Hoarseness or severe stridor indicates damage to the laryngeal nerve. Difficulty swallowing does not indicate postoperative bleeding.
CN: Physiological integrity; CNS: Physiological adaptation; CL: Apply

81. 4. Hypersecretion of growth hormone causes pituitary gigantism. The nurse would question giving TSH as this is not the area of concern for the client. Octreotide and pegvisomant are injections used to treat pituitary gigantism. Thyroid function studies are monitored in these clients.
CN: Physiological integrity; CNS: Physiological adaptation; CL: Apply

82. 3. Clients with hyperthyroidism are typically anxious, diaphoretic, nervous, and fatigued; they need a calm, restful environment in which to relax and get adequate rest. Clients with hyperthyroidism are usually warm and need a cool environment. Activity should not be increased. If a client is exhibiting dyspnea, the client would benefit from high Fowler's position.
CN: Safe, effective care environment; CNS: Management of care; CL: Apply

83. 1. Immediate treatment for a client who develops hypocalcemia and tetany after thyroidectomy is calcium gluconate. Potassium chloride and sodium bicarbonate are not indicated. Sodium phosphorus would not be given because phosphorus levels are already elevated.
CN: Physiological integrity; CNS: Pharmacological and parenteral therapies; CL: Apply

84. 1, 2, 3, 5. Natural iodine content is highest in seafood and shellfish. It is also found in smaller amounts in bread, milk, eggs, meat, and spinach. Fruit and peanut butter are not good sources of iodine.
CN: Physiological integrity; CNS: Basic care and comfort; CL: Apply

85. The nurse is providing education for a client about insulin. The health care provider has prescribed regular insulin 6 units U100. Which statement(s) by the client indicates the education has been effective? Select all that apply.
1. "This insulin is cloudy in the vial."
2. "I will shake the vial before drawing insulin into the syringe."
3. "I will give myself 6 units of insulin with each dose."
4. "I should rotate my injection sites."
5. "The insulin should be drawn up in a tuberculin syringe."

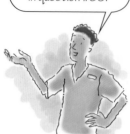

Remember to "select all that apply" in question #85.

85. 3, 4. There are 100 units of insulin in each milliliter of U100 insulin, and it should be drawn up in a U100 syringe (orange needle cap). Six units are to be administered. Subcutaneous injection sites require rotation to avoid breakdown and/or buildup of subcutaneous fat, either of which can interfere with insulin absorption in the tissue. Regular insulin is clear. Cloudy insulin has a zinc precipitate that must be evenly distributed in the solution. Insulin vials should be rolled in the hands to mix, not shaken vigorously. Insulin syringes are the only type of syringe used for drawing up insulin.
CN: Physiological integrity; CNS: Pharmacological and parenteral therapies; CL: Apply

86. The nurse is caring for a postpartum client with Hashimoto's thyroiditis. While educating the client, the nurse will include which statement?
1. "You may notice excessive weight loss over the next several months."
2. "If you notice any pedal edema, call your health care provider."
3. "You may feel a flushed sensation most of the time."
4. "You will need to take levothyroxine to control symptoms."

86. 2. Hashimoto's thyroiditis is the most common form of thyroiditis. It is believed to be an autoimmune disorder that develops in response to some stressor. Levothyroxine is generally used to treat Hashimoto's thyroiditis. Clients with Hashimoto's often experience weight gain, edema of the extremities, and cold intolerance.
CN: Physiological integrity; CNS: Physiological adaptation; CL: Apply

87. A healthy 50-year-old client with a history of type 2 diabetes mellitus has gone to the immunization clinic. The client reports no known allergies and no immunizations for the last 5 years. Which vaccine(s) will the nurse administer to the client? Select all that apply.
1. Influenza vaccine
2. Human papillomavirus vaccine
3. Rotavirus vaccine
4. Pneumococcal polyvalent vaccine
5. Respiratory syncytial virus immune globulin

87. 1, 4. Influenza vaccine is recommended annually for all people older than 6 months of age. Pneumococcal polyvalent vaccine is recommended for people over age 65 and people 2 to 64 years who have chronic conditions such as diabetes. Human papillomavirus vaccine is not recommended after 26 years of age. Rotavirus vaccine and respiratory syncytial virus immune globulin are recommended for infants.
CN: Health promotion and maintenance; CNS: None; CL: Apply

88. A client tells the nurse that two recent, fasting blood glucose results were 132 mg/dL (7.33 mmol/L) and 146 mg/dL (8.10 mmol/L). The nurse will expect which actions to occur?
1. These are normal results; no further action is needed
2. These results indicate diabetes; further follow-up is needed
3. The fasting blood glucose tests should be repeated two more times
4. The client should be scheduled for an HbA1C test

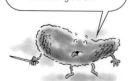

High blood glucose means something's out of whack with production of or sensitivity to insulin—what condition does that remind you of?

88. 2. A fasting blood glucose of 126 mg/dL (6.99 mmol/L) or more, on at least two occasions, is indicative of diabetes. These are not normal results. Further tests to make a definitive diagnosis of diabetes should be random blood glucose or glucose tolerance tests, not a fasting blood glucose or HbA1C.
CN: Physiological integrity; CNS: Reduction of risk potential; CL: Analyze

89. A client has diabetic ketoacidosis secondary to infection. As the condition progresses, which manifestations will the nurse expect to assess?
   1. Kussmaul's respirations and a fruity odor on the breath
   2. Shallow respirations and severe abdominal pain
   3. Decreased respirations and increased urine output
   4. Cheyne-Stokes respirations and foul-smelling urine

90. In caring for a client with insulin-dependent diabetes mellitus, the nurse identifies the client may require which change to the daily routine during periods of infection?
   1. No changes
   2. Less insulin
   3. More insulin
   4. Oral antidiabetic agents

91. The nurse is preparing to administer 4 units of regular insulin subcutaneously to a client with type 1 diabetes. Which equipment will the nurse need to administer the insulin? Select all that apply.
   1. Medication administration record
   2. Nursing assessment sheet
   3. 27-gauge, 1/2-inch needle
   4. 22-gauge, 1/2-inch needle
   5. 27-gauge, 1-inch needle
   6. 22-gauge, 1-inch needle

Sometimes nursing requires you to take your best shot.

92. After falling off a ladder and suffering a brain injury, a client develops syndrome of inappropriate antidiuretic hormone (SIADH). Which finding(s) indicates to the nurse the effectiveness of the client's treatment? Select all that apply.
   1. Decrease in body weight
   2. Rise in blood pressure and drop in heart rate
   3. Absence of wheezes in the lungs
   4. Increased urine output
   5. Decreased urine osmolarity

93. A client is seen in the clinic with suspected parathyroid hormone (PTH) deficiency. Which electrolyte level(s) will the nurse expect to be abnormal in this client? Select all that apply.
   1. Sodium
   2. Potassium
   3. Calcium
   4. Chloride
   5. Phosphorus

89. **1.** Coma and severe acidosis are ushered in with Kussmaul's respirations (very deep but not labored respirations) and a fruity odor on the breath (acidemia). Shallow respirations and severe abdominal pain may be symptoms of pancreatitis. Decreased respirations and increased urine output are not symptoms related to diabetic ketoacidosis. Cheyne-Stokes respirations and foul-smelling urine do not result from diabetic ketoacidosis.
CN: Physiological integrity; CNS: Physiological adaptation; CL: Apply

90. **3.** During periods of infection or illness, insulin-dependent clients may need even more insulin, rather than reducing the levels or not making any changes in their daily insulin routines, to compensate for increased blood glucose levels. Clients usually are not switched from injectable insulin to oral antidiabetic agents during periods of infection.
CN: Physiological integrity; CNS: Pharmacological and parenteral therapies; CL: Apply

91. **1, 3.** To administer medication, the nurse needs the medication administration record to verify the correct client, medication, dose, time, and route. A subcutaneous injection, such as insulin, is administered with a 25-gauge to 27-gauge, 5/8-inch to 1/2-inch needle. The nursing assessment sheet is not necessary for administering insulin. A 22-gauge needle is too large for a subcutaneous injection. A 1-inch needle would deliver the medication into muscle rather than subcutaneous tissue.
CN: Physiological integrity; CNS: Pharmacological and parenteral therapies; CL: Apply

92. **1, 4, 5.** SIADH is an abnormality in which there is an abundance of antidiuretic hormone. The predominant feature is water retention, accompanied by oliguria, edema, and weight gain. Evidence of successful treatment includes a reduction in weight, an increase in urine output, and a decrease in the urine's concentration (urine osmolarity). SIADH does not manifest as symptoms associated with blood pressure, heart rate, or abnormal breath sounds.
CN: Physiological integrity; CNS: Physiological adaptation; CL: Analyze

93. **3, 5.** A client with PTH deficiency has abnormal serum calcium and phosphorus levels because PTH regulates these two electrolytes. PTH deficiency does not affect sodium, potassium, or chloride.
CN: Physiological integrity; CNS: Physiological adaptation; CL: Apply

94. A client is admitted with a diagnosis of diabetic ketoacidosis. An insulin drip is initiated with 50 units of insulin in 100 mL of normal saline solution. The intravenous fluid is being infused via an infusion pump, and the pump is correctly set at 10 mL/hour. The nurse determines the client is receiving how many units of insulin each hour? Record your answer using a whole number.

_____ units

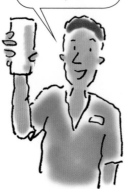

Cheers to you! You finished the chapter.

94. 5.
Use the formula below:

$$\frac{units}{hour} = dose\ on\ hand\,(units/mL) \times drip\ rate\,(mL/hour)$$

$$\frac{units}{hour} = \frac{50\ units}{100\ mL} \times \frac{10\ mL}{hr} = \frac{500}{100} = 5\ units/hr$$

CN: Physiological integrity; CNS: Pharmacological and parenteral therapies; CL: Apply

Chapter 10

Genitourinary Disorders

Genitourinary refresher

Acute poststreptococcal glomerulonephritis

Inflammation of the kidney tubules (glomeruli) that occurs after infection with certain strains of *Streptococcus* bacteria

Key signs and symptoms
- Azotemia
- Fatigue
- Oliguria
- Hematuria
- Edema

Key test results
- Blood tests show elevated serum creatinine and potassium levels
- 24-hour urine sample shows low creatinine clearance and impaired glomerular filtration
- Urinalysis typically reveals proteinuria, albuminuria, and hematuria; red blood cells (RBCs), white blood cells, and mixed cell casts are common findings in urinary sediment
- Kidney–ureter–bladder (KUB) x-rays show bilateral kidney enlargement
- Biopsy to confirm the cause

Key treatments
- Bed rest
- Diuretics: metolazone, furosemide
- Antihypertensive: hydralazine
- If residual infection is present: antibiotic therapy
- Fluid restriction
- High-calorie, low-sodium, low-potassium, low-protein diet

Key interventions
- Check vital signs.
- Monitor intake and output and daily weight.
- Watch for signs of acute kidney failure (oliguria, azotemia, and acidosis).
- Provide good nutrition, use good hygienic technique, and prevent contact with infected people.

- Encourage necessary bed rest during the acute phase.
- Encourage client to gradually resume normal activities as symptoms subside.

Acute kidney injury

Sudden loss of kidney function which can be reversible if detected and treated early

Key signs and symptoms
- Sudden onset of urine output less than 400 mL/day
- Weight gain

Key test results
- Creatinine clearance is low
- Blood tests show azotemia
- Glomerular filtration rate is:
  - 16 to 59 mL/minute (renal insufficiency)
  - less than 16 mL/minute (chronic kidney disease)

Key treatments
- Identify and reverse cause of injury
- Early continuous kidney replacement therapy or hemodialysis to assist with renal insufficiency
- Low-protein; high-carbohydrate; moderate-fat; and moderate-calorie diet with potassium, sodium, and phosphorus intake regulated according to serum levels
- Inotropic agent: dopamine, initially low-dose to improve renal perfusion
- Diuretics: furosemide, metolazone, bumetanide

Key interventions
- Monitor fluid balance and respiratory, cardiovascular, and neurologic status.
- Monitor and record vital signs, intake and output, and daily weight.
- Maintain the client's diet.

Benign prostatic hyperplasia

Noncancerous enlargement of the prostate gland

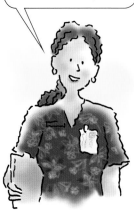

For more information about genitourinary system disorders, visit the Web site of the National Institute of Diabetes and Digestive and Kidney Diseases at www.niddk.nih.gov/.

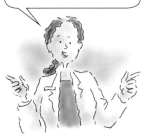

Reduced urine output is a key sign of acute kidney failure.

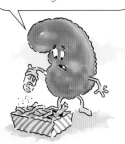

I know it's bad for me, but it just tastes so good.

231

Key signs and symptoms
- Decreased force and amount of urine
- Difficulty starting a urine flow or dribbling following urination
- Nocturia
- Urgency, frequency, and burning on urination

Key test results
- Increased prostate specific antigen (PSA) level
- Digital rectal examination shows enlarged prostate gland.
- Cystoscopy shows enlarged prostate gland, obstructed urine flow, and urinary stasis

Key treatments
- Forcing fluids
- Transurethral resection of the prostate (TURP) or prostatectomy

Key interventions
- Force fluids.
- Give alpha reductase inhibitors: finasteride.
- Provide postoperative care.
- Maintain continuous bladder irrigation.

Bladder cancer
Malignancy of the bladder

Key signs and symptoms
- Frequent urination
- Painless hematuria
- Urgency of urination
- Urinary obstruction
- Urinary retention

Key test results
- Biopsy and cytology examination are positive for malignant cells
- Cystoscopy reveals a bladder mass

Key treatments
- Surgery, depending on the location and progress of the tumor

Key interventions
- Provide postoperative care:
  - closely monitor urine output
  - observe for hematuria (reddish tint to gross bloodiness) or infection (cloudy, foul smelling, with sediment)
  - maintain continuous bladder irrigation, if indicated
  - assist with turning, coughing, deep breathing, and incentive spirometry
  - apply a sequential compression device while client is on bed rest
  - if placed, assessment of an ileal conduit.
- Force fluids.

Breast cancer
Malignancy involving the breast

Key signs and symptoms
- Cervical, supraclavicular, or axillary lymph node lump or enlargement on palpation
- Painless lump or mass in the breast or thickening of breast tissue
- Skin changes of the breast

Key test results
- Mammography and MRI detect a tumor
- Fine-needle aspiration and excisional biopsy provide histologic cells that confirm diagnosis

Key treatments
- Bone marrow and peripheral stem cell therapy for advanced breast cancer
- Surgery: lumpectomy, skin-sparing mastectomy, partial mastectomy, total mastectomy, or a modified radical mastectomy
- Antineoplastics: cyclophosphamide, methotrexate, fluorouracil, doxorubicin
- Hormonal therapy: tamoxifen, raloxifene, fulvestrant, megestrol
- Radiation therapy: internal or external

Key interventions
- Note the client's feelings about the illness, and determine what the client knows about breast cancer and client expectations.
- Provide routine postoperative care.
- Perform comfort measures.
- Administer analgesics as prescribed and monitor their effectiveness.
- Watch for treatment-related complications, such as nausea, vomiting, anorexia, leukopenia, thrombocytopenia, gastrointestinal ulceration, and bleeding.
- Educate client on how to care for mastectomy site.

Cervical cancer
Malignancy of the cervix

Key signs and symptoms
- Preinvasive: absence of symptoms
- Invasive: abnormal vaginal discharge (yellowish, blood-tinged, and foul-smelling)
- Postcoital pain and bleeding

Key test results
- Colposcopy determines the source of the abnormal cells seen on Papanicolaou (Pap) test
- Cone biopsy identifies malignant cells

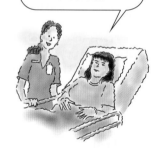

For any client with a urinary disorder, monitoring of fluid intake and output is essential.

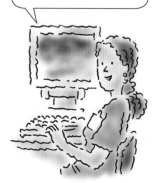

What key signs of cervical cancer will you instruct your client to look for?

Key treatments

- Preinvasive: cryosurgery, loop electrosurgical excision procedure (LEEP)
- Invasive: radiation therapy (internal, external, or both), radical hysterectomy

Key interventions

- Promote pelvic rest.
- Encourage client to use relaxation techniques.
- Watch for complications related to therapy.
- Provide postoperative care.

Chlamydia

Sexually transmitted infection caused by the bacteria *Chlamydia trachomatis*

Key signs and symptoms

In women
- Dyspareunia
- Mucopurulent discharge
- Pelvic pain

In men
- Dysuria
- Erythema
- Tenderness of the meatus
- Urethral discharge
- Urinary frequency

Key test results

- Antigen detection methods are diagnostic tests of choice for identifying chlamydia:
  - enzyme-linked immunosorbent assay
  - direct fluorescent antibody test
- Nucleic acid amplification test (NAAT)
- Tissue cell cultures for specific diagnosis

Key treatments

- Antibiotics: doxycycline, azithromycin
- For pregnant women with chlamydial infections, azithromycin, in a single 1-g dose

Key interventions

- Practice standard and contact precautions when caring for a client with a chlamydial infection.
- Make sure client fully understands dosage requirements of any prescribed medications for this infection.
- Obtain appropriate specimens for diagnostic testing.
- Provide client education on importance of protected sex.

Chronic glomerulonephritis

Long-standing kidney disease affecting the glomeruli

Key signs and symptoms

- Edema
- Hematuria
- Hypertension
- Azotemia

Key test results

- Kidney biopsy identifies the underlying disease and provides data needed to guide therapy
- Blood studies reveal rising blood urea nitrogen (BUN) and serum creatinine levels, which indicate advanced renal insufficiency
- Urinalysis reveals proteinuria, hematuria
- Morphological analysis of urine sediment reveals cylindruria and RBC casts

Key treatments

- Blood pressure management
- Dialysis
- Kidney transplant

Key interventions

- Client care is primarily supportive, focusing on continual observation and sound client teaching.
- Accurately monitor vital signs, intake and output, and daily weight.
- Observe for signs of fluid and electrolyte imbalances.
- Administer medications.
- Provide good skin care.

Chronic kidney disease

Long-standing damage to kidneys, preventing them from removing wastes from the body

Key signs and symptoms

- Azotemia
- Decreased urine output
- Indications of heart failure
- Lethargy
- Pruritus
- Weight gain

Key test results

- Glomerular filtration rate is less than 16 mL/minute
- Blood chemistry shows:
  - increased BUN, creatinine, potassium, phosphorus, and lipid levels
  - decreased calcium, carbon dioxide, and albumin levels

Key treatments

- Limited fluids
- Low-protein, low-sodium, low-potassium, low-phosphorus, high-calorie, and high-carbohydrate diet

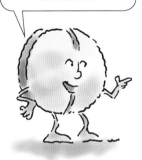

Many sexually transmitted infections, including chlamydia, respond well to antibiotics.

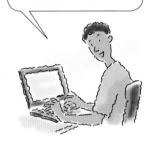

Hematuria is a key sign of chronic glomerulonephritis. Do you remember what this term means?

- Peritoneal dialysis or hemodialysis
- Antacid: aluminum hydroxide gel
- Antiemetic: prochlorperazine, metoclopramide
- Calcium supplement: calcium carbonate
- Cation exchange resin: sodium polystyrene sulfonate
- Diuretics: furosemide, bumetanide
- Antianemics: epoetin

Key interventions

- Monitor renal, respiratory, and cardiovascular status and fluid balance.
- Check dialysis access for bruit and thrill.
- Follow standard precautions.
- Restrict fluids.

Cystitis

Inflammation of the bladder usually caused by infection

Key signs and symptoms

- Dark, odoriferous urine
- Frequency of urination
- Urgency of urination
- Pain in pelvic area

Key test results

- Urine culture and sensitivity positively identifies organisms (*Escherichia coli*, *Proteus vulgaris*, and *Streptococcus faecalis*)
- Cystoscopy

Key treatments

- Diet: increased intake of fluids and vitamin C

Key interventions

- Monitor vital signs.
- Monitor intake and output.
- Force fluids (cranberry or orange juice) to 3 qt (2.8 L)/day.
- Instruct client to decrease intake of carbonated beverages.
- Instruct client to avoid coffee, tea, and alcohol.

Gonorrhea

Sexually transmitted infection caused by *Neisseria gonorrhoeae*

Key signs and symptoms

- Dysuria
- Purulent urethral or cervical discharge
- Itching, burning, and pain

Key test results

- A culture from site of infection (urethra, cervix, rectum, or pharynx) is used to establish diagnosis by isolating the organism

Key treatments

- Antibiotics: ceftriaxone, azithromycin
- Prophylactic antibiotic: 1% silver nitrate or erythromycin eye drops to prevent infection in neonates

Key interventions

- Before treatment, establish whether client has any drug sensitivities.
- Follow standard and contact precautions.

Herpes simplex

Vesicular skin rash caused by herpes virus (type 1 simplex: oral; type 2 simplex: genital)

Key signs and symptoms

- Blisters, which may form on any part of the mouth
- Dysuria (genital herpes)
- Erythema
- Flulike symptoms
- Fluid-filled blisters (genital herpes)
- Inguinal lymphadenopathy (genital herpes)

Key test results

- Confirmation requires:
  - isolation of the virus from local lesions
  - histologic biopsy/culture

Key treatments

- Antiviral agents: idoxuridine, trifluridine, or vidarabine
- 5% acyclovir ointment (possible relief to clients with genital herpes or to immunosuppressed clients with *Herpesvirus hominis* skin infections; IV acyclovir to help treat more severe infections)

Key interventions

- Follow standard and contact precautions; for clients with extensive cutaneous, oral, or genital lesions, institute contact precautions.
- Administer pain medication and prescribed antiviral agents as prescribed.
- Provide supportive care, as indicated (oral hygiene, nutritional supplementation, antipyretics for fever).

Neurogenic bladder

Lack of bladder control due to a brain or spinal cord injury

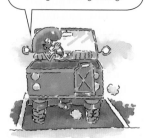

I prefer to keep things moving along!

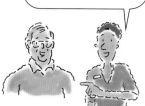

Be sure to check with your client about any drug sensitivities before administering medications.

Key symptoms
- Altered micturition
- Decreased bladder sensations

Key test results
- Voiding cystourethrography evaluates bladder neck function, vesicoureteral reflux, and continence.

Key treatments
- Indwelling urinary catheter insertion (including teaching client self-catheterization techniques)
- Voiding schedule

Key interventions
- Use strict sterile technique during insertion of an indwelling urinary catheter (a temporary measure to drain the incontinent client's bladder); do not interrupt the closed drainage system for any reason.
- Clean catheter insertion site with soap and water at least twice a day.
- Clamp tubing or empty the catheter bag before transferring client to a wheelchair or stretcher.
- Watch for signs of infection (fever, cloudy or foul-smelling urine).

Ovarian cancer
Malignancy of the ovary(ies)

Key signs and symptoms
- Abdominal distention
- Pelvic discomfort
- Abdominal bloating
- Weight loss

Key test results
- Abdominal ultrasonography, computed tomography (CT) scan, or x-ray may delineate tumor size

Key treatments
- Resection of the involved ovary
- Total abdominal hysterectomy and bilateral salpingo-oophorectomy with tumor resection, omentectomy, and appendectomy
- Antineoplastics: carboplatin, chlorambucil, cyclophosphamide, dactinomycin, doxorubicin, fluorouracil, paclitaxel, topotecan
- Analgesics: morphine, fentanyl

Key interventions
Before surgery
- Thoroughly explain:
  - all preoperative tests
  - expected course of treatment
  - surgical and postoperative procedures.

After surgery
- Monitor vital signs frequently.
- Monitor intake and output while maintaining good catheter care.
- Check dressing regularly for excessive drainage or bleeding.
- Watch for signs of infection.
- Encourage coughing, deep breathing, and incentive spirometry hourly during the waking hours.
- Reposition client often.
- Encourage client to walk shortly after surgery.

Prostate cancer
Malignancy of the prostate gland

Key signs and symptoms
- Decreased size and force of urinary stream
- Difficulty and frequency of urination
- Hematuria
- Urine retention

Key test results
- Digital rectal examination reveals palpable firm nodule in gland or diffuse induration in posterior lobe
- Prostatic-specific antigen (PSA) is increased
- Biopsy

Key treatments
- Radiation implant
- Radical prostatectomy (for localized tumors without metastasis)
- Transurethral resection of the prostate (TURP) to relieve obstruction in metastatic disease
- Luteinizing hormone-releasing hormone agonists: goserelin acetate, leuprolide acetate
- Antiandrogens: bicalutamide, flutamide, nilutamide

Key interventions
- Monitor and record vital signs.
- Monitor intake and output.
- Check for signs of infection.
- Monitor the client's pain and note the effectiveness of analgesia.
- Maintain the client's diet.
- Maintain the patency of the urinary catheter and note drainage.

Renal calculi
Solid piece or pieces of material that form in the kidney from substances in the urine, known as kidney stones

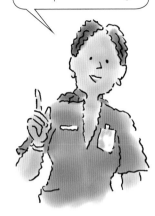

Neurogenic bladder typically occurs as a result of an injury to which part of the body?

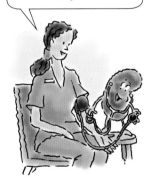

Don't forget to monitor those vital signs.

Key signs and symptoms
- Flank pain
- Frequent urination
- Hematuria

Key test results
- Excretory urography reveals stones
- KUB x-ray reveals stones

Key treatments
- Diet:
  - for calcium stones, acid-ash with limited intake of calcium and milk products
  - for oxalate stones, alkaline-ash with limited intake of foods high in oxalate (cola, tea)
  - for uric acid stones, alkaline-ash with limited intake of foods high in purine
- Encourage fluids
- Extracorporeal shock wave therapy (ESWT)
- Surgery to remove the stone if other measures are not effective (type of surgery depends on location of the stone)

Key interventions
- Monitor the client's urine for evidence of renal calculi.
- Strain all urine and save all solid material for analysis.
- Force fluids to 3 qt (2.8 L)/day.
- If surgery was performed:
  - check dressings regularly for bloody drainage and report excessive amounts of bloody drainage to health care provider
  - use sterile technique to change dressing
  - maintain nephrostomy tube or indwelling urinary catheter if indicated
  - monitor incision site for signs of infection.

Syphilis

Chronic infection caused by a spirochete, *Treponema pallidum*. Most commonly transmitted through sexual contact but can also be transmitted congenitally

Key signs and symptoms

Primary syphilis
- Chancres on the genitalia, anus, fingers, lips, tongue, nipples, tonsils, or eyelids

Secondary syphilis
- Symmetrical mucocutaneous lesions
- Malaise
- Anorexia
- Weight loss
- Slight fever

Tertiary syphilis
- Organ failure

Key test results
- Fluorescent treponemal antibody-absorption test:
  - identifies antigens of *T. pallidum* in tissue, ocular fluid, cerebrospinal fluid, tracheobronchial secretions, and exudates from lesions
  - most sensitive test available for detecting syphilis in all stages
  - once reactive, it remains so permanently
- Venereal Disease Research Laboratory (VDRL) slide test and rapid plasma reagin test:
  - both tests detect nonspecific antibodies
  - both tests, if positive, become reactive within 1 to 2 weeks after the primary lesion appears or 4 to 5 weeks after infection begins

Key treatments
- Antibiotics: penicillin G benzathine; if allergic to penicillin, doxycycline or tetracycline

Key interventions
- Check for a history of drug sensitivity before administering first dose of penicillin.
- Urge the client to seek VDRL testing after 3, 6, 12, and 24 months.
- Client treated for latent or late syphilis should receive blood tests at 6-month intervals for 2 years.

Testicular cancer

Malignancy of the testicle(s)

Key signs and symptoms
- Firm, painless, smooth testicular mass varying in size (sometimes producing a sense of testicular heaviness)

In advanced stages
- Ureteral obstruction
- Abdominal mass
- Weight loss
- Fatigue
- Back pain
- Pallor

Key test results
- Testicular palpation during routine physical examination may detect testicular tumors
- Surgical excision and biopsy of the tumor and testes permits histologic verification of the tumor cell types

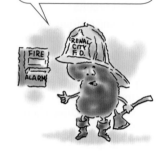

Flank pain is an alarm that often means you have kidney stones.

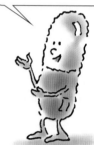

If syphilis is your villain, try killin' it with penicillin.

Key treatments

- Surgery: orchiectomy (testicle removal; most surgeons remove the testicle but not the scrotum to allow for a prosthetic implant)
- High-calorie diet provided in small, frequent feedings
- IV fluid therapy
- Antineoplastics: bleomycin, carboplatin, cisplatin, dactinomycin, etoposide, ifosfamide, plicamycin, vinblastine
- Analgesics: morphine, fentanyl
- Antiemetics: trimethobenzamide, metoclopramide, ondansetron

Key interventions

- Develop a treatment plan that addresses the client's psychological and physical needs.
- Provide client education on sperm banking prior to surgery.
- After orchiectomy:
  - for first day after surgery, apply an ice pack to the scrotum and provide an analgesic
  - check for excessive bleeding, swelling, and signs of infection
  - give an antiemetic, as needed
  - encourage small, frequent meals.

thePoint® You can download tables of drug information to help you prepare for the NCLEX®! View Generic Drug Names, Drug Classifications, Drug Actions, and Nursing Implications for the drugs discussed in this refresher at **http://thePoint.lww.com**

Genitourinary questions, answers, and rationales

1. A client has an applicator of radioactive material placed in her vagina for cervical cancer treatment. Which action concerns the nurse?
1. The client is placed on strict bed rest
2. The head of the bed is elevated to 15 degrees
3. The client gets a complete bed bath each morning
4. The health care provider checks applicator placement

2. The nurse is educating a group of clients about sexually transmitted infections. Which client statement indicates to the nurse the need for further teaching?
1. "Genital warts cannot be cured by a procedure or with medication."
2. "A newborn can receive medication to prevent contracting gonorrhea."
3. "Medication can be taken when a symptom of herpes simplex first appears."
4. "If someone has syphilis and a penicillin allergy, they have no treatment options."

3. The nurse is caring for a client with gonorrhea. Which finding(s) will **most** concern the nurse? Select all that apply.
1. Burning on urination
2. Green vaginal discharge
3. Diffuse skin rash
4. Painless chancre
5. Vesicular rash

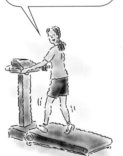

Remember: Slow and steady wins the race. Now, let's get started.

1. 3. The client should not receive a complete bed bath while the applicator is in place. In fact, she should not be bathed below the waist because of the risk of radiation exposure to the nurse. During this treatment, the client should remain on strict bed rest with the head of the bed raised no higher than a 15-degree angle. The nurse should check the applicator's position every 4 hours to ensure that it remains in the proper place.
CN: Safe, effective care environment; CNS: Safety and infection control; CL: Apply

2. 4. Other treatment options for syphilis are doxycycline or tetracycline. Genital warts are not curable, and a client will always be at risk for a flare-up. Newborns are typically given erythromycin eye drops to prevent gonorrhea infections in the eyes. Acyclovir is a treatment option for herpes, which can be taken as soon as a sign or symptom occurs.
CN: Physiological integrity; CNS: Physiological adaptation; CL: Apply

3. 3, 4, 5. The nurse will be most concerned when the client exhibits findings not related to gonorrhea. A diffuse rash may indicate secondary stage syphilis. A painless chancre is the hallmark of primary syphilis. It appears wherever the organisms enter the body, such as on the genitalia, anus, or lips. A vesicular rash may indicate herpes simplex virus (HSV). Burning on urination may be a symptom of gonorrhea or a urinary tract infection. A purulent discharge may be a sign of gonorrhea.
CN: Safe, effective care environment; CNS: Management of care; CL: Apply

CN: Client needs category   CNS: Client needs subcategory   CL: Cognitive level

4. A male client is admitted with penile discharge, burning upon urination, and a fever. What health care provider prescription will the nurse question?
   1. Perform a nucleic acid amplification test.
   2. Administer azithromycin 1 g orally.
   3. Obtain a consent for a biopsy of the prostate.
   4. Provide education on abstinence from sex.

5. The nurse is educating a client with genital herpes about treatment options. Which statement by the client indicates to the nurse that education has been effective?
   1. "I can take a medication to assist with managing symptoms."
   2. "I will not need pain medication as the blisters are painless."
   3. "Medications are given to help kill the virus and prevent invasion."
   4. "I can pour hydrogen peroxide and water over my lesions."

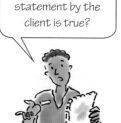

In other words, in question #5, which statement by the client is true?

6. The nurse educates a client prescribed furosemide on adverse reactions. Which client statement indicates to the nurse the client accurately understandings the education?
   1. "I will eat foods like as apricots, dates, and citrus fruits."
   2. "I need to avoid consuming magnesium-rich foods."
   3. "I will watch for, and report signs of, hypercalcemia."
   4. "I need to stop taking my antihypertensive tablet."

7. The nurse knows which female client is at **most** risk for developing breast cancer?
   1. A nulligravida, 20-year-old client of Asian heritage whose menstrual cycle began when she was 10 years of age
   2. A 30-year-old Native American/First Nations client with a mother who had breast cancer and who has unprotected sex
   3. A 45-year-old Caucasian client who has been taking oral contraceptives for 15 years and drinks alcohol regularly
   4. A postmenopausal, 50-year-old client of African decent who breastfed two children for 1.5 years each

4. **3.** A biopsy of the prostate is not indicated for chlamydia. Chlamydia is a sexually transmitted infection which causes penile discharge, burning, and a fever in men. Chlamydia is diagnosed by a nucleic acid amplification test and treatment consists of azithromycin. The client should be educated on abstinence from sex until the infection clears.
CN: Physiological integrity; CNS: Reduction of risk potential; CL: Apply

5. **1.** Medication can be taken to help with symptom management such as pain and flare-ups of the virus. The blisters are painful and usually require pain medication. Antiviral medication helps by preventing replication of the virus, not killing the virus. The use of hydrogen peroxide and water on the lesions is not recommended.
CN: Physiological integrity; CNS: Pharmacological and parenteral therapies; CL: Apply

6. **1.** Because furosemide is a potassium-wasting diuretic, the client should eat potassium-rich foods, such as apricots, dates, and citrus fruits, to prevent potassium depletion. The other client statements have no relationship to potassium balance. The client may consume magnesium-rich foods as desired. The client should watch for signs of adverse reactions to furosemide such as hypocalcemia—not hypercalcemia. The client should take furosemide with an antihypertensive drug only if prescribed; the combination may produce hypotension but does not cause potassium depletion.
CN: Physiological integrity; CNS: Pharmacological and parenteral therapies; CL: Apply

7. **3.** Risk factors for developing breast cancer consist of early menarche (before 12 years old), increasing age, ethnicity (Caucasian at highest risk), history of breast cancer or family history of breast cancer, use of oral contraceptives, first pregnancy after age 30, consuming alcohol, and a late menopause (after 55 years). Breastfeeding children will decrease the risk of developing breast cancer. The client in option 3 has four risk factors: gender, ethnicity, oral contraceptive use, and alcohol consumption. The client in option 1 has two risk factors: gender and early menarche. The client in option 2 has two risk factors: gender and family history. The client in option 4 has one risk factor: gender.
CN: Health promotion and maintenance; CNS: None; CL: Apply

8. The nurse examines the laboratory values, noted in the chart exhibit below, of a client with chronic kidney failure. Which value indicates to the nurse that hemodialysis is effective for this client?

Laboratory Test	Value
Red blood cell count	5.2 mm³ (5.2 ×10¹²/L)
White blood cell count	8,000 mm³ (8,000 ×10⁹/L)
Calcium	8.7 mEq/L (2.17 mmol/L)
Blood urea nitrogen	8 mg/dL (3.21 mmol/L)

1. Red blood cells
2. White blood cells
3. Calcium
4. Blood urea nitrogen

9. The nurse provided disease prevention education to a female client diagnosed with genital herpes. Which client action indicates to the nurse the education is successful?
1. The client applies saline soaked gauze to affected area
2. The client keeps her fingernails long and painted
3. The client wears tight-fitting jeans and satin underwear
4. The client washes hands before and after touching lesions

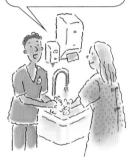

Frequent hand hygiene is the No. 1 way to prevent infections.

10. A client who has a recent history of strep throat is reporting general fatigue and pedal edema. The client's laboratory values are indicated in the chart exhibit below. Which nursing intervention is **priority** for this client?

Laboratory results	
Blood urea nitrogen	30 mg/dL (10.7 mmol/L)
Creatinine	2.0 mg/dL (176.8 µmol/L)
Blood in urine	Positive

1. Check the client's blood pressure.
2. Obtain a dry weight using a bed scale.
3. Send the client for an x-ray of the kidneys.
4. Place the client on immediate bed rest.

11. The nurse is caring for a client with candidiasis. Which question(s) will the nurse ask the client during admission? Select all that apply.
1. "Have you taken an antibiotic recently?"
2. "Do you still have your menstrual cycle?"
3. "Are you taking or have taken prednisone?"
4. "Are you currently taking an oral contraceptive?"
5. "Do you use any herbal remedies or supplements?"

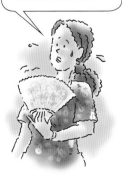

I'm way too young to be having hot flashes ... aren't I?

8. 4. The blood urea nitrogen (BUN) level reflects the amount of urea and nitrogenous waste products in the blood. Dialysis removes excess amounts of these elements from the blood, which is reflected in a lower BUN level. Hemodialysis does not affect red or white blood cell counts. Calcium levels are usually low in clients with chronic kidney failure. These levels are corrected by giving calcium supplements, not through hemodialysis.
CN: Physiological integrity; CNS: Physiological adaptation; CL: Apply

9. 4. Because hand-to-body contact is a common method of transmitting the herpes simplex virus, the client should wash the hands before and after touching the lesions to prevent the spread of the disease. To promote lesion healing and client comfort, the client should keep the affected area dry. To prevent scratching of the lesions, the client should keep the fingernails short instead of long, and nail polish can harbor bacteria. Because tight-fitting and satin clothes retain heat and moisture, which can delay healing and cause discomfort, the client should wear loose-fitting garments.
CN: Safe, effective care environment; CNS: Safety and infection control; CL: Apply

10. 1. The client is experiencing acute poststreptococcal glomerulonephritis. Management of hypertension is a priority for this individual as hypertension can cause further kidney injury. Obtaining a dry weight for the client would be completed but not by using a bed scale. The client would also need bed rest and an x-ray, but after blood pressure is assessed and treated if needed.
CN: Health promotion and maintenance; CNS: None; CL: Analyze

11. 1, 3, 4. The use of antibiotics increases the risk of candidiasis. Small numbers of the fungus *Candida albicans* commonly inhabit the vagina. Because corticosteroids decrease host defense, they increase the risk of candidiasis. Candidiasis is rare before menarche and after menopause. The use of hormonal contraceptives increases the risk of candidiasis. Over-the-counter herbal medications do not increase the incidence of candidiasis.
CN: Health promotion and maintenance; CNS: None; CL: Apply

CN: Client needs category   CNS: Client needs subcategory   CL: Cognitive level

12. The nurse is caring for a client diagnosed with gonorrhea. Which treatment regimen(s) will the nurse anticipate? Select all that apply.
  1. Ceftriaxone
  2. Azithromycin
  3. Amoxicillin
  4. Ampicillin
  5. Sulfamethoxazole–trimethoprim

12. 1, 2. Treatment for gonorrhea includes ceftriaxone and azithromycin to prophylactically treat for chlamydia. Amoxicillin, ampicillin, and sulfamethoxazole–trimethoprim are not recommended in the treatment of gonorrhea.
CN: Physiological integrity; CNS: Pharmacological and parenteral therapies; CL: Apply

13. A client underwent a left mastectomy yesterday and has a saline lock for intermittent intravenous access in the lower right arm. Which technique is **most** appropriate for the nurse to use when obtaining a blood pressure reading on this client?
  1. Using the right arm, and placing the cuff above the saline lock insertion site
  2. Using the left arm, and pumping the cuff only as high as necessary
  3. Using the leg, and placing the cuff on the client's upper thigh
  4. Using the right arm, and placing the cuff below the saline lock insertion site

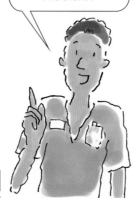

Question #13 is tricky. What's the most important consideration when taking a blood pressure reading for this client?

13. 1. To obtain a blood pressure reading, the nurse should always use the arm opposite the side of the mastectomy. The nurse should never take a blood pressure reading in the arm on the affected side without a health care provider's prescription. Blood pressure readings may be taken in the leg in some cases, but doing so is not necessary in this case. It is not necessary to place the cuff below the saline lock to obtain a blood pressure reading.
CN: Health promotion and maintenance; CNS: None; CL: Apply

14. The nurse is administering an antiseptic douche to a client scheduled for a vaginal hysterectomy. Place the procedure steps in the order in which the nurse will perform them. Use all answer choices once.

1. Clean the vaginal orifice.
2. Insert the douche nozzle 2 in (5 cm).
3. Separate the labia.
4. Administer 100°F (37.7°C) solution.

14. Ordered Response:

3. Separate the labia.
1. Clean the vaginal orifice.
2. Insert the douche nozzle 2 in (5 cm).
4. Administer 100°F (37.7°C) solution.

CN: Safe, effective care environment; CNS: Safety and infection control; CL: Apply

15. A client who is crying reports to the nurse she has an abnormal Papanicolaou (Pap) smear and asks if she has cervical cancer. Which statement by the nurse is **most** appropriate?
  1. "Before you worry, know the results could be false and not indicate cancer."
  2. "Your health care provider will need to take a biopsy from your cervix."
  3. "Once the Pap smear results are further analyzed, you will have a diagnosis."
  4. "If you had the human papilloma virus (HPV) vaccine, then you do not have cancer."

15. 2. An abnormal Pap smear should be followed up with a colposcopy and a biopsy for confirmation of cancer. Although results may be false, confirmation will still be needed. The HPV vaccine assists in decreasing a woman's risk of developing cervical cancer from the virus, but it will not prevent development of cancer.
CN: Safe, effective care environment; CNS: Management of care; CL: Apply

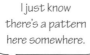

I just know there's a pattern here somewhere.

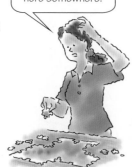

16. The nurse is caring for a client newly diagnosed with benign prostatic hyperplasia (BPH). Which assessment finding will the nurse report to the health care provider?
  1. Pain and burning with urination
  2. Waking frequently during the night to void
  3. Prostate specific antigen (PSA) level 6 ng/dL (6 µg/L)
  4. Difficulty starting a urine stream

16. 1. The nurse would report pain and burning with urination to the health care provider. This often indicates a bladder infection or nephrolithiasis. BPH is classified by the common report of difficulty starting a stream of urine, nocturia, weak stream, and dribbling after urination. PSA levels can increase with BPH and prostate cancer.
CN: Safe, effective care environment; CNS: Management of care; CL: Analyze

17. The nurse is teaching a client about home care following an abdominal hysterectomy. Which teaching topic(s) will the nurse include in the session? Select all that apply.
1. Notify the health care provider if temperature is above 100.4°F (38°C).
2. Avoid having any sexual intercourse for at least 6 weeks.
3. Light house work such as vacuuming the carpet is recommended.
4. Do not drive a vehicle for at least 6 weeks following your surgery.
5. Do not pick up heavy objects until cleared by your health care provider.

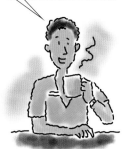

Stay focused and keep moving. You've got this.

17. 1, 2, 4, 5. Following an abdominal hysterectomy, a client should monitor for infection (fever), avoid heavy lifting, avoid any pushing or pulling exercises, practice pelvic rest, and refrain from driving until cleared by the health care provider. Vacuuming a carpet will cause the client to pull on the surgical site and possibly lead to evisceration or dehiscence.
CN: Physiological integrity; CNS: Reduction of risk potential; CL: Apply

18. A client has a spinal cord injury. Upon palpation, the nurse notes a distended bladder. What nursing intervention is **priority**?
1. Perform a bladder scan.
2. Insert an in-and-out catheter.
3. Obtain a blood pressure.
4. Administer furosemide.

18. 2. A client with a spinal cord injury may be at risk for neurogenic bladder. A bladder that is palpable indicates the client is not voiding or not completely emptying the bladder. A bladder scan will confirm the presence of urinary retention, which is already determined by the distended bladder. Insertion of an in-and-out catheter will release the urine and decrease bladder distention. A blood pressure will not address the full bladder, and giving furosemide will not assist the client in voiding.
CN: Physiological integrity; CNS: Pharmacological and parenteral therapies; CL: Analyze

19. The nurse is caring for a client with breast cancer. The client is prescribed intravenous methotrexate, intravenous fluorouracil, and oral cyclophosphamide. Which statement made by the client will cause the nurse to intervene?
1. "I will wash any surfaces that come in contact with my pills with soap and water."
2. "If I get any bodily waste on my skin, I will wash the area for 5 minutes."
3. "I cannot crush or chew the pills. If I cannot swallow them, I will tell my health care provider."
4. "When I am flushing the toilet, the toilet lid can be placed up or down."

19. 4. While taking chemotherapy medications, clients must follow safety precautions to protect themselves and family. The toilet lid should be closed when flushing bodily waste to prevent splashing. All surfaces should be washed with soap and water. If the client's skin comes in contact with a chemotherapeutic agent, the area should be wasted with soap and water for 5 minutes. The client should then watch that area for the next 7 days and notify the health care provider of any irritation. Cyclophosphamide should not be crushed or chewed.
CN: Safe, effective care environment; CNS: Safety and infection control; CL: Apply

20. The nurse is providing education to a client diagnosed with renal calculi. Which statement by the client indicates to the nurse the need for further teaching?
1. "I should contact my health care provider if I develop flank pain again."
2. "I should contact my health care provider if I see blood in my urine."
3. "I should avoid foods high in sodium, like canned and processed foods."
4. "I do not need to limit my fluid intake and can have soda, tea, or water."

20. 4. A client with a history of renal calculi should notify the health care provider if the client develops flank pain or blood in the urine. Foods high in sodium can cause calcium stones. Colas and teas can lead to the development of oxalate stones, which are the most common form of renal calculi.
CN: Physiological integrity; CNS: Reduction of risk potential; CL: Apply

CN: Client needs category   CNS: Client needs subcategory   CL: Cognitive level

21. The nurse is assessing a client who has a prescription for placement of a condom catheter. During the assessment, the nurse notes irritation, excoriation, and swelling of the client's penis. Which nursing intervention is **most** appropriate?
1. Ask the client when the findings started.
2. Apply the condom catheter as prescribed.
3. Immediately notify the health care provider.
4. Ask another nurse to assess the client's penis.

21. 1. The nurse should determine how long the client has been experiencing the symptoms, then inform the health care provider of the baseline data because a condom catheter should not be used on a client with penile irritation, excoriation, swelling, or discoloration. Further inflammation and ulceration may occur if the catheter is applied. The nurse should be confident in the findings and not need another nurse to assess the client.

CN: Safe, effective care environment; CNS: Management of care; CL: Analyze

Don't forget to stop for potty breaks.

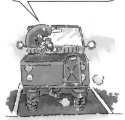

22. Which intervention(s) will the nurse include while caring for a client with chronic glomerulonephritis? Select all that apply.
1. Administer hydralazine.
2. Limit intake of potassium.
3. Measure urine output hourly.
4. Draw blood urea nitrogen (BUN) and creatinine levels.
5. Report any hematuria noted.

22. 1, 2, 3, 4. Chronic glomerulonephritis must be monitored and treated carefully to preserve kidney function. Close monitoring of BUN, creatinine, blood pressure, and urine output should be performed to identify changes in kidney function. Blood pressure should be kept within normal range by hydralazine, and the client should limit intake of potassium because the kidneys will not be able to excrete potassium. Hematuria is an expected finding and does not require reporting.

CN: Health promotion and maintenance; CNS: None; CL: Apply

23. The nurse is planning to insert an in-and-out catheter to drain an uncircumcised male client's bladder. Place the steps in the correct order the nurse will complete them. Use all answer choices once.

| 1. Remove the catheter. |
| 2. Provide perineal care. |
| 3. Insert the catheter into the urinary meatus. |
| 4. Let the container fill with urine. |
| 5. Lubricate the catheter. |
| 6. Cleanse the penis. |
| 7. Pull back the foreskin. |

23. Ordered Response:

| 2. Provide perineal care. |
| 7. Pull back the foreskin. |
| 6. Cleanse the penis. |
| 5. Lubricate the catheter. |
| 3. Insert the catheter into the urinary meatus. |
| 4. Let the container fill with urine. |
| 1. Remove the catheter. |

CN: Safe, effective care environment; CNS: Safety and infection control; CL: Apply

24. The nurse is caring for client prescribed tamoxifen for breast cancer. The nurse reviews the client's laboratory data in the chart exhibit below. Which nursing intervention is **priority**?

Laboratory Test	Value
Calcium	10.2 mEq/L (2.55 mmol/L)
Red blood cell (RBC) count	4.2 mm³ (4.2 × 10¹²/L)
White blood cell (WBC) count	6,500 mm³ (6,500 × 10⁹/L)
Thrombocyte count	25,000 mm³ (25 × 10⁹/L)

1. Place the client on fall precautions.
2. Initiate neutropenic precautions.
3. Request a prescription for a blood transfusion.
4. Administer intravenous fluids.

24. 1. The nurse will place the client on fall precautions due to the presence of thrombocytopenia. Neutropenic precautions are initiated for neutropenia, but this client's WBC count is within normal range. A blood transfusion is not needed because this client has a normal RBC count. Intravenous fluids can help decrease hypercalcemia; however, this client's calcium level is within normal range. Tamoxifen can cause thrombocytopenia, leukopenia, and hypercalcemia.

CN: Safe, effective care environment; CNS: Safety and infection control; CL: Analyze

CN: Client needs category   CNS: Client needs subcategory   CL: Cognitive level

25. The nurse is caring for a client with a continuous bladder irrigation following a transurethral resection of the prostate (TURP). Which action(s) will the nurse take while caring for this client? Select all that apply.
1. Increase the rate of irrigation flow for dark red urine.
2. Administer hyoscyamine orally for bladder spasms.
3. Empty the catheter bag and measure urine every hour.
4. Hang a bag of room temperature normal saline for irrigation.
5. Perform manual irrigation if clots are noted in drainage system.

25. 1, 2, 3, 4, 5. The irrigation rate is increased for dark red urine or clots to prevent obstruction. Administration of hyoscyamine is recommended for bladder spasms, and the urine bag should be emptied and measured every hour to maintain accurate intake and output records. Normal saline or sterile water may be used for irrigation and should be stored at room temperature to prevent bladder spasms. Manual irrigation may be needed if clots interfere with drainage.
CN: Physiological integrity; CNS: Basic care and comfort; CL: Apply

26. A client admitted for acute kidney injury is prescribed oral metolazone. Which nursing intervention is appropriate?
1. Monitor the client for hyperkalemia.
2. Check the client's blood pressure before administration.
3. Encourage the client to take increase sun exposure.
4. Give metolazone daily, 1 hour before bed.

In other words, in question #26, which is an appropriate action for the medication?

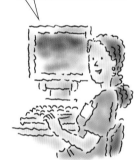

26. 2. Metolazone is an antihypertensive and diuretic medication. The nurse would monitor the client's blood pressure before administration, as well as check weight and intake and output daily. The client is at risk for hypokalemia and should increase consumption of foods high in potassium. Metolazone can cause photosensitivity; the client should limit sun exposure and take precautions when exposed (sunscreen). Metolazone should be taken in the morning to limit sleep interruption.
CN: Physiological integrity; CNS: Physiological adaptation; CL: Apply

27. The nurse is caring for a client who reports abdominal pain. Which potential diagnosis will the nurse anticipate for this client? Select all that apply.
1. Urinary tract infection
2. Internal hemorrhoids
3. Appendicitis
4. Renal calculi
5. Bronchitis

27. 1, 3, 4. Renal calculi typically produce flank pain but can also cause abdominal pain. Appendicitis often causes right lower quadrant abdominal pain. Urinary tract infections often cause lower abdominal pain. Hemorrhoids cause rectal pain and pressure. Bronchitis can cause chest discomfort and coughing.
CN: Health promotion and maintenance; CNS: None; CL: Apply

28. A client is taking vancomycin to treat an infection. Which laboratory result(s) indicate to the nurse a complication with this medication? Select all that apply.
1. Blood urea nitrogen (BUN) 45 mg/dL (16.1 mmol/L)
2. Creatinine 0.5 mg/dL (44.2 μmol/L)
3. White blood cells (WBC) 13,000/mm³ (13 × 10⁹/L)
4. Alanine transaminase (ALT) 3 U/L (0.5 μkat/L)
5. Glomerular filtration rate (GFR) of 20 mL/minute

28. 1, 5. Vancomycin is an aminoglycoside. These medications can cause kidney failure if not closely monitored. A sign that this medication is causing a problem would be an indication of kidney failure or injury. Increased BUN and a low GFR show signs of renal insufficiency. A decreased creatinine does not indicate a complication from the medication. Increased WBCs would be expected as the client is being treated for an infection. A decreased ALT (liver enzyme) does not indicate a problem from the medication.
CN: Physiological integrity; CNS: Pharmacological and parenteral therapies; CL: Analyze

29. The nurse is caring for a client with cervical polyps being treated with cryosurgery. Which discharge education will the nurse provide to the client? Select all that apply.
   1. Avoid douching for 2 weeks.
   2. Complete all antibiotics as prescribed.
   3. Use intravaginal antibiotic cream.
   4. Use a peri-pad as needed.
   5. Avoid sexual intercourse for 24 hours.

30. The nurse is caring for a client who has internal radiation pellets placed in the vagina. Which statement made by the client **most** concerns the nurse?
   1. "I will need to eat while I am lying flat in the bed."
   2. "My small children are coming for a visit today."
   3. "The catheter is placed to help keep my bladder empty."
   4. "The nursing staff all wear small badges to monitor exposure."

31. On which health issue will the nurse provide education to a female client who is sexually active with multiple partners? Select all that apply.
   1. Bartholinitis
   2. Candidiasis
   3. Chlamydia
   4. Trichomoniasis
   5. Gonorrhea

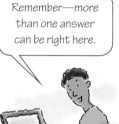

Remember—more than one answer can be right here.

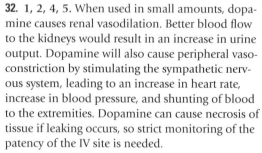

32. The nurse is caring for a client with acute kidney injury prescribed dopamine. Which finding(s) will the nurse expect for this client? Select all that apply.
   1. Increase in hourly urine output
   2. Elevation in heart rate
   3. Decrease in blood pressure
   4. Warmth of extremities
   5. Blood return from the IV site

33. A male client comes to the emergency room with dysuria and a temperature of 101.5°F (38.6°C). The client has a history of recurrent urinary tract infections (UTIs). Which health care provider prescription will the nurse question?
   1. Obtain a clean catch urine culture.
   2. Obtain a consent for orchiectomy.
   3. Administer fluoroquinolone IV.
   4. Apply a scrotal support.

29. 1, 2, 3, 4. Intravaginal antibiotic cream is commonly used to aid healing and prevent infection. Anytime prescribed antibiotics, the client should complete the prescription. Oral antibiotics are used for clients with acute cervicitis or perimetritis. Douching and sexual intercourse are generally avoided for 2 weeks. Peri-pads should be used, not tampons, if needed for the first 2 weeks.
CN: Physiological integrity; CNS: Reduction of risk potential; CL: Apply

30. 2. Clients with internal radiation pellets need to limit exposure to others, especially small children. Staff caring for the client will wear a badge to monitor the exposure amount during each rotation. Clients having internal radiation pellets are on strict bed rest, with the head of the bed elevated no more than 15 degrees to avoid displacing the radiation source. An indwelling urinary catheter is used to prevent urine from distending the bladder and changing the position of tissues relative to the radiation source.
CN: Physiological integrity; CNS: Reduction of risk potential; CL: Apply

31. 3, 4, 5. Chlamydia, trichomoniasis, and gonorrhea are common sexually transmitted infections requiring treatment to prevent continued spread of the infection. Bartholinitis results from obstruction of a duct and is not transmitted sexually. Candidiasis is a yeast infection that commonly occurs as a result of antibiotic use.
CN: Health promotion and maintenance; CNS: None; CL: Understand

32. 1, 2, 4, 5. When used in small amounts, dopamine causes renal vasodilation. Better blood flow to the kidneys would result in an increase in urine output. Dopamine will also cause peripheral vasoconstriction by stimulating the sympathetic nervous system, leading to an increase in heart rate, increase in blood pressure, and shunting of blood to the extremities. Dopamine can cause necrosis of tissue if leaking occurs, so strict monitoring of the patency of the IV site is needed.
CN: Physiological integrity; CNS: Pharmacological and parenteral therapies; CL: Apply

33. 2. The client is experiencing symptoms of prostatitis. Recurrent UTIs is a clinical sign of prostatitis. The nurse would expect the health care provider to prescribe a urine culture, antibiotic such as fluoroquinolone IV, and scrotal support for edema. The client would not need a consent for an orchiectomy (removal of the testicles); this is not a treatment for inflammation of the prostate.
CN: Safe, effective care environment; CNS: Management of care; CL: Apply

34. The nurse is caring for a client with metastatic prostate cancer prescribed hydrocodone with acetaminophen. Which finding(s) will the nurse report to the health care provider? Select all that apply.
1. Urine output of 100 mL in 6 hours
2. Two bowel movements in 8 hours
3. Client report of having unusual dreams
4. Vomiting four times in 5 hours
5. Temperature of 98.9°F (37.2°C)

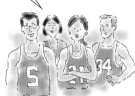

Providing excellent care requires teamwork—don't forget to collaborate.

34. 1, 4. Vomiting is an adverse reaction to the drug that should be reported because it impairs the client's quality of life and places him at risk for dehydration. A decrease in urine output should be reported to a health care provider. Taking the medication with food may prevent vomiting. If not, other opiate analgesics may be better tolerated. Two bowel movements within 8 hours is a normal finding. Unusual dreams are a common side effect but do not need to be reported unless bothersome to the client. The nurse should report temperature over 100.4°F (38°C).
CN: Physiological integrity; CNS: Pharmacological and parenteral therapies; CL: Analyze

35. The nurse is preparing a client the morning of surgery for a right orchiectomy. Which preoperative question(s) will the nurse include during the assessment? Select all that apply.
1. "Have you had anything at all to eat or drink this morning?"
2. "Did you stop taking your clopidogrel as prescribed by the surgeon?"
3. "Have you and the health care provider discussed implantation of a prosthesis?"
4. "Can you describe the procedure you are having completed this afternoon?"
5. "Were you able to preserve some of your semen in a sperm bank?"

35. 1, 2, 3, 4. Preoperative care should include assessing if the client has had anything to eat or drink and which medications a client has taken. Clopidogrel will increase the risk of bleeding and should be stopped prior to the scheduled surgery. Food or oral liquid can increase the risk of aspiration during surgery and should be addressed prior to the surgery. The nurse would address all aspects of the procedure, including the use of a prosthesis. Ensuring the client can describe the procedure indicates the client fully understands what will occur. The client having a right orchiectomy will have only the right testicle removed. Sperm banking is only needed for removal of both testicles or radiation to the testicles.
CN: Physiological integrity; CNS: Basic care and comfort; CL: Apply

36. The nurse is preparing to discuss administration of a vaginal irrigation with a client. Which step is appropriate to have the client perform?
1. Insert the nozzle about 3 in (7.6 cm) into the vagina.
2. Direct the tip of the nozzle toward the client's sacrum.
3. Instill the solution in a constant flow over 5 to 10 minutes.
4. Raise the solution at least 24 in (61 cm) above the client's hip level.

36. 2. The normal position of the vagina slants up and back toward the sacrum. Directing the tip of the nozzle toward the sacrum allows it to follow the normal slant of the vagina and minimizes tissue trauma. The nozzle should be inserted about 2 in (5.1 cm). The fluid can be instilled intermittently and, for best therapeutic results, over 20 to 30 minutes. The container should be no higher than 24 in (61 cm) above the client's hip level to avoid forcing fluid and bacteria through the cervical os into the uterus.
CN: Safe, effective care environment; CNS: Safety and infection control; CL: Apply

37. The nurse is assigned to care for four clients. Which client will the nurse see **first**?
1. A client with chronic kidney failure whose potassium level is 5.6 mEq/dL (5.6 mmol/L) awaiting dialysis
2. A client with an acute kidney injury whose current blood pressure is 88/60 mm Hg and urine output is 20 mL/hour
3. A client on peritoneal dialysis reporting clear fluid draining into the drainage bag and feeling fatigued
4. A female client experiencing burning, frequency, and urgency with a pain level of "5" upon urination

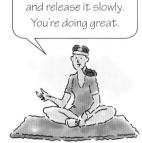

Take a deep breath and release it slowly. You're doing great.

37. 2. The client who has a low urine output and blood pressure should be seen first, as this client is at risk for developing acute kidney injury. The client with chronic kidney disease will have dialysis for the expected high potassium level. Clear drainage into the drainage bag with peritoneal dialysis is an expected finding. The client with burning, frequency, and pain upon urination has indications of a urinary tract infection.
CN: Safe, effective care environment; CNS: Management of care; CL: Analyze

CN: Client needs category   CNS: Client needs subcategory   CL: Cognitive level

38. A male client is admitted for chest pain. The nurse is reviewing the client's medication history. Which medication will the nurse verify before administering nitroglycerin?
1. Sildenafil citrate
2. Aspirin
3. Hydrocodone
4. Ampicillin

39. The nurse knows which female client is at **highest** risk for developing cervical cancer?
1. The client who is currently being treated for syphilis and is 25 lb (11.3 kg) underweight
2. The client who had human papillomavirus (HPV) 10 years ago and smokes cigarettes daily
3. The client who has had gonorrhea multiple times in the past 15 years
4. The client who drinks alcohol a few times a month and takes oral contraceptives

40. A client is scheduled for a stereotactic breast biopsy of the right breast. Which position will the nurse place the client in for the procedure?
1. Left lateral Sims
2. Supine
3. Prone
4. High Fowler's

41. The registered nurse (RN) is observing an assistive personal (AP) insert a urinary catheter on a male client. Which action(s) by the AP causes the RN to intervene? Select all that apply.
1. Pulls back the client's foreskin before cleaning
2. Dons sterile gloves before touching items in the sterile kit
3. Lubricates the urinary catheter before inserting into the penis
4. Keeps all sterile items and the sterile drape at waist level
5. Inflating the balloon before visualizing urine flow

42. The nurse is caring for a client with nephrotic syndrome. Which assessment finding(s) will the nurse expect? Select all that apply.
1. Periorbital edema
2. Weight gain
3. Anasarca
4. Hypertension
5. Fatigue

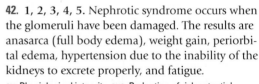

Check out these symptoms carefully. Which ones are abnormal and concerning in this situation?

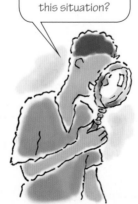

38. 1. The use of erectile dysfunction medications such as sildenafil should be verified prior to administration of nitrates. The combination of nitrates and sildenafil citrate will cause the client's blood pressure to decrease. Nitroglycerin can be used in combination with aspirin, hydrocodone, and ampicillin.
CN: Physiological integrity; CNS: Pharmacological and parenteral therapies; CL: Apply

39. 2. This client has two risk factors. HPV has a high association with causing cervical cancer in females, as well as smoking. Syphilis, being underweight, gonorrhea, and alcohol consumption are not risk factors in developing cervical cancer. Other risk factors for cervical cancer include being overweight, being immunosuppressed, history of chlamydia, family history of cervical cancer, long-term oral contraceptive use, having three or more full-term pregnancies, and prior use of diethylstilbestrol (DES). The other clients have zero or one risk factor.
CN: Physiological integrity; CNS: Reduction of risk potential; CL: Analyze

40. 3. A stereotactic breast biopsy requires the client lay prone and place the breast through an opening on the table. The client would not be placed in high Fowler's, supine, or left lateral Sims as these positions would not allow the breast to be placed through the opening for needle biopsy.
CN: Safe, effective care environment; CNS: Safety and infection control; CL: Understand

41. 5. The nurse should intervene if the AP begins to inflate the balloon prior to visualizing the flow of urine. In a male client the catheter may not be in the bladder without urine confirmation due to an enlarged prostate. The proper steps of urinary catheter insertion include pulling back the foreskin and cleaning the penis, donning sterile gloves before handling items in the sterile field, lubricating the urinary catheter before insertion, and keeping all sterile items at waist level.
CN: Safe, effective care environment; CNS: Safety and infection control; CL: Apply

42. 1, 2, 3, 4, 5. Nephrotic syndrome occurs when the glomeruli have been damaged. The results are anasarca (full body edema), weight gain, periorbital edema, hypertension due to the inability of the kidneys to excrete properly, and fatigue.
CN: Physiological integrity; CNS: Reduction of risk potential; CL: Apply

43. A client reports tea-colored urine following an intensive cardio workout. Which response by the nurse is **priority**?
  1. "You need to refrain from working out for the next 2 weeks."
  2. "You need to be seen by your primary health care provider."
  3. "You need to increase your intake of water significantly."
  4. "If these symptoms persist for 24 hours, go to the emergency room."

44. The nurse understands which client has the **highest** risk of developing urinary retention?
  1. A male client who reports burning upon urination
  2. A female client with a history of renal calculi
  3. A male client with recurrent urinary tract infections
  4. A female client with a blood pressure of 90/56 mm Hg

45. The nurse is educating a group of women on risk factors that contribute to bacterial vaginosis. Which risk factor(s) will the nurse include in the education? Select all that apply.
  1. Frequent douching
  2. Multiple sex partners
  3. Chlamydia
  4. Smoking
  5. Tampon usage

46. The clinic nurse is caring for a client with primary syphilis. Which health care provider prescription will the nurse question?
  1. Document client's recent sexual partners and notify.
  2. Administer benzathine penicillin G intramuscularly.
  3. Schedule client for repeat venereal disease research laboratory (VDRL) testing in 3 months.
  4. Notify the local public health agency.

47. A client comes to the clinic and states to the nurse, "I have firm masses in my breasts that change in size with my menstrual cycle. What do you think this is?" Which response by the nurse is appropriate?
  1. "If the masses are painful, I think it is breast cancer."
  2. "Nodules present during your menses are fibrocystic changes."
  3. "I am not sure, but to be safe you need to see an oncologist."
  4. "Breast cancer lumps are related to the increased secretion of hormones."

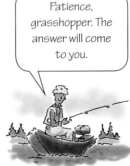

Patience, grasshopper. The answer will come to you.

43. **2.** The nurse would suspect rhabdomyolysis, which can occur following an intensive workout. Tea-color urine is a result of the breakdown of skeletal muscle being filtered out by the kidney. The client needs aggressive intravenous fluid replacement and should be seen right away, not in 24 hours. The client may need to refrain from workouts and increase oral intake, but these are not priority.
CN: Safe, effective care environment; CNS: Management of care; CL: Analyze

44. **2.** The retention of urine in the bladder occurs by a blockage or spinal cord injury. Renal calculi (kidney stones) are a common source of urinary retention. Burning upon urination indicates a possible infection or sexually transmitted infection. Recurrent urinary tract infection could be a complication from having urinary retention but would not be a cause of the urinary retention. A low blood pressure reading could cause acute kidney injury but not retention of urine.
CN: Safe, effective care environment; CNS: Management of care; CL: Apply

45. **1, 2, 3, 4.** Bacterial vaginosis has several risk factors including multiple sexual partners, sexually transmitted infections, frequent douching, and smoking. The use of tampons is not directly related to the development of vaginosis as this does not cause a change in the normal bacteria found in the vagina.
CN: Physiological integrity; CNS: Physiological adaptation; CL: Apply

46. **1.** The nurse will question documenting and notifying the client's recent sexual partners. This would be recommended for the client to perform. IM benzathine penicillin G is the treatment of choice for syphilis. VDRL testing is recommended at 3, 6, 9, and 12 months following treatment. The local public health agency must be notified in the United States and Canada.
CN: Safe, effective care environment; CNS: Safety and infection control; CL: Apply

47. **2.** Masses associated with fibrocystic disease of the breast, not breast cancer, are firm and increase in size before menstruation. They may be bilateral in a mirror image and are typically well demarcated and freely movable. Breast cancer is typically not painful. The nurse would notify the clinic health care provider before determining if the client needs to be referred to an oncologist.
CN: Health promotion and maintenance; CNS: None; CL: Apply

CN: Client needs category   CNS: Client needs subcategory   CL: Cognitive level

48. The registered nurse (RN) is caring for four clients. Which task will the RN appropriately delegate to the assistive personal (AP)?
1. Obtain a clean catch specimen from a client with a possible infection.
2. Turn the irrigation fluid down on a client following a transurethral prostate resection.
3. Ambulate a client for the first time following an abdominal hysterectomy.
4. Educate a client on hemodialysis about food choices low in potassium.

48. 1. A AP could safely perform a clean catch specimen on a client with an infection. The AP should not educate a client on food choices and should not ambulate a client for the first time as this requires nursing assessment. Irrigation is considered a medication and requires nursing judgment task, so the nurse should not delegate this task to the AP.
CN: Physiological integrity; CNS: Reduction of risk potential; CL: Apply

49. The nurse will monitor which client for possible prerenal acute kidney failure?
1. A client prescribed aminoglycosides
2. A client with decreased cardiac output
3. A client diagnosed with prostatic hyperplasia
4. A client with a history of rhabdomyolysis

49. 2. Prerenal acute kidney failure refers to kidney failure due to an interference with renal perfusion. Decreased cardiac output causes a decrease in renal perfusion, which leads to a lower glomerular filtration rate. Aminoglycosides and rhabdomyolysis are intrarenal causes of acute kidney failure. Prostatic hyperplasia would be an example of a postrenal cause of acute kidney failure.
CN: Physiological integrity; CNS: Physiological adaptation; CL: Apply

50. The nurse is assessing a client with chronic kidney disease prior to dialysis treatment. Which finding(s) will the nurse report to the health care provider? Select all that apply.
1. Crackles
2. Pruritus
3. Blood pressure 92/54 mm Hg
4. Jugular vein distention
5. Tachypnea

Chronic kidney disease. What is that condition again?

50. 3. Due to the inability to eliminate fluid and waste, the client would present with hypertension instead of hypotension. Dialysis may further decrease the client's blood pressure; therefore, the health care provider should be notified prior to the procedure. Prior to a dialysis treatment, a client is expected to show signs of fluid volume overload such as crackles, jugular vein distention, hypertension, and tachypnea. Clients with chronic kidney disease have pruritus due to the uremic crystals forming on the skin from the inability to excrete waste.
CN: Safe, effective care environment; CNS: Management of care; CL: Apply

51. A client presents with nephrotic syndrome. Which treatment regimen will the nurse question?
1. Furosemide IV daily
2. Methylprednisolone IV daily
3. Enalapril IV twice a day
4. Gentamicin IV twice a day

51. 4. A client with nephrotic syndrome requires management of blood pressure, decreasing inflammation, and fluid volume overload. Medications such as enalapril, furosemide, and methylprednisolone will be used for this client. Gentamicin would cause further renal complications. Gentamicin is an aminoglycoside and can cause further renal damage.
CN: Physiological integrity; CNS: Reduction of risk potential; CL: Apply

52. A client has been admitted with rhabdomyolysis. Which health care provider prescription will the nurse anticipate?
1. Administer furosemide IV twice daily.
2. Give 4 L normal saline boluses.
3. Potassium IV 40 mEq (40 mmol) once today.
4. Dopamine at a renal maintenance dose.

52. 2. The treatment of rhabdomyolysis begins with aggressive fluid resuscitation. The kidneys need to be flushed out. Furosemide is not the recommended diuretic; mannitol will be used. In rhabdomyolysis the potassium level is high and additional potassium replacement is not needed. Dopamine would increase renal blood flow, but the issue is the skeletal muscle being broken down and excreted. The excess needs to be flushed out of the kidneys to prevent acute injury.
CN: Health promotion and maintenance; CNS: None; CL: Apply

53. The nurse is educating a client about home care of an ileal conduit. Which client statement indicates to the nurse a need for further education?
1. "I will be able to self-cath at home and not have to wear a bag."
2. "My health care provider should be called if my stoma turns purple."
3. "When changing the device, I should only use warm water on the stoma."
4. "The bag should be emptied when half full to avoid spills or leaks."

53. 1. The client will need to wear a bag and will not be able to self-cath. This would be for a Kock pouch, not an ileal conduit. The stoma should be red and moist, indicating adequate blood flow. A dusky or cyanotic stoma indicates insufficient blood supply and is an emergency needing prompt intervention. Using warm water is appropriate as soap will cause irritation and dry the stoma. To avoid leaks the ostomy bag should emptied frequently and when half full.
CN: Physiological integrity; CNS: Reduction of risk potential; CL: Apply

54. The nurse is providing discharge education for a female client with cystitis. Which information will the nurse include? Select all that apply.
1. Bathe in a bathtub.
2. Wear cotton underwear.
3. Use a feminine hygiene spray.
4. Encourage intake of cranberry juice.
5. Douche once a week.

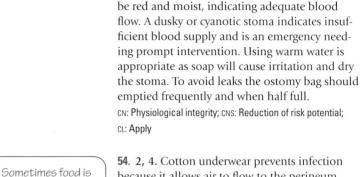

Sometimes food is the best medicine.

54. 2, 4. Cotton underwear prevents infection because it allows air to flow to the perineum. Cranberry juice helps prevent cystitis because it increases urine acidity and prevents *E. coli* from sticking to the urinary tract; alkaline urine supports bacterial growth. Women should shower instead of taking a tub bath to prevent infection. Feminine hygiene spray can act as an irritant. Douching is not recommended in women unless recommended by a health care provider.
CN: Health promotion and maintenance; CNS: None; CL: Apply

55. The nurse is reviewing laboratory results, seen in the chart exhibit below, for a client diagnosed with chronic kidney failure. Which result will the nurse report to the health care provider **first**?

Laboratory Test	Value
Potassium	6.2 mEq/L (6.2 mmol/L)
Sodium	134 mEq/L (134 mmol/L)
Glomerular filtration rate	17
Creatinine	2.1 mg/dL (185.6 µmol/L)

1. Potassium
2. Sodium
3. Glomerular filtration rate
4. Creatinine

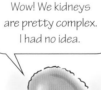
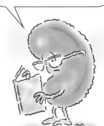

Wow! We kidneys are pretty complex. I had no idea.

55. 1. The kidneys are responsible for excreting potassium. In kidney failure, the kidneys can no longer excrete potassium, resulting in hyperkalemia. A level of 6.2 mEq/L (6.2 mmol/L) requires immediate intervention. Generally, hyponatremia would occur because of the dilutional effect of water retention. A glomerular filtration rate of 17 indicates kidney failure, which the client is diagnosed with already. Creatinine is also excreted by the kidneys and levels would rise with kidney failure.
CN: Safe, effective care environment; CNS: Management of care; CL: Analyze

56. Which client will the nurse monitor closely for the development of a urinary tract infection (UTI)?
1. A female client with incomplete emptying of the bladder and fecal incontinence
2. A male client with an increase in urine acidity and a temperature of 101.6°F (38.7°C)
3. A female client diagnosed with congenital shortening of the urethra
4. A male client diagnosed with a kidney stone who has a history of gonorrhea

56. 1. The client with incomplete emptying of the bladder, perineal soiling from incontinence, and female gender has three risk factors. The male client with increased urine acidity and a fever has no risk factors. Acidic urine impedes bacterial growth. A fever is associated with a UTI; however, there are a multitude of rationales for a client having a fever beyond a UTI. The female client with congenital shortening of the urethra has two risk factors. Urinary tract anomalies can increase a client's risk of developing a UTI; and female gender is a risk factor. The male client with a kidney stone and a history of gonorrhea has one risk factor. A history of sexually transmitted infections does not increase risks for a UTI. Blockages in the urinary tract do increase risks.
CN: Physiological integrity; CNS: Reduction of risk potential; CL: Apply

57. The nurse is caring for a client diagnosed with a urinary tract infection (UTI). Which manifestation(s) will **most** concern the nurse? Select all that apply.
1. Dysuria
2. Azotemia
3. Hematuria
4. Urinary frequency
5. Fever

58. A client received a kidney transplant 2 months ago and is admitted to the hospital with the diagnosis of acute rejection. Which finding(s) will the nurse expect to assess in this client? Select all that apply.
1. Blood pressure 150/96 mm Hg
2. Temperature 101 °F (38.3 °C)
3. White blood cell (WBC) 3,000 mm³ (3 × 10⁹/L)
4. Blood urea nitrogen (BUN) 43 mg/dL (15.4 mmol/L)
5. Creatinine 3.6 mg/dL (274.5 µmol/L)

59. The nurse is caring for a client receiving peritoneal dialysis treatments. The treatment amount instilled to dwell is 1.5 L. Which finding will the nurse report to the health care provider?
1. Cloudy peritoneal drainage in the drainage bag
2. Removal of 1,300 mL of clear drainage
3. Report of abdominal tension when the fluid is instilled
4. After fluid instillation, shortness of breath when lying flat

60. A client has a continuous bladder irrigation following a transurethral prostatectomy for benign prostatic hyperplasia (BPH). The client's output in the catheter bag is clear. Which action will the nurse perform **first**?
1. Measure the total output and subtract the irrigation insertion to obtain the urine output.
2. Stop the irrigation and call the health care provider to discontinue the irrigation.
3. Slow down the current rate of the irrigation infusing into the client's bladder.
4. Retrieve a new irrigation bag to hang once the current one infusing is finished.

61. The nurse is assessing a client diagnosed with chronic glomerulonephritis when the hospital's fire alarm begins to sound. Which action will the nurse take **next**?
1. Close the door to the client's room.
2. Report to the nurse's station.
3. Escort the client out of the facility.
4. Determine the best evacuation route.

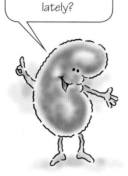

Your kidneys work hard every day for you. Have you thanked them lately?

57. 2. Azotemia is not associated with UTIs; it is associated with complications such as acute poststreptococcal glomerulonephritis. Clients with a UTI will need to use the bathroom frequently. Blood may be present in the urine and the client could have a fever. Painful urination is common.
CN: Safe, effective care environment; CNS: Management of care; CL: Apply

58. 1, 2, 4, 5. In a client with acute renal graft rejection, evidence of deteriorating renal function, including elevated BUN and creatinine levels, is expected. The client would most likely have acute hypertension. The nurse would see elevated, not decreased, WBC counts as well as fever because the body is recognizing the graft as foreign and is attempting to fight it.
CN: Physiological integrity; CNS: Reduction of risk potential; CL: Analyze

59. 1. Cloudy peritoneal fluid indicates possible peritonitis and should be reported to the health care provider. If less fluid is removed than put in, the client should be turned on the side first to fully drain the fluid. Once the fluid is instilled and dwelling the client will need to stay elevated to prevent shortness of breath, and slight abdominal tension is normal with fluid placed into the abdomen.
CN: Safe, effective care environment; CNS: Safety and infection control; CL: Apply

60. 3. If the urine or output in the catheter bag is clear, then the irrigation is infusing too rapidly and needs to be decreased. The irrigation should not be stopped as long as the catheter is draining because clots will form. Measuring the total urine output is required but not the first task of the nurse. A new irrigation bag will need to be started once the old one is finished, but currently the irrigation is infusing too fast.
CN: Safe, effective care environment; CNS: Management of care; CL: Analyze

61. 1. First, the nurse would close the door to the client's room. Hospital doors are generally fire retardant, providing a layer of protection. The nurse would then determine if clients need to be evacuated and follow the facility's procedure accordingly.
CN: Safe, effective care environment; CNS: Safety and infection control; CL: Analyze

CN: Client needs category   CNS: Client needs subcategory   CL: Cognitive level

62. The nurse is caring for a client with an ileal conduit. Place the steps in the order the nurse will complete them when changing an ostomy device. Use all answer choices once.

| **1.** Apply the wafer to the new collection device. |
| **2.** Cut the wafer at least 0.33 in (0.85 cm) larger than the stoma. |
| **3.** Cleanse the client's skin and stoma. |
| **4.** Empty and remove the old collection device. |
| **5.** Add paste to the client's skin to hold the collection device. |

62. Ordered Response:

| **4.** Empty and remove the old collection device. |
| **3.** Cleanse the client's skin and stoma. |
| **2.** Cut the wafer at least 0.33 in (0.85 cm) larger than the stoma. |
| **5.** Add paste to the client's skin to hold the collection device. |
| **1.** Apply the wafer to the new collection device. |

CN: Safe, effective care environment; CNS: Safety and infection control; CL: Apply

63. A registered nurse (RN) and an assistive personnel (AP) are caring for a client with an indwelling urinary catheter. Which intervention performed by the AP will require the RN to intervene?
1. Placing the indwelling urinary catheter below the level of the client's bladder after moving
2. Disconnecting the urinary catheter from the client's drainage bag to empty
3. Performing perineal care and cleaning around the meatus while bathing
4. Emptying the catheter system when it becomes full and measuring output

63. 2. Disconnecting the urinary catheter from the drainage bag opens the system and increases the risk of infection. The catheter bag should be placed below the client's waist and perineal care should be performed every shift. Draining the catheter tubing by gravity and eliminating dependent loops will decrease the risk of infection and help the system better drain the bladder.

CN: Safe, effective care environment; CNS: Safety and infection control; CL: Apply

64. A client is being discharged home following a kidney transplant. Which information will the nurse include in the client's discharge teaching?
1. "A slight elevation in your temperature is normal following surgery."
2. "Your urine output will be less than normal but there is no need to monitor it."
3. "You will need to take antirejection medication for the rest of your life."
4. "Drinking fluids is not important because a return to your normal kidney function will be delayed."

Educating your client is a huge job with extreme importance.

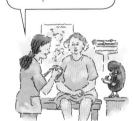

64. 3. A client should be aware that antirejection medication will be needed for life and should be strictly adhered to. A slight elevation in temperature is very important as the medication taken for rejection can suppress the response. Temperature indicates possible rejection of the kidney. Urine output should return to normal and is a good indicator of how the kidney is functioning. The client should drink plenty of fluids to keep the kidneys flushed.

CN: Health promotion and maintenance; CNS: None; CL: Apply

65. A client is admitted with severe nausea, vomiting, and diarrhea, and is hypotensive. The client is experiencing severe oliguria with elevated blood urea nitrogen (BUN) and creatinine levels. Which prescription will the nurse anticipate from the health care provider?
1. Peritoneal dialysis with a catheter
2. Hemodialysis using an arteriovenous shunt
3. Insertion of a temporary dialysis access device
4. Rapid fluid resuscitation via central line

65. 4. The client is experiencing prekidney failure secondary to hypovolemia. IV fluids should be given to rehydrate the client. The client is not fluid overloaded and would not require dialysis at this time.

CN: Safe, effective care environment; CNS: Management of care; CL: Analyze

66. The nurse is providing instructions for a client taking furosemide. Which education will the nurse include? Select all that apply.
1. Take your furosemide every morning.
2. High doses of furosemide can cause hearing loss.
3. Notify your health care provider if you cannot void.
4. Drink an 8-oz glass of grapefruit juice daily.
5. You should eat foods high in potassium.

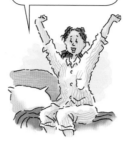

Yay! I slept through the whole night without having to get up to pee.

66. 1, 2, 3. A diuretic such as furosemide given in the morning has time to work throughout the day. Diuretics given at nighttime will cause the client to get up to go to the bathroom frequently, interrupting sleep. High doses of furosemide can cause hearing loss. Clients should notify their health care provider if they are unable to void. When taking furosemide, clients should avoid grapefruit and foods high in potassium.
CN: Physiological integrity; CNS: Pharmacological and parenteral therapies; CL: Apply

67. Which dietary choice is appropriate for the nurse to recommend for client with a chronic kidney disease?
1. Chopped steak, rice, bananas, and a glass of milk
2. Garden salad with carrots, frozen popsicle, and water
3. Turkey sandwich, potato chips, and orange juice
4. Canned tomato soup. Greek yogurt, and apple juice

67. 2. Chronic kidney disease clients should avoid foods high in potassium like bananas and oranges. They should also avoid foods high in sodium such as canned foods and potato chips. These clients should also limit their intake of protein.
CN: Physiological integrity; CNS: Basic care and comfort; CL: Apply

68. A client has just returned from kidney surgery. Which nursing intervention is **priority**?
1. Administration of IV fluids
2. Drawing blood urea nitrogen (BUN) and creatinine labs
3. Frequently monitoring urine output
4. Restriction intake of protein

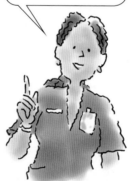

When looking for the priority intervention, think, "If I can only do one thing, what will I do?".

68. 1. A client returning from surgery is at risk for bleeding and dehydration. Starting IV fluids early will assist in preventing acute kidney injury. Drawing BUN and creatinine labs would alert the nurse to a problem once the problem has developed. Monitoring urine output will also alert the nurse to a possible complication but not prevent the injury. Restriction of protein is only required once a renal issue exists.
CN: Physiological integrity; CNS: Reduction of risk potential; CL: Analyze

69. The nurse is caring for a client with urinary retention. Which catheter will the nurse obtain for insertion for this client?
1. Straight
2. Coudé
3. Indwelling
4. Three-way

69. 1. Urine retention is usually a temporary problem. A straight catheter is generally used for the client with urine retention. The three-way catheter is used for clients who need bladder irrigation, such as after a prostate resection. A Coudé catheter is used only when it is difficult to insert a standard catheter, often because of an enlarged prostate. An indwelling catheter is used for longer-term bladder problems.
CN: Physiological integrity; CNS: Basic care and comfort; CL: Apply

70. When making assignments for the shift, which client will the registered nurse (RN) assign to the licensed practical nurse (LPN)?
1. A client with new onset acute poststreptococcal glomerulonephritis with periorbital edema
2. A client with benign prostatic hyperplasia who is reporting dribbling following urination
3. A client diagnosed with breast cancer who just returned from having a total mastectomy
4. A client with ovarian cancer prescribed fluorouracil treatment starting today

70. 2. Dribbling following urination is expected in a client with benign prostatic hyperplasia. A client with a new onset of any disorder will require education, which cannot be delegated to the LPN. An immediate postoperative client and a client beginning a new antineoplastic agent will require frequent assessment for complications as well as additional education.
CN: Safe, effective care environment; CNS: Management of care; CL: Apply

71. A 50-year-old female client asks the nurse about the best screening tool for detecting breast cancer. Which response by the nurse is **most** appropriate?
1. "The best thing for you to do is perform breast self-exams each month."
2. "It is recommended for you to have a mammogram at your age to look for breast cancer."
3. "We recommend women have a magnetic resonance imaging (MRI) every 2 years."
4. "Your primary health care provider can make the best recommendation for you."

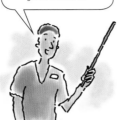

Know the best methods of breast examination for your clients.

71. 2. The best screening tool to detect breast cancer is a mammogram. Current recommendation by the American Cancer Society is: annual mammogram from age 45 to 54, mammogram every other year for women aged 55 and older. Current recommendation by the Canadian Cancer Society is: need/frequency for mammogram determined by health care provider from age 40 to 49, mammogram every other year for women aged 50 to 74. Breast self-exams are no longer recommended by the American Cancer Society. A MRI would only be used to further view a section of the breast if the mammogram found an area to investigate or if the client is at very high risk. Telling the client the health care provider can make the best recommendation does not address the client's concern.
CN: Physiological integrity; CNS: Reduction of risk potential; CL: Apply

72. A male client diagnosed with chronic kidney failure (CKF) is admitted to the urology unit. Which diagnostic test results will the nurse report to the health care provider? Select all that apply.
1. Increased pH with increased hydrogen ions
2. Serum calcium level 17 mEq/L (8.5 mmol/L)
3. Blood urea nitrogen (BUN) level 100 mg/dL (35.7 mmol/L)
4. Serum creatinine level 6.5 mg/dL (495.6 µmol/L)
5. Uric acid level of 3.5 mg/dL (28.2 µmol/L)
6. Phenolsulfonphthalein (PSP) excretion of 75%

72. 1, 2. The client's pH, hydrogen ions, and calcium levels are unexpected for a diagnosis of CKF. CKF causes decreased pH and increased hydrogen ions, not vice versa. CKF also increases serum levels of potassium, magnesium, and phosphatase, and decreases serum levels of calcium. A BUN level of 100 mg/dL (35.7 mmol/L) and a serum creatinine level of 6.5 mg/dL (495.6 µmol/L) are reflective of CKF and the kidneys' decreased ability to remove nonprotein nitrogen waste from the blood. The normal BUN level is 10 to 20 mg/dL (3.57 to 7.14 mmol/L), and the normal serum creatinine level is 0.7 to 1.4 mg/dL (53.4 to 106.75 µmol/L). A uric acid level of 3.5 mg/dL (28.2 µmol/L) falls within the normal range of 3.4 to 7.0 mg/dL (202.25 to 416.4 µmol/L) for males; PSP excretion of 75% also falls within the normal range of 60% to 75%.
CN: Safe, effective care environment; CNS: Management of care; CL: Analyze

73. A client is scheduled for a procedure requiring radiographic contrast medium. The client's blood urea nitrogen (BUN) and creatinine levels are slightly elevated. Which nursing intervention is **priority** following the procedure?
1. Notify the health care provider.
2. Start IV fluids to flush out the dye.
3. Administer a binding agent for the dye.
4. Observe the client for an allergic reaction.

73. 2. Due to the client's elevated renal labs, the client will need IV fluid to help with flushing out the dye. This is priority for this client. Once the IV fluids are running then the client would be given a binding agent. The health care provider should be notified prior to the procedure of the client's laboratory values, and observing the client for an allergic reaction would occur during the procedure.
CN: Safe, effective care environment; CNS: Management of care; CL: Apply

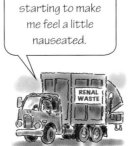

All this waste is starting to make me feel a little nauseated.

74. The nurse is caring for a client with kidney failure who is reporting nausea. The nurse understands which factor is responsible for the client's nausea?
1. Oliguria
2. Gastric ulcer
3. Electrolyte imbalance
4. Accumulation of metabolic wastes

74. 4. Although a client with kidney failure can develop stress ulcers, nausea is usually related to the poisons of metabolic wastes that accumulate when the kidneys cannot eliminate them. The client may have electrolyte imbalances and oliguria, but these conditions do not directly cause nausea.
CN: Physiological integrity; CNS: Physiological adaptation; CL: Understand

CN: Client needs category   CNS: Client needs subcategory   CL: Cognitive level

75. The nurse is educating a client who is scheduled for a biopsy of the bladder. Which medication(s) will the nurse anticipate the client will discontinue taking prior to the procedure? Select all that apply.
1. Warfarin
2. Antibiotic
3. Aspirin
4. Lisinopril
5. Furosemide

76. The nurse is caring for a client following a radical mastectomy. Which assessment finding **most** concerns the nurse?
1. The surgical bandage is saturated with bright red drainage
2. The client reports pain, swelling, and warmth in the left calf
3. The client's pain rating is an 8 on a 10-point pain scale
4. A reddened area on the client's coccyx that blanches

77. The nurse is caring for a client with urinary calculus. What information will the nurse provide to this client?
1. "You need to save any stones that are larger than 0.25 cm (0.1 in)."
2. "Strain the urine, limit oral fluids, and take pain medication as needed."
3. "Drink plenty of fluids, strain the urine, and save all calculi passed."
4. "You will need an indwelling urinary catheter to adequately assess output."

78. The nurse is obtaining data from a client with a urinary tract infection (UTI). Which statement(s) will the nurse expect the client to make? Select all that apply.
1. "I urinate large amounts."
2. "I need to urinate frequently."
3. "It burns when I urinate."
4. "My urine smells sweet."
5. "I need to urinate urgently."

79. The nurse is completing an intake and output record for a client who is receiving continuous bladder irrigation after transurethral resection of the prostate (TURP). How many milliliters of urine will the nurse record as output for the shift if the client received 1,800 mL of normal saline irrigating solution and the output in the urine drainage bag is 2,400 mL? Record your answer as a whole number.

_____ mL

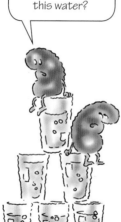

I know it's supposed to keep the stones away, but how are we going to drink all this water?

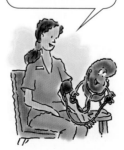

Your blood pressure is 112/73—that's good news for both of us!

75. 1, 3. The client needs to take an antibiotic as prescribed. Anticoagulants and aspirin should be discontinued for 3 to 5 days before the procedure due to the risk of increased bleeding. Lisinopril and furosemide do not interfere with this procedure and should be taken as prescribed.
CN: Physiological integrity; CNS: Reduction of risk potential; CL: Apply

76. 1. The saturated dressing indicates the client is bleeding. Pain is expected following surgery. A deep vein thrombosis and potential early stages of a pressure injury would cause alarm but bleeding is priority.
CN: Safe, effective care environment; CNS: Management of care; CL: Analyze

77. 3. Encouraging fluids and straining all urine, saving all calculi, including "flecks," is the appropriate intervention. Pain medications are taken as needed because renal calculi are extremely painful. Indwelling urinary catheters usually are not needed.
CN: Physiological integrity; CNS: Basic care and comfort; CL: Apply

78. 2, 3, 5. Typical assessment findings for a client with a UTI include urinary frequency, burning on urination, and urinary urgency. The client with a UTI typically reports voiding frequently in small amounts, not large amounts. The client with a UTI reports foul-smelling, not sweet-smelling, urine.
CN: Physiological integrity; CNS: Physiological adaptation; CL: Apply

79. 600.
To calculate urine output, subtract the amount of irrigation solution infused into the bladder from the total amount of fluid in the drainage bag. For this client:

$$2,400 \ mL - 1,800 \ mL = 600 \ mL.$$

CN: Physiological integrity; CNS: Reduction of risk potential; CL: Apply

80. The nurse is collecting a sterile urine specimen for a culture and sensitivity test from an indwelling urinary catheter. Identify the area on the indwelling urinary catheter where the nurse will insert the sterile syringe to obtain the urine specimen.

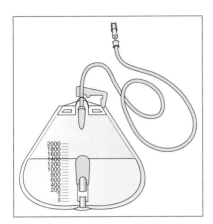

80. A sterile urine specimen is obtained from an indwelling urinary catheter by clamping the catheter briefly, cleaning the rubber port with an alcohol wipe, and using a sterile syringe to withdraw the urine.

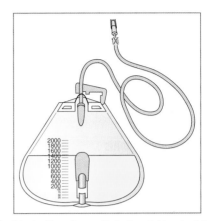

CN: Physiological integrity; CNS: Reduction of risk potential; CL: Apply

81. A client with chronic kidney failure wants to receive a kidney transplant. The client is a poor candidate for transplant because of chronic uncontrolled hypertension and diabetes. Now, the client tells the nurse, "I want to go off dialysis. I would rather not live than be on this treatment for the rest of my life." Which nursing action(s) is **most** appropriate? Select all that apply.
1. Take a seat next to the client and sit quietly.
2. State, "We all have days when we do not feel like going on."
3. Leave the room to allow the client to collect thoughts.
4. State, "You are feeling upset about the news you got about the transplant."
5. State, "The treatments are only 3 days a week. You can live with that."

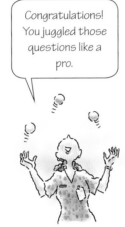

Congratulations! You juggled those questions like a pro.

81. 1, 4. Silence is a therapeutic communication technique that allows the nurse and client to reflect on what has been said or taken place. By waiting quietly and attentively, the nurse encourages the client to initiate and maintain conversation. By reflecting the client's implied feelings, the nurse promotes communication. Using such platitudes as "We all have days when we do not feel like going on" fails to address the client's needs. The nurse should not leave the client alone because he or she may harm oneself. Minimizing the treatment frequency does not address the client's feelings.

CN: Psychosocial integrity; CNS: None; CL: Apply

CN: Client needs category   CNS: Client needs subcategory   CL: Cognitive level

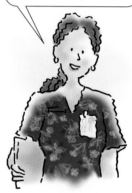

So, you think caring for a client with a skin disorder isn't your strong suit, eh? Check out this Web site before taking on this chapter: www.aad.org. Enjoy!

Chapter 11

Integumentary Disorders

Integumentary refresher

Atopic dermatitis

Itchy skin that is warm, red, and tender

Key signs and symptoms

- Erythematous lesions that eventually become scaly and lichenified
- Excessively dry skin
- Hyperpigmentation
- Skin eruptions

Key test results

- Serum immunoglobulin E levels are commonly elevated (not a confirmation the client has atopic dermatitis)

Key treatments

- Antihistamines: diphenhydramine
- Corticosteroid: hydrocortisone

Key interventions

- Help client set up an individual schedule and plan for daily skin care.
- Instruct client to bathe in plain water (bathing may have to be limited according to severity of lesions).
- Instruct client to bathe with special nonfatty soap and tepid water (96° F [35.6° C]).
- Instruct client to avoid using soap when lesions are acutely inflamed.
- Instruct client to limit baths and showers to 5 to 7 minutes.
- For scalp involvement, advise client to shampoo frequently and to apply corticosteroid solution to scalp afterward.
- Lubricate skin after a shower or bath.

Burns

Injury caused by exposure to heat, flame or electricity

Key signs and symptoms

- Superficial partial-thickness burn
  - Erythema, edema, pain, blanching
- Deep dermal partial-thickness burn
  - Pain, oozing, fluid-filled vesicles
  - Erythema
  - Shiny and wet subcutaneous layer after vesicles rupture

- Full-thickness burn
  - Eschar, edema, little or no pain

Key test results

- Visual inspection allows examiner to estimate extent of the burn (determined by the Rule of Nines and the Lund and Browder chart)

Key treatments

- IV therapy: hydration and electrolyte replacement using a fluid replacement formula such as the Parkland formula
- Skin grafts
- Analgesic: morphine
- Antianxiety agent: lorazepam
- Antibiotic: gentamicin
- Anti-infectives: mafenide, silver sulfadiazine, silver nitrate
- Anti-tetanus: tetanus toxoid
- Colloid: albumin 5%

Key interventions

- Maintain airway and monitor respiratory status.
- Monitor fluid status.
- Maintain IV fluids.
- Administer oxygen.
- Monitor total parenteral or enteral feedings.
- Maintain protective precautions.

Herpes zoster

Vesicular rash caused by herpesvirus, also known as shingles

Key signs and symptoms

- Neuralgia
- Severe, deep pain
- Unilaterally clustered skin vesicles along peripheral sensory nerves on the trunk, thorax, or face

Key test results

- A skin study identifies the organism
- Visual inspection identifies vesicles along the peripheral sensory nerves

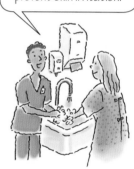

Clients with dermatitis may need to lay off the soap to prevent skin irritation.

Key treatments

- Analgesics: acetaminophen, codeine
- Antianxiety agents: lorazepam, hydroxyzine
- Antipruritic: diphenhydramine
- Antiviral agents: acyclovir, valacyclovir, famciclovir
- Vaccine: zoster vaccine, live

Key interventions

- Monitor neurologic status.
- Monitor pain and note the effectiveness of analgesics.
- Prevent scratching and rubbing of affected areas.

Pressure injury

Injury to the skin caused by prolonged pressure

Key signs and symptoms

- Signs are determined by stage of ulceration

Key treatments

- High-protein, high-calorie diet in small, frequent feedings
- Parenteral or enteral feedings if client is unable or unwilling to take adequate nutrients orally
- Topical wound care according to facility protocol
- Wound debridement; tissue flap

Key interventions

- Monitor skin integrity and watch for signs of infection.
- Monitor any bedridden client for possible changes in skin color, turgor, temperature, and sensation.
- Reposition client every 1 to 2 hours.
- Provide meticulous skin care and check bony prominences.
- Maintain client's diet and encourage oral fluid intake.

Psoriasis

Autoimmune disease characterized by itchy, red, scaly patches on the skin

Key signs and symptoms

- Itching
- Lesions (red and usually well-defined patches)
- Pustules (with secondary infection)

Key test results

- Skin biopsy is positive for the disorder

Key treatments

- Antipsoriatic agents: calcipotriene
- Corticosteroid ointments: hydrocortisone, clobetasol propionate
- Topical retinoids: tazarotene
- Ultraviolet light to retard cell production; may be used in conjunction with psoralens (psoralen plus ultraviolet A [PUVA] therapy)

Key interventions

- Make sure client understands prescribed therapy.
- Provide written instructions.
- Watch for adverse reactions, especially:
  - allergic reactions to anthralin
  - atrophy and acne from steroids
  - burning, itching, nausea, and squamous cell epitheliomas from PUVA therapy.
- Caution client receiving PUVA therapy to:
  - stay out of the sun on day of treatment
  - protect eyes with sunglasses that screen UVA for 24 hours after treatment
  - wear goggles during any exposure to this light.

Skin cancer

Malignancy involving any layer of the skin

Key signs and symptoms

- Change in color, size, or shape of preexisting lesion
- Irregular, circular bordered lesion with hues of tan, black, or blue (melanoma)
- Small, red, nodular lesion that begins as an erythematous macule or plaque with indistinct margins (squamous cell carcinoma)
- Waxy nodule with telangiectasis (basal cell epithelioma)

Key test results

- A skin biopsy shows cytology positive for cancer cells

Key treatments

- Chemosurgery with zinc chloride
- Cryosurgery with liquid nitrogen
- Curettage and electrodesiccation
- Antimetabolite: fluorouracil

Key interventions

- Monitor treated lesion sites.
- Administer medications as prescribed.
- Provide postchemotherapy and postradiation nursing care.

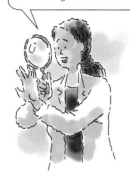

Routine self-checks can help detect skin irregularities.

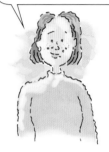

Great, I've got zits. Aren't I too old for this?

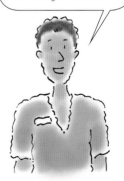

Your client comes in concerned a skin lesion might be cancerous. What signs should you look for?

Integumentary questions, answers, and rationales

1. A client is admitted to the emergency department with a deep partial-thickness burn on the arm after a fire in the workplace. Which finding(s) will the nurse expect to assess? Select all that apply.
  1. Pain and superficial redness
  2. Blisters on the arm
  3. Minimal damage to the epidermis
  4. Necrotic tissue through all layers of skin
  5. Necrotic tissue through most of the dermis

2. A client reports being exposed to lice and thinks she may have them. Which finding made by the nurse indicates the client needs to be treated for lice?
  1. Diffuse, pruritic wheals
  2. Oval, white dots stuck to the hair shafts
  3. Pain, redness, and edema with an embedded stinger
  4. Pruritic nodules and linear burrows of the finger and toe webs

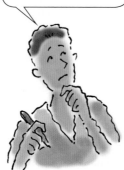

What you're looking for are the lice's eggs. Hmm… what do tiny eggs look like?

3. The nurse is admitting a client who states, "I think a brown recluse spider bit me." Which assessment finding confirms the client's statement for the nurse?
  1. Bull's-eye rash
  2. Painful rash around a necrotic lesion
  3. Herald patch of oval lesions
  4. Line of papules and vesicles

4. The nurse is instructing a client after the administration of a Mantoux test. Which statement from the client indicates an accurate understanding of the nurse's teaching?
  1. "A Mantoux test will confirm if I have active tuberculosis."
  2. "I will return to the office in 2 to 3 days to have the results read."
  3. "If the site itches, I should apply an anti-itch cream."
  4. "I should rub the area for 10 seconds after it is injected."

5. A client arrives to the clinic with reports of a rash. During assessment, the nurse notes the client has 0.5 cm papules. What is the **best** way for the nurse to document this finding?
  1. A 0.5 cm fluid-filled lesion
  2. A 0.5 cm red, flat pinpoint rash
  3. A 0.5 cm elevated area
  4. A 0.5 cm erosion

1. **2, 5.** A deep, partial-thickness burn causes necrosis of the epidermal and dermal layers. Blisters may be noted. Redness and pain are characteristics of a superficial injury. Superficial burns cause slight epidermal damage. With deep burns, the nerve fibers are destroyed, and the client does not feel pain in the affected area. Necrosis through all skin layers is seen with full-thickness injuries.
CN: Physiological integrity; CNS: Physiological adaptation; CL: Apply

2. **2.** Nits, the eggs of lice, are seen as white, oval dots. Diffuse, itchy wheals indicate an allergy. Stings from bees are associated with a stinger, pain, and redness. Pruritic nodules and linear burrows are diagnostic of scabies.
CN: Physiological integrity; CNS: Physiological adaptation; CL: Understand

3. **2.** Necrotic, painful rashes are associated with the bite of a brown recluse spider. A bull's-eye rash located primarily at the site of the bite is a classic sign of Lyme disease. A herald patch—a slightly raised, oval lesion about 2 to 6 cm in diameter that appears anywhere on the body—is indicative of pityriasis rosea. A linear, papular, vesicular rash is characteristic of exposure to poison ivy.
CN: Physiological integrity; CNS: Physiological adaptation; CL: Apply

4. **2.** The results of a Mantoux test should be read 48 to 72 hours after placement by measuring the diameter of the induration that develops at the site. The test confirms if a client has ever been exposed and developed immunity for tuberculosis (TB), not that active TB is present. Additional testing is needed to confirm active TB. Rubbing the site of an intradermal injection could cause leakage from the injection site. Avoid applying anti-itch creams directly to the site.
CN: Physiological integrity; CNS: Reduction of risk potential; CL: Apply

5. **3.** Papules are elevated up to 0.5 cm, and nodules and tumors are masses elevated more than 0.5 cm. Erosions are characterized by loss of the epidermal layer. Macules and patches are nonpalpable, flat changes in skin color. Fluid-filled lesions are vesicles and pustules.
CN: Health promotion and maintenance; CNS: None; CL: Understand

CN: Client needs category   CNS: Client needs subcategory   CL: Cognitive level

6. The nurse is caring for a client with a burn injury. Which statement **best** describes the client's nutritional state?
1. The client needs 100 cal/kg throughout hospitalization
2. The hypermetabolic state after a burn injury leads to poor healing
3. Controlling the environmental temperature decreases caloric demands
4. Maintaining a hypermetabolic rate decreases the risk of infection

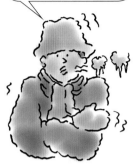

Make sure the client doesn't expend energy trying to stay warm.

6. 2. A burn injury causes a hypermetabolic state resulting in protein and lipid catabolism that affects wound healing adversely. Caloric intake must be 1½ to 2 times the basal metabolic rate, with at least 1.5 to 2 g of protein per kilogram of body weight daily. An environmental temperature within normal range lets the body function efficiently and devote caloric expenditure to healing and normal physiologic processes. If the temperature is too warm or too cold, the body devotes energy to warming or cooling, which takes away from energy used for tissue repair. High metabolic rates increase the risk of infection.
CN: Physiological integrity; CNS: Basic care and comfort; CL: Apply

7. A client is brought to the emergency department with partial-thickness and full-thickness burns on the left arm, left anterior leg, and anterior trunk. Using the Rule of Nines, the nurse will determine which percentage of the client's total body surface area has been burned?
1. 9%
2. 18%
3. 34%
4. 36%

7. 4. The Rule of Nines divides body surface into percentages that, when totaled, equal 100%. According to the Rule of Nines, the arms account for 9% each, the anterior legs account for 9% each, and the anterior trunk accounts for 18%. Therefore, this client's burns cover 36% of the body surface area.
CN: Physiological integrity; CNS: Physiological adaptation; CL: Apply

8. A client comes to the clinic with pruritic, dark red lesions on the hands, wrist, and waistline that are bleeding. Which nursing instruction is appropriate?
1. Press on the lesions.
2. Apply heat to the skin.
3. Tightly bandage the lesions.
4. Wash the lesions with a bleach solution.

Ugh! My foot is itching like crazy. How can I make it stop?

8. 1. Pressing the skin stimulates nerve endings and can reduce the sensation of itching. Pressing the skin does not promote breaks in the skin. Applying heat would increase the itching. The nurse and health care provider should assess the lesions before a bandage is applied. A bleach solution would further damage and irritate the client's skin.
CN: Physiological integrity; CNS: Physiological adaptation; CL: Analyze

9. The nurse is caring for a female client who is planning to start isotretinoin in 3 months. The client expresses a desire to have a baby. Which statement will the nurse include in the medication teaching?
1. "You need to start some form of contraceptive."
2. "This is the perfect time to become pregnant."
3. "Isotretinoin is safe for you to take while pregnant."
4. "Isotretinoin can cause you to become infertile."

9. 1. Even small amounts of isotretinoin are associated with severe birth defects. Most female clients are also prescribed oral contraceptives to prevent pregnancy. Isotretinoin does not cause infertility in women.
CN: Physiological integrity; CNS: Pharmacological and parenteral therapies; CL: Apply

10. The nurse is caring for an adolescent client with a diagnosis of atopic dermatitis. Which action(s) are **most** appropriate for the nurse to include in the client's care? Select all that apply.
1. Help the client develop a daily skin care routine.
2. Lubricate the skin after bathing.
3. Scrub the areas for 10 minutes while inflamed.
4. Shampoo often if the scalp is involved.
5. Take a shower in hot water every day.

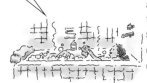

A long soak followed by some moisturizing lotion is a great way to care for your integument.

10. 1, 2, 4. Tepid baths and moisturizers are indicated for eczema to keep the infected areas clean and to minimize itching. Clients should lubricate the skin directly after bathing to reduce dryness and pruritus. Clients should shampoo their scalp frequently. Hot baths can exacerbate the condition and increase itching. Tepid baths are indicated for these clients, not hot showers. Clients should not scrub the areas while inflamed.
CN: Physiological integrity; CNS: Physiological adaptation; CL: Apply

11. The nurse is caring for a client with thrush who has been prescribed nystatin mouthwash. Which instruction will the nurse provide this client?
1. Take the drug right after meals.
2. Take the drug with a glass of water.
3. Mix the drug with small amounts of food.
4. Take half the dose before and half after meals.

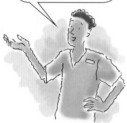

Timing matters when taking medication for thrush.

11. 1. Nystatin oral solution should be swished around the mouth after eating for the best contact with mucous membranes. Taking the drug before or with meals does not allow for the best contact with the mucous membranes. The drug should not be taken with a glass of water or mixed with small amounts of food.
CN: Physiological integrity; CNS: Pharmacological and parenteral therapies; CL: Apply

12. A client is examined and found to have pinpoint, pink-to-purple, nonblanching macular lesions 1 to 3 mm in diameter. How will the nurse document the findings?
1. Ecchymosis
2. Hematoma
3. Petechiae
4. Purpura

12. 3. Petechiae are small macular lesions 1 to 3 mm in diameter. Ecchymosis is a purple-to-brown bruise, macular or papular, that varies in size. A hematoma is a collection of blood from ruptured blood vessels that is more than 1 cm in diameter. Purpura are purple macular lesions larger than 1 cm.
CN: Physiological integrity; CNS: Physiological adaptation; CL: Understand

13. The nurse notes several areas of ecchymosis on a client's arms and is informed by the client that she is being abused by her partner. Which nursing intervention is **most** appropriate?
1. Immediately inform the health care provider.
2. Refer the client for counseling.
3. Notify the local law enforcement.
4. Ask whether the client has a safe place to go if needed.

13. 4. Because there are physical indicators of violence, ensuring the client's safety is a priority. Therefore, the nurse should make sure the client has a safe place to go if needed. Calling the local police or the health care provider right away are inappropriate options because they undermine the trust the client has placed in the nurse; safety could be jeopardized if the secret is revealed to the health care provider or legal authorities without permission. A referral to counseling is not the priority, as this does not directly address the client's safety.
CN: Psychosocial integrity; CNS: None; CL: Analyze

14. The nurse is caring for a client diagnosed with herpes zoster. Which finding **most** concerns the nurse?
1. A clustered rash following the sensory nerves
2. Lesions noted bilaterally on the inner aspect of the client's thighs
3. Deep pain at the site of the rash
4. Pruritus

14. 2. Herpes zoster causes a painful vesicular rash that follows a sensory nerve. The rash is unilateral and clustered. Clients often report itching at the site. Lesions on the inner thighs are not expected and would most concern the nurse.
CN: Safe, effective care environment; CNS: Management of care; CL: Analyze

15. Which nursing intervention will **best** maintain skin integrity in an adult client?
1. Placing powder on the axillae, groin, beneath the breasts, and between the toes
2. Applying an antiperspirant immediately after shaving under the arms
3. Thoroughly drying the client's skin folds after a bath
4. Using an alcohol solution when rubbing the client's skin

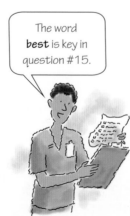

*The word **best** is key in question #15.*

15. 3. Thoroughly drying the skin decreases skin breakdown and prevents bacterial growth. To reduce moisture, the nurse can apply a nonirritating dusting powder, such as cornstarch, to the client's axillae and groin, beneath the breasts, and between the toes after those areas are dry. Deodorants and antiperspirants should not be applied to the skin immediately after shaving because they may cause irritation. The nurse should use lotion if rubbing the skin because alcohol dries the skin and can irritate it.
CN: Physiological integrity; CNS: Basic care and comfort; CL: Analyze

CN: Client needs category   CNS: Client needs subcategory   CL: Cognitive level

16. The nurse is caring for a client with suspected psoriasis. Which nursing interventions are **most** appropriate for this client? Select all that apply.
1. Assessing for red, well-defined lesions
2. Preparing the client for a skin biopsy
3. Giving the client information on antiviral medications
4. Cautioning the client on long-term corticosteroid ointment use
5. Administering psoralen plus ultraviolet A (PUVA) therapy

17. The nurse is caring for a client diagnosed with ringworm. Which medication will the nurse anticipate the primary health care provider prescribing?
1. Gentamicin
2. Hydrocortisone cream
3. Bleach solution
4. Ketoconazole

18. A client has thick, discolored nails with splintered hemorrhages, easily separated from the nail bed. There are also "ice pick" pits and ridges. The nurse will anticipate providing the client care for which condition?
1. Paronychia
2. Psoriasis
3. Seborrhea
4. Scabies

19. A client is diagnosed with a fungal infection of the scalp. The nurse knows the client understands the treatment plan when which statement(s) is made? Select all that apply.
1. "I should throw away my combs and hats."
2. "I will need to take all of my medication."
3. "I can scratch the areas as long as I wash my hands."
4. "It is not possible to spread the infection to other people."
5. "I can use a steroid cream if the rash begins to itch."

20. A client has been admitted with burns on both legs. Which nursing intervention is **priority** for this client?
1. Apply knee splints.
2. Elevate the foot of the bed.
3. Hyperextend the client's palms.
4. Perform shoulder range-of-motion (ROM) exercises.

16. 1, 2, 4, 5. Psoriasis causes well-defined patches on the skin. Skin biopsy is used to confirm the diagnosis. The use of corticosteroids for long periods of time can cause thinning of the client's skin, increasing the risk for infection. PUVA therapy may be used as a treatment. Antiviral medications are not appropriate for this client.
CN: Physiological integrity; CNS: Physiological adaptation; CL: Apply

17. 4. Antifungals, such as ketoconazole, are the treatment of choice for clients diagnosed with ringworm (fungal rash). Antibiotics (gentamicin) and corticosteroids (hydrocortisone) do not treat fungal infections and often make them worse. A bleach solution would irritate and damage the skin.
CN: Physiological integrity; CNS: Pharmacological and parenteral therapies; CL: Apply

18. 2. Psoriasis, a chronic skin disorder with an unknown cause, can make fingernails thick and discolored with splintered hemorrhages, and the nails can become easily separated from the nail bed with pits and ridges. A paronychia is a bacterial infection of the nail bed. Seborrhea is a chronic inflammatory dermatitis known as cradle cap. Scabies are mites that burrow under the skin, generally between the webbing of the fingers and toes.
CN: Physiological integrity; CNS: Physiological adaptation; CL: Apply

Grrr! All this stress is making me break out in a rash.

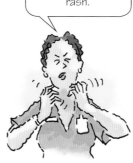

19. 1, 2. Tinea capitis is a fungal infection of the scalp. Over-the-counter steroid cream is not an appropriate treatment for fungal rashes, as they often make the rash worse. Fungal infections can be spread via a fomite transmission, so combs and hats should be discarded. Medications should be taken as prescribed even if the rash is gone. The client should not scratch the areas, as this would lead to skin breakdown and a potential infection.
CN: Physiological integrity; CNS: Physiological adaptation; CL: Apply

20. 1. Applying knee splints prevents leg contractures by holding the joints in a position of function. Elevating the foot of the bed cannot prevent contractures because this action does not hold the joints in a position of function. Hyperextending a body part for an extended time is inappropriate because it can cause contractures. Performing shoulder ROM exercises can prevent contractures in the shoulders but not in the legs.
CN: Safe, effective care environment; CNS: Management of care; CL: Analyze

CN: Client needs category   CNS: Client needs subcategory   CL: Cognitive level

21. The nurse is reviewing a newly admitted client's chart. Based on the chart exhibit below, the nurse will suspect which condition?

Progress notes	
10/04	Client was admitted from the ED after having
1830	been found unconscious at home. Client
	is unresponsive to painful stimuli. Blood
	pressure is 90/60 mm Hg. Heart rate is 110
	beats/minute in sinus rhythm. Respiratory
	rate is 14 breaths/minute. Nail beds and all
	mucous membranes appear cherry red.
	—Lily Sue, RN

1. Spider bite
2. Aspirin ingestion overdose
3. Hydrocarbon ingestion
4. Carbon monoxide poisoning

22. A client has just arrived at the emergency department after sustaining both full-thickness and partial-thickness burns. Which treatment(s) will the nurse anticipate the primary health care provider prescribing? Select all that apply.
1. Intravenous (IV) fluids
2. Morphine
3. Tdap injection
4. IV antibiotic therapy
5. Oxygen

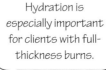

Hydration is especially important for clients with full-thickness burns.

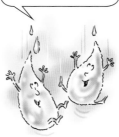

23. The nurse is caring for a client with a third-degree burn. Which medication(s) will the nurse anticipate administering to this client? Select all that apply.
1. Intravenous (IV) fluid
2. Morphine
3. Mafenide
4. Malathion
5. Diazepam
6. Aspirin

24. The nurse is caring for an older adult client who is bedridden from a recent stroke. Which intervention(s) will the nurse include while caring for this client? Select all that apply.
1. Turn the client every 1 to 2 hours.
2. Provide protein-rich meals.
3. Request an air mattress.
4. Splint the affected extremities.
5. Apply lotion during morning care.

Remember to select all that apply.

STOP

21. 4. Cherry-red skin indicates exposure to high levels of carbon monoxide. Spider bite reactions are usually localized to the area of the bite. Nausea and vomiting and pale skin are symptoms of aspirin ingestion overdose. Hydrocarbon or petroleum ingestion usually causes respiratory symptoms and tachycardia.
CN: Physiological integrity; CNS: Physiological adaptation; CL: Analyze

22. 1, 2, 5. Administering IV fluids and maintaining fluid status are imperative for clients with full-thickness burns. Morphine should be administered to relieve the client's pain. A Tdap injection would not be needed for burns. IV antibiotics may be prescribed if a secondary infection develops but should not be anticipated as an initial treatment. Oxygen should be administered to this client to maintain oxygenation and tissue perfusion.
CN: Physiological integrity; CNS: Physiological adaptation; CL: Analyze

23. 1, 2, 3, 5. IV therapy is a priority in clients with burns to replace fluid loss. The opioid analgesic morphine is used to help control pain in clients with burns. The topical antibiotic mafenide is prescribed to prevent infection in clients with second- and third-degree burns. Malathion is a pediculicide used to treat lice infestation. Diazepam is an antianxiety agent that may be administered to clients with burns. Aspirin is not routinely prescribed to burn clients.
CN: Physiological integrity; CNS: Pharmacological and parenteral therapies; CL: Apply

24. 1, 2, 3, 5. The nurse would be concerned about skin breakdown for this client. Turning the client every 1 to 2 hours is a priority nursing intervention to prevent skin breakdown over bony prominences. A high-protein diet helps promote healing and blood supply. An air mattress provides movement to promote blood supply and movement of the client when turning is not performed. Applying lotion keeps the skin moist and reduces the risk of skin breakdown. There is no need to splint the client's extremities.
CN: Physiological integrity; CNS: Basic care and comfort; CL: Apply

25. The nurse is caring for a postoperative client and notes the dressing was not changed on the previous shift even though the health care provider prescribed a dressing change each shift. Which nursing action is **priority**?
 1. Change the client's dressing.
 2. Put a sign above the head of the client's bed.
 3. Report the finding to the nurse manager.
 4. Notify the health care provider.

25. 1. It is priority for the nurse to provide the needed care to the client. The nurse would first change the client's dressing. A sign could be placed as a reminder, according to facility policy. The nurse should first notify the nurse from the previous shift of the incident and not the nurse manager or health care provider.
CN: Safe, effective care environment; CNS: Management of care; CL: Apply

26. A postoperative client has just been admitted to the surgical unit from the postanesthesia care unit. The client asks the nurse to change the dressing. Which nursing action is appropriate?
 1. Have the assistive personnel change the dressing.
 2. Gather supplies and change the client's dressing.
 3. Inform the client the dressing cannot be changed until tomorrow.
 4. Tell the client the health care provider will change the first dressing.

26. 4. The health care provider always performs the first postoperative dressing change. Generally, the health care provider changes the dressing and assesses the wound the day following admission during rounds. The dressing should not need to be changed at this time. If the first dressing becomes saturated, it may be secured with additional tape or bandages.
CN: Physiological integrity; CNS: Basic care and comfort; CL: Apply

27. The nurse is monitoring clients for impaired wound healing. Which client(s) will the nurse monitor **most** closely? Select all that apply.
 1. A 65-year-old client with chronic hypertension
 2. A 60-year-old client with impaired mobility following a cerebrovascular accident
 3. A 58-year-old client with asthma
 4. A 75-year-old client with poorly controlled diabetes
 5. A 60-year-old client with elevated cholesterol

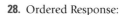

Washing your hands before and after working with an infected wound helps prevent spreading disease.

27. 2, 4. Limited mobility and poorly controlled diabetes are serious risk factors for impaired wound healing. Other factors that impair wound healing include advanced age, inadequate blood supply, nutritional deficiencies, and obesity. Elevated blood pressure, asthma, or high cholesterol would not impair wound healing.
CN: Safe, effective care environment; CNS: Management of care; CL: Analyze

28. A client is suspected of having a postoperative wound infection and the health care provider prescribes a wound culture. Place the steps the nurse will complete to obtain a wound culture in chronological order. Use all options.
 1. Properly label the collection tube.
 2. Gently roll the sterile swab in the center of the wound.
 3. Properly identify the client.
 4. Wash hands thoroughly.

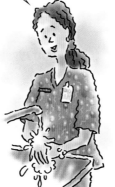

28. Ordered Response:

4. Wash hands thoroughly.
3. Properly identify the client.
1. Properly label the collection tube.
2. Gently roll the sterile swab in the center of the wound.

CN: Safe, effective care environment; CNS: Safety and infection control; CL: Apply

29. The nurse is assessing a client with an abdominal incision and suspects delayed wound healing. Which observation **most** supports the nurse's suspicion?
 1. Sutures that are dry and intact
 2. Wound edges in close approximation
 3. Purulent drainage on a soiled wound dressing
 4. Sanguineous drainage in a wound collection drainage bag

29. 3. Purulent drainage contains white blood cells, which fight infection. The sutures from a wound that is draining purulent secretions would pull away with an infection. Wound edges cannot approximate in an infected wound. Sanguineous drainage indicates bleeding, not infection. The other answers refer to wounds that should heal properly.
CN: Physiological integrity; CNS: Physiological adaptation; CL: Apply

CN: Client needs category   CNS: Client needs subcategory   CL: Cognitive level

30. The nurse is working with a kidney transplant client diagnosed with herpes zoster. Which precaution(s) will the nurse apply before caring for this client? Select all that apply.
1. Shoe covers
2. Gown
3. Gloves
4. Mask
5. No precautions are needed

31. The nurse is caring for a client with a pressure injury. Which nursing intervention(s) is appropriate for this client? Select all that apply.
1. Slide the client when turning the client.
2. Turn and reposition the client at least every 2 hours.
3. Apply lotion after bathing the client and vigorously massage the skin.
4. Post a turning schedule at the client's bedside.
5. Adapt position changes to the client's situation.
6. Apply an egg crate mattress to the client's bed.

32. The nurse is caring for a client who recently had a skin graft. Which information is **most** important for the nurse to include when educating the client?
1. Continue physical therapy.
2. Protect the graft from direct sunlight.
3. Use cosmetic camouflage techniques.
4. Apply lubricating lotion to the graft site.

33. The nurse is educating a client on how to prevent development of basal cell epithelioma. Which information is **most** important for the nurse to include in the teaching?
1. Avoid thermal burns.
2. Avoid exposure to sun.
3. Avoid immunosuppression.
4. Avoid exposure to radiation.

34. The nurse observes an older client's skin turgor and finds inelasticity present. What will the nurse do **next**?
1. Limit the client's oral intake.
2. Apply protective sleeves to extremities.
3. Document the finding.
4. Call the health care provider.

35. A client received burns to the entire back and left arm. Using the Rule of Nines, the nurse calculates that the client sustained burns to what percentage of the body? Record your answer using a whole number.

_____%

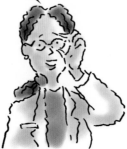

Stay focused. You're more than halfway done.

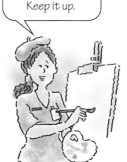

Beautiful work! Keep it up.

30. 2, 3, 4. Immunocompromised clients with herpes zoster require health care professionals to use airborne precautions until the lesions are crusted over. These precautions include wearing a gown, gloves, and a mask. Shoe covers are not needed. CN: Safe, effective care environment; CNS: Safety and infection control; CL: Analyze

31. 2, 4, 5, 6. A turning schedule with a signing sheet ensures that the client gets turned. When moving a client, lift rather than slide, to avoid shearing. A client in bed for prolonged periods should be turned every 1 to 2 hours. Apply lotion to keep the skin moist but refrain from vigorous massage to avoid damaging capillaries. Egg crate mattresses help to reduce pressure injuries. Adapting position changes to the client's situation helps ensure the client's comfort and prevents injury to the client. CN: Safe, effective care environment; CNS: Safety and infection control; CL: Apply

32. 2. To avoid burning and sloughing, the client must protect the graft from direct sunlight. The other three interventions are all helpful to the client and the client's recovery but are not as important. CN: Safe, effective care environment; CNS: Management of care; CL: Analyze

33. 2. The sun is the best known and most common cause of basal cell epithelioma. Thermal burns, immunosuppression, and radiation are less common causes. CN: Physiological integrity; CNS: Reduction of risk potential; CL: Apply

34. 3. The nurse should simply document the finding because inelastic skin turgor is a normal part of aging. Limiting oral fluids is not appropriate; overly hydrated skin would appear edematous and spongy. Protective sleeves and calling the health care provider is not indicated for expected findings. CN: Physiological integrity; CNS: Basic care and comfort; CL: Apply

35. 27. According to the Rule of Nines, the posterior trunk, anterior trunk, and legs are each 18% of the total body surface. The head, neck, and arms are each 9% of total body surface, and the perineum is 1%. In this case, the client received burns to the back (18%) and one arm (9%), totaling 27% of the body. CN: Physiological integrity; CNS: Reduction of risk potential; CL: Analyze

CN: Client needs category   CNS: Client needs subcategory   CL: Cognitive level

36. The nurse is caring for a client receiving psoralen plus ultraviolet A (PUVA) treatment. Which statement by the client indicates a proper understanding of this treatment?
1. "On the day of treatment, I need to stay out of the sun."
2. "Protective eyewear during the UV light treatment is not necessary."
3. "I need to wear sunglasses for 4 hours after the treatment."
4. "PUVA therapy is the use of UV light with topical ointments."

36. **1.** On the day of treatment, the client should stay out of the sun. Clients should wear sunglasses for 24 hours after treatment. The client should wear goggles during any exposure to UV light. PUVA therapy is UV light used with psoralens.
CN: Physiological integrity; CNS: Basic care and comfort; CL: Apply

37. The nurse is examining the back of a client who was admitted with stage III pressure injuries on the sacral area. Which illustration shows a stage III pressure injury?

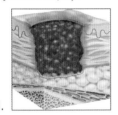
1.

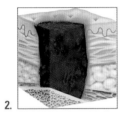
2.

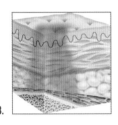
3.

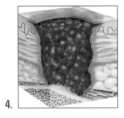
4.

37. **1.** In a stage III pressure injury, there is full-thickness skin loss along with damage or necrosis of the subcutaneous tissue. It may or may not extend down to (but not through) the fascia. Undermining may be present. Option 2 shows an unstageable pressure injury. In an unstageable pressure injury, the true stage of the injury cannot be determined until the base of the wound is exposed. Option 3 shows suspected deep tissue injury, which presents as a purple or maroon localized area of intact skin or blood-filled blister. Option 4 shows a stage IV pressure injury. In a stage IV pressure injury, there is full-thickness skin loss with extensive tissue destruction, tissue necrosis, or damage to the muscle, bone, or support structures.
CN: Physiological integrity; CNS: Physiological adaptation; CL: Apply

38. The nurse is caring for a client with a pressure injury on the sacrum. When educating the client about dietary intake, which food(s) will the nurse emphasize as **most** important for the client to consume? Select all that apply.
1. Quinoa
2. Whole-grain products
3. Fruits
4. Vegetables
5. Lean meats
6. Low-fat milk

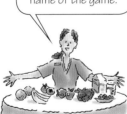
When it comes to healing injuries, proteins are the name of the game.

38. **1, 5, 6.** Although the client should eat a balanced diet with foods from all food groups, the diet should emphasize foods that supply complete protein, such as lean meats, quinoa, soy, beans, and low-fat milk. Protein helps build and repair body tissue, which promotes healing. Whole-grain products supply incomplete proteins and carbohydrates. Fruits and vegetables provide mainly carbohydrates.
CN: Physiological integrity; CNS: Basic care and comfort; CL: Apply

39. A client develops wound evisceration following abdominal surgery. Which nursing intervention is **priority**?
1. Give prophylactic antibiotics as prescribed.
2. Administer intravenous fluids.
3. Explain to the client what is happening.
4. Cover the organs with sterile saline-soaked gauze.

39. **4.** Evisceration requires emergency surgical repair. Covering the wound with sterile gauze moistened with sterile saline is essential to prevent the organs from drying. The gauze and saline must be sterile to reduce the risk of infection. Antibiotics are usually prescribed and started as soon as possible but are not the priority. The nurse should administer intravenous fluids, but covering the wound takes priority. While the nurse works quickly to prepare the client for surgery, explaining to the client what is happening would help reduce the client's anxiety, but it is not the priority for this client.
CN: Safe, effective care environment; CNS: Management of care; CL: Analyze

40. The nurse is preparing to perform a dressing change on a client with a stage III decubitus injury. Put the steps in the chronological order the nurse will perform them. Use all options.

1. Don gloves.

2. Wash hands thoroughly.

3. Apply a new dressing to the site.

4. Slowly remove the soiled dressing.

5. Observe the site for the amount, type, and odor of drainage.

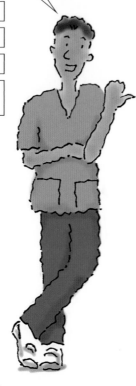

This question is all about putting the steps in the right order.

40. Ordered Response:

2. Wash hands thoroughly.

1. Don gloves.

4. Slowly remove the soiled dressing.

5. Observe the site for the amount, type, and odor of drainage.

3. Apply a new dressing to the site.

CN: Physiological integrity; CNS: Basic care and comfort; CL: Apply

41. Which nursing action is **priority** to prevent complications in an immobilized client?
1. Provide a high-protein diet.
2. Turn every 1 to 2 hours.
3. Assess the skin each shift.
4. Keep the client supine.

41. 2. Turning the client every 1 to 2 hours prevents pressure areas from developing and helps prevent atelectasis and other pulmonary complications. A high-protein diet aids in healing skin but does not prevent complications. Assessing the skin aids in finding areas of concern but does not prevent complications. The client should spend time supine according to the turning schedule (not be kept supine indefinitely). During that period, the head of the bed should be raised to prevent the client from aspirating.
CN: Physiological integrity; CNS: Basic care and comfort; CL: Analyze

42. The nurse is instructing a client regarding hypersensitivity after administering a skin test. Which instruction is **most** important for the nurse to include when discussing the skin test?
1. Wash the sites daily with a mild soap.
2. Read the sites on the correct date.
3. Keep the skin test areas moist with a mild lotion.
4. Stay out of direct sunlight until the tests are read.

42. 2. An important facet of evaluating skin tests is to read the skin test results at the proper time. Evaluating the skin test too late or too early gives inaccurate, unreliable results. There is no need to wash the test sites with soap. The sites should be kept dry. Direct sunlight is not prohibited.
CN: Health promotion and maintenance; CNS: None; CL: Apply

43. A client is brought to the emergency department with partial-thickness and full-thickness burns over 15% of the body. Admission vital signs are: blood pressure of 100/50 mm Hg, heart rate of 130 beats/minute, and respiratory rate of 26 breaths/minute. Which nursing intervention(s) is appropriate for this client? Select all that apply.
1. Clean the burns with hydrogen peroxide.
2. Cover the burns with saline-soaked towels.
3. Begin an intravenous (IV) infusion of lactated Ringer's solution.
4. Place ice directly on the burn areas.
5. Administer 6 mg of morphine IV.
6. Administer tetanus prophylaxis, as prescribed.

43. 3, 5, 6. Immediate interventions for this client should aim to stop the burning and relieve the pain. The nurse should begin IV therapy with a crystalloid, such as lactated Ringer's solution, to prevent hypovolemic shock and to maintain cardiac output. Typically, 2 to 25 mg of morphine are administered IV in small increments to treat pain. Tetanus prophylaxis should also be administered, as prescribed. Hydrogen peroxide and povidone-iodine solution could further damage tissue, and saline-soaked towels could lead to hypothermia. Ice placed directly on burn wounds could cause further thermal damage.
CN: Physiological integrity; CNS: Physiological adaptation; CL: Apply

44. A client is prescribed methotrexate 25 mg by mouth as a single weekly dose. The pharmacy dispenses 2.5 mg scored tablets. How many tablets will the nurse instruct the client to take to achieve the prescribed dose? Record your answer using a whole number.

_____ tablets

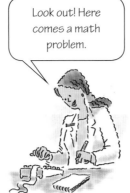

Look out! Here comes a math problem.

44. 10.

The correct formula to calculate a drug dose is:

$$\frac{Dose\ on\ hand}{Quantity\ on\ hand} = \frac{Dose\ desired}{X}$$

The health care provider prescribes 25 mg, which is the dose desired. The pharmacy dispenses 2.5-mg tablets, which is the dose on hand.

$$\frac{2.5\ mg}{1\ tablet} = \frac{25\ mg}{X}$$

$$X = 10\ tablets$$

CN: Physiological integrity; CNS: Pharmacological and parenteral therapies; CL: Apply

45. A client who is 5 ft 4 in (1.63 m) and weighs 145 lb (66 kg) is admitted to the long-term care facility. The admitting nurse takes this report: "The client sits for long periods in a wheelchair and has bowel and bladder incontinence. The client has a fair appetite, eating best at breakfast, and is often observed to be crying and depressed. Medications include daily use of sedatives." The nurse knows which factors place the client at risk for developing a pressure injury? Select all that apply.
1. Weight
2. Incontinence
3. Sitting for long periods
4. Sedation
5. Crying and depression
6. Decreased appetite

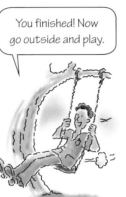

You finished! Now go outside and play.

45. 2, 3, 4. Inactivity, immobility, incontinence, and sedation are all risk factors for developing pressure injuries. The client's weight and poor eating habits at lunch and dinner are not directly related to the risk of developing pressure injuries, but a calorie count should be taken to see whether the client is getting adequate calories and fluids because poor nutrition can contribute to pressure injuries. The fact that the client cries and is depressed has no direct bearing on this client's risk for developing a pressure injury. However, clients with depression are commonly not as active, so this client's activity levels should be monitored closely to minimize inactivity.

CN: Physiological integrity; CNS: Reduction of risk potential; CL: Analyze

Part III

Care of the Psychiatric Client

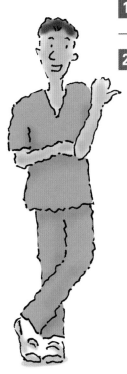

Part III

Care of the Psychiatric Client

Chapter 12

Somatic Symptom & Related Disorders

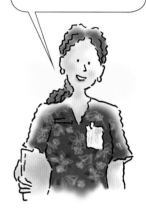

Can't remember much about a particular somatic symptom disorder? Type this address into your Internet browser: www.emedicine.com. Then search for the disorder. Cool!

Somatic symptom & related disorders refresher

Conversion disorder (Functional neurologic symptoms disorder)

When physiologic symptoms appear as a result of a psychological condition

Key signs and symptoms
- La belle indifference (a lack of concern about the symptoms or limitation on functioning)

Key test results
- Absence of expected diagnostic findings can confirm the disorder

Key treatments
- Individual therapy

Key interventions
- Establish supportive relationship that communicates acceptance of the client but keeps focus away from symptoms
- Review all laboratory and diagnostic study results
- Neurologic examination

Pain disorder

Presence of chronic or severe pain that is not supported by a physiologic condition

Key signs and symptoms
- May be attributed to a combination of factors
- Anger, frustration, and depression
- Drug-seeking behavior in an attempt to relieve pain
- History of frequent visits to multiple health care providers to seek pain relief
- Insomnia

Key test results
- Test results do not support client reports

Key treatments
- Individual therapy
- Tricyclic antidepressants: amitriptyline, imipramine, doxepin

Key interventions
- Acknowledge client's pain
- Encourage client to recognize situations that precipitate pain

Sleep–wake disorders

Characterized by impaired sleep quality or quantity

Key signs and symptoms
Insomnia disorder
- History of light or easily disturbed sleep, or difficulty falling asleep
- Insomnia

Breathing-related sleep disorder
- Obstructive sleep apnea hypopnea
- Central sleep apnea
- Sleep-related hypoventilation

Narcolepsy
- Cataplexy (bilateral loss of muscle tone triggered by strong emotion)
- Generalized daytime sleepiness
- Hypnagogic hallucination (intense dreamlike images)
- Irresistible attacks of refreshing sleep
- Hypocretin deficiency

Key test results
- Polysomnography is diagnostic for individual sleep disorder

Key treatments
- Hypnotic: zolpidem

Key interventions
Insomnia disorder and circadian rhythm disturbance
- Encourage client to discuss concerns that may be preventing sleep.
- Schedule regular sleep and awakening times.

Breathing-related sleep disorder
- Administer continuous positive airway pressure (CPAP).

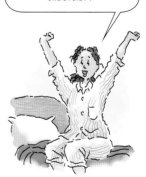

Is trouble getting out of bed in the morning a sleep disorder?

Neurodevelopmental disorders

Characterized by developmental delays in personal, social, academic, or occupational functioning

Key signs and symptoms

Autism spectrum disorder
- Impaired social interaction skills
- Communication impairment
- Stereotypical behavioral patterns
- Little eye contact
- Few facial expressions to others

Tic disorders
- Rapid, recurring motor movement or vocal sounds
- Blinking, clearing the throat, sniffing, snorting, barking
- Repetition of words, coprolalia (use of socially inappropriate words)
- Palilalia (repeating one's own sounds or words)
- Echolalia (repeating last word or phrase said)

Key test results

Autism spectrum disorder
- Generally identified by 18 months of age and should be identified by no later than 3 years of age
- Behavioral testing for definitive diagnosis

Tic disorders
- Magnetic resonance imaging
- Behavioral observation

Key treatments

Autism spectrum disorder
- Individualized treatment
- Special education and language therapy
- Cognitive behavioral therapy
- Antipsychotics: haloperidol, risperidone

Tic disorders
- Antipsychotics: risperidone, olanzapine

Key interventions

Autism spectrum disorder
- Prevent injury.
- Promote learning and development.

Tic Disorders
- Encourage client to get plenty of rest.
- Assist with stress management.

Attention deficit hyperactivity disorder (ADHD)

Neurobehavioral disorder that interferes with a person's ability to stay on task and to exercise age-appropriate inhibition (cognitive alone or both cognitive and behavioral).

Key signs and symptoms

- Inability to sit still
- Difficult for child to carry on a conversation
- Behavioral immaturity
- Labile mood with temper tantrums
- Poor judgment and decision making

Key test results

- Behavioral observation

Key treatments

- Central nervous system stimulants: methylphenidate, amphetamine
- Antidepressants such as atomoxetine
- Antihypertensives such as clonidine

Key interventions

- Ensure safety
- Structure the daily routine
- Support for family members

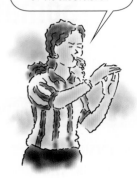

Time out! Can you list some of the key signs and symptoms of tic disorders?

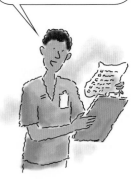

Can you name some of the common medications used to treat ADHD?

thePoint® You can download tables of drug information to help you prepare for the NCLEX®! View Generic Drug Names, Drug Classifications, Drug Actions, and Nursing Implications for the drugs discussed in this refresher at **http://thePoint.lww.com**

Somatic symptom & related disorders questions, answers, and rationales

1. Which statement will the nurse include when teaching clients who have somatic symptom disorder?
1. "They usually seek medical attention."
2. "They have organic pathologic disorders."
3. "They regularly attend psychotherapy sessions."
4. "They are eager to learn the reasons for their physical symptoms."

1. 1. A client with a somatic symptom disorder usually seeks medical attention. These clients have a history of reporting multiple physiologic symptoms without associated demonstrable, organic pathologic causes. The expected behavior for this type of disorder is to seek treatment from several medical health care providers for somatic symptoms, not psychiatric evaluation.
CN: Psychosocial integrity; CNS: None; CL: Apply

CN: Client needs category   CNS: Client needs subcategory   CL: Cognitive level

2. The health care provider has prescribed methylphenidate. Which finding(s) in the client's medical history concerns the nurse about this therapy? Select all that apply.
1. The client has a history of alcoholism.
2. The client has a familial history of hypoglycemia.
3. The client has type 1 diabetes mellitus.
4. The client has a history of gallbladder disease.
5. The client's history indicates a recent myocardial infarction.

3. Which question asked by the nurse **best** assesses for possible trigger of physical symptoms in a client diagnosed with a somatic symptom disorder?
1. "Have you ever been told you were expressing delusional thinking?"
2. "Are you comfortable being the center of attention in social situations?"
3. "Are you currently experiencing symptoms of anxiety or depression?"
4. "Are your family members a source of support for you?"

4. The nurse is talking with a client who has been taking amphetamine salt combo for the past 3 weeks. Which statement(s) by the client indicate the medication is having the desired effects? Select all that apply.
1. "I feel jittery in the morning."
2. "I have been sleeping well at night."
3. "My appetite is somewhat reduced."
4. "I feel increasingly focused at work."
5. "I am feeling less depressed."

5. A client reports of chronic pain to the nurse during the assessment. The client's history reveals numerous visits to the health care provider for pain relief. Which nursing intervention(s) will be effective in caring for this client? Select all that apply.
1. Low-dose narcotic analgesics
2. Behavioral therapy
3. Relaxation techniques
4. Hypnosis
5. Tricyclic antidepressants

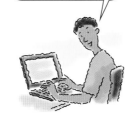

Remember to "select all that apply" in question #2.

2. **1, 5.** Methylphenidate is addictive. Any history of alcohol or drug use past or current would warrant concern for the administration of this medication. The medication may be contraindicated in the presence of cardiac disorders. Health concerns such as hypoglycemia, diabetes, and gallbladder disease are not contraindications for the use of methylphenidate.
CN: Physiological integrity; CNS: Pharmacological and parenteral therapies; CL: Apply

3. **3.** Anxiety and depression commonly occur in somatic symptom disorders. The client prevents or relieves symptoms of anxiety by focusing on physical symptoms. Somatic delusions are not characteristic of somatic symptom disorders but rather occur in schizophrenia. The symptoms allow the client to avoid unpleasant activity, not to seek individual attention. Somatization in dysfunctional families shifts the open conflict to the client's illness, thus providing some stability for the family, not the client. Such a family dynamic is not likely to be a trigger for the symptoms but rather a secondary gain.
CN: Psychosocial integrity; CNS: None; CL: Apply

4. **2, 4.** Amphetamine salt combo is used to treat attention deficit hyperactivity disorder (ADHD). Individuals with this condition experience difficulty focusing on tasks. Amphetamine salt combo will modify the brain's chemistry and promote increased abilities to focus on tasks. Improvements in sleep patterns may also be noted with this medication. Feeling jittery may occur with the medication and is considered a side effect, not a desired effect. Appetite changes may occur but are not associated with the desired effects of the medication. Mood alteration is not the intended outcome of medication therapy with this drug.
CN: Physiological integrity; CNS: Pharmacological and parenteral therapies; CL: Apply

5. **2, 3, 4, 5.** When caring for the client with chronic pain the focus should be on promoting skills to improve the client's coping with regard to the discomfort. The use of narcotic medications should be avoided. They are habit forming and problematic when managing chronic pain disorders. Behavioral therapies focusing on stress reduction and coping are recommended. Relaxation techniques should be taught to the client. Hypnosis may also be employed. Pharmacologic therapies may include tricyclic antidepressants.
CN: Physiological integrity; CNS: Reduction of risk potential; CL: Apply

6. Parents of an 8-year-old child inform the school nurse they believe their child has attention deficit hyperactivity disorder (ADHD). Which statement(s) made by the parents supports the suspected diagnosis? Select all that apply.
   1. "My child cries a lot and frequently states 'Momma, I am unhappy.'"
   2. "It is concerning that my child has missed so much school because of stomach aches."
   3. "It is embarrassing that my child is never still and always fidgets."
   4. "My child has a temper and throws tantrums daily."
   5. "It worries me that my child will go up and talk to anyone even total strangers."

7. The nurse observes a child with autism banging his head against the floor repetitively. Which nursing action is **priority**?
   1. Apply a helmet on the child.
   2. Administer risperidone to the child.
   3. Place restraints on the child.
   4. Allow the child to continue the behavior.

8. A parent of a child with autism asks the nurse, "Will my child ever get better?" Which statement(s) will be included in the response by the nurse? Select all that apply.
   1. "Most likely, your child will always be like this."
   2. "This is chronic and your child's behavior will get worse."
   3. "With behavioral therapy, your child's symptoms may get better."
   4. "Since your child cannot recover, institutionalization will likely be needed".
   5. "Medication therapies may help to improve your child's condition."

9. A client is exhibiting anxiety. The nurse notes muscle tension, distractibility, and increased heart rate and blood pressure. Which nursing intervention is **priority**?
   1. Remain with the client, using a soft voice and reassuring approach.
   2. Assist the client to identify factors that contribute to anxiety.
   3. Educate the client on relaxation techniques.
   4. Administer antianxiety medications as appropriate.

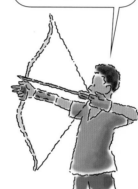

Looks like you're right on target. Keep up the good work.

6. 3, 5. One of the hallmark characteristic behaviors of a child with ADHD is that the child has difficulty sitting or standing still. This behavior makes it difficult for the child to succeed in school. The child is not usually sad or withdrawn or prone to temper tantrums but is likely to be outgoing and talkative. It is not a characteristic of ADHD for children to be absent from school with reports of vague stomach problems.
CN: Physiological integrity; CNS: Physiological adaptation; CL: Apply

7. 1. The priority for all clients is their safety. A helmet should be applied to this child with autistic disorder so that the child will not sustain a head injury. It is not necessary to administer risperidone at this time to the child. Restraining the child will increase the behavior and cause more anxiety and stress reactions. The child may continue the behavior but should be protected.
CN: Safe, effective care environment; CNS: Safety and infection control; CL: Analyze

8. 3, 5. Autism may improve when children begin to use speech to communicate. It will require a considerable commitment from the parents to assist the child with improving behaviors and, in some instances, special programs and schools. Medication therapies are commonly incorporated into the plan of care. The behavior usually does not get worse unless these programs are not utilized. There is no reason that the child will require institutionalization.
CN: Health promotion and maintenance; CNS: None; CL: Apply

9. 1. The priority nursing intervention is to remain with the client and use a soft voice and reassuring approach. Remaining with the client provides for his or her safety, and a soft voice is calming and reassuring, which will add to the client's feelings of safety and protection. Interventions such as identifying factors that contribute to anxiety, teaching relaxation techniques, and administering antianxiety medications are included in the client's care plan but should be addressed later.
CN: Safe, effective care environment; CNS: Management of care; CL: Apply

10. A client has been diagnosed with a tic disorder. Which information will the nurse provide to help the client reduce the frequency of the tics? Select all that apply.
1. Increase medications following tics.
2. Be sure to get plenty of rest.
3. Avoid extremes in temperature.
4. Decrease the amount of protein in the diet.
5. Reduce the level of stress in your life.

11. The nurse is providing teaching for a client prescribed triazolam. Which statement made by the client indicates an understanding of the information provided?
1. "I should take the medication with citrus juice."
2. "I should not confuse this medication with haloperidol."
3. "It is okay to take a short drive after taking the medication."
4. "It is okay to smoke while I take this medication."

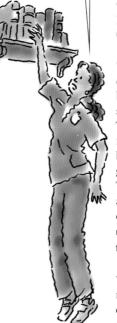

Hmm. What was that I read about reducing tic frequency?

12. A client has been diagnosed with a conversion disorder after presenting with reports of new-onset paralysis in a lower extremity. When providing education about this phenomenon to a group of nurses, which information will the nurse include? Select all that apply.
1. Symptom onset may be due to psychological stressors.
2. The onset of the symptoms is normally gradual.
3. Many symptoms will reoccur in one year.
4. Most symptoms will resolve.
5. Ignoring the manifestations is recommended.

13. A client is diagnosed with conversion disorder with paralysis of the legs. Which is the **best** nursing intervention for this client?
1. Discuss with the client ways to live with the paralysis.
2. Focus interactions on results of medical tests.
3. Encourage the client to move the legs as much as possible.
4. Avoid focusing on the client's physical limitations.

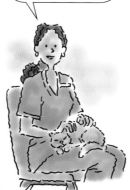

Relax. You're doing fine.

14. A client reports difficulty falling and staying asleep to the nurse. Which statement will the nurse include when educating this client?
1. "Behavior therapy techniques like aversion therapy are effective in managing insomnia."
2. "I will arrange for you to get literature on the effects of biofeedback and muscle relaxation."
3. "Group therapy will introduce you to others with similar sleep related problems."
4. "While insight-oriented psychotherapy is time consuming, it will best help your sleep."

10. 2, 5. It is important that the client gets ample rest and uses stress reduction techniques to control the tics or motor responses. Stress and fatigue are shown to increase these symptoms. The client should not increase any medication without a health care provider's prescription. Avoiding extreme temperatures and decreasing the amount of protein in the diet do not have any effect on the tics.
CN: Physiological integrity; CNS: Physiological adaptation; CL: Apply

11. 2. Triazolam is an antipsychotic that is used for clients with psychoses, Tourette's syndrome, severe behavioral problems in children, and emergency sedation of severely agitated, psychotic clients. Triazolam is one of a group of sedative-hypnotic medications that can be used only for a limited time because of the risk of dependency. Grapefruit and grapefruit juices can alter the absorption of triazolam. The client should avoid driving and tasks that require alertness or motor skills because the medication may cause drowsiness. Smoking reduces drug effectiveness.
CN: Physiological integrity; CNS: Pharmacological and parenteral therapies; CL: Apply

12. 1, 4. A conversion disorder results in the manifestation of physiologic symptoms that have developed in response to psychological stressors. The disorder usually suddenly occurs. A full recovery is normal. Approximately 25% of those affected will experience a reoccurrence of symptomatology. Ignoring the physical manifestations is not recommended.
CN: Physiological integrity; CNS: Physiological adaptation; CL: Apply

13. 4. The paralysis is used as an unhealthy way of expressing unmet psychological needs. The nurse should avoid speaking about the paralysis to shift the client's attention to the mental aspect of the disorder. The other interventions focus too much on the paralysis, instead of recognizing the underlying psychological motivations.
CN: Psychosocial integrity; CNS: None; CL: Apply

14. 2. Biofeedback, relaxation therapy, and psychopharmacology are appropriate treatments for sleep disorders. Biofeedback can be useful in identifying and managing muscle tension that interferes with effective sleep. Behavior therapy, group therapy, and insight-oriented psychotherapy are treatments related to somatic symptom disorders and are not generally associated with the treatment of sleep related disorders.
CN: Physiological integrity; CNS: Basic care and comfort; CL: Apply

15. What information will the nurse include when educating a client newly diagnosed with cataplexy?
1. Cataplexy causes an irresistible need to sleep especially during the day.
2. This sleep disorder is sometimes the result of a neuropeptide deficiency.
3. Intense, vivid dreams are a characteristic of this sleep disorder.
4. Emotions can trigger a loss of muscle tone, resulting in a fall.

16. The nurse is planning care for a client with a psychophysiologic disorder. The nurse will include nursing interventions to address which symptoms?
1. The physical symptoms that are life-threatening.
2. The physical symptoms that are distressing the client.
3. Physical symptoms and psychosocial and spiritual problems.
4. The psychosocial symptoms that are concerning to the client.

17. Which client statement(s) will cause the nurse to assess the client for insomnia? Select all that apply.
1. "I am really a very light sleeper."
2. "I wake up at least 4 times a night."
3. "It takes hours for me to fall asleep."
4. "I have such vivid dreams every night."
5. "I generally only sleep 5 hours each night."

18. The nurse is caring for a client being evaluated for a diagnosis of conversion disorder manifested by paralysis in the left arm. Which nursing intervention(s) is appropriate for this client? Select all that apply.
1. Perform neurological assessments as prescribed and warranted.
2. Perform routine physical tasks for the client to foster a sense of caring.
3. Encourage the client to describe the impact of the physical limitations.
4. Review laboratory and diagnostic study results as they become available.
5. Demonstrate acceptance of the client as an individual with a physical problem.

How many sheep do I have to count to fall asleep? Curse you, mocha latte!

15. 4. Cataplexy is a form of narcolepsy that results in the bilateral loss of muscle tone that is triggered by any form of strong emotion. Irresistible attacks of sleep are associated with narcolepsy. Narcolepsy can be a result of a deficiency of hypocretin. A hypnagogic hallucination is an intense dream-like experience.
CN: Physiological integrity; CNS: Basic care and comfort; CL: Apply

16. 3. Physical, psychosocial, and spiritual problems are thoroughly and continuously assessed with each client. The nurse must include all symptoms, even those that are not life-threatening, and consider all physical symptoms, even those the client does not find distressing. Psychosocial symptoms should be considered, but all three areas must be assessed to provide a thorough care plan.
CN: Psychosocial integrity; CNS: None; CL: Apply

17. 1, 2, 3. Insomnia is characterized by a history of light or easily disturbed sleep, waking multiple times during the night, and a history of difficulty falling asleep. Vivid dreams are associated with hypnagogic hallucinations, not insomnia. Although sleeping only 5 hours per night may not allow for sufficient rest, it is not a factor related to insomnia.
CN: Physiological integrity; CNS: Basic care and comfort; CL: Analyze

18. 1, 4, 5. The nature of the physiological symptom requires regular neurological assessment to best insure client safety and minimize risk for injury. The review of laboratory and diagnostic study results are necessary to manage potential physiological injury risks. The diagnosis of conversion disorder as the cause of the physiological symptom, depends on the realization that the diagnostic results fail to provide a physiological cause for the symptom. Establishment of a supportive relationship with the client is based on caring and respect; in this situation caring and respect must include an acceptance of the client's problem as being real. The nurse should support the client in being as independent as possible and intervene only when the client requires assistance thus encouraging the client to perform physical activities to the greatest extent possible. The nurse should not focus on the disability but rather support the client in discussing the factors that may be contributing to the emotional trauma that is triggering the physical symptoms.
CN: Psychosocial integrity; CNS: None; CL: Apply

19. Which statement by the nurse reflects an understanding of the key intervention for a client diagnosed with a breathing-related sleep disorder?
1. "It is important to manage stress because it may be interfering with your sleep."
2. "Let us discuss the possible side effects of your prescribed zolpidem."
3. "Bedtime should be at the same scheduled time even on the weekends."
4. "Remember to clean your CPAP machine regularly."

20. The parent of a client approaches the nurses' station in tears and says she is upset about her child's diagnosis of conversion disorder. Which nursing response is **best**?
1. "Tell me what it is that upsets you the most."
2. "Are you afraid your child will never get well?"
3. "Her behavior is typical for conversion disorder."
4. "Let me give you some information about the illness."

21. Which outcome is **most** appropriate for the nurse to set for a teenager who is irritable, has not slept well in 6 months, and has dropped out of social activities?
1. The client will sleep well at night and remain focused during the day.
2. The parents will stop worrying about the client's behavior.
3. The client will obtain appropriate mental health services.
4. The parents will impose behavior guidelines for the client to follow.

22. Which nursing intervention will be included for an anxious client who reports difficulty settling down for sleep?
1. Educate the client on time management skills.
2. Educate the client on conflict resolution skills.
3. Educate the client on progressive muscle relaxation.
4. Educate the client on adverse effects of antipsychotic medication.

23. How will the nurse describe conversion disorder to a newly diagnosed client?
1. "Conversion disorder symptoms are voluntarily created by the client."
2. "The trigger of conversion disorder symptoms is psychological in nature."
3. "Medications are the most viable treatment option for clients with conversion disorder."
4. "Conversion disorder symptoms are often gastrointestinal or cardiac in nature."

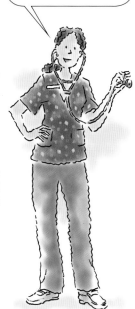

When your client is upset, practice your listening skills.

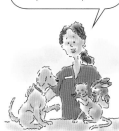

Feeling stressed? Take a break and try some pet therapy.

19. 4. A continuous positive airway pressure (CPAP) machine is the key intervention prescribed for breathing-related sleep disorders. Stress management, the medication zolpidem, and regularly scheduled sleep and awakening times are helpful when managing insomnia and circadian rhythm disorders.
CN: Physiological integrity; CNS: Basic care and comfort; CL: Apply

20. 1. Asking the parent an open-ended question permits the nurse to collect data reported in the parent's own words. The other responses narrow the data collection process prematurely. Also, it is important to hear what the parent has to say without planting suggestions about the child's condition.
CN: Psychosocial integrity; CNS: None; CL: Apply

21. 3. Mental health services can protect the client and offer the best means of regaining mental health. The client could reestablish a healthy sleeping pattern without addressing underlying issues. The parents' worry is unrelated to the child's immediate need for help. The child's behavior suggests the need for professional mental health services, not disciplinary measures.
CN: Psychosocial integrity; CNS: None; CL: Apply

22. 3. Progressive muscle relaxation is a systematic tensing and relaxing of separate muscle groups. As the technique is mastered, relaxation results. Time management skills and conflict resolution skills are helpful in an overall effort to reduce stress and anxiety, but do not provide immediate relief in an effort to sleep. Antipsychotic medications are not usually used to treat anxiety or difficulty with sleep.
CN: Psychosocial integrity; CNS: None; CL: Apply

23. 2. A conversion disorder occurs when physiological symptoms are a result of a psychological condition. In conversion disorders, the client is not conscious of intentionally producing symptoms that cannot be self-controlled. The symptoms are characterized by one or more neurologic symptoms. Understanding the principles and conflicts behind the symptoms can prove helpful during a client's individualized cognitive and behavioral therapy. Medication is not generally effective for this condition but can be prescribed for comorbid conditions such as depression.
CN: Psychosocial integrity; CNS: None; CL: Understand

24. Which statement made by the parent of a child being treated for attention deficit hyperactivity disorder (ADHD) demonstrates to the nurse an understanding of the child's needs?
1. "He is happiest when he is allowed to do what he wants."
2. "We keep him on a regular sleeping and eating schedule."
3. "He is medicated when his behavior is really out of control."
4. "We allow him to make his own decisions, to encourage autonomy."

25. The nurse will include information on which potential side effect associated with risperidone when educating the parents of a 15-month-old diagnosed with autism spectrum disorder?
1. Loss of appetite
2. Involuntary motions of the head or extremities
3. Frequent bouts of nausea and vomiting
4. Severe disruption of normal sleep patterns

26. The nurse will expect to assess which classic behavior in a client diagnosed with pain disorder?
1. Reports hopelessness.
2. Has difficulty sleeping.
3. Tends to socially isolate.
4. Has multiple health care providers.

27. The parents of a child with attention deficit hyperactivity disorder (ADHD) say they are concerned because the child is losing weight. Which recommendation(s) will the nurse give to the parents? Select all that apply.
1. Have high-calorie finger foods available for the child to eat.
2. Decrease the amount of medications being taken.
3. Force the child to sit for three meals a day with the family.
4. Administer an appetite stimulant to the child daily.
5. Encourage the child to eat small, frequent meals.

28. Which nursing action will **best** help a client with conversion disorder blindness to eat?
1. Direct the client to independently locate items on the tray and feed himself.
2. See to the needs of the other clients in the dining room, and then feed this client last.
3. Establish a "buddy" system with other clients who can feed the client at each meal.
4. Expect the client to feed himself after explaining the location of food on the tray.

24. 2. ADHD interferes with a person's ability to stay on task and to exercise age-appropriate inhibition related to cognition and behavior. A structured daily routine provides support for the individual. Decision making requires intervention because judgment is often impaired. Medication therapy is prescribed to be used on a regular basis, not to be introduced only when behavior becomes uncontrollable or dangerous.
CN: Psychosocial integrity; CNS: None; CL: Analyze

25. 2. The treatment plan for autism spectrum disorder generally includes an antipsychotic medication such as risperidone. Risperidone can cause extrapyramidal effects that include involuntary motions of the head, neck, arms, body, or eyes. Clonidine, atomoxetine, and methylphenidate are generally prescribed as a part of the treatment plan for attention deficit hyperactivity disorder (ADHD) and can cause the other side effects mentioned.
CN: Psychosocial integrity; CNS: None; CL: Apply

26. 4. A client diagnosed with pain disorder is likely to have a long history of establishing relationships with a multitude of health care providers. Insomnia, social isolation, and depression-induced hopelessness may occur but are not unique to pain disorders.
CN: Psychosocial integrity; CNS: None; CL: Apply

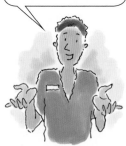

Sometimes lifestyle changes are the best way to meet a client's needs.

27. 1, 5. Because it is difficult for children with ADHD to sit still while eating, it is acceptable to keep high-calorie finger foods available to avoid the weight loss that can accompany this disorder. Small, frequent meals promote continuous intake throughout the day. The medication should not be decreased without a health care provider's prescription. The child should not be forced to sit at the table. An appetite stimulant is not necessary if foods are offered.
CN: Health promotion and maintenance; CNS: None; CL: Apply

28. 4. The client is expected to maintain some level of independence by feeding himself. At the same time, the nurse should be supportive in a matter-of-fact way. Feeding the client leads to dependence.
CN: Physiological integrity; CNS: Basic care and comfort; CL: Apply

CN: Client needs category   CNS: Client needs subcategory   CL: Cognitive level

29. When the nurse is speaking with a client diagnosed with conversion disorder, which nursing statement(s) will be **most** helpful? Select all that apply.
1. "Tell me why you think you are having vision trouble."
2. "I am going to sit with you while you are watching television."
3. "Can you describe to me how you are feeling today?"
4. "Explain how you are going to live alone if you cannot feel your left leg."
5. "You need to talk about the accident if you ever want to feel better."

30. The nurse expects which behavior in a client with a suspected conversion disorder?
1. Client states, "I am the only one who can solve the world's problems."
2. Client frequently observed crying whenever left alone.
3. Client reports sudden episodes of unexplainable dread.
4. Client reports, "All of a sudden, I could not see."

31. A client diagnosed with conversion disorder has a nursing diagnosis of Interrupted Family Processes related to the disability. Which goal will the nurse set for this client?
1. The client will resume former roles and tasks.
2. The client will take over roles of other family members.
3. The client will rely on family members to meet all client needs.
4. The client will focus energy on problems occurring in the family.

32. The nurse is reviewing the medical record of a client hospitalized with a conversion disorder. Which finding(s) will the nurse expect? Select all that apply.
1. A history of depression.
2. A history of sexual abuse.
3. Frequent use of marijuana.
4. A history of hypothyroidism.
5. Increased weight gain.

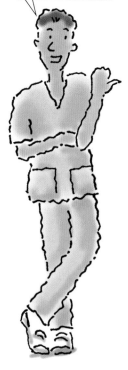

In conversion disorder, it's better to distract from than to emphasize symptoms.

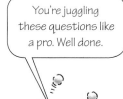

You're juggling these questions like a pro. Well done.

29. 2, 3. Establishing a supportive relationship that communicates acceptance of the client but keeps the focus away from symptoms is key in working with clients with conversion disorder. Using therapeutic communication techniques such as offering self and using open-ended questions is a way to establish a supportive relationship. Requesting an explanation, such as asking why, and probing are both nontherapeutic communication techniques. The focus of the care should not be on the loss of independence. This line of communication would not be therapeutic.
CN: Psychosocial integrity; CNS: None; CL: Apply

30. 4. Symptoms of conversion disorders are neurologic in nature (paralysis, blindness). Delusional disorders are characterized by delusions. Mood disorders are characterized by abnormal feelings of depression or euphoria. Anxiety is characterized by a feeling of dread.
CN: Health promotion and maintenance; CNS: None; CL: Apply

31. 1. The client who uses somatization has typically adopted a sick role in the family, characterized by dependence. Increasing independence—not relying on family members to meet all needs—and resumption of former roles are necessary to change this pattern. The client should not be expected to take on the roles or responsibilities of other family members. The client's treatment goal should focus on improving the client's condition, which is what is interrupting his family's processes, not on problems occurring in the family, which may or may not relate to his conditions.
CN: Psychosocial integrity; CNS: None; CL: Apply

32. 1, 2. A conversion disorder is a neurologic disorder in which psychological stressors are manifested with the display of physical disorders for which there is not a related cause. Conversion disorders are more common in those with a history of psychological disorders, including mood disorders. A history of neglect or sexual abuse may be noted in the medical record. Drug use is not tied to conversion disorders. Hypothyroidism and weight gain are not associated with conversion disorders.
CN: Psychosocial integrity; CNS: None; CL: Apply

33. Which question(s) are appropriate for the nurse to ask while assessing a client with a suspected tic disorder? Select all that apply.
1. "Do you have a habit of making unusual sounds in public?"
2. "Have you ever found yourself involuntary saying obscene words?"
3. "Have you ever dropped to the floor because your legs got weak?"
4. "Are you experiencing bladder or bowel incontinence?"
5. "Do you regularly repeat what others say to you?"

34. The nurse is preparing an educational program for new graduate nurses. Which information about conversion disorder will the nurse include? Select all that apply.
1. Work to establish a therapeutic relationship with the client.
2. Set limits on time spent discussing the client's symptoms.
3. *La belle indifference* is a key symptom in conversion disorder.
4. The focus of care needs to be on the client's symptoms.
5. Individualized therapy is the key treatment for this disorder.

35. Which client statement indicates to the nurse the goal of stress management has been attained?
1. "Both of my arms have been hurting occasionally the past few days."
2. "I am able to find joy in being dependent on others around me."
3. "I do not really understand what I am doing in this place."
4. "My muscles feel relaxed after progressive relaxation exercise."

36. The health care provider prescribes secobarbital sodium 75 mg by mouth at bedtime for a client with insomnia. The nurse has secobarbital sodium 25 mg tablets on hand. How many tablets will the nurse administer to the client? Record your answer using whole numbers.

_____ tablets

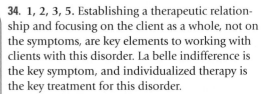

In conversion disorder, psychological concerns are "converted" to physical symptoms such as paralysis and blindness.

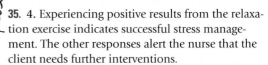

33. 1, 2, 5. Tic disorder is often characterized by involuntary barking, snorting, coprolalia (the use of socially inappropriate words), and echolalia (repeating the last word or phrase said). Neither drop seizures nor incontinence is associated with tic disorder.

CN: Psychosocial integrity; CNS: None; CL: Apply

34. 1, 2, 3, 5. Establishing a therapeutic relationship and focusing on the client as a whole, not on the symptoms, are key elements to working with clients with this disorder. La belle indifference is the key symptom, and individualized therapy is the key treatment for this disorder.

CN: Psychosocial integrity; CNS: None; CL: Apply

35. 4. Experiencing positive results from the relaxation exercise indicates successful stress management. The other responses alert the nurse that the client needs further interventions.

CN: Physiological integrity; CNS: Basic care and comfort; CL: Analyze

36. 3.
Each tablet contains 25 mg of the medication. The correct formula to calculate this drug dose is:

$$Dose\ of\ each\ tablet \times X = Prescribed\ dose,$$

where X is the number of tablets.

$$25\ mg/tablet \times X = 75\ mg.$$

$$X = 75\ mg \div 25\ mg/tablet.$$

$$X = 3\ tablets.$$

CN: Physiological integrity; CNS: Pharmacological and parenteral therapies; CL: Apply

37. Which intervention will the nurse recommend to the parents of a child with attention deficit hyperactivity disorder (ADHD) to help the child achieve daily tasks?
1. "Change the routine of the child daily to avoid repetition."
2. "Repeat information to the child several times during the day."
3. "Give general direction for the task to be completed."
4. "Break up each task given to the child into smaller steps."

38. A nurse is teaching the family of a client diagnosed with a pain disorder. Which statement made by the nurse **most** accurately describes this disorder?
1. "It is a preoccupation with pain in the absence of physical disease."
2. "It is physical or somatic symptoms without any demonstrable organic findings."
3. "It is neurologic symptoms associated with psychological conflict or need."
4. "It is anxiety related to health issues that have no physical cause."

39. The nurse is caring for a client diagnosed with narcolepsy. The nurse understands that which client action(s) will assist the client in managing this condition? Select all that apply.
1. Drink a glass of red wine each evening.
2. Limit daily caffeine intake.
3. No smoking.
4. Exercise 1 hour before going to bed.
5. Maintain a regular sleep and rest schedule.

40. The nurse is caring for a 3-year-old client diagnosed with autism spectrum disorder. Which behavior(s) will the nurse expect to observe in this client? Select all that apply.
1. Becomes easily upset with changes to routine.
2. Rocks back and forth while sitting.
3. Does not make eye contact when held.
4. Speaks in short, two- to three-word sentences.
5. Smiles when the mother walks into the room.

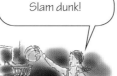

Slam dunk!

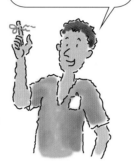

Remember: If physiological evidence for pain is present, it's not pain disorder.

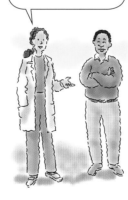

Don't forget to educate your client on lifestyle changes that can improve his condition.

37. 4. For the child to be able to complete daily tasks, it helps to break the tasks into smaller steps. This action makes it easier for the child to focus. The parents should provide specific, not general, directions and describe exactly what needs to be done. They do not need to be repetitive with information. The child should respond more effectively to a routine than to change.
CN: Physiological integrity; CNS: Physiological adaptation; CL: Apply

38. 1. Pain disorder is a preoccupation with pain in the absence of physical disease. A physical or somatic symptom refers to somatic symptom disorders in general. Neurologic symptoms are associated with conversion disorders. Anxiety related to health issues that have no physical cause is illness anxiety disorder.
CN: Psychosocial integrity; CNS: None; CL: Understand

39. 2, 3, 5. Narcolepsy is a chronic sleep disorder. Individuals having this disorder experience excessive sleepiness. They may find themselves falling asleep without warning and at frequent intervals. Caffeine intake and smoking have stimulating effects and can disrupt sleep. It is important that individuals with narcolepsy have activities that promote quality rest and sleep periods. A regular schedule of sleep and rest is important to ensure obtaining adequate rest. Exercise is recommended in the management of narcolepsy but it should be completed about 4 to 5 hours prior to bedtime. Drinking a glass of wine each evening is not associated with improving sleep quality.
CN: Health promotion and maintenance; CNS: None; CL: Apply

40. 1, 2, 3. Common symptoms of autism spectrum disorder include an inability to "handle" changes in routines or schedules. These individuals may become extremely agitated when these changes occur. Rocking back and forth is also often noted. Social skill impairments are common with the disorder. These impairments may include an inability to make eye contact. Other symptoms include limited to no verbal interaction; two- to three-word sentences would not be common in this disorder at this age. Limited facial expressions are also common. The client smiling at his mother would not be common, either.
CN: Physiological integrity; CNS: Physiological adaptation; CL: Apply

CN: Client needs category   CNS: Client needs subcategory   CL: Cognitive level

41. A client with a tic disorder has tried to use stress reduction techniques without success. Which antipsychotic medication will the nurse anticipate the health care provider will prescribe for this client?
 1. Methylphenidate
 2. Clonidine
 3. Atomoxetine
 4. Risperidone

42. A client informs the nurse that they have difficulty sleeping. Which question(s) will the nurse ask the client to determine factors inhibiting adequate sleep patterns? Select all that apply.
 1. "Is shift work required at your job?"
 2. "Have you been diagnosed with sleep apnea?"
 3. "Have you reduced your external stimuli?"
 4. "How much caffeine do you ingest each evening?"
 5. "Do you follow a consistent bedtime routine?"
 6. "Do you experience excessive worrying or anxiety?"

43. The nurse is caring for a client diagnosed with pain disorder. When reviewing the chart, which finding will cause the nurse to question this diagnosis?
 1. Reports of back pain, with spinal x-ray indicating no significant findings.
 2. Narcotic medications prescribed by three different health care providers.
 3. The client has had twenty-two emergency department visits in the past 60 days.
 4. Reports hip pain, with CT scan showing significant degenerative changes to the joint.

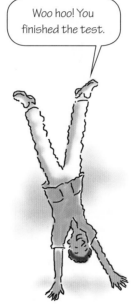

Woo hoo! You finished the test.

41. 4. The atypical antipsychotic drug risperidone is effective in reducing tics. The other medications are not effective for this disorder. Clonidine is a centrally acting alpha-agonist while atomoxetine is a selective norepinephrine reuptake inhibitor. Methylphenidate belongs to a class of drugs known as stimulants.
CN: Physiological integrity; CNS: Pharmacological and parenteral therapies; CL: Understand

42. 1, 2, 4, 6. Shift work can disrupt the circadian rhythm. Sleep apnea can cause a reduction in oxygen to the brain, which can reduce the quality of rest. Caffeine is a stimulant and, if taken too close to bedtime, it can interfere with falling asleep. Excessive worry or anxiety causes an increase in adrenaline, which enhances alertness and reduces sleepiness. A consistent bedtime routine and reduction of external stimuli promote good sleep.
CN: Health promotion and maintenance; CNS: None; CL: Analyze

43. 4. Pain disorder is the presence of chronic or severe pain that is not supported by a physiologic condition. A computed tomography (CT) scan showing degenerative changes to the site of pain may not support the diagnosis of pain disorder. A report of back pain with no underlying physiologic condition, seeking medications from multiple health care providers, and multiple visits to health care facilities **do** support the diagnosis of pain disorder.
CN: Physiological integrity; CNS: Physiological adaptation; CL: Apply

Chapter 13

Anxiety, Obsessive-Compulsive, Stress-Related, & Mood Disorders

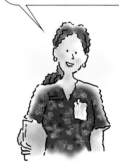

Want more information on anxiety, obsessive-compulsive, stress-related, and mood disorders to help you prepare for the NCLEX®? Check out the Web site of the National Alliance for the Mentally Ill at www.nami.org/.

Anxiety, obsessive-compulsive, stress-related, & mood disorders refresher

Bipolar disorder

Manic and depressive episodes

Key signs and symptoms

During periods of mania
- Euphoria and hostility
- Feelings of grandiosity
- Inflated sense of self-worth
- Increased energy (feeling of being charged up)

During periods of depression
- Altered sleep patterns
- Anorexia and weight loss
- Helplessness
- Irritability
- Lack of motivation
- Low self-esteem
- Sadness and crying

Key test results
- EEG is abnormal during:
  - depressive episodes of bipolar I disorder
  - major depression

Key treatments
- Individual therapy
- Family therapy
- Antimanic agents: lithium carbonate, lithium citrate
- Antipsychotic agents: risperidone
- Anticonvulsants: valproic acid, divalproex, lamotrigine

Key interventions

Manic phase
- Decrease environmental stimuli by behaving consistently and supplying external controls.
- Ensure a safe and supportive environment.
- Define and explain acceptable behaviors and then set limits.
- Monitor drug levels, especially lithium.

Depressive phase
- Ensure a safe and supportive environment for the client.
- Evaluate the risk of suicide and formulate a safety contract with the client, as appropriate.
- Observe the client for medication compliance and adverse effects.
- Encourage the client to identify current problems and stressors.

Generalized anxiety disorder

Excessive or disproportionate anxiety about several aspects of life, such as work, social relationships, or financial matters

Key signs and symptoms
- Easy startle reflex
- Excessive worry and anxiety
- Fatigue
- Fears of grave misfortune or death
- Motor tension
- Muscle tension

Key test results
- Laboratory tests rule out physiologic causes

Key treatments
- Individual therapy focusing on coping skills
- Anxiolytics: alprazolam, lorazepam, clonazepam, buspirone

Key interventions
- Help the client identify and explore coping mechanisms used in the past.
- Observe for signs of mounting anxiety.

Major depression

Persistent feeling of sadness and loss of interest

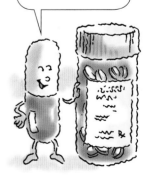

Compliance is key. Medications should only be used as directed.

Key signs and symptoms
- Altered sleep patterns
- Anorexia and weight loss
- Helplessness
- Irritability
- Lack of motivation
- Low self-esteem
- Sadness and crying

Key test results
- Beck Depression Inventory indicates depression

Key treatments
- Selective serotonin reuptake inhibitors (SSRIs): paroxetine, fluoxetine, sertraline, escitalopram, bupropion, citalopram, venlafaxine
- Tricyclic antidepressants (TCAs): imipramine, desipramine, amitriptyline, clomipramine, doxepin, nortriptyline
- Other antidepressants: mirtazapine, nefazodone
- Electroconvulsive therapy (ECT) for chronic depression or major depression that has not responded to classic treatment.

Key interventions
- Ensure safe, supportive environment for the client.
- Evaluate the risk of suicide and formulate a safety contract with client.
- Observe client for medication compliance and adverse effects.

Obsessive-compulsive disorder

Unreasonable thoughts and fears (obsessions) that lead to repetitive behaviors (compulsions)

Key signs and symptoms
- Compulsive behavior
  - repetitive touching or counting
  - doing and undoing small tasks
  - any other repetitive activity
- Obsessive thoughts
  - thoughts of contamination
  - repetitive worries about impending tragedy
  - repeating and counting images or words

Key test results
- Positron emission tomography shows increased activity in the frontal lobe of the cerebral cortex

Key treatments
- Behavioral therapy
- Individual therapy

- Anxiolytics: alprazolam, lorazepam, clonazepam
- SSRIs: fluoxetine, fluvoxamine, paroxetine, sertraline

Key interventions
- Encourage client to express feelings.
- Encourage client to identify situations that produce anxiety and precipitate obsessive-compulsive behavior.
- Work with client to develop appropriate coping skills.

Panic disorder

Debilitating anxiety and fear arising frequently and without reasonable cause

Key signs and symptoms
- Diminished ability to focus, even with direction from others
- Edginess or impatience
- Loss of objectivity
- Severely impaired rational thought
- Uneasiness and tension

Key test results
- Medical tests rule out physiologic causes

Key treatments
- Individual therapy
- Anxiolytics: alprazolam, lorazepam, clonazepam

Key interventions
- During panic attacks:
  - Distract the client from the attack.
  - Approach the client calmly and unemotionally.
  - Use short, simple sentences.

Phobia

Extreme or irrational fear of, or aversion to, something

Key signs and symptoms
- Panic when confronted with the feared object
- Persistent fear of specific thing, place, or situation

Key test results
- No specific test is available to diagnose a phobia

Key treatments
- Family therapy
- Supportive therapy
- Benzodiazepines: alprazolam, lorazepam, clonazepam

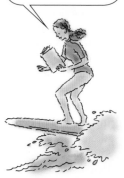

Some people think I'm obsessive-compulsive about studying.

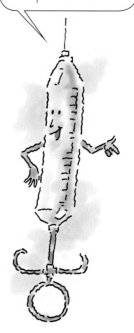

A lot of people have a phobia of me.

Key interventions
- Provide a safe and supportive environment.
- Collaborate with client to identify the feared object or situation.
- Assist in desensitizing the client.

Posttraumatic stress disorder (PTSD)

Persistent mental and emotional stress occurring as a result of injury or severe psychological shock, typically involving disturbance of sleep and constant vivid recall of the experience, with dulled responses to others and to the outside world

Key signs and symptoms
- Anxiety
- Flashbacks of the client's traumatic experience
- Nightmares about the traumatic experience
- Poor impulse control
- Social isolation
- Survivor guilt

Key test results
- No specific tests are available to identify or confirm posttraumatic stress disorder

Key treatments
- Individual therapy
- Group therapy
- Systematic desensitization
- Benzodiazepines: alprazolam, lorazepam, clonazepam
- Tricyclic antidepressants (TCAs): imipramine, amitriptyline
- SSRIs: sertraline, paroxetine

Key interventions
- Work with client to identify stressors.
- Provide safe, supportive environment.
- Encourage client to explore the traumatic event and the meaning of the event.
- Assist client with problem solving and resolving guilt.

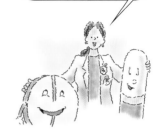

Altogether, now! Medication and therapy can work together to treat anxiety and related disorders.

thePoint® You can download tables of drug information to help you prepare for the NCLEX®! View Generic Drug Names, Drug Classifications, Drug Actions, and Nursing Implications for the drugs discussed in this refresher at **http://thePoint.lww.com**

Anxiety, obsessive-compulsive, stress-related, & mood disorders questions, answers, and rationales

1. A client has been taking lithium carbonate for 6 months and recently developed symptoms of arthritis. The client asks the nurse for ibuprofen for pain. Which nursing response is **best**?
1. "Ibuprofen will cause lithium level to drop very low and arthritis symptoms may return."
2. "Let me assess your pain, then I may be able to give you a dose of acetaminophen."
3. "Naproxen would be best for you because ibuprofen can elevate your lithium blood level."
4. "You will have to stop taking the lithium if you take any pain medication."

2. A client experiencing an extremely severe form of obsessive-compulsive disorder (OCD) wants to know whether the scheduled neurosurgical procedure will alleviate symptoms. Which nursing response is **best**?
1. "The neurosurgical procedure has a very low likelihood of successfully treating OCD."
2. "Most clients experience no further symptoms with the rest being significantly improved."
3. "It has high rate of success and is the preferred method of treating OCD."
4. "You need to trust your health care provider and not question the recommendation."

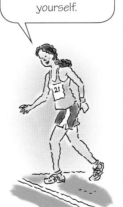

Here we go. Remember to pace yourself.

1. 2. It is best to avoid NSAIDs while taking lithium, and acetaminophen is a safe alternative to NSAIDs for these clients. Ibuprofen and naproxen are NSAIDs, which increase renal lithium carbonate reabsorption. Stronger analgesics are not necessary for mild arthritis. Not all pain medications are contraindicated while on lithium. Ibuprofen does not cause the lithium level to fall too low.
CN: Physiological integrity; CNS: Pharmacological and parenteral therapies; CL: Apply

2. 2. Neurosurgical treatment is extremely rare for cases of obsessive-compulsive disorder. Such treatment is typically reserved for only the most severe cases of the disease. The surgery involves making a series of lesions to interrupt the efferent tracts from the frontal cortex to the limbic and basal ganglia structures. In a recent study, 65% of people who underwent this procedure were completely symptom free of obsessive-compulsive disorder, with no further need for treatment.
CN: Psychosocial integrity; CNS: None; CL: Apply

CN: Client needs category   CNS: Client needs subcategory   CL: Cognitive level

3. The nurse caring for a client with panic disorder will expect which assessment finding?
 1. A systolic blood pressure recording of 20 mm Hg below the client's baseline.
 2. The client reports a headache and nausea occurring intermittently.
 3. The client denies feeling any appreciable anxiety between episodes.
 4. The client reports difficulty falling asleep at night.

4. A client sees a spider while raking leaves. Immediately, the client's heart begins beating rapidly and the client breaks into a sweat. The client asks the nurse, "What just happened to me?" Which statement made by the nurse is **best**?
 1. "What you felt were anxiety-triggered responses to the spider that were worsened by sustained physical exertion."
 2. "What you experienced is a common reaction many people have when coming into contact with spiders."
 3. "Your behavior was an example of anxiety triggered by reliving a previous experience with a spider."
 4. "The fear reaction was triggered by your autonomic system responding to suddenly seeing the spider."

5. A nurse is providing education to a client prescribed lamotrigine. Which adverse effect(s) will the nurse instruct the client to report to the health care provider? Select all that apply.
 1. Muscle weakness
 2. Insomnia
 3. Blurred vision
 4. Skin rashes
 5. Headache
 6. Polycythemia

6. A client informs the nurse he lives alone and never leaves the bedroom because the bedroom is a calm and relaxed environment. If the client leaves the room, extreme panic occurs. The nurse will **best** explain this client's behavior to the health care provider using which statement?
 1. "The client is manifesting this disorder based on a fear of becoming helpless and incurring a panic attack."
 2. "The client is manifesting this disorder based on unreasonable fear of specific objects and a need to repeat behavior."
 3. "This client is not manifesting any anxiety disorder. This behavior is within the range of cultural norms."
 4. "This client is manifesting agoraphobia related to a previous diagnosis of generalized anxiety disorder."

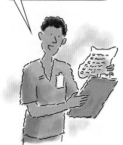

To answer question #3, you need to remember the difference between panic disorder and generalized anxiety disorder.

3. 3. Most people who experience panic attacks have little or no residual anxiety between attacks. In some individuals, the panic attacks are reproducibly provoked by exposure to certain stimuli. In others, they appear unexpectedly or are most likely to occur in specific settings. The nurse would expect the blood pressure to increase, not decrease. A headache, nausea, and difficulty falling asleep are associated with generalized anxiety disorder. CN: Psychosocial integrity; CNS: None; CL: Apply

4. 4. The client's response is an example of fear because it is triggered by a known, specific object, the spider. The autonomic responses of the pounding heart and hair standing on end are directly related to the sight of the spider. A person experiencing anxiety would have a sense of dread without having a specific source or reason for the emotion. While many people experience a spider phobia, it is not considered a common reaction. CN: Psychosocial integrity; CNS: None; CL: Apply

5. 3, 4, 5. Blurred vision, headache, and skin rashes are common adverse effects of lamotrigine. The client will not develop insomnia, muscle weakness, or polycythemia (increased RBC count) as a result of taking the medication. CN: Physiological integrity; CNS: Pharmacological and parenteral therapies; CL: Apply

6. 1. Nursing interventions would be based on the client manifesting this disorder because of a fear of becoming helpless and incurring a panic attack; this disorder is not from fear of specific objects, this behavior is not normal, and the client is not experiencing agoraphobia. CN: Psychosocial integrity; CNS: None; CL: Apply

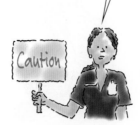

True panic attacks occur without reasonable cause, but life-threatening conditions, such as heart attack, can also cause panic and should be ruled out.

Caution

7. A nurse is providing education to a client who has been prescribed buspirone for long-term treatment of anxiety. The nurse determines the education has been effective when the client makes which statement?
   1. "I will take the buspirone before I have an anxiety attack."
   2. "I do not need to take this medication with my meals."
   3. "I will not stop taking this medicine if I become pregnant."
   4. "I will not take the medicine with grapefruit juice."

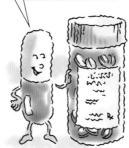

Careful what you mix us drugs with … sometimes we don't get along well with other substances.

7. 4. Clients who are taking buspirone should be instructed to avoid grapefruit juice. It can increase the effects of buspirone. Instruct clients to take buspirone with food to decrease nausea, to avoid taking it during pregnancy, and to take on a regular basis—not "as needed."
CN: Physiological integrity; CNS: Pharmacological and parenteral therapies; CL: Apply

8. The nurse is caring for a client experiencing a panic attack. Which nursing intervention is **most** appropriate?
   1. Tell the client to take deep breaths.
   2. Allow the client privacy during the attack.
   3. Encourage the client to verbalize feelings.
   4. Ask the client about the cause of the attack.

8. 1. During a panic attack, a client may experience symptoms of dizziness, shortness of breath, and feelings of suffocation. The nurse should remain with the client and direct any statements toward changing the physiologic response, such as taking deep breaths. During an attack, the client is unable to talk about anxious situations and is not able to address feelings, especially uncomfortable feelings and frustrations. While having a panic attack, the client is also unable to focus on anything other than the symptoms, so the client will not be able to discuss the cause of the attack.
CN: Safe, effective care environment; CNS: Management of care; CL: Analyze

9. The nurse is discussing the incidence of obsessive-compulsive disorder (OCD) with a client. Which statement made by the client demonstrates to the nurse an understanding of the education?
   1. "OCD is an extremely uncommon disorder."
   2. "OCD seldom occurs in young adults."
   3. "OCD is more common than bipolar depression."
   4. "OCD only occurs among alcoholics and drug abusers."

9. 3. Obsessive-compulsive disorder is said to occur more frequently than bipolar depression, and yet clients frequently hide their symptoms from family and health care providers. Most cases of this disorder begin in at a young age, often during young adulthood or before. OCD does not only occur among people with alcohol or substance use disorders.
CN: Psychosocial integrity; CNS: None; CL: Understand

10. The nurse provides care for a postpartum client's follow-up visits at 2, 4, and 6 weeks' postpartum. Which method is **best** for the nurse to use to screen the client for postpartum depression?
   1. Using the Edinburgh Postnatal Depression Scale during each of the three visits
   2. Engaging in general conversation and observation beginning 4 weeks' postpartum
   3. Using the Beck Depression Inventory beginning 6 weeks' postpartum
   4. Interviewing the father of the child during each of the three visits

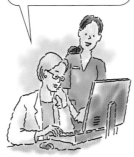

Frequent depression screenings in the postpartum period are key in detecting postpartum depression.

10. 1. The nurse would best assess for postpartum depression using the Edinburgh Postnatal Depression Scale during each of the three visits. This scale is a commonly used short screening instrument that has been shown to perform well in detecting postpartum depression. Screening should begin at the first postpartum visit, not the second or third, as signs and symptoms of postpartum depression may be present by 2 weeks' postpartum. Moreover, the Edinburgh Postnatal Depression Scale is more specific to screening for postpartum depression than is the Beck Depression Inventory. Interviewing the father of the child, who may or may not be aware of signs and symptoms of postpartum depression in the mother, would most likely be less effective than screening with a formal, evidence-based tool.
CN: Psychosocial integrity; CNS: None; CL: Understand

CN: Client needs category   CNS: Client needs subcategory   CL: Cognitive level

11. A client is newly diagnosed with generalized anxiety disorder. Which nursing intervention will **best** meet the needs of this client?
1. Conducting individual psychotherapy for the client.
2. Administering antianxiety medications as needed.
3. Providing education regarding prescribed medications.
4. Leading exposure therapy sessions for the client.

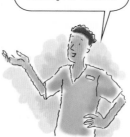

Don't miss out on opportunities to teach your clients.

11. 3. Teaching the client about antianxiety medications would best meet the needs of a client newly diagnosed with generalized anxiety disorder. Because the client is newly diagnosed, explaining about the medications should be a greater priority for the nurse than just administering them. Teaching the client skills dealing with cognitive restructuring and initiating supportive therapy are appropriate nursing interventions for this client but not as important as teaching the client about prescribed medications.
CN: Psychosocial integrity; CNS: None; CL: Analyze

12. The nurse is caring for a client who is in the panic level of anxiety. Which nursing action is **priority**?
1. Encourage the client to discuss feelings.
2. Provide for the client's safety needs.
3. Decrease environmental stimuli.
4. Assist the client to complete hygiene care.

12. 2. A client in the panic level of anxiety does not comprehend and cannot follow instructions or care for basic needs. The client is unable to express feelings due to the level of anxiety. Decreased environmental stimulus is needed but only after the client's safety needs and other basic needs are met. Although the nurse should assist the client with completing personal care, the client's safety is the priority.
CN: Safe, effective care environment; CNS: Management of care; CL: Analyze

13. Which nursing intervention is appropriate when caring for a client diagnosed with panic disorder?
1. Identify childhood trauma.
2. Monitor nutritional intake.
3. Institute suicide precautions.
4. Decrease episodes of disorientation.

13. 3. Clients with panic disorder are at risk for suicide. Childhood trauma is associated with posttraumatic stress disorder, not panic disorder. Nutritional problems do not typically accompany panic disorder. Clients with panic disorder are not typically disoriented; they may have a temporarily altered sense of reality, but that lasts only for the duration of the attack.
CN: Psychosocial integrity; CNS: None; CL: Apply

14. The nurse is caring for a client newly diagnosed with a phobia of dogs. Which treatment(s) will the nurse anticipate the health care provider prescribing for this client? Select all that apply.
1. Cognitive behavioral therapy
2. A magnetic resonance imaging (MRI) scan
3. Benzodiazepines, prescribed three times a day
4. Education about relaxation techniques
5. A buccal smear for genetic testing

14. 1, 4. Cognitive behavioral and exposure therapies have been shown to be the best treatments for specific phobias. An MRI is not indicated for clients with a phobia. Medications, unless being used to treat a related illness such as depression, have not been conclusively shown to be effective. Moreover, administering benzodiazepines several times a day could lead to a decreased level of consciousness or even respiratory compromise. Educating the client on relaxation techniques may help the client cope with anxiety and stress caused by the phobia. Although phobias may be genetic, genetic testing is not indicated at this time.
CN: Psychosocial integrity; CNS: None; CL: Apply

15. Which statement made by a client diagnosed with bipolar disorder suggests to the nurse the client is experiencing mania?
1. "I know nothing can stop me today."
2. "I have never seen a more beautiful day."
3. "I have slept really well these last three nights."
4. "It felt great to get compliments on my hair."

15. 1. The client may be in the manic phase of bipolar disorder when expressing feelings of invincibility. Mania presents with insufficient sleep patterns. The remaining statements are expressions of pleasure, not mania.
CN: Psychosocial integrity; CNS: None; CL: Apply

16. A nurse performing group therapy understands which intervention is **priority** for a client with panic disorder?
1. Explore how secondary gains are derived from the disorder.
2. Discuss new ways of thinking and feeling about panic attacks.
3. Work to eliminate manipulative behavior used for meeting needs.
4. Learn the risk factors and other demographics associated with panic disorder.

16. 2. Discussion of new ways of thinking and feeling about panic attacks can enable others to learn and benefit from a variety of intervention strategies. There are usually no secondary gains obtained from having a panic disorder. People with panic disorder are not using the disorder to manipulate others. Learning the risk factors could be accomplished in another format such as a psychoeducational program.
CN: Psychosocial integrity; CNS: None; CL: Apply

17. Which intervention is **most** appropriate for the nurse to implement when caring for a client experiencing the effects of a mild panic attack?
1. Distracting the client by having them take deep, slow breaths
2. Helping them remove any tight-fitting clothing
3. Identifying possible triggers for the anxiety
4. Moving the client to a low stimulus environment

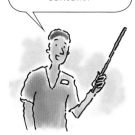

The timing of your teaching can be just as important as the content.

17. 1. The client will best pay attention to instructions if the client is experiencing mild anxiety. With mild anxiety, the client is alert and there is an increase in the perceptual field, making it possible to follow instructions such as breathing deeply. Removing the client's tight-fitting clothing and moving the client to a low stimulus environment will not help in minimizing or managing the anxiety. Identifying the client's triggers is only possible once the anxiety has been resolved.
CN: Psychosocial integrity; CNS: None; CL: Apply

18. A client is diagnosed with panic disorder associated with a phobia. Which client statement **best** indicates to the nurse the client is responding favorably to treatment?
1. "I spent last Saturday listening to a podcast lecture at home."
2. "I am getting better at knowing when I am going to hyperventilate."
3. "Today, I have decided not to stop taking my medication."
4. "Last night, I read my favorite poem to my support group."

18. 4. Clients with panic disorder associated with phobias may be experiencing fear of speaking in public. Reading a poem to a support group would be an example of desensitization therapy. While positive statements, none of the remaining options deal with a therapy directed at phobia management.
CN: Psychosocial integrity; CNS: None; CL: Analyze

19. The nurse is caring for a client who has been diagnosed as having social anxiety disorder. Which coping skill is appropriate for the nurse to encourage the client to develop?
1. Being in situations where the client is alone
2. Speaking or performing before large groups
3. Being surrounded by other people in crowded places
4. Having to shake hands and be exposed to others' germs

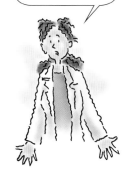

Sometimes it's best to just face your fears.

19. 2. The client experiencing a social anxiety disorder is suffering from a social phobia. This type of phobia is a profound fear of public speaking. The nursing care plan would focus on social skills training and exposure to social situations. Coping skills would be directed toward assisting the client with developing skills related to speaking or performing in public, meeting new people, or taking tests.
CN: Psychosocial integrity; CNS: None; CL: Apply

20. A client on the sixth floor of a psychiatric unit has a morbid fear of elevators. The client is scheduled to attend occupational therapy, which is located on the ground floor of the hospital. The client refuses to take the elevator, insisting that the stairs are safer. Which nursing action is **best**?
1. Insist that the client take the elevator.
2. Offer a reward if the client rides the elevator.
3. Hold therapy until the client can ride the elevator.
4. Allow the client to take the stairs to therapy.

20. 4. This client has a phobia and must not be forced to ride the elevator because of the risk of panic-level anxiety, which can occur if forced to contact the phobic object. This client cannot control the fear; therefore, stating that the client must take the elevator or promising a reward will not work. Occupational therapy is a treatment the client needs, not a reward.
CN: Psychosocial integrity; CNS: None; CL: Apply

21. The nurse is caring for a client experiencing dreams and flashbacks related to past experiences of sexual abuse and feelings of isolation. Which psychosocial disorder does this behavior indicate to the nurse?
1. Phobia
2. Panic disorder
3. Posttraumatic stress disorder (PTSD)
4. Obsessive-compulsive disorder (OCD)

22. Which statement made by the nurse is appropriate when providing education for a client and family about phobias and the need for a strong support system?
1. "The use of a family support system is only temporary."
2. "The need to be assertive can be reinforced by the family."
3. "The family must set limits on inappropriate behaviors."
4. "The family plays a role in promoting client independence."

23. The nurse is assessing a client recently diagnosed with obsessive-compulsive disorder (OCD). Which assessment question is **most** appropriate for the nurse to include when caring for this client?
1. "Would you like to discuss the results of your brain x-rays?"
2. "Have you experienced any manic behavior since starting treatment?"
3. "Have you been regularly attending your cognitive therapy sessions?"
4. "What are the possible side effects of lorazepam?"

24. Which nursing intervention(s) is appropriate in assisting a client to cope with stress? Select all that apply.
1. Teach relaxation exercises.
2. Develop a plan of care for the client.
3. Minimize environmental stimuli.
4. Encourage verbalization of feelings.
5. Encourage increase in workload.
6. Establish a trusting relationship.

25. A client was the lone survivor of a train crash 6 months ago. Which client statement indicates to the nurse the client has a maladaptive response to the trauma?
1. "I do not need to talk about the train wreck."
2. "I am able to concentrate on reading a book."
3. "I have finally started to sleep through the night."
4. "I jump at train whistles because it reminds me of the wreck."

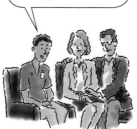

Educating the family can be just as important as educating the client when it comes to phobias.

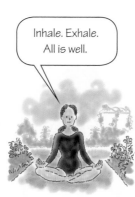

Inhale. Exhale. All is well.

21. 3. The client is most likely suffering from posttraumatic stress disorder. Individuals with this disorder have been exposed to an event that threatened the person's physical integrity. In this situation, the experience of sexual abuse was perceived as a threat to the client's physical integrity. Flashbacks are often experienced when an individual suffers from this disorder but are not associated with phobias, panic disorder, or OCD.
CN: Psychosocial integrity; CNS: None; CL: Understand

22. 4. The family plays a vital role in supporting the client in treatment and preventing the client from using the phobia to obtain secondary gains. Family support must be ongoing, not temporary. The family can be more helpful by focusing on effective handling of anxiety rather than focusing energy on developing assertiveness skills. People with phobias are already restrictive in their behavior; more restrictions are not necessary.
CN: Psychosocial integrity; CNS: None; CL: Apply

23. 4. The client diagnosed and being treated for obsessive-compulsive disorder (OCD) will be prescribed an antianxiety medication such as alprazolam, lorazepam, or clonazepam. Confirming medication education would be an appropriate intervention. Manic behavior is not associated with OCD. Positron emission tomography (PET) scan, not a brain x-ray, shows increased activity in the frontal lobe of the cerebral cortex often associated with OCD. Behavioral, not cognitive, therapy is often a part of the treatment plan for this disorder.
CN: Psychosocial integrity; CNS: None; CL: Analyze

24. 1, 3, 6. People use adaptive measures to deal directly with a stressful situation or the symptoms the situation produces; these measures require minimal expenditure of energy and include relaxation exercises, minimization of environmental stimuli, and support networks. Developing a plan of care and encouraging verbalization of feelings are appropriate interventions but do not directly help the client cope with stress. Encouraging an increase in workload would tend to increase a person's stress, not help cope with it.
CN: Psychosocial integrity; CNS: None; Apply

25. 1. Denial is used as a protective response to posttraumatic stress. Concentration and sleeping through the night indicate resolution of conflicts. Startling sounds can provoke anxiety in a client with posttraumatic stress disorder, but this client expresses understanding of why this is happening.
CN: Psychosocial integrity; CNS: None; CL: Apply

26. A client diagnosed with severe posttraumatic stress disorder (PTSD) is prescribed imipramine. Which outcome will the nurse monitor for to determine success with the prescribed regimen?
1. The client does not have hyperactivity and purposeless movements.
2. The client has an increase in the ability to concentrate.
3. The client does not experience the reenactment of the trauma.
4. The client no longer experiences the grieving process.

27. Which nursing intervention will be included in a care plan for a client diagnosed with posttraumatic stress disorder (PTSD) who has lost several jobs because of "a bad temper"?
1. Encourage the client to seek less stressful employment.
2. Assist the client in identifying triggers resulting in anger.
3. Work with the client to forget the traumatic memories.
4. Help the client recognize the situation as a part of life that can be controlled.

28. Which medication will the nurse advise the client to avoid while taking isocarboxazid?
1. Acetaminophen
2. Ibuprofen
3. Guaifenesin
4. Meperidine

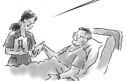

Before administering any medication to a client, be sure to confirm the client's identity.

29. The nurse is obtaining data from a group of clients diagnosed with depression. The nurse knows that which client population will **most** benefit from electroconvulsive therapy (ECT)?
1. Clients who are having suicidal or homicidal thoughts.
2. Clients who are aggressive or acting out and depressed.
3. Clients with physical problems resulting in depression.
4. Clients who do not respond positively to medication therapy.

30. The nurse is providing education for a client taking a monoamine oxidase inhibitor (MAOI). Which dietary choice(s) will the nurse tell the client to avoid? Select all that apply.
1. Smoked fish
2. A ripe avocado
3. Wine
4. Cottage cheese
5. Grilled chicken

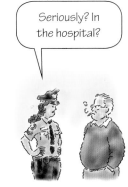

Seriously? In the hospital?

26. 3. Imipramine, a tricyclic antidepressant medication, decreases the frequency of reenactment of the trauma for the client. It helps memory problems and sleeping difficulties and decreases numbing. The medication will not prevent hyperactivity and purposeless movements nor increase the client's concentration. No medication facilitates the grieving process.
CN: Physiological integrity; CNS: Pharmacological and parenteral therapies; CL: Apply

27. 2. The client must define and identify the triggers for the behaviors that are associated with anger. The management of poor impulse control is not entirely focused on stress management. The traumatic experiences must be addressed and dealt with; this trauma is not a controllable factor but one that can be managed with therapy.
CN: Psychosocial integrity; CNS: None; CL: Apply

28. 4. Clients taking monoamine oxidase inhibitors (MAOIs) should avoid meperidine. Other medications to avoid include tricyclic antidepressants, fluoxetine, amphetamines, and amphetamine-like medications, including all sympathomimetics.
CN: Physiological integrity; CNS: Pharmacological and parenteral therapies; CL: Apply

29. 4. ECT is highly effective in helping clients who are severely depressed and do not respond to medication therapy. Many studies on ECT and depression indicate efficacy rates for ECT as high as 90%, in comparison to medications (tricyclic antidepressants and monoamine oxidase inhibitors). The other client groups listed may benefit from ECT but are not as likely to benefit from it as those who do not respond positively to medication therapy.
CN: Psychosocial integrity; CNS: None; CL: Apply

30. 1, 2, 3. Foods to be avoided are those containing tyramine and alcohol, such as smoked fish, ripe avocados, and wine. A client taking MAOIs can consider cottage cheese and chicken safe foods.
CN: Psychosocial integrity; CNS: None; CL: Apply

31. A client diagnosed with bipolar disorder is experiencing mania with labile mood changes. The client is threatening to assault staff members and other clients. Which nursing response is **best**?
1. "Hitting others will only make things worse. Why would you want to hit someone?"
2. "You will be put in solitary seclusion and kept there if you threaten anyone else."
3. "Do not hit other clients or me. If you cannot control your behavior, we will help you."
4. "That is enough! You know we do not tolerate this type of behavior and you will be punished."

32. The nurse is caring for a client diagnosed with posttraumatic stress disorder (PTSD), and the family informs the nurse that loud noises cause a serious anxiety response. Which explanation made by the nurse will help the family understand the client's response?
1. "Environmental triggers can cause the client to react emotionally."
2. "Clients commonly experience extreme fear of normal environmental stimuli."
3. "After a trauma, the client cannot respond to stimuli in an appropriate manner."
4. "The response indicates another emotional problem needs investigation."

33. During the assessment, a client diagnosed with depression tells the nurse, "I take St. John's wort daily." Which statement will the nurse include when discussing this medication with the client?
1. "It is a nonstandard preparation, so the amount of hypericum may vary among manufacturers."
2. "It has a much more expensive cost of preparation than other commonly prescribed drugs."
3. "Blood testing is required every week for dyscrasias associated with taking St. John's wort."
4. "Great! St. John's wort has been shown to be more effective than prescription medications."

34. The nurse is assessing a client being treated for major depression and the client states, "I am unable to brush my teeth and comb my hair by myself." What will the nurse do **next**?
1. Begin planning care to address the client's ADL needs.
2. Contact the health care provider to change the client's medication.
3. Assess the client for other self-care deficits that may be present.
4. Continue to monitor the client for other related health needs.

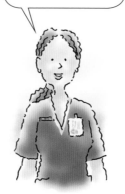

Clients with bipolar disorder may need help establishing appropriate boundaries.

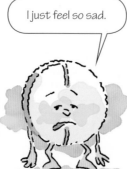

I just feel so sad.

31. 3. The correct response is to set limits in a simple, concrete sentence to de-escalate the situation. Asking the client why he would want to hit someone asks a question that the client cannot answer. Suggesting the client will be put in seclusion threatens the client and that is assault. Yelling at the client that the behavior will not be tolerated does not help the client stop the behavior.
CN: Psychosocial Integrity; CNS: None; CL: Apply

32. 1. Repeated exposure to environmental triggers can cause the client to experience a hyperarousal state because there is a loss of physiologic control of incoming stimuli. After experiencing a trauma, the client may have strong reactions to stimuli similar to those that occurred during the traumatic event. However, not all stimuli cause an anxiety response. The client's anxiety response is typically seen after a traumatic experience and does not indicate the presence of another problem.
CN: Psychosocial integrity; CNS: None; CL: Apply

33. 1. St. John's wort (hypericum), which is an over-the-counter medication for depression, may have a nonstandard preparation and the amount of hypericum may vary among manufacturers. Other disadvantages of St. John's wort include reduced effectiveness compared to prescription drug therapy or cognitive therapy. In addition, drug interactions can occur and may be significant. Dyscrasias are not associated with taking St. John's wort, and its cost of preparation is not more expensive than prescription drugs.
CN: Psychosocial integrity; CNS: None; CL: Apply

34. 3. When the client begins to be unable to care for basic physical and personal needs, the nurse needs to assess the client regarding self-care deficits. The remaining options are appropriate but require the additional assessment to identify the existence of such problems.
CN: Psychosocial integrity; CNS: None; CL: Analyze

35. The nurse assessing a client on admission suspects the client may be depressed. Which self-rating scales will the nurse have the client complete?
1. Stanford and the WISC
2. Beck and Zung
3. Miller and GRE
4. Rorschach and MMPI

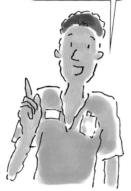

What key test is used to assess for depression?

35. 2. The two most common self-rating scales used with clients who may be depressed are the Beck Depression Inventory and the Zung Self-Rating Depression Scale. The Beck Depression Inventory is a 21-item scale used with individuals aged 13 and older. It measures the severity of depression. The Zung Self-Rating Depression Scale is a 20-item scale that measures four common characteristics of depression. The other tests listed are not self-rating scales for depression.
CN: Psychosocial integrity; CNS: None; CL: Understand

36. Which principles will be kept in mind when the nurse evaluates a client's progress in managing depression?
1. Grieving resulting from significant loss should never exceed 2 months.
2. To be considered successful, all the identified outcomes should show progress.
3. The client's view of the changes since the beginning of therapy is not objective.
4. Significant energy and a conscious effort are required by the client to maintain perspective.

36. 4. When evaluating, the nurse needs to remind the client that managing depression often requires significant energy, and a conscious effort on the client's part to balance emotions and maintain perspective. It is also important to remember that depression resulting from a significant loss, such as loss of a loved one, may take many weeks or months to overcome; the client will need sensitive nursing care to adapt to the new situations and roles that accompany such a loss. Success does not require that all identified outcomes show progress. The client's objectivity related to progress should not be a significant a concern of the nurse.
CN: Psychosocial integrity; CNS: None; CL: Apply

37. The nurse is caring for a client being treated for major depression who is concerned about urinary retention and constipation. What education will the nurse provide to the client regarding these complications?
1. The adverse effects of medications currently prescribed
2. The effects of exercise on the processes of elimination
3. The need to consume sufficient fluids to avoid dehydration
4. The importance of good dietary choices on proper elimination

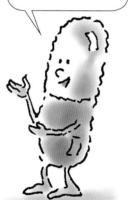

Sometimes we drugs have negative unintended effects ... sorry about that.

37. 1. In this client's situation, urinary retention and constipation would most likely be caused by medications. Educating the client on side effects of the medication addresses both constipation and urinary retention. Constipation can be related to dehydration, poor diet, and lack of exercise, but these factors are less likely to be of concern to this client than the medications.
CN: Physiological integrity; CNS: Pharmacological and parenteral therapies; CL: Apply

38. The nurse is directing a therapy session for a group of adolescents who witnessed the violent death of a peer. Which outcome **best** meets the needs of the students?
1. Learning violence prevention strategies
2. Talking about appropriate expression of anger
3. Discussing the effect of the trauma on their lives
4. Developing trusting relationships among their peers

38. 3. By discussing the effect of the trauma on their lives, the adolescents can grieve and develop effective coping strategies. Learning violence prevention strategies is not the most immediate concern after a trauma occurs, nor is working on developing healthy relationships. It is appropriate to talk about expressing anger after the trauma is addressed.
CN: Psychosocial integrity; CNS: None; CL: Apply

39. Which statement indicates a client diagnosed with generalized anxiety disorder (GAD) understands the nurse's nutritional education?
1. "I have stopped drinking so much diet cola."
2. "I have reduced my intake of carbohydrates."
3. "I now eat less at dinner and before bedtime."
4. "I have cut back on my use of dairy products."

39. 1. Clients with GAD can decrease anxiety by eliminating caffeine from their diets. It is not necessary for clients with generalized anxiety to decrease their carbohydrate intake, eat less at dinner or before bedtime, or cut back on their use of dairy products.
CN: Physiological integrity; CNS: Basic care and comfort; CL: Apply

40. The nurse is caring for a hospitalized client diagnosed with posttraumatic stress disorder (PTSD) who is experiencing a frightening flashback. Which action will the nurse complete **first**?
   1. Have the client talk about the traumatic event.
   2. Assess for maladaptive and coping strategies.
   3. Stay in the hospital room with the client.
   4. Acknowledge feelings of guilt or self-blame

41. Which nursing behavior demonstrates caring to a client with a diagnosis of anxiety disorder?
   1. Verbalize concern about the client.
   2. Arrange group activities for clients.
   3. Ask client to sign the treatment plan.
   4. Arrange for an educational group on medications.

42. Which finding will the nurse expect to assess when talking about school with a child diagnosed with a generalized anxiety disorder (GAD)?
   1. The child has been fighting with peers for the past month.
   2. The child cannot stop lying to parents and teachers.
   3. The child has gained 15 lb (6.8 kg) in the past month.
   4. The child expresses concern about current grades.

43. The nurse is assessing a client with suspected generalized anxiety disorder (GAD). Which finding indicates to the nurse that the client is experiencing GAD?
   1. The client reports, "I do not rest well at night."
   2. Muscle wasting noted in the bilateral lower extremities.
   3. The client reports, "I have noticed my heart skipping beats."
   4. Excessive startle reflex noted in client in response to noises.

44. During a conversation with a client, the nurse recognizes a delusion of grandeur. Which nursing action is **priority**?
   1. Ask the client to expand on the comment.
   2. Redirect the conversation back to reality.
   3. Engage the client and enter the delusion.
   4. Dispute the reality of the delusion.

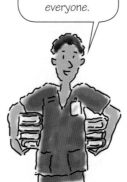
School can be a big source of anxiety for everyone.

40. 3. The nurse should stay with the client during periods of flashbacks and nightmares, offer reassurance of safety and security, and assure the client that these symptoms are not uncommon following a severe trauma. Encouraging the client to talk about the traumatic event, observing for maladaptive and coping strategies, and acknowledging feelings of guilt or self-blame may be carried out in the future. The nurse's top priority during the flashback is to stay with the client.
CN: Psychosocial integrity; CNS: None; CL: Apply

41. 1. The nurse who verbally expresses concern about a client's well-being is acting in a caring and supportive manner. Arranging for group activities may be an action where the nurse has no direct client contact and therefore cannot demonstrate caring to clients. Asking a client to sign the treatment plan may not be viewed as a sign of caring. An educational group on medications may be viewed by clients as an educational experience, as opposed to a sign of caring, because the nurse may have limited interaction with the client.
CN: Health promotion and maintenance; CNS: None; CL: Apply

42. 4. Children with GAD worry about how well they are performing in school. Children with GAD do not tend to be involved in conflict. They are more oriented toward good behavior. Children with GAD do not tend to lie to others. They would want to do their best and try to please others. A weight gain of 15 lb (6.8 kg) is not a typical characteristic of a child with anxiety disorder.
CN: Psychosocial integrity; CNS: None; CL: Analyze

43. 4. GAD presents with a heightened state of arousal that results in being easily startled. Although anxiety may affect sleep, it is not generally characterized by insomnia. Muscle tension, not wasting, is observed, and cardiac dysrhythmia is not a symptom of GAD.
CN: Psychosocial integrity; CNS: None; CL: Apply

44. 2. The priority action is for the nurse to redirect the conversation back to reality. The nurse should never ask the client to expand on the comment, enter the delusion, or argue with the client over the reality of the delusion.
CN: Psychosocial integrity; CNS: None; CL: Apply

45. The nurse assesses a client diagnosed with depression who reports fatigue, sadness, insomnia, powerlessness, and social isolation. What is the **priority** area for the nurse to focus on to ensure meeting the needs of the client while forming an effective nurse-client relationship?
1. Fatigue, so that the client has energy to work on other symptoms.
2. Sadness, to reduce or eliminate the need for suicide precautions.
3. The symptoms that the client identifies as being the most urgent.
4. All of the identified symptoms simultaneously in a coordinated manner.

46. A health care provider increases a client's prescription of sertraline to 150 mg daily to help manage the client's major depressive disorder (MDD). The medication is available in 50 mg scored tables. How many tablets will the nurse administer to the client during a 24-hour period? Record your answer using a whole number.

_____ tablets

47. Which statement by a middle-aged adult client with a diagnosis of generalized anxiety disorder (GAD) indicates to the nurse that anxiety has been a long-standing condition?
1. "I was, and still am, an extremely impulsive person."
2. "I have always been hyperactive but not in useful ways."
3. "When I was in college, I never thought I would finish."
4. "All my life, I have had intrusive dreams and scary nightmares."

48. While assessing a client diagnosed with major depression, the nurse associates which finding(s) with this diagnosis? Select all that apply.
1. The client reports, "I feel like I have no control over my life."
2. The client states, "I am a failure at most of the things I have tried."
3. The client demonstrates irritation at the length of time the assessment requires.
4. The client expresses remorse regarding employment decisions made over the years.
5. The client reports, "I feel a lot of guilt about how I acted while I was married."

Working with clients with mood disorders can be a real adventure. Make sure you're armed with all the right tools.

Don't get restless. You'll figure this one out.

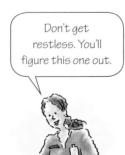

45. 3. The nurse knows that the best practice is to focus on the symptoms that the client identifies as the most urgent. This approach would indicate to the client that the nurse cares about the client's feelings and perception of the problem. By focusing on the symptoms that the client feels are most urgent, the nurse can build a trusting relationship with the client.
CN: Psychosocial integrity; CNS: None; CL: Analyze

46. 3.
The correct formula to calculate a drug dose is:

$$\frac{Dose\ on\ hand}{Quantity\ on\ hand} = \frac{Dose\ desired}{X}$$

For this situation, the nurse should calculate:

$$\frac{50\ mg}{1\ tablet} = \frac{150\ mg}{X}$$

$$X = 3\ tablets$$

CN: Physiological integrity; CNS: Pharmacological and parenteral therapies; CL: Apply

47. 3. For many people who have GAD, the age of onset is during young adulthood. The symptoms of impulsiveness and hyperactivity are not commonly associated with a diagnosis of GAD. The symptom of intrusive dreams and nightmares is associated with posttraumatic stress disorder (PTSD) rather than GAD.
CN: Psychosocial integrity; CNS: None; CL: Apply

48. 1, 2, 3. Helplessness, low self-esteem, and irritability are signs associated with major depression. Remorse and guilt are not generally associated with this mood disorder.
CN: Psychosocial integrity; CNS: None; CL: Apply

49. When caring for a client with generalized anxiety disorder, which intervention is **most** important for the nurse to include?
1. Encourage the client to engage in activities that increase self-esteem.
2. Promote the client's interaction and socialization with others.
3. Assist the client to make plans for regular periods of leisure time.
4. Encourage the client to use a diary to record what triggers anxiety.

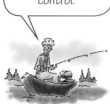

Being outdoors helps me keep my stress under control.

50. The nurse's assessment is focused on the early life of a client diagnosed with posttraumatic stress disorder (PTSD). Which client statement correlates with this diagnosis?
1. "I had an overprotective, ever-present mother."
2. "I saw many incidences of physical violence as a child."
3. "I had a rigid, consistent daily schedule of activities."
4. "I had an intact family that was stoic and emotionally reserved."

51. The nurse is educating a client experiencing considerable anxiety about an impending surgical procedure. Which nursing intervention is **most** appropriate?
1. Reassure the client that there are many treatments for the problem.
2. Calmly ask the client to describe the procedure that is to be done.
3. Tell the client that the nursing staff will help in any way they can.
4. Tell the client not to internalize personal feelings about the procedure.

52. A client with a diagnosis of generalized anxiety disorder (GAD) wants to stop taking lorazepam. Which possible outcome(s) will the nurse discuss with the client about discontinuing lorazepam? Select all that apply.
1. Muscle cramps
2. Memory loss
3. Insomnia
4. Depression
5. Anxiety

53. A client diagnosed with chronic anxiety disorder reports chest pain. Which nursing intervention will the nurse complete **first**?
1. Notify the health care provider.
2. Stay at the client's bedside.
3. Obtain the client's vital signs.
4. Administer an antianxiety medication.

49. 4. One of the nurse's goals is to help the client with generalized anxiety disorder associate symptoms with an event, thereby beginning to learn appropriate ways to eliminate or reduce distress. A diary can be a beneficial tool for this purpose. Although encouraging the client to engage in activities that increase self-esteem, promoting interaction and socialization with others, and assisting the client to make plans for regular periods of leisure time may be appropriate, they are not the priority.
CN: Psychosocial integrity; CNS: None; CL: Apply

50. 2. When obtaining a history about the early life of individuals with PTSD, one would most likely find a violent experience. None of the other options is directly associated with violence or PTSD.
CN: Psychosocial integrity; CNS: None; CL: Apply

51. 2. An appropriate nursing intervention is to ask the client to repeat to the nurse the major points of the procedure. By asking the client to describe the procedure, the nurse can assess the client's level of understanding and address anxiety by providing necessary education. Reassuring the client that there are many treatments; informing the client the nursing staff will help; and telling the client not to internalize feelings do not address the client's current anxiety or lack of knowledge about the procedure.
CN: Psychosocial integrity; CNS: None; CL: Apply

52. 1, 3, 4, 5. Abruptly stopping antianxiety drugs such as benzodiazepines can cause the client to have withdrawal symptoms that include anxiety, insomnia, muscle cramps, and depression. Memory loss is not generally associated with lorazepam withdrawal.
CN: Physiological integrity; CNS: Pharmacological and parenteral therapies; CL: Apply

53. 3. Although the client with chronic anxiety disorder may have somatic symptoms, physiologic causes for chest pain must be thoroughly assessed. Notifying the health care provider may be necessary after assessing the client. Staying with the client may be therapeutic but obtaining vital signs would take precedence. Administering antianxiety agents might mask signs of cardiac problems.
CN: Psychosocial integrity; CNS: None; CL: Analyze

54. A client prescribed alprazolam reports light-headedness while getting out of bed. Which action will the nurse incorporate to help ensure client safety?
1. Encourage the client to change positions slowly.
2. Report the symptom to the client's health care provider.
3. Teach the client to regularly monitor his or her blood pressure.
4. Have the client take the medication daily with the noon meal.

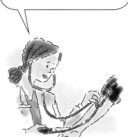

Watch out for those adverse effects.

54. 1. The nurse should encourage the client to change positions slowly because orthostatic hypotension is a side effect of this medication. It is not necessary to report the symptom if effective instructions are provided. Administration of the medication with food does not eliminate the side effect. Monitoring blood pressure is appropriate but does not focus on client safety.
CN: Physiological integrity; CNS: Reduction of risk potential; CL: Apply

55. Which nursing statement demonstrates the understanding of communication guidelines when talking with a client experiencing a panic attack?
1. "I will not leave you."
2. "What can I do to help you?"
3. "Let us try some deep breathing."
4. "Tell me what is causing this feeling."

55. 1. A panicked client is best communicated with using short, simple sentences. During a panic attack, the client is unable to focus on questions being asked or on taking instructions.
CN: Psychosocial integrity; CNS: None; CL: Apply

56. The client is scheduled for electroconvulsive therapy (ECT). The client says to the nurse, "My health care provider has discussed ECT with me, but could you remind me of some of the adverse effects I may experience?" Which adverse effect(s) will the nurse include when educating this client? Select all that apply.
1. Headache
2. Confusion
3. Dementia
4. Muscle pain
5. Short-term memory loss

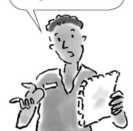

Be prepared to review the adverse effects of a treatment with your client.

56. 1, 2, 4, 5. A client may temporarily experience headache, confusion, muscle pain, and short-term memory loss. Dementia is not a side effect of ECT; dementia would signal a long-term, irreversible condition.
CN: Physiological integrity; CNS: Physiological adaptation; CL: Apply

57. A client who just had electroconvulsive therapy (ECT) asks for a drink of water. Which nursing intervention is **priority**?
1. Check the client's blood pressure.
2. Assess the client's gag reflex.
3. Obtain a body temperature.
4. Determine level of consciousness.

57. 2. The nurse must check the client's gag reflex before allowing the client to have a drink after an ECT procedure. Blood pressure and body temperature do not influence whether the client may have a drink after the procedure. The client is obviously conscious if requesting a glass of water.
CN: Physiological integrity; CNS: Physiological adaptation; CL: Apply

58. A client experiencing grandiose delusions states, "I am very powerful and only I can fix the world's problems; that is why the government hates me." Which nursing response is **most** empathic?
1. "That sounds frightening."
2. "You cannot sleep?"
3. "This cannot be true."
4. "You are having a delusion."

58. 1. The most empathic response would be to acknowledge that the delusion sounds frightening. This response would address the client's feelings. The other three options do not address feelings or demonstrate that the nurse is caring.
CN: Psychosocial integrity; CNS: None; CL: Apply

59. A client reports headache, agitation, and indigestion. Which behavior associated with bipolar disorder does the nurse suspect this client is experiencing?
1. Depression
2. Cyclothymia
3. Hypomania
4. Mania

59. 4. Headache, agitation, and indigestion are symptoms that suggest mania in a client with a history of bipolar disorder. These symptoms are not suggestive of depression, cyclothymia, or hypomania.
CN: Physiological integrity; CNS: Physiological adaptation; CL: Understand

60. A client diagnosed with bipolar disorder has abruptly stopped taking prescribed medications. Which behavior indicates to the nurse the client is experiencing a complication associated with mania?
1. Worries about "things going wrong"
2. Demonstrates severe irritability
3. Cries whenever limits are set
4. Paces almost constantly

61. What nursing intervention will help the client with bipolar disorder to maintain adequate nutrition?
1. Assess the client for favorite foods.
2. Recognize that the client will eat when hungry.
3. Provide high-calorie finger foods and beverages.
4. Request that total parenteral nutrition (TPN) be started.

62. The nurse is providing education to a client being discharged on lithium. The client demonstrates an understanding of lithium when stating that he or she will notify the health care provider of which adverse effect?
1. Black tongue
2. Increased lacrimation
3. Periods of disorientation
4. Persistent gastrointestinal upset

63. Which activity will the nurse encourage a client with a diagnosis of bipolar disorder to engage in during the manic phase of this disorder?
1. Card games
2. Basketball
3. Board games
4. Painting

A warm foot soak before bed is one of my favorite routines.

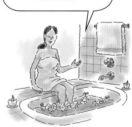

64. A client diagnosed with bipolar disorder is having difficulty sleeping. Which behavior modification technique will the nurse recommend to the client?
1. Taking a sleep medication
2. Working on solving a problem
3. Exercising before bedtime
4. Developing a sleep ritual

65. Which explanation will the nurse give to a client who does not understand why frequent blood work is necessary while taking lithium?
1. "Keeping track of your lithium levels helps your health care provider to avoid damaging your liver."
2. "Tracking your lithium levels help assure you are taking a therapeutic dosage of the medication."
3. "Lithium levels indicate whether the drug is effectively making it through the blood-brain barrier."
4. "You will not need to monitor your lithium levels once you have proven you are taking your medications correctly."

60. 4. Manic behavior is a complication that clients with bipolar disorder may experience if they abruptly stop taking medications. Signs of manic behavior include increased energy, often manifested in pacing. Irritability and crying are associated with depression, whereas generalized worrying is a characteristic of anxiety.
CN: Psychosocial integrity; CNS: None; CL: Apply

61. 3. By giving the client high-calorie food and beverages that can be consumed while active, the nurse facilitates the client's nutritional intake. While assessing for favorite foods is appropriate, that does not help assure adequate nutrition. The client cannot be relied upon to recognize the need to eat and drink when in a manic state. An invasive intervention such as TPN is not necessary.
CN: Psychosocial integrity; CNS: None; CL: Apply

62. 4. Persistent gastrointestinal upset indicates a mild-to-moderate toxic reaction. Black tongue is an adverse reaction of mirtazapine, not lithium. Increased lacrimation is not an adverse effect of lithium. Periods of disorientation do not tend to occur with the use of lithium.
CN: Physiological integrity; CNS: Pharmacological and parenteral therapies; CL: Apply

63. 4. An activity that promotes minimal stimulation, such as painting, is the best choice. Activities such as cards, basketball, or a board game may escalate hyperactivity and should be avoided.
CN: Psychosocial integrity; CNS: None; CL: Apply

64. 4. A sleep ritual or nighttime routine helps the client to relax and prepare for sleep. Obtaining sleep medication is a temporary solution. Working on problem solving may excite rather than tire the client. Exercise before retiring is stimulating and not conducive to sleep.
CN: Physiological integrity; CNS: Reduction of risk potential; CL: Apply

65. 2. Measurement of lithium levels in the blood determines whether an effective dose of lithium is being given to maintain a therapeutic level of the drug. The drug is contraindicated for clients with renal, cardiac, or liver disease. Lithium levels are not measured to determine if the drug passes through the blood-brain barrier. Taking the drug as prescribed does not eliminate the need for blood work.
CN: Physiological integrity; CNS: Pharmacological and parenteral therapies; CL: Apply

66. The nurse is providing education for a client with bipolar disorder. Which statement by the client indicates the nurse's education on coping strategies was effective?
1. "I can decide what to do to prevent family conflict."
2. "I can handle problems without asking for any help."
3. "I can stay away from my friends when I feel distressed."
4. "I can ignore things that go wrong instead of getting upset."

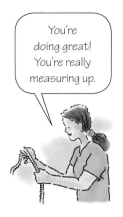

You're doing great! You're really measuring up.

67. A client is prescribed alprazolam 0.5 mg orally TID for panic disorder. The nurse has 0.25 mg tablets available. How many tablets will the nurse administer per dose? Record your answer using a whole number.
_____ tablets

68. The nurse assesses a client who reports daily insomnia, fatigue, and depression. The client states, "It has been like this since I was a child." Which behaviors demonstrated by the client indicate to the nurse the client has dysthymic disorder?
1. Having insomnia for several years, accompanied by fatigue.
2. The triad of insomnia, fatigue, and depression over several years.
3. Experiencing a depressed mood for at least 2 years.
4. Episodes of depression over time with no evidence of suicidal ideation.

69. When the nurse is developing a no-suicide contract with a client, what will the nurse include in the contract?
1. To increase client accountability, ask the client to promise the nurse or friends and family to avoid harming others.
2. Communicate belief in the client and establish a minimum time frame of 1 week for the first contract.
3. Make the agreement official and binding, and have the document typed, signed by the client, and notarized.
4. Have a detailed action plan with names and phone numbers of persons to call and the suicide crisis hotline to call if needed.

66. 1. The client should be focusing on strengths and abilities to prevent family conflict. Not asking for help is problematic and not a good coping strategy. Avoiding problems is also not a good coping strategy. It is better to identify and handle problems as they arise. Ignoring situations that cause discomfort will not facilitate solutions or allow the client to demonstrate effective coping skills.
CN: Psychosocial integrity; CNS: None; CL: Apply

67. 2.
The correct formula to calculate a drug dose is:

$$\frac{Dose\ on\ hand}{Quantity\ on\ hand} = \frac{Dose\ desired}{X}$$

For this situation, the nurse should calculate:

$$\frac{0.25\ mg}{1\ tablet} = \frac{0.5\ mg}{X}$$

$$X = 2\ tablets$$

CN: Physiological integrity; CNS: Pharmacological and parenteral therapies; CL: Apply

68. 3. To be diagnosed with a dysthymic disorder, a person must experience a depressed mood for at least 2 years. The individual often feels depressed—most of the day, for more days than not. A person with dysthymic disorder must also have at least two of the following symptoms: appetite disturbances, sleep disturbances, fatigue, low self-esteem, poor concentration or difficulty making decisions, and feelings of hopelessness.
CN: Psychosocial integrity; CNS: None; CL: Apply

69. 4. A no-suicide contract should include a promise to not harm oneself, not others; to maintain the contract no matter what happens; and to talk to someone if thoughts of suicide return. In addition, there should be a detailed plan of action with the names and phone numbers of persons to call and the number of the local suicide crisis hotline to call if experiencing suicidal thoughts. The nurse should not include a time frame in the agreement. It is not necessary to have the agreement notarized.
CN: Psychosocial integrity; CNS: None; CL: Analyze

70. Which client statement **best** indicates to the nurse manifestations of generalized anxiety?
1. "I am too worried about what might go wrong to enjoy family vacation."
2. "I seem to always make social mistakes, especially around strangers."
3. "My parents have always said I have a lack of motivation and self-esteem."
4. "My college years were terrible; I failed almost every course I took."

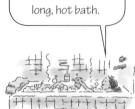

My favorite stress reliever is a long, hot bath.

70. 1. General anxiety is an excessive amount of worry that severely affects one's normal activities, such as engaging in family time. Anxiety is not a common trigger for poor social skills. Depression is likely to affect concentration, motivation, and self-esteem in a negative manner.
CN: Psychosocial integrity; CNS: None; CL: Apply

71. A client asks about how various medications are prescribed to treat anxiety disorders. What is the **best** response by the nurse?
1. Benzodiazepines are the treatment of choice for short-term management of acute anxiety.
2. Selective serotonin reuptake inhibitors (SSRIs) are used to treat acute panic attacks.
3. Beta-blockers are used for long-term treatment to manage generalized anxiety disorder.
4. Buspirone is the medication of choice to treat obsessive-compulsive disorder (OCD).

71. 1. Benzodiazepines have established short-term effectiveness in the control of anxiety symptoms. They are the treatment choice for acute episodes of anxiety, such as during crises. SSRIs are used to treat major depression, OCD, and posttraumatic stress disorder but not panic disorder; benzodiazepines are used to treat panic disorder. Beta-blockers are used to treat hypertension, not generalized anxiety disorder. Buspirone is used to treat generalized anxiety disorder, not OCD.
CN: Psychosocial integrity; CNS: None; CL: Apply

72. A client is diagnosed with postpartum depression. It is important for the nurse to monitor the client for which manifestation(s) of this mood disorder? Select all that apply.
1. Feelings of worthlessness
2. Poor bonding with the newborn
3. Suicidal or infanticidal ideations
4. Inability to care for the newborn
5. Uncontrollable crying

72. 1, 2, 3, 4, 5. Postpartum depression may lead to serious disturbances in mother-infant bonding; feelings of guilt, inadequacy, or worthlessness; uncontrollable crying; breastfeeding ineffectiveness; and disruption in family functioning. In severe circumstances, postpartum depression may result in psychosis and suicidal or infanticidal ideations. Postpartum depression is a true form of depression that requires interventions.
CN: Psychosocial integrity; CNS: None; CL: Apply

73. An adolescent who is depressed and having difficulty in school is brought to the community mental health center to be evaluated. The nurse will assess the client for which other health problem?
1. Anxiety disorder
2. Behavioral difficulties
3. Cognitive impairment
4. Labile moods

In other words, which statement by the client should cause the most concern?

73. 2. Adolescents tend to demonstrate severe irritability and behavioral problems rather than simply a depressed mood. Anxiety disorder is more commonly associated with small children rather than adolescents. Cognitive impairment is typically associated with delirium or dementia. Labile mood is more characteristic of a client with cognitive impairment or bipolar disorder.
CN: Psychosocial integrity; CNS: None; CL: Apply

74. The nurse is educating a client about taking lorazepam. Which statement by the client indicates to the nurse a need for further education?
1. "I should get up slowly from a sitting or lying position."
2. "I should not stop taking this medicine abruptly."
3. "I usually drink a beer every night to help me sleep."
4. "If I have a sore throat, I will report it to the health care provider."

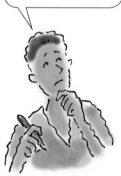

74. 3. The client should not consume alcohol or any other central nervous system depressant while taking this drug. The other statements indicate that the client understands the nurse's education.
CN: Physiological integrity; CNS: Pharmacological and parenteral therapies; CL: Apply

75. A nurse is providing education for the parents of a teenage client about the warning signs of potential adolescent suicide. Which sign will the nurse include?
1. Recently changing from one set of friends to another set of friends
2. Reclaiming of possessions previously given to friends and loved ones
3. Making statements such as not being around much longer
4. Having an increased interest in personal appearance and hygiene

76. A client has been receiving treatment for depression for 3 weeks. Which behavior suggests to the nurse the client's treatment is effective?
1. Talking about the difficulties of returning to college
2. Spending most of the day sitting alone in the room
3. Wearing a hospital gown instead of street clothes
4. Showing no emotion when visitors leave

77. The nurse is educating a client about newly prescribed lithium. The nurse instructs the client that a lack of dietary salt intake can have which effect on lithium levels?
1. Causes a marked decrease
2. Results in an increase
3. Causes an increase, then a decrease
4. Results in no effect at all

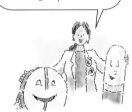

With drugs, it's best to remember the nursing implications.

78. A client diagnosed with bipolar disorder has been taking lithium for 3 years. Today, family members brought the client to the hospital reporting the client has not slept, bathed, or changed clothes for 4 days, has lost 10 lb (4.5 kg) in the past month, and woke the entire family at 0400 with plans to fly them to Hawaii. What does the nurse suspect?
1. The family is not supportive of the client.
2. The client has stopped taking lithium.
3. The client has not accepted the bipolar disorder diagnosis.
4. The client's lithium level needs to be assessed.

79. A client taking antidepressants for major depression for about 3 weeks is expressing "feeling better." The nurse will monitor the client for which complication?
1. Bipolar disorder
2. Potential for violence
3. Substance use disorder
4. Suicidal ideation

75. 3. The warning signs of potential adolescent suicide include statements such as not being around much longer, restlessness, pacing, poor impulse control, making arrangements or putting personal affairs in order, and giving away personal possessions, especially treasured items.
CN: Psychosocial integrity; CNS: None; CL: Apply

76. 1. By talking about returning to college, the client is demonstrating an interest in making plans for the future, which is a sign of beginning recovery from depression. Decreased socialization, lack of interest in personal appearance, and lack of emotion are all symptoms of depression.
CN: Physiological integrity; CNS: Reduction of risk potential; CL: Apply

77. 2. There is an inverse relationship between the amount of salt and the plasma levels of lithium. Lithium plasma levels increase when there is a decrease in dietary salt. An increase in dietary salt causes the opposite effect of decreasing lithium plasma levels. It is important that the nurse monitors adequate dietary sodium.
CN: Physiological integrity; CNS: Pharmacological and parenteral therapies; CL: Apply

78. 4. Measuring the lithium level is the best way to evaluate the effectiveness of lithium therapy and begin to assess the client's current status. The client's unsupportive family, stopping the medication, and not accepting the diagnosis may all have contributed to the manic episode, but the nurse cannot assume anything until after assessing the client and family more fully.
CN: Physiological integrity; CNS: Reduction of risk potential; CL: Apply

79. 4. After a client has been on antidepressants and is feeling better, the client commonly then has the energy for self-harm. Bipolar disorder is not treated with antidepressants. Nothing in the client's history suggests a potential for violence. There are no signs or symptoms suggesting substance use disorder.
CN: Psychosocial integrity; CNS: None; CL: Apply

80. The nurse is caring for a client diagnosed with posttraumatic stress disorder (PTSD). Which therapeutic nursing approach will have the **best** client outcome?
1. Ignoring client behaviors unless they are threatening.
2. Identifying the client's expressed fears as being unfounded.
3. Teaching the client about the details of the diagnosis.
4. Assisting the client to adopt improved problem-solving skills.

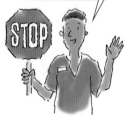

Check out that word "best" in question #80. It's kind of important.

81. A client on the psychiatric unit is receiving lithium and has a lithium level of 1 mEq/L (1 mmol/L). The nurse notes that the client has fine tremors of the hands. Which nursing action is **priority**?
1. Withhold the client's next lithium dose.
2. Notify the health care provider immediately.
3. Repeat the lithium level measurement.
4. Realize that a fine tremor is expected.

82. The nurse preparing to administer an injection observes that the client appears very hyperalert and is clenching both fists. Perspiration is noticeably present on the client's brow. Which nursing statement is **most** appropriate?
1. "Are you nervous about getting an injection?"
2. "Let me help you relax the muscles in your upper arm."
3. "Would you prefer getting this medication in pill form?"
4. "I suggest distracting yourself while I give this injection."

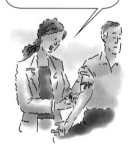

Injections can be a source of anxiety for both the client and the nurse.

83. The nurse is caring for a client who reports feeling very "stressed." When assessing the client, which physiologic correlating manifestation(s) will the nurse expect? Select all that apply.
1. Irritability
2. Nausea
3. Increased breathing
4. Confusion
5. Insomnia
6. Headache

84. A client arrives at the health clinic and informs the nurse, "I have been doubling my daily dose of bupropion to get better faster." The nurse notes the client was prescribed 100 mg three times per day. The nurse will closely monitor the client for which complication?
1. Orthostatic hypotension
2. Weight gain
3. Seizure activity
4. Insomnia

80. 4. Assisting the client in improving problem-solving skills would provide the client with coping skills. The nurse should not attempt to talk the client out of unfounded fears as this will merely lead to the client becoming more defensive. Helping the client to cope is more important than simply providing information to the client. The nurse should provide feedback to the client's behaviors, as often the client does not realize how he or she comes across to others.
CN: Psychosocial integrity; CNS: None; CL: Apply

81. 4. Fine tremors of the hands are considered normal with lithium therapy. The lithium level is within normal limits so there is no need to withhold a dose, notify the health care provider, or repeat the blood work.
CN: Psychosocial integrity; CNS: None; CL: Apply

82. 2. The client is experiencing anxiety over the impending injection. The nurse demonstrates an understanding of the impact this anxiety will have on the injection by assisting the client in relaxing the muscles of the injection site. Suggesting an oral form of medication is not a likely option in this situation. While assessing for nervousness and suggesting distraction are both appropriate interventions, neither will impact the administration of the medication as directly as will helping the client relax the injection site.
CN: Psychosocial integrity; CNS: None; CL: Apply

83. 2, 3, 6. Nausea, increased breathing, and headache are physiologic signs and symptoms of stress. Insomnia is a behavioral sign and symptom of stress; confusion is a cognitive sign and symptom of stress; and irritability is a psychological sign and symptom of stress.
CN: Psychosocial integrity; CNS: None; CL: Apply

84. 3. Seizure activity is common in dosages greater than 450 mg daily. Bupropion is an atypical antidepressant and does not cause orthostatic hypotension. It frequently causes weight loss, and insomnia is an adverse effect, but seizure activity causes a greater client risk.
CN: Physiological Integrity; CNS: None; CL: Apply

85. The nurse interviews the family of a client hospitalized with severe depression and suicidal ideation. Which information about the family is essential for the nurse to obtain to assist in formulating an effective care plan? Select all that apply.
1. Physical pain
2. Personal responsibilities
3. Employment skills
4. Communication patterns
5. Role expectations
6. Current family stressors

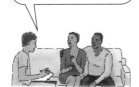

Family members can be a valuable source of information about a client with depression.

85. 4, 5, 6. When working with the family of a depressed client, it is helpful for the nurse to be aware of the family's communication style, the role expectations for its members, and current family stressors. This information can help identify family difficulties and teaching points that could benefit the client and the family. Information concerning physical pain, personal responsibilities, and employment skills is not directly related to the experience of having a depressed family member. CN: Psychosocial integrity; CNS: None; CL: Apply

86. The nurse is providing discharge instructions to a client prescribed sertraline. The nurse will monitor the client for which adverse drug effect(s)? Select all that apply.
1. Agitation
2. Agranulocytosis
3. Sleep disturbance
4. Intermittent tachycardia
5. Dry mouth
6. Seizure

86. 1, 3, 5. Common adverse effects of sertraline include agitation, sleep disturbance, and dry mouth. Agranulocytosis, intermittent tachycardia, and seizures are adverse effects of clozapine. CN: Physiological integrity; CNS: Pharmacological and parenteral therapies; CL: Apply

87. The health care provider prescribes olanzapine 15 mg orally once per day for bipolar mania. Available is olanzapine 7.5 mg. How many tablets will the nurse administer the client per dose? Record your answer using a whole number.
_____ tablets

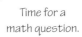

Time for a math question.

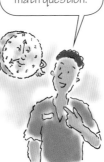

87. 2.
The correct formula to calculate a drug dose is:

$$\frac{Dose\ on\ hand}{Quantity\ on\ hand} = \frac{Dose\ desired}{X}$$

For this situation, the nurse should calculate:

$$\frac{7.5\ mg}{1\ tablet} = \frac{15\ mg}{X}$$

$$X = 2\ tablets$$

CN: Physiological integrity; CNS: Pharmacological and parenteral therapies; CL: Apply

88. An adolescent client is diagnosed with a phobia disorder. What statement made by the client informs the nurse that the client understands the disorder?
1. "I will need to start desensitization therapy."
2. "I will likely outgrow most of my fears."
3. "I had specific testing to determine my diagnosis."
4. "I have this problem because I do not always pay attention."

88. 1. Individuals with phobias respond with panic when confronted with a feared object or situation. Phobias are often treated with desensitization therapy, which involves exposing the client to the object of fear and helping them to overcome the fear. There is no specific test to diagnose a phobia. The client is not likely to outgrow the irrational fear. Not paying attention is not a sign or symptom of this disorder. CN: Psychosocial integrity; CNS: None; CL: Apply

89. A client insists the nurse place four sheets of newspaper beneath the nursing bag and that all supplies be returned to their original place after being counted three times. This behavior **most** suggests which disorder to the nurse?
1. Bipolar disorder
2. Depression
3. Schizophrenia
4. Obsessive-compulsive disorder

89. 4. The client's insistence indicates a compulsive behavior, which may include repetitive touching or counting, doing and undoing small tasks, or any other repetitive behavior. The behavior is not indicative of the other disorders listed. CN: Psychosocial integrity; CNS: None; CL: Apply

CN: Client needs category   CNS: Client needs subcategory   CL: Cognitive level

90. A client informs the nurse, "Last week I felt sad, had a poor appetite, and did not want to go out, but this week I feel better because my child asked me to come to dinner." What does this client behavior indicate to the nurse?

1. Normal fluctuation
2. Clinical depression
3. Predisposition to psychotic depression
4. Precursor to bipolar disorder

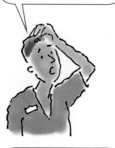

Some days I feel like the king of the world; other days I feel worthless. What's wrong with me?

91. A rape victim is being prepared for discharge. The nurse is aware that the client is at risk for posttraumatic stress disorder (PTSD) and instructs the client that it is important to report which symptom(s) associated with PTSD? Select all that apply.

1. Recurrent, intrusive nightmares
2. Gingival and dental problems
3. Sleep disturbances
4. Flight of ideas
5. Unusual talkativeness
6. Difficulty concentrating

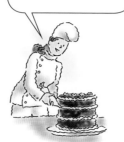

Congratulations! You finished the test.

90. 1. Feelings of sadness are normal for most individuals at some time. Losses and stresses far less profound than death can make an individual sad, but the feelings are usually fleeting, lasting a few hours to a few days. Even though the client felt fatigue and sadness, and had a poor appetite, the mood changed when the client's child invited the client to dinner. This behavior does not indicate psychotic behavior, clinical depression, or bipolar disorder.

CN: Psychosocial integrity; CNS: None; CL: Analyze

91. 1, 3, 6. Clients diagnosed with PTSD typically experience recurrent, intrusive recollections or nightmares, sleep disturbances, difficulty concentrating, chronic anxiety or panic attacks, memory impairment, and feelings of detachment or estrangement that destroy interpersonal relationships. Gingival and dental problems are associated with bulimia. Flight of ideas and unusual talkativeness are characteristic of the acute manic phase of bipolar affective disorder.

CN: Psychosocial integrity; CNS: None; CL: Apply

Chapter 14

Cognitive Disorders

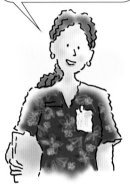

This chapter covers a host of cognitive disorders. Are your own cognitive powers ready? OK, let's go!

Cognitive disorders refresher

Alzheimer's disease

Progressive, non-curable disorder characterized by memory loss, decline of cognitive function, and eventual loss of motor skills

Key signs and symptoms

Stage 1 (mild symptoms)
- Confusion and short-term memory loss
- Disorientation to time and place
- Difficulty performing routine tasks
- Changes in personality and judgment

Stage 2 (moderate symptoms)
- Anxiety
- Obvious memory loss
- Suspicion
- Agitation
- Wandering
- Difficulty recognizing family members

Stage 3 (moderate-to-severe symptoms)
- Increasing loss of expressive language skills
- Loss of reasoning ability
- Loss of ability to perform activities of daily living

Stage 4 (severe symptoms)
- Absent cognitive abilities
- Disorientation to time and place
- Impaired or absent motor skills
- Bowel and bladder incontinence

Key test results
- Cognitive assessment scale demonstrates cognitive impairment
- Functional dementia scale shows the degree of the dementia
- Magnetic resonance imaging (MRI) shows apparent structural and neurologic changes
- The Mini-Mental State Examination reveals disorientation and cognitive impairment

Key treatments
- Group therapy
- Anticholinesterase agents: donepezil, rivastigmine, galantamine
- *N*-methyl-D-aspartate receptor: memantine

Key interventions
- Remove hazardous items or potential obstacles from client's environment.

- Communicate verbally and nonverbally with the client in a consistent, structured way.
- Increase client's social interaction.
- Encourage the use of community resources.

Amnesic disorder

Group of disorders characterized by impairments in memory in the absence of other cognitive dysfunction

Key signs and symptoms
- Confusion, disorientation, and lack of insight
- Inability to learn and retain new information
- Tendency to remember the remote past better than more recent events

Key test results
- The Mini-Mental State Examination shows:
  - client is disoriented
  - client has difficulty recalling events and information

Key treatments
- Correction of the underlying medical cause
- Group therapy
- Family therapy

Key interventions
- Ensure client's safety.
- Encourage the client to explore his or her feelings.
- Provide simple, clear medical information.

Delirium

Presents with a loss of mental clarity; may be associated with physical or psychological causative factors

Key signs and symptoms
- Altered psychomotor activity (e.g., apathy, withdrawal, agitation)
- Bizarre, destructive behavior that is worse at night
- Disorganized thinking
- Distractibility
- Impaired decision making
- Inability to complete tasks

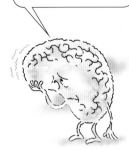

"Where did I leave my keys?" Persistent memory loss can be an indicator of cognitive disorder.

- Insomnia or daytime sleepiness
- Poor impulse control
- Rambling, bizarre, or incoherent speech

Key test results

- Laboratory results indicate that the delirium is a result of:
  - physiologic condition
  - intoxication
  - substance withdrawal
  - toxic exposure
  - prescribed medicines
  - combination of these factors
- The Mini-Mental Status Examination shows that the client has difficulty with:
  - attention
  - cognition
  - awareness

Key treatments

- Correction of the underlying physiologic problem
- Antipsychotic agent: risperidone

Key interventions

- Minimize excessive sensory stimuli.
- Create a structured, safe, and supportive environment.
- Keep a light on in client's room.

Vascular dementia

Loss of cognitive function associated with a reduction in blood perfusion to the brain

Key signs and symptoms

- Depression
- Difficulty following instructions
- Emotional lability
- Inappropriate emotional reactions
- Memory loss
- Wandering and getting lost in familiar places

Key test results

- Cognitive assessment scale shows a deterioration in cognitive ability
- Global Deterioration Scale signifies degenerative dementia
- The Mini-Mental Status Examination reveals that the client is:
  - disoriented
  - has difficulty recalling information

Key treatments

- Carotid endarterectomy to remove blockages in the carotid artery
- Treatment of the underlying condition (hypertension, high cholesterol, or diabetes)
- Antiplatelet aggregate drugs: aspirin, ticlopidine

Key interventions

- Orient client to his surroundings.
- Monitor client's environment.
- Encourage client to express feelings of sadness and loss.

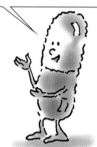

I'm an antipsychotic agent that is used to treat delirium. Do you know my name?

thePoint® You can download tables of drug information to help you prepare for the NCLEX®! View Generic Drug Names, Drug Classifications, Drug Actions, and Nursing Implications for the drugs discussed in this refresher at **http://thePoint.lww.com.**

Cognitive disorders questions, answers, and rationales

1. A client is being seen for a routine physical exam. The client is concerned because her parent has been diagnosed with dementia and the client fears "getting it" when getting older. Which nursing response is **most** appropriate?

1. "I understand your concern. Dementia is a scary condition that is a concern for all of us as we age."
2. "Because there are no known familial factors associated with dementia, you have no reason to worry."
3. "Even though aging and a family history elevate your risk, there is no guarantee that you will develop dementia."
4. "Your worries should be limited because most dementia occurs because of a history of head injury."

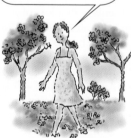

Take a deep breath and stretch your legs. You'll be done with this test before you know it.

1. **3.** Dementia has risk factors, which include a family history and aging. Although aging is a risk factor, describing dementia as something to be feared when aging is not the best response by the nurse because it does not address the client's concerns. Although family history is a risk factor, it does not mean it will be "passed down" to the client. Dementia is not linked to a single incidence of head injury. If the trauma is severe, the client is diagnosed with traumatic brain injury, not dementia.

CN: Health promotion and maintenance; CNS: None; CL: Apply

2. A client has been prescribed donepezil. Which client statement(s) indicate to the nurse the client understands the medication? Select all that apply.
1. "This medication works by halting the progression of Alzheimer's disease."
2. "It will take a few weeks for this medication to begin improving my condition."
3. "Some nausea and vomiting may be experienced when I begin donepezil."
4. "If donepezil impacts my ability to rest at night, I will call my health care provider."
5. "After a year, I may need to change from donepezil to another medication."

3. The nurse is discussing a recent diagnosis of Alzheimer's disease with a client and immediate family. Which statement(s) by the family indicate to the nurse the need for further instruction? Select all that apply.
1. "Alzheimer's disease is commonly caused by cerebral abscesses."
2. "Alcohol use disorder plays a role in the development of Alzheimer's disease."
3. "Multiple small brain infarctions typically lead to Alzheimer's disease."
4. "The cause of Alzheimer's disease is currently unknown."
5. "Not all causes of memory losses are the result of Alzheimer's disease."

4. A client suddenly begins to exhibit symptoms of dementia. The nurse will assess the client for which condition that can cause symptoms like those of dementia?
1. Multiple sclerosis
2. Electrolyte imbalance
3. Multiple small brain infarctions
4. Human immunodeficiency virus (HIV)

5. Which assessment data obtained by the nurse indicates a client is exhibiting impairment in abstract thinking and reasoning? Select all that apply.
1. The client is unable to repeat the sentence, "Mary had a little lamb."
2. The client states, "You know 2 plus 2 equals 22."
3. When asked who the current American president is, the client states, "Reagan."
4. The client failed to correctly identify the triangles among several different geometric shapes.
5. When shown a group of words, the client is unable to decide which word does not belong.

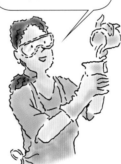

Hard work and a positive attitude are the perfect formula for success. Now let's get down to business.

2. 2, 3, 4. Donepezil is prescribed for Alzheimer's disease. The medication is used to reduce confusion and may improve memory. The medication does not halt the progression of or cure Alzheimer's disease. The medication will take a few weeks to begin to work. Some gastrointestinal symptoms may be noted. These symptoms will gradually subside. The medication is normally taken at bedtime. If this impacts the ability to obtain rest the client may confer with the prescriber to review the timing of dosages. This medication varies in duration of effectiveness from individual to individual, so there is not a standard, predetermined time at which the client will change to another medication.
CN: Physiological integrity; CNS: Pharmacological and parenteral therapies; CL: Apply

3. 1, 2, 3. Several hypotheses suggest genetic factors, trauma, accumulation of aluminum, alterations in the immune system, or alterations in acetylcholine as contributing to the development of Alzheimer's disease, but the exact cause is unknown. Alcohol use disorder has not been associated with the development of Alzheimer's disease, nor has the presence of cerebral abscess or small brain infarction. Alzheimer's disease is not the lone cause of memory loss.
CN: Health promotion and maintenance; CNS: None; CL: Apply

4. 2. Electrolyte imbalance is a correctable metabolic abnormality that may present with dementia-type symptomatology. Multiple sclerosis presents with neuromuscular changes, not dementia. Small brain infarctions do not present with dementia-like symptoms. HIV does not present with dementia.
CN: Physiological integrity; CNS: Physiological adaptation; CL: Apply

5. 4, 5. Abstract thinking is assessed by noting similarities and differences between related words or objects. Not being able to do a simple calculation or repeat a sentence shows a client's inability to concentrate and focus on thoughts. Not knowing the name of the president of the United States is a deficiency in general knowledge.
CN: Psychosocial integrity; CNS: None; CL: Apply

CN: Client needs category   CNS: Client needs subcategory   CL: Cognitive level

6. While caring for a client with delirium, which nursing intervention is **priority**?
1. Provide a safe environment.
2. Offer recreational activities.
3. Provide a structured environment.
4. Institute measures to promote sleep.

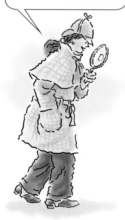

Which symptoms would most cause you to suspect Alzheimer's disease?

7. A client is suspected of experiencing early-stage Alzheimer's disease. Which symptom(s) documented by the nurse correlate with this suspicion? Select all that apply.
1. Dilated pupils bilaterally
2. Constant rambling speech
3. Elevated blood pressure
4. Significant recent memory loss
5. Having difficulty grocery shopping

8. A Mini-Mental State Examination has been scheduled for a client experiencing episodes of memory impairment. Which information will the nurse provide to the client about this test? Select all that apply.
1. The level of a client's education may impact overall scoring.
2. The test results will decline as a normal part of aging.
3. Lower test scores are associated with dementia.
4. The test will be completed over several appointments.
5. The test is used to diagnose Alzheimer's disease.

9. When planning care for the client with Alzheimer's disease, which nursing action is **priority**?
1. Provide the client with a list of activities to complete.
2. Assist the client in establishing a daily routine.
3. Place pictures of family in the care environment.
4. Review safeguards that will limit client wandering.

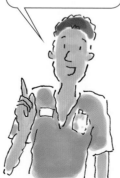

Remember–clients with Alzheimer's disease respond to your demeanor.

10. Which nursing intervention will assist a client diagnosed with Alzheimer's disease to perform activities of daily living?
1. Urge the client to perform all basic care without help.
2. Tell the client that morning care must be done by 0900.
3. Give the client a written list of activities to perform.
4. Provide ample time for the client to complete basic tasks.

6. **1.** The nurse's priority when caring for a client with delirium is to ensure client safety. Offering recreational activities, providing a structured environment, and promoting sleep are all appropriate interventions after safety measures are in place.
CN: Safe, effective care environment; CNS: Management of care; CL: Analyze

7. **4, 5.** Significant recent memory loss, indicated by the inability to verbalize remembrances after several minutes to an hour, can be assessed in the early stages of Alzheimer's disease. During the early stages of Alzheimer's disease there is increasing difficulty performing simple tasks such as shopping or dressing. Dilated pupils, elevated blood pressure, and rambling speech are expected symptoms of delirium.
CN: Physiological integrity; CNS: Physiological adaptation; CL: Apply

8. **1, 3.** The Mini-Mental State Examination is used to assess cognition. Areas assessed include global cognition, orientation, and visuospatial ability. The assessment does not provide a definitive diagnosis but is a tool in the process. Clients with higher levels of education may score higher on the test. Test results do not decline with aging. The test can be completed in a short period of time and does not take multiple appointments. Lower scores are consistent with cognitive impairment.
CN: Health promotion and maintenance; CNS: None; CL: Apply

9. **4.** Protection of the client, such as by reviewing safeguards that limit wandering, is the priority. The other activities listed would be beneficial to the client with Alzheimer's disease but are not as important as the client's safety.
CN: Safe, effective care environment; CNS: Safety and infection control; CL: Apply

10. **4.** Clients with Alzheimer's disease respond to the demeanor of those around them. A gentle, calm approach is comforting and nonthreatening, whereas a tense, hurried approach may agitate the client. The client has problems performing tasks independently; expecting him or her to perform self-care independently may lead to frustration.
CN: Physiological integrity; CNS: Basic care and comfort; CL: Apply

CN: Client needs category   CNS: Client needs subcategory   CL: Cognitive level

11. Which medication(s) will the nurse anticipate administering to a client with Alzheimer's disease? Select all that apply.
1. Bupropion
2. Haloperidol
3. Donepezil
4. Triazolam
5. Divalproex

12. The nurse places an object in the hand of a client diagnosed with Alzheimer's disease and asks the client to identify the object. The client is unable to identify the object. Which nursing action is **most** appropriate?
1. Notify the client's family.
2. Document the finding.
3. Repeat the test in 1 hour.
4. Give the client a different object.

13. Which nursing intervention will assist a client diagnosed with progressive memory deficit function **most** effectively?
1. Label cupboards and drawers with simple descriptions of their contents.
2. Arrange for meals to be delivered by a community social service agency.
3. Suggest that family members alternate spending nights with the client.
4. Discuss the advantages of elder care services with the client and family.

14. When caring for a client diagnosed with Alzheimer's disease, which nursing intervention is **priority**?
1. Providing social contact opportunities
2. Addressing nutritional needs
3. Providing enough sensory stimulation
4. Addressing physical safety issues

15. Which nursing intervention is **priority** when caring for a client diagnosed with Alzheimer's disease?
1. Placing an identification bracelet on the client's wrist
2. Making sure the client is involved in making clothing choices
3. Arranging for recreational experiences to stimulate the client
4. Providing support to the client in performing activities of daily living

16. The nurse is caring for a client diagnosed with dementia who is agitated, violent, and experiencing bizarre thoughts. Which medication will the nurse expect the health care provider to prescribe this client?
1. Diazepam
2. Ergoloid
3. Haloperidol
4. Donepezil

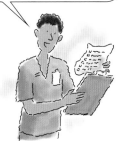

What are the key signs and symptoms of stage 3 Alzheimer-type dementia?

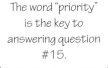

The word "priority" is the key to answering question #15.

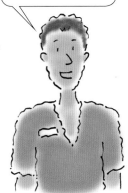

11. 3. Donepezil is used to improve cognition and functional autonomy in mild-to-moderate dementia of the Alzheimer's type. Bupropion is used for depression. Haloperidol is used for agitation, aggression, hallucinations, thought disturbances, and wandering. Triazolam is used for sleep disturbances. Divalproex is an anticonvulsant used to treat disorders such as bipolar disorder.
CN: Physiological integrity; CNS: Pharmacological and parenteral therapies; CL: Apply

12. 2. Agnosia is the inability to recognize familiar objects and usually occur in stage 3 of Alzheimer's disease. The nurse would document this expected finding. The client's family can be updated when visiting. There is no need to repeat the test later or to conduct the test using a different object.
CN: Health promotion and maintenance; CNS: None; CL: Apply

13. 1. Clients with cognitive impairment should assume responsibility for as many tasks as they can. By labeling cupboards and drawers, the client may be able to manage self-care tasks such as dressing despite memory deficiencies. All the remaining options, although appropriate, do not support the client's autonomy.
CN: Safe, effective care environment; CNS: Safety and infection control; CL: Apply

14. 4. Whenever client safety is at risk, attention to appropriate interventions is a priority. Although the other options are appropriate, safety is the nurse's priority.
CN: Safe, effective care environment; CNS: Management of care; CL: Apply

15. 1. Providing for client safety is the number-one priority when caring for any client, but particularly when a client is already compromised and at greater risk for injury. Properly identifying the client would be helpful in case of wandering. Although the remaining options are appropriate, interventions related to safety have priority.
CN: Safe, effective care environment; CNS: Safety and infection control; CL: Apply

16. 3. Haloperidol is an antipsychotic medication that decreases the symptoms of agitation, violence, and bizarre thoughts. Diazepam is used for anxiety and muscle relaxation. Ergoloid is an adrenergic blocker used to block vascular headaches. Donepezil is used for improvement of cognition.
CN: Physiological integrity; CNS: Reduction of risk potential; CL: Apply

CN: Client needs category   CNS: Client needs subcategory   CL: Cognitive level

17. A client diagnosed with Alzheimer's disease states, "Today I have a luncheon date with my child." The nurse knows that the child is not visiting today. Which response by the nurse is **most** appropriate?
1. "Tell me where you are planning to have your luncheon."
2. "You are confused and do not know what you are talking about."
3. "I think you need some more medication, and I will bring it to you."
4. "Today is Monday, March 8, and we will be eating lunch in the dining room."

18. The nurse is caring for a client diagnosed with a cognitive disorder. Which assessment finding will the nurse anticipate the client will exhibit?
1. Catatonia
2. Depression
3. Feeling of dread
4. Memory deficit

19. Which degenerative disorder will the nurse expect an older adult client with progressive deterioration in cognition to exhibit while assessing?
1. Delirium
2. Dementia
3. Neurosis
4. Psychosis

20. The nurse is educating the family of a client diagnosed with dementia. Which statement will the nurse include in the education?
1. "Personal neglect in self-care is common in clients with dementia."
2. "Dementia often causes poor judgment, especially in social situations."
3. "Memory loss begins to occur due to a natural consequence of aging."
4. "It causes a loss of intellectual abilities that impairs the ability to perform basic care."

21. The nurse is reviewing the medical record of a client who has a primary diagnosis of vascular dementia. Which findings(s) in the medical record supports this diagnosis? Select all that apply.
1. Uncontrolled diabetes
2. Hypotension
3. Obesity
4. Mitral valve prolapse
5. History of addiction to opiates

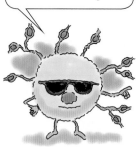

The word "degenerative" is key to answering question #19 correctly.

17. 4. The best nursing response is to reorient the client to the date and environment. Confrontation can provoke an outburst. Medication will not provide immediate relief for memory impairment. The nurse should not encourage the misconception.
CN: Psychosocial integrity; CNS: None; CL: Apply

18. 4. Cognitive disorders represent a significant change in cognition or memory from a previous level of functioning. Catatonia is a type of schizophrenia characterized by periods of physical rigidity, negativism, excitement, and stupor. Depression is a feeling of sadness and apathy and is part of major depressive and other mood disorders. A feeling of dread is characteristic of an anxiety disorder.
CN: Physiological integrity; CNS: Physiological adaptation; CL: Apply

19. 2. Dementia is progressive and commonly associated with aging or underlying metabolic or organic deterioration. Delirium is characterized by abrupt, spontaneous cognitive dysfunction with an underlying organic mental disorder. Neurosis and psychosis are psychological diagnoses.
CN: Physiological integrity; CNS: Physiological adaptation; CL: Apply

20. 4. The ability to perform self-care is an important measure of the progression of dementia. Personal neglect and poor judgment typically occur in dementia but are not considered defining characteristics. Memory loss reflects underlying physical, metabolic, and pathologic processes.
CN: Physiological integrity; CNS: Physiological adaptation; CL: Apply

21. 1, 3. Vascular dementia is an impairment in brain function that results from an alteration in perfusion to the organ. Risk factors for vascular dementia include diabetes and obesity. Elevation in blood pressure, not hypotension, is a risk factor. Cardiovascular rhythm disorders, not mitral valve prolapse, are associated with this condition. The use or misuse of opiates is not associated with vascular dementia.
CN: Physiological integrity; CNS: Physiological adaptation; CL: Apply

22. The nurse is assessing a client with suspected dementia disorder. Which factor is **most** important for the nurse to determine when assessing for this diagnosis?
1. Prognosis
2. Genetic information
3. Degree of impairment
4. Implications for treatment

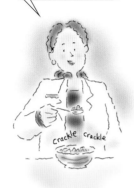

Can you remember what you had for breakfast this morning?

crackle crackle

23. The nurse asks a client with a suspected dementia disorder to recall what was eaten for breakfast. What is the nurse's assessment focus regarding this client?
1. Food preferences
2. Recent memory
3. Remote memory
4. Speech capacity

24. A client has been prescribed donepezil. Which instruction will the nurse include in the client education?
1. Take the medication every other day.
2. Take the medication with milk.
3. Take the medication in the evening.
4. Crush and take in pudding or applesauce.

25. The nurse is assessing a client diagnosed with vascular dementia. Which finding(s) will the nurse expect to assess in this client? Select all that apply.
1. The family reports that the client sleeps most of the day.
2. The client lacks upper body strength.
3. When awake, the client spends much time pacing.
4. The client ambulates using a shuffling, small-stepped gait.
5. The client consistently refers to a glass as a shoe.

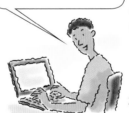

Can you remember what the key signs and symptoms of vascular dementia are?

26. The spouse of a client diagnosed with vascular dementia asks the nurse if this is the same as having Alzheimer's disease. Which response by the nurse is **most** appropriate?
1. "Yes, vascular dementia is another term used for Alzheimer's disease."
2. "There are similarities in the conditions, but they are not the same condition."
3. "Vascular dementia is actually much more severe than Alzheimer's disease."
4. "No, they are not the same. Alzheimer's disease is more successfully treated."

27. The nurse is caring for a client diagnosed with a cognitive disorder. Which nursing action is **priority**?
1. Promote increased socialization.
2. Maintain optimal physical health.
3. Provide frequent changes in personnel.
4. Provide an overstimulating environment.

22. 4. The progression of biological impairment in the central nervous system is a function of the underlying pathologic states, so it is important to collect data and treat the underlying cause. Prognosis is not the most important factor when making a diagnosis. Genetic information is not relevant. The degree of impairment is necessary information for developing a care plan.
CN: Health promotion and maintenance; CNS: None; CL: Apply

23. 2. Persons with dementia have difficulty with recent memory or learning, which may be a key to early detection. Assessing food preferences may be helpful in determining what the client likes to eat, but this assessment has no direct correlation in assessing dementia. Speech difficulties, such as rambling, irrelevance, and incoherence, may be related to delirium.
CN: Health promotion and maintenance; CNS: None; CL: Apply

24. 3. Donepezil is a medication used in the treatment of Alzheimer's disease. The medication should be taken daily in the evening close to bedtime. It is administered whole and with a glass of water.
CN: Physiological integrity; CNS: Pharmacological and parenteral therapies; CL: Apply

25. 2, 4, 5. Focal neurologic signs commonly seen with vascular dementia include weakness of the limbs, small-stepped gait, and difficulty with speech. Hypersomnolence, insomnia, and restlessness are symptoms related to delirium.
CN: Physiological integrity; CNS: Physiological adaptation; CL: Apply

26. 2. Vascular dementia differs from Alzheimer's disease in that it has a more abrupt onset and runs a highly variable course. Both conditions are characterized by losses in cognitive function. Both are severe conditions. Although treatments are available, neither condition can be cured nor the damages be reversed.
CN: Physiological integrity; CNS: Physiological adaptation; CL: Apply

27. 2. A client's cognitive impairment may hinder self-care abilities. More socialization, frequent changes in staff members, and an overstimulating environment would only increase anxiety and confusion.
CN: Health promotion and maintenance; CNS: None; CL: Apply

CN: Client needs category   CNS: Client needs subcategory   CL: Cognitive level

28. A client is brought to the emergency department by a spouse, who reports the client has become increasingly confused over a period of 3 to 4 days. The spouse reports there is no history of confusion. Which initial question by the nurse is **most** appropriate?
1. "Is there a family history of dementia-related conditions?"
2. "What medications and supplements are being taken?"
3. "How has your spouse been sleeping the last few days?"
4. "Have there been any recent stressors at home?"

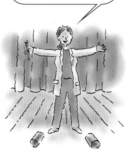

You really perform well under pressure. Bravo!

28. 2. Delirium refers to a rapid onset of a loss of cognitive abilities. There are a variety of potential causative factors. Obtaining a history is the most important action. Many cases of delirium can be attributed to medication therapies. Rest and sleep can play a factor, but not with delirium lasting for nearly a week. Stress at home may intensify conditions but is not the underlying cause. Dementia and delirium are not the same condition, so asking about a family history of dementia would be inappropriate.
CN: Physiological integrity; CNS: Physiological adaptation; CL: Apply

29. Memantine has been prescribed to a client. When discussing the planned therapy with the client's spouse, which statement(s) by the spouse indicates to the nurse a correct understanding of how to prevent or manage side effects of the medication? Select all that apply.
1. "I plan to add fiber-rich snacks to the daily menu."
2. "I may need to help my spouse get up."
3. "This medication will need to be taken with milk."
4. "Monitoring my spouse's weight will be necessary."
5. "We need to maintain sleep and nap routines."

29. 1, 2, 4, 5. Memantine is a medication used in the treatment of Alzheimer's disease. The medication may result in constipation. Fiber-rich snacks are helpful in preventing this side effect. The medication is associated with dizziness. Assistance with position changes is beneficial in preventing falls. Weight gain is a side effect of the medication, so it is important to monitor weight. Sleeplessness may result, so it is important to maintain organized sleep periods. There is no need to administer this medication with milk.
CN: Physiological integrity; CNS: Pharmacological and parenteral therapies; CL: Apply

30. The nurse is preparing to administer ticlopidine to a client hospitalized with vascular dementia. The client questions the nurse about how this medication will help the condition. Which information will be included in the nurse's response? Select all that apply.
1. "Ticlopidine promotes an increase in the blood flow to your brain."
2. "Ticlopidine works by reducing the blockages caused by platelets."
3. "Enzymes that regulate impulse controls are increased by ticlopidine."
4. "Plaques responsible for confusion are lessened by ticlopidine."
5. "Ticlopidine makes transmitters of impulses in your brain more effective."

30. 1, 2. Ticlopidine is used to reduce platelet aggregation, which promotes increased perfusion to the brain. Enzymes and neurotransmitters are not impacted by ticlopidine. Plaques that are associated with Alzheimer's disease are not impacted by this medication.
CN: Physiological integrity; CNS: Pharmacological and parenteral therapies; CL: Apply

31. During a routine physical exam the client reports concerns about getting older and losing cognitive abilities. Which nursing response is **most** appropriate?
1. "Aging is a risk for cognitive changes, but it does not always happen."
2. "Research has failed to show that age has a bearing on mental function."
3. "You should not be anxious as nothing can be done about this concern."
4. "It is unwise to worry about these changes before they occur."

31. 1. Aging is a risk factor for the loss of cognitive function and related disease processes, but not all older adults experience delirium or dementia-related conditions. So, the risk, although present, is not absolute. There are recommended steps an individual can take to reduce losses in cognitive function. These include activities that challenge the mind and promote memory. Concern for and prevention of health problems is wise for all individuals.
CN: Health promotion and maintenance; CNS: None; CL: Apply

32. The nurse is preparing to care for a client with amnesia. Which nursing action **best** meets the needs of this client?
1. Provide the client with lots of space to test independence.
2. Promote activities to keep the client busy throughout the day.
3. Use short, simple commands when providing instruction.
4. Spend time with the client, asking questions about the client's recent life.

33. Which finding(s) warrant **immediate** nursing intervention in a client taking memantine? Select all that apply.
1. Weakness
2. Bradycardia
3. Dizziness
4. Hallucinations
5. Tachycardia

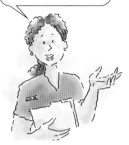

In question #33, keep in mind that "bradycardia" and "tachycardia" are opposites, so only one can be correct. Which is it?

34. A client has been diagnosed with an amnesic disorder. Which change(s) will the nurse anticipate with this condition? Select all that apply.
1. Impaired speech patterns or slurring
2. Being easily distracted from the task at hand
3. Diminished ability to complete word games
4. Inability to recall recent activities from earlier in the day
5. Lapses of memory from periods of time in the past

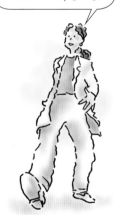

Looks like you're making great strides. Keep going!

35. Which nursing action is **best** to help a client diagnosed with mild Alzheimer's disease remain functional?
1. Obtain a health care provider's prescription for a mild anxiolytic.
2. Point out mistakes so the client can be quickly corrected.
3. Advise the client to move into a retirement center.
4. Maintain a stable, predictable environment and daily routine.

36. The nurse is providing care to a client diagnosed with Alzheimer's disease. Which nursing intervention is **priority**?
1. Establish a daily routine that supports the client's former habits.
2. Maintain physical surroundings that are cheerful and pleasant.
3. Maintain an exact routine from day to day for the client.
4. Control the environment by providing structure, boundaries, and safety.

32. 3. Disruptions in the ability to perform basic care, along with confusion and anxiety, are commonly apparent in clients with amnesia. Offering simple directions to promote daily functions and reduce confusion helps increase feelings of safety and security. Giving this client lots of space may make her feel insecure. There is no significant rationale for keeping her busy all day with no rest periods; the client may become more tired and less functional at other basic tasks. Asking her many questions that she will not be able to answer would just intensify her anxiety level. CN: Safe, effective care environment; CNS: Management of care; CL: Apply

33. 1, 2, 3, 4. Memantine is used in the treatment of Alzheimer's disease. This medication is typically initiated at a low dosage and then progressively increased in dosage as needed. Manifestations associated with overdose include slowed movements, weakness, bradycardia, dizziness, and hallucinations. Tachycardia is not a side effect of this medication. CN: Physiological integrity; CNS: Pharmacological and parenteral therapies; CL: Analyze

34. 4, 5. The primary area affected in amnesia is memory. This includes both short-term and long-term memory. Other areas of cognition are not impacted. CN: Physiological integrity; CNS: Physiological adaptation; CL: Apply

35. 4. Clients in the early stages of Alzheimer's disease remain fairly functional with familiar surroundings and a predictable routine. They become easily disoriented with surprises and social overstimulation. Anxiolytics can impair memory and worsen function. Calling attention to the client's mistakes is unproductive and lowers self-esteem. Moving the client to an unfamiliar environment would heighten agitation and confusion. CN: Psychosocial integrity; CNS: None; CL: Apply

36. 4. By controlling the environment and providing structure and boundaries, the nurse is helping to keep the client safe and secure, which is a priority nursing measure. Establishing a routine that supports former habits and maintaining cheerful, pleasant surroundings and an exact routine foster a supportive environment; however, keeping the client safe and secure takes priority. CN: Safe, effective care environment; CNS: Management of care; CL: Apply

CN: Client needs category   CNS: Client needs subcategory   CL: Cognitive level

37. The nurse finds a client with Alzheimer's disease wandering in the hall at 0300. The client has removed clothing and says to the nurse, "I am just taking a stroll through the park." What is the **priority** nursing action?
1. Immediately help the client back to the client's room and help client get dressed.
2. Inform the client that this type of behavior will not be tolerated.
3. Tell the client it is too early in the morning to be taking a stroll in the park.
4. Ask the client if the client would like to go back to the room and put on clothing.

37. 1. The nurse should not allow the client to embarrass self in front of others, regardless of the time of day. Intervene as soon as the behavior is observed. Scolding the client is not helpful because it is not something the client can understand. Do not engage the client in social chatter; the interaction should be concrete and specific. Do not ask the client to choose unnecessarily. The client may not be able to make appropriate choices.
CN: Psychosocial integrity; CNS: None; CL: Apply

38. The nurse is caring for a client admitted with Alzheimer's dementia and a history of wandering behavior at night. Which nursing action is **priority**?
1. Use a bed check monitor device.
2. Use vest and extremity restraints as needed.
3. Place the call light within the client's reach.
4. Use a sitter during the night hours.

38. 4. Providing a safe, effective care environment takes priority in this case. A sitter can remain with the client to limit the opportunities to get up unattended. Monitors are useful but do not prevent the client from getting up. The use of the call light is important but does not stop the client from getting out of bed unattended. Restraints are to be avoided.
CN: Safe, effective care environment; CNS: Management of care; CL: Apply

39. The nurse is reviewing home administration for a client prescribed rivastigmine. Which response by the client indicates to the nurse the need for further instruction?
1. "If I miss a dose by more than an hour, I will wait until the next day to take it."
2. "I need to take this medication as close to the same time every day as possible."
3. "I may take this medication with a small glass of water or juice."
4. "This medication needs to be taken with meals."

39. 1. Rivastigmine is used to promote improved cognition in affected clients. The medication slows the breakdown of neurotransmitters in the brain. When taking the medication, a missed dose may be taken when noted unless it is almost time for the next dose. An hour is not an excessive amount of time. The medication may be taken with or without a small glass of water, cold fruit juice, or soda. It should be taken with meals. Taking the medication at the same time each day is recommended.
CN: Physiological integrity; CNS: Pharmacological and parenteral therapies; CL: Apply

40. A client is admitted to the acute care facility diagnosed with an amnesic disorder. Which intervention **best** demonstrates the nurse's understanding of this client's needs?
1. Frequently reinforce the unit's rules with the client.
2. Contact the health care provider to prescribe donepezil.
3. Monitor the client for signs of cardiac dysrhythmias.
4. Use distraction if the client displays inappropriate behaviors.

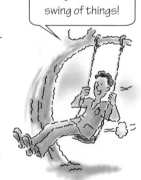

Now you're in the swing of things!

40. 1. Amnesic disorders affect a client's ability to learn and retain new information, requiring frequent reinforcement. Donepezil is prescribed for Alzheimer's disease. Amnesia is not associated with cardiac comorbid conditions nor is the client likely to behave inappropriately.
CN: Physiological integrity; CNS: Physiological adaptation; CL: Apply

41. The nurse will anticipate the health care provider prescribing which test for a client diagnosed with amnesic disorder?
1. Angiography
2. Cardiac catheterization
3. Electrocardiography
4. Mini-Mental State screening

41. 4. An amnesic disorder is characterized by impairment in memory. The Mini-Mental State Examination screens for difficulty recalling events and information. None of the other tests is related to memory assessment.
CN: Health promotion and maintenance; CNS: None; CL: Understand

42. A nurse is working with the family of a client who has been diagnosed with Alzheimer's disease. The nurse notes that the client's spouse is too exhausted to continue providing care alone. The adult children live too far away to provide relief on a weekly basis. Which nursing intervention(s) is appropriate? Select all that apply.
1. Tell the children they must participate in helping provide care to the client.
2. Suggest the spouse seek counseling to help cope with the feelings of exhaustion.
3. Recommend community resources for adult day care and respite care to the spouse.
4. Talk to the spouse about the difficulties of caring for someone with Alzheimer's disease.
5. Ask whether friends or church members can help with providing care or running errands.
6. Recommend that the spouse consider placing the client in a long-term care facility.

42. **3, 4, 5.** Many community services exist for clients with Alzheimer's disease and their families. Encouraging use of these resources may make it possible for the client to stay at home and alleviate the spouse's exhaustion. The nurse can also support the caregiver by urging her to talk about the difficulties she is facing in caring for a spouse with Alzheimer's disease. Friends and church members may be able to help provide care to the client, allowing the caregiver time for rest, exercise, or an enjoyable activity. Telling the children to participate more would probably be ineffective and may evoke anger or guilt. Counseling may be helpful, but it would not alleviate the caregiver's physical exhaustion and would not address the client's immediate needs. A long-term care facility is not an option until the family is ready to make that decision.
CN: Psychosocial integrity; CNS: None; CL: Apply

43. The nurse is assigned to care for a client diagnosed with early-stage Alzheimer's disease. Which nursing intervention(s) will be included in the client's care plan? Select all that apply.
1. Change the client's day-to-day routine often.
2. Engage the client in complex discussions.
3. Place familiar possessions in the client's room.
4. Assist the client with activities of daily living (ADLs) as needed.
5. Assign the client tasks by giving simple steps.

43. **3, 4, 5.** A client with Alzheimer's disease experiences progressive deterioration in cognitive functioning. Familiar possessions may help to orient the client. The client should be encouraged to perform ADLs but may need assistance with certain activities. Using a step-by-step approach helps the client complete tasks independently. A client with Alzheimer's disease functions best with consistent routines. Complex discussions do not improve the memory of a client with Alzheimer's disease.
CN: Psychosocial integrity; CNS: None; CL: Apply

44. The nurse is assessing a client with suspected dementia or depression. Which finding(s) will cause the nurse to suspect dementia rather than depression? Select all that apply.
1. The progression of the client's symptoms is slow.
2. The client answers questions with, "I do not know."
3. The client always acts apathetic and pessimistic.
4. The family cannot identify when the symptoms first appeared.
5. The family states that the client's personality has changed.
6. The client has great difficulty paying attention to others.

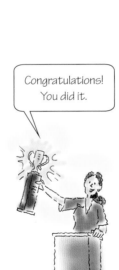

Congratulations! You did it.

44. **1, 4, 5, 6.** Common characteristics of dementia include a slow onset of symptoms, difficulty identifying when the symptoms first occurred, noticeable changes in the client's personality, and impaired ability to pay attention to other people. Answering questions with "I do not know" and displays of pessimism and apathy are symptoms of depression, not dementia.
CN: Psychosocial integrity; CNS: None; CL: Analyze

Chapter 15

Personality Disorders

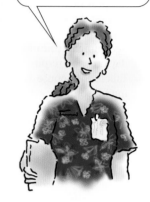

No, this chapter doesn't cover quirks of the rich and famous. It's all about mental disorders affecting the personality. Have a blast!

Personality disorders refresher

Antisocial personality disorder

Disregard for the needs or well-being of others

Key signs and symptoms

- Destructive tendencies
- General disregard for the rights and feelings of others
- Lack of remorse
- Sudden or frequent changes in job, residence, or relationships

Key test results

- The Minnesota Multiphasic Personality Inventory–2 reveals an antisocial personality disorder

Key treatments

- Behavioral therapy
- Antimanic: lithium carbonate
- Beta-blocker: propranolol for controlling aggressive outbursts
- Selective serotonin reuptake inhibitor (SSRI): paroxetine

Key interventions

- Help the client to identify manipulative behaviors.
- Establish a behavioral contract with the client.
- Hold the client responsible for his or her behavior.

Borderline personality disorder

Erratic, unstable emotions and difficulty maintaining relationships

Key signs and symptoms

- Destructive behavior
- Impulsive behavior
- Inability to develop a healthy sense of self
- Inability to maintain relationships
- Moodiness
- Self-mutilation

Key test results

- Standard psychological tests reveal a high degree of dissociation

Key treatments

- Individual therapy
- Antimanic: valproate sodium, lithium carbonate
- Anxiolytic: buspirone
- SSRIs: paroxetine, fluoxetine, sertraline

Key interventions

- Recognize the behaviors that the client uses to manipulate others.
- Set limits on behavior.
- Provide a positive role model.

Dependent personality disorder

- Abnormal and excessive need to be dependent/reliant on others

Key signs and symptoms

- Clinging, demanding behavior
- Fear and anxiety about losing the people on whom the client is dependent
- Hypersensitivity to potential rejection and decision making
- Inability to make decisions
- Low self-esteem

Key test results

- Laboratory tests rule out any underlying medical condition

Key treatments

- Behavior modification through assertiveness training
- Individual therapy
- Benzodiazepines: alprazolam, lorazepam, clonazepam
- SSRIs: paroxetine, sertraline

Key interventions

- Support the client in accepting increased decision making (e.g., balancing the checkbook, planning meals, paying bills).
- Help the client to identify manipulative behaviors, focusing on specific examples.

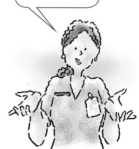

Finally, a chapter with personality! Let's dive in.

316

Paranoid personality disorder

Distrust in others

Key signs and symptoms
- Feelings of being deceived
- Hostility
- Major distortions of reality
- Social isolation
- Suspicion and mistrust of friends and relatives

Key treatments
- Possible drug-free treatment to reduce the chance of causing increased paranoia

- Individual therapy
- Antipsychotic agents: olanzapine, risperidone, chlorpromazine, haloperidol, quetiapine

Key interventions
- Establish a therapeutic relationship by listening and responding to the client.
- Avoid supporting the client's paranoid delusions without minimizing the client's concerns.
- Instruct the client in, and help the client to practice, strategies that facilitate the development of social skills.

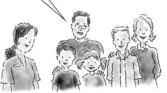

Personality disorders can make it challenging to maintain healthy relationships.

thePoint® You can download tables of drug information to help you prepare for the NCLEX®! View Generic Drug Names, Drug Classifications, Drug Actions, and Nursing Implications for the drugs discussed in this refresher at **http://thePoint.lww.com.**

Personality disorders questions, answers, and rationales

1. A client tells the nurse, "My coworkers are plotting to steal my identity." When the nurse attempts to engage in a discussion about the claim, which nursing response is **most** appropriate to initiate the conversation?
1. "Identity theft seems to be a common occurrence these days."
2. "What makes you think they are planning to steal your identity?"
3. "It must be very frightening to think about your identity being stolen."
4. "Have you told your employer about your concerns of identity thief?"

2. The nurse observes a client being mistrustful and showing hostile behavior toward others. The nurse will anticipate the client being diagnosed with which personality disorder?
1. Antisocial
2. Avoidant
3. Borderline
4. Paranoid

The behavior of clients with personality disorders doesn't always compute.

3. The nurse is caring for a client diagnosed with paranoid personality disorder. Which behavior will the nurse expect to assess in this client?
1. The client cannot follow limits set on behavior.
2. The client is afraid another person will harm the client.
3. The client avoids responsibility for personal health care.
4. The client depends on others to make important decisions.

1. 3. Establishing a therapeutic relationship with a client experiencing paranoid delusions is priority. Encouraging the client to share his or her feelings demonstrates caring without supporting the paranoid thoughts. None of the other options provides the needed support and may allow the client to focus on the delusions during the conversation.
CN: Psychosocial integrity; CNS: None; CL: Analyze

2. 4. Paranoid individuals have a need to constantly scan the environment for signs of betrayal, deception, and ridicule, appearing mistrustful and hostile. They expect to be tricked or deceived by others. The extreme suspiciousness is lacking in antisocial personalities, who tend to be more arrogant and self-assured despite their vigilance and mistrust. Individuals with avoidant personality disorders are guarded, fearing interpersonal rejection and humiliation. Clients with borderline personality disorders behave impulsively and tend to manipulate others.
CN: Psychosocial integrity; CNS: None; CL: Apply

3. 2. A client with paranoid personality disorder is afraid others will inflict harm on him or her. A client with antisocial personality disorder is not able to follow the limits set on behavior. A client with an avoidant personality might avoid responsibility for health care because the client tends to scan the environment for threatening things. A client with dependent personality disorder is likely to want others to make important decisions for him or her.
CN: Psychosocial integrity; CNS: None; CL: Apply

CN: Client needs category   CNS: Client needs subcategory   CL: Cognitive level

4. Which statement made by a client will the nurse document as being typical for a client with paranoid personality disorder?
1. "I understand you are to blame."
2. "I must be seen first; it is not negotiable."
3. "I see nothing humorous in this situation."
4. "I wish someone would select the outfit for me."

5. The nurse shares with a client diagnosed with borderline personality disorder that they will be meeting for 1 hour every week on Mondays at 1 p.m. Which statement **best** describes the proper rationale for the nurse providing this information to the client?
1. Telling the client helps the client clarify limits.
2. It encourages the client to be manipulative.
3. It gives the nurse leverage against unacceptable behavior.
4. It provides an opportunity for the client to assess the situation.

6. The nurse will expect to observe which behavior in a client diagnosed with paranoid personality disorder?
1. The wearing of sexually revealing clothing
2. Placing a personal journal in a locked box
3. Spending over a thousand dollars on comic books
4. Refusing to be compliant with a treatment plan for type 2 diabetes

7. The nurse is talking with the spouse of a client suspected to have a paranoid personality disorder. Which statement(s) made by the client's spouse indicates to the nurse support for the client's diagnosis? Select all that apply.
1. "My spouse is terribly forgetful and unreliable all the time."
2. "Whenever he can, my spouse seems to take advantage of others."
3. "My spouse is always convinced that something negative is going to happen."
4. "Establishing friendships is hard for my spouse because he does not trust anyone."
5. "My spouse is so flirtatious, and he does not care that it is hurtful to me."

8. Which short-term goal is **most** appropriate for a client diagnosed with paranoid personality disorder with impaired social skills?
1. Attend five social events in the community.
2. Discuss anxiety-provoking situations.
3. Address positive and negative feelings about self.
4. Identify personal feelings that hinder social interaction.

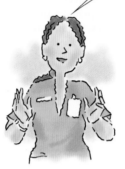

Clients with borderline personality disorder often need help in establishing boundaries.

4. 3. Clients with paranoid personality disorder tend to be extremely serious and lack a sense of humor. Clients with borderline personality disorder tend to blame others for their problems. Clients with narcissistic personality disorders have a sense of self-importance and entitlement. Clients with dependent personality disorder want others to make their decisions.
CN: Psychosocial integrity; CNS: None; CL: Apply

5. 1. Clarifying limits and clearing up any of the client's misconceptions helps the client establish boundaries, which fosters a therapeutic, trusting relationship between the nurse and the client. The nurse should never encourage manipulation or attempt to gather leverage against the client, which would be unprofessional. The client must understand the client's own behavior patterns before he or she can start assessing the situation.
CN: Psychosocial integrity; CNS: None; CL: Apply

6. 2. Clients diagnosed with paranoid personality disorder tend to be secretive. Clients with histrionic personality disorder tend to be exhibitionists, and those with borderline personality disorder tend to be impulsive and self-destructive.
CN: Psychosocial integrity; CNS: None; CL: Apply

7. 3, 4. People with paranoid personality disorder are hypersensitive to perceived threats. This can be demonstrated by reports that something bad has happened or will happen. This can impair the ability to establish trusting relationships. There is not a loss of cognitive abilities, so forgetfulness is not supportive of this diagnosis. Clients with narcissistic personality disorder are interpersonally exploitative to enhance themselves or to indulge their own desires. A client with histrionic personality disorder can be extremely seductive when in search of stimulation and approval.
CN: Psychosocial integrity; CNS: None; CL: Analyze

Clients with paranoid personality disorder need help discovering the source of their problematic social interactions.

8. 4. The client must address the feelings that impede social interactions before developing ways to address impaired social skills or attending social events. Discussion of anxiety-provoking situations is important but does not help the client with impaired social skills. Addressing the client's positive and negative feelings about himself or herself will not directly influence impaired social skills.
CN: Psychosocial integrity; CNS: None; CL: Apply

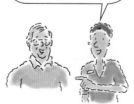

CN: Client needs category   CNS: Client needs subcategory   CL: Cognitive level

9. A client diagnosed with paranoid personality disorder is discussing current problems with a nurse. Which nursing intervention(s) is appropriate when caring for this client? Select all that apply.
1. Encourage the client to look at sources of frustration.
2. Ask the client to focus on ways to interact with others.
3. Urge the client to discuss the use of defense mechanisms.
4. Suggest the client clarify thoughts and beliefs about an event.
5. Help the client identify actions to promote better outcomes.

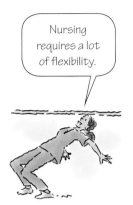

Nursing requires a lot of flexibility.

9. **4, 5.** Clarifying thoughts and beliefs helps the client avoid misinterpretations. Clients with paranoid personality disorder tend to be aggressive and argumentative rather than frustrated. They tend to mistrust people and do not see interacting with others as a way to handle problems. The client's priority must be to interpret thoughts and beliefs realistically rather than discuss defense mechanisms. A paranoid client focuses on defending himself or herself rather than acknowledging the use of defense mechanisms.
CN: Psychosocial integrity; CNS: None; CL: Apply

10. A client diagnosed with a paranoid personality disorder makes an inappropriate and unreasonable report to the nurse. Which communication technique is **best** for the nurse to use?
1. Express disagreement using a matter-of-fact approach.
2. Confront the client about the stated misperception.
3. Use nonverbal communication to address the issue.
4. Use logic to address the client's concern.

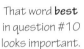

That word **best** in question #10 looks important.

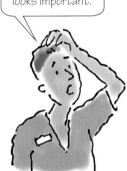

10. **1.** When the nurse tells the client that the nurse does not agree with the client's interpretation, it helps the client differentiate between realistic and emotional thoughts and conclusions. When the nurse uses logic to respond to a client's inappropriate statement, the nurse risks creating a power struggle with the client. It is unwise to confront a client with a paranoid personality disorder because the client will immediately become defensive. The use of nonverbal communication would probably be misinterpreted and arouse the client's suspicion.
CN: Psychosocial integrity; CNS: None; CL: Apply

11. The nurse observes a client diagnosed with histrionic personality disorder tearing pages out of the books in the unit library and putting them into the ventilation system. Which nursing intervention(s) is appropriate? Select all that apply.
1. Place the client in a safe, secluded environment.
2. Help the client develop acceptable methods to gain attention.
3. Withdraw attention from the client.
4. Matter-of-factly identify inappropriate behaviors to the client.
5. Discuss the client's sources of frustration.

11. **1, 4, 5.** If the client begins destroying property or presenting potential harm to self or others, it may be necessary to immediately place the client in a safe, secluded environment. When the client regains control and ceases the behavior, then the nurse can attempt a conversation to explore more acceptable ways of handling frustration and expressing feelings. Lack of attention from the nurse would not reduce the client's attention-seeking behaviors. When the client regains control and ceases the behavior, the nurse must make it clear which behaviors are inappropriate.
CN: Safe, effective care environment; CNS: Safety and infection control; CL: Apply

12. The nurse is caring for a client diagnosed with a paranoid personality disorder. The client has had several confrontations with the nursing staff as a result of misinterpretation of events on the unit. Which nursing action(s) will be therapeutic for this client? Select all that apply.
1. Speak in simple messages without details when interacting with the client.
2. Allow the client the opportunity to ask questions as questions arise.
3. Limit contact between the client and staff.
4. Address only the client's problems and causes of distress.
5. Explore anxious situations and offer reassurance to the client.

12. **1, 2.** The nurse who speaks to the client using clear, simple messages lessens the chance that information will be misinterpreted. Allowing the client time to ask questions will promote understanding of information provided. Contact between the client and staff should not be limited because it would interfere with working on identified treatment goals. Discussing complex topics creates additional information for the client to misinterpret. The nurse who addresses only problems and specific stressors makes it difficult to establish a trusting relationship.
CN: Psychosocial integrity; CNS: None; CL: Apply

13. A client diagnosed with paranoid personality disorder responds aggressively to something another client said during a psychoeducational group session. Which question is **most** appropriate for the nurse to ask the client based on the interaction?
1. "Are you interested in participating in this group?"
2. "What makes you take that comment personally?"
3. "Do you find these sessions particularly frustrating?"
4. "Is your anger a result of some physical trauma you have experienced?"

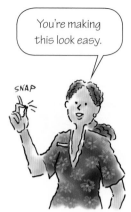

You're making this look easy.

SNAP

13. 2. Clients with paranoid personality disorder tend to be hypersensitive and take what other people say as a personal attack on their character. The client is driven by the suspicion that others will inflict harm. The client's participation in group therapy would be minimal because the client is directing energy toward emotional self-protection. Clients with a paranoid personality disorder tend to be rigid and guarded rather than impulsive and rebellious. The client with a paranoid personality disorder is acting to defend himself, not handle emotional distress.
CN: Psychosocial integrity; CNS: None; CL: Apply

14. A client has been prescribed lithium carbonate in extended-release tablets. Which client statement(s) indicates to the nurse that teaching was effective? Select all that apply.
1. "I should take this medication at the same times each day."
2. "I can crush the tablet and add it to applesauce or pudding."
3. "It will take a few weeks for this medication to help me feel calmer."
4. "Muscle tremors and weakness are common side effects of lithium."
5. "Taking this medication with orange juice will promote its absorption."

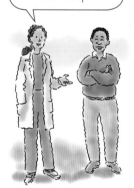

Getting your client with paranoid personality disorder to drop his guard is a key first step.

14. 1, 3. Lithium carbonate is prescribed to manage manic behaviors. Extended-release tablets cannot be chewed or crushed. Taking the medication at the same time each day is important to maintain therapeutic medication levels. It will take 1 to 3 weeks for the client to begin to experience a relief of symptomology. Muscle tremors and weakness are not normal adverse effects and may signal a problem. If they occur, the medication should be held, and the health care provider should be contacted. Taking the medication with a citrus beverage does not impact the absorption of the drug.
CN: Physiological integrity; CNS: Pharmacological and parenteral therapies; CL: Apply

15. Which characteristic of a client diagnosed with a paranoid personality disorder makes it difficult for the nurse to establish an interpersonal relationship?
1. Belief that "the whole world is falling apart."
2. Insists upon "never sitting with my back to the door."
3. Attitude that a diagnosed heart condition is "no big deal."
4. Demonstrates pride when sharing, "I am addicted to sex."

15. 2. Clients with paranoid personality disorder think others will harm, deceive, or exploit them in some way, and they are commonly guarded and ready to defend themselves from actual or perceived attacks. They do not tend to be dysphoric, indifferent, or promiscuous.
CN: Psychosocial integrity; CNS: None; CL: Apply

16. The nurse understands that which action(s) will likely cause distress to clients diagnosed with paranoid personality disorders? Select all that apply.
1. Talking to another client in the corner of the lounge
2. Shutting the door after entering the staff's break room
3. Requiring all clients to participate in group sessions
4. Laughing and smiling with a group of clients
5. Checking vital signs of clients on the unit each morning

16. 1, 2, 4. Clients with paranoid personality disorder tend to interpret any discussion that does not include them as evidence of a plot against them. The nurse laughing and smiling with a group, talking with another client, or interacting with others in what appears to be a secretive manner can increase feelings of paranoia in these clients. Neither requiring all clients to participate in group sessions nor checking vital signs of each client on the unit would alarm a client with paranoid personality disorder because such activities also involve them.
CN: Psychosocial integrity; CNS: None; CL: Analyze

17. The health care provider prescribed olanzapine for a client. Which statement by the client indicates to the nurse the medication is having the desired effect?
1. "I feel more comfortable talking with others."
2. "I am feeling rested when I wake up each morning."
3. "I can tell my appetite is getting better now."
4. "It is getting easier for me to rest at night."

18. Which statement made by a client diagnosed with paranoid personality disorder indicates to the nurse the education provided on social relationships was effective?
1. "As long as I live, I will not abide by social rules."
2. "Sometimes I can see what causes relationship problems."
3. "I will find out what problems others have so I will not repeat them."
4. "I do not have problems in social relationships; I never really did."

19. Which statement made by a client diagnosed with borderline personality disorder demonstrates to the nurse the client has made an improvement in relating to peers?
1. "My church group are people I can actually trust to be there for me."
2. "My friends are people who do not care what others think about them."
3. "My new friends know I do not drive; they always offer to pick me up."
4. "I have been spending time with a group of people who like me for being me."

20. Which behavior by a client diagnosed with antisocial personality disorder alerts the nurse to the need for education related to interaction skills?
1. Frequent crying
2. Failure to follow social norms
3. Frequent panic attacks
4. Avoidance of social activities

21. The family of a client diagnosed with paranoid personality disorder is trying to understand the client's behavior. Which intervention will the nurse implement to help the client's family?
1. Help the family manage the client's eccentric actions.
2. Help the family find appropriate ways to handle stress.
3. Explore the possibility of finding the client respite care.
4. Encourage the family to focus on the client's strengths.

17. 1. Olanzapine is used in the treatment of paranoid personality disorders. If effective, the medication will help the client have control of symptoms, such as paranoia, that impair interactions with others. Restful sleep is not a goal of this medication. Appetite changes do not reflect that the medication is therapeutic.
CN: Physiological integrity; CNS: Pharmacological and parenteral therapies; CL: Apply

18. 2. Progress is shown when the client addresses behaviors that negatively affect relationships. Clients with paranoid personality disorder struggle to understand and express their feelings about social rules. Knowing other people's problems is not useful; the client must focus on his or her own issues. Clients with paranoid personality disorder tend to have impaired social relationships and are very uncomfortable in social settings. By not recognizing the problem, the client indicates that he or she is in denial.
CN: Psychosocial integrity; CNS: None; CL: Apply

19. 4. A statement reflecting being liked for being yourself demonstrates a healthy sense of self; a goal for the client diagnosed with borderline personality disorder. Being able to trust demonstrates improvement related to paranoid thoughts. Not being concerned with the opinions of others is related to antisocial tendencies. Always relying on others is a characteristic of dependent personality disorder.
CN: Psychosocial integrity; CNS: None; CL: Apply

20. 2. Failure to abide by social norms influences the client's ability to interact in a healthy manner with peers. Clients with antisocial personality disorders do not have frequent crying episodes or panic attacks. Avoiding social activities is more likely observed in an avoidant personality type.
CN: Psychosocial integrity; CNS: None; CL: Analyze

21. 1. The family needs to know how to handle the client's symptoms and eccentric behaviors. All people need to learn strategies for handling stress, but the focus must be on helping the family learn how to handle symptoms. There is no need to find respite care for a client with a paranoid personality disorder. Focusing on the client's strengths is a positive action, but the family in this situation must learn how to manage the client's eccentric behavior.
CN: Psychosocial integrity; CNS: None; CL: Apply

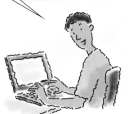

The word "improvement" is the key to answering question #19 correctly.

---

22. A client diagnosed with antisocial personality disorder is trying to convince the nurse that the client deserves special privileges and an exception to the rules should be made. Which response by the nurse is appropriate?
1. "I believe we need to sit down and talk about this."
2. "What you are asking me to do is unacceptable."
3. "Do you not know better than to try to bend the rules?"
4. "Why do you not bring this request to the group meeting?"

23. A client diagnosed with antisocial personality disorder tells the nurse, "My life has been full of problems since childhood." Which finding(s) will the nurse anticipate discovering during the assessment? Select all that apply.
1. Angry outbursts
2. Birth defects
3. Easy distractibility
4. Hypoactive behavior
5. Substance use

24. The nurse is caring for a client diagnosed with antisocial personality disorder who knowingly breaks unit rules. Which statement by the nurse **most** appropriately addresses the client's behavior?
1. "You have lost gym privileges as the consequence for breaking the rules."
2. "Let us talk about your tendency to frequently make poor decisions."
3. "Tell me what your punishment should be for breaking unit rules."
4. "Everyone on the unit must obey the rules and that includes you."

25. A client diagnosed with antisocial personality disorder is aggressively confronting both staff and other clients. Verbal de-escalation has been ineffective. Which nursing action is appropriate for this client?
1. Administer propranolol as prescribed.
2. Apply wrist and ankle restraints.
3. Place a sitter continuously at the bedside.
4. Put the client in solitary isolation.

26. Which is the **initial** nursing intervention for a client who has been diagnosed with an antisocial personality disorder and has a history of polysubstance use?
1. Perform human immunodeficiency virus (HIV) testing.
2. Obtain an electrolyte panel and urine specimen for a urinalysis.
3. Use an anxiety screening tool to assess the client's anxiety level.
4. Have the client undergo psychological testing immediately.

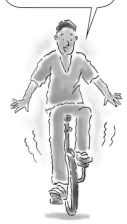

Impressive performance! Keep going.

22. 2. Clients with antisocial personality disorder commonly try to manipulate the nurse to get special privileges or make exceptions to the rules on their behalf. By informing the client directly when actions are inappropriate, the nurse helps the client learn to control unacceptable behaviors by setting limits. By sitting down to talk about the request, the nurse is telling the client there is room for negotiation when there is not. Implying that the client wants to bend the rules humiliates him. The client's request is unacceptable and should not be brought to a community meeting.
CN: Psychosocial integrity; CNS: None; CL: Apply

23. 1, 5. Clients with antisocial personality disorder commonly experience angry outbursts and start engaging in substance use during childhood. They do not have a higher incidence of birth defects than other people. Clients with antisocial personality disorder are commonly manipulative and are no more distracted from issues than others. They tend to be *hyperactive*, not hypoactive.
CN: Psychosocial integrity; CNS: None; CL: Apply

24. 1. Clients diagnosed with antisocial personality disorder must learn how to take responsibility for their actions. Matter-of-factly providing a consequence for breaking the rules is the most appropriate manner of addressing this client's behavior. None of the other options provide an appropriate consequence for this act of defiance and disregard to rules.
CN: Psychosocial integrity; CNS: None; CL: Apply

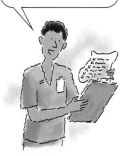

Hint: a history of polysubstance use means the client probably engages in other high-risk behaviors.

25. 1. Propranolol is a beta blocker that can be effective in treating aggressive behavior. Restraints should be used only as a last resort. Neither placing a sitter at the client's bedside nor placing the client in isolation will effectively address the aggressive behavior.
CN: Safe, effective care environment; CNS: Safety and infection control; CL: Apply

26. 1. A client who engages in high-risk behaviors such as polysubstance use should undergo HIV testing. This client would benefit from an entire chemistry profile as part of a complete medical examination, rather than a single test for electrolytes. An anxiety screen is not needed for a client with antisocial personality disorder. Information from psychological testing is valuable when developing a treatment plan but is not an immediate concern.
CN: Safe, effective care environment; CNS: Management of care; CL: Apply

CN: Client needs category   CNS: Client needs subcategory   CL: Cognitive level

27. When reviewing a client's chart, the nurse notes the chart exhibit below. Which nursing statement about the client's condition is **most** accurate?

Progress notes	
9/4	Client, age 28, admitted to unit with a
1130	diagnosis of antisocial personality disorder
	and suicide attempt after cutting the right
	wrist. Right wrist dressing appears dry and
	intact. Client states, "I do not want to be
	here and I am not following your treatment
	plan or any of your rules. I am going to tell
	everyone here not to follow your rules."
	—Elana Knight, RN

1. "The client may not be motivated to change personal behavior or lifestyle."
2. "The client requires psychotropic drugs to treat the condition but is refusing."
3. "The client manipulates other clients but has not tried to manipulate family."
4. "The client could quickly make behavior changes if encouraged appropriately."

27. 1. Clients with antisocial personality disorder feel nothing is wrong with their behavior and have no desire to change. These clients do not benefit from psychotropic drug therapy. They attempt to manipulate all people with whom they come in contact. A quick behavior change is not a realistic expectation for clients with this disorder.

CN: Psychosocial integrity; CNS: None; CL: Apply

28. Which short-term goal is appropriate for the nurse to set for a client diagnosed with an antisocial personality disorder who acts out when distressed?
1. The client will develop four goals for personal improvement.
2. The client will identify situations that are out of the client's control.
3. The client will identify ways to make traumatic life events positive.
4. The client will understand how to express feelings nondestructively.

28. 4. By working on appropriate expression of feelings, the client learns how to talk about what is stressful, rather than hurt oneself or others. The most pressing need is to learn to cope and talk about problems rather than act out. Developing goals for personal improvement is a long-term goal, not a short-term one. Although it is important to differentiate what is and is not under the client's control, the most important goal for handling distress is to talk about feelings appropriately. The identification of traumatic life events will occur only after the client begins to express feelings appropriately. However, it is not appropriate to expect a client to make such events a positive memory.

CN: Psychosocial integrity; CNS: None; CL: Apply

29. Which goal is appropriate for the nurse to set for a client diagnosed with antisocial personality disorder who possesses a high risk of violence directed at others?
1. The client will discuss the desire to hurt others rather than act.
2. The client will be given something to destroy to displace the anger.
3. The client will develop a list of resources to use when anger escalates.
4. The client will understand the difference between anger and physical symptoms.

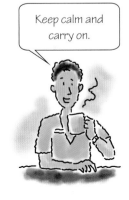

Keep calm and carry on.

29. 1. By discussing the desire to be violent toward others, the nurse can help the client get in touch with the pain associated with the angry feelings. It is not helpful to give the client something to destroy. The client needs to talk about strong feelings in a nonviolent manner, not refer to a list of crisis resources. Helping the client understand the relationship between feelings and physical symptoms can be done after discussing the desire to hurt others.

CN: Psychosocial integrity; CNS: None; CL: Apply

CN: Client needs category   CNS: Client needs subcategory   CL: Cognitive level

30. The nurse notices other clients on the unit are avoiding a client diagnosed with antisocial personality disorder. When discussing appropriate behavior in group therapy, which comment made by peers about this client will the nurse expect?
1. "He is no one who can be trusted."
2. "He is always so irrational."
3. "He yells and is threatening."
4. "He has to be the center of attention."

30. 1. Clients with antisocial personality disorder tend to engage in acts of dishonesty, shown by lying. These clients do not tend to be irrational or threatening. Clients with histrionic personality disorder tend to overreact to frustrations and disappointments, have temper tantrums, and seek attention.
CN: Psychosocial integrity; CNS: None; CL: Apply

31. During a family meeting for a client with an antisocial personality disorder, which statement will the nurse expect from an exasperated family member?
1. "Today I am the enemy, but tomorrow I will be a saint to him."
2. "When he is wrong, he never apologizes or even acts sorry."
3. "Sometimes I cannot believe how he exaggerates about everything."
4. "There are times when his compulsive behavior is too much to handle."

A client's personality disorder affects everyone in the family.

31. 2. The client with antisocial personality disorder has no remorse. The client with a borderline personality disorder shows splitting. The client with an antisocial personality disorder does not tend to exaggerate about life events or to be compulsive.
CN: Psychosocial integrity; CNS: None; CL: Apply

32. A client diagnosed with antisocial personality disorder states, "I can get anyone to do what I want them to do." Which response by the nurse is **most** appropriate?
1. "Do you get excited or a thrill out of being manipulative?"
2. "Let us talk about strategies that do not involve manipulation."
3. "Do you feel your parents manipulated you as a child?"
4. "Being manipulative makes it hard to have good relationships."

Family members often contribute to a client's negative behaviors without even realizing it.

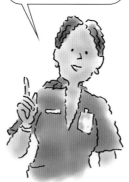

32. 2. By considering options or strategies, the client gains skills to overcome ineffective behaviors. The questions are less appropriate because they do not provide the client with needed skills. Although it is true that manipulative behavior is a stress on relationships, the client benefits most from learning and implementing alternative strategies and behaviors.
CN: Psychosocial integrity; CNS: None; CL: Apply

33. Which goal for the family of a client diagnosed with antisocial disorder will the nurse stress in the education process?
1. The family must assist the client to decrease ritualistic behavior.
2. The family must learn to cope with the client's impulsive behavior.
3. The family must stop reinforcing inappropriate negative behavior.
4. The family must start to use negative reinforcement of the client's behavior.

33. 3. The family needs help learning how to stop reinforcing inappropriate client behavior. Clients with antisocial personality disorder do not show ritualistic behaviors. The family can set limits and reinforce consequences when the client shows shortsightedness and poor planning. Negative reinforcement is an inappropriate strategy for the family to use to support this client.
CN: Psychosocial integrity; CNS: None; CL: Apply

34. A client diagnosed with dependent personality disorder is expressing concerns about the impending death of a parent. Which statement by the client will the nurse recognize as **most** characteristic of the diagnosis?
1. "I am afraid of losing my mother and being all alone."
2. "I am not really sure it is true that she is dying."
3. "I am not ready to lose either of my parents."
4. "I find it difficult to even think about death and dying."

34. 1. The client diagnosed with a dependent personality disorder would express great concern about being alone. Paranoia might be the cause of doubting the truth concerning the impending death. For many people, not being ready to lose a parent, or even thinking about death, is a normal emotional reaction to the subject.
CN: Psychosocial integrity; CNS: None; CL: Apply

CN: Client needs category   CNS: Client needs subcategory   CL: Cognitive level

35. A client is suspected of having antisocial personality disorder tendencies. Which finding by the nurse supports this diagnosis?
1. Delusional thinking
2. Not having finished high school
3. Disorganized thoughts
4. Multiple criminal charges

36. The nurse on the psychiatric unit is caring for a client diagnosed with antisocial personality disorder. Which client behavior is the nurse **most** likely to assess?
1. Demonstrates a need for immediate gratification
2. Learns how to correct mistakes from past experiences
3. Expresses feelings of anxiety regarding behavior
4. Regularly defers to authority figures for decisions

37. Which finding will the nurse recognize as characteristic of a client diagnosed with antisocial personality disorder?
1. Having been fired from five jobs in the last 2 years
2. Being prescribed an antianxiety medication
3. Being treated for both chronic cardiac and renal disease
4. Frequently refers to self as a "loser"

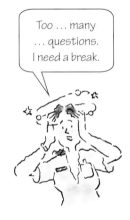

Too … many … questions. I need a break.

38. Which behavior indicates to the nurse a client diagnosed with antisocial personality disorder is beginning to exhibit socially acceptable behaviors in group settings?
1. Fewer panic attacks
2. Acceptance of reality
3. Improved self-esteem
4. Fewer physical symptoms

39. The nurse is taking a health history on a client diagnosed with borderline personality disorder. Which finding will the nurse expect to assess?
1. A negative sense of self
2. A tendency to be compulsive
3. A problem with communication
4. An inclination to be philosophical

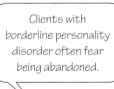

Clients with borderline personality disorder often fear being abandoned.

40. The nurse knows which characteristic or situation can precipitate a crisis in a client diagnosed with borderline personality disorder?
1. Antisocial behavior
2. Relationship problems
3. Paranoid behavior
4. Auditory hallucinations

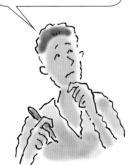

35. 4. Clients with antisocial personality disorder are commonly sent for treatment by the court after multiple crimes or for the use of illegal substances. Clients with antisocial personality disorder do not tend to have delusional or disorganized thinking. Lack of education is not generally considered a risk factor.
CN: Psychosocial integrity; CNS: None; CL: Apply

36. 1. Because of the lack of scruples and underlying powerlessness of the client with antisocial personality disorder, the nurse expects to see manipulation, shallowness, impulsivity, and self-centered behavior. This client does not profit from mistakes or learn from past experiences, lacks anxiety and guilt, and is unable to accept authority and discipline.
CN: Psychosocial integrity; CNS: None; CL: Apply

37. 1. Clients with a diagnosis of antisocial personality disorder tend to have problems in their job roles and poor work histories. They do not have severe anxiety disorders, severe physical health problems, or low self-esteem.
CN: Psychosocial integrity; CNS: None; CL: Apply

38. 3. When clients with antisocial personality disorder begin to practice socially acceptable behaviors, they also commonly experience a more positive sense of self. Clients with antisocial personality disorder do not tend to have panic attacks, alteration in their perception of reality, or somatic manifestations of their illness.
CN: Psychosocial integrity; CNS: None; CL: Apply

39. 1. Clients with a borderline personality disorder have low self-esteem and a negative sense of self. They have little or no problem expressing themselves and communicating with others. Although they tend to be impulsive, they usually are not compulsive or philosophical.
CN: Psychosocial integrity; CNS: None; CL: Apply

40. 2. Relationship problems can precipitate a crisis because they bring up issues of abandonment. Clients with borderline personality disorder are not usually suspicious or paranoid; they are more likely to be depressed or highly anxious. They do not have symptoms of antisocial behavior or auditory hallucinations.
CN: Psychosocial integrity; CNS: None; CL: Apply

CN: Client needs category   CNS: Client needs subcategory   CL: Cognitive level

41. A client with a diagnosis of borderline personality disorder is admitted to the hospital after a self-inflicted wrist wound. Which goal is **most** appropriate for the nurse to set for this client?
1. Identify whether splitting is present in the client's thoughts.
2. Establish a therapeutic relationship with the client.
3. Discuss acting out and self-destructive tendencies.
4. Encourage the client to understand why the client blames others.

42. Which nursing intervention will help a client diagnosed with a borderline personality disorder identify appropriate behaviors?
1. Scheduling a family meeting
2. Placing the client in seclusion
3. Formulating a behavioral contract
4. Assessing the client's mental status

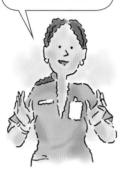

Contracts with clients help outline what's appropriate and what's not.

43. The nurse understands that which statement is typical of a client diagnosed with borderline personality disorder who has recurrent suicidal thoughts?
1. "I cannot believe how everyone has suddenly stopped believing in me."
2. "I do not care what other people say, I know how bad I look to them."
3. "I will not stop until I have gotten revenge on all those people who blamed me."
4. "I might as well check out because my boyfriend does not want me anymore."

44. The nurse is assessing a client diagnosed with borderline personality disorder. Which finding will the nurse determine is relevant to this diagnosis?
1. Abrasions in various healing stages
2. Intermittent episodes of hypertension
3. Alternating tachycardia and bradycardia
4. Mild state of euphoria with disorientation

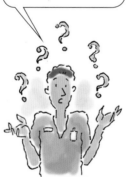

Your client has just been diagnosed with borderline personality disorder. What behavior should you expect to see?

45. Which intervention(s) is important to include in an education plan for the family of a client diagnosed with borderline personality disorder? Select all that apply.
1. Educate the family about various methods for handling the client's anxiety.
2. Explore family behaviors that can reinforce the client's undesirable behaviors.
3. Encourage the family to have the client express intense emotions as they arise.
4. Help the family to pressure the client to improve current negative behaviors.
5. Educate the family about the client's diagnosis of borderline personality disorder.

41. 2. After promoting client safety, the nurse establishes a rapport with the client to facilitate appropriate expression of feelings. At this time, the client is not ready to address unhealthy behaviors. A therapeutic relationship must be established before the nurse can effectively work with the client on splitting, self-destructive tendencies, and blaming others.
CN: Safe, effective care environment; CNS: Management of care; CL: Apply

42. 3. The use of a behavioral contract establishes a framework for healthier functioning and places responsibility for actions back on the client. Seclusion reinforces the fear of abandonment found in clients with borderline personality. Performing a mental status assessment or scheduling a family meeting would not help the client identify appropriate behaviors.
CN: Psychosocial integrity; CNS: None; CL: Apply

43. 4. The client with borderline personality disorder who is suicidal typically exhibits a tendency toward all-or-nothing thinking. The first statement indicates the client has experienced a credibility problem; the second statement indicates the client is extremely embarrassed; and the third statement indicates the client has an antisocial personality disorder.
CN: Safe, effective care environment; CNS: Safety and infection control; CL: Apply

44. 1. Clients with borderline personality disorder tend to self-mutilate and have abrasions in various stages of healing. Intermittent episodes of hypertension, alternating tachycardia and bradycardia, or a mild state of euphoria with disorientation do not tend to occur with this disorder.
CN: Psychosocial integrity; CNS: None; CL: Apply

45. 1, 2, 5. The family needs to learn how to handle the client's intense stress and low tolerance for frustration. Family members need to understand how they can impact behaviors of the client. Education about the disorder is paramount to the success of their involvement in the plan of care. Clients with borderline personality disorder already maintain intense emotions, and it is not safe to encourage further expression of them. The family does not need to pressure the client to change behavior; this approach will only cause inappropriate behavior to escalate.
CN: Psychosocial integrity; CNS: None; CL: Apply

CN: Client needs category   CNS: Client needs subcategory   CL: Cognitive level

46. Which short-term goal is appropriate for the nurse to set for a client diagnosed with borderline personality disorder displaying low self-esteem?
1. Write in a journal daily.
2. Express fears and feelings.
3. Stop obsessive-compulsive behaviors.
4. Decrease dysfunctional family conflicts.

47. Which statement made to the nurse by a client with borderline personality disorder indicates a history of dysfunctional relationships?
1. "I will not get involved in another relationship."
2. "I am determined to look for the perfect partner."
3. "I am going to be an equal partner in a relationship."
4. "I have decided to learn better communication skills."

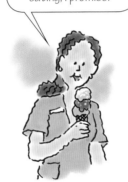

Just one more triple-scoop ice cream cone—then I'll stop eating, I promise.

48. The nurse recognizes which client behavior as characteristic for borderline personality disorder?
1. Eating two whole pizzas at a unit party
2. Failing to remember what day it is
3. Demonstrating interest in joining a "street gang"
4. Frequently stating, "The government is afraid of me; that is why I am here."

49. The nurse is caring for a client diagnosed with borderline personality disorder. Which intervention will the nurse implement?
1. Encourage the client to assess current behaviors.
2. Work with the client to develop outgoing behavior.
3. Limit the client's interactions to family members only.
4. Encourage the client to approach others for interactions.

50. Which statement is an example of a common defense mechanism the nurse will **most** likely hear when having a conversation with a client diagnosed with borderline personality disorder?
1. "I am not good at spelling, but I am great at math."
2. "When I am angry I go for a 5- or 6-mile run."
3. "I have always been one of the popular kids at school."
4. "I did not know the rules; no one told me I could not smoke here."

46. 2. Acknowledging fears and feelings can help clients identify parts of themselves that make them uncomfortable, and they can begin to work on developing a positive sense of self. Writing in a daily journal is not a short-term goal to enhance self-esteem. A client with borderline personality disorder does not struggle with obsessive-compulsive behaviors. Decreasing dysfunctional family conflicts is a long-term goal.
CN: Psychosocial integrity; CNS: None; CL: Apply

47. 2. Clients with borderline personality disorder look for a perfect partner. This characteristic is a result of the dichotomous manner in which these clients view the world. They go from relationship to relationship without taking responsibility for their behavior. It is unlikely an unsuccessful relationship would cause these clients to change. Because they tend to blame others for problems, it is unlikely they would express a desire to learn communication skills. They tend to be demanding and impulsive in relationships. There is no thought given to what one wants or needs from a relationship.
CN: Psychosocial integrity; CNS: None; CL: Analyze

48. 1. Clients with borderline personality disorder are likely to develop dysfunctional coping and act out in self-destructive ways, such as binge eating. They are not prone to develop memory loss or delusional thinking. Joining a group may be seen in some clients with antisocial personality disorder.
CN: Psychosocial integrity; CNS: None; CL: Apply

49. 1. Self-assessment of behavior enables the client to look inward and identify social behaviors that need to be changed. Clients with borderline personality disorder do not tend to have difficulty approaching and interacting with other people. It is unrealistic to limit clients with borderline personality disorder to interactions with family members only. Clients with borderline personality disorder tend to be demanding and enjoy being the center of attention. It is not useful for these clients to develop outgoing behavior.
CN: Psychosocial integrity; CNS: None; CL: Apply

50. 4. Clients with borderline personality disorder tend to blame others and project their feelings and inadequacies onto others. They do not identify with other people or use compensation to handle distress. Clients with borderline personality disorder are impulsive and tend to react immediately. It is unlikely the client would channel anger in a constructive manner.
CN: Psychosocial integrity; CNS: None; CL: Apply

CN: Client needs category   CNS: Client needs subcategory   CL: Cognitive level

51. On which client statement will the nurse place **priority** when providing care for a client diagnosed with borderline personality disorder?
    1. "I do whatever I want, whenever I want to."
    2. "I have been in and out of jail most of my adult life."
    3. "I have been told I have frequent mood changes."
    4. "I have been a loner pretty much my entire life."

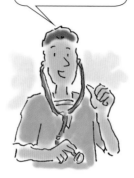

What's the priority statement in question #51?

51. 1. Clients with borderline personality disorder are erratic, emotionally unstable, and often destructive and impulsive. All these characteristics pose safety issues especially when the client is defiant. Reasonable limits must be set and enforced by staff to help assure the safety of the client and others. The other options reflect less problematic characteristics of the disorder.
CN: Safe, effective care environment; CNS: Management of care; CL: Analysis

52. Which action by a client diagnosed with borderline personality disorder indicates to the nurse adequate learning about personal behavior?
    1. Smiles while making demands
    2. Freely talks about intense anger
    3. Promises never to engage in conflict
    4. Takes control of personal finances

52. 2. Learning has occurred when anger is discussed rather than acted out in unhealthy ways by the client with borderline personality disorder. The behavior to change would be the demands placed on others. Smiling while making these demands shows manipulative behavior. Not engaging in conflict is unrealistic. It is important to help this client slowly develop financial responsibility rather than just stopping the family from monitoring the client's tendency to overspend.
CN: Psychosocial integrity; CNS: None; CL: Apply

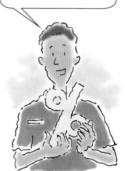

Looks like you're giving 150% on this test. Way to go!

53. The nurse will **most** closely monitor for behaviors associated with which condition while caring for a client diagnosed with borderline personality disorder?
    1. Avoidance
    2. Depression
    3. Delirium
    4. Disorientation

53. 2. Chronic feelings of emptiness and sadness predispose this client to depression. About 40% of people with borderline personality disorder struggle with depression. They tend to disregard boundaries and limits. Avoidance is not an issue with these clients. They do not tend to develop delirium or become disoriented. These conditions are only a possibility if the client becomes intoxicated.
CN: Safe, effective care environment; CNS: Management of care; CL: Understand

54. The nurse is assessing a client for dependent personality disorder. Which statement made by the client **best** indicates this diagnosis to the nurse?
    1. "I do not feel safe in my home because I live alone."
    2. "It is so very lonely and boring living by myself."
    3. "I have been so depressed since my parents died."
    4. "I leave all the decision-making to my spouse."

54. 4. Dependent personality disorder is characterized by an excessive need to rely on others. Deferring to a spouse to make decisions is an example of such a behavior. The other options are more associated with expected emotions, such as loneliness, depression, and a concern for safety.
CN: Psychosocial integrity; CNS: None; CL: Analyze

55. The nurse will expect a client diagnosed with borderline personality disorder to exhibit which behavioral trait(s)? Select all that apply.
    1. Repeatedly asking the nurse if the nurse will return upon leaving the room
    2. A propensity to act out when feeling afraid, alone, or devalued
    3. An inability to make decisions independently
    4. A belief in deserving special privileges not accorded to others
    5. A display of inappropriately seductive appearance and behavior

55. 1, 2. Clients with borderline personality disorder have an intense fear of abandonment, so they act out when feeling afraid, alone, or devalued. These clients are able to make decisions independently. A person who feels deserving of special privileges is characteristic of narcissistic personality disorder. Inappropriate seductive appearance and behavior are characteristics of someone with histrionic personality disorder.
CN: Psychosocial integrity; CNS: None; CL: Apply

CN: Client needs category   CNS: Client needs subcategory   CL: Cognitive level

56. A client is admitted to a medical–surgical unit for treatment of an orthopedic injury. During the assessment, the nurse notes the client has a history of borderline personality disorder with episodes of self-mutilation. Which type of behavior(s) will the nurse expect to be present? Select all that apply.
1. No presence of cuts or burns located on the client's body
2. Bruises where the client can explain how they were obtained
3. A knife or razor located in the client's personal belongings
4. Insistence on wearing a long-sleeved shirt in warm temperatures
5. Overly hesitant behavior when the nurse attempts to assist with bathing

57. The nurse is caring for a client with dependent personality disorder. Which nursing action is appropriate for this client?
1. Orient the client to the current surroundings.
2. Reassure the client regarding personal safety.
3. Ask questions to help the client recall problems.
4. Distinguish between positive and negative feedback.

58. Which short-term goal is appropriate for the nurse to set for a client with dependent personality disorder experiencing excessive dependency needs?
1. Verbalize self-confidence in own abilities.
2. Decide relationships do not take energy to sustain.
3. Discuss feelings related to frequent mood swings.
4. Stop obsessive thinking that impedes daily social functioning.

59. While assessing a client diagnosed with impulse control disorder who is displaying violent, aggressive, and assaultive behavior, what will the nurse expect to discover about the client? Select all that apply.
1. The client functions well in other areas of life.
2. The degree of aggressiveness is out of proportion to the stressor.
3. The client typically uses a stressor to justify violent behavior.
4. The client has a history of parental alcoholism.
5. The client shows no remorse about the inability to control behaviors.

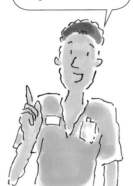

Expect clients with dependent personality disorder to be hypersensitive to your comments.

56. 3, 4, 5. The client who self-mutilates can be expected to have numerous small cuts on the body, unexplained frequent injuries, and possibly a knife or razor in his or her possession. The client may wear long-sleeved shirts even in warm weather to prevent anyone from seeing self-inflicted cuts or burns. The client may be overly hesitant for medical personnel to assist with bathing or dressing due to the presence of cuts or burns over the body. Occasional bruising that the client can accurately account for is not a sign of borderline personality disorder.
CN: Psychosocial integrity; CNS: None; CL: Apply

57. 4. Clients with dependent personality disorder tend to view all feedback as criticism; they commonly misinterpret another's remarks. Clients with dependent personality disorder do not need orientation to their surroundings. Personal safety is not an issue because these clients typically are not self-destructive. Memory problems are not associated with this disorder, so asking questions to stimulate memory is not necessary.
CN: Psychosocial integrity; CNS: None; CL: Apply

58. 1. Individuals with dependent personalities believe they must depend on others to be competent for them. They need to gain more self-confidence in their own abilities. The client must realize relationships take energy to develop and sustain. Clients with dependent personality disorder usually do not have mood swings or obsessive thinking that interferes with their socialization.
CN: Psychosocial integrity; CNS: None; CL: Apply

59. 1, 2, 4. A client with an impulse control disorder who displays violent, aggressive, and assaultive behaviors generally functions well in other areas of life. The degree of the client's aggressiveness is disproportionate to the stressor, and the client commonly has a history of parental alcoholism as well as a chaotic family life. The client usually verbalizes sincere guilt and remorse for the aggressive behavior and does not typically use a stressor to justify violent behavior.
CN: Psychosocial integrity; CNS: None; CL: Apply

CN: Client needs category   CNS: Client needs subcategory   CL: Cognitive level

60. A client diagnosed with dependent personality disorder is planning to get a part-time job. Which nursing intervention is **most** appropriate for this client?
1. Helping the client develop strategies to control impulsive actions
2. Explaining that there are consequences for inappropriate behaviors
3. Helping the client to decrease the use of regression as a defense mechanism
4. Encouraging the client to work to sustain healthy interpersonal relationships

61. A client diagnosed with dependent personality disorder has difficulty expressing personal concerns. Which communication technique is **best** for the nurse to teach the client?
1. Questioning
2. Reflection
3. Silence
4. Touch

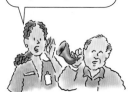

If your client seems confused about instructions you are giving, try rephrasing them.

62. A nurse is evaluating the effectiveness of an assertiveness group for a client with dependent personality disorder. Which client statement indicates to the nurse the group is beneficial for the client?
1. "It is okay that I cannot do the things other people do."
2. "I plan to become more organized like other people."
3. "I want to talk about something that is bothering me."
4. "I just do not want people in my family to fight anymore."

63. While caring for a client diagnosed with a dependent personality disorder, the nurse will monitor for which comorbid condition?
1. Psychotic disorder
2. Acute stress disorder
3. Alcohol-related disorder
4. Posttraumatic stress disorder (PTSD)

64. After a family visit, a client with dependent personality disorder becomes anxious. The nurse will suspect which event is the cause of the client's anxiety?
1. Being subjected to criticism from the family
2. Having a discussion regarding family rules
3. Being asked personal questions by siblings
4. The family monitoring for eccentric behavior

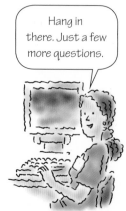

Hang in there. Just a few more questions.

60. 4. Sustaining healthy relationships will help the client be comfortable with peers in the job setting. Clients with dependent personality disorder do not usually have trouble with impulse control or offensive behavior that would lead to negative consequences. They do not usually use regression as a defense mechanism. It is common to see denial and introjection used.
CN: Psychosocial integrity; CNS: None; CL: Apply

61. 1. Questioning is a way to learn to identify feelings and express self. The use of reflection is not a communication technique that will help the client with dependent personality disorder to express personal feelings and concerns. Using silence will not help the client identify and discuss personal concerns. If touch is used to express feelings and personal concerns, it must be used very judiciously.
CN: Psychosocial integrity; CNS: None; CL: Apply

62. 3. By asking to talk about a bothersome situation, the client with dependent personality disorder has taken the first step toward assertive behavior. Noting an inability to do things other people do reflects a lack of self-confidence; it is not assertive. Making plans to be more organized is not assertive. To smooth over or minimize troubling events such as family fights is not an assertive action.
CN: Psychosocial integrity; CNS: None; CL: Apply

63. 2. Because they have placed their own needs in the hands of others, clients with dependent personalities are extremely vulnerable to acute stress disorder. They do not tend to have coexisting problems of psychotic disorder, alcohol-related disorder, or PTSD.
CN: Psychosocial integrity; CNS: None; CL: Understand

64. 1. Clients with dependent personality disorder are extremely sensitive to criticism and can become very anxious when they feel interpersonal conflict or tension. When they have discussions about family rules, they try to become submissive and please others rather than become anxious. When they are asked personal questions, they do not necessarily become anxious. Clients with dependent personality disorder do not tend to behave eccentrically.
CN: Psychosocial integrity; CNS: None; CL: Apply

65. A client undergoing treatment for paranoia refuses to take risperidone, stating, "I think it is poisoned." Which nursing action is **most** appropriate?
1. Hold the dose and immediately notify the health care provider.
2. Tell the client an injection will be prescribed if the pill is refused.
3. Put the medication in the client's juice without informing the client.
4. Allow the client to open and examine each risperidone tablet.

66. While in the dayroom, a client with a history of paranoia becomes increasingly agitated and appears to be experiencing auditory hallucinations. Which nursing intervention(s) is appropriate? Select all that apply.
1. Prepare to either restrain or place the client in seclusion.
2. Reinforce to the client that the staff are there to keep everyone safe.
3. Directly ask the client, "Are you hearing voices?"
4. Minimize environmental stimulation by turning off the television.
5. Call security to assist in keeping the environment safe.
6. Talk to the client calmly using simple and concise language.

67. A client is diagnosed with borderline personality disorder. Which behavior(s) is the nurse likely to assess in this client? Select all that apply.
1. Recurrent suicidal behaviors, gestures, or threats
2. Chronically depressed affect and slowed thinking
3. Frantic attempts to avoid real or imagined abandonment
4. Stating chronic feelings of emptiness since childhood
5. Fluctuations between binging and purging

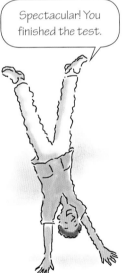

The client won't let you help him. What should I do?

Spectacular! You finished the test.

65. **1.** The nurse's best response is to hold the dose and notify the health care provider. Insisting that the client take the medication would only increase paranoia and agitation. Forcing injections and tricking a client into taking medication by putting it in juice are illegal. A rational approach to irrational ideas, such as allowing the client to examine the medication, seldom works.
CN: Safe, effective care environment; CNS: Management of care; CL: Analyze

66. **2, 3, 4, 6.** While using a calm voice, the nurse should provide reassure that the client is safe and provide simple, concise instructions. It is appropriate to attempt to confirm that the client is hearing voices and, if so, ask if they are suggesting harm to the client or to others. Minimizing environmental stimuli is appropriate. Although the client is agitated, no evidence exists that the client is at risk for harming self or others; it is premature to prepare to restrain the client, place the client in seclusion, or to alert security.
CN: Psychosocial integrity; CNS: None; CL: Apply

67. **1, 3, 4.** Recurrent suicidal behaviors, gestures, or threats; frantic attempts to avoid real or imagined abandonment; and chronic feelings of emptiness are typical with borderline personality disorder. Chronically depressed affect and slowed thinking are more indicative of a mood disorder. Binging and purging are consistent with an eating disorder.
CN: Psychosocial integrity; CNS: None; CL: Apply

Chapter 16

Schizophrenia Spectrum & Other Psychotic Disorders

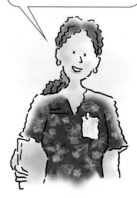

It's no delusion. You'll *do* great on this chapter if you use your nursing skills—knowledge, experience, compassion, insight …

Schizophrenia spectrum & other psychotic disorders refresher

Schizophrenia

Disturbances in thought content and form, perception, emotions and affect, movements and behavior; they result in difficulty thinking clearly, managing emotions, making decisions, and relating to others.

Key signs and symptoms

Positive or hard symptoms
- Hallucinations (auditory, visual, tactile)
- Delusions
- Bizarre behavior
- Thought disorders (disorganized thinking)
- Agitated movements (psychomotor agitation)
- Echopraxia (involuntary imitation of another person's movements and gestures)
- Loose associations

Negative or soft symptoms
- Catatonia (psychomotor slowing)
- Flat or blunted affect
- Alogia (speak very little)
- Anhedonia (lack of pleasure in things that used to bring pleasure)
- Lack of focus

Key test results
- Magnetic resonance imaging (MRI) shows possible enlargement of lateral ventricles, enlarged third ventricle, and enlarged sulci
- Impaired performance on neuropsychological and cognitive tests

Key treatments
- Milieu therapy
- Supportive psychotherapy
- Social skills training
- Antipsychotic medication therapy: haloperidol, aripiprazole, olanzapine, risperidone, quetiapine, fluphenazine, paliperidone, clozapine

Key interventions
- Monitor client for adverse effects of antipsychotic drugs, such as dystonic reactions, tardive dyskinesia, and akathisia.
- Be aware of client's personal space; use gestures and touch judiciously.
- Provide appropriate measures to ensure client's safety.
- Collaborate with client to identify anxious behaviors as well as probable causes.
- Help client meet basic needs for food, comfort, and a sense of safety.
- During an acute psychotic episode, remove any potentially hazardous items from client's environment.
- If client experiences hallucinations, ensure safety and provide comfort and support.
- Encourage client to participate in one-on-one interactions and then help client progress to small groups.
- Provide positive reinforcement for socially acceptable behavior, such as an effort to improve hygiene and table manners.
- Encourage client to express feelings about the hallucinations experienced.
- Set limits on aggressive behavior.
- Maintain a low level of stimuli.
- Provide reality-based diversional activities.
- Provide a safe environment.
- Reorient the client to time and place when appropriate.

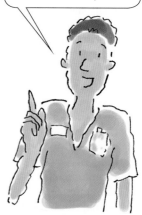

No, you're not hallucinating … this really is the psychotic disorders chapter.

Schizoaffective disorder

Psychosis occurring with a mood disturbance at the same time

Key signs and symptoms
- Client is extremely ill, with symptoms of psychotic behavior as well as mood symptoms
- Symptoms may alternate between the psychotic behavior and the mood symptoms

Key treatments
- Milieu therapy
- Atypical antipsychotics, mood stabilizers, and antidepressants are first-line medications for treatment

Key interventions
- Supportive psychotherapy
- Milieu therapy

Delusional disorder

Psychotic disorder characterized by delusions (false, fixed beliefs); these delusions can be plausible or bizarre and impossible

Key signs and symptoms
- Delusions (false, fixed beliefs)
- Inability to trust
- Projection

Key test results
- Blood and urine tests eliminate an organic or chemical cause.

- Endocrine function tests rule out hyperadrenalism, pernicious anemia, and thyroid disorders.
- Neurologic evaluations rule out an organic cause.

Key treatments
- Milieu therapy
- Supportive psychotherapy
- Antipsychotics: chlorpromazine, clozapine, fluphenazine, haloperidol, olanzapine, risperidone, aripiprazole

Key interventions
- Explore events that trigger delusions.
- Do not directly attack the delusion.
- After the dynamics of the delusions are understood, discourage repetitious talk about delusions and refocus the conversation on the client's underlying feelings.
- Recognize the delusion as the client's perception of the environment.

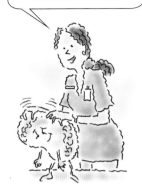

Direct confrontation of a client's delusions should be avoided.

Schizophrenia spectrum & other psychotic disorders questions, answers, and rationales

1. A client diagnosed with schizophrenia tells the nurse, "I am scheduled to meet the King of Samoa at a special time," making it impossible for the client to leave the room for dinner. Which response by the nurse is **most** appropriate?
1. "It is dinner time. Let us go so you can eat."
2. "The King of Samoa told me to take you to dinner."
3. "You are expected to follow the unit's schedule."
4. "People who do not eat are not being cooperative."

2. The nurse is monitoring a client who appears to be hallucinating and notes paranoid content in the client's speech. The client appears agitated, gesturing at a figure on the television. Which nursing intervention(s) is appropriate? Select all that apply.
1. Instruct the client to stop the behavior.
2. Reassure the client that there is no danger.
3. Acknowledge the presence of the hallucinations.
4. Instruct other staff to ignore the client's behavior.
5. Immediately apply physical restraints.
6. Use a calm voice and simple commands.

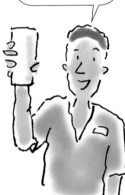

Here's to you—you're off to a fine start.

1. 1. A delusional client is so wrapped up in the false beliefs that there tends to be a disregard for activities of daily living, such as nutrition and hydration. The client needs clear, concise, firm directions from a caring nurse to meet needs. Telling the client a false story belittles and tricks the client, possibly leading to the client no longer trusting the nurse. Talking about the health care provider's expectations evades the issue of meeting the client's basic needs. Telling the client that not eating equates to being uncooperative is demeaning and does not address the delusion.
CN: Psychosocial integrity; CNS: None; CL: Analyze

2. 2, 3, 6. Using a calm voice, the nurse should reassure the client of his or her safety. Do not challenge the client; rather, acknowledge the hallucinatory experience. It is not appropriate to request that the client stop the behavior or instruct other staff to ignore the client's behavior. Implementing restraints is not warranted at this time. Although the client is agitated, no evidence exists that there is a risk for harming self or others.
CN: Psychosocial integrity; CNS: None; CL: Apply

CN: Client needs category   CNS: Client needs subcategory   CL: Cognitive level

3. The nurse is caring for a client newly diagnosed with schizophrenia. Which nursing intervention is **priority**?
1. Teach the client about schizophrenia.
2. Initiate a behavioral contract with the client.
3. Ensure the client attends all unit functions.
4. Provide a consistent, predictable environment.

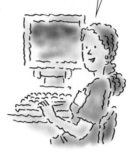

Check out that word "priority" in question #3—it looks important.

4. A client diagnosed with schizophrenia was admitted during the night. The next morning, the client begins to call the nurse by the client's sister's name. Which nursing intervention is **best**?
1. Assess the client for potential violent behaviors.
2. Take the client back to his or her private room.
3. Assume the misidentification helps the client.
4. Correct the misidentification and orient the client.

5. A client is diagnosed with schizoaffective disorder. When working with the interdisciplinary team on developing a treatment plan for the client, the nurse will ask which assessment question(s) to confirm this diagnosis? Select all that apply.
1. "Do you hear voices that no one else seems to hear?"
2. "Have you ever thought of yourself as being depressed?"
3. "How does it feel when you are not getting the attention you want?"
4. "When did you last make yourself purge a meal?"
5. "How do you feel when you have to leave your home?"

6. A client demonstrates no change in emotion when sharing details of intimate partner violence. When documenting this observation, the nurse will describe it using which term?
1. Regression
2. Blunted affect
3. Anhedonia
4. Denial

3. 4. A consistent, predictable environment helps the client remain as functional as possible and prevents sensory overload. Teaching the client about the illness is important but not a priority. A behavioral contract and required attendance at all functions are not particularly effective for clients diagnosed with schizophrenia.
CN: Safe, effective care environment; CNS: Management of care; CL: Apply

4. 4. Misidentification can contribute to anxiety, fear, aggression, and hostility. Orienting a new client to the hospital unit, staff, and other clients, along with establishing a nurse-client relationship, can decrease these feelings and help the client feel in control. Assessing for potential violence is an important nursing function for any psychiatric client, but a perceived supportive environment reduces the risk of violence. Withdrawing to the room, unless interpersonal relationships have become nontherapeutic, encourages the client to remain in the fantasy world.
CN: Psychosocial integrity; CNS: None; CL: Apply

5. 1, 2. A client diagnosed with schizoaffective disorder experiences signs and symptoms of a mood disorder (major depression, mania, or mixed episode) along with signs and symptoms of schizophrenia. Therefore, the treatment plan would need to address these signs and symptoms. Personality disorder (histrionic personality), eating disorder, and anxiety disorder (agoraphobia) are not involved with schizoaffective disorder.
CN: Safe, effective care environment; CNS: Management of care; CL: Apply

6. 2. Affect refers to behaviors, such as facial expression, that can be observed when a person is expressing and experiencing feelings. Blunted affect refers to a reduction in the intensity of an individual's emotional response. If the client's affect does not reflect the expected emotional content of the statement, the affect is considered inappropriate. Regression is a psychological defense mechanism in which a person abandons age-appropriate coping strategies in favor of earlier, more childlike patterns of behavior. Anhedonia is the lack of pleasure in things that used to bring pleasure. Denial is a defense mechanism in which confrontation with a personal problem or with reality is avoided by denying the existence of the problem or reality.
CN: Psychosocial integrity; CNS: None; CL: Understand

7. The nurse is caring for a client diagnosed with delusional disorder who is experiencing somatic sensations. The nurse suspects the client is currently experiencing such a delusion when the client makes which statement?
1. "There are bugs swarming all around me and drilling holes in my skin."
2. "No one else at this place has hair as beautiful as mine."
3. "My mother has always been terribly envious of my physical beauty."
4. "The President calls me all the time to be sure that I am feeling better."

I think I'm a great artist, but my sister says I'm delusional.

7. **1.** Somatic delusions involve bodily functions or sensations such as insects invading the skin. This type of delusion is often accompanied by tactile hallucinations, such as the intense itching or burning voiced by the client. Grandiose delusions reflect the belief that the person has some great, unrecognized talent; made some important discovery; or has a special relationship with a prominent person. Jealous delusions involve unfaithfulness or infidelity of a spouse or significant other and are based on incorrect inferences on the part of the client. Erotomanic delusions involve the belief that the client is loved intensely by another who is, under normal circumstances, is out of the client's usual environment.
CN: Psychosocial integrity; CNS: None; CL: Apply

8. Which behavior observed by the nurse indicates a client diagnosed with schizophrenia is experiencing echopraxia?
1. Observes the nurse to see when it is appropriate to speak during a therapy session.
2. Consistently imitates the nurse as medications are being administered.
3. Insists that the food being served at the facility is poisoned.
4. Turns the light off and on 34 times before going to sleep.

8. **2.** Echopraxia, observed in clients diagnosed with schizophrenia, is the involuntary copying of another's behaviors and is the result of the loss of ego boundaries. Modeling is the conscious copying of someone's behaviors. Paranoia is an unfounded fear often associated with possible harm. Ritualistic behaviors are repetitive and compulsive. Modeling, paranoia, or ritualistic behaviors are associated with echopraxia.
CN: Psychosocial integrity; CNS: None; CL: Apply

9. The nurse is caring for a client admitted with suspected schizophrenia. Which statement made by the nurse is appropriate regarding the anticipated treatment regimen?
1. "The magnetic resonance imaging (MRI) will help determine the size of your brain's lateral ventricle."
2. "The x-rays of your brain will help determine if your brain is receiving a sufficient blood supply."
3. "Your health care provider will evaluate the results of your endocrine function tests to determine treatment."
4. "The amount of paliperidone found in your blood will help determine if the dose is sufficient to manage your symptoms."

9. **1.** An MRI would support a possible diagnosis of schizophrenia if it confirmed the enlargement of the lateral or third ventricle or sulci (a groove or furrow on the surface of the brain). X-rays will not effectively confirm the status of cerebral blood flow. Endocrine function tests as well as blood and urine testing are used in diagnosing delusional disorders. Paliperidone is used to treat schizophrenia and schizoaffective disorders and may be prescribed once a diagnosis is confirmed.
CN: Physiological integrity; CNS: Reduction of risk potential; CL: Apply

10. The nurse is assessing a client recently prescribed risperidone. The nurse recognizes the medication is effective if the client reports relief of which symptom(s)? Select all that apply.
1. Apathy
2. Delusions
3. Social withdrawal
4. Attention impairment
5. Disorganized speech

10. **1, 3, 4.** Apathy, social withdrawal, and attention impairment are part of the category of negative symptoms, which also includes affective flattening, restricted thought and speech, and anhedonia. These symptoms are more responsive to the atypical antipsychotics, such as clozapine, risperidone, and olanzapine. Positive symptoms, such as delusions, hallucinations, thought disorder, and disorganized speech, respond to traditional antipsychotic drugs.
CN: Physiological integrity; CNS: Pharmacological and parenteral therapies; CL: Apply

11. A client, involuntarily hospitalized after the adult child filed a petition for safety reasons, is angry and refuses to talk with the family. The child is frustrated and states, "I feel so guilty about my decision." Which nursing response to this client's child is **most** empathic?

1. "Your parent is here because the parent desperately needs our help."
2. "Your parent will feel differently about you as the parent gets better."
3. "This is a stressful time, but you will feel better as the parent gets well."
4. "It is common to feel this way. Can we talk about your feelings?"

12. A client prescribed an antipsychotic medication regimen for several years is now being treated for a urinary tract infection with antibiotic therapy. Which nursing action is **most** appropriate?

1. Plan for possible hospitalization if the client is unable to adhere to the new therapy.
2. Arrange for a home health nurse to give the medication to reduce the risk for nonadherence.
3. Give instruction on the medication, possible adverse effects, and a return demonstration.
4. Develop a psychoeducational program to address any emotional and physical problems.

13. While caring for a client receiving antipsychotic therapy, the nurse suspects the client is experiencing tardive dyskinesia based on which client statement?

1. "I cannot keep my feet from tapping."
2. "It is difficult to read since my vision is blurry."
3. "I am so restless; I cannot seem to sit quietly anymore."
4. "Check my temperature; suddenly I feel feverish."

14. A client diagnosed with schizophrenia is prescribed clozapine. On a follow-up visit, which finding(s) are **most** concerning to the nurse? Select all that apply.

1. Sore throat
2. Pill-rolling movements
3. Polyuria
4. Fever
5. Polydipsia
6. Orthostatic hypotension

11. 4. This response is most empathic because it focuses on the adult child and helps the child understand that he or she is not alone. In addition, asking the child to tell the nurse more about the child's feelings helps the child to discuss and deal with feelings. Unresolved feelings of guilt, shame, isolation, and loss of hope impact the family's ability to manage the crisis and be supportive of the client. The other responses offer premature reassurance and cut off the opportunity for the adult child to discuss feelings.

CN: Psychosocial integrity; CNS: None; CL: Apply

12. 3. The client has been successful and reliable in carrying out current medication regimen. The nurse should assume the competency includes self-administration of antibiotics if the instructions are understood. No evidence exists that the client is having a relapse as a result of the infection, so the client would not need a psychoeducational program or hospitalization. Arranging for a community nurse to give the medication encourages dependency as opposed to self-care.

CN: Safe, effective care environment; CNS: Management of care; CL: Apply

13. 1. Symptoms of tardive dyskinesia include tongue protrusion, lip smacking, chewing, blinking, grimacing, choreiform movements of limbs and trunk, and foot tapping. Blurred vision is a common adverse reaction of antipsychotic drugs and usually disappears after a few weeks of therapy. Restlessness is associated with akathisia. Sudden fever may be a symptom of a malignant neurologic disorder.

CN: Physiological integrity; CNS: Reduction of risk potential; CL: Apply

14. 1, 4. Sore throat, fever, and sudden onset of other flulike symptoms are signs of agranulocytosis, an adverse effect of clozapine caused by an insufficient number of granulocytes. This causes the client to be susceptible to infection. The client's white blood cell count should be monitored at least weekly throughout the course of treatment. Pill-rolling movements can occur in those experiencing extrapyramidal adverse effects associated with antipsychotic medication that is prescribed for much longer than a medication such as clozapine. Polydipsia (excessive thirst) and polyuria (increased urine) are common adverse effects of lithium. Orthostatic hypotension is an adverse effect of tricyclic antidepressants.

CN: Physiological integrity; CNS: Pharmacological and parenteral therapies; CL: Apply

CN: Client needs category   CNS: Client needs subcategory   CL: Cognitive level

15. The nurse is leading an inpatient therapy group which has an average attendance of nine clients. Which nursing action is **priority** when attempting to provide effective treatment?
   1. Cancel the therapy group.
   2. Continue the group as scheduled.
   3. Consult with the unit's nurse manager.
   4. Combine the group with another group.

16. A client recently admitted to the emergency department is hypervigilant while reporting, "They want to hurt me and I cannot stop them." Which intervention is the nurse's **priority**?
   1. Attempt to rule out real threats as causing the client's stress.
   2. Determine whether the client has a history of mental illness.
   3. Promise the client that nothing bad will happen to him or her.
   4. Ask the health care provider for a prescription for haloperidol.

17. A client admitted to an inpatient unit approaches the nurse and states, "I am descended from a long line of people of a 'super-race.'" Which nursing action is appropriate?
   1. Smile and walk into the staff breakroom.
   2. Sit down with the client in the dayroom.
   3. Inform the client this is an inaccurate belief.
   4. Listen for hidden messages in themes of delusion.

18. The nurse understands which finding **most** suggests a client is demonstrating a behavior associated with schizophrenia?
   1. Speaking loudly in conversation
   2. Ignoring comments by the nurse
   3. Limiting responses to the same person
   4. Randomly tilting the head to one side

19. A nurse is performing morning care when a client begins demonstrating behavior characteristic of depersonalization. Which client statement suggests this psychotic state to the nurse?
   1. "My body is changing and disintegrating because I am not of this world!"
   2. "That television newscaster is talking just to me."
   3. "The towels are white, and I am white from the cold."
   4. "Do not touch me! You need to get away from me now."

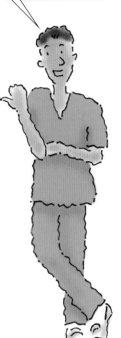

I wonder what the client means by "They want to hurt me?" Something to look into, for sure.

15. 2. The ideal number of clients to have in an inpatient group is 7 to 10. The nurse would not need to cancel or combine the group, because an ideal number of clients are participating. A consultation is not needed.
CN: Psychosocial integrity; CNS: None; CL: Analyze

16. 1. Of the options presented, ruling out the possibility of real treats to the client's safety has priority. The nurse should never make promises to the client that may not be able to be fulfilled. A history of mental illness is not relevant to the client's safety initially. Medication may be prescribed, but an assessment is required first.
CN: Psychosocial integrity; CNS: None; CL: Apply

17. 2. The first goal is to establish a relationship with the client, which includes creating psychological space for the creation of trust. The nurse should sit and be available, reflecting concern and interest. Walking into the nurse's station would indicate disinterest and lack of concern about the client's feelings. Delusions are firmly maintained false beliefs and attempts to dismiss or challenge them do not work. After establishing a relationship and lessening the client's anxiety, the nurse can orient the client to reality, clarify the meaning of the delusion, listen to concerns and fears, and try to understand the feelings reflected in the delusions.
CN: Safe, effective care environment; CNS: Management of care; CL: Apply

18. 4. Audio hallucinations are common manifestations associated with schizophrenia. A client who is having auditory hallucinations may tilt the head to one side, as if listening to someone or something. Speaking loudly, ignoring comments, and responding only to one person are indicative of hearing deficit, anxiety, and paranoid behavior, respectively.
CN: Psychosocial integrity; CNS: None; CL: Apply

19. 1. Depersonalization is a state in which the client feels unreal or believes parts of the body are being distorted. Ideas of reference are beliefs unrelated to situations and hold special meaning for the individual. The phrase "looseness of association" refers to sentences that have a vague connection to one another. Paranoid ideations are beliefs that others intend to harm the client in some way.
CN: Psychosocial integrity; CNS: None; CL: Apply

20. When assessing a client diagnosed with schizophrenia, the nurse notes the client is exhibiting opposing emotions simultaneously. How will the nurse document this finding?
1. Double bind
2. Ambivalence
3. Loose associations
4. Inappropriate affect

20. 2. Ambivalence, one of the symptoms associated with schizophrenia, immobilizes the person from acting. A double bind presents two conflicting messages—for example, saying that you trust someone but not allowing the person in your room. Loose association involves rapid shifts of ideas from one subject to another in an unrelated manner. Inappropriate affect refers to an observable expression of emotion incongruent with the emotion felt.
CN: Psychosocial integrity; CNS: None; CL: Understand

21. An adolescent client with a diagnosis of schizophrenia has been newly admitted to the hospital for stabilization of dysfunctional thought processes. What nursing intervention is **priority**?
1. Schedule attendance in unit orientation groups.
2. Arrange for one-on-one interaction with staff.
3. Introduce activities that focus on socialization.
4. Work on critical thinking and problem-solving skills.

21. 2. The psychotic client should first be involved in one-on-one interactions and then gradually advanced to small groups as psychotic symptoms subside. Once the client is stabilized, attention can be focused on socialization and other necessary skills.
CN: Psychosocial integrity; CNS: None; CL: Analyze

22. A client approaches the nurse frantically pointing at the sky stating, "The alien men are coming in spaceships to kill me." Which nursing response is **most** therapeutic?
1. "Why do you think the men are coming here to harm you?"
2. "Remember you are safe here; we will not let anyone harm you."
3. "It seems like the world is pretty scary for you, but you are safe here."
4. "There are no bad men in the sky because no one lives close to Earth."

22. 3. Explaining the world is scary but that the client is safe acknowledges the client's fears and feelings and offers a sense of security as the nurse tries to understand the symbolism. The nurse reflects these concerns to the client, along with reassurance of safety. The first response validates the delusion, not the feelings and fears, and does not orient the client to reality. The second response gives false reassurance; since the nurse is not sure of the symbolism, the nurse cannot make this promise. The last response rejects the client's feelings and does not address the fears.
CN: Psychosocial integrity; CNS: None; CL: Apply

23. Which assessment question demonstrates the nurse's understanding of the unique effects of schizoaffective disorder?
1. "Are you currently having suicidal ideations?"
2. "Can you tell me if you are actively hallucinating?"
3. "When did you begin having feeling of mistrust?"
4. "Do you have a history of generalized anxiety?"

23. 1. Schizoaffective disorder includes both psychosis and mood disturbance at the same time. Hallucinations are a part of schizoaffective disorder, but they are not the unique effect. This disorder does not always involve paranoia or anxiety.
CN: Psychosocial integrity; CNS: None; CL: Apply

24. A client asks the nurse, "Do you hear someone talking to me?" Which nursing response is **best**?
1. "Stop asking about voices. No one is in your room except you."
2. "Yes, I hear the voices too, but I refuse to listen to the voices."
3. "We all hear voices once in a while. What is your voice saying?"
4. "No, I do not hear anything, but I know you do. What are they saying?"

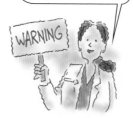

Remember to "keep it real" when discussing a client's hallucination. Lying is a violation of the therapeutic relationship.

24. 4. The nurse who admits not hearing the voice but is interested in what has been said points out reality and shows concern and support for the client. Attempting to argue the client out of the belief might entrench the client more firmly in the belief, making the client feel more out of control because of the negative and fearful nature of hallucinations. The other two responses violate the trust of the therapeutic relationship because they do not maintain reality orientation.
CN: Psychosocial integrity; CNS: None; CL: Apply

25. The nurse is educating a client newly pre-scribed chlorpromazine. Which response by the client indicates to the nurse the client understands the education?
1. "I can reduce the dosage when I begin to feel better."
2. "It is okay if I have an occasional alcoholic drink."
3. "I will stop taking it if I experience adverse effects."
4. "I need to schedule appointments for routine checks."

26. A client is referred to a mental health clinic for a possible delusional disorder. The nurse will assess the client for which health concern during the admission assessment?
1. Type 2 diabetes
2. Pernicious anemia
3. Lupus erythematosus
4. Polycystic ovary syndrome

27. The nurse will educate a homebound client prescribed clozapine to notify the health care provider immediately if which symptom(s) is experienced? Select all that apply.
1. Weakness
2. Sore throat
3. Tachycardia
4. Hypotension
5. Sudden fever
6. Bleeding gums

28. The nurse understands which client is expressing sentiments associated with delusional thinking?
1. The client who points to the nurse's stetho-scope and yells, "It is a snake!"
2. The client who tells the nurse, "I do not think life is worth living anymore."
3. The client who repeatedly refers to the night nurse as, "Mother."
4. The client who reports, "I hear the wolves howling outside my window again."

29. The nurse is planning care for a client experi-encing hallucinations. Which nursing intervention will the nurse include in the plan?
1. Confine the client to his or her room until the client feels better.
2. Provide a competing stimulus that distracts from the hallucinations.
3. Allow the client regular opportunities to dis-cuss the hallucinations.
4. Support perceptual distortions until the client gives them up on own accord.

25. 4. Ongoing assessment by a health care pro-vider is important to assess for adverse reactions to chlorpromazine and continued therapeutic effectiveness. The dosage should be cut only after checking with the health care provider. Alcoholic beverages are contraindicated while taking an antipsychotic drug. Adverse reactions should be reported immediately to determine if the drug should be discontinued.
CN: Physiological integrity; CNS: Pharmacological and parenteral therapies; CL: Apply

26. 2. Pernicious anemia is an endocrine disorder, which should be ruled out as a cause of delusional thinking. B_{12} deficiency can cause almost any psychiatric symptom, from anxiety and panic to depression and delusional thinking. While the other conditions are associated with the endocrine system, they lack a connection with B_{12} deficiency; thus, they are not associated with delusional thinking.
CN: Psychosocial integrity; CNS: None; CL: Apply

27. 1, 2, 3, 4, 5, 6. These are all symptoms of agranulocytosis, which is both an adverse effect of clozapine and a medical emergency. The client should stop the medication and see the health care provider immediately for any indication of agranulocytosis.
CN: Physiological integrity; CNS: Pharmacological and parenteral therapies; CL: Apply

28. 3. A delusion is a fixed belief. An illusion is a misinterpretation of an actual sensory stimula-tion. A wish to die is expressed through a suicidal ideation. A hallucination is a false sensory percep-tion without a stimulus.
CN: Psychosocial integrity; CNS: None; CL: Apply

29. 2. Providing a competing stimulus acknowledges the presence of the hallucinations and teaches the client ways to decrease their frequency. The other nursing actions support and maintain hallucination occurrence or deny its existence.
CN: Safe, effective care environment; CNS: Management of care; CL: Apply

30. A client diagnosed with schizophrenia is noted to have a problem with social isolation. Which nursing intervention is appropriate for this client?
1. Encourage the client to join in a group game.
2. Ask the client to participate in a group sing-along.
3. Name the client the leader of the client support group.
4. Suggest the client play solitaire in the therapy room.

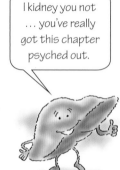

I kidney you not ... you've really got this chapter psyched out.

31. A client diagnosed with schizophrenia, admitted to the hospital 2 days ago, is prescribed haloperidol. When reviewing the client's chart, the nurse notes the entry below. Which finding will the nurse report to the health care provider **immediately**?

Progress notes	
6/22	Client is pale and diaphoretic, with warm skin.
1345	Client has tremors and difficulty speaking.
	Vital signs: Temp, 102.6° F (39.2° C);
	BP, 160/98 mm Hg; heart rate, 94 beats/
	minute; respiratory rate, 22 breaths/minute.
	Laboratory results received: CK, 500 units/L
	(500 U/L); WBC, 15,000/μ mm³ (15.0 × 10⁹/L);
	HCT, 38% (0.38); Hb, 14 g/dL (140 g/L)

1. Difficulty speaking
2. Respiratory rate
3. CK and WBC
4. HCT and Hb

32. A client is admitted with a diagnosis of acute exacerbation of schizophrenia. The nurse anticipates which therapy to be prescribed by the health care provider?
1. Counseling
2. Drug therapy
3. Biofeedback
4. Electroconvulsive therapy

33. The nurse is interacting with a client experiencing delusions. Which intervention is **most** appropriate for the nurse to implement?
1. Tell the client the delusions are not real.
2. Explain the delusion to the client.
3. Encourage the client to remain delusional.
4. Identify the meaning of the delusion.

30. 2. Inviting the client to participate in a noncompetitive group activity such as a sing-along does not require individual participation and will not present a threat to the client with schizophrenia. Games can become competitive and can lead to anxiety or hostility. The client probably does not have the social skills to lead a group at this time. Playing solitaire does not encourage socialization.
CN: Psychosocial integrity; CNS: None; CL: Apply

31. 3. The client's symptoms and elevated CK level and WBC count indicate possible neuroleptic malignant syndrome (NMS), a potentially fatal reaction to antipsychotic medications. Signs and symptoms of NMS include elevated blood pressure, hyperthermia, muscle rigidity, diaphoresis, and pale skin. HCT and Hb are within normal range.
CN: Physiological integrity; CNS: Pharmacological and parenteral therapies; CL: Analyze

32. 2. Drug therapy is usually successful in normalizing behavior and reducing or eliminating hallucinations, delusions, thought disorder, affect flattening, apathy, avolition, and asociality. Counseling to produce insight into the client's behavior usually is not effective in an acute schizophrenic reaction. Biofeedback reduces anxiety and modifies behavioral responses but is not the major component in the treatment of schizophrenia. Electroconvulsive therapy might be considered for schizoaffective disorder (which has a mood component) and is a treatment of choice for clinical depression.
CN: Psychosocial integrity; CNS: None; CL: Apply

33. 4. Identifying the meaning of the delusion helps the client understand and begin to develop strategies for dealing with these thought processes. Never argue with or try to talk the client out of a delusion. The delusions are very real to the client. Explaining the delusions helps the nurse, not the client. Encouraging the client to remain delusional is not therapeutic.
CN: Psychosocial integrity; CNS: None; CL: Apply

34. A client states to the nurse, "The voices are telling me to do terrible things." Which action will the nurse do **next**?
1. Find out what the voices are saying.
2. Allow the client sit in a private room.
3. Talk to the client about an unrelated topic.
4. Remind the client the voices are not real.

34. **1.** For safety purposes, the nurse must find out whether the voices are directing the client to harm himself or others. Further assessment can help identify appropriate therapeutic interventions. Isolating a person during this intense sensory confusion commonly reinforces the psychosis. Changing the topic indicates that the nurse is not concerned about the client's fears. Dismissing the voices shuts down communication between the client and the nurse.
CN: Safe, effective care environment; CNS: Safety and infection control; CL: Apply

35. The nurse recognizes the newly admitted client diagnosed with schizophrenia is exhibiting paranoid delusions when the client makes what statement?
1. "Space travelers are planning to take me back with them if they find me."
2. "I am a prophet just like Jacob and Abraham of the Old Testament."
3. "I can heal heart problems by merely touching your chest."
4. "My lover is infested with worms and needs to take medication."

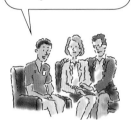

No, Mrs. Williams, I'm not an operative with the CIA. I'm just your nurse.

35. **1.** This client is exhibiting paranoid delusions, which are excessive or irrational suspicions or distrust of others. A religious delusion is the belief that one is favored by a higher being or is an instrument of a higher being. A grandiose delusion is the belief that one possesses greatness or special powers. A somatic delusion is the belief that one's body or body parts are distorted or diseased.
CN: Psychosocial integrity; CNS: None; CL: Apply

36. A client prescribed risperidone states, "I noticed I have a decreased sex drive." Which nursing statement is **most** appropriate?
1. "Unfortunately, this is an adverse effect you should expect."
2. "Stop the medication and notify your health care provider now."
3. "The effect will wear off and your libido will return to normal."
4. "Alert your health care provider but do not discontinue the medication."

36. **4.** Risperidone can cause sexual dysfunction in the form of a decreased sex drive. The condition should be discussed with the health care provider, but the medication should not be discontinued without provider knowledge. None of the other responses sufficiently address the educational issue.
CN: Physiological integrity; CNS: Pharmacological and parenteral therapies; CL: Apply

37. A nurse is assessing a client diagnosed with schizophrenia. Which statement made by the client will the nurse recognize as supporting this diagnosis?
1. "I keep getting these thoughts of hurting myself."
2. "There is no hope; I should just die."
3. "I am the best painter there ever was."
4. "I do not like people; I much rather be left alone."

37. **4.** Schizophrenia is a brain disease characterized by a variety of symptoms, including hallucinations, delusions, and asociality. Clients with obsessive-compulsive disorder experience intrusive thoughts and ritualistic behaviors. Feelings of helplessness and hopelessness are pivotal symptoms of clinical depression. Unstable moods and delusions of grandeur are characteristics of bipolar affective disorder.
CN: Psychosocial integrity; CNS: None; CL: Apply

38. A client is being discharged with a prescription for fluphenazine. Which statement made by the client indicates an understanding of medication education provided by the nurse?
1. "It is good to know this medication is not likely to cause extrapyramidal symptoms."
2. "I will need to have my eyes checked regularly for cataracts."
3. "I am told that this medication can cause my heart to beat dangerously slow."
4. "I realize it is important to keep my appointments for scheduled blood work."

38. **4.** Routine blood counts are advisable during therapy because blood dyscrasias, including leukopenia and agranulocytosis, have been observed in clients taking fluphenazine. The side effects most frequently reported with phenothiazine compounds are extrapyramidal symptoms. Glaucoma, not cataracts, has been noted in some clients. The effects on the heart tend to be tachycardia or dysrhythmias.
CN: Psychosocial integrity; CNS: Pharmacological and parenteral therapies; CL: Apply

39. During the initial interview, a client diagnosed with schizophrenia responds to questions with one-word answers, if answering at all. The nurse suspects the client is experiencing which condition?
   1. Avolition
   2. Anhedonia
   3. Alogia
   4. Flat affect

39. 3. Alogia, also called poverty of speech, is a decrease in the amount of richness of speech. A flat affect is absence of emotional expression. Anhedonia is the loss of pleasure in things that are usually pleasurable. Avolition is the lack of motivation.

CN: Psychosocial integrity; CNS: None; CL: Understand

40. A client prescribed quetiapine BID has not been experiencing the expected results of this therapy. Which recommendation by the nurse is likely to help the client experience the maximum benefit from the medication?
   1. "The medication should not be taken with food."
   2. "Take the medication at the same times each day."
   3. "Take the medication as soon as you notice any symptoms."
   4. "Avoid taking the medication within 2 hours of bedtime."

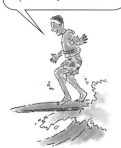

I don't know what my therapist is talking about ... I feel perfectly balanced.

40. 2. Quetiapine is known as an antipsychotic drug (atypical type). It works by helping to restore the balance of certain natural substances (neurotransmitters) in the brain. Taking this medication regularly provides the most benefit. Quetiapine should be taken daily with or without food. Taking the medication at bedtime may improve sleep.

CN: Physiological integrity; CNS: Pharmacological and parenteral therapies; CL: Apply

41. The nurse will include which statement when educating the family of a client diagnosed with schizophrenia?
   1. "Relapse can be prevented if the client takes medication as prescribed."
   2. "Support is available to help family members meet their own needs."
   3. "Improvement should occur if the client has a stimulating environment."
   4. "Stressful situations in the family can precipitate a relapse in the client."

41. 2. Because family members of a client diagnosed with schizophrenia face difficult situations and great stress, the nurse should inform them of support services that can help them cope. The nurse should also teach them that medication cannot prevent relapses and that environmental stimuli may precipitate symptoms. Although stress can trigger symptoms, the nurse should not make the family feel responsible for the client's relapses.

CN: Health promotion and maintenance; CNS: None; CL: Apply

42. The nurse on an inpatient unit is having a discussion with a client diagnosed with schizophrenia about a new prescription for olanzapine. It is appropriate for the nurse to ask the client which question(s) prior to administering olanzapine? Select all that apply.
   1. "Are you allergic to dairy products?"
   2. "Have you been told you have cataracts?"
   3. "How many packs of cigarettes do you smoke each day?"
   4. "Do you have a history of seizures?"
   5. "When was the last time you got a cold or the flu?"

42. 3, 4, 5. Olanzapine belongs to a class of drugs called atypical antipsychotics. It works by helping to restore the balance of certain natural substances in the brain. Because they are contraindications, history of smoking, seizures, and low white blood cell count resulting in infections are all conditions that are of importance when olanzapine is prescribed. Dairy allergies are not a known risk factor. Glaucoma, not cataracts, is a risk factor as well.

CN: Psychosocial integrity; CNS: Pharmacological and parenteral therapies; CL: Apply

43. The nurse anticipates the health care provider will prescribe which medication therapy **first** for a client being treated for schizoaffective disorder?
   1. Antiseizure medication
   2. Antianxiety medication
   3. Typical antipsychotic medication
   4. Atypical antipsychotic medication

43. 4. Atypical antipsychotics, mood stabilizers, and antidepressants are first-line medication treatments for schizoaffective disorder.

CN: Physiological integrity; CNS: Pharmacological and parenteral therapies; CL: Apply

44. Which statement made by a client diagnosed with delusional disorder demonstrates personal self-reflection for managing the disorder?
1. "I need to distract myself when I start focusing on my delusion."
2. "The medication I am taking will help control my delusions."
3. "My delusion could be true, but it is not likely that it is."
4. "I have been told that my delusion is a perception of my surroundings."

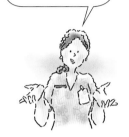

I come up with neo worgs all the time … do you think it's anything to be consterned about?

44. 1. After the initial discussion regarding the dynamics of the delusion is understood, repetitious talk about the belief should be avoided. While the other statements are true, none relate to self-awareness and the personal management of the delusional disorder.
CN: Psychosocial integrity; CNS: None; CL: Apply

45. A client diagnosed with schizophrenia has been taking haloperidol for 1 week when a nurse observes the client continuously staring at the ceiling. Which action will the nurse take **next**?
1. Continue to monitor the client.
2. Notify the health care provider.
3. Obtain a stat complete blood count.
4. Administer another dose of haloperidol.

45. 2. The client is experiencing an oculogyric crisis, which is spasmodic movements of the eyeballs into fixed positioning, typically in an upward gaze. The condition is generally caused by medications or occurs secondary to various neurological conditions where dopamine production is affected. Treatment includes reducing or withdrawing causative medications or replacing neurotransmitters when dopamine is lacking. The nurse needs to contact the health care provider to discuss possible change in medication administration. Continuing to monitor the client provides no relief. A complete blood count is not necessary. Administering more haloperidol may potentiate the effect.
CN: Physiological integrity; CNS: Pharmacological and parenteral therapies; CL: Analyze

46. A client diagnosed with schizophrenia becomes agitated and confronts the nurse with clenched fists. Which nursing action is **priority**?
1. Lead the client by the hand to the activity room for a card game.
2. Step up to the client and state that this behavior is inappropriate.
3. Request for a member of security to take the client to a seclusion room.
4. Speak with a quiet voice and offer medication to help with de-escalation.

46. 4. Always use the least restrictive means to calm a client. Never touch an agitated client; touch can be misinterpreted as a threat and further escalate the situation. Stepping up to an agitated client can be seen as an aggressive act. Seclusion is a last resort.
CN: Safe, effective care environment; CNS: Safety and infection control; CL: Apply

47. A client is prescribed aripiprazole and is given discharge instructions. Which statement by the client indicates to the nurse the discharge education was successful?
1. "I need to take an afternoon nap."
2. "I need to stay out of the sun."
3. "I cannot eat any aged cheese."
4. "I will monitor for weight loss."

47. 1. Aripiprazole is an antipsychotic drug that can cause tiredness; an afternoon nap could prove helpful. Clients taking aripiprazole do not need to avoid cheeses or the sun. Weight gain is a side effect of this medication.
CN: Physiological integrity; CNS: Pharmacological and parenteral therapies; CL: Apply

48. The nurse observes a client engaging in behaviors that suggest reoccurring auditory hallucinations. What is the **priority** basis for the nurse inviting the client to join in a game of cards?
1. Provides for a positive form of socialization
2. Demonstrates caring on the part of the nurse
3. Allows the nurse to confirm the hallucination
4. Provides a distraction for the client on which to focus

48. 4. Joining the nurse and playing a game provides a distraction that competes with the hallucinations. While playing cards with the nurse is a form of socialization and can be viewed as caring, neither of these outcomes is the basis for the intervention. Playing a game with the nurse allows for additional assessment but will not confirm hallucinations.
CN: Psychosocial integrity; CNS: None; CL: Analyze

49. While looking out the window, a client diagnosed with schizophrenia remarks, "That school across the street has creatures in it that are waiting for me." Which nursing action is the **most** appropriate?
1. Ask the client why the creatures are waiting.
2. Acknowledge the client's fears and insecurities.
3. Explain that there are no creatures in the school.
4. Redirect the client to group activities.

50. The nurse notes in the medical record that a client diagnosed with schizophrenia has been experiencing hallucinations. What statement by the client will support this documentation?
1. The client frequently tells staff, "A vampire is living under my bed."
2. The client states, "I hear voices telling me that you are evil and deserve to die."
3. The client states, "My mom was here but it started to rain; the door swung open and I sang."
4. The client states, "The newspaper's comics are really messages from a deceased friend."

51. A health care provider prescribes a client haloperidol. Based on the nurse's understanding of possible adverse effects, which measure(s) will the nurse take when administering haloperidol to the client? Select all that apply.
1. Review subcutaneous injection techniques.
2. Closely monitor the client's vital signs.
3. Provide the client the opportunity to pace.
4. Monitor the client's blood glucose levels.
5. Provide the client with sugar-free hard candy.
6. Monitor for signs and symptoms of urticaria.

49. 2. Acknowledging the client's fears and insecurities helps to establish a trusting relationship and increase feelings of safety. Asking the client why the creatures are waiting only serves to reinforce the delusional thoughts. Challenging the client's delusion may lead to agitation. Ignoring the remark does not reassure the client. A delusional client cannot participate in group activities.

CN: Psychosocial integrity; CNS: None; CL: Analyze

50. 2. Hallucinations are sensory experiences like hearing voices that are misrepresentations of reality or have no basis in reality. Delusions are beliefs not based in reality. Disorganized speech is characterized by jumping from one topic to the next or using unrelated words. An idea of reference is a belief that an unrelated situation holds special meaning for the client.

CN: Psychosocial integrity; CNS: None; CL: Apply

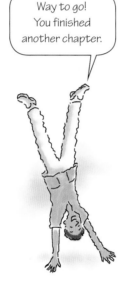

Way to go! You finished another chapter.

51. 2, 3, 5. Neuroleptic malignant syndrome is a life-threatening extrapyramidal adverse effect of antipsychotic medications such as haloperidol. It is associated with a rapid increase in temperature. The most common extrapyramidal adverse effect, akathisia, is a form of psychomotor restlessness that can commonly be relieved by pacing. The anticholinergic medications provided to alleviate the extrapyramidal effects of haloperidol can result in dry mouth. Providing the client with sugarless hard candy to suck on can help alleviate this problem. Haloperidol is not given subcutaneously and does not affect blood glucose levels. Urticaria isn't usually associated with haloperidol.

CN: Physiological integrity; CNS: Pharmacological and parenteral therapies; CL: Apply

Chapter 17

Substance Use Disorders

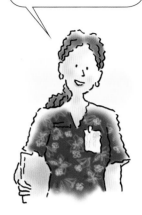

Substance use is serious business—as is answering these questions carefully and thoughtfully.

Substance use disorders refresher

Alcohol use disorder

Problem drinking that becomes severe whether it be use or dependency

Key signs and symptoms
- History of alcohol intake
- History of blackouts
- Pathologic intoxication
- Symptoms of withdrawal

Key test results
- CAGE questionnaire responses indicate alcoholism
- Michigan Alcoholism Screening Test results indicate alcoholism

Key treatments
- Alcoholics Anonymous
- Individual therapy
- Rehabilitation
- Antidepressants: bupropion
  - maximum daily dosage should not exceed 450 mg/day, in up to 4 divided doses; a single dose should not exceed 150 mg
- Anxiolytics: chlordiazepoxide, diazepam, lorazepam
- Disulfiram to prevent relapse into alcohol use
  - client must be alcohol-free for 12 hours before administering this drug
- Naltrexone to prevent relapse into alcohol use
- Selective serotonin reuptake inhibitors (SSRIs): fluoxetine, paroxetine

Key interventions
- Evaluate the client's use of alcohol as a coping mechanism.
- Set limits on denial and rationalization.
- Ask client to formulate goals for actions that will help the client maintain a lifestyle free from substance use.

Cocaine use disorder

When use of cocaine harms a person's health or social functioning, or when a person has physical withdrawal symptoms when attempting to discontinue use of the drug

Key signs and symptoms
- Elevated energy and mood
- Grandiose thinking
- Impaired judgment

Key test results
- A drug screening is positive for cocaine

Key treatments
- Detoxification
- Rehabilitation (inpatient or outpatient)
- Narcotics Anonymous
- Individual therapy
- Anxiolytics: lorazepam, alprazolam
- Dopamine agent: bromocriptine
- Selective serotonin reuptake inhibitors (SSRIs): fluoxetine, paroxetine

Key interventions
- Establish a trusting relationship with client.
- Provide client with well-balanced meals.
- Set limits on client's attempts to rationalize behavior.

Opioid use disorder

When use of opioid harms a person's health or social functioning, or when a person has physical withdrawal symptoms when attempting to discontinue use of the drug

Key signs and symptoms
- Chronic constipation
- Sweating
- Euphoria
- Small pupils
- Nausea
- Slurred speech
- General discontent

Key test results
- A drug screening is positive for opioids

Key treatments
- Detoxification
- Rehabilitation (inpatient or outpatient)
- Narcotics Anonymous
- Individual therapy

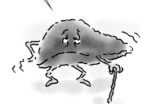

I've definitely been working too hard!

345

- Opioid agonists: buprenorphine, methadone
- Opioid antagonist: naloxone

Key interventions
- Establish a trusting relationship with client.
- Provide client with well-balanced meals.
- Set limits on client's attempts to rationalize behavior.

Other substance use disorders

Use or dependence on a drug leading to consequences that are negative to the individual's physical and/or mental health, and/or the well-being of others

Key signs and symptoms
- Blaming others for problems
- Development of physiologic or psychological need for a substance
- Dysfunctional anger
- Feelings of grandiosity
- Impulsiveness

- Use of denial and rationalization to explain consequences of behavior

Key test results
- A drug screening is positive for the used substance

Key treatments
- Individual therapy
- Clonidine for opiate withdrawal symptoms
- Methadone maintenance for opiate addiction detoxification
- Naloxone for opiate overdose

Key interventions
- Ensure a safe, quiet environment free from stimuli.
- Monitor for withdrawal symptoms, such as tremors, seizures, and anxiety.
- Help the client understand the consequences of substance use.
- Encourage the client to vent fear and anger.

> Discussing substance use is especially important during pregnancy, as many drugs can harm the fetus.

thePoint® You can download tables of drug information to help you prepare for the NCLEX®! View Generic Drug Names, Drug Classifications, Drug Actions, and Nursing Implications for the drugs discussed in this refresher at **http://thePoint.lww.com.**

Substance use disorders questions, answers, and rationales

1. To **best** prepare family members to support a client who has an alcohol use disorder, the nurse will suggest which intervention?
   1. Accepting they have no control over their family member's addiction
   2. Attending a support group that focuses on family members
   3. Providing financial support while the family member is in therapy
   4. Being the caregiver during the family member's detoxification period

2. The health care provider has prescribed oral diazepam 50 mg daily. The drug is available as oral suspension with a strength of 25 mg/5 mL. How many milliliters will the nurse administer per dose? Record your answer as a whole number.
_____ mL

> With substance use, the whole family needs to be involved in treatment.

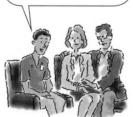

1. **2.** Dealing with a loved one's alcohol use disorder can be a difficult, long-term endeavor. It is vital that the family have effective support in dealing with the challenges the addiction will present. While the other interventions are appropriate, they are all issues that are addressed by family-focused support groups like Al-Anon.
CN: Psychosocial integrity; CNS: None; CL: Analyze

2. **10.**
The correct formula to calculate a drug dose is:

$$\frac{Dose\ on\ hand}{Quantity\ on\ hand} = \frac{Dose\ desired}{X}$$

The health care provider prescribes 50 mg, which is the dose desired. The drug available is 25 mg/5 mL, which is the dose on hand.

$$\frac{25mg}{5mL} = \frac{50mg}{X}$$

$$X = 10mL$$

CN: Physiological integrity; CNS: Pharmacological and parenteral therapies; CL: Apply

CN: Client needs category   CNS: Client needs subcategory   CL: Cognitive level

3. A client with a history of an alcohol use disorder tells the nurse, "I am merely a social drinker. Many of my friends drink much more than I do." Which nursing response is **most** appropriate?
1. "Social drinking can lead to serious alcohol use."
2. "How does social drinking affect your friends' lives?"
3. "What do you believe it means to be a social drinker?"
4. "You need to avoid alcohol; that includes social drinking."

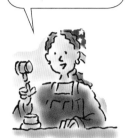

Avoid being judgmental with clients struggling with addiction problems.

3. **3.** Asking the client to define what is meant by "social drinker" will allow the conversation to be founded upon an understanding of the client's definition of the term. Social drinking does not always lead to alcohol use disorder. The conversation should focus on the client's experiences, not friends' experiences. The statement about avoiding all alcohol, while true, is likely to shut down communication between the client and nurse.
CN: Psychosocial integrity; CNS: None; CL: Apply

4. The nurse is observing a client for signs of alcohol withdrawal. Which observation will the nurse expect to assess if the client last consumed alcohol 6–12 hours ago?
1. The client is found crying in the client's room.
2. The client states, "I feel really, really nauseated."
3. The client's blood pressure is 88/50 mm Hg.
4. The client reports difficulty falling and staying asleep.

4. **2.** Nausea and subsequent vomiting are early signs of alcohol withdrawal, noted within 6–12 hours of a client last consuming alcohol. Depression and hypotension are not associated with alcohol withdrawal (hypertension is). Insomnia is noted 48 hours after last consuming alcohol.
CN: Psychosocial integrity; CNS: None; CL: Apply

5. Which response by the nurse is **most** appropriate when a client demands, "You cannot discuss my drinking problems with my children!"?
1. "Do you really think your children do not already know you have a drinking problem?"
2. "Do you not think your children deserve to know about your alcohol use?"
3. "They need to be told the truth about your drinking, but they need to hear it from you."
4. "You seem concerned about what will happen when you tell them you have a problem."

5. **4.** A client struggling with addiction problems commonly believe people will be judgmental, rejecting, and uncaring if they are told that the client is recovering from alcohol use disorder. The first response challenges the client and will put the client on the defensive. The second response will also make the client defensive and apt to construct rationalizations about why the children do not need to know. The third response is valid, but it is not appropriate to ask a client who is afraid to tell others about the addiction until the client is ready.
CN: Psychosocial integrity; CNS: None; CL: Analyze

6. The nurse will focus on which assessment when admitting a client with prolonged, chronic alcohol intake to determine the existence of a physical complication of alcohol use disorder?
1. Palpating the abdomen
2. Inspecting the nasal passages
3. Determining muscle mass of the legs
4. Identifying any feeling of tingling in the hands

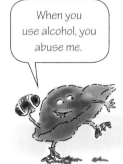

When you use alcohol, you abuse me.

6. **1.** A major effect of alcohol on the body is liver impairment, and an enlarged liver is a common physical finding. Nasal irritation is commonly seen in clients who snort cocaine or opioids. Muscle wasting and limb paresthesia do not tend to occur in clients who use alcohol.
CN: Physiological integrity; CNS: Physiological adaptation; CL: Apply

7. A client diagnosed with alcohol use disorder experiences tremors, loss of appetite, and disordered thinking 8 hours after alcohol consumption. Which nursing action is **priority**?
1. Obtain a prescription for lorazepam.
2. Administer disulfiram as prescribed.
3. Provide muscle-relaxation exercises.
4. Initiate constant one-on-one monitoring.

7. **1.** A client in alcohol withdrawal should be medicated with a benzodiazepine, such as lorazepam, to prevent progression of symptoms to delirium tremens, a life-threatening withdrawal syndrome. Disulfiram is used during early recovery, not during detoxification. Muscle relaxation exercises are not particularly effective during withdrawal. Close monitoring during withdrawal is appropriate after the client has been medicated for withdrawal symptoms.
CN: Psychosocial integrity; CNS: None; CL: Analyze

CN: Client needs category   CNS: Client needs subcategory   CL: Cognitive level

8. A client tells the nurse, "Alcohol helps me sleep." Which nursing response is **most** appropriate?
1. "Drinking alcohol does not help promote sleep."
2. "Continued alcohol consumption causes insomnia."
3. "One glass of alcohol a night can induce sleep."
4. "Alcohol can make one drowsy enough to fall asleep."

9. A client withdrawing from alcohol is prescribed fluoxetine. Which response by a family member indicates to the nurse the family understands the education provided?
1. "Short-term use of fluoxetine can lead to dependency."
2. "Fluoxetine can exacerbate the symptoms of withdrawal."
3. "A dry mouth needs to be reported immediately."
4. "The family needs to be alert for mood changes."

10. The nurse is providing information concerning disulfiram to a client about to be discharged after alcohol detoxification. Which statement made by the client indicates to the nurse a need for further instruction?
1. "I need to take disulfiram every day as prescribed."
2. "This medication is not a cure, but it can help me stay sober."
3. "Chest pain can occur if I take this medication improperly."
4. "Disulfiram will minimize the risk of symptoms if I relapse."

11. Which symptom(s) suggests to the nurse a client with a history of alcohol use disorder is experiencing cirrhosis of the liver? Select all that apply.
1. Icterus noted bilaterally
2. Numerous bruises
3. Weight loss of 15 lb (6.8 kg)
4. Admission of suicidal ideations
5. Chronic constipation

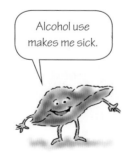

Alcohol use makes me sick.

12. Which question is **most** appropriate for the nurse to ask a female client with depression to assess for a common associated problem?
1. "Have you ever been sexually abused?"
2. "Have you ever been told that you anger easily?"
3. "When did you have your last menstrual period?"
4. "Could you tell me what you ate for breakfast today?"

8. 2. Alcohol use may initially promote sleep but, with continued use, it causes insomnia. Evidence shows that alcohol does not facilitate sleep. One glass of alcohol a night will not induce sleep. Stating that alcohol can make one drowsy enough to fall asleep does not give information about how alcohol adversely affects sleep. It encourages the client to think using alcohol to induce sleep is an appropriate strategy.
CN: Psychosocial integrity; CNS: None; CL: Apply

9. 4. Fluoxetine, a selective serotonin reuptake inhibitor (SSRI), is an antidepressant that may be prescribed to help manage withdrawal-induced depression. The major safety risk is the development of mood changes that can result in suicide. Fluoxetine is not associated with dependency or exacerbation of withdrawal symptoms and signs. A dry mouth is a rare adverse reaction, but it does not require immediate intervention.
CN: Physiological integrity; CNS: Pharmacological and parenteral therapies; CL: Apply

10. 4. Disulfiram is used to treat chronic alcohol use. It causes unpleasant effects when even small amounts of alcohol are consumed. These effects include flushing of the face, headache, nausea, vomiting, chest pain, weakness, blurred vision, mental confusion, sweating, choking, breathing difficulty, and anxiety. Disulfiram comes in tablets to be taken by mouth. It should be taken once a day. Disulfiram is not a cure for alcohol use disorder but discourages drinking.
CN: Physiological integrity; CNS: Pharmacological and parenteral therapies; CL: Apply

11. 1, 2, 3. Cirrhosis of the liver presents with jaundice, icterus (yellowing of the sclera of the eye), easy bruising, and weight loss. While they may be present, neither severe depression nor constipation is generally associated with this liver disorder.
CN: Physiological integrity; CNS: Reduction of risk potential; CL: Apply

12. 1. Many women diagnosed with substance use problems also have a history of physical or sexual abuse. Alcohol use is not a common finding in a woman showing defiant behavior or experiencing amenorrhea. Short-term memory loss is not expected in a woman dealing with alcohol use.
CN: Psychosocial integrity; CNS: None; CL: Apply

13. A client is currently enrolled in an alcohol recovery program. The nurse educates the client about addressing nutritional needs. Which client statement suggests to the nurse the client needs additional information?
1. "Eating a balanced diet is not as bad as I thought it would be."
2. "I have been watching my carbs, so my blood sugar does not spike."
3. "I do not like protein drinks, but I drink one daily because I have to."
4. "I will discuss with a nutritionist what I should and should not eat."

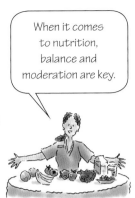

When it comes to nutrition, balance and moderation are key.

13. 3. The client must be involved in the decision to supplement daily dietary intake and should not be forced to drink protein drinks daily when other protein supplements are available. Clients who use alcohol are commonly malnourished and need help to follow a balanced diet. Monitoring carbohydrate intake is especially important because episodes of hypoglycemia and hyperglycemia may occur due to the high sugar content of alcohol. The statements about eating healthy and talking with a nutritionist are positive statements and do not require follow-up.
CN: Physiological integrity; CNS: Basic care and comfort; CL: Apply

14. A client being treated for alcohol withdrawal is prescribed bupropion 150 mg QID. Which finding is **most** concerning to the nurse?
1. The client has a history of depression.
2. The daily dosage of bupropion prescribed.
3. The client took isocarboxazid 2 months ago.
4. The client has type 2 diabetes mellitus.

14. 2. To minimize the risk of seizures, the maximum recommended dose of bupropion must not be exceeded (450 mg/day). Bupropion is safe for clients with a history of depression. Bupropion should not be taken if a monoamine oxidase inhibitor (MAOI), such as isocarboxazid, was taken in the past 14 days. The client's glucose level needs to be monitored closely as adverse reactions to bupropion include hypo- and hyperglycemia; however, the risk of seizures is more concerning.
CN: Physiological integrity; CNS: Pharmacological and parenteral therapies; CL: Analyze

15. A client in the emergency department is suspected of experiencing an opiate overdose. Which medication does the nurse prepare to administer?
1. Naloxone
2. Flumazenil
3. Acetylcysteine
4. Protamine sulfate

15. 1. The antidote for opiate overdose is naloxone. Flumazenil is used to reverse the effects of benzodiazepine sedatives. Acetylcysteine may be given for acetaminophen overdose. Protamine sulfate is given for heparin overdose.
CN: Physiological integrity; CNS: Pharmacological and parenteral therapies; CL: Apply

16. A home health nurse is caring for a client who typically consumes 15 to 20 beers per week and is extremely defensive about alcohol intake. The client admits to experiencing blackouts and has had three alcohol-related motor vehicle accidents. What is the **best** nursing action for this client?
1. Monitor the client's daily alcohol intake.
2. Tell the client to switch to low-alcohol wine coolers.
3. Have the client limit intake to 3 or less beers daily.
4. Encourage the client to abstain from alcohol consumption.

16. 4. This client demonstrates behaviors consistent with addiction. Once addicted, the only way to control intake is to abstain altogether—monitoring or limiting intake or switching to low-alcoholic drinks will not work for this client.
CN: Psychosocial integrity; CNS: None; CL: Apply

17. Which goal is the **priority** for the nurse to set for a client experiencing alcohol withdrawal?
1. The client will commit to a drug-free lifestyle.
2. The client will work with the nurse to remain safe.
3. The client will drink plenty of fluids daily.
4. The client will make a personal inventory of strengths.

17. 2. The most important goal is client safety. Although drinking enough fluids, identifying personal strengths, and committing to a drug-free lifestyle are important goals, promoting client safety must be the nurse's priority.
CN: Psychosocial integrity; CNS: None; CL: Analyze

18. A client, admitted for management of alcohol withdrawal, tells the nurse, "I do not have a drinking problem. I just have a really bad case of the flu." The nurse recognizes the client is relying on which defense mechanism(s) to manage the situation? Select all that apply.
1. Projection
2. Denial
3. Rationalization
4. Suppression
5. Repression

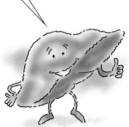

Encourage clients with alcohol use disorder to seek treatment. Their livers will thank you.

18. 2, 3. The client is using denial and rationalization. Denial is the unconscious disclaimer of unacceptable thoughts, feelings, needs, or certain external factors. Rationalization is the unconscious effort to justify intolerable feelings, behaviors, and motives. The client is not using projection, suppression, or repression. Emotions, behavior, and motives, which are consciously intolerable, are denied and then attributed to others in projection. Suppression is a conscious effort to control and conceal unacceptable ideas and impulses into the unconscious. Repression is the unconscious placement of unacceptable feelings into the unconscious mind.
CN: Physiological integrity; CNS: Physiological adaptation; CL: Understand

19. Which client statement demonstrates to the nurse an understanding of the effects of chronic alcohol use?
1. "I make a conscious effort to eat a well-balanced diet every single day."
2. "It is important that I have a good relationship with my health care provider."
3. "Getting sufficient rest is a very important part of my lifestyle routine now."
4. "Attending a weekly aerobic exercise class has helped me feel so much better."

19. 2. It is important for the client to maintain a cooperative relationship with a health care provider so that existing and further health issues can be identified and managed effectively. While diet, exercise, and rest are important to good health, they are not sufficient to deal with the chronic and acute problems alcohol use can cause.
CN: Safe, effective care environment; CNS: Management of care; CL: Analysis

20. A nurse is assigned to care for a recently admitted client who has attempted suicide. Which is the **priority** nursing action?
1. Search the client's belongings and room.
2. Tell the client the nurse trusts that he or she will not to attempt self-harm again.
3. Respect the client's need for and right to privacy.
4. Remind all staff members to frequently check on the client.

20. 1. Because a client who has attempted suicide could try again, the nurse should search the client's belongings and room to remove any items that could be used in another suicide attempt; the need to maintain a safe environment supersedes the client's right to privacy. Expressing trust that the client will not cause self-harm may increase the client's guilt and pain if the client cannot live up to that trust. Frequent checks by staff members are not enough because the client may attempt suicide between checks.
CN: Safe, effective care environment; CNS: Safety and infection control; CL: Apply

21. A client, who started consuming alcohol 30 years ago, now self-identifies as drinking "way too much." The client asks the nurse if the client's immune system has suffered permanent damage. Which assessment question will **best** assist the nurse in addressing the client's concern?
1. "How many times have you been prescribed an antibiotic in the last 3 years?"
2. "Can you describe for me what your weekly diet mostly consists of?"
3. "How many times a week do you drink enough to be considered drunk?"
4. "When did you start consuming enough alcohol to be considered a heavy drinker?"

21. 1. Chronic alcohol use can permanently depress the immune system and cause increased susceptibility to infections. Determining the frequency of prescribed antibiotic therapy will help determine the frequency of non–self-resolving infections. A nutritionally well-balanced diet that includes foods high in protein and B vitamins will help develop a strong immune system, but it will not likely offset the effects of excessive alcohol consumption on the immune system. Assessing sobriety is appropriate but has limited impact on determining the effect it has on the client's immune system. Drinking alcohol may put the client at risk for immune system problems at any time in life.
CN: Physiological integrity; CNS: Physiological adaptation; CL: Apply

22. A client experiencing alcohol withdrawal expresses concern about experiencing hallucinations. Which nursing intervention is **priority**?

1. Pointing out that the sensation does not exist
2. Allowing the client to talk about the experience
3. Determining if the client has a cognitive impairment
4. Encouraging the client to return to his or her room and rest

23. What will the nurse **initially** ask a client recovering from an alcohol use disorder to facilitate stress management?

1. "Tell me how you usually handle a stressful situation."
2. "What type of stress management would you like to focus on?"
3. "May we talk about ways to avoid conflict at work and at home?"
4. "Please tell me what types of situations stress you out the most."

24. A client struggling with alcohol use disorder tells the nurse, "I do not need to be preached to; I get enough of that from my family." What nursing response is **most** appropriate?

1. "You sound frustrated and maybe even angry."
2. "Do not worry, I will not insult you by preaching."
3. "Your family is concerned about your alcohol problem."
4. "Tell me when you are ready to talk about your drinking."

25. A client voluntarily enters an alcohol treatment program. During the first visit with the nurse, the client insists there is no problem with alcohol and states, "I am only here because my spouse is threatening to divorce me if I do not come." What is the **best** response by the nurse?

1. "I wonder why your spouse would issue such a drastic ultimatum."
2. "Because you came voluntarily, you are free to leave anytime you wish."
3. "You sound pretty definite about not having a problem with alcohol."
4. "From your point of view, what is most important for me to know about you?"

26. Which characteristic indicates to the nurse a client recovering from alcohol use disorder has relationship problems?

1. The client is prone to panic attacks.
2. The client has poor problem-solving skills.
3. The client does not pay attention to details.
4. The client ignores the need to relax and rest.

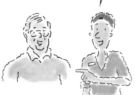

When your client expresses concern about his symptoms, listen up!

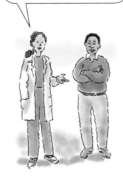

Alcohol use disorder is a disease. Listen empathetically to your client.

22. 2. The client needs to talk about the periodic hallucinations to prevent them from becoming triggers to aggressive behaviors and possible self-injury. The client's experience of sensory-perceptual alterations must be acknowledged. Determining if the client has a cognitive impairment and encouraging the client to rest do not address the problem of periodic hallucinations.
CN: Psychosocial integrity; CNS: None; CL: Apply

23. 1. The client needs help identifying a successful coping behavior and developing ways to incorporate that behavior into daily functioning. Initially, the nurse should assess the client's usual coping skills for both effectiveness and appropriateness. While the other options are appropriate, they are not effective until an initial assessment of coping skills is done.
CN: Psychosocial integrity; CNS: None; CL: Analyze

24. 1. Blaming or preaching to the client should be avoided because the negativity created prevents the client from hearing what the nurse has to say. Opening the conversation with an empathic or validating response is most effective. The remaining statements are not likely to initiate a conversation because they tend to avoid the client's feelings or postpone a conversation.
CN: Psychosocial integrity; CNS: None; CL: Apply

25. 4. Asking the client what is most important for the nurse to know allows the nurse to collect more information. Wondering why the spouse would issue an ultimatum focuses on the spouse, not the client. Telling the client he or she is free to leave is abrasive and blocks communication. Telling the client he or she sounds definite about not having an alcohol problem does not allow for further exploration of the problem.
CN: Psychosocial integrity; CNS: None; CL: Apply

26. 2. To have satisfying relationships, a person must be able to communicate and problem-solve. Relationship problems do not predispose people to panic attacks any more than other psychosocial stressors. Paying attention to details is not a major concern when addressing the client's relationship difficulties. Although ignoring the need for rest and relaxation is unhealthy, it should not pose a major relationship problem.
CN: Psychosocial integrity; CNS: None; CL: Apply

CN: Client needs category   CNS: Client needs subcategory   CL: Cognitive level

27. The nurse suggests to a client struggling with an alcohol use disorder to commit to keeping a daily journal. Which statement by the client **best** demonstrates an understanding of the nurse's intervention?
1. "Keeping a journal will help me to reflect on my stressors and how I cope."
2. "Journaling will help me improve my writing and communication skills."
3. "My journal will serve to remind me how much alcohol has affected my life."
4. "I will keep a journal to channel my frustrations away from family and friends."

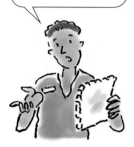

In question #27, you are looking for the best rationale for the suggested intervention.

27. 1. Keeping a journal enables the client to identify problems and patterns of coping. From this information, the difficulties the client faces can be addressed. Although journaling may relate to all the remaining statements, the best option addresses problem and skill evaluation.
CN: Psychosocial integrity; CNS: None; CL: Analyze

28. A client being treated for an alcohol use disorder is prescribed diazepam. What assessment finding **most** concerns the nurse?
1. The client is a 71-year-old man.
2. Non-adherent with previous alcohol use disorder treatment.
3. History of lung cancer; currently in remission.
4. The client currently takes omeprazole daily.

28. 1. Diazepam is known to cause an increased risk of falls in older adults. Clients taking omeprazole along with benzodiazepines should be monitored to determine if the dosages need to be adjusted due to a slight risk of an interaction. However, safety is priority. None of the other findings are problematic among clients taking diazepam.
CN: Physiological integrity; CNS: Pharmacological and parenteral therapies; CL: Apply

29. The nurse is preparing to provide education for a group of clients who are beginning an alcohol recovery program. Which statement will the nurse use to initiate the first session?
1. "Let us start with what brings each of you here today."
2. "We will start by introducing ourselves to the group."
3. "This group will focus on keeping each of you sober."
4. "These sessions are most effective when everyone participates."

29. 1. It is important to know if the client's current situation helps or hinders the potential to learn. Knowing what motivates the client will be vital in providing the support needed to master the skills needed to maintain sobriety. Although the other statements reflect the facts associated with such therapeutic groups, none provide the information needed to help assure individual success.
CN: Psychosocial integrity; CNS: None; CL: Apply

30. Which statement made by a member of an alcoholic support group **most** concerns the nurse?
1. "I miss the fun I had with my drinking buddies."
2. "I struggle every day with the need for a drink."
3. "Alcohol has been a part of my life for a long time."
4. "It is difficult making time to come to these meetings."

Asking appropriate questions is a key communication skill for nurses.

30. 1. Changing the client's old habits is essential for sustaining a sober lifestyle. The feelings about friends and drinking are the greatest concern of the statements made. This statement shows insight: the client recognizes the struggle sobriety causes and the effects alcohol has had on one's life. The remaining statements reflect common feelings associated with alcohol use.
CN: Psychosocial integrity; CNS: None; CL: Analyze

31. What assessment question is **priority** for the nurse to ask when educating a client prescribed buprenorphine?
1. "Have you ever taken this medication before?"
2. "Are you likely to drink alcohol when you leave?"
3. "Have you ever had a seizure or aneurysm?"
4. "Do you think you will keep your follow-up appointments"

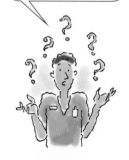

31. 2. A client, prescribed buprenorphine as a part of therapy for opioid use disorder, must avoid all alcohol to best support therapeutic effect and avoid adverse effects. Buprenorphine is not known to cause seizures or aneurysms. It is important to know if the client has taken buprenorphine before and if the client plans to keep follow-up appointments; however, these are not priority.
CN: Physiological integrity; CNS: Pharmacological and parenteral therapies; CL: Analyze

32. The nurse is meeting with a client who uses alcohol and the client's family. While listening to the family, which finding **most** concerns the nurse?
  1. The repeated use of descriptive jargon
  2. Disapproval of the client's behaviors
  3. Avoidance of issues that cause conflict
  4. The expression of nonverbal communication

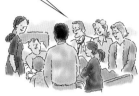

Families that suffer together also need to heal together.

33. A client with alcohol use disorder begins individual therapy with the nurse. Which nursing goal is **priority** for the client?
  1. Learning to express feelings
  2. Establishing new family roles
  3. Determining new socializing strategies
  4. Decreasing fixation with physical health

34. A client asks the nurse, "Why does my health care provider want me to take methadone?" Which nursing response is **most** appropriate?
  1. "Methadone has relatively few side effects and drug interactions."
  2. "Your health care provider believes this is the best course of action for you."
  3. "It will help with the muscle-related pain associated with opiate withdrawal."
  4. "Methadone reduces withdrawal symptoms without producing a narcotic 'high.'"

35. A client diagnosed with alcohol use disorder has just completed a residential treatment program. Which information will the nurse provide the client and the family to help manage expectations for future sobriety?
  1. There will likely be a need to initially support the client financially.
  2. Ways to help minimize triggers that have caused the client to drink in the past.
  3. Accept the possibility that the client may relapse and use alcohol again.
  4. Insist that the client consume alcohol in moderation and on rare occasions.

32. 3. The interaction pattern of a family with a member who uses alcohol commonly revolves around denying the problem, avoiding conflict, or rationalizing the addiction. Health care providers are more likely to use jargon. The family generally will struggle with setting limits and expressing disapproval of the client's behavior. Nonverbal communication usually gives the nurse insight into family dynamics.
CN: Psychosocial integrity; CNS: None; CL: Analyze

33. 1. The client must address issues, learn ways to cope effectively with life stressors, and express needs appropriately. Only after the client establishes sobriety can the possibility of taking on new roles become a reality. Determining new strategies for socializing is not the priority goal for an addicted client. Usually, these clients need to change unhealthy socializing habits. Clients with alcohol use disorder do not tend to be preoccupied with physical health problems.
CN: Safe, effective care environment; CNS: Management of care; CL: Apply

34. 4. Methadone is used to prevent withdrawal symptoms in clients who are dependent on opiate drugs and are enrolled in treatment programs to stop taking or continue not taking the drugs without causing the "high" associated with the drug addiction. The major hazards of methadone are respiratory depression and, to a lesser degree, systemic hypotension. Respiratory arrest, shock, cardiac arrest, and death have occurred. The most frequently observed adverse reactions include light-headedness, dizziness, sedation, nausea, vomiting, and sweating. Numerous drug interactions exist for methadone. Stating that the provider believes methadone to be the best course of action is not the best nursing response because it provides no information to the client. While methadone is prescribed for severe chronic pain, that is not the advantage for the client with opioid use disorder.
CN: Physiological integrity; CNS: Pharmacological and parenteral therapies; CL: Apply

35. 2. Helping the client avoid drinking triggers will best support the client's goal of sobriety. Addiction is a relapsing illness. Knowledge of this realization is appropriate but is not directed at promoting sobriety. The client may well need financial support, but helping to meet this need has only minimal impact on assure future sobriety. A client with a history of alcohol use disorder cannot consume alcohol in moderation.
CN: Psychosocial integrity; CNS: None; CL: Apply

36. The nurse is assessing a client to rule out poly-substance use. Which finding does the nurse find **most** indicative?
1. The absence of acute signs and symptoms of drug toxicity
2. Appointments with five different health care providers last week
3. The presence of agitation and impaired judgment
4. The client admittedly expresses denial of drug addiction

37. Which client statement(s) will the nurse consider when determining positive responses to the CAGE Questionnaire screening tool? Select all that apply.
1. "I feel bad for my children when I get drunk and yell at them."
2. "It makes me really angry when my family nags me about my drinking."
3. "I usually handle my hangovers by starting the day with a shot of whiskey."
4. "I know I drink too much but I never seem to be able to cut back on alcohol."
5. "I find myself looking forward to spending the weekends drinking with friends."

38. The nurse suspects a client is using cocaine. Which client statement supports the nurse's concern?
1. "I think the dangers of cocaine are overdramatized."
2. "Alcohol is more problematic that snoring a little cocaine."
3. "Several of my friends use cocaine and they are just fine."
4. "Using cocaine just gives you energy and a sense of power."

39. A seizure-prone client receives alprazolam to manage alcohol withdrawal. Which client statement demonstrates understanding of the risks associated with alprazolam?
1. "Alprazolam can make me really depressed."
2. "I could gain weight while taking alprazolam."
3. "I can have seizures if I stop taking alprazolam."
4. "Alprazolam may cause me to develop a rash."

40. The nurse assessing a client prescribed paroxetine will place **priority** on asking which question(s)? Select all that apply.
1. "Have you developed any problems sleeping?"
2. "Are you having any symptoms of depression?"
3. "Do you have any concerns with sexual performance?"
4. "Has your energy level decreased since starting paroxetine?"
5. "Have you experienced any auditory or visual hallucinations?"

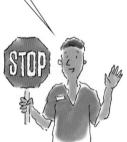

Remember that "select all that apply" questions can have one correct answer, a few correct answers, or even all of the answers correct.

36. 2. Clients with polysubstance use often see many different health care providers to obtain various prescriptions. Symptoms of toxicity do not necessary confirm consistent use of multiple drugs. Impaired judgment and agitation can be a result of a variety of causes. Denial of an addition is not a reliable indicator.
CN: Psychosocial integrity; CNS: None; CL: Apply

37. 1, 2, 3, 4. The CAGE Questionnaire asks questions concerning cutting down on drinking, being annoyed by criticisms related to personal drinking, feeling guilty about drinking, and drinking to manage hangovers. The questionnaire does not address pleasure related to drinking.
CN: Psychosocial integrity; CNS: None; CL: Apply

38. 4. Cocaine use is associated with both elevated energy and mood. This statement infers the client knows this from personal experience with the drug. The remaining statements relate to perceptions regarding cocaine use but not necessarily personal experience.
CN: Psychosocial integrity; CNS: None; CL: Analyze

39. 3. Alprazolam is an anxiolytic that depresses the central nervous system (CNS) to suppress seizure activity. Abrupt withdrawal from the medication can cause seizures. The other statements are associated with the selective serotonin reuptake inhibitor (SSRI) fluoxetine.
CN: Physiological integrity; CNS: Pharmacological and parenteral therapies; CL: Apply

40. 3, 5. The antidepressant paroxetine can increase or cause psychosis and sexual dysfunctions. None of the other questions are associated with adverse effects of paroxetine.
CN: Physiological integrity; CNS: Pharmacological and parenteral therapies; CL: Apply

41. The parent of an adolescent who smokes marijuana asks the nurse if the use of marijuana can be addicting. Which nursing response is **best**?
   1. "The use of marijuana is a stage many adolescents go through."
   2. "The use of marijuana can lead to psychological dependence."
   3. "Many people use marijuana and do not use other street drugs."
   4. "It is difficult to answer that question, as I do not know your child."

42. Which laboratory test will the nurse anticipate being ordered for a client with a history of opioid use who is exhibiting behavior changes?
   1. Antibody testing
   2. Glucose monitoring
   3. Hepatic levels
   4. Urine toxicology

43. Which assessment question will the nurse ask to assist in identifying a significant risk for injury for a client prescribed methadone?
   1. "Have you ever been prescribed methadone before?"
   2. "Do you have trouble swallowing pills?"
   3. "Do you have a history of asthma?"
   4. "Are you going to take your medication as prescribed?"

44. The registered nurse (RN) and an assistive personnel (AP) are caring for a client admitted for cocaine detoxification. The RN will appropriately delegate which task to the AP?
   1. Giving the client a lunch tray
   2. Monitoring the client's anxiety
   3. Giving the client bromocriptine
   4. Determining the client's readiness for therapy

45. Which client will the nurse refer to Al-Anon for treatment?
   1. A wife affected by her husband's alcohol use disorder
   2. A client demonstrating clinical depression
   3. A client dealing with the personal effects of alcohol use disorder
   4. A son trying to cope with his mother's opioid use

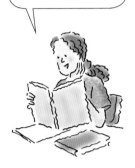

Do you remember which body system opioids are most likely to affect?

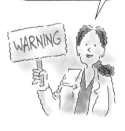

Clients recovering from substance use disorder are at risk for experiencing depression.

41. 2. Marijuana can cause psychological dependence. There is controversy over whether physiologic dependency to marijuana can occur and whether it is a "gateway" drug leading to the use of more potent drugs. Marijuana use is not part of a developmental stage that adolescents go through. It is not important that the nurse know the child to address this question.
CN: Psychosocial integrity; CNS: None; CL: Apply

42. 4. A urine toxicology screen would show the presence of an opioid in the body. Antibody, glucose, or hepatic screening would not show the presence of opioids in the body.
CN: Psychosocial integrity; CNS: None; CL: Apply

43. 3. Methadone may cause serious or life-threatening breathing problems, especially during the first 24 to 72 hours of treatment and any time the dose is increased. A history of respiratory problems such as asthma would increase the risk for injury. While assessing for a previous history of methadone use is appropriate, it is not directly associated with a significant risk for injury. Difficulty swallowing and proper usage, although risk factors, are not as significant as a history of respiratory problems.
CN: Physiological integrity; CNS: Reduction of risk potential; CL: Apply

44. 1. It is appropriate for the RN to delegate meal tray distribution to the AP, which is an unchanging procedure. The AP cannot assess or administer medications. The RN needs to assess the client to determine if the client is capable to attend therapy.
CN: Psychosocial integrity; CNS: None; CL: Apply

45. 1. Al-Anon offers hope and recovery to all people affected by the alcohol use of a loved one or friend, whether the person of concern is still drinking or not. Alcoholic Anonymous or Cocaine Anonymous are better suited to meet the needs of the recovering individual. Dual Recovery Anonymous is focused on those individuals with diagnoses that include both a chemical dependency and an emotional or psychiatric illness.
CN: Safe, effective care environment; CNS: Management of care; CL: Apply

CN: Client needs category   CNS: Client needs subcategory   CL: Cognitive level

46. The nurse will monitor for which short-term adverse effect(s) in a client with a heroin use disorder? Select all that apply.
1. Chills
2. Agitation
3. Disorientation
4. Nausea and vomiting
5. Heart rate 43 beats/minute

46. 3, 4, 5. The common short-term adverse effects that may occur with heroin use include nausea, vomiting, disorientation, and bradycardia. Agitation and chills are not short-term characteristics of heroin use.
CN: Psychosocial integrity; CNS: None; CL: Apply

47. The nurse is planning care for clients known to be abusing oxycodone. Which nursing intervention(s) will the nurse include for the management of overdose? Select all that apply.
1. Naloxone
2. Portable oxygen
3. Intubation tray
4. Intravenous fluids
5. Portable electrocardiogram (EKG) machine

47. 1, 2, 3, 4, 5. Naloxone is an opioid antagonist, meaning that it binds to opioid receptors and can reverse and block the effects of other opioids. It can very quickly restore normal respiration to a person whose breathing has slowed. The remaining options are all used to either support the client's respiratory function and to assess, monitor, and stabilize the cardiovascular system.
CN: Physiological integrity; CNS: Physiological adaptation; CL: Apply

48. Which statement made by a client who is a known substance user suggests to the nurse the presence of long-term opioid use disorder?
1. "I feel like I sleep all the time."
2. "I seem to be hungry all the time"
3. "It seems like I am always constipated."
4. "I have had this rash on my legs for weeks."

48. 3. People who use opioids long term may develop chronic constipation and insomnia. Neither a rash nor hunger is associated with opioid use disorder.
CN: Physiological integrity; CNS: Pharmacological and parenteral therapies; CL: Apply

49. A family member of a client with cocaine use disorder for several years asks the nurse, "Why can't my aunt just quit using cocaine?" Which nursing response is appropriate?
1. "Repetitive cocaine use leads to an impaired ability to resist dangerous urges."
2. "Cognitive abilities are altered significantly when someone uses cocaine for a long time."
3. "Memories are lost with cocaine use, making it tough for your aunt to remember the good times in her life."
4. "Your aunt's ability to think critically has been severely diminished by the effects of cocaine."

49. 1. Cocaine use, especially repetitive use, can alter systems associated with pleasure, memory, and decision making but when someone is addicted, the ability to resist urges becomes impaired, making it harder to quit. This inability to manage urges is the primary factor affecting the cessation of cocaine use. References to cognitive abilities, memory loss, and critical thinking do not adequately explain why cocaine use is difficult to stop.
CN: Psychosocial integrity; CNS: None; CL: Apply

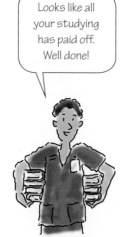

Looks like all your studying has paid off. Well done!

50. A nurse is caring for a client being treated for cocaine use disorder. Which nursing intervention(s) is pertinent? Select all that apply.
1. Measure temperature.
2. Assess apical heart sounds.
3. Monitor urine output.
4. Inspect skin for jaundice.
5. Monitor for seizure activity.

50. 1, 2, 4, 5. Cocaine use disorder increases the risk for weakened immune system, heart arrhythmia, seizures, and hepatitis. While such an addiction is a strain on all body systems, the effect on the renal system would be indirect.
CN: Physiological integrity; CNS: Physiological adaptation; CL: Analyze

51. Which question will the nurse ask a client to **best** determine a client's risk for an alcohol use disorder?
1. "Do you have a family history of alcohol use?"
2. "When did you have your first alcoholic drink?"
3. "What is your preferred type of alcohol?"
4. "How much alcohol do you drink each day?"

51. 4. The most relevant assessment question regarding alcohol use disorders would be one directed at the amount of alcohol the client regularly consumes. While there appears to be a pattern of alcohol use among some families, such a history does not focus on the individual being assessed. The remaining statements are too general.
CN: Psychosocial integrity; CNS: None; CL: Apply

CN: Client needs category   CNS: Client needs subcategory   CL: Cognitive level

52. The family of a client who is recovering from heroin use disorder asks the nurse why the client is receiving naltrexone. Which nursing response is correct?
1. "It is used to block the effects or 'high' produced by heroin."
2. "It is used to keep the client sedated during withdrawal."
3. "It takes the place of methadone during detoxification."
4. "It is given to decrease the client's memory of withdrawal."

52. 1. Naltrexone is an opioid antagonist that is used to help maintain sobriety by blocking and reversing the effects of opioids. Keeping the client sedated during withdrawal is not the reason for giving this drug. The drug is not used in place of methadone during detoxification and does not decrease the client's memory of the withdrawal experience.
CN: Physiological integrity; CNS: Reduction of risk potential; CL: Apply

53. Which nursing intervention is an important component for a client in a treatment program for cocaine use disorder?
1. Facilitating the client's finding ways to be happy and competent
2. Fostering the creative use of self in community activities
3. Educating the client about handling stresses in the work setting
4. Helping the client acknowledge the current level of dependency

53. 1. The major component of a treatment program for a client with cocaine use disorder is to help the client discover ways to feel happy and competent without using the drug. Because clients typically credit cocaine for their achievements, helping them discover ways of achieving happiness and success without the drug are paramount. Fostering the creative use of self in community activities may encourage cocaine use because the client has not yet discovered drug-free ways of engaging in challenging activities. Educating the client about handling stress at work is appropriate but is not the major component of treatment. Helping the client acknowledge the current level of dependency is not a major treatment component because the client must first work on remaining drug-free.
CN: Psychosocial integrity; CNS: None; CL: Apply

54. To which client(s) will the nurse anticipate administering clonidine? Select all that apply.
1. A 59-year-old diagnosed with hypertension
2. A 42-year-old being treated for acute depression
3. A 37-year-old demonstrating signs of opioid withdrawal
4. A 26-year-old diagnosed with an eating disorder that involves purging
5. A 16-year-old demonstrating severe signs of antisocial personality disorder

54. 1, 3. Clonidine works by blocking chemicals in the brain that trigger sympathetic nervous system activity. Clonidine belongs to a class of medicines known as antihypertensives. It is frequently prescribed to help with the symptoms of opioid withdrawal. Clonidine is not effective in the treatment of acute depression, eating, or antisocial personality disorders.
CN: Physiological integrity; CNS: Pharmacological and parenteral therapies; CL: Analyze

55. The nurse is assessing a client with a history of cocaine use by various forms. Which statement by the client indicates the existence of a common complication?
1. "I am so tired and I need a nap several times a day."
2. "I have gained 10 lb (4.5 kg) within the past 2 months."
3. "My ears feel 'full' and I feel a lot of pressure behind them."
4. "I have had a nose bleed and this whistling noise when I breathe."

55. 4. The client who snorts cocaine commonly develops a perforated nasal septum. Cocaine use results in insomnia and weight loss as a result of the cocaine's stimulant effects. Ear problems are not generally triggered by injecting, ingesting, snorting, or smoking cocaine.
CN: Physiological integrity; CNS: Physiological adaptation; CL: Apply

56. Which statement **most** concerns the nurse regarding alcohol use by a 20-year-old client?
1. "I drank so much on prom night I cannot remember getting home."
2. "I go out drinking with my friends and coworkers most weekends."
3. "I have been drinking since I was 15 years old."
4. "I am too young to worry about how my drinking is affecting my health."

57. A family expresses concern that a relative who stopped using amphetamines 3 months ago is demonstrating paranoid behavior. What question will the nurse ask to **best** address the family's concerns?
1. "What is most concerning about your family member's behavior?"
2. "Can you give me some examples of the behaviors that concern you?"
3. "Has your family member always been a bit suspicious of others?"
4. "Can we talk about your general feelings concerning your family member?"

58. Which assessment question is **priority** for the nurse to address when caring for a client with a history of alcohol use disorder?
1. "Do you ever feel guilty about your drinking?"
2. "Do people criticize or nag you about your drinking?"
3. "Do you ever drive while or after you have been drinking?"
4. "Have you ever felt you should cut down on the amount you drink?"

59. A client returns to the psychiatric unit after returning from a 6-hour leave. The nurse observes that the client is agitated and is ataxic with nystagmus and general muscle hypertonicity. The nurse suspects the client used which drug while away from the unit?
1. Phencyclidine (PCP)
2. Crack cocaine
3. Opioid
4. Marijuana

60. The nurse has developed a therapeutic relationship with a client who has an addiction problem. Which information indicates the nurse-client interaction is in the working stage? Select all that apply.
1. The client addresses how addiction has contributed to family distress.
2. The client reluctantly shares a family history of addiction.
3. The client verbalizes difficulty identifying personal strengths.
4. The client discusses financial problems related to the addiction.
5. The client expresses uncertainty about meeting with the nurse.
6. The client acknowledges the addiction's effects on the children.

CN: Client needs category   CNS: Client needs subcategory   CL: Cognitive level

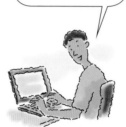

Stuck on a question? Try to eliminate as many incorrect answer choices as you can before answering.

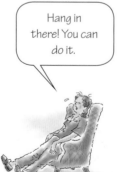

Hang in there! You can do it.

56. 1. Blackouts are a serious event, regardless of the age of the drinker. Although the other statements present issues that are problematic regarding the client's habits and attitudes related to alcohol consumption, blacking out demonstrates a possible symptom of alcohol use disorder.
CN: Psychosocial integrity; CNS: None; CL: Apply

57. 2. The conversation concerning the family's concerns should begin with a definition of what the family considers paranoid behavior. Although the remaining questions cover appropriate topics, they will not effectively address the issue of whether the client is truly demonstrating paranoid characteristics.
CN: Psychosocial integrity; CNS: None; CL: Analyze

58. 3. Addressing driving while under the influence is priority because this is a safety concern. All the remaining questions focus on the personal or individual impact of an alcohol use disorder.
CN: Psychosocial integrity; CNS: None; CL: Apply

59. 1. The client's behavior suggests the use of PCP. Crack cocaine intoxication is characterized by euphoria, grandiosity, aggressiveness, paranoia, and depression. Opioid use is characterized by euphoria, followed by sleepiness. Marijuana intoxication is characterized by a panic state and visual hallucinations.
CN: Psychosocial integrity; CNS: None; CL: Apply

60. 1, 4, 6. Addressing how the addiction has contributed to family distress, discussing financial problems related to addiction, and acknowledging the addiction's effects on the children are examples of the nurse-client working phase of an interaction. In the working phase, the client explores, evaluates, and determines solutions to identified problems. Reluctant sharing of family addiction history, difficulty identifying personal strengths, and expressing uncertainty about meeting with the nurse are examples of what happens during the *introductory* phase of the nurse-client interaction.
CN: Psychosocial integrity; CNS: None; CL: Apply

61. A client with a history of substance use is recovering from an appendectomy. The client is alert, ambulatory, and reporting pain. The nurse is planning to administer an analgesic medication to the client. List in ascending chronological order the steps the nurse will take to administer the oral analgesic. Use all the options.

1. Check two client identifiers with the medication administration record.

2. Stay with the client while the client takes the medication.

3. Document that the medication has been given.

4. Administer the medication.

5. Check the prescription with the medication administration record to see if it is time for the medication.

6. Place the correct medication and dose in a medication cup.

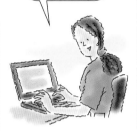

Bravo! You finished another chapter.

61. Ordered Response:

5. Check the prescription with the medication administration record to see if it is time for the medication.

6. Place the correct medication and dose in a medication cup.

1. Check two client identifiers with the medication administration record.

4. Administer the medication.

2. Stay with the client while the client takes the medication.

3. Document that the medication has been given.

The first step is to check the health care provider's prescription to ensure accuracy. The nurse should check for the appropriate time because this is a PRN prescription. Once the correct medication and dose are obtained and placed in a medication cup, the nurse would go to the client with the medication prescription and check the client's two identifiers. Medication is always administered after establishing the correct identity of the client. Because this client has a history of substance use, the nurse should remain with the client as he takes the medication; check the mouth to be sure it has been swallowed, and then document the medication administration on the medication sheet.

CN: Safe, effective care environment; CNS: Management of care; CL: Apply

Chapter 18

Dissociative Disorders

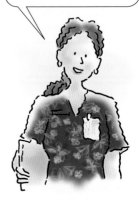

Caring for clients with dissociative disorders can be challenging and rewarding. Get ready . . . this chapter is a real out-of-body experience.

Dissociative disorders refresher

Depersonalization/Derealization disorder

Feelings of being detached or disconnected from one's own thoughts or body, often described as feeling as if a person is "outside of one's own body" or living in a dream; the person does not lose touch with reality

Key signs and symptoms
- Fear of "going insane"
- Impaired occupational functioning
- Impaired social functioning
- Persistent or recurring feelings of detachment from mind and body

Key test results
- Standard dissociative disorder tests demonstrate a high degree of dissociation. These tests include:
  - diagnostic drawing series
  - dissociative experience scale
  - dissociative interview schedule
  - structured clinical interview for dissociative disorders

Key treatments
- Benzodiazepines: alprazolam, lorazepam, clonazepam

Key interventions
- Encourage the client to recognize that depersonalization is a defense mechanism used to deal with anxiety and trauma.
- Assist the client in establishing supportive relationships.

Dissociative amnesia

An inability to remember important personal information, often resulting from a stressful or traumatic event

Key signs and symptoms
- Altered identity
- Low self-esteem

- No conscious recollection of a traumatic event, yet colors, sounds, sites, or odors of the event may trigger distress or depression
- Sudden onset of amnesia and inability to recall personal information

Key test results
- Standard dissociative disorder tests demonstrate a degree of dissociation. These tests include:
  - diagnostic drawing series
  - dissociative experience scale
  - dissociative interview schedule
  - structured clinical interview for dissociative disorders

Key treatments
- Individual therapy
- Benzodiazepines: alprazolam, lorazepam
- Selective serotonin reuptake inhibitors (SSRIs): paroxetine

Key interventions
- Encourage the client to verbalize feelings of distress.
- Encourage the client to recognize that memory loss is a defense mechanism used to deal with anxiety and trauma.

Dissociative identity disorder

Disturbance in a person's identity, with the development of two or more distinct personalities or identities, called "alters," that control the person's behavior at different times; formerly called multiple personality disorder

Key signs and symptoms
- Guilt and shame
- Lack of recall (beyond ordinary forgetfulness)
- Presence of two or more distinct identities or personality states

Key test results
- Standard dissociative disorder tests demonstrate a degree of dissociation. These tests include:

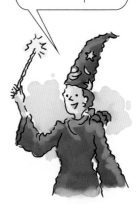

There are no magic cures for dissociative identity disorder, but benzodiazepines and psychotherapy can help.

- ○ diagnostic drawing series
- ○ dissociative experience scale
- ○ dissociative interview schedule
- ○ structured clinical interview for dissociative disorders
- EEG readings may vary markedly among the different identities

Key treatments

- Long-term reconstructive psychotherapy

- Benzodiazepines: alprazolam, lorazepam, clonazepam
- SSRIs: paroxetine
- Tricyclic antidepressants: imipramine, desipramine

Key interventions

- Assist the client in identifying each personality.
- Encourage the client to identify emotions that occur under duress.

thePoint® You can download tables of drug information to help you prepare for the NCLEX®! View Generic Drug Names, Drug Classifications, Drug Actions, and Nursing Implications for the drugs discussed in this refresher at **http://thePoint.lww.com.**

Dissociative disorders questions, answers, and rationales

1. The nurse is assessing a client with dissociative identity disorder (DID). Which statement will the nurse **most** likely hear from the client?
   1. "My mother was so busy she had little time for me."
   2. "I told myself I was not the one with the problem."
   3. "I thought everyone had parents who yelled at them a lot."
   4. "My father said he loved me but did not show it when we were alone."

Several answers to question #1 could be true, but you are looking for the one that is *most* likely.

2. The nurse is caring for a client diagnosed with depersonalization/derealization disorder. Which finding is **priority** for the nurse to address?
   1. Ritualistic behavior
   2. Out-of-body experiences
   3. History of sexual abuse
   4. Inability to give a personal history

3. The nurse caring for a client diagnosed with dissociative identity disorder (DID) will set which goal for the client?
   1. The client will be able to confront the abuser.
   2. The client will attend the unit's milieu meetings.
   3. The client will prevent alter personalities from emerging.
   4. The client will report less anger about childhood traumas.

1. **4.** Repeated exposure to a childhood environment that alternates between highly stressful and then loving and supportive can be a factor in the development of DID. Many children grow up in a dysfunctional household but do not develop DID. Clients with DID commonly have low self-esteem.
   CN: Psychosocial integrity; CNS: None; CL: Apply

2. **2.** Out-of-body experiences are commonly associated with depersonalization/derealization disorder and must be addressed as the priority for this client. Ritualistic behavior is seen with obsessive-compulsive disorders. DID is theorized to develop as a protective response to traumatic experiences such as sexual abuse. An inability to give a personal history would be more often associated with DID or dissociative amnesia.
   CN: Safe, effective care environment; CNS: Management of care; CL: Apply

3. **2.** The desired outcome would be that the client attends milieu meetings. Doing so decreases feelings of isolation and shows that the client has begun to trust the nurse. Typically, the abuser was a part of the client's childhood, and confrontation in adulthood may not be possible or therapeutic. The client with DID is commonly unaware of alter personalities and thus cannot prevent them from emerging. Clients with DID have dissociated from painful experiences, so the host personality usually does not have negative feelings about such experiences.
   CN: Psychosocial integrity; CNS: None; CL: Apply

4. The nurse is caring for a client diagnosed with dissociative identity disorder (DID) who is newly admitted to the psychiatric facility. Which potential complication of DID is **priority** for the nurse to monitor?
  1. Delusional ideations
  2. Possibility for self-harm
  3. Alternate identity
  4. Feelings of shame and guilt

5. The nurse is caring for a client diagnosed with dissociative identity disorder (DID). Which nursing intervention is **priority** for this client?
  1. Administering antipsychotic medications as prescribed
  2. Maintaining consistency when interacting with the client
  3. Confronting the client about having alter personalities
  4. Preventing the client from interaction with others on the unit

6. A nurse is caring for a client diagnosed with dissociative amnesia who is exhibiting signs of low self-esteem. The nurse determines the interventions have been successful when the client demonstrates which behavior?
  1. Participation in new activities
  2. Sleeping without interruption at night
  3. Consumes sufficient food to meet daily requirements
  4. Greater time spent interacting with the nurse

7. A nurse is caring for a client with a diagnosis of dissociative identity disorder (DID). Which client behavior will the nurse identify as a safety risk?
  1. The client is frequently unable to account for hours of time.
  2. The client writes a detailed plan on "making my pain go away."
  3. The client tells the nurse about having "never felt happier."
  4. The client reports hearing voices when alone.

8. A client is admitted with suspected dissociative identity disorder (DID). Which statement made by the client indicates an understanding of how diagnostic testing will help confirm the diagnosis?
  1. "A chronic infection can cause DID so blood work will help rule out such an infection."
  2. "I understand that a brain scan will tell if a congenital malformation is causing my alternates."
  3. "The CAGE screening tool will help determine if alcohol use triggered my symptoms."
  4. "Performing an electroencephalogram will show if I have alternate identities."

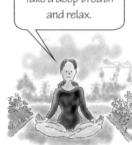

Feeling stressed? Take a deep breath and relax.

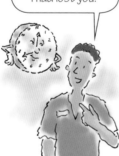

Oh—there you are! I thought I had lost you.

4. **2.** A common reason clients with DID are admitted to a psychiatric facility is because one of the alternate personalities is trying to kill another personality, thus the risk for self-harm. Delusions and hallucinations are commonly associated with schizophrenia. The presence of alternate identities and feelings of shame and guilt are expected in DID.
CN: Safe, effective care environment; CNS: Management of care; CL: Apply

5. **2.** Using consistency to establish trust and support is important when interacting with a client with DID. Most of these clients have had few healthy relationships. Medication has not proven effective in the treatment of DID. Confronting the client about the alter personalities would be ineffective because the client has little, if any, knowledge of the presence of these other personalities. Isolating the client would not be therapeutic.
CN: Safe, effective care environment; CNS: Management of care; CL: Apply

6. **1.** Interventions for persons with dissociative amnesia and low self-esteem would be demonstrated by participation in new activities. There is not an issue related to either sleep or nutrition. Spending more time with the nurse would be inappropriate. The client needs to participate in new activities with others.
CN: Psychosocial integrity; CNS: None; CL: Apply

7. **2.** The nurse needs to initiate safety precautions to prevent self-harm. The sensation of lost periods of time is not a safety issue. Being glad to be in the unit indicates a feeling of security. The client with DID hearing voices does not indicate a psychotic episode.
CN: Safe, effective care environment; CNS: Safety and infection control; CL: Apply

8. **4.** DID is characterized by the presence of two or more distinct personality identities, often referred to as alternate identities. An EEG may show marked differences in brain activities among the different identities. CAGE is a screening tool directed at diagnosis of alcohol use disorder; it is not associated with the triggering of DID symptoms. DID is usually a reaction to trauma that helps a person to avoid bad memories. It is not related to an infection or congenital anomaly.
CN: Psychosocial integrity; CNS: None; CL: Apply

CN: Client needs category   CNS: Client needs subcategory   CL: Cognitive level

9. The nurse is assessing a client suspected to have dissociative identity disorder (DID). Which client statement indicates to the nurse the client does have DID?
1. "I have a close relationship with my mother."
2. "I never did well in my classes in school."
3. "I cannot recall certain events or experiences."
4. "I can perform a skill or task consistently."

9. 3. Clients with DID commonly experience bouts of amnesia when alter personalities are in control. Clients with DID have learned in childhood how to live in two separate worlds: one in the daytime, in which they are able to perform well in school and have friendships, and one at nighttime, when the abuse occurs. The alter personalities may vary in the ability and type of skills and tasks performed. A close relationship with a parent is unlikely because of probable abuse in childhood.
CN: Psychosocial integrity; CNS: None; CL: Apply

10. A hospitalized client diagnosed with dissociative identity disorder (DID) tells the nurse about "hearing my alters arguing, again." Which nursing intervention is **priority** for the client?
1. Determine how many voices are heard.
2. Request haloperidol for the client.
3. Notify the client's health care provider.
4. Play a game of checkers with the client.

10. 4. Because many clients diagnosed with DID hear voices, it is appropriate to acknowledge the voices and then attempt to distract the client from focusing on them. Determining how many voices the client is hearing is not priority and does not help the situation. The health care provider would not be notified because the client's statement reflects an expected finding of DID. An antipsychotic medication such as haloperidol would not be prescribed for the client diagnosed with DID.
CN: Safe, effective care environment; CNS: Management of care; CL: Apply

11. A client diagnosed with dissociative identity disorder (DID) reports hearing voices and asks the nurse if, "that means I am crazy." Which nursing response is **most** therapeutic?
1. "Can you tell me what the voices tell you?"
2. "Sometimes people with DID report hearing voices."
3. "Do not say that. Why would you think you are crazy?"
4. "Hearing voices is typically a symptom of schizophrenia."

11. 2. The most therapeutic response is to give the client the correct information, that people with DID sometimes hear voices. Asking what the voices tell the client would be changing the topic without answering the question. Asking "why" questions can put the client on the defensive. Schizophrenia is not the only cause of hearing voices, and this response suggests the client may have schizophrenia.
CN: Psychosocial integrity; CNS: None; CL: Apply

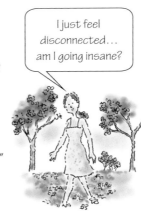

I just feel disconnected... am I going insane?

12. A client is diagnosed with depersonalization/derealization disorder. Which statement(s) made by the client confirms this diagnosis to the nurse? Select all that apply.
1. "I really feel as though I am going crazy."
2. "It is like I am outside my body looking down on it."
3. "Everything around me seems to be so real."
4. "I know what is real, but I feel disconnected."
5. "I do not remember ever being in a fire."

12. 1, 2, 4. Clients with depersonalization/derealization disorder exhibit feelings of being detached or disconnected from their body or thoughts. They often report feeling like they are going crazy or looking down on their body from the outside. Clients with this disorder often report feeling like everything around them is unreal and experience a disconnectedness, but they are in touch with reality. The inability to remember a traumatic event is most likely to occur with dissociative amnesia.
CN: Psychosocial integrity; CNS: None; CL: Apply

13. Which medication(s) will the nurse expect the health care provider to prescribe for a client diagnosed with depersonalization/derealization? Select all that apply.
1. Alprazolam
2. Lorazepam
3. Clonazepam
4. Paroxetine
5. Imipramine

13. 1, 2, 3. Depersonalization/derealization disorder may be treated with benzodiazepines such as alprazolam, lorazepam, or clonazepam. Paroxetine may be prescribed for dissociative amnesia or dissociative identity disorder. Imipramine may be prescribed to treat dissociative identity disorder.
CN: Physiological integrity; CNS: Pharmacological and parenteral therapies; CL: Understand

14. A client diagnosed with dissociative identity disorder (DID) requires hospitalization. Which intervention will the nurse **most** likely include in caring for this client?
1. Arrange to have staff check on the client every 15 to 30 minutes.
2. Place the client in a quiet room away from the nurses' station.
3. Do not allow visitation from family members or friends for 72 hours.
4. Ensure the staff knows the client will be placed on seizure precautions.

14. 1. A common reason for hospitalization in clients with DID is suicidal ideations or gestures. For the client's safety, frequent checks should be done. Family interactions might be therapeutic for the client, and the family may be able to provide a more thorough history because of the client's dissociation from traumatic events. Seizure activity is not an expected symptom of DID. Because of the possibility of suicide, the client's room should be close to the nurses' station.
CN: Safe, effective care environment; CNS: Safety and infection control; CL: Apply

15. A client, being treated at a community mental health clinic, is suspected to have depersonalization disorder. Which client statement will the nurse report to the health care provider as indicative of this diagnosis?
1. "I have a fear that I am crazy and will not get better."
2. "I have been told I was raped, but I do not remember it."
3. "I really do not think I am worth much to anybody."
4. "I believe I can change personalities at any time."

15. 1. The fear of going insane is commonly expressed among clients diagnosed with depersonalization disorder. Dissociative amnesia is characterized with the inability to remember details, especially traumatic ones. Low self-esteem is noted in many mental health disorders. Displaying characteristics of several personalities is associated with dissociative identity disorder.
CN: Psychosocial integrity; CNS: None; CL: Apply

16. The nurse is interacting with a hospitalized client diagnosed with a dissociative identity disorder (DID). Which statement does the nurse expect the client to make?
1. "Hello there, my name is Suzanne. Do I know you?"
2. "I cannot remember the accident so why talk about it?"
3. "We have talked about defense mechanisms before; I am bored."
4. "I do not like being here; I want to leave and go home."

> Working with a client with dissociative identity disorder is like working a puzzle. It's hard to figure out how all the pieces fit together.

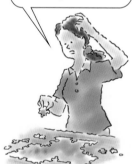

16. 1. DID involves the existence of alternate personalities; this statement appears to be made by such an "alter." A lack of memory of a traumatic event is associated with dissociative amnesia. Not wanting education and wanting to leave are common feelings among hospitalized clients.
CN: Psychosocial integrity; CNS: None; CL: Analyze

17. The spouse of a client reports the client often disappears for days at a time, not showing up for work, and then returning with no memory of anything unusual occurring. Which scenario(s) will the nurse suspect? Select all that apply.
1. The client is experiencing sleep terror disorder.
2. The client is taking a hallucinogenic medication.
3. The client is experiencing dissociative fugue.
4. The client has a severe dissociative identity disorder.
5. The client has a neurologic disorder.

17. 3, 4. Dissociative fugue is a type of dissociative identity disorder (DID) characterized by sudden, unexpected travel away from home, with the inability to recall what took place during this time frame. DIDs are considered severe, chronic identity disorders. Sleep terror disorder involves recurrent episodes in which the client awakens abruptly from sleep and experiences feelings of panic. Use of hallucinogenic drugs is unlikely, because drugs would not explain the inability to recover lengthy periods of lost time such as this client experiences. A serious neurologic disorder is possible, but not likely because there are no other physiologic symptoms and the predominant report from the spouse is more characteristic of a severe dissociative disorder.
CN: Psychosocial integrity; CNS: None; CL: Analyze

18. The nurse provides education to a client diagnosed with dissociative identity disorder (DID). The nurse determines the client understands the need to continue therapy when the client makes which statement?
 1. "Participating in therapy will help eliminate my family problems."
 2. "Therapy will help me integrate all my alter personalities into one."
 3. "I must continue going to outpatient treatment for the next 2 months."
 4. "Once therapy is complete, I will not have traits of my alter personalities."

18. 2. The main goal of therapy of clients with DID is to integrate the alter personalities. Complete elimination of personalities may not be possible. Therapy is usually long term. Through therapy, the client can learn how to cope with family problems.
CN: Psychosocial integrity; CNS: None; CL: Analyze

19. A client with depersonalization/derealization disorder asks the nurse, "Why have I not been offered hypnotic therapy?" Which nursing response is **most** appropriate?
 1. "Where did you learn that hypnosis could help your condition?"
 2. "Unfortunately, hypnosis rarely is effective for your condition."
 3. "Hypnosis is prescribed when traditional therapies fail."
 4. "Hypnosis has not proven to be effective, but let us talk about medication therapy."

19. 4. Depersonalization/derealization disorder is typically not treated with hypnosis. The mainstay of treatment usually includes medication therapy that includes a benzodiazepine or an antidepressant if either condition exists. The first response could place the client on the defensive. Hypnosis is used in a variety of psychiatric conditions; however, it is not used with depersonalization/derealization disorder.
CN: Psychosocial integrity; CNS: None; CL: Apply

20. When caring for a client diagnosed with dissociative identity disorder (DID), which nursing intervention is appropriate?
 1. Establish an empathic relationship with each emerging personality.
 2. Remind the alter personalities that they are part of the host personality.
 3. Limit contact with the client to when the host personality is in control.
 4. Give positive support to the client when calm alter personalities are present.

Working with clients' alter personalities can go a long way toward soothing their symptoms.

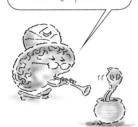

20. 1. Establishing an empathic relationship with each emerging personality, including those that may seem unpleasant, provides a therapeutic environment in which to care for the client. This is a priority intervention. As time goes on, it may be appropriate to remind the alter personalities that they are part of the host. Interacting with the client only when the host personality is in control is inappropriate because the client has limited, if any, control or awareness when alter personalities are in control.
CN: Psychosocial integrity; CNS: None; CL: Apply

21. Which information noted in the client's medical record suggests to the nurse an adverse effect of imipramine?
 1. The client is reporting a dull headache.
 2. After falling, the client stated, "I got really dizzy."
 3. The client refused lunch due to "feeling nauseated."
 4. The client has an oral temperature of 101°F (38.8°C).

21. 4. Imipramine is a tricyclic antidepressant (TCA) and can trigger leukopenia that results in an increased risk for infection. Benzodiazepines like alprazolam can trigger ataxia. The TCA desipramine is associated with nausea and headache.
CN: Physiological integrity; CNS: Pharmacological and parenteral therapies; CL: Apply

22. The nurse is caring for a client diagnosed with dissociative identity disorder (DID). Which behavior reported by a family member indicates to the nurse the client's therapy is effective?
 1. The client is asking for frequent orientation cues.
 2. The client is sleeping through the night.
 3. The client is eating meals with the family.
 4. The client can recognize when voices are heard.

22. 2. Because clients with DID often have sleep disorders, sleeping through the night is a sign of effective therapy. Forgetfulness, difficulty forming relationships, and hallucinations are signs of unsuccessful treatment. None of the remaining statements indicate effective treatment.
CN: Psychosocial integrity; CNS: None; CL: Apply

CN: Client needs category   CNS: Client needs subcategory   CL: Cognitive level

23. While the nurse is interacting with a client diagnosed with dissociative identity disorder (DID), an alter takes control. The client suddenly becomes angry and shouts, "I am so mad because no one ever listens to me." Which nursing response is **most** appropriate in managing this situation?

1. "I need to know who I am talking to."
2. "Please do not shout, I am listening to you."
3. "Please tell me about what is making you so angry."
4. "I cannot help you if you are not able to talk calmly."

24. The nurse knows which client is demonstrating findings associated with dissociative fugue?

1. A 30-year-old with a history of family-inflicted physical and sexual abuse that lasted 20 years.
2. A 45-year-old found a great distance from the nearest town who cannot remember name.
3. A 50-year-old who displays four different personalities of differing ages and genders.
4. A 60-year-old who often says, "I am going insane" and "I feel like I am separated from my body."

25. The nurse interrupts a client attempting to commit suicide. Which nursing action is **priority**?

1. Seclude the client with visual checks every 15 minutes.
2. Dedicate a staff member to remain with the client.
3. Require the client stay with the group at all times.
4. Transfer the client to a semi-private room.

26. The nurse provides discharge education for a client diagnosed with dissociative identity disorder (DID). Which statement by the client indicates to the nurse teaching was successful?

1. "I need to continue psychotherapy for a long time."
2. "I need to confront my abuser before I can get well."
3. "I am going to name my alter egos Carson and Alejandro."
4. "It is important to take my prescribed antipsychotic drugs."

27. Which client will the nurse assess **first** for a possible diagnosis of dissociative amnesia?

1. A chronic alcoholic experiencing blackouts
2. An immigrant from Syria seeking asylum
3. A skier who experienced a severe concussion
4. A client diagnosed with Lewy body dementia

23. 3. Asking the client how he or she is feeling now encourages integration and discourages dissociation. When interacting with clients with DID, the nurse always wants to remind the client that the alter personalities are a component of one person. Responses reinforcing interaction with only one alter personality instead of trying to interact with the individual as a single person are not appropriate. Asking "why" questions can put the client on the defensive and impede further communication. Focusing on the client's angry display will be a barrier to further communication.
CN: Psychosocial integrity; CNS: None; CL: Apply

24. 2. Dissociative fugue is one or more episodes of amnesia in which an individual cannot recall some or all of the past. Either the loss of one's identity or the formation of a new identity may occur with sudden, unexpected, purposeful travel away from home. Long-term abuse is often a trigger for depersonalization disorder; that condition does not include amnesia but is often characterized as "going insane" and feeling outside one's body. Dissociative identity disorder is associated with alternate personalities.
CN: Psychosocial integrity; CNS: None; CL: Apply

25. 2. Implementing a one-to-one staff-to-client ratio is the nurse's highest priority because it provides constant visual supervision of the client. Doing so allows the client to maintain self-esteem and remain safe. Seclusion could damage the client's self-esteem and is not close enough supervision. Forcing the client to stay with the group and refusing to let the client stay in a private room will not guarantee safety.
CN: Safe, effective care environment; CNS: Safety and infection control; CL: Apply

26. 1. Clients with DID need long-term psychotherapy to improve and maintain their mental health. The client with DID has repressed the abuse and would be unable to confront the abuser. The client naming subpersonalities is nontherapeutic. Antipsychotic drugs are not prescribed for DID.
CN: Psychosocial integrity; CNS: None; CL: Apply

27. 2. Dissociative amnesia typically occurs after the person has experienced a significantly stressful, traumatic situation, such as a living in a war zone. Alcoholism, concussion, and Lewy body dementia all share physiological not psychological causes.
CN: Psychosocial integrity; CNS: None; CL: Analyze

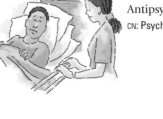

Before discharging clients, make sure they have an accurate understanding of the course of treatment they face.

28. After educating a client on alprazolam, the nurse determines the teaching was successful when the client states to avoid which substance(s)? Select all that apply.

1. Alcohol
2. Nicotine
3. Grapefruit juice
4. St. John's wort
5. Root vegetables
6. Dairy products

28. **1, 2, 3, 4.** Alprazolam can interact with alcohol, causing additive effects on the central nervous system. Nicotine may decrease the effectiveness of alprazolam and should be discouraged. Grapefruit juice may increase alprazolam levels whereas St. John's wort may decrease drug levels. Alprazolam does not interact with root vegetables or dairy products.

CN: Physiological integrity; CNS: Pharmacological and parenteral therapies; CL: Apply

29. A client diagnosed with dissociative identity disorder (DID) is admitted to an inpatient psychiatric unit. The nurse manager meets with the nurses caring for the client. Which education is **priority** for the nurse manager to provide the nurses?

1. Review the facility's restraint protocol with the nurses.
2. Tell the nurses no one can refuse to care for the client.
3. Warn the staff this client may be difficult to care for.
4. Allow nurses to discuss concerns about caring for this client.

29. **4.** Allowing all staff members to meet may prevent them from splitting into groups of those who believe the diagnosis is valid and those who do not. Unless this client shows behaviors harmful to self or others, restraints are not needed. Telling the staff that no one should refuse to work with the client or that this client will probably be difficult sets a negative tone for the staff as they develop a plan of care for the client and implement it.

CN: Safe, effective care environment; CNS: Management of care; CL: Apply

30. The nurse is caring for a client diagnosed with depersonalization disorder. Which nursing intervention is **priority**?

1. Assist the client in identifying individuals to include in his or her support system.
2. Help the client to use defense mechanisms to manage the triggering trauma.
3. Provide the client with the opportunity to explore his or her individual personality.
4. Encourage the client to be adherent to the planned treatment modality.

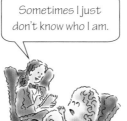

Sometimes I just don't know who I am.

30. **1.** Depersonalization disorder contributes to an individual's sense of isolation and detachment from reality. Having an effective support system is vital to the management of this disorder. The disorder is based on the ineffective reliance of defense mechanisms. While understanding one's personality is positive, in this case it does not have priority. Being adherent to treatment is also important in the management of any disorder.

CN: Psychosocial integrity; CNS: None; CL: Apply

31. A client is awake and sitting quietly in a chair but does not respond to verbal or tactile stimuli. There are repeated episodes of staring into the distance, seemingly oblivious to events or persons in the immediate vicinity. When the client emerges from these episodes, life continues as usual. Which nursing consideration(s) are accurate based on assessment findings? Select all that apply.

1. The client has entered a state of self-induced hypnosis.
2. The client is involved in ritual activity leading to a trancelike state.
3. The client is demonstrating signs of a dissociative trance disorder.
4. The client is currently in a state of factitious disease.
5. The client is demonstrating psychotic behavior and decompensation.
6. The client has no control over personal behaviors.

31. **3, 6.** The client is demonstrating typical signs of a dissociative trance that is not consciously induced. There is no basis to assume the client is in a state of self-induced hypnosis or has any involvement in ritual activities that would account for this behavioral state. There is no evidence to suggest that factitious disease is a reasonable explanation. The client, though not responsive, does come out of the trances and demonstrates normal behavior, so psychosis with decompensation can be ruled out.

CN: Psychosocial integrity; CNS: None; CL: Analyze

CN: Client needs category   CNS: Client needs subcategory   CL: Cognitive level

32. The nurse is providing care to a client who just experienced an episode of dissociative fugue. Which nursing statement demonstrates the **priority** focus for nursing care of this client?
1. "It must be troubling to not remember anything about the time you were missing."
2. "Please tell me what that experience was like for both you and your family."
3. "It is very important for your safety that you do not disappear like that again."
4. "It seems to me that you have deep-seated problems that we need to discuss."

33. Which statement made by a client's mother will the nurse flag as a possible trigger for the client's dissociative identity disorder (DID)?
1. "My son has an extensive history of food and environment-related allergies."
2. "It is very hard for my son to find a good job in the small town we live in."
3. "We have two distant relatives who have been diagnosed with mental illnesses."
4. "A family friend sexually abused my son when he was a young child."

34. A client is experiencing recurrent episodes of dissociative fugue. Which client statement indicates to the nurse an ability to reduce these recurrent episodes?
1. "I can promise you that I will not run away again."
2. "I meditate daily, especially when I am stressed."
3. "I really enjoy attending my support group sessions."
4. "It will be hard, but I will try to confront my fears."

35. Which nursing intervention is **priority** for the nurse caring for a client with a dissociative disorder?
1. Encourage the client to participate in unit activities and meetings.
2. Question the client about the events triggering the dissociative disorder.
3. Allow the client to remain in the room when experiencing feelings of dissociation.
4. Encourage the client to form friendships with other clients in therapy groups.

Decreasing a sense of isolation is a key goal for clients with dissociative disorders.

32. 1. An episode of dissociative fugue can be a frightening experience; discussing fears will help establish a plan for coping with them. The client rarely remembers the events during the fugue episode and asking the client to recall them can increase anxiety. Promising not to disappear again has little effect because a dissociative fugue episode is not something the client consciously wants. Discussing the cause of the behavior is not initially the focus of care.
CN: Psychosocial integrity; CNS: None; CL: Apply

33. 4. The best description of the cause of a dissociative disorder is that the brain tries to protect the person from severe stress. This stress is most dangerous when experienced during childhood. There is no known association between allergies and DID. Neither a family history of mental illness nor being of a low socioeconomic level is considered a risk factor for DID.
CN: Psychosocial integrity; CNS: None; CL: Apply

34. 2. Dissociative fugue is precipitated by stressful situations. Helping the client identify coping resources could prevent recurrences. When the dissociative fugue episode is over, the client returns to normal functioning; the client would not be an elopement risk. While support groups can be helpful, stress management is most important in preventing recurrent fugue events. Clients commonly have amnesia about the events during the dissociative fugue episode; therefore, asking them to share or remember their experiences or confronting them about running away from their problems can increase their anxiety.
CN: Psychosocial integrity; CNS: None; CL: Apply

35. 1. Individuals with certain dissociative disorders feel detached from their environment and can experience impaired social functioning. Attending unit activities and meetings helps decrease the client's sense of isolation. Often, the client cannot recall the events that triggered the dissociative disorder, so the client would need to be isolated from others only if the client could not interact appropriately. A client with a dissociative disorder has typically had few healthy relationships. Forming friendships with others in therapy could result in the client establishing unhealthy relationships.
CN: Safe, effective care environment; CNS: Management of care; CL: Apply

36. A client is admitted with suspected depersonalization disorder. Which information from the client's admission interview indicates to the nurse support for this diagnosis?
1. Describes personal life as existing in a dream
2. Has no memory of recently being physically assaulted and robbed
3. Was found 100 miles (160 kilometers) away from home with no memory of the trip
4. Frequently presents with a female alternative identity named Susan

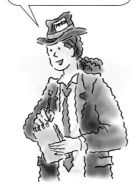

Word on the street is that you are dominating this test. Care to comment?

36. 1. The primary symptom of depersonalization disorder is a distorted perception of the body. The person might feel like he or she is a robot or in a dream. Dissociative amnesia commonly occurs after a person has experienced a traumatic event. Dissociative fugue is one or more episodes of amnesia in which either the loss of one's identity or the formation of a new identity may occur with sudden, unexpected, purposeful travel away from home. Dissociative identity disorder is the coexistence of two or more personalities within the same individual.
CN: Psychosocial integrity; CNS: None; CL: Apply

37. The nurse is caring for a client who was in an automobile accident in which a 3-year-old boy was killed. The client is now experiencing dissociative amnesia. The nurse determines the client demonstrates understanding of treatment if which client statement is made?
1. "I will not be driving an automobile again for at least one year."
2. "I will attend hypnotic therapy sessions my health care provider prescribed."
3. "I plan to take my lorazepam whenever I feel upset about this situation."
4. "I will visit the child's grave as soon as I am released from the hospital."

37. 2. Hypnosis can be beneficial to this client because it allows repressed feelings and memories to surface. Visiting the child's grave upon release from the hospital may be too traumatic and could encourage continuation of the amnesia. The client needs to learn coping mechanisms other than taking a highly addictive drug such as lorazepam. The client may be ready to drive again, and circumstances may dictate the client drives again before one year has passed.
CN: Psychosocial integrity; CNS: None; CL: Apply

38. A nurse is discussing the teaching plan with a client diagnosed with dissociative identity disorder (DID). Which statement by the client indicates to the nurse the education has been effective?
1. "I will probably never be able to regain my memories of the fire."
2. "I have problems with my memory due to abusing tranquilizers."
3. "If I concentrate hard enough, I can regain memories of the car accident."
4. "My brain has temporarily hidden my memories of the rape to protect me."

38. 4. One of the cardinal features of DID is that the person has loss of memory of a traumatic event. With this disorder, the loss of memory is a protective function performed by the brain and is not within the person's conscious control. With therapy and time, the person will probably be able to recall the traumatic event. This type of amnesia is not related to substance use.
CN: Psychosocial integrity; CNS: None; CL: Apply

39. A client diagnosed with dissociative disorder has threatened to commit suicide. When assessing the client, which set of circumstances will the nurse identify as indicating the **highest** risk of suicide?
1. Suicide plan, the ability to carry out the plan, and history of previous attempt
2. Preoccupation with morbid thoughts, history of depression, and limited support system
3. Suicidal ideation, active suicide planning, and a family history of suicide
4. Threats of suicide, recently experiencing the loss of a job, and an intact support system

39. 1. A lethal plan with a handy means of carrying it out along with a previous attempt poses the highest risk and requires immediate intervention. Although all the remaining risk factors can lead to suicide, they are not considered as high a risk as a formulated, lethal plan and the means at hand. However, a client exhibiting any of these risk factors should be taken seriously and considered at risk for suicide.
CN: Safe, effective care environment; CNS: Management of care; CL: Apply

40. A client diagnosed with dissociative amnesia says, "You must think it is really odd that I have no recollection of the accident." Which nursing response is **most** appropriate?
1. "Why would I think it is odd for you to have no memory?"
2. "It is very likely that your memories will return one day."
3. "You will be fine soon. Do not worry about your memory loss."
4. "The brain sometimes protects us by repressing traumatic events."

41. Which statement leads the nurse to suspect a client is experiencing a depersonalization/derealization disorder?
1. "I need you to tell me what day it is and where I am."
2. "I feel like I am watching a movie of my life."
3. "Why can't I remember how and why I ended up here?"
4. "Everything about my life is so messed up; I am really scared."

42. The nurse is caring for a client diagnosed with depersonalization/derealization disorder who is prescribed clonazepam. Which comorbid condition will the nurse expect to improve because of this medication therapy?
1. Chronic depression with a history of suicide attempts
2. Seizure disorder with a history of panic attacks
3. Alcohol use disorder with a history of allergic asthma
4. Bulimia and a history of migraine headaches

43. Based on the provided information, the nurse will monitor which client(s) diagnosed with depression for dissociative identity disorder (DID)? Select all that apply.
1. The client denying any history of alcohol or illicit drug use
2. The client frequently unable to remember home address and telephone number
3. The client stating, "I do not want to talk about my childhood; it was painful."
4. The client stating, "I single-handedly saved the poor children in my neighborhood."
5. The client whose sleep is often disrupted by dreams of "going insane"

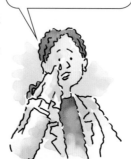

Being depressed without any memory of traumatic events could be a sign of dissociative identity disorder.

40. 4. The nurse's response that the brain sometimes does not let humans remember traumatic events as a means of protection provides a simple explanation for the client. The use of "why" questions can make the client become defensive. Telling the client he or she will be fine soon or that his or her memories will return gives false reassurance.

CN: Psychosocial integrity; CNS: None; CL: Apply

41. 2. In depersonalization/derealization disorder, the client feels detached from the client's body and mental processes. The client is usually oriented to time, place, and person. Unexpected and sudden travel to another location is one of the characteristics of dissociative fugue. Feelings of depression and despair are common but are secondary to the feelings of detachment.

CN: Psychosocial integrity; CNS: None; CL: Apply

42. 2. Clonazepam is an antianxiety medication in the benzodiazepine family that acts by enhancing the effects of gamma-aminobutyric acid (GABA) in the brain. GABA is a neurotransmitter that inhibits brain activity. Clonazepam is primarily used for treating panic disorder and preventing certain types of seizures. None of the other medical conditions would benefit from clonazepam's effect on GABA and the brain.

CN: Physiological integrity; CNS: Pharmacological and parenteral therapies; CL: Analyze

43. 2, 5. A dissociative disorder is a persistent state of being disconnected from the totality of one's personhood, particularly painful emotions. With dissociative disorder, the inability to recall personal information is far more extensive than ordinary forgetfulness. Posttraumatic symptoms, such as flashbacks, nightmares, and an exaggerated startle response, are also signs and symptoms of DID. The symptoms occur apart from any chemical inducement, and the individual does not have the ability to consciously separate from painful emotions or topics. A sense of grandiosity is not a characteristic of this disorder.

CN: Psychosocial integrity; CNS: None; CL: Analyze

44. A client has a diagnosis of depersonalization/derealization disorder. The nurse will expect the client to demonstrate which behavior resulting from the condition's associated perceptual impairment?
1. Requires frequent re-orientation to time and place
2. Is prone to falling because of impaired balance
3. Frequently makes verbal threats to both staff and other clients
4. Spends most to the day sitting on the dayroom sofa in a dreamlike state

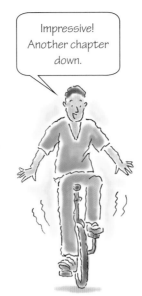

Impressive! Another chapter down.

44. 4. Depersonalization/derealization disorder can result in an altered perception. This impairment can be demonstrated by spending time in a dreamlike state. A neurological or cardiac disorder is more likely the cause of impaired balance. Memory impairment is more of a problem with other dissociative disorders, such as dissociative identity disorder and dissociative amnesia. While aggressive behavior can be a result of various physiological and psychological disorders, it is not generally associated with depersonalization/derealization disorder.

CN: Safe, effective care environment; CNS: Safety and infection control; CL: Apply

Chapter 19

Sexual Dysfunctions & Gender Dysphoria

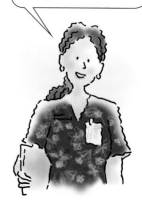

This chapter will test your knowledge of disorders of a highly sensitive nature. You'll do great. Good luck!

Sexual dysfunctions & gender dysphoria refresher

Gender dysphoria

Conflict between a person's physical gender and the gender he or she identifies with

Key signs and symptoms
- Dreams of cross-gender identification
- Finding one's own genitals "disgusting"
- Persistent distress about sexual orientation
- Preoccupation with appearance
- Self-hatred

Key test results
- Psychological testing may reveal cross-gender identification or behavior patterns

Key treatments
- Group and individual psychotherapy
- Hormonal therapy
- Gender reassignment surgery

Key interventions
- Assess with PLISSIT clinical tool.
- Demonstrate a nonjudgmental attitude.
- Help the client to identify positive aspects of self.

Paraphilic disorders

Sexual arousal and satisfaction that depend on engaging in, and fantasizing about, sexual behaviors that are uncharacteristic and risky

Key signs and symptoms
- Development of a hobby or change in occupation that makes the paraphilia more accessible
- Recurrent paraphilic fantasies
- Social isolation
- Troubled social or sexual relationships

Key treatments
- Individual therapy
- Medication therapy: leuprolide

Key interventions
- Demonstrate a nonjudgmental attitude.
- Institute safety precautions as needed according to facility protocol.
- Initiate a discussion about how emotional needs for self-esteem, respect, love, and intimacy influence sexual expression.
- Encourage the client to identify feelings (such as pleasure, reduced anxiety, increased control, and shame) associated with sexual behavior and fantasies.

Sexual dysfunction

Any physical or psychological problem that prevents the client or partner from getting sexual satisfaction

Key signs and symptoms
Female sexual interest/arousal disorder and genito-pelvic pain/penetration disorder
- Anxiety
- Decreased sexual desire
- Delayed or absent orgasm
- Depression
- Pain with sexual intercourse

Male sexual dysfunction
- Anxiety
- Inability to maintain an erection
- Premature ejaculation

Key test results
Female sexual interest/arousal disorder and genito-pelvic pain/penetration disorder
- Diagnostic tests are used to rule out a physiologic cause for the dysfunction.

Male sexual dysfunction
- Diagnostic tests are used to rule out a physiologic cause for the dysfunction.

Key treatments
Female sexual interest/arousal disorder and genito-pelvic pain/penetration disorder
- Individual therapy

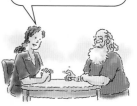

A nonjudgmental attitude is essential when discussing sensitive issues with clients.

Male sexual dysfunction
- Individual therapy
- Hormone replacement therapy; testosterone
- Sildenafil, tadalafil, vardenafil for impotence

Key interventions

Female sexual interest/arousal disorder and genito-pelvic pain/penetration disorder
- Take assessment with PLISSIT clinical tool.
- Encourage client to discuss feelings and perceptions about sexual function.

- Offer client suggestions about alternative ways of expressing her affection.
- Encourage client to seek evaluation and therapy from a qualified professional.

Male sexual dysfunction
- Take assessment with PLISSIT clinical tool.
- Encourage client to discuss feelings and perceptions about his sexual dysfunction.
- Teach client and his partner alternative ways of expressing their affection.
- Encourage client to seek evaluation and therapy from a qualified professional.

the **Point**® You can download tables of drug information to help you prepare for the NCLEX®! View Generic Drug Names, Drug Classifications, Drug Actions, and Nursing Implications for the drugs discussed in this refresher at **http://thePoint.lww.com**

Sexual dysfunctions & gender dysphoria questions, answers, and rationales

1. A 65-year-old male client underwent surgery for repair of an abdominal aortic aneurysm and now seeks information regarding the resulting impotence. Which nursing response is **best**?
1. "This must be very difficult for you to talk about."
2. "Your age is likely contributing to your impotence."
3. "Tell me about the sexual problem you are experiencing."
4. "There are different approaches to managing this problem."

2. Which statement made by the nurse is **most** effective in initiating a conversation concerning a client's history of paraphilic disorder?
1. "Let us discuss your primary sexual fantasies."
2. "I bet it is really hard for you to discuss your sexual health."
3. "I cannot image how hard it is to deal with such feelings."
4. "What do you think is the cause of this inappropriate behavior."

3. The nurse will question an initial prescription for vardenafil 10 mg once daily as needed if written for which client(s)? Select all that apply.
1. A 17-year-old diagnosed with erectile dysfunction
2. A 66-year-old male with a history psoriasis
3. A 48-year-old diagnosed with Peyronie's disease
4. A 51-year-old being treated with an alpha blocker
5. A 32-year-old who is deaf in the left ear

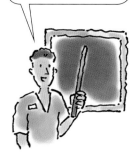

Don't forget to cover sexual function considerations during discharge, when needed.

1. **3.** Erectile dysfunction and retrograde ejaculation are sexual dysfunctions commonly experienced after abdominal aortic aneurysm repair. The initial step in discussing the client's concern should begin with identifying the existing dysfunction and then discussing how the client feels about the problem. The nurse should approach the discussion in a matter-of-fact manner. Age may be a contributing factor but that is not the initial concern. Managing the problem will be approached after the problem is thoroughly identified.
CN: Psychosocial integrity; CNS: None; CL: Apply

2. **1.** Paraphilia involves sexual arousal and satisfaction that depend on engaging in, and fantasizing about, sexual behaviors that are uncharacteristic and risky. The discussion initiated in a matter-of-fact, nonjudgmental manner is most appropriate. The other statements inappropriately include the nurse's emotional response to the disorder.
CN: Psychosocial integrity; CNS: None; CL: Apply

3. **1, 2, 4.** Vardenafil relaxes muscles of the blood vessels and increases blood flow to particular areas of the body. Vardenafil is given to treat impotence but is not approved for men younger than 18 years old. Clients over the age of 65 or those with a history of alpha blocker therapy should be prescribed vardenafil 5 mg daily as needed. A history of Peyronie's disease would not require a decreased initial dose of the medication but rather consideration for possible painful erection. A sudden loss of hearing would possibly be associated with a serious effect of vardenafil therapy; a chronic hearing loss is not an acknowledged reason for a decrease in initial dosing.
CN: Physiological integrity; CNS: Pharmacological and parenteral therapies; CL: Analyze

4. During an assessment, the nurse learns the client is taking tadalafil. It is **priority** for the nurse to monitor this client for which complication?
1. Hypotension
2. Nausea
3. Back pain
4. Pyrosis

5. A female client diagnosed with chronic obstructive pulmonary disease (COPD) tells the nurse, "I no longer have enough energy to make love to my spouse." Which nursing intervention is **most** appropriate?
1. Refer the couple to a sex therapist.
2. Suggest ways to conserve energy.
3. Refer the client to a gynecologist.
4. Have the client discuss it with her spouse.

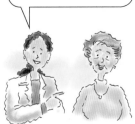

Be open and honest when discussing sexual dysfunction with your client—just as you would with any other condition.

6. A client with an ileostomy asks the nurse, "Will I still be able to have an erection?" The nurse will address the client's concern with which response?
1. "Unfortunately, it is unlikely you will regain sexual function."
2. "The results of the x-rays you have had will help determine if function will return."
3. "You should ask your health care provider to explain long-term outcomes."
4. "Impotence is rarely associated with postsurgical outcomes of an ileostomy."

7. The nurse is caring for a female client reporting vaginal pain during coitus. Which nursing statement is **most** appropriate?
1. "Are you taking an antidepressant medication?"
2. "Do you want to have vaginal intercourse?"
3. "When was your last pelvic examination?"
4. "Have you ever given birth vaginally?"

8. A 60-year-old client is taking antihypertensive medication and tells the nurse he cannot have sexual intercourse with his spouse anymore. Which potential cause will the nurse discuss with this client?
1. Advancing age
2. Blood pressure
3. Anxiety level
4. Medications

9. The nurse will consider which client finding a likely trigger for chronic depression and substance use disorders?
1. Experienced childhood sexual abuse
2. Manages anxiety through ritual behavior
3. Expresses delusional thinking
4. Describes having frequent periods of manic behavior

4. 1. When a client is receiving tadalafil, the nurse should monitor the client's blood pressure carefully because of the risk of hypotension. All other complications are common adverse reactions that are not priority.
CN: Physiological integrity; CNS: Pharmacological and parenteral therapies; CL: Apply

5. 2. Sexual dysfunction in clients with COPD is the direct result of dyspnea and reduced energy levels. Measures to reduce physical exertion, enhance oxygenation, and accommodate decreased energy levels may aid sexual activity. If the problem persists, a consult with a sex therapist might be necessary. A gynecologic consult is not necessary. Discussing this with the client's spouse may not resolve the problem.
CN: Physiological integrity; CNS: Reduction of risk potential; CL: Apply

6. 4. Sexual dysfunction is uncommon after an ileostomy; psychological causes of impotence are more likely. An abdominal x-ray is not indicated for sexual dysfunction and would not provide useful information. It is inappropriate for the nurse to refer the client to the health care provider for such assurance as this is not within the scope of nursing.
CN: Psychosocial integrity; CNS: None; CL: Apply

7. 3. The nurse will begin with a thorough physical assessment that includes asking about the client's history. It is most appropriate for the nurse to determine if there is a known physical cause for the pain. The remaining questions suggest physical or psychological causes that would be explored after any physical cause was ruled out.
CN: Psychosocial integrity; CNS: None; CL: Analyze

8. 4. Antihypertensive medication can cause impotence in men. Blood pressure itself does not cause impotence, but its treatment does. Stress may cause erectile dysfunction, but there is no evidence that the client is under stress. Men are usually able to have an erection throughout their lives.
CN: Physiological integrity; CNS: Pharmacological and parenteral therapies; CL: Understand

9. 1. Childhood sexual abuse is closely linked to the development of depression and substance use disorders. Although it is possible, victims of childhood sexual abuse are not predisposed to developing bipolar, narcissistic, or obsessive-compulsive disorders.
CN: Psychosocial integrity; CNS: None; CL: Apply

CN: Client needs category   CNS: Client needs subcategory   CL: Cognitive level

10. A 30-year-old client's medical record identifies that the client has a diagnosis of menorrhagia. Which client statement supports this diagnosis?
1. "I have a menstrual period every 2 weeks and it lasts for 7 days."
2. "My menstrual period just stopped about 1 year ago."
3. "I am in so much pain I cannot go to work when I am having my menstrual period."
4. "It is not unusual for me to have vaginal bleeding between menstrual periods."

11. The nurse is caring for a client who recently had female-to-male gender reassignment surgery. Which client statement indicates to the nurse a need for additional counseling?
1. "I have concerns about learning how to live successfully as a man."
2. "I know it is too late to have second thoughts now that I had the surgery."
3. "I am not sure how I will react when I see my new penis for the first time."
4. "I am concerned about how my parents will react to having a son instead of a daughter."

12. A client must undergo a hysterectomy for uterine cancer. Which nursing action **best** meets the woman's needs?
1. Ask her if she is having pain.
2. Refer her to a psychotherapist.
3. Do not discuss the subject with her.
4. Encourage her to verbalize her feelings.

13. A client with a history of atherosclerosis and depression was just diagnosed with erectile dysfunction. The client asks the nurse, "Did my poor health cause my erectile dysfunction?" Which nursing response is appropriate?
1. "It is likely your erectile dysfunction is caused by impaired blood flow to the penis because of atherosclerosis."
2. "I would say the presence of depression has led to the development of your erectile dysfunction."
3. "Erectile dysfunction is caused by rigid blood vessels in the penis, which is not related to your other health problems."
4. "Your erectile dysfunction has probably stemmed from impaired oxygenation caused by your atherosclerosis."

14. The nurse will monitor which client for an increased risk for sexual impotence?
1. A client with a family history of diabetes
2. A client who runs 25 miles a week
3. A client prescribed metoprolol
4. A client diagnosed with asthma

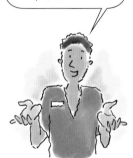

Caring for a client's psychological health following surgery can be just as important as caring for physical health.

10. 1. Menorrhagia is an excessive menstrual period. Amenorrhea is lack of menstruation. Dyspareunia is painful intercourse. Metrorrhagia is uterine bleeding from a cause other than menstruation.
CN: Physiological integrity; CNS: Reduction of risk potential; CL: Apply

11. 2. The nurse must observe for any indication that the client is experiencing doubts about the decision to proceed with the surgery. The client requires counseling to identify doubts and to work through the uncertainty. All the other statements demonstrate normal concerns about adjusting to the surgery.
CN: Psychosocial integrity; CNS: None; CL: Apply

12. 4. Encourage the client to verbalize her feelings because loss of reproductive organs may bring on feelings of loss related to body image and sexuality. Pain is a concern after surgery, but it has no bearing on body image. Referring the client to a psychotherapist may be premature; the client should be given time to work through her feelings. Avoiding the subject is not a therapeutic nursing intervention.
CN: Psychosocial integrity; CNS: None; CL: Apply

13. 1. Atherosclerosis causes the blood vessels to become clogged, thus diminishing blood flow required to bring about an erection. Arteriosclerosis results in a thickening and hardening of the blood vessels. While both depression and cognitive decline can result from the effects of atherosclerosis, neither is a direct factor in the development of erectile dysfunction.
CN: Physiological integrity; CNS: Physiological adaptation; CL: Apply

14. 3. Beta blockers like metoprolol can be the cause of impotence. A diagnosis of diabetes, not a family history, is also a possible factor in impotence. Neither asthma nor exercise is directly related to impotence.
CN: Psychosocial integrity; CNS: None; CL: Apply

15. A client scheduled for gender reassignment therapy asks the nurse, "What change(s) will the androgen therapy cause in my body?" Which change(s) will the nurse include in the response? Select all that apply.
  1. Shrinking of the laryngeal prominence
  2. Increased body hair distribution
  3. Increased muscle mass
  4. Increased fat deposits
  5. Deepening of the voice

16. A client tells the nurse, "I have never had an orgasm and my partner is upset that he cannot meet my needs." Which assessment question **best** demonstrates the nurse's ability to initially address the client's concern?
  1. "How do you feel about not experiencing orgasms?"
  2. "How long have you and your partner been together?"
  3. "What other problems do you and your partner have?"
  4. "Have you and your partner ever seen a counselor?"

17. A client is in the emergency department after being sexually assaulted by a stranger. Which nursing intervention is **priority**?
  1. Assist in identifying which behaviors placed the client at risk for the attack.
  2. Make the client a follow-up appointment at a sexual assault crisis center.
  3. Determine how the client was able to get away from the attacker.
  4. Assist in identifying family or friends who can provide immediate support.

18. A female client states she has had difficulty conceiving. Which statement made by the client does the nurse find **most** significant?
  1. "I have used oral contraceptives for approximately 2 years."
  2. "I had gonorrhea that went untreated for about 3 months."
  3. "I was diagnosed with iron deficiency anemia"
  4. "I was told I am borderline for developing osteoporosis."

19. Which statement by a male client leads the nurse to suspect the client is experiencing feelings associated with gender dysphoria?
  1. "I do not believe I have to identify with a particular gender."
  2. "I have a strong desire to live and be treated as a woman."
  3. "I preview sex with members of my own gender."
  4. "I believe I have a hormone imbalance."

15. 2, 3, 5. Androgen therapy involving testosterone would result in an increase in body hair and muscle mass, and deepening of the voice to more closely mimic male characteristics. Hormonal therapy for male-to-female gender reassignment involve estrogen and result in the remaining options.
CN: Physiological integrity; CNS: Pharmacological and parenteral therapies; CL: Apply

16. 1. Assessing the couple's perception of the problem will define it and assist the couple and the nurse in understanding it. Understanding the problem from the woman's perspective is the initial step to dealing with the couple's concerns. None of the other questions will provide insight into the feelings and values of the woman.
CN: Psychosocial integrity; CNS: None; CL: Apply

17. 4. The client who has been sexually assaulted by a stranger needs tremendous support to help get through this ordeal. Assisting the client in identifying behaviors that were risk factors for the attack places the blame on the client. A follow-up appointment is needed but is not priority. Determining how the client was able to get free is not priority.
CN: Psychosocial integrity; CNS: None; CL: Apply

18. 2. If left untreated, some sexual transmitted infections (STIs) can interfere with fertility. A history of taking oral contraceptives does not lead to infertility. Anemia does not lead to infertility; however, correcting this condition can increase fertility and help maintain a pregnancy. Osteoporosis is a condition in which bone loss occurs; the risk of developing osteoporosis increases after menopause.
CN: Health promotion and maintenance; CNS: None; CL: Apply

19. 2. A persistent, cross-gender identification and dissatisfaction with one's assigned gender are major characteristics of gender dysphoria. Gender fluid is the term used to identify a person who feels no fixed gender. Homosexuality is an attraction to members of the same sex. Hormone imbalances are not relevant to the diagnosis of gender dysphoria.
CN: Psychosocial integrity; CNS: None; CL: Apply

20. The nurse will question which prescription(s) for a client prescribed sildenafil? Select all that apply.
1. Nitroglycerin as needed
2. Erythromycin BID for 7 days
3. Multivitamin once daily
4. Atazanavir one tablet daily
5. Ketoconazole once daily

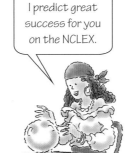

I predict great success for you on the NCLEX.

21. Which statement by a client diagnosed with paraphilia warrants additional monitoring by the nurse?
1. "I guess I will attend outpatient therapy."
2. "I will try to attend all therapy sessions."
3. "I will stay away from my old drinking buddies."
4. "I think taking leuprolide acetate will help."

22. A client is preparing for female-to-male gender reassignment surgery. The nurse will prepare to educate the client on which medication?
1. Estrogen
2. Sildenafil
3. Vardenafil
4. Testosterone

23. A client diagnosed with chronic ulcerative colitis has recently had a colostomy. The client tells the nurse, "I do not think I can ever have another sexual relationship." Which nursing intervention is **most** appropriate?
1. Offer to refer the client to a support group.
2. Encourage the client to express concerns.
3. Offer to research statistics on this topic.
4. Educate the client on the treatment regimen.

24. Which goal is **priority** for the nurse to set for a client diagnosed with pedophilia?
1. Attend and participate in all therapy meetings on the unit.
2. Learn personal triggers for pedophilic feelings to avoid sexual behaviors.
3. The client will inform the employer of the diagnosis and treatment.
4. Verbalize appropriate methods to meet sexual needs before discharge.

20. **1, 2, 4, 5.** Using sildenafil and nitroglycerin concurrently may cause hypotension; therefore, it is contraindicated to use nitrates. Macrolide antibiotics (erythromycin) and antiviral (atazanavir) and antifungal (ketoconazole) medications should be avoided while taking sildenafil. Sildenafil is not contraindicated with the use of multivitamins.
CN: Physiological integrity; CNS: Pharmacological and parenteral therapies; CL: Apply

21. **3.** Alcohol is not necessarily a factor in paraphilia relapse. A lack of insight into the problem may indicate a potential for relapse for this client. Attending all therapy sessions and outpatient therapy demonstrates compliance with the treatment. Leuprolide acetate is an antiandrogenic that lowers testosterone levels and decreases the libido.
CN: Psychosocial integrity; CNS: None; CL: Apply

22. **4.** Female-to-male gender reassignment will require testosterone therapy to stimulate tissue development associated with the male body. Estrogen would be required with male-to-female gender reassignment. Sildenafil and vardenafil are prescribed for erectile dysfunction.
CN: Physiological integrity; CNS: Pharmacological and parenteral therapies; CL: Understand

23. **2.** Encouraging the client to express concerns is a therapeutic first step. Referring to a support group is premature. Offering to research statistics or to explore positive aspects of treatment negates the emotional aspect of this problem, and the client might conclude that it is not acceptable to discuss feelings.
CN: Physiological integrity; CNS: Reduction of risk potential; CL: Apply

24. **4.** Upon discharge, the client should be able to verbalize an alternative, appropriate method to meet sexual needs, as well as effective strategies to prevent relapse. These alternatives must not involve sexual contact with an underage individual. It is not imperative that the client attend all meetings on the unit, but it is important that the client attend the required group sessions. A client with pedophilia should recognize triggers that initiate inappropriate sexual behavior and learn ways to direct impulses, but this is not priority at this time in treatment. The client determines what discussions about the disorder and treatment are appropriate.
CN: Psychosocial integrity; CNS: None; CL: Analyze

25. A client recently diagnosed with human papillomavirus (HPV) infection comes to the health clinic and is both anxious and tearful. Which nursing intervention is **most** appropriate?
  1. Engage the client and discuss the client's concerns.
  2. Educate the client on HPV symptoms and treatment.
  3. Refer the client to a specialized health care provider.
  4. Discuss the dangers of multiple sex partners.

25. 1. Encouraging the client to discuss concerns establishes a nonjudgmental, therapeutic relationship and would be the best initial response. Other interventions might be appropriate at some point. After a therapeutic relationship is established, the nurse should discuss the dangers of multiple sex partners in a nonjudgmental manner.
CN: Psychosocial integrity; CNS: None; CL: Apply

26. A client admitted for treatment of pedophilia tells the nurse, "I do not want to talk about my sexual behaviors." Which response from the nurse is **most** appropriate?
  1. "I need to ask you a few admission questions."
  2. "It is your right not to answer any of my questions."
  3. "Okay, I will just put 'no comment' for answers."
  4. "I know this process must be difficult for you."

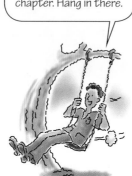

Hey—you're halfway through the chapter. Hang in there.

26. 4. Telling the client that talking about the condition must be difficult acknowledges the client's feelings and opens communication. Insisting that the form must be completed does not open communication or acknowledge the client's feelings. Clients have rights, but data collection is necessary so that help with the problem can be offered. Writing "no comment" alone would be inappropriate and not therapeutic.
CN: Psychosocial integrity; CNS: None; CL: Apply

27. While assessing a client admitted after being sexually assaulted, the nurse suspects the client is in denial of the event. The nurse's suspicion is based on which client behavior or statement?
  1. Appears relaxed and is calmly talking to a relative.
  2. Is crying loudly while pounding the wall.
  3. Repeatedly states, "I should not have gone alone."
  4. Is found rocking and softly crying.

27. 1. The client is demonstrating the defense mechanism of denial. Denial is the refusal to accept reality or fact, acting as if a painful event, thought, or feeling did not exist. Anger is demonstrated by crying and fist pounding. Self-blame occurs when one assumes responsibility for another's inappropriate behavior. Regression is a psychological defense mechanism in which a person abandons age-appropriate coping strategies in favor of earlier, more childlike patterns of behavior.
CN: Psychosocial integrity; CNS: None; CL: Apply

28. A client admitted with a diagnosis of pedophilia tells the roommate about the diagnosis. The roommate runs down the hall yelling to the nurse, "I do not want to be in here with a child molester!" Which response from the nurse is **most** appropriate?
  1. "You need to stop acting out right now."
  2. "Calm down and go back to your room."
  3. "Your roommate is not a child molester."
  4. "I see you are upset. Let us sit down and talk."

28. 4. Acknowledging the client is upset and sitting down and talking with the client allows the client to verbalize feelings. Telling the client to stop acting out is not a therapeutic response. It would not be therapeutic or safe to keep these clients together without intervention if one is agitated or anxious about the presence of the other. Stating that the client with pedophilia is not a child molester does not acknowledge the roommate's feelings.
CN: Psychosocial integrity; CNS: None; CL: Apply

29. A male client is suspected to have voyeurism. Which statement made by the client to the nurse supports this diagnosis?
  1. "I get aroused when I secretly watch others engage in sex."
  2. "I have always liked the feel of silky underwear."
  3. "The urge to rub up against a stranger is very hard to resist."
  4. "All my orgasms are associated with foot and shoe fantasies."

29. 1. Voyeurism is sexual arousal from secretly observing someone who is engaging in intimate behavior. Transvestic fetishism describes the enjoyment of cross-dressing (e.g., a male wearing female underwear). Rubbing against someone who is nonconsenting is referred to as frottage. Using objects for sexual arousal such as shoes or the human foot is an example of fetish.
CN: Psychosocial integrity; CNS: None; CL: Apply

CN: **Client needs category**   CNS: **Client needs subcategory**   CL: **Cognitive level**

30. A client being treated for infertility confides to the nurse about not telling the client's partner about a past sexually transmitted infection. What is the **most** therapeutic response for the nurse to give the client?
1. "What concerns do you have about sharing this information with your partner?"
2. "Do you think withholding this information is the basis for a trusting relationship?"
3. "Don't you think your partner deserves to know about your past health concerns?"
4. "I absolutely understand why you would want to keep this information private."

31. The nurse will monitor a client prescribed tadalafil for an adverse effect when the client makes what report?
1. "There is a red, itchy rash on my arms."
2. "My erections are always so painful."
3. "I have been having trouble with constipation."
4. "I have a history of benign prostatic hyperplasia."

32. A client diagnosed with a sexual arousal disorder asks the nurse if taking sildenafil is the only method to treat erectile dysfunction. What is the **best** response by the nurse?
1. "It is not the only treatment, but it is the best treatment for sexual arousal."
2. "Do you have some concerns about being prescribed sildenafil?"
3. "Group therapy has also been shown to be successful in many cases."
4. "Would you like to discuss treatment options with your health care provider?"

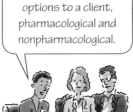

Remember to present all treatment options to a client, pharmacological and nonpharmacological.

33. A nurse is conducting a sexual awareness group for clients diagnosed with pedophilia. What is **priority** for the nurse to include in the education?
1. Socialization
2. Cognitive restructuring
3. Feeling of guilt
4. Punishment

34. Which client will the nurse assess **first** after receiving 0700 shift report?
1. A client with gender dysphoria prescribed testosterone at 0800
2. A client with genito-pelvic pain requesting help with bathing
3. A client taking vardenafil with a pulse rate of 75 beats/minute
4. A client with a paraphilic disorder waiting to be admitted

30. 1. Asking about the client's concerns over sharing the information encourages the client to verbalize the concerns in a safe environment and begin to choose a course of action for dealing with this issue. Telling the client that withholding information may cause distrust in a relationship or that the partner deserves to know conveys negative judgments. The nurse who supports withholding of information does not encourage discussion or problem solving.
CN: Psychosocial integrity; CNS: None; CL: Apply

31. 2. Tadalafil is prescribed for erectile dysfunction and may cause persistent and painful erections of the penis called priapism. Benign prostatic hyperplasia (BPH) is a cause of erectile dysfunction. Neither a red rash nor constipation is associated with the administration of tadalafil.
CN: Psychosocial integrity; CNS: None; CL: Understand

32. 3. Group therapy is a successful treatment to reduce the anxiety connected with erectile dysfunction. Sildenafil is not the only treatment option for erectile dysfunction. While discussing client concerns is appropriate, the client's question is not one of concern but rather information gathering. The nurse can and should address the question rather than suggesting a discussion with another health care provider.
CN: Psychosocial integrity; CNS: None; CL: Apply

33. 2. The nurse's focus is on education. The priority is to obtain an awareness of the sexual behaviors and the consequences. Cognitive restructuring is used to change the individual's maladaptive behaviors. Socialization is not a problem associated with pedophilia. Although feelings of guilt and punishment may be addressed in a group setting, neither is the primary focus of a sexual awareness group.
CN: Psychosocial integrity; CNS: None; CL: Apply

34. 4. The nurse will first assess the client waiting to be admitted so baseline information can be obtained and the level of care needed can be determined. Next, the nurse would administer the testosterone. A client with genito-pelvic pain should be able to bathe independently and needs encouragement. A pulse rate of 75 beats/minute is a normal finding, so medication administration is not impacted.
CN: Psychosocial integrity; CNS: None; CL: Analyze

CN: Client needs category   CNS: Client needs subcategory   CL: Cognitive level

35. A nurse is assessing a client admitted with a diagnosis of paraphilic disorder. Which intervention(s) **best** demonstrate the appropriate nursing care for this client? Select all that apply.
1. Provide care to the client with a nonjudgmental attitude.
2. Institute safety precautions as needed according to facility protocol.
3. Inform the client that behaviors like "that" will not be tolerated.
4. Encourage the client to identify feelings related to the diagnosis.
5. Initiate a contract with the client to no longer have inappropriate sexual feelings.

35. 1, 2, 4. The nurse should always maintain a nonjudgmental attitude when caring for any client. Safety precautions should be taken for the client as well as other clients. Informing a client that behaviors will not be tolerated is threatening behavior and the nurse should abstain from making this type of statement. Encouraging the client to identify feelings is a key factor in attempting a behavior change. It is unrealistic to expect a client to suppress feelings without therapeutic interventions.
CN: Psychosocial integrity; CNS: None; CL: Apply

36. A parent brings their 14-year-old son to the psychiatric crisis room and states, "He is always dressing in female clothing. There must be something wrong with him." Which response from the nurse is **most** appropriate?
1. "Cross-dressing is a fad many teens experiment with."
2. "I would like to schedule a meeting with your family."
3. "You seem to be upset. Would you like to talk?"
4. "How often does he dress in female clothing?"

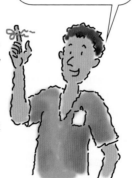

Remember— you're looking for the *most appropriate* response in question #36.

36. 3. Acknowledging the parent's feelings and offering an opportunity to verbalize concerns provides a forum for open communication. How often this behavior occurs is not the primary focus at this time. The remaining statements minimize the parent's concerns and thus are not appropriate.
CN: Psychosocial integrity; CNS: None; CL: Apply

37. A client is undergoing hormone therapy in preparation for future gender reassignment surgery. Which assessment question is **best** directed at identifying concerns?
1. "What do we need to discuss together today?"
2. "Have you noticed any physical changes yet?"
3. "Are you having any medication reactions?"
4. "Do you have any doubts about continuing therapy?"

37. 1. A client working toward gender reassignment surgery is likely to have feelings, perceptions, and concerns that need to be addressed. Providing the client with the opportunity to pick the topic will provide support in a positive, therapeutic manner. The other questions are close-ended, which will limit discussion and learned information.
CN: Psychosocial integrity; CNS: None; CL: Analyze

38. A client taking antidepressant medication reports a decreased sex drive, which is causing significant marital stress. Which response by the nurse is **most** appropriate?
1. "Do not stop taking your antidepressant medication."
2. "What are your thoughts on how you can handle this?"
3. "Does your spouse know the importance of your medication?"
4. "Have you discussed this with your health care provider?"

38. 2. Encouraging the client to verbalize thoughts will help to problem-solve. Telling the client not to stop taking the medication is too direct and does not encourage exploration on the part of the client. Asking the client if the spouse understands the importance of taking the medication conveys negative judgment. Asking if the client has discussed the issue with a health care provider might be appropriate, but it may also give the impression that the nurse does not want to discuss the problem with the client.
CN: Psychosocial integrity; CNS: None; CL: Apply

39. The nurse is developing an education plan on rape prevention. On which guideline will the nurse place **priority** during the education session?
1. Avoid drinking at a party.
2. Limit walking outside at night.
3. Learn methods of physical defense.
4. Take the shortest driving route home.

39. 3. Learning a self-defense method helps protect an individual in various situations. Drinking in moderation and not leaving a drink unattended are commonly included in teaching. Limiting walking outside at night may not be appropriate for the client. The shortest driving route might take an individual through a high-crime neighborhood; one should learn alternative routes to have options if safety seems compromised.
CN: Health promotion and maintenance; CNS: None; CL: Apply

CN: Client needs category   CNS: Client needs subcategory   CL: Cognitive level

40. The nurse is assessing a client with the potential diagnosis of male gender dysphoria. The nurse will monitor the client for which sign or symptom?
  1. The presence of impotence
  2. The presence of a micropenis
  3. Reluctance to engage in heterosexual intercourse
  4. Any symptom associated with schizophrenia

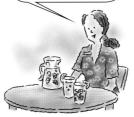

Sweet. You've already finished 40 questions.

40. 1. Diagnostic criteria for male gender dysphoria include a pervasive identification with femaleness and feelings of discomfort or inappropriateness with maleness. These feelings cause significant distress and disturbances in functioning such as impotence and are not simply a rejection of sex-role stereotypes. Gender dysphoria does not usually occur because of an intersex condition such as a micropenis and rarely occurs along with a diagnosis of schizophrenia.
CN: Psychosocial integrity; CNS: None; CL: Apply

41. A group of college students were walking back to their dorm at night when someone suddenly jumped out and exposed himself. One of the students was extremely upset and went to the clinic. Which response by the nurse is **most** appropriate?
  1. "I can see that you are upset about this."
  2. "Can you imagine a flasher on campus?"
  3. "I will call campus security right away."
  4. "Can you describe this person to me?"

41. 1. Acknowledging the client's emotions is the best initial step in helping the client talk about concerns. Making a comment about a flasher on campus is not therapeutic. Calling security and asking for the flasher's description are appropriate interventions but do not help the student deal with the emotional reaction.
CN: Psychosocial integrity; CNS: None; CL: Apply

42. Which statement made by an adolescent diagnosed with gender dysphoria indicates to the nurse the client's therapy was effective?
  1. "I can now better manage my tendency to focus on pornography."
  2. "I am looking into the possibility of gender reassignment surgery."
  3. "I am so happy that my friends and family understand me."
  4. "I just wish this was not such a huge problem for others."

42. 2. Conflict between a person's physical gender and the gender identified with is referred to as gender dysphoria. Preparing to have gender reassignment surgery demonstrates a goal of effective treatment of the condition. Pornography is not a factor in gender dysphoria. The remaining statements are general to most problems.
CN: Psychosocial integrity; CNS: None; CL: Apply

43. A male client who has been married for 10 years arrives at the psychiatric clinic stating, "I cannot live this lie anymore. I wish I were a woman. I do not want my wife. I need a man." Which nursing intervention is **most** appropriate?
  1. Call the primary health care provider.
  2. Encourage the client to speak to his wife.
  3. Refer the client to group therapy sessions.
  4. Have the client talk about his feelings.

43. 4. Sitting down with the client and exploring his feelings allows the nurse to assess him. The primary health care provider should not be notified until an assessment is made. The client should not speak to his wife until he has processed his feelings. Referring the client to group therapy does not address the issue in the current situation.
CN: Psychosocial integrity; CNS: None; CL: Apply

44. A client states little or no sexual desire and says this is causing great distress in his marriage. What further information is **most** useful to help the nurse assess the situation? Select all that apply.
  1. Existence of chronic prostate problems
  2. When the problem first appeared
  3. Current medications and dosages
  4. Report of recent bladder issues
  5. Any potential contributing factors

44. 2, 3, 5. In assessing this situation, it would be most useful to know when the problem first appeared and what contributed to it. These questions provide an opportunity to gather a great deal of useful information to better understand the client's current condition. Knowing the client's medications and dosages is very important because certain medications profoundly affect sexual desire. Neither chronic prostate problems nor recent bladder issues would affect sexual desire, though they could affect sexual performance.
CN: Psychosocial integrity; CNS: None; CL: Apply

45. A male client is receiving court-ordered treatment after being released from jail for actions indicating pedophilia. Which statement made by the client causes the nurse concern regarding a relapse?
1. "I am just so ashamed of how I behaved."
2. "I am determined not to go back to jail."
3. "I have got a good job that I can do from home."
4. "I am happy my old friends still like me."

46. A client's family is upset after learning the client was diagnosed with exhibitionism. The nurse informs the family about the current theories related to the cause of the paraphilia. Which statement indicates the nurse needs to provide additional education to the family?
1. "The person who does this must have abnormal levels of hormones."
2. "This behavior must result from not developing correctly."
3. "Maybe the person who has this behavior was sexually abused."
4. "Exposing oneself to others is caused by a sexual dysfunction."

47. The nurse uses the PLISSIT model to help clients with gender issues or sexual problems. Which statement or question is associated with the first step of the tool?
1. "Do you have a particular therapist you want to be referred to?"
2. "I want you to know there are several therapy options you can consider."
3. "What concerns do you have about your sexuality or behaviors?"
4. "Let us discuss what may be causing your concerns."

48. Which client statement indicates to the nurse the client is experiencing fetishism?
1. "The best sex is with 9-year-old girls."
2. "Sex is not exciting unless I am tied up."
3. "Watching an unsuspecting person masturbate is the best."
4. "I am only interested in having sex with life-sized dolls."

49. A homosexual client tells the nurse "my family is not supportive." What is the **best** nursing response?
1. "What do you mean by 'not supportive'?"
2. "When did you come out to them?"
3. "Tell me how your family treats you."
4. "Would you like to arrange for counseling?"

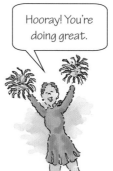

Hooray! You're doing great.

45. 3. Pedophilia is a disorder characterized by a strong sexual attraction to prepubescent children. Social isolation supports the behaviors; working from home would likely support such isolation. None of the other statements relate to supporting a relapse in a direct way.
CN: Psychosocial integrity; CNS: None; CL: Apply

46. 4. Sexual dysfunction is not thought to be a causative factor for paraphilia. The person with a sexual dysfunction has a disturbance in one or more phases of the sexual response cycle, and interventions assist the client to identify the stressors that interfere with the normal sexual response cycle. The other statements are accurate when discussing exhibitionism.
CN: Psychosocial integrity; CNS: None; CL: Apply

47. 4. The first step involves giving the client permission to initiate a discussion related to the sexually associated concerns. Step 2 relates to providing limited information about treatment options. Step 3 provides specific suggestions after an evaluation has been made, whereas Step 4 involves intensive therapy options.
CN: Psychosocial integrity; CNS: None; CL: Apply

48. 4. A client with fetishism uses sexually arousing objects as part of sexual activity. Sexual arousal by and preference for a prepubescent child are characteristic of pedophilia. Masochism is the recurrent urge or behavior of wanting to be humiliated, beaten, bound, or otherwise made to suffer. Voyeurism refers to viewing others, who are unaware they are being observed, in intimate situations.
CN: Psychosocial integrity; CNS: None; CL: Apply

49. 1. By asking the client to define "not supportive," the nurse is encouraging the client to talk about the difficulty and the feelings connected to the client's perception. Learning when the family became aware of the client's sexual preference is irrelevant to the client's stated concern. Asking the client to discuss how the family acts focuses the discussion on the family and does not give the client the opportunity to explore the meaning of not feeling supported by family. Asking a closed-ended question about counseling would focus on the client's perceptions before initiating a solution to the problem.
CN: Psychosocial integrity; CNS: None; CL: Apply

CN: Client needs category   CNS: Client needs subcategory   CL: Cognitive level

50. A client in the behavioral health unit with a history of noncoercive paraphilia is experiencing an auditory hallucination. What is the **priority** nursing action?

1. Remain with the client.
2. Call the health care provider.
3. Give the client medication.
4. Alert the staff on the unit.

51. A client confides to a nurse, "I have urges and desires to have sex with children." What is the **most** appropriate nursing action?

1. Ask the client, "Have you ever acted on these desires?"
2. Ask the client, "Are you able to control these thoughts?"
3. Explain that these thoughts are unacceptable and therapy is needed.
4. Inform child protective services about the situation.

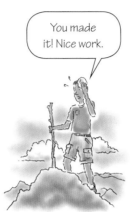

You made it! Nice work.

50. **1.** Staying with the client, listening, and offering methods of controlling the hallucinations will calm the client. This will be an effective action to keep the client and others safe. Calling the health care provider is not necessary at this time. The nurse can initiate interventions to assist the client to cope with the hallucinations. Giving the client medication may be useful, but the nurse should begin with the least restrictive interventions. Alerting the staff is not a priority.
CN: Psychosocial integrity; CNS: None; CL: Analyze

51. **1.** If a client reports a desire for pedophilia, then it is important to assess if the client ever acted upon these thoughts; the best predictor of future behaviors is past behaviors. Humans may have sexual fantasies, but it is their behavior by which they are judged. No human thoughts are unacceptable, but therapy is required if the client is dystonic. Informing child protective services is premature; the nurse has not obtained information whether the client has acted on these thoughts.
CN: Psychosocial integrity; CNS: None; CL: Apply

Chapter 20

Eating Disorders

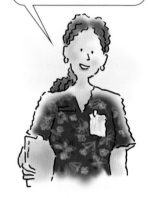

New information about eating disorders is released continuously. Start educating yourself by considering these questions carefully!

Eating disorders refresher

Anorexia nervosa

Obsession for thinness achieved by self-starvation

Key signs and symptoms
- Decreased blood volume, evidenced by lowered blood pressure and orthostatic hypotension
- Electrolyte imbalance, evidenced by muscle weakness, seizures, or dysrhythmias
- Low body weight for developmental stage
- Need to achieve and please others
- Obsessive rituals concerning food
- Refusal to eat
- Persistent behavior that interferes with weight gain

Key test results
- Eating Attitude Test suggests eating disorder.
- Electrocardiogram reveals nonspecific ST-segment changes and a prolonged PR interval.
- Laboratory tests show elevated blood urea nitrogen (BUN) level and electrolyte imbalances.
- Female clients exhibit low estrogen levels.
- Male clients exhibit low serum testosterone levels.

Key treatments
- Psychotherapy: individual, family-based, group
- Nutritional counseling
- Antianxiety agents: lorazepam, alprazolam
- Antidepressants: amitriptyline, imipramine
- Selective serotonin reuptake inhibitors (SSRIs): paroxetine, fluoxetine

Key interventions
- Contract for specific amount of food to be eaten at each meal.
- Provide one-on-one support before, during, and after meals.
- Prevent client from using the bathroom for 2 hours after eating.
- Help client identify coping mechanisms for dealing with anxiety.
- Weigh client once or twice a week at the same time of day using the same scale.
- Help client understand the cycle of anorexia.

Bulimia nervosa

Uncontrolled consumption of large amounts of food followed by compensatory behaviors to prevent weight gain

Key signs and symptoms
- Alternating episodes of binge eating and purging
- Constant preoccupation with food
- Disruptions in interpersonal relationships
- Eroded tooth enamel
- Extreme need for acceptance and approval
- Irregular menses
- Russell's sign (bruised knuckles due to induced vomiting)
- Sporadic, excessive exercise

Key test results
- Beck Depression Inventory may reveal depression.
- Eating Attitude Test suggests eating disorder.
- Metabolic acidosis may occur from diarrhea caused by enemas and excessive laxative use.
- Metabolic alkalosis may occur from frequent vomiting.

Key treatments
- Cognitive therapy to identify triggers for binge eating and purging
- SSRIs: paroxetine, fluoxetine

Key interventions
- Explain the purpose of a nutritional contract.
- Avoid power struggles about food.
- Prevent client from using the bathroom for 2 hours after eating.
- Provide one-on-one support before, during, and after meals.
- Weigh client once or twice per week at the same time of day using the same scale.
- Help client identify cause of the disorder.
- Point out cognitive distortions.

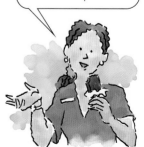

My relationship with food is complicated.

the**Point**® You can download tables of drug information to help you prepare for the NCLEX®! View Generic Drug Names, Drug Classifications, Drug Actions, and Nursing Implications for the drugs discussed in this refresher at **http://thePoint.lww.com**

Eating disorders questions, answers, and rationales

1. The nurse is caring for a client suspected of having an eating disorder. Which client comment indicates to the nurse the client does have such a disorder?

  1. "I do not have control over when or what I eat."
  2. "I have several friends who binge and purge."
  3. "I would really like to look good in my clothes."
  4. "I usually eat to make myself feel better."

2. A nurse is caring for an adolescent client. After reviewing the chart exhibit below, which condition does the nurse suspect?

Progress notes	
1/25	Received 15-year-old female admitted with
1015	diagnosis of bulimia nervosa. Vital signs: blood
	pressure, 100/70 mm Hg; heart rate,
	82 beats/minute; respiratory rate,
	20 breaths/minute; temperature, 98° F
	(36.7° C). Laboratory results: Na, 136 mEg/L
	(136 mmol/L); K, 3.0 mEg/L (3.0 mmol/L);
	Cl, 104 mEg/L (104 mmol/L); Ca, 9.5 mg/dL
	(2.38 mmol/L); fasting blood glucose, 90 g/dL
	(5 mmol/L). Health care provider notified.
	—Emma Smith, RN

  1. Hypocalcemia
  2. Hypoglycemia
  3. Hypokalemia
  4. Hyponatremia

3. The nurse knows a client with a diagnosis of bulimia and a history of purging by vomiting requires which intervention(s)? Select all that apply.

  1. Frequent glucose monitoring
  2. Asking, "How many times have you vomited today?"
  3. Assessing apical pulse for rhythm
  4. Asking, "How difficult is it for you to swallow solid food?"
  5. Frequent monitoring of body temperature

4. A nurse is assessing a client diagnosed with bulimia for possible substance use. Which question is **best** for the nurse to ask the client?

  1. "Have you ever used diet pills?"
  2. "Where would you go to buy drugs?"
  3. "At what age did you start drinking?"
  4. "Do your peers ever offer you drugs?"

1. **1.** A person diagnosed with bulimia nervosa expresses a lack of control over eating during an eating-purging episode. The other statements express eating-related values or concerns but none are associated with the involuntary aspect of the disorder.

CN: Psychosocial integrity; CNS: None; CL: Apply

2. **3.** Clients who are bulimic have hypokalemia (decreased potassium levels) due to purging behaviors. Hyponatremia, hypoglycemia, and hypocalcemia do not tend to occur in clients with bulimia nervosa; all the lab results are at normal levels for this client.

CN: Physiological integrity; CNS: Physiological adaptation; CL: Apply

3. **2, 3, 4.** People who purge by vomiting are at increased risk for electrolyte imbalance and resulting cardiac dysrhythmias as well as for esophageal erosion. Bulimia and purging are not disease producing, so monitoring for diabetes and infections like septicemia is not necessary.

CN: Physiological integrity; CNS: Reduction of risk potential; CL: Apply

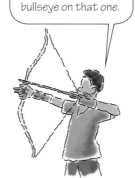

Nice. You hit the bullseye on that one.

4. **1.** Some clients with bulimia nervosa have a history of, or actively use, amphetamines to control weight. The use of alcohol and street drugs is also common. All the other questions can be answered by the client without revealing drug use.

CN: Psychosocial integrity; CNS: None; CL: Apply

CN: Client needs category   CNS: Client needs subcategory   CL: Cognitive level

5. Which statement about the binge–purge cycle demonstrates to the nurse that the client understands the triggers?

1. "I know midterm exams are a bad time for me."
2. "I know if I start eating pizza I would be able to stop."
3. "When I binge I know I will feel better once I purge."
4. "I binge when I am really hungry; then I cannot stop eating."

6. A client with a diagnosis of bulimia nervosa is working on relationship issues. Which nursing intervention is **most** important?

1. Assist the client to work on developing appropriate social skills.
2. Facilitate the client's ability to identify feelings about associations.
3. Help the client identify how relationships can lead to bulimic behavior.
4. Discuss ways to prevent getting overinvolved in relationships.

7. A young adult client diagnosed with bulimia nervosa wants to lessen feelings of powerlessness. Which short-term goal is **most** important for the nurse to set initially?

1. Learning problem-solving skills
2. Decreasing symptoms of anxiety
3. Performing self-care activities
4. Stating how to set limits with others

8. A client diagnosed with bulimia nervosa tells a nurse, "My parents do not know about my eating disorder." Which goal is appropriate for the client to set for this client and family?

1. Decreasing the chaos in the family unit
2. Learning effective communication skills
3. Spending time together in social situations
4. Discussing the client's need to be responsible

9. When the nurse is discussing self-esteem with a client diagnosed with bulimia nervosa, which area of focus is **most** important?

1. Assess personal fears.
2. Identify family strengths.
3. Discuss negative thinking patterns.
4. Reduce environmental stimuli.

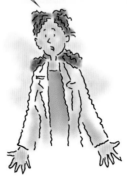

Ack! I'm so stressed. I need a doughnut … or six.

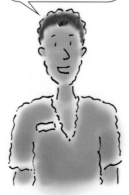

Changing the way a client thinks is half the battle with eating disorders.

5. **1.** It is important for the client to understand the emotional triggers for bingeing, such as disappointment, depression, and anxiety. Physiologic hunger does not predispose a client to bingeing behaviors. Purging is triggered by bingeing; it is an extension of the disorder. "Cannot stop" is an expression used to describe a love for a certain food.

CN: Psychosocial integrity; CNS: None; CL: Apply

6. **2.** The client must address personal feelings about associations, especially uncomfortable ones, because they may trigger bingeing behavior. Social skills are important to a client's well-being, but they are not typically a major problem for the client with bulimia nervosa. Relationships do not cause bulimic behaviors. It is the inability to handle stress or conflict that arises from interactions that causes the client to be distressed. The client is not necessarily overinvolved in relationships; the issue may be the lack of satisfying relationships in the client's life.

CN: Psychosocial integrity; CNS: None; CL: Apply

7. **1.** When the client can learn effective problem-solving skills, the client will gain a sense of control and power over life. Development of these skills is essential to recovery. Anxiety is commonly caused by feelings of powerlessness. Performing daily self-care activities will not reduce one's sense of powerlessness. Verbalizing how to set limits to protect oneself from the intrusive behavior of others is a necessary life skill, but problem-solving skills take priority in this case.

CN: Psychosocial integrity; CNS: None; CL: Analyze

8. **2.** A major goal for the client with bulimia nervosa and family is to learn to communicate directly and honestly in a peaceful environment. To change the chaotic environment, the family must first learn to communicate effectively. Families with a member who has an eating disorder are commonly enmeshed and do not need to spend more time together. Before discussing the client's level of responsibility, the family needs to establish effective ways of communicating with one another.

CN: Psychosocial integrity; CNS: None; CL: Apply

9. **3.** Clients with bulimia nervosa need to work on identifying and changing their negative thinking and distortion of reality. Personal fears are related to negative thinking. Exploring family strengths is not a priority; it is more appropriate to explore the client's strengths. Environmental stimuli do not cause bulimic behaviors.

CN: Psychosocial integrity; CNS: None; CL: Analyze

10. The nurse is caring for a client with bulimia nervosa. Which finding will the nurse report to the health care provider immediately?
1. Serum calcium 7.1 mg/dL (1.77 mmol/L)
2. Heart rate 60 beats/minute
3. Serum potassium 3.8 mEq/L (3.8 mmol/L)
4. Respiratory rate 16 breaths/minute

10. **1.** Electrolyte imbalance such as hypocalcemia (low serum calcium) is a serious complication of bulimia nervosa due to purging behaviors. A serum calcium level of 7.1 mg/dL (1.77 mmol/L) is dangerously low (normal is 8.5 to 10.2 mg/dL or 2.13 to 2.55 mmol/L). Normal serum potassium is 3.5 to 5 mEq/L (3.5 to 5 mmol/L). A heart rate of 60 beats/minute is at the low border of normal. A respiratory rate of 16 breaths/minute is within the normal range.
CN: Physiological integrity; CNS: Reduction of risk potential; CL: Apply

11. A nurse is talking to a client diagnosed with bulimia nervosa about possible comorbid conditions associated with bulimia? Which result will the nurse use to identify a potential associated condition?
1. Blood urea nitrogen (BUN)
2. Occult stool screening
3. Eating Attitude Test
4. Beck's Depression Inventory

11. **4.** A serious complication of bulimia is depression. While not impossible, renal failure and gastrointestinal bleeding are not commonly associated with bulimia. The Eating Attitude Test is used to suggest an eating disorder.
CN: Physiological integrity; CNS: Physiological adaption; CL: Apply

12. Which statement made by a client diagnosed with bulimia right after lunch will **most** concern the nurse?
1. "It is crazy, but I still feel hungry."
2. "I do not think I will be hungry for dinner."
3. "I ate way too many calories for lunch."
4. "I am going to go take a shower now."

Only one of the statements in question #12 will yield the most valuable information from the client.

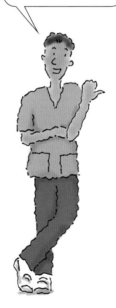

12. **4.** A client diagnosed with bulimia may resort to purging and should not be allowed privacy in the bathroom for at least 2 hours after a meal. The client still feeling hungry and not being hungry for dinner are less concerning when considering bulimia nervosa. The client worrying about calorie intake would be more concerning for a client diagnosed with anorexia nervosa.
CN: Psychosocial integrity; CNS: None; CL: Apply

13. The nurse is caring for an adolescent client prescribed a selective serotonin reuptake inhibitor (SSRI) as part of the treatment plan for anorexia nervosa. Which nursing action is **priority**?
1. Monitor for suicidal thoughts.
2. Weigh the client daily.
3. Monitor for nausea and diarrhea.
4. Explore the client's strengths.

13. **1.** There is an increased risk of suicidal ideation and behavior in children, adolescents, and young adults (18 to 24 years of age) when taking antidepressants. Weighing the client and exploring the client's strengths are important interventions but do not relate to the SSRI administration. Nausea and diarrhea are common adverse reactions.
CN: Physiological integrity; CNS: Pharmacological and parenteral therapies; CL: Analyze

14. A client diagnosed with anorexia is prescribed imipramine. Which assessment finding suggests to the nurse the client is experiencing an adverse reaction?
1. Oral temperature 100.8°F (38.2°C)
2. Apical heart rate 90 beats/minute
3. Client states, "My vision is blurry."
4. Client states, "My nose is really stuffy."

14. **1.** Imipramine, an antidepressant, can cause a decrease in the functioning of the immune system. A fever would indicate a possible infection, confirming such an effect. A heart rate of 90 beats/minute is within normal limits. Imipramine is not associated with blurry vision or nasal congestion.
CN: Physiological integrity; CNS: Pharmacological and parenteral therapies; CL: Apply

15. The nurse is caring for a client with a diagnosis of bulimia. The health care provider has prescribed 20 mEq of potassium chloride oral solution to be administered today. The label on the oral solution states potassium chloride oral solution 40 mEq/15 mL. How many milliliters will the nurse administer per dose? Record your answer using one decimal place.

_____ mL

16. A client diagnosed with bulimia has been hospitalized after experiencing diarrhea for 2 days. The nurse reviews the laboratory data in the chart exhibit below. Which finding(s) will the nurse expect to assess in this client? Select all that apply.

Laboratory results	
4/2	Sodium 130 mEq/L (130 mmol/L)
1650	Chloride 98 mEq/L (98 mmol/L)
	Albumin 3.5 g/dL (35 g/L)
	pH 7.25
	PaO_2 95 mm Hg (12.64 kPa)
	$PaCO_2$ 34 mm Hg (4.79 kPa)
	HCO_3 20 mEq/L (2.66 kPa)
	SaO_2 96% (0.96)

1. Fine tremors in the hands
2. Tingling in the face
3. Intermittent muscle cramping in legs
4. Respiratory rate 28 breaths/minute
5. 250 mL of emesis in 2 hours

17. The nurse is working with a client diagnosed with bulimia. Which statement made by the client will support the dynamics generally demonstrated by such families?
1. "My grandfather was diagnosed with schizophrenia when he was in his early 20s and my aunt was diagnosed in her 30s."
2. "My brother died in a car accident just months before my mother was diagnosed with terminal breast cancer."
3. "Several members of my extended family are being treated for varying degrees of anxiety, including panic attacks."
4. "I cannot leave my children alone with either grandparent since both abuse alcohol and pain medication."

Now you're cooking.

15. 7.5.
The correct formula to calculate a drug dose is:

$$\frac{Dose\ on\ hand}{Quantity\ on\ hand} = \frac{Dose\ desired}{X}$$

The health care provider prescribes 20 mEq, which is the dose desired. The available solution states 40 mEq/15 mL, which is the dose on hand.

$$\frac{40\ mEq}{15\ mL} = \frac{20\ mEq}{X}$$

$$40x = 300$$

$$X = 7.5\ mL$$

CN: Physiological integrity; CNS: Pharmacological and parenteral therapies; CL: Apply

16. 4, 5. The client is experiencing metabolic acidosis based on the $PaCo_2$ (less than 35), pH (less than 7.35), and HCO_3 (less than 22). Metabolic acidosis is characterized by hyperpnea and vomiting. Metabolic alkalosis is characterized by hand tremors, facial numbness, and muscle spasms.

CN: Physiological integrity; CNS: Physiological adaptation; CL: Analyze

17. 2. Families with a member who has bulimia usually struggle with multiple losses. Mental illness, chronic anxiety, and substance use do not tend to be themes in the family background of the client with bulimia.

CN: Psychosocial integrity; CNS: None; CL: Apply

CN: Client needs category   CNS: Client needs subcategory   CL: Cognitive level

18. A client diagnosed with bulimia tells a nurse, "My major problem is eating too much food in a short period of time and then vomiting." Which short-term goal is **most** important for the nurse to set for this client?
1. Helping the client understand every person has a satiety level
2. Encouraging the client to verbalize fears and concerns about food
3. Determining the amount of food the client will eat without purging
4. Obtaining a therapy appointment to look at the emotional contributors

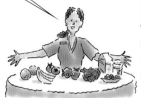

Encourage clients with bulimia to eat small portions of healthy food.

18. 3. The client must meet nutritional needs to prevent further complications and identify the amount of food that can be eaten without purging as a first short-term goal. Determining satiety level and verbalizing fears and feelings about food are not priority goals for this client. All clients must first take steps to meet their nutritional needs. Therapy is an important part of dealing with this disorder, but it is not the first step.
CN: Physiological integrity; CNS: Reduction of risk potential; CL: Apply

19. Which statement indicates to the nurse treatment has been effective for the client diagnosed with bulimia?
1. "I have learned that talking helps when I get upset."
2. "I know I will have this problem with eating forever."
3. "I started asking my family to watch me eat each meal."
4. "My friend will bring me home from parties if I want to purge."

19. 1. The client who verbalizes feelings and interacts with people instead of turning to food for comfort shows signs of progress. Feeling that the eating problem will last forever indicates the client needs more information on how to handle the disorder. Having another person watch the client eat is not a helpful strategy, as the client will depend on others to help control food intake. Asking a friend to take the client home from parties to purge indicates the client is in denial about the severity of the problem.
CN: Psychosocial integrity; CNS: None; CL: Apply

20. A client with a diagnosis of bulimia asks the nurse, "How can I ask for help from my family?" Which nursing response is **most** appropriate?
1. "When you ask for help, make sure you really need it."
2. "Have you ever asked your family for help in the past?"
3. "Ask family members to have meals with you."
4. "Think about how you can handle this situation without help."

20. 2. The nurse should determine whether the client has ever been successful in asking for help because previous experiences affect the client's ability to ask for help now. The client needs to be able to ask for help at any time without analyzing the level of need. Asking other people to be present at mealtime is not the only way to ask for help. Developing a support system is imperative for this client, not trying to handle the situation independently.
CN: Psychosocial integrity; CNS: None; CL: Apply

21. The nurse will expect the health care provider to prescribe a combination of which medication(s) for a client diagnosed with anorexia nervosa? Select all that apply.
1. Amitriptyline
2. Alprazolam
3. Imipramine
4. Paroxetine
5. Lorazepam
6. Fluoxetine

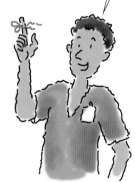

Remember, all answer choices may be right in "select all that apply" questions.

21. 1, 2, 3, 4, 5, 6. Each medication may be prescribed to a client diagnosed with anorexia nervosa.
CN: Physiological integrity; CNS: Pharmacological and parenteral therapies; CL: Apply

22. A client diagnosed with bulimia tells the nurse, "I had a really bad argument with my mom this morning." Which nursing intervention is **most** appropriate for this client?
1. Suggest the client attend today's family therapy counseling session.
2. Initiate a conversation about the relationship between feelings and eating.
3. Provide the client with information on anger management skills.
4. Offer to assist the client with practicing stress management techniques.

22. 2. The client must understand his or her feelings and their effect on eating. Such stressors can trigger the binge-purge cycle for this client. While the other actions may prove helpful, initially the client must understand the connection between the disorder and feelings.
CN: Psychosocial integrity; CNS: None; CL: Apply

CN: Client needs category   CNS: Client needs subcategory   CL: Cognitive level

23. Which statement made by a client with bulimia indicates to the nurse a need for additional education?
1. "If I have a relapse, it is only a temporary setback."
2. "If I follow my treatment plan, relapse is unlikely to occur."
3. "A relapse teaches me important information about my illness."
4. "A relapse is not good, but it does not mean my situation is hopeless."

23. **2.** The client with bulimia should be prepared to accept that relapses can occur and that relapse is not a sign of hopelessness; rather, relapses are temporary and provide valuable information about triggers and treatment needs. All other statements indicate successful education.
CN: Psychosocial integrity; CNS: None; CL: Apply

24. A client diagnosed with bulimia has a history of severe gastrointestinal problems. Based on this finding, the nurse will be prepared to include which intervention(s) in the client's plan of care to address likely physiological complications? Select all that apply.
1. Straining the client's urine
2. Administrating antibiotic as prescribed
3. Instituting seizure precautions
4. Testing all stools for occult blood
5. Monitoring the client's temperature frequently

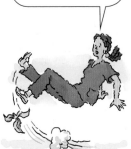

Don't let this question trip you up. Slow down and read it again.

24. **1, 2, 4, 5.** A client with bulimia who has severe gastrointestinal problems has probably experienced excessive purging. This history increases the client's risk for esophageal tears and irritation, or esophagitis. These conditions increase the risk for infection and thus require monitoring for early signs like fever and the administration of prescribed antibiotics. In addition, clients with eating disorders may develop renal calculi that require the straining of the client's urine. Purging by excessive laxative use can result in rectal bleeding identified by occult blood screening of the client's stool. Focal seizures are not related to severe gastrointestinal problems.
CN: Physiological integrity; CNS: Reduction of risk potential; CL: Apply

25. Which statement made by the nurse demonstrates an understanding of the **priority** intervention when caring for a client diagnosed with an eating disorder?
1. "You can exercise for 10 minutes twice a day."
2. "I have filled out your menu cards for your meals."
3. "Let us discuss how you try to distract staff during meals."
4. "You need to use the same scale each time you are weighed."

25. **3.** Clients with eating disorders commonly use manipulative ploys and countertransference to resist weight gain (if they restrict food intake) or maintain purging practices (if they have bulimia). They commonly play staff members against one another and exploit their caretaker's vulnerabilities. Exercise is proper but should be controlled so it is not a way to inappropriately burn off calories. The nurse should not assume control over the client's food selections but rather work with the client in making selections. While it is important to use the same scale, doing so does not have priority over managing unhealthy behaviors.
CN: Safe, effective care environment; CNS: Management of care; CL: Apply

26. The nurse caring for a client diagnosed with anorexia nervosa determines which goal is **priority**?
1. The client will establish adequate daily nutritional intake.
2. The client will make a contract with the nurse for a target weight.
3. The client will identify unrealistic self-perceptions about body size.
4. The client will verbalize the physiologic consequences of self-starvation.

26. **1.** According to Maslow's hierarchy of needs, all humans need to meet basic physiologic needs first. Because a client with anorexia nervosa eats little or nothing, the nurse must plan to help the client meet this basic, immediate, physiologic need first. The nurse may give lower priority to goals that address long-term plans, self-perception, and potential complications.
CN: Safe, effective care environment; CNS: Management of care; CL: Analyze

27. A client diagnosed with anorexia nervosa is prescribed lorazepam for anxiety. The nurse concludes the teaching has been effective when the client makes which statement(s)? Select all that apply.
1. "It is okay for me to drive after I have taken this medication."
2. "I will not stop lorazepam without notifying my health care provider."
3. "I only need to take lorazepam until I learn to manage my anxiety."
4. "I should avoid drinking alcohol while taking this medication."
5. "I can take this medication without worrying about becoming addicted."

28. Which statement made by a client being treated for anorexia nervosa suggests to the nurse the client is demonstrating a cognitive distortion related to the illness?
1. "I will never be as slender as I would like to be."
2. "If I eat that sandwich I will look grossly fat."
3. "I envy people who can eat anything and not gain weight."
4. "I exercise twice a day so I can keep my weight under control."

29. A client with anorexia nervosa attended psychoeducational sessions on the principles of adequate nutrition. Which statement by the client indicates to the nurse a need for further education?
1. "I should eat slowly and focus on how my food tastes."
2. "I should eat several small meals spread out over the entire day."
3. "I should view eating with my family and friends as a positive thing."
4. "Eating a strict vegetarian diet is a good way to control my weight."

30. Which statement made by a client diagnosed with anorexia nervosa demonstrates effective communication with the nurse?
1. "It is raining cats and dogs outside today."
2. "I went out shopping with friends last night."
3. "I really enjoyed spending time with you today."
4. "I am interested in what you have to say about the movie."

31. Which statement made by a parent of a teenager diagnosed with anorexia nervosa is characteristic of the parent-child relationship?
1. "I expect my teen to be the very best she can be."
2. "I know how hard it is to be a teenager today."
3. "I am not an emotional person, but she knows I love her."
4. "I work long hours to give her everything she needs and wants."

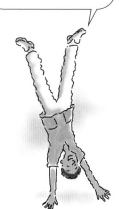

Clients with anorexia nervosa have a distorted view of their bodies.

Woo-hoo! You've finished 30 questions.

27. **2, 3, 4.** Lorazepam is a benzodiazepine and is known to cause drowsiness and sedation. Activities that require alertness, like driving a car, should be avoided while taking this drug. The drug should be tapered, not stopped abruptly. These drugs are only recommended for short-term use. Long-term use can result in dependency. Alcohol use with the benzodiazepines will cause an additive central nervous system depression, so alcohol should be avoided.
CN: Physiological integrity; CNS: Pharmacological and parenteral therapies; CL: Apply

28. **2.** The client with anorexia nervosa pursues thinness and has a distorted view of self. This is demonstrated in the belief that eating a sandwich will result in gross obesity. The remaining statements express rational beliefs concerning weight and weight control.
CN: Psychosocial integrity; CNS: None; CL: Apply

29. **4.** While a vegetarian diet can be a healthy nutritional plan, it should not be viewed as a way to control weight, especially by a client with an eating disorder. The remaining statements show learning of sensible eating information.
CN: Health promotion and maintenance; CNS: None; CL: Apply

30. **3.** Clients with anorexia nervosa commonly communicate on a superficial level and avoid expressing feelings. Identifying feelings and learning to express them are initial steps in decreasing isolation. Clients with anorexia nervosa are usually able to discuss abstract and concrete issues. None of the other statements demonstrate effective communication of personal feelings.
CN: Psychosocial integrity; CNS: None; CL: Analyze

31. **1.** Clients with anorexia nervosa typically come from a family with parents who are controlling and overprotective. These clients use eating to gain control of an aspect of their lives and to manage the stress they are feeling. None of the other statements demonstrate that high level of control or protectiveness.
CN: Psychosocial integrity; CNS: None; CL: Apply

CN: Client needs category   CNS: Client needs subcategory   CL: Cognitive level

32. The nurse is talking to the family of a client diagnosed with anorexia nervosa. Which statement made by a family member suggests a characteristic family situation?
  1. "My siblings have always been very competitive with each other."
  2. "My family approaches all problems with yelling and screaming."
  3. "My parents never argue but their marriage should have ended years ago."
  4. "My family members seldom spend time together, even on holidays."

33. The nurse is assessing a client diagnosed with anorexia nervosa and notes mild acrocyanosis with capillary refill less than 3 seconds. Which nursing action will be completed **next**?
  1. Continue to monitor the client.
  2. Notify the health care provider.
  3. Transfuse 2 units of blood.
  4. Give ferrous sulfate daily.

34. A client diagnosed with anorexia nervosa is discharged from the hospital after gaining 12 lb (5.5 kg). Which client statement(s) best indicates the nurse's discharge education was effective? Select all that apply.
  1. "I plan to eat two small meals a day once I am discharged."
  2. "I will need to work on my eating disorder for a long time."
  3. "This is scary, so I am going to write about it in my journal."
  4. "I have to cut back on my calorie intake to limit weight gain."
  5. "To stay healthy, I will need to attend therapy sessions."

35. A client with a diagnosis of anorexia nervosa tells a nurse about always feeling fat. Which nursing intervention is **best** for this client?
  1. Educate about the dynamics of the disorder.
  2. Talk about how the client is different from peers.
  3. Identify positive characteristics to boost self-esteem.
  4. Have the client honestly evaluate his or her body in a mirror.

36. The grandparents of a client diagnosed with anorexia nervosa want to support the client but are not sure what they should do. Which intervention is **best** for the nurse to educate the grandparents about?
  1. Encourage positive expressions of affection.
  2. Encourage behaviors that promote socialization.
  3. Discuss how eating disorders create powerlessness.
  4. Discuss the meaning of hunger and body sensations.

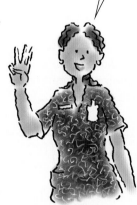

Don't give up. The answer will come to you.

32. 3. In many families with a member suffering from anorexia nervosa, there is marital conflict and parental disagreement. Sibling rivalry is common and not specific to a family with a member who suffers from anorexia nervosa. In these families, the members tend to be enmeshed and dependent on each other. The family with an anorexic member is usually one that looks good to the outside observer. Emotions are overcontrolled, and there is difficulty with appropriately expressing negative feelings.
CN: Psychosocial integrity; CNS: None; CL: Apply

33. 1. The client's acrocyanosis is probably caused by decreased blood volume. The client's capillary refill is within normal limits, so the nurse will continue to monitor the client. The nurse may notify the health care provider to get a prescription for ferrous sulfate or a blood transfusion if the client becomes symptomatic.
CN: Physiological integrity; CNS: Physiological adaption; CL: Analyze

34. 2, 3, 5. The client is planning to attend therapy after discharge, and this shows an understanding of the need for continued counseling. Recovery from eating disorders may take years and clients may relapse. Eating only two small meals a day is an unrealistic plan for meeting nutritional needs. Feeling insecure when leaving a controlled environment is a common response to discharge; however, writing about feelings in a journal would be therapeutic. Gaining 12 lb (5.5 kg) indicates that the client's nutritional needs are being met at the present caloric intake levels.
CN: Psychosocial integrity; CNS: None; CL: Analyze

35. 1. The client can benefit from understanding the underlying dynamics of the eating disorder. The client with anorexia nervosa has low self-esteem and will not believe the positive statements. Looking in a mirror is not the best intervention because the client still has an incorrect perception of him- or herself. Pointing out differences will only diminish already low self-esteem.
CN: Psychosocial integrity; CNS: None; CL: Apply

36. 1. Clients with eating disorders need emotional support and expressions of affection from family members. It would not be appropriate for the grandparents to promote socialization. Clients with eating disorders feel powerless, but it is better to have the grandparents focus on something positive. Talking about hunger and other body sensations is not a useful strategy.
CN: Psychosocial integrity; CNS: None; CL: Apply

CN: Client needs category   CNS: Client needs subcategory   CL: Cognitive level

37. The nurse is planning care for a client diagnosed with anorexia nervosa. Which nursing intervention will **best** support the client to address the physiological problems experienced during treatment?
1. Educating the client regarding prescribed antianxiety medication
2. Comparing the client's previous electrocardiogram results
3. Encouraging the client to engage in moderate exercise
4. Scheduling regular nutritional counseling sessions

38. An adolescent client with anorexia nervosa tells a nurse about outstanding academic achievements and thoughts about suicide. Which factor will the nurse consider when developing a care plan for this client?
1. Self-esteem
2. Physical illnesses
3. Paranoid delusions
4. Relationship avoidance

39. When reviewing prescriptions for a client diagnosed with bulimia nervosa, the nurse anticipates which medication(s) to be prescribed? Select all that apply.
1. Alprazolam
2. Amitriptyline
3. Imipramine
4. Fluoxetine
5. Lorazepam

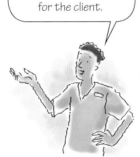

When developing a care plan, don't forget to include measures that have previously worked well for the client.

40. The nurse caring for a client diagnosed with an eating disorder suspects the client is demonstrating cognitive distortions. Which statement made by the client supports this suspicion?
1. "I have been told my weight–height ratio is within normal limits, but I know I am way too fat."
2. "I do not think vomiting is all that uncomfortable or unhealthy for younger people."
3. "Everyone here just wants to make me eat so I can get even fatter and be grossly obese."
4. "I bet you have never seen arms and legs as grossly fat as mine in your career."

41. How can the nurse **best** assess a client for Russell's sign?
1. Ask, "How often do you have your menstrual period?"
2. Examine the client's knuckles for bruising.
3. Evaluate the client's teeth for eroded tooth enamel.
4. Ask, "When did this red rash on your lips first become apparent?"

37. 4. The client receiving nutritional counseling will be assisted in making dietary choices that support physical recovery. Antianxiety medication therapy will help address specific psychosocial issues. Cardiac monitoring will help identify but not address associated physical health issues. Moderate exercise, while appropriate, is not as important as sound nutrition to clients diagnosed with eating disorders because the trigger for the physiological problems is nutritionally based.
CN: Physiological integrity; CNS: Reduction of risk potential; CL: Apply

38. 1. The client lacks self-esteem, which contributes to the client's level of depression and feelings of personal ineffectiveness, which, in turn, may lead to suicidal thoughts. Physical illnesses are common with clients with anorexia nervosa, but they do not relate to this situation. Paranoid delusions refer to an individual's false idea that others want to cause harm. No evidence exists that this client is socially isolated.
CN: Psychosocial integrity; CNS: None; CL: Apply

39. 4. Selective serotonin reuptake inhibitors (SSRIs), such as paroxetine and fluoxetine, are used to treat bulimia nervosa. Alprazolam and lorazepam are antianxiety medications and amitriptyline and imipramine are antidepressants. These four medications are used to treat clients with anorexia nervosa.
CN: Physiological integrity; CNS: Pharmacological and parenteral therapies; CL: Apply

40. 1. A cognitive distortion is a way that the mind convinces people of something that is not true. A selective or biased perception is the tendency not to notice and more quickly forget stimuli that cause emotional discomfort and contradict prior beliefs. A paranoid delusion is the fixed, false belief that one is being harmed or persecuted by a person or group of people. An optical illusion is characterized by visually perceived images that are deceptive or misleading.
CN: Psychosocial integrity; CNS: None; CL: Apply

41. 2. Russell's sign involves the presence of bruised knuckles resulting from the use of fingers to induce vomiting. None of the other assessments are associated with Russell's sign.
CN: Physiological integrity; CNS: Physiological adaptation; CL: Apply

CN: Client needs category   CNS: Client needs subcategory   CL: Cognitive level

42. A client diagnosed with anorexia nervosa has been prescribed fluoxetine. The nurse will include which question when assessing the client?
1. "Have you experienced any heartburn?"
2. "Are you experiencing any headaches?"
3. "How much liquid are you drinking each hour?"
4. "Are you having thoughts about hurting yourself?"

43. A client diagnosed with anorexia nervosa is worried about rectal bleeding. Which question by the nurse is **most** appropriate?
1. "How often you are using laxatives?"
2. "How many days ago did you stop vomiting?"
3. "Are you eating anything that causes irritation?"
4. "Do you bleed before or after exercise?"

44. The nurse is caring for a client with a diagnosis of anorexia nervosa. Which nursing intervention(s) is appropriate for this client? Select all that apply.
1. Provide small, frequent feedings throughout the day.
2. Monitor the client's weight frequently, but randomly.
3. Let the client skip meals until antidepressant levels are therapeutic.
4. Encourage the client to journal to promote the expression of feelings.
5. Encourage the client to eat three substantial meals per day.

45. Which characteristic(s) will the nurse expect to assess in a client diagnosed with anorexia nervosa? Select all that apply.
1. The intense fear of gaining weight
2. Weight 70% or less of ideal body weight
3. Awareness of the problem but refusal to admit it
4. Self-esteem that is dependent on personal looks
5. Weight loss accomplished using diet pills

46. A client is being evaluated for bulimia nervosa. Which assessment data indicate to the nurse support for this diagnosis? Select all that apply.
1. Heart rate of 72 beats/minute and irregular.
2. Severe enamel erosion noted on front teeth.
3. Client reports, "I am hot regardless of the weather."
4. Hands are both cold to the touch and mottled in color.
5. Swelling noted at the site of salivary glands bilaterally.
6. Client reports difficulty falling and staying asleep.

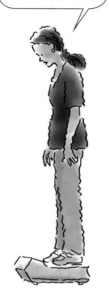

Repeat after me: my weight is not my identity.

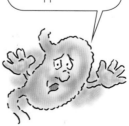

In bulimia, I don't function the way I'm supposed to.

42. 4. Fluoxetine is a selective serotonin reuptake inhibitor (SSRI). It is important to monitor the client for mood changes and suicidal tendencies when prescribed this classification of medication. While the other questions may be appropriate during assessment, they are not associated with effective care of a client prescribed fluoxetine.
CN: Physiological integrity; CNS: Pharmacological and parenteral therapies; CL: Apply

43. 1. Excessive use of laxatives will cause gastrointestinal irritation and rectal bleeding. If the client stopped vomiting but is still using laxatives, rectal bleeding can occur. Clients with anorexia eat very little, and what they eat would not cause rectal bleeding. Exercise does not cause rectal bleeding.
CN: Health promotion and maintenance; CNS: None; CL: Apply

44. 1, 2, 4. Smaller, more frequent meals may be better tolerated by the client and will gradually increase daily caloric intake. Weight should be monitored randomly to prevent the client from water loading, or drinking excessive water and not urinating prior to being weighed. Clients with anorexia are emotionally restrained and afraid of their feelings, so journaling can be a powerful tool that assists in recovery. Clients with anorexia are obsessed with gaining weight and will skip all meals if given the opportunity, so encouraging the client to skip meals is not therapeutic. Because of self-starvation, clients with anorexia seldom tolerate large meals three times per day.
CN: Safe, effective care environment; CNS: Management of care; CL: Apply

45. 1, 4. Individuals with anorexia are intensely afraid of gaining weight. Self-esteem depends on how the person looks. The diagnostic criteria state that a person has anorexia when weight is 85% below the expected weight for height. Individuals with the disorder typically do not believe they have a problem and do not consider their behavior abnormal. They do not accomplish weight loss with diet pills, but through avoidance of food and with excessive exercise.
CN: Psychosocial integrity; CNS: None; CL: Apply

46. 1, 2, 4, 5, 6. Constant bingeing and purging behaviors can cause severe electrolyte imbalances resulting in cardiac irregularities, erosion of tooth enamel from constant exposure to gastric acids, swelling and circulatory issues with the hands and feet, swelling of the salivary glands, and problems sleeping. Feeling cold, not hot, is typically associated with bulimia nervosa.
CN: Physiological integrity; CNS: Physiological adaptation; CL: Apply

CN: Client needs category   CNS: Client needs subcategory   CL: Cognitive level

47. The nurse is caring for a client with bulimia nervosa requiring IV fluids for dehydration and electrolyte imbalances. The primary health care provider has prescribed 1,000 mL of 0.9% sodium chloride with 40 mEq of potassium chloride to infuse over 6 hours. The drop factor of the IV tubing is 10 drops per milliliter. How many drops per minute will the nurse infuse? Record the answer as a whole number.

_____ drops/min

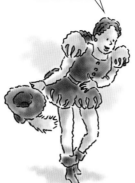

Take a bow.
You deserve it.

47. 28.
The correct formula to calculate a drug dose is:

$$\frac{drops}{min} = \frac{drops}{mL} \times \frac{Dose\ desired}{Time\ desired} \times \frac{1\ hr}{60\ min}$$

$$\frac{10\ drops}{mL} \times \frac{1000\ \cancel{mL}}{6\ \cancel{hrs}} \times \frac{1\ \cancel{hr}}{60\ min} = \frac{10000}{360}$$

$$= 27.7 = 28\ drops/min$$

CN: Physiological integrity; CNS: Pharmacological and parenteral therapies; CL: Apply

Maternal–Neonatal Care

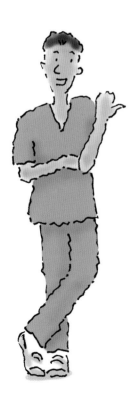

Chapter 21

Antepartum Care

Looking for information about antepartum care before tackling this chapter? Visit www.obgyn.net/, an independent Web site dedicated to obstetric and gynecologic health problems.

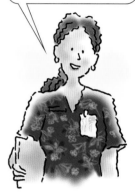

Antepartum care refresher

Acquired immunodeficiency syndrome (AIDS)

Condition caused by the human immunodeficiency virus (HIV); infection places the client at high risk for opportunistic infections, unusual cancers, and other abnormalities

Key signs and symptoms
- Diarrhea
- Fatigue
- Kaposi sarcoma
- Mild flulike symptoms
- Opportunistic infections, such as toxoplasmosis, oral and vaginal candidiasis, herpes simplex, *Pneumocystis jiroveci*, and *Candida esophagitis*
- Weight loss

Key test results
- CD4+ T-cell level is less than 200 cells/μL
- Enzyme-linked immunosorbent assay shows positive HIV antibody titer
- Western blot test is positive

Key treatments
- Treatment depends upon clinical situation
- Anti-HIV medications should be a combination of at least three medications: two nucleoside reverse transcriptase inhibitor class (one should be azidothymidine) and either one nonnucleoside reverse transcriptase inhibitor class or one protease inhibitor

Key interventions
- Determine whether the client will be able to care for her infant after the birth.

Adolescent pregnancy

Pregnancy that occurs in females between the ages of 11 to 19 years; the pregnant adolescent is considered high-risk due to the physical and psychological demands associated with her own growth and development along with the demands of pregnancy

Key signs and symptoms
- Denial of pregnancy, which may deter the client from seeking medical attention early in pregnancy

Key test results
- Positive indicators of pregnancy: presence of a fetal heartbeat, fetal movement, visualization of the fetus
- Pregnancy test is positive (probable indicator of pregnancy)

Key treatments
- Diet with caloric intake that supports the growing adolescent and developing fetus

Key interventions
- Monitor client's weight gain.
- Provide psychological support.
- Inform client of appropriate support agencies and groups.
- Educate client on expected physiological changes during pregnancy.
- Advise client of her options, including:
    ○ terminating the pregnancy
    ○ continuing the pregnancy and giving up the infant for adoption
    ○ continuing the pregnancy and keeping the infant

Gestational diabetes

Endocrine disorder that involves problems of glucose metabolism; women who enter pregnancy and develop diabetes during pregnancy are diagnosed with gestational diabetes

Key signs and symptoms
- Hypoglycemia
- Hyperglycemia
- Glycosuria
- Ketonuria
- Polyuria
- Oligohydramnios
- Fetal macrosomia

I don't know about you, but drinking lots of coffee always gives me polyuria.

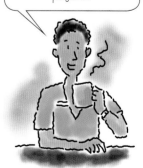

Key test results

- Diagnosed if the client has two or more of the following results during a 3-hour glucose tolerance test:
  ○ fasting blood sugar level at or above 95 mg/dL
  ○ three-hour glucose tolerance test reveals 1-hour level at or above 180 mg/dL
  ○ three-hour glucose tolerance test reveals 2-hour level at or above 155 mg/dL
  ○ three-hour glucose tolerance test reveals 3-hour level at or above 140 mg/dL

Key treatments

- 1,800- to 2,200-calorie diet divided into three meals and three snacks
- Diet should be low in fat and cholesterol and high in fiber
- Administration of insulin or glyburide after the first trimester as needed

Key interventions

- Encourage adherence to dietary regulations.
- Encourage client to exercise moderately.
- Prepare the client for antepartum fetal surveillance testing, including:
  ○ oxytocin challenge or nipple stimulation stress testing
  ○ amniotic fluid index
  ○ biophysical profile
  ○ non-stress test.

Ectopic pregnancy

Pregnancy in which the fertilized ovum implants outside the uterine cavity; although implantation can occur on the ovarian surface, on the intestine, or in the cervix, the most common site of implantation is the fallopian tube.

Key signs and symptoms

- Irregular vaginal bleeding
- Dull abdominal pain on the affected side early in pregnancy
- Positive Cullen's sign (bluish discoloration around the umbilicus)
- Rupture of the affected tube, causing sudden and severe abdominal pain, syncope, and referred shoulder pain as the abdomen fills with blood

Key test results

- Human chorionic gonadotropin (HCG) titers are abnormally low when compared to a normal pregnancy
- Transvaginal ultrasound confirms pregnancy placement

Key treatments

- Laparotomy to ligate the bleeding vessels and remove or repair damaged fallopian tube
- If the tube has not ruptured, methotrexate followed by leucovorin to stop the trophoblastic cells from growing (therapy continues until negative HCG levels are achieved)

Key interventions

- Monitor for signs of rupturing ectopic pregnancy, such as:
  ○ severe abdominal pain
  ○ orthostatic hypotension
  ○ tachycardia
  ○ dizziness.
- Maintain IV fluid replacement.
- Monitor blood product administration.
- Assess psychological status.

Heart disease

A pregnant woman with heart disease is at high risk for complications due to the physiologic changes that occur during pregnancy, primarily the increase in circulating blood volume

Key signs and symptoms

- Crackles at the base of the lungs
- Diastolic murmur at the heart's apex
- Dyspnea
- Fatigue
- Tachycardia

Key test results

- Echocardiography, electrocardiography, and chest x-ray may reveal cardiac abnormalities, dysrhythmias, impaired cardiac function, increased workload on the heart, and cardiovascular decompensation

Key treatments

Class III and class IV disease
- Anticoagulants: heparin
- Antiarrhythmics: digoxin, procainamide, beta-blockers
- Thiazide diuretics and furosemide to control heart failure if activity restriction and reduced sodium intake do not prevent it

Key interventions

- Monitor cardiovascular and respiratory status.
- Administer oxygen by nasal cannula or face mask during labor.
- Position client on her left side with her head and shoulders elevated during labor.

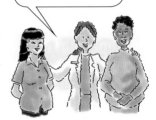

I have great expectations for this chapter ... it's pregnant with possibilities.

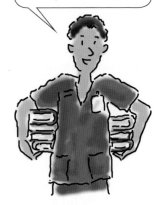

Do you remember where the fertilized egg implants in an ectopic pregnancy?

Hydatidiform mole

Abnormal growth and degeneration of the trophoblastic villi cells; cells become fluid-filled vesicles and the embryo fails to develop (also known as gestational trophoblastic disease)

Key signs and symptoms

- Intermittent or continuous bright red or brownish vaginal bleeding by the 12th week of gestation
- Uterine size greater than expected for dates
- Absence of fetal heart tones

Key test results

- HCG levels much higher than normal
- Ultrasound fails to reveal a fetal skeleton or heart tone

Key treatments

- Therapeutic abortion (suction and curettage) if spontaneous abortion does not occur
- Weekly monitoring of HCG levels until they remain normal for 3 consecutive weeks
- Periodic follow-up for 1 year because of increased risk of neoplasm

Key interventions

- Monitor vaginal bleeding.
- Send contents of uterine evacuation to laboratory for analysis.
- Recommend client does not become pregnant again for 12 months due to risk of neoplasm.

Hyperemesis gravidarum

Nausea and vomiting that persist past the 12th week of pregnancy or that are so severe that they interfere with the pregnant woman's nutrition.

Key signs and symptoms

- Continuous, severe nausea and vomiting
- Dehydration
- Oliguria
- Significant weight loss (≥5% prepregnancy weight)

Key test results

- Arterial blood gas analysis reveals metabolic alkalosis
- Hemoglobin and hematocrit levels are elevated
- Serum sodium level reveals hyponatremia
- Serum potassium level reveals hypokalemia

Key treatments

- Restoration of fluid and electrolyte balance

- Antiemetic or antihistamine H_1 receptor blocker medication

Key interventions

- Monitor fundal height and client's weight.
- NPO until vomiting controlled, then slowly advance diet to provide small, frequent, bland meals.
- Monitor intake and output.
- Monitor urine for ketones.
- Maintain IV fluid replacement and total parenteral nutrition.

Hypertension in pregnancy

High blood pressure during pregnancy (termed gestational hypertension if condition develops during pregnancy)

Key signs and symptoms

Gestational hypertension
- Systolic blood pressure ≥140 mm Hg or diastolic blood pressure ≥90 mm Hg after 20 weeks' gestation taken on two separate occasions at least 4 hours apart
- No proteinuria or multisystem disturbances consistent with preeclampsia

Preeclampsia
- Systolic blood pressure ≥140 mm Hg or diastolic blood pressure ≥90 mm Hg taken on two separate occasions at least 4 hours apart
- Proteinuria (300 mg protein in 24-hour specimen) or any of the following disturbances: thrombocytopenia, impaired liver function, new development of renal insufficiency, pulmonary edema, or cerebral or visual disturbance
- Presence of HELLP syndrome (hemolysis, elevated liver enzymes, and low platelet count) may be noted
- Hyperreflexia, nausea, vomiting, irritability, and epigastric pain may be noted
- Severe features of preeclampsia include: BP 160/110 or above on two separate occasions at least 4 hours apart, thrombocytopenia (platelets less than 100,000), impaired liver function (serum transaminases twice normal value), new development of renal insufficiency (serum creatinine greater than 1.1 mg/dL or doubling of serum creatinine), pulmonary edema, or cerebral or visual disturbance

Key test results

- Blood chemistry reveals:
  - increased blood urea nitrogen, creatinine, and uric acid levels
  - thrombocytopenia
  - elevated liver function studies

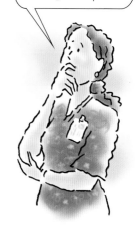

A client has continuous bright red bleeding in her 12th week of gestation, no fetal heart tones are heard, and HCG levels are sky-high. What condition would you suspect?

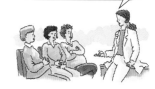

"Hyperemesis gravidarum" is just a fancy way of saying "lots of nausea and vomiting when you're pregnant."

Key treatments

- Bed rest in a left lateral position
- Birth:
  - of uncomplicated preeclampsia with no severe features: when fetus is mature and safe induction is possible
  - with severe features: regardless of gestational age
- High-protein diet with restriction of excessively salty foods
- With preeclampsia:
  - hydralazine hydrochloride, labetalol hydrochloride, or nifedipine to control blood pressure
  - betamethasone to accelerate fetal lung maturation
  - magnesium sulfate to reduce the amount of acetylcholine produced by motor nerves, thereby preventing seizures

Key interventions

All clients

- Evaluate client for multisystem disturbances.
- Maintain seizure precautions in hospitalized clients.
- Encourage bed rest in a left lateral recumbent position.
- Monitor blood pressure.

Severe features of preeclampsia

- Monitor maternal blood pressure at least every 4 hours, more frequently if unstable.
- Be prepared to obtain a blood sample for typing and cross-matching.
- Keep calcium gluconate (antidote to magnesium sulfate) nearby for administration at first sign of magnesium sulfate toxicity (elevated serum levels, decreased deep tendon reflexes, muscle flaccidity, clonus, central nervous system depression, and decreased respiratory rate and renal function).

Multifetal pregnancy

Pregnancy with more than one fetus present in the uterus

Key signs and symptoms

- More than one set of fetal heart sounds
- Uterine size greater than expected for dates

Key test results

- Alpha-fetoprotein (AFP) levels are elevated
- Human chorionic gonadotropin (HCG) levels are elevated
- Ultrasonography is positive for multifetal pregnancy

Key treatments

- Bed rest if early dilation occurs before or at 24 to 28 weeks' gestation
- Biweekly non-stress test to document fetal growth, beginning at the 28th week of gestation
- Increased intake of calories, iron, folate, and vitamins
- Ultrasound examinations monthly to document fetal growth

Key interventions

- Monitor fetal well-being.
- Monitor maternal vital signs and weight.
- Monitor maternal cardiovascular and pulmonary status.

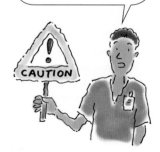

If your client has high blood pressure, proteinuria, and severe headaches, suspect preeclampsia.

Placenta previa

Abnormal implantation of the placenta in the uterus; a common cause of painless bleeding during the second half of pregnancy

Key signs and symptoms

- Painless, bright red vaginal bleeding, especially during third trimester

Key test results

- Early ultrasound evaluation reveals placenta implanted in the lower uterine segment

Key treatments

- Depends on gestational age, when first episode occurs, and amount of bleeding
- If gestational age less than 34 weeks, hospitalize client and restrict her to bed rest to avoid preterm labor
- Surgical intervention by cesarean birth depending on placental placement and maternal and fetal stability

Key interventions

- Avoid rectal or vaginal examinations unless equipment is available for vaginal and cesarean birth.

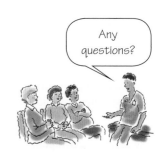

Any questions?

thePoint® You can download tables of drug information to help you prepare for the NCLEX®! View Generic Drug Names, Drug Classifications, Drug Actions, and Nursing Implications for the drugs discussed in this refresher at **http://thePoint.lww.com**

Antepartum care questions, answers, and rationales

1. A pregnant client who is in her third trimester calls the clinic nurse and states, "Sometimes I feel faint and light-headed while I am watching television." Which question is **most** important for the nurse to ask the client?
1. "What position are you in while watching television?"
2. "Do you have a history of asthma or difficulty breathing?"
3. "How many times a day do you feel faint and light-headed?"
4. "What was your weight at your last antepartum appointment?"

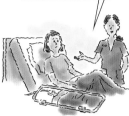

Watch out for that vena cava. If your client starts feeling light-headed while supine, it might be time to roll over.

1. 1. The nurse should determine the client's position, as these are symptoms of superior vena cava syndrome. As the enlarging uterus increases pressure on the inferior vena cava, it compromises venous return, which can cause the client to feel faint, dizzy, or light-headed when the client is supine. The nurse should then tell the client to lie on her left side to relieve the pressure on the vena cava and restore venous return. Breathing difficulties and weight gain are not related to the client's symptoms. Determining how many times the client feels this way in one day does not help the nurse determine whether the client is experiencing superior vena cava syndrome.
CN: Safe, effective care environment; CNS: Safety and infection control; CL: Apply

2. A nurse is educating a client about the signs of labor. The nurse determines the client has an accurate understanding of the instructions when the client makes which statement?
1. "I will not come to the hospital until my contractions are 1 minute apart."
2. "I will know I am in true labor if my membranes rupture."
3. "I will come to the hospital if my contractions are occurring in my abdomen."
4. "Contraction pain that goes from my back to my stomach indicates labor."

2. 4. True labor contractions move from the back to the front of the abdomen, are regular, and are not relieved by walking. False labor contractions are usually felt in the abdomen, are irregular, and are typically relieved by walking.
CN: Health promotion and maintenance; CNS: None; CL: Apply

3. Alpha-fetoprotein (AFP) testing of a client at 17 weeks' gestation with twins reveals that one twin has a high level of AFP. Which nursing intervention is appropriate for this client?
1. Schedule the client for repeat testing at 25 weeks' gestation.
2. Recommend the client terminate the pregnancy this trimester.
3. Inform the client that the results of this test are often inaccurate.
4. Provide emotional support to the client and significant other.

3. 4. The nurse should provide emotional support and answer any questions the client and significant other may have at this time. AFP testing performed from 16 to 18 weeks' gestation is highly accurate. AFP testing can be done only from 14 to 20 weeks' gestation. A high AFP level indicates a potential neural tube or esophageal defect or an unclosed fetal abdomen. The client should be scheduled for a diagnostic ultrasound to confirm the diagnosis. The nurse should not tell the client what to do, such as terminate the pregnancy.
CN: Safe, effective care environment; CNS: Management of care; CL: Apply

4. The labor and delivery nurse is admitting a 42-year-old pregnant client at 34 weeks' gestation who reports moderate amounts of painless vaginal bleeding. What will the nurse do **next**?
1. Notify the health care provider.
2. Place the client in a side-lying position.
3. Determine when the bleeding started.
4. Obtain the client's vital signs.

4. 2. The nurse should suspect that the client has a placenta previa due to the painless vaginal bleeding during the third trimester and place the client in a side-lying position to best facilitate uterine blood flow. The nurse should also obtain vital signs, determine when the bleeding started and the amount being lost, and notify the health care provider, but these are not priority.
CN: Safe, effective care environment; CNS: Management of care; CL: Analyze

CN: Client needs category   CNS: Client needs subcategory   CL: Cognitive level

5. A client with painless vaginal bleeding is suspected of having placenta previa. The nurse will assist in preparing the client for which procedure?
1. Amniocentesis
2. Speculum examination
3. External fetal monitoring
4. Ultrasound

6. A client is diagnosed with placenta previa at 24 weeks' gestation. Which education will the nurse provide to the client? Select all that apply.
1. Do not engage in sexual intercourse.
2. Call the health care provider if vaginal bleeding occurs.
3. You will be on bed rest for the rest of the pregnancy.
4. You may need to deliver via a cesarean section.
5. You need to have a non-stress test (NST) weekly.
6. Use a peri-pad if vaginal bleeding occurs, not tampons.

7. A client is diagnosed with hyperemesis gravidarum after coming to the antepartum unit with persistent vomiting, weight loss, and hypovolemia. Which assessment finding will the nurse expect with this client?
1. Presence of trophoblastic disease
2. Maternal age older than 35 years
3. History of chronic malnutrition
4. Low human chorionic gonadotropin (HCG) levels

8. A nurse is educating a client who is at 29 weeks' gestation. The nurse determines the client understands the education when she states she will **immediately** report which symptom(s)? Select all that apply.
1. Hemorrhoids
2. Blurred vision
3. Dyspnea on exertion
4. Elevated temperature
5. Increased vaginal mucus

9. The nurse will monitor which client **most** cautiously for the development of a hydatidiform mole?
1. A 17-year-old Asian client with a history of a molar gestation
2. A 26-year-old Caucasian client with a history of diabetes
3. A 30-year-old primigravida of African descent
4. A 45-year-old client of European descent pregnant with triplets

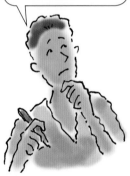

What is the best way to find out whether the placenta is implanted in the wrong spot?

5. **4.** When the mother and fetus are stabilized, ultrasound evaluation of the placenta should be done to determine the cause of the bleeding. Amniocentesis is contraindicated in placenta previa. A digital or speculum examination should not be done, as this may lead to severe bleeding or hemorrhage. External fetal monitoring cannot detect a placenta previa, although it can detect fetal distress, which may result from blood loss or placental separation.
CN: Physiological integrity; CNS: Reduction of risk potential; CL: Apply

6. **1, 2, 4, 6.** Clients with placenta previa are instructed to practice pelvic rest (nothing inserted into the vagina). The health care provider should be notified if vaginal bleeding occurs to assess the well-being of the client and fetus. A cesarean section may be indicated depending on the location of the placenta at the time of birth. The client would not have to be on bed rest or have weekly NSTs unless complications of the placenta previa developed.
CN: Physiological integrity; CNS: Reduction of risk potential; CL: Apply

7. **1.** Trophoblastic disease is associated with hyperemesis gravidarum. Obesity and maternal age younger than 20 years are risk factors for developing hyperemesis gravidarum. Malnutrition has no association with hyperemesis gravidarum. High levels of estrogen and HCG, not low, have been associated with hyperemesis.
CN: Physiological integrity; CNS: Reduction of risk potential; CL: Apply

8. **2, 4.** During pregnancy, blurred vision may be a danger sign of preeclampsia or eclampsia, complications that require immediate attention because they can cause severe maternal and fetal consequences. An elevated temperature could indicate an infection, which can lead to fetal complications. Although hemorrhoids may occur during pregnancy, they do not require immediate attention. Dyspnea on exertion and increased vaginal mucus are common discomforts caused by the physiologic changes of pregnancy.
CN: Safe, effective care environment; CNS: Management of care; CL: Apply

9. **1.** A previous molar gestation increases a woman's risk for developing a subsequent molar gestation by four to five times. Women who are of Asian descent, younger than 15 years, or older than 45 years are also at increased risk for molar pregnancies. Primigravida status, diabetes, and multiple fetuses are not risk factors for molar pregnancies.
CN: Safe, effective care environment; CNS: Management of care; CL: Apply

10. The nurse is caring for a client at 9 weeks' gestation with a history of a hydatidiform mole. Which finding(s) will the nurse report to the health care provider as indicative of another hydatidiform mole? Select all that apply.
1. Heavy, bright red bleeding
2. Absence of a fetal heart tone
3. Dense growth noted on an ultrasound
4. Fundus felt 3 cm above the symphysis pubis
5. High human chorionic gonadotropin (HCG) levels

10. **2, 3, 4, 5.** Clients with a hydatidiform mole do not have a fetal heart tone, as there is no fetus. Dense growth is noted on an ultrasound, and the chorionic villi of a molar pregnancy often resemble a "snowstorm" pattern. The uterus expands more quickly than expected due to the rapid growth of trophoblast cells, therefore reaching fundal landmarks more quickly than expected. HCG levels are also exceedingly high. Heavy, bright red bleeding would need to be reported, but not as indicating a molar pregnancy. Bleeding with a hydatidiform mole is generally dark brown and may be accompanied by clear fluid-filled vesicles.
CN: Physiological integrity; CNS: Reduction of risk potential; CL: Analyze

11. The nurse is caring for a 26-year-old client who is reporting abdominal cramping and vaginal spotting. During the assessment, the nurse notes a blood pressure reading of 90/56 mm Hg, pulse rate of 119 beats/minute, rigid abdomen, and Cullen's sign. What will the nurse do **next**?
1. Administer an intravenous (IV) bolus.
2. Monitor the client's hemoglobin level.
3. Check the client's oxygen saturation level.
4. Immediately notify the health care provider.

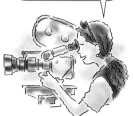

Looking good! You're putting on quite a performance.

11. **1.** The nurse should suspect that the client has a ruptured ectopic pregnancy. The client has symptoms consistent with substantial blood loss and would need intravenous fluids first to quickly replenish circulating volume. The nurse should subsequently perform the other interventions after starting the IV bolus.
CN: Safe, effective care environment; CNS: Management of care; CL: Analyze

12. A client who is at 38 weeks' gestation presents to labor and delivery with severe abdominal pain and vaginal bleeding after being physically assaulted by her significant other. The nurse places external monitors on the client and notes a fetal heart rate of 100 beats/minute and uterine contractions every 5 minutes, with a resting tone of 30 mm Hg. What will the nurse do **next**?
1. Obtain the client's vital signs.
2. Administer intravenous butorphanol.
3. Notify the local law enforcement agency.
4. Give pamphlets on intimate partner violence.

12. **1.** To help determine the amount of blood lost, the nurse should assess the client's vital signs. A client experiencing a placental abruption may present with uterine tenderness, abdominal pain, vaginal bleeding, a rigid abdomen, uterine contractions, and an increased uterine resting tone. A uterine tone greater than 20 mm Hg requires evaluation. The fetus would start to show signs of distress, with decelerations in the heart rate or even fetal death with a large placental separation. Administering pain medication and providing education are not priority concerns. The nurse would only contact law enforcement if the client requested.
CN: Physiological integrity; CNS: Reduction of risk potential; CL: Apply

13. The nurse reviews the results of a female client's lab work, shown in the chart exhibit below. Based on the findings, what diagnosis does the nurse expect for this client?

Test	Result
Human chorionic gonadotropin (HCG)	1400 mIU/mL (1400 IU/L)
Luteinizing hormone (LH)	1.0 mIU/mL (1.0 IU/L)
Follicle stimulating hormone (FSH)	3.5 mIU/mL (3.5 IU/L)
Progesterone	11.2 ng/mL (35.62 nmol/L)

1. Subfertility
2. Pregnancy
3. Polycystic ovarian syndrome
4. Gestational trophoblastic disease

13. **2.** The client's hormone levels indicate the client is pregnant. HCG levels greater than 25 mIU/mL (greater than 25 IU/L), LH levels less than 1.5 mIU/mL (less than 1.5 IU/L), FSH levels from 3 to 10 mIU/mL (3 to 10 IU/L), and elevated progesterone levels—11.2 to 90 ng/mL (35.62 to 286.20 nmol/L)—are indicative of pregnancy, not of subfertility, polycystic ovarian syndrome, or gestational trophoblastic disease.
CN: Health promotion and maintenance; CNS: None; CL: Apply

CN: Client needs category   CNS: Client needs subcategory   CL: Cognitive level

14. The registered nurse (RN) and an assistive personnel (AP) are preparing a 16 weeks' gestation client for an amniocentesis. Which intervention is **most** appropriate for the RN to delegate to the AP?
  1. Monitor the fetal heart rate.
  2. Tell the client about the procedure.
  3. Determine the client's rhesus factor.
  4. Assist the client to the bathroom to void.

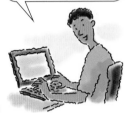

Remember—amniocentesis involves inserting a needle into the client's uterus to remove amniotic fluid from very near the bladder.

15. A client at 27 weeks' gestation arrives at the clinic reporting fever, nausea, vomiting, malaise, unilateral flank pain, and costovertebral angle tenderness. Which nursing intervention is **most** appropriate?
  1. Determine if this is the client's first pregnancy.
  2. Send a vaginal specimen to the lab.
  3. Provide education on pyelonephritis.
  4. Obtain urine for a culture.

16. A pregnant client presents with tiny, blanched, slightly raised arterioles on her face, neck, arms, and chest. Which nursing action is **most** appropriate?
  1. Tell the client to see a dermatologist.
  2. Place the client in strict isolation.
  3. Notify the health care provider.
  4. Document the findings in the client's chart.

17. A nurse is collecting data as part of an initial history on a pregnant client. The client asks about the chances of having dizygotic twins. Which statement by the nurse about dizygotic twins is **most** accurate?
  1. They occur most frequently in women of Asian descent.
  2. There is a decreased risk with increased parity.
  3. There is an increased risk with increased maternal age.
  4. Use of fertility drugs poses no additional risk.

18. The nurse is caring for a 10 weeks' gestation client with hyperemesis gravidarum. The client has vomited 5 times over the past 2 hours. Which order is **priority** for the nurse to complete?
  1. Give lactated Ringer's IV.
  2. Perform daily weights.
  3. Monitor intake and output.
  4. Administer ondansetron 4 mg PRN nausea.

14. 4. It would be most appropriate for the AP to assist the client to void. Before an amniocentesis, the client should void to empty the bladder, reducing the risk of bladder perforation. The RN cannot delegate monitoring fetal heart tones or educating clients. The RN, not the AP, should review the client's medical records to assess the client's rhesus factor and for any potential complications.
CN: Safe, effective care environment; CNS: Management of care; CL: Analyze

15. 3. The symptoms indicate acute pyelonephritis, a serious condition in a pregnant client. The nurse will notify the health care provider and provide education to the client. Determining the client's obstetrical history is not necessary at this time as it does not relate to the symptoms. The client's symptoms do not include vaginal discharge or urinary symptoms; therefore, vaginal and urine specimens are not indicated.
CN: Physiological integrity; CNS: Reduction of risk potential; CL: Apply

16. 4. Dilated arterioles that occur during pregnancy are due to the elevated level of circulating estrogen and are called telangiectasias. Telangiectasias are very common during pregnancy and generally disappear within weeks after birth. The client does not need a referral or to be placed in isolation as this is a very common condition during pregnancy and not contagious. Since these are common, the health care provider does not need to be notified.
CN: Health promotion and maintenance; CNS: None; CL: Apply

17. 3. Dizygotic twinning is influenced by race (most frequent in women of African descent and least frequent in women of Asian descent), age (increased risk with increased maternal age), parity (increased risk with increased parity), and fertility drugs (increased risk with the use of fertility drugs, especially ovulation-inducing drugs). The incidence of monozygotic twins is not affected by race, age, parity, heredity, or fertility medications.
CN: Health promotion and maintenance; CNS: None; CL: Understand

18. 1. Excessive vomiting in clients with hyperemesis gravidarum commonly causes weight loss and fluid, electrolyte, and acid–base imbalances. Administering IV fluids to restore hydration and increase fetal perfusion is priority for this client. The nurse would then administer ondansetron as needed followed by monitoring intake and output and weights.
CN: Safe, effective care environment; CNS: Management of care; CL: Analyze

19. The nurse is reviewing the laboratory data, shown in the chart exhibit below, for a client who is 24 weeks' gestation. Which result(s) will the nurse report to the health care provider? Select all that apply.

Hemoglobin	8 g/dL (80 g/L)
Hematocrit	31% (0.31)
White blood cell count	12,000 mm³ (12 × 10⁹/L)
Platelet count	250,000 mm³ (250 × 10⁹/L)
Fasting glucose	110 mg/dL (6.1 mmol/L)

1. Hemoglobin
2. Hematocrit
3. White blood cell count
4. Platelet count
5. Fasting glucose

19. 1, 2. The nurse should report the hemoglobin and hematocrit results. The client's levels are indicative of anemia. All other laboratory values are within normal range for a pregnant client. White blood cell count rises during pregnancy to compensate for the pregnant woman's decreased immune response.

CN: Safe, effective care environment; CNS: Management of care; CL: Analyze

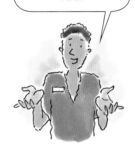

Glucose level is like a golf score ... try to keep it under 100.

20. The nurse is educating a client just diagnosed with gestational diabetes. The nurse will plan to educate the client on which treatment method as the primary intervention?
1. Diabetic diet regimen
2. Subcutaneous insulin
3. Oral hypoglycemic agents
4. Daily exercise routines

20. 1. Clients with gestational diabetes are usually managed by diet alone to control their glucose intolerance. Insulin usually is not needed for blood glucose control in the client with gestational diabetes. Oral hypoglycemic drugs are contraindicated in pregnancy. Exercise may be recommended to assist with diet control but would be secondary to it.

CN: Safe, effective care environment; CNS: Management of care; CL: Apply

21. While caring for a 32 weeks' gestation client diagnosed with preeclampsia, the nurse reviews the report from the nurse on the previous shift, shown below. Which finding will the nurse report to the health care provider **immediately**?

Progress notes	
11/25	Client reported not feeling well, blurred
1750	vision, headache, and "seeing spots."
	Upon assessment, vital signs were:
	temperature, 98.9° F (37.2° C); blood
	pressure, 168/118 mm Hg; heart rate,
	120 beats/min; respiratory rate,
	20 breaths/min. No contractions were noted.
	Fetal heart rate was 120 beats/min
	with moderate variability. Client had a grand
	mal seizure and diazepam 5 mg given IV
	slowly. Client is resting in bed following
	seizure.
	— L. Roman, RN

1. Respiratory rate
2. Occurrence of seizure
3. Fetal heart rate
4. "Seeing spots"

21. 2. The nurse should report the occurrence of seizure immediately to the health care provider. The client's status has changed to eclampsia. The primary difference between preeclampsia and eclampsia is the occurrence of seizures, which occur when the client develops eclampsia. Headaches, blurred vision, weight gain, increased blood pressure, and edema of the hands and feet are all indicative of preeclampsia. The client's respirations and fetal heart rate are within normal range.

CN: Safe, effective care environment; CNS: Safety and infection control; CL: Apply

CN: Client needs category   CNS: Client needs subcategory   CL: Cognitive level

22. While assessing a pregnant client, the nurse notes the following: blood pressure 158/96 mm Hg, pulse rate 89 beats/minute, respiratory rate 22 breaths/minute, O_2 saturation level 96% on room air, and a reading of 3+ on a urine dipstick for protein. Which order will the nurse anticipate from the health care provider?
1. Administer magnesium sulfate IV.
2. Administer oral nifedipine.
3. Insert an indwelling Foley catheter.
4. Apply oxygen via a nasal cannula.

23. The nurse is monitoring a pregnant client during an oxytocin challenge test (OCT). The nurse notes moderate fetal heart rate variability and no decelerations in a 10-minute period during which the client experienced three contractions. What will the nurse do?
1. Notify the health care provider.
2. Prepare the client for a cesarean birth.
3. Continue the OCT for another 10 minutes.
4. Document the results in the medical record.

24. A pregnant client at 12 weeks' gestation comes to the clinic for a follow-up visit and tells the nurse she is "feeling really constipated." Which nursing response(s) is appropriate? Select all that apply.
1. "Make sure that you attempt to move your bowels regularly."
2. "Try increasing the amount of fruits and vegetables in your diet."
3. "Be sure to increase the amount of fluids that you drink each day."
4. "Use mineral oil as a gentle laxative to get things moving."
5. "An enema once a week should give you adequate relief."

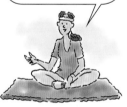

What do pregnant women and nurses have in common? A need to relax and de-stress.

25. A 31-week-gestation client with preeclampsia is receiving an intravenous infusion of magnesium sulfate. The nurse's assessment findings are in the chart exhibit below. Which order will the nurse complete **first**?

Progress notes	
5/15	Client is lying in bed, with minimal response to
1348	verbal stimuli. Fetal heart rate is 133 beats/min
	with moderate variability. No contractions are
	noted. Vital signs: temperature, 100.6° F (38.1° C);
	blood pressure, 110/64 mm Hg; heart rate,
	52 beats/min; respiratory rate, 8 breaths/min.
	Deep tendon reflexes (DTRs) are 0. Urine
	output is 95 mL in the last 6 hours.

1. Give 500 mg acetaminophen orally.
2. Insert an indwelling Foley catheter.
3. Give 1 g calcium gluconate intravenously.
4. Administer 12 mg betamethasone intramuscularly.

22. 1. The nurse should anticipate the health care provider ordering magnesium sulfate for preeclampsia. Magnesium sulfate is believed to depress seizure foci in the brain and peripheral neuromuscular blockade, thus preventing eclampsia. Hydralazine and labetalol are generally prescribed before nifedipine for hypertension. A Foley catheter and oxygen are not needed for this client.

CN: Physiological integrity; CNS: Pharmacological and parenteral therapies; CL: Apply

23. 4. The nurse should document the results of the client's normal OCT. An OCT measures the fetal response to uterine contractions. For a normal OCT, a client must have three contractions in a 10-minute period with moderate fetal heart rate variability and no decelerations from uterine contractions. There are no indications to call the health care provider, prepare for a cesarean section, or continue the OCT.

CN: Health promotion and maintenance; CNS: None; CL: Apply

24. 1, 2, 3. For constipation during pregnancy, appropriate suggestions would include making sure to attempt to move one's bowels regularly (i.e., making time to have a bowel movement), ingesting more foods high in fiber (such as fruits and vegetables), and increasing the amount of fluid ingested each day. Mineral oil interferes with the absorption of fat-soluble vitamins and should be avoided. Enemas also should be avoided during pregnancy.

CN: Physiological integrity; CNS: Basic care and comfort; CL: Apply

25. 3. The client is exhibiting signs of magnesium toxicity. Calcium gluconate is the antidote for magnesium toxicity and should be administered immediately to increase the client's respiratory rate, DTRs, and urine output. All other orders would be completed after the client is stabilized.

CN: Physiological integrity; CNS: Pharmacological and parenteral therapies; CL: Analyze

26. The nurse is gathering information from the chart of a pregnant client. Which finding is **least** concerning to the nurse?
1. Cardiac tamponade
2. Heart failure
3. Endocarditis
4. Systolic murmur

27. A client with preeclampsia is prescribed magnesium sulfate. The nurse is reviewing the results of the client's serum magnesium level and determines the client's level is therapeutic based on which result?
1. 6.8 mEq/L (3.4 mmol/L)
2. 9.2 mEq/L (4.6 mmol/L)
3. 11.5 mEq/L (5.75 mmol/L)
4. 16 mEq/L (8 mmol/L)

28. The nurse is caring for multiple preeclamptic clients, all receiving magnesium sulfate intravenously. Which assessment finding(s) will the nurse report to the health care provider? Select all that apply.
1. Reports of epigastric pain
2. 35 mL of urine output in 2 hours
3. 4+ deep tendon reflexes (DTRs)
4. Respiratory rate of 8 breaths/minute
5. Platelet level of 100,000 mm³ (100 × 10⁹/L)

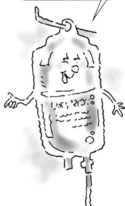

When you're administering me, get ready for a lot of trips to the bathroom.

29. A pregnant client is screened for varicella and rubella immunity during her first prenatal visit. The results are equivocal for both varicella and rubella. Which statement will the nurse include in the client's education?
1. "You will receive the varicella and rubella vaccinations during the last trimester."
2. "You are immune to both varicella and rubella, so no additional vaccinations are needed."
3. "You should receive both vaccinations while you are in the hospital after your birth."
4. "You can get the varicella vaccination now and the rubella after you deliver your baby."

26. 4. Systolic murmur is heard in up to 90% of pregnant clients, and the murmur disappears soon after the birth. Cardiac tamponade, which causes effusion of fluid into the pericardial sac, is not normal during pregnancy. Despite the increases in intravascular volume and workload of the heart associated with pregnancy, heart failure is not normal in pregnancy. Endocarditis is most commonly associated with IV drug use and is not a normal finding in pregnancy.
CN: Health promotion and maintenance; CNS: None; CL: Apply

27. 1. The therapeutic level of magnesium for clients with preeclampsia ranges from 3 to 7 mEq/L (1.5 to 3.5 mmol/L). A serum magnesium level of 8 to 10 mEq/L (4 to 5 mmol/L) may cause the absence of reflexes in the client. Serum levels of 10 to 12 mEq/L (5 to 6 mmol/L) may cause respiratory depression. Serum levels of magnesium greater than 15 mEq/L (7.5 mmol/L) may result in respiratory paralysis, and serum levels greater than 25 mEq/L (12.5 mmol/L) may result in cardiopulmonary arrest.
CN: Physiological integrity; CNS: Pharmacological and parenteral therapies; CL: Understand

28. 1, 2, 3, 4, 5. The nurse should report all findings as all are abnormal. Epigastric pain and thrombocytopenia could indicate that the client is experiencing HELLP syndrome. Magnesium is excreted through the kidneys, so a decreased urine output may result in retention of magnesium, which can accumulate to toxic levels. Urine output should be monitored closely and be greater than 30 mL/h. Magnesium infusions may cause depression of DTRs, not hyperreflexia. A client with 4+ DTRs is at high risk of having a seizure. Respiratory depression can occur when serum magnesium levels reach approximately 10 mEq/L (5 mmol/L).
CN: Physiological integrity; CNS: Pharmacological and parenteral therapies; CL: Analyze

29. 3. An equivocal result is one that is inconclusive; in such cases, the client should be assumed to be nonimmune and in need of the vaccinations. The client should be offered the vaccinations following birth to assist in protecting the woman and any future fetuses. Varicella and rubella vaccinations should not be administered to a pregnant client because the fetus would be at risk from exposure to the viruses as these vaccinations contain live, weakened virus strands.
CN: Health promotion and maintenance; CNS: None; CL: Apply

CN: Client needs category   CNS: Client needs subcategory   CL: Cognitive level

30. A nurse is teaching a group of pregnant adolescents about the anatomy and physiology of reproduction. The nurse determines that the teaching was effective when the adolescents correctly identify the area where fertilization occurs. Mark the correct area on the illustration.

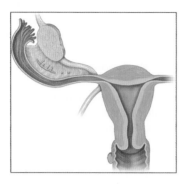

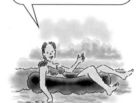

Floating around in a warm, comfortable environment with not a care in the world … life as a fetus sounds pretty good!

30. After ejaculation, the sperm travel by flagellar movement through the fluids of the cervical mucus into the fallopian tube to meet the descending ovum in the ampulla, where fertilization occurs.

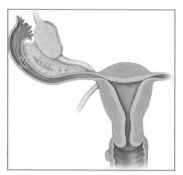

CN: Health promotion and maintenance; CNS: None; CL: Apply

31. The nurse is educating a 27-week-gestation client whose blood type is A-negative. The nurse notes the following prescription for the client: Rho(D) immune globulin to be administered subcutaneously. Which action will the nurse complete **first**?
1. Administer Rho(D) immune globulin as prescribed.
2. Contact the health care provider for clarification.
3. Obtain consent from the client for the medication.
4. Educate the client on the medication.

31. 2. Rho(D) is given intramuscularly, not subcutaneously. The nurse would first contact the health care provider to clarify the prescription. After the prescription is corrected, the nurse would educate the client, obtain consent, and administer the medication.

CN: Safe, effective care environment; CNS: Safety and infection control; CL: Analyze

32. A pregnant client develops iron-deficiency anemia and is prescribed supplemental iron along with prenatal vitamins. After reviewing possible adverse effects of iron supplementation with the client, the nurse determines the education was successful when the client identifies which adverse effect(s)? Select all that apply.
1. Gastric upset
2. Bright red blood in stools
3. Constipation
4. Anorexia
5. Metallic taste
6. Nausea and vomiting

32. 1, 3, 4, 5, 6. Adverse effects of iron supplementation include gastric upset, nausea, vomiting, anorexia, diarrhea, metallic taste, and constipation. Typically, iron makes stools appear black and tarry. Bright red blood in the stools is not associated with iron therapy.

CN: Physiological integrity; CNS: Pharmacological and parenteral therapies; CL: Apply

33. A client at 30 weeks' gestation is hospitalized for preterm labor. The nurse notes contractions of varying frequency, occurring every 10 to 25 minutes, and a fetal heart rate of 148 beats/minute. Which nursing intervention is **most** appropriate?
1. Administer oxytocin at 1 mU/min.
2. Place the client on bed rest.
3. Give intravenous and oral fluids.
4. Perform intermittent fetal and contraction monitoring.

Supplemental iron helps treat anemia but can cause adverse effects. That's what I call iron-y.

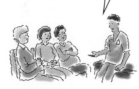

33. 3. Adequate hydration may help decrease or stop labor contractions. Administering oxytocin would promote contractions. Bed rest may help decrease contractions but is not supported by strong evidence. The fetus and client should be monitored continuously, not intermittently.

CN: Physiological integrity; CNS: Reduction of risk potential; CL: Apply

34. A pregnant woman provides the nurse with the following obstetrical history: she delivered a daughter, now 14 years old, at 41 weeks' gestation; delivered a son, now 12 years old, at 39 weeks' gestation; and had an abortion at 10 weeks' gestation 5 years ago. Which listing will the nurse document to portray the client's gravity and parity?
1. G4 P2012
2. G3 P2012
3. G4 P2102
4. G3 P0213

34. 1. Gravida refers to the number of times a client has been pregnant; para refers to the number of viable children born. GTPAL, meaning gravida, term, preterm, abortion, and living, is a more comprehensive system that gives information about each infant from prior pregnancies. This client has been pregnant three previous times and is currently pregnant, for a total gravida of 4. She has delivered 2 term babies and no preterm babies, had 1 abortion, and has 2 living children.
CN: Health promotion and maintenance; CNS: None; CL: Analyze

35. A client is diagnosed with an unruptured ectopic pregnancy. Which medication will the nurse expect to administer to the client?
1. Methotrexate
2. Labetalol
3. Magnesium sulfate
4. Indomethacin

Some of these conditions in question #36 are notorious for increasing the risk for complications. Can you remember which ones?

35. 1. Unruptured ectopic pregnancies can be treated with medication therapy, most commonly methotrexate. Labetalol is used to treat hypertension. Magnesium sulfate is used to treat preeclampsia and eclampsia. Indomethacin would be used to slow contractions of preterm labor.
CN: Physiological integrity; CNS: Pharmacological and parenteral therapies; CL: Apply

36. The nurse is performing the initial interview on a client at 7 weeks' gestation. Which finding(s) increase the client's risk for perinatal complications? Select all that apply.
1. The client is 45 years old.
2. The client is a G2 P1.
3. The client has type 1 diabetes.
4. The client is employed as a welder.
5. The client had a molar pregnancy.
6. The fetal heart rate is 158 beats/minute.

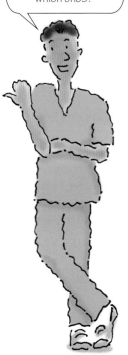

36. 1, 3, 4, 5. Advanced maternal age, a history of diabetes, frequent exposure to high heat (welder), and a history of a gestational trophoblastic disease all increase the risk for perinatal complications. This client would need to be closely monitored throughout the pregnancy. Low gravida and a fetal heart rate of 158 are not risk factors.
CN: Safe, effective care environment; CNS: Management of care; CL: Analyze

37. The nurse is caring for a client at 39 weeks' gestation. When the client was admitted 8 hours ago, she was having contractions every 12 to 15 minutes and her cervix was 4 cm dilated. She is now having contractions every 8 to 10 minutes, and her cervix is 5 cm dilated. The nurse will anticipate which prescription from the health care provider?
1. Monitor contractions intermittently.
2. Insert an in-and-out catheter.
3. Administer butorphanol intravenously.
4. Start oxytocin intravenously at 1 mU/minute.

37. 4. The nurse should anticipate oxytocin being prescribed to augment labor. Oxytocin is the hormone responsible for stimulating uterine contractions and may be given to clients to induce or augment uterine contractions. The nurse should expect to monitor contractions continuously, not intermittently, because the client is not progressing well. A full bladder can hinder uterine contractions, but the client should be allowed to void if possible. Butorphanol is for pain, and the client has not expressed pain.
CN: Physiological integrity; CNS: Pharmacological and parenteral therapies; CL: Apply

38. A client, 8 weeks' pregnant, comes to the emergency department with reports of severe, stabbing, lower abdominal pain. The nurse will suspect the client has a ruptured ectopic pregnancy based on which finding(s)? Select all that apply.
1. Thready, rapid pulse
2. Increased blood pressure
3. Scant vaginal bleeding
4. Abdominal tenderness with distention
5. Referred shoulder pain

38. 1, 3, 4, 5. Signs and symptoms associated with an ectopic pregnancy include a rapid, thready pulse and decreased blood pressure due to internal bleeding, scant vaginal bleeding, abdominal tenderness with distention, and referred shoulder pain due to irritation of the phrenic nerve.
CN: Physiological integrity; CNS: Physiological adaptation; CL: Apply

CN: Client needs category   CNS: Client needs subcategory   CL: Cognitive level

39. A client at 34 weeks' gestation has come to the clinic for a routine checkup. Which education is appropriate for the nurse to provide to the client? Select all that apply.
1. Signs of true labor versus false labor
2. Use of the left side-lying position
3. How to perform fetal kick counts
4. Forms of permanent birth control
5. What to do if client's membranes rupture

40. A pregnant client calls the clinic and states, "I am not sure my fetus has moved much today and I am worried." Which nursing response is **most** appropriate?
1. "You need to drink a caffeinated beverage to get the baby to start moving."
2. "Eating cold foods, such as ice cream or frozen yogurt, should stimulate the fetus to move."
3. "Lie down and count your baby's movements. You should feel at least 4 movements per hour."
4. "Do not worry. When you are busy, it is easy to not know whether your baby has moved much."

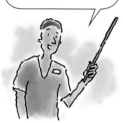

Helping your client become more attuned to fetal movement can help calm fears.

41. The nurse is caring for a 15-year-old client at 9 weeks' gestation. Which nursing intervention is **priority**?
1. Schedule the client for a maternal serum alpha-fetoprotein screening.
2. Educate the client on nutritional needs during pregnancy.
3. Teach the client about signs of true labor versus false labor.
4. Monitor the fetus for signs and symptoms of chromosomal anomalies.

42. A client in her early second trimester tells the nurse she is experiencing a significant amount of pyrosis. Which recommendation(s) is appropriate for the nurse to provide? Select all that apply.
1. Eat small, frequent meals.
2. Eat crackers before getting out of bed.
3. Drink a preparation of salt and vinegar.
4. Drink orange juice frequently.
5. Keep the head of the bed elevated.
6. Consume spicy and fatty foods.

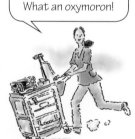

"Non-stress test"? What an oxymoron!

43. A client is scheduled to undergo a non-stress test (NST) and asks the nurse why this test is being performed. Which nursing response is **most** appropriate?
1. "NSTs detect fetal genetic anomalies."
2. "NSTs determine contraction frequency."
3. "NSTs are done to check placental function."
4. "NSTs monitor fetal well-being."

39. 1, 2, 3, 5. During the third trimester, it is appropriate for the nurse to educate the client on signs of true labor, correct positions to best facilitate placental blood flow, how to monitor fetal well-being, and what to do if her amniotic membranes rupture. This is not the best time to discuss permanent birth control unless the client specifically requests this information, as the client is overwhelmed with preparing for labor and the arrival of a new baby.
CN: Health promotion and maintenance; CNS: None; CL: Apply

40. 3. The nurse should have the woman perform fetal kick count measurements. Instructing the client to lie down allows her to concentrate on detecting fetal movement. If the woman does not feel the fetus move appropriately, she would need to come to the office. Consuming a caffeinated beverage or cold foods is not an appropriate method to monitor fetal well-being. Telling the client not to worry is not therapeutic.
CN: Psychosocial integrity; CNS: None; CL: Apply

41. 2. Nutritional counseling must be emphasized as part of the prenatal care for adolescent clients. Adolescents need to meet nutritional needs for this rapid period of growth and development. The needs are further increased due to the pregnancy. Maternal serum alpha-fetoprotein screening is done from 14 to 20 weeks' gestation. Signs of true labor and monitoring for anomalies are not priority during the first trimester.
CN: Safe, effective care environment; CNS: Management of care; CL: Apply

42. 1, 5. Eating small, frequent meals and keeping the head of the bed elevated place less pressure on the esophageal sphincter, reducing the likelihood of the regurgitation of stomach contents into the lower esophagus. Eating crackers, drinking a salt and vinegar solution, drinking orange juice, and consuming spicy and fatty foods have not been shown to decrease heartburn.
CN: Physiological integrity; CNS: Basic care and comfort; CL: Apply

43. 4. An NST is based on the theory that a healthy fetus has transient fetal heart rate accelerations with fetal movement. An NST cannot detect genetic anomalies in a fetus, contraction frequency, or placental function.
CN: Physiological integrity; CNS: Reduction of risk potential; CL: Apply

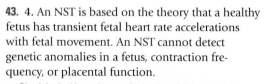

44. The nurse will monitor an obese pregnant client closely for the development of which condition?
1. Hyperemesis gravidarum
2. Placenta previa
3. Preeclampsia
4. Incompetent cervix

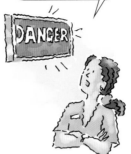

Obesity is a critical risk factor for a serious blood pressure–related condition.

44. 3. The incidence of preeclampsia in obese clients is significantly greater than in pregnant clients who are not obese. Hyperemesis gravidarum, placenta previa, and an incompetent cervix are not associated with increased incidence in pregnant clients who are obese.
CN: Safe, effective care environment; CNS: Management of care; CL: Apply

45. A pregnant client is diagnosed with gestational diabetes. When reviewing the client's fasting blood glucose levels, which value indicates to the nurse the client's disease is controlled?
1. 45 mg/dL (2.5 mmol/L)
2. 85 mg/dL (4.7 mmol/L)
3. 120 mg/dL (6.67 mmol/L)
4. 136 mg/dL (7.56 mmol/L)

45. 2. The recommended fasting blood glucose level in the pregnant client with diabetes is 60 to 95 mg/dL (3.33 to 5.28 mmol/L). A fasting blood glucose level of 45 mg/dL (2.5 mmol/L) is low and may result in symptoms of hypoglycemia. A blood glucose level below 120 mg/dL (6.67 mmol/L) is recommended for 2-hour postprandial values. A blood glucose level above 136 mg/dL (7.56 mmol/L) in a pregnant client indicates hyperglycemia.
CN: Health promotion and maintenance; CNS: None; CL: Apply

46. The nurse is reviewing the non-stress test (NST) results of a 38-week-gestation client with gestational diabetes. The 20-minute NST strip showed three fetal heart rate accelerations that exceeded the baseline by 15 beats/minute and lasted longer than 15 seconds. What will the nurse do?
1. Continue the NST for an additional 20 minutes.
2. Apply an acoustic stimulator to the woman's abdomen.
3. Document the results as normal in the client's medical record.
4. Notify the health care provider immediately of the results.

46. 3. The results are normal; therefore, the nurse would document the results. A normal finding on a non-stress test is two or more fetal heart rate accelerations that exceed baseline by at least 15 beats/min and last longer than 15 seconds within a 20-minute period. A lack of accelerations in the fetal heart rate with fetal movement over a 40-minute timeframe would be an abnormal finding on an NST. An acoustic stimulator is used if the fetus is not moving appropriately.
CN: Physiological integrity; CNS: Reduction of risk potential CL: Apply

47. A client is pregnant with triplets. The nurse will educate the client about the signs and symptoms of which potential complication(s)? Select all that apply.
1. Placenta previa
2. Preterm labor
3. Anemia
4. Hypertension of pregnancy
5. Hydatidiform mole

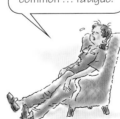

Another thing pregnant women and nurses have in common … fatigue!

47. 1, 2, 3, 4. Women with multifetal pregnancies are at greater risk for complications such as hypertension of pregnancy, placenta previa, preterm labor, and anemia. They are not considered to be at greater risk for the development of a hydatidiform mole.
CN: Physiological integrity; CNS: Reduction of risk potential; CL: Apply

48. A client at 28 weeks' gestation undergoes a 3-hour glucose tolerance test. The nurse will flag which result for the health care provider?
1. A fasting glucose level of 90 mg/dL (5 mmol/L)
2. A 1-hour glucose level of 170 mg/dL (9.44 mmol/L)
3. A 2-hour glucose level of 140 mg/dL (7.78 mmol/L)
4. A 3-hour glucose level of 155 mg/dL (8.61 mmol/L)

48. 4. The nurse would flag the 3-hour glucose level. Gestational diabetes is diagnosed when a 3-hour glucose tolerance test has two abnormal values. The normal glucose values are: fasting ≤ 95 mg/dL (5.27 mmol/L), 1-hour ≤ 180 mg/dL (10 mmol/L), 2-hour ≤ 155 mg/dL (8.61 mmol/L), 3-hour ≤ 140 mg/dL (7.78 mmol/L).
CN: Safe, effective care environment; CNS: Management of care; CL: Apply

49. A client who is 15 weeks' pregnant admits to using cocaine. Which condition will the nurse closely monitor the client for?
1. Abruptio placentae
2. Gestational diabetes
3. Placenta previa
4. Anemia

50. A client comes to the clinic for a follow-up visit and reports swelling in her feet and ankles. Which nursing response is **most** appropriate?
1. "You should only drink two 8-ounce glasses of water a day."
2. "You need to take at least two breaks a day to elevate your feet."
3. "Take a furosemide tablet daily to see if that relieves the swelling."
4. "Feet and ankle swelling is not concerning as it is normal during pregnancy."

51. The nurse is ordering a meal tray for a client at 32 weeks' gestation diagnosed with preeclampsia. Which meal is **best** for the nurse to order the client?
1. Grilled chicken breast, side salad, and pineapple chunks
2. Tomato soup, grilled cheese sandwich, and apple slices
3. Sushi, roasted potatoes with ranch topping, and an orange
4. Rare steak, macaroni and cheese, and a cluster of grapes

52. A pregnant client in the second trimester is scheduled for an amniocentesis. What will the nurse do to prepare the client for the procedure? Select all that apply.
1. Ask the client to void.
2. Have the client drink 1 L of fluid.
3. Ask the client to lie on her left side.
4. Assess the fetal heart rate.
5. Insert an intravenous catheter.
6. Monitor maternal vital signs.

53. A woman with acquired immunodeficiency syndrome (AIDS) is pregnant. She tells the nurse she is concerned her baby will be born with AIDS. Which response by the nurse is **most** appropriate?
1. "Unfortunately, your baby will most likely be infected with the virus."
2. "It is very important for you to take your medications to reduce the baby's risk."
3. "As long as you agree to have a cesarean birth, your baby will be fine."
4. "It is important to keep your viral load up as much as possible."

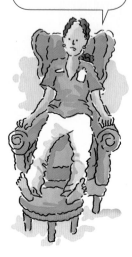

I wish someone would tell me to put my feet up and rest a while.

49. 1. The use of cocaine greatly increases the client's chance of developing abruptio placentae. The client is not at a higher risk for developing gestational diabetes, placenta previa, or anemia.
CN: Safe, effective care environment; CNS: Management of care; CL: Apply

50. 2. Sitting down and putting the feet up at least twice daily helps to promote venous return in the pregnant client and, therefore, decrease edema. Limiting fluid intake is not recommended unless there are additional medical complications such as heart failure. Diuretics are not recommended during pregnancy because it is important to maintain adequate circulatory volume. Telling the client this is a normal finding is correct but does not address the client's concern or provide relief.
CN: Physiological integrity; CNS: Basic care and comfort; CL: Apply

51. 1. The best meal for a pregnant client with preeclampsia is one that is high in protein and low in sodium. Tomato soup, cheese, and ranch dressing are high in sodium. Sushi and rare cooked meats should not be consumed during pregnancy due to the risk of coliform bacteria, toxoplasmosis, and salmonella.
CN: Physiological integrity; CNS: Basic care and comfort; CL: Analyze

52. 1, 4, 6. To prepare a client for amniocentesis, the nurse should ask her to empty her bladder to reduce the risk of bladder perforation. Before the procedure, the nurse should also assess the fetal heart rate and maternal vital signs to establish baselines. The client should be asked to drink 1 L of fluid before a transabdominal ultrasound, not amniocentesis. The client should be supine during an amniocentesis; afterward, she should be placed on her left side to avoid supine hypotension, promote venous return, and ensure adequate cardiac output. Intravenous access is not necessary for this procedure.
CN: Safe, effective care environment; CNS: Safety and infection control; CL: Apply

53. 2. Drug therapy is an important part of treatment for pregnant women with AIDS to reduce the woman's viral load as much as possible, thus decreasing the risk of transmission to the fetus. Although cesarean birth performed before the onset of labor and rupture of membranes aids in reducing the risk of perinatal transmission, it alone does not reduce the risk of transmission to the fetus. The baby may or may not become infected with the virus. The key is reducing, not increasing, the woman's viral load.
CN: Psychosocial integrity; CNS: None; CL: Apply

CN: Client needs category   CNS: Client needs subcategory   CL: Cognitive level

54. The nurse is discussing nutrition with a primigravida. The client states that she knows calcium is important during pregnancy, but she and her family do not consume many milk or dairy products. Which nursing statement is appropriate for this client?

1. "Prenatal vitamins satisfy all dietary requirements."
2. "You can take 1,800 mg of over-the-counter calcium tablets daily."
3. "You need to consume other nondairy foods that are high in calcium."
4. "Calcium is not as important after 14 weeks of pregnancy."

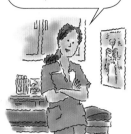

Congratulations! You've delivered another healthy test performance.

54. 3. Food is considered the ideal source of nutrients. However, milk and dairy are not the only food sources of calcium. The client should consume other nondairy foods that are high in calcium, such as dark green leafy vegetables. Although prenatal vitamins are generally recommended, they do not satisfy all requirements. The calcium requirement for pregnancy is 1,300 mg/day. Over-the-counter supplements are not always safe and should be specifically recommended by the health care provider. Although it is true that all fetal organs are formed by the end of the first trimester, development continues throughout pregnancy. Calcium requirements remain at 1,300 mg/day throughout pregnancy.

CN: Heath promotion and maintenance; CNS: None; CL: Apply

Intrapartum care refresher

Abruptio placentae

Premature separation of the placenta from the uterus; a common cause of third trimester bleeding

Key signs and symptoms

- Acute abdominal pain and a rigid abdomen
- Hemorrhage with dark red vaginal bleeding

Key test result

- Ultrasonography locates the placenta and may reveal a clot or hematoma

Key treatments

- Transfusion: packed red blood cells (RBCs), platelets, and fresh frozen plasma if necessary
- Cesarean birth

Key interventions

- Avoid pelvic or vaginal examinations and enemas
- Monitor administration of packed RBCs, platelets, or fresh frozen plasma
- Position client in a left lateral recumbent position

Amniotic fluid embolism

Amniotic fluid entering the maternal circulation through some break in the normal barrier mechanism; the fluid contains debris such as hair, skin, and vernix, subsequently causing obstruction of the pulmonary vessels and resulting in severe respiratory distress

Key signs and symptoms

- Cyanosis and chest pain
- Tachypnea and sudden dyspnea
- Coughing with pink, frothy sputum
- Increasing restlessness and anxiety

Key test result

- Electronic fetal monitor reveals fetal distress (during the intrapartum period)

- Arterial blood gas results (ABG) reveal hypoxemia

Key treatments

- Oxygen therapy: face mask, cannula, or endotracheal (ET) intubation and mechanical ventilation if respiratory arrest occurs
- Cardiopulmonary resuscitation (CPR) if client is apneic and pulseless
- Emergency birth using forceps or by cesarean birth

Key interventions

- Monitor respiratory and cardiovascular status.
- Monitor fetal heart rate (FHR).
- Perform CPR if necessary.
- Assist with immediate birth of neonate.

Disseminated intravascular coagulation (DIC)

Clotting system is abnormally activated and leads to increased coagulation along with a bleeding defect.

Key signs and symptoms

- Abnormal bleeding (petechiae, hematomas, ecchymosis, cutaneous oozing)
- Oliguria

Key test result

- Coagulation studies reveal:
  - decreased fibrinogen level
  - positive D-dimer test specific for disseminated intravascular coagulation (DIC)
  - prolonged prothrombin time (PT)
  - prolonged partial thromboplastin time (PTT).
- Hematology studies reveal decreased platelet count.

Key treatments

- Transfusion therapy: packed RBCs, fresh frozen plasma, platelets, and cryoprecipitate
- Treatment of the underlying condition
- Immediate birth of the fetus

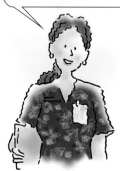

The antepartum and postpartum periods are important to know about. However, the intrapartum period— that's where the action is! This chapter covers the intrapartum period, perhaps the most critical of the three.

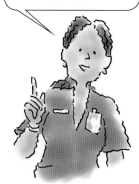

Take a deep breath and bear down...this chapter will be a labor of love.

Key interventions

- Monitor cardiovascular, respiratory, neurologic, GI, and renal status.
- Monitor vital signs frequently.
- Closely monitor intake and output.
- Monitor client closely for signs and symptoms of a transfusion reaction.
- Monitor the results of serial blood studies.

Dystocia

Difficult or abnormal labor that results from a myriad of factors; typically associated with a slow and abnormal progression of labor

Key signs and symptoms

- Arrested descent
- Hypotonic contractions

Key test result

- Ultrasonography shows fetal malposition or malformation.

Key treatments

- Birth of fetus by cesarean if labor fails to progress and mother or fetus shows signs of distress
- Oxytocic agent: oxytocin if contractions are ineffective

Key interventions

- Monitor vital signs.
- Assist the client to a left side-lying position.
- Monitor the effectiveness of oxytocin therapy and watch for complications.

Emergency birth

Situation in which immediate birth of the fetus is necessary to reduce the risk of injury and death to the mother, fetus, or both

Key signs and symptoms

Prolapsed umbilical cord
- Cord visible at the vaginal opening
- Cord palpable during vaginal examination
- Variable decelerations or bradycardia noted on fetal monitor strip

Uterine rupture
- Abdominal pain and tenderness, especially at the peak of a contraction, or the feeling that "something ripped"
- Excessive external bleeding
- Late decelerations, reduced fetal heart rate (FHR) variability, tachycardia followed by bradycardia, cessation of FHR
- Palpation of the fetus outside the uterus

Amniotic fluid embolism
- Chest pain
- Coughing with pink, frothy sputum
- Increasing restlessness and anxiety
- Sudden dyspnea
- Tachypnea

Key test result

Prolapsed umbilical cord
- Ultrasonography confirms that the cord is prolapsed.

Uterine rupture
- Ultrasonography may reveal absence of the amniotic cavity within the uterus.

Amniotic fluid embolism
- ABG analysis reveals hypoxemia.

Key treatments

- Administration of oxygen by nasal cannula or mask (endotracheal intubation and mechanical ventilation may be necessary in the case of amniotic fluid embolism).
- Emergency cesarean birth

Key interventions

- Monitor maternal vital signs, pulse oximetry, and intake and output as well as FHR.
- Administer maternal oxygen by face mask at 8 to 10 L/minute.
- Maintain IV fluid replacement.
- Place client in left lateral recumbent position.
- Obtain blood samples to determine hematocrit (HCT), hemoglobin (Hgb) level, PT and PTT, fibrinogen level, and platelet count, and to type and cross-match blood.
- Monitor administration of blood products as necessary.
- Prepare client and her family for possibility of cesarean birth.

Fetal distress

Signs exhibited by fetus that indicate an inability to cope with the demands of labor, as evidenced by changes in fetal heart rate and rhythm

Key signs and symptoms

- Change in FHR

Key test result

- Fetal scalp blood sampling reveals acidosis.

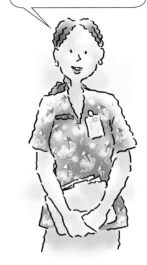

Your client is exhibiting signs of dystocia. What will you do?

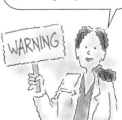

The umbilical cord being visible at the vaginal opening is a critical sign of a prolapsed cord, and an indication for an emergency birth.

Key treatments

- Supplemental oxygen by face mask, typically at 6 to 10 L/minute
- IV fluid administration
- Stop or decrease oxytocin administration as applicable
- Emergent fetal birth by cesarean

Key interventions

- Monitor FHR, fetal activity, and fetal heart variability.
- Assist client to a left side-lying position.

Inverted uterus

Uterine fundus prolapses to, or through, the cervix, causing the uterus to turn inside out after birth.

Key signs and symptoms

- Large, sudden gush of blood from vagina
- Severe uterine pain

Key test result

- Hematology tests reveal decreased Hgb levels and HCT.

Key treatments

- Fluid resuscitation with IV fluids and blood products
- Supplemental oxygen administration
- Immediate manual replacement of uterus
- Possible emergency hysterectomy

Key interventions

- Administer supplemental oxygen.
- Monitor vital signs frequently.
- Closely monitor intake and output.

Laceration

Injury to the vaginal tissue during labor; can range from a tear involving only the lining or the tissue of the vagina to a tear involving the vaginal lining, submucosal tissues, anal sphincter, and rectal lining

Key signs and symptoms

- Increased vaginal bleeding after delivery of placenta

Key test result

- Hematology studies may reveal decreased levels of Hgb and HCT.

Key treatments

- Laceration repair
- Analgesics: ibuprofen, acetaminophen and oxycodone, acetaminophen

Key interventions

- Monitor vital signs, including temperature.
- Monitor laceration site for signs of infection.

Precipitate labor

Abrupt onset of strong contractions that occur in a short period of time, instead of the typical gradually increasing contractions associated with labor

Key signs and symptoms

- Cervical dilation greater than 5 cm/hour in a nulliparous woman; more than 10 cm/hour in a multiparous woman

Key test result

- No key test result specific to this complication

Key treatments

- Controlled birth to prevent maternal and fetal injury
- May administer a tocolytic

Key interventions

- Monitor FHR and variability.

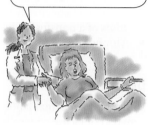

Wow—you're progressing rapidly. This must be a case of precipitate labor.

Premature rupture of membranes

Membrane ruptures before client goes into labor

Key signs and symptoms

- Amniotic fluid gushing or leaking from vagina
- Uterine tenderness

Key test result

- Nitrazine or ferning test is positive
- Vaginal probe ultrasonography allows detection of amniotic sac tear or rupture

Key treatments

- Hospitalization to monitor for maternal fever, leukocytosis, and fetal tachycardia if pregnancy is between 28 and 34 weeks; if infection is confirmed, labor must be induced
- Oxytocic agent: oxytocin for labor induction if term pregnancy and if labor does not result within 24 hours after membrane rupture
- Betamethasone administered IM to increase fetal lung maturity if gestational age is 24 to 34 weeks

Key interventions

- Monitor for signs of infection or fetal distress.
- Administer antibiotics as prescribed.
- Encourage client to express her feelings and concerns.

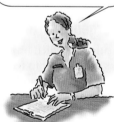

Immediately after birth, there is a large, sudden gush of blood from your client's vagina and she complains of severe uterine pain. What's going on?

Preterm labor

Labor that occurs before the end of the 37th week of gestation; involves regular uterine contractions in conjunction with cervical effacement and dilation

Key signs and symptoms

- Feeling of pelvic pressure or abdominal tightening
- Increased blood-tinged vaginal discharge
- Intestinal cramping
- Uterine contractions that result in cervical dilation and effacement

Key test results

- External or internal uterine monitoring confirms contractions.
- Vaginal examination confirms cervical effacement and dilation.

Key treatments

- Betamethasone administered IM at regular intervals over 48 hours to increase fetal lung maturity in a fetus expected to be delivered preterm
- Magnesium sulfate to maintain uterine relaxation
- Tocolytic agents, such as terbutaline, to inhibit uterine contractions

Key interventions

- Monitor maternal vital signs.
- Continuous uterine contractions and FHR monitoring.
- Monitor for magnesium sulfate toxicity and ensure calcium gluconate is available.

Prolapsed umbilical cord

Umbilical cord protrusion alongside, or ahead of, the fetal presenting part; occlusion of the cord can lead to impaired fetal perfusion

Key signs and symptoms

- Cord visible at the vaginal opening

- Variable decelerations or bradycardia noted on fetal monitor strip

Key test result

- Ultrasonography may reveal the cord as the presenting part

Key treatment

- Immediate birth of the fetus

Key interventions

- Manually elevate fetal head off cord with continuous upward pressure.
- Place client in Trendelenburg position (client's hips higher than head in a knee-to-chest position).
- Monitor FHR and variability.

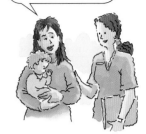

Proper care helps to ensure birth of a healthy baby.

Uterine rupture

Uterus tears and opens into the abdominal cavity; site of the rupture is usually a previous scar.

Key signs and symptoms

- Abdominal pain and tenderness, especially at the peak of a contraction, or the feeling that "something ripped"
- Late decelerations, reduced FHR variability, tachycardia followed by bradycardia, cessation of FHR

Key test result

- Hematology tests reveal decreased levels of Hgb and HCT.

Key treatments

- Fluid resuscitation: IV fluids and blood products via rapid infusion
- Surgery to remove the fetus and repair the tear or hysterectomy if necessary
- Oxytocic agent: oxytocin to help contract the uterus

Key interventions

- Monitor vital signs frequently.
- Prepare client for immediate surgery.

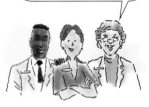

If you suspect uterine rupture, call the doctor STAT—a cesarean birth may be in order.

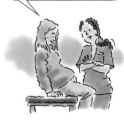

Expectant mothers should discuss any concerns with their health care provider.

Intrapartum care questions, answers, and rationales

1. A 32-week-gestation client calls to the nursing station, stating, "I think my water just broke." Which nursing action is **priority**?

1. Prepare the client for an amnioinfusion.
2. Assess the fluid to determine whether it is amniotic fluid.
3. Immediately assess the fetal heart rate and pattern.
4. Check the client's cervical dilation and effacement status.

2. A client who is 36 weeks' pregnant comes into the labor and delivery unit with mild contractions. While the nurse is assessing the client, which finding(s) indicates to the nurse the client is experiencing abruptio placentae? Select all that apply.

1. Spontaneous rupture of membranes
2. Dark red vaginal bleeding
3. Emesis
4. Temperature 102.5°F (39.2°C)
5. Rigid abdomen
6. Sharp, stabbing pain high in abdomen

3. The health care provider prescribes oxytocin intravenously (IV) at 3 mU/min to augment a client's labor. The pharmacy sends 1,000 mL of normal saline with 10 U of oxytocin. The nurse will set the pump to infuse at what rate? Record your answer using one decimal place.

_____ mL/min

4. A laboring client receiving intravenous oxytocin asks the nurse why her urine output has to be measured. Which nursing response is correct?

1. "I need to monitor your intake and output because oxytocin can cause water intoxication."
2. "We measure the urine output on all laboring clients, not just those receiving oxytocin."
3. "Oxytocin can be toxic to the kidneys, so I need to make sure they are working appropriately."
4. "Oxytocin has a diuretic effect, so I need to make sure you do not lose too much fluid."

5. A laboring client is prescribed an amniotomy. Which outcome will the nurse identify as **priority** for this client?

1. The client will have increased knowledge about amniotomy.
2. The fetus will maintain adequate tissue perfusion.
3. The fetus will display no signs of infection.
4. The client's labor will begin to progress adequately.

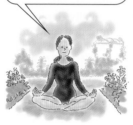

Staying calm will help your client stay calm. Remember to manage your own breathing while helping manage hers.

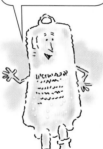

Careful with your calculation—it helps me know how fast to flow.

1. **3.** Immediately assessing the fetal heart rate helps determine whether a prolapsed cord has occurred. The client is at a higher risk because the fetus is preterm. An amnioinfusion may be needed if cord prolapse has occurred, but this must first be determined by assessing the fetal heart rate. If the fetal heart rate is stable, the nurse would then assess the fluid and cervical status.
CN: Safe, effective care environment; CNS: Management of care; CL: Apply

2. **2, 5, 6.** A client with abruptio placentae would most likely exhibit a rigid abdomen, intense pain at the abruption site, and dark red vaginal bleeding. Sudden rupture of membranes, emesis, and fever are not associated with abruptio placentae.
CN: Physiological integrity; CNS: Reduction of risk potential; CL: Apply

3. **0.3.**
The answer is found by setting up a ratio and following through with the calculations shown below. Each unit of oxytocin contains 1,000 mU. Therefore, 10 U of oxytocin is equivalent to 10,000 mU. Thus 1,000 mL of IV fluid contains 10,000 mU (10 U) of oxytocin. Use the following equation:

$$10,000/1,000 = 3/X;$$
$$10,000X = 3,000;$$
$$X = 0.3 \ mL/min.$$

CN: Physiological integrity; CNS: Pharmacological and parenteral therapies; CL: Analyze

4. **1.** The nurse should monitor fluid intake and output because prolonged oxytocin infusion may cause severe water intoxication, leading to seizure, coma, and death. Urine output is not routinely measured on all laboring clients. Oxytocin has no nephrotoxic or diuretic effects; in fact, it produces an antidiuretic effect.
CN: Physiological integrity; CNS: Pharmacological and parenteral therapies; CL: Apply

5. **2.** Amniotomy increases the risk of umbilical cord prolapse, which would impair the fetal blood supply and tissue perfusion. Because the fetus's life depends on the oxygen carried by that blood, maintaining fetal tissue perfusion takes priority over goals related to increased knowledge, infection prevention, and labor progression.
CN: Safe, effective care environment; CNS: Management of care; CL: Analyze

CN: Client needs category   CNS: Client needs subcategory   CL: Cognitive level

6. A client is receiving oxytocin to augment her labor. The nurse notes the client's contractions have recurrently remained intense for 60 or more seconds. Which action will the nurse take **first**?
1. Stop the oxytocin infusion.
2. Notify the health care provider.
3. Continue to monitor the client.
4. Turn the client on her left side.

6. 1. A contraction that remains strong for 60 seconds or more with no sign of letting up signals impending tetany and could cause rupture of the uterus. Oxytocin stimulates contractions and should be stopped. The nurse should continue to monitor the client and fetus and notify the health care provider but only after stopping the oxytocin. If the client isn't already on her left side, the nurse would turn her to facilitate placental perfusion; again, only after stopping the oxytocin.
CN: Safe, effective care environment; CNS: Management of care; CL: Analyze

7. A 40 weeks' gestation client is experiencing contractions every 4 minutes. When reviewing the client's medical record, the nurse will monitor the client closely for fetal distress based on which finding?
1. Total weight gain of 30 lb (13.6 kg)
2. Client age of 32 years
3. Initial blood pressure of 146/90 mm Hg
4. Treatment for syphilis at 15 weeks' gestation

7. 3. A blood pressure of 146/90 mm Hg may indicate gestational hypertension. Over time, gestational hypertension reduces blood flow to the placenta and can cause intrauterine growth retardation and other problems that make the fetus less able to tolerate the stress of labor. A weight gain of 30 lb is within expected parameters for a healthy pregnancy. A woman at the age of 32 years does not have a greater risk of complications if she is healthy before pregnancy. Increased risk of complications begins around the age of 35 years. Syphilis that has been treated does not pose an additional risk.
CN: Physiological integrity; CNS: Reduction of risk potential; CL: Analyze

8. A client at 42 weeks' gestation is having strong contractions every 3 to 4 minutes that last 45 to 60 seconds each and is 4 cm dilated and 50% effaced. Fetal heart rate (FHR) has been 130 to 135 beats/minute. The nurse notes on the external fetal monitor the FHR is now ranging from 170 to 190 beats/minute and the client states her baby is more active than normal. What will the nurse do **next**?
1. Request an internal fetal monitor be placed.
2. Apply oxygen via a face mask at 10 L.
3. Prepare the client for a cesarean section.
4. Decrease the client's intravenous fluid rate.

8. 2. Fetal tachycardia and excessive fetal activity are the first signs of fetal hypoxia. To increase fetal oxygenation, the nurse would administer oxygen to the client. Internal fetal monitoring is not needed because the external monitor is working. The client may need a cesarean section, but increasing fetal oxygenation is priority. The nurse would actually increase the fluid rate, not decrease it.
CN: Physiological integrity; CNS: Reduction of risk potential; CL: Apply

9. A client at 31 weeks' gestation reports contractions. The nurse notes uterine irritability on the external monitor, and the client is prescribed nifedipine. The nurse will include which statement when educating this client?
1. "This medicine will make it easier for you to breathe."
2. "Let me know if your mouth gets dry or you start to feel thirsty."
3. "Nifedipine may make you feel warm and like your heart is racing."
4. "You will need to have a daily non-stress test done while taking nifedipine."

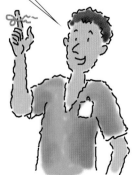

Don't forget to inform your client of any side effects associated with prescribed medications.

9. 3. Maternal tachycardia and flushing are common adverse reactions to nifedipine. The drug is being given to this client to reduce the client's uterine irritability, not relieve bronchospasm. Dry mouth, feelings of thirst, and daily NSTs are not common with this drug.
CN: Physiological integrity; CNS: Pharmacological and parenteral therapies; CL: Apply

CN: Client needs category   CNS: Client needs subcategory   CL: Cognitive level

10. The nurse is caring for a primigravida client diagnosed with gestational hypertension who is receiving magnesium sulfate intravenously (IV). During assessment, the nurse notes the following: blood pressure, 160/102 mm Hg; heart rate, 96 beats/minute; respiratory rate, 8 breaths/minute; and urine output, 15 mL/hour. Which nursing action is **most** appropriate?
1. Assess the client's deep tendon reflexes (DTRs).
2. Request a STAT serum magnesium level.
3. Call the rapid response team to the client's room.
4. Stop the IV magnesium sulfate infusion.

11. Upon vaginal examination of a client in labor, the nurse notes the fetus's diamond-shaped fontanel is toward the anterior portion of the client's pelvis. How will the nurse interpret this finding?
1. The client can expect a brief and intense labor, with potential for lacerations.
2. The client is at risk for uterine rupture and needs constant monitoring.
3. The client may need interventions to ease her back labor and change the fetal position.
4. The client must be told that birth of the fetus will require forceps or a vacuum extractor.

12. A laboring primigravida client is requesting an epidural for pain control. The nurse reviews the client's laboratory data, shown in the chart exhibit below. Which laboratory result **most** concerns the nurse?

Test	Result
Hemoglobin	12 g/dL (120 g/L)
Hematocrit	35% (0.35)
White blood cell count	20,000 mm³ (20 × 10⁹/L)
Platelet count	100,000 mm³ (100 × 10⁹/L)

1. Hemoglobin
2. Hematocrit
3. White blood cell count
4. Platelet count

13. The nurse assesses a laboring client's cervix and states it is 6 cm dilated and 70% effaced. The client asks what effacement means. The nurse will include which description(s) when responding to the client? Select all that apply.
1. Thinning
2. Shortening
3. Widening
4. Lowering
5. Engaging

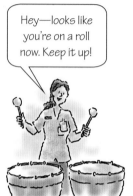

Hey—looks like you're on a roll now. Keep it up!

10. 4. Magnesium sulfate should be withheld if the client's respiratory rate or urine output falls or if reflexes are diminished or absent, two of which are true for this client. The client may also show other signs of impending toxicity, such as flushing and feeling warm. Assessing the client's DTRs would not resolve the low respiratory rate and urine output. The rapid response team is not needed at this time. The client is already showing central nervous system depression because of excessive magnesium sulfate, so requesting a serum level is not priority.
CN: Physiological integrity; CNS: Pharmacological and parenteral therapies; CL: Analyze

11. 3. The fetal position is occiput posterior, a position that commonly produces intense back pain during labor. Most of the time, the fetus rotates during labor to occiput anterior position. Positioning the client on her side can facilitate this rotation. An occiput posterior position would most likely result in prolonged labor. Occiput posterior position alone does not create a risk of uterine rupture. Forceps or a vacuum extractor would be necessary only if the fetus did not rotate spontaneously.
CN: Safe, effective care environment; CNS: Safety and infection control; CL: Apply

12. 4. The client's platelet count should most concern the nurse and needs to be reported to the health care provider. The client would not be a candidate for an epidural due to the risk of bleeding. An elevated white blood cell count is expected during the labor process. The hemoglobin level and hematocrit are in normal range.
CN: Physiological integrity; CNS: Reduction of risk potential; CL: Analyze

13. 1, 2. Cervical effacement refers to a thinning and shortening of the cervix. Dilation refers to the widening of the cervix. Both facilitate opening the cervix in preparation for birth. Lowered is not a term used to describe a pregnant woman's cervix. Engagement refers to the movement of the fetal head into the mother's pelvis and is unrelated to changes in the woman's cervix.
CN: Health promotion and maintenance; CNS: None; CL: Apply

14. The nurse is assessing the fetal position of a laboring client. Which position is **least** concerning to the nurse?
1. Vertex
2. Transverse lie
3. Footling breech
4. Face presentation

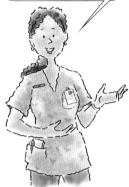

Well, "easy passage" might be stretching it (literally), but one of these positions is better than the others.

14. 1. Vertex position (flexion of the fetal head) is the optimal position for passage through the birth canal in a vaginal birth. All remaining positions are recommended for cesarean sections. Transverse lie positioning generally results in poor labor contractions and an unacceptable fetal position for birth. Footling breech positioning, in which a foot presents first, is a difficult birth. Face presentation positioning makes it difficult for the fetus to progress through the birth canal.
CN: Health promotion and maintenance; CNS: None; CL: Apply

15. The nurse is caring for a client in labor. The client is 6 cm dilated, 80% effaced, +1 station, and having uterine contractions every 3 minutes that last for 40 to 50 seconds. Which stage of labor will the nurse document the client as being in currently?
1. First
2. Second
3. Third
4. Fourth

15. 1. The first stage of labor begins with the onset of labor and ends with complete cervical dilation. The first stage is also divided into three distinct phases: latent, active, and transition. This client is in the active phase of the first stage. The second stage of labor begins with complete dilation and ends with the expulsion of the fetus. The third stage of labor begins immediately following the birth of the neonate and ends with the expulsion of the placenta. The fourth stage of labor is the first 4 hours' postpartum, following placental expulsion.
CN: Health promotion and maintenance; CNS: None; CL: Apply

16. The nurse is admitting a laboring client. Which nursing action(s) is **most** appropriate? Select all that apply.
1. Determining the estimated date of birth
2. Estimating the size of the fetus
3. Taking maternal and fetal vital signs
4. Asking about the client's menstrual history
5. Administering an analgesic to the client
6. Determining the frequency and duration of contractions

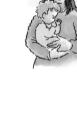

The labor in the hospital is nothing compared to the labor over the next 18 years or so.

16. 1, 3, 6. The nurse should ask about the estimated date of birth and then compare the response to the information in the prenatal record. If the fetus is preterm, special precautions and equipment are necessary. The nurse should obtain maternal and fetal vital signs to evaluate the well-being of the client and fetus. Determining the frequency and duration of contractions provides valuable baseline information. The nurse does not estimate the size of the fetus. It would not be appropriate at this time for the nurse to ask about the client's menstrual history; this information would be collected at the first prenatal visit. It would be premature to administer an analgesic, which could slow or stop labor contractions.
CN: Health promotion and maintenance; CNS: None; CL: Apply

17. After admitting a client in the latent phase of labor, who received no prenatal care, the nurse begins completing prescriptions from the primary health care provider. Which prescription(s) is **priority** for the nurse to complete? Select all that apply.
1. Obtain the client's blood type.
2. Determine the estimated date of birth.
3. Apply an external fetal heart rate monitor.
4. Assess the client for any known allergies.
5. Administer meperidine intravenously for contraction pain.

17. 1, 2, 3, 4. It is priority for the nurse to determine the client's blood type because the risk of blood loss is always a potential complication during the labor and birth process. Determining the gestational age of the fetus is priority to plan newborn care. Applying a fetal monitor will provide information on the well-being of the fetus. The nurse must know the client's allergies before any medications can be administered. Pain management is considered psychosocial and not priority for this client.
CN: Safe, effective care environment; CNS: Management of care; CL: Analyze

CN: Client needs category   CNS: Client needs subcategory   CL: Cognitive level

18. The nurse is assessing the fetal heart rate of a client at 39 weeks' gestation who is in labor. Which finding(s) require follow-up from the nurse? Select all that apply.
1. 88 beats/minute
2. 100 beats/minute
3. 135 beats/minute
4. 150 beats/minute
5. 180 beats/minute

19. The nurse is assessing a client in the early stages of labor who has an external fetal heart rate monitor applied. The nurse understands the monitor data as indicative of which finding?
1. Gender of the fetus
2. Fetal position
3. Labor progress
4. Oxygenation

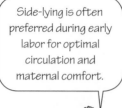

Side-lying is often preferred during early labor for optimal circulation and maternal comfort.

20. Which nursing intervention is **priority** for a laboring client requesting epidural analgesia?
1. Insert an indwelling Foley catheter.
2. Obtain the client's heart rate.
3. Administer a 500-mL intravenous bolus.
4. Monitor the client's hemoglobin level.

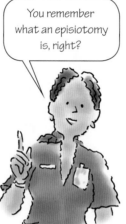

You remember what an episiotomy is, right?

21. A client in labor requires an episiotomy to facilitate birth. Which nursing intervention is priority for this client during the fourth stage of labor?
1. Administer 100 mg of docusate.
2. Clean the site with warm water.
3. Teach the client how to do a sitz bath.
4. Monitor the site for infection.

22. A client in labor tells the nurse, "I have been having golden yellow discharge from my breasts." Which nursing action is appropriate?
1. Assess the client's temperature.
2. Complete a thorough breast examination.
3. Send a specimen to the lab for a culture.
4. Tell the client the discharge is normal.

18. 1, 2, 5. A fetal heart rate of 110 to 160 beats/minute is appropriate for filling the heart with blood and pumping it out to the system. A fetal heart rate of 135 and 150 beats/minute falls within this range. Faster or slower rates do not accomplish perfusion adequately and require further nursing assessment.
CN: Health promotion and maintenance; CNS: None; CL: Apply

19. 4. Oxygenation of the fetus may be indirectly determined through fetal monitoring by closely examining the fetal heart rate strip. Accelerations in the fetal heart rate indicate normal oxygenation, whereas decelerations in the fetal heart rate sometimes indicate abnormal fetal oxygenation. The fetal heart rate monitor cannot determine the gender or position of the fetus. Labor progress can be directly monitored only through cervical examination.
CN: Physiological integrity; CNS: Reduction of risk potential; CL: Understand

20. 3. One of the major adverse effects of epidural administration is hypotension. Therefore, a 500-mL fluid bolus is usually administered to help prevent hypotension in the client who wishes to receive an epidural for pain relief. A Foley catheter would be inserted after the client receives the epidural to limit discomfort. Obtaining the client's heart rate is important for baseline data, but is not a priority over maintaining the client's blood pressure. Monitoring maternal hemoglobin level is not necessary.
CN: Physiological integrity; CNS: Reduction of risk potential; CL: Apply

21. 2. Cleaning the site is priority to prevent infection. The nurse would administer docusate to prevent the client from having to strain with bowel movements, which would be painful and could break sutures. The client would need to apply ice to the site for the first 24 hours to decrease edema and then heat to promote healing. Monitoring for infection would not be priority immediately following the procedure.
CN: Physiological integrity; CNS: Basic care and comfort; CL: Analyze

22. 4. After the fourth month of pregnancy, colostrum may be noticed. Colostrum appears as either clear or golden to dark yellow in color. The breasts normally produce colostrum for the first few days after birth. Milk production begins 1 to 3 days' postpartum. A complete breast examination is not required. The client's statement does not indicate infection, so a culture or temperature assessment is not warranted.
CN: Health promotion and maintenance; CNS: None; CL: Apply

CN: Client needs category   CNS: Client needs subcategory   CL: Cognitive level

23. The nurse is reviewing a client's assessment data. Which finding will the nurse highlight for the health care provider?
  1. Urine output of 100 mL every 2 hours after epidural placement
  2. Increase in blood pressure to 154/96 mm Hg during contractions
  3. Decrease in respirations to 12 breaths/minute at the acme of contractions
  4. Increase in temperature from 98°F to 99.6°F (36.7°C to 37.6°C)

24. A client asks the nurse about the pinkish "stretch marks" on her abdomen. Which nursing response is appropriate?
  1. "They will go away completely in a few months."
  2. "They will not disappear, but they will fade over time."
  3. "You need to use an emollient cream to remove them."
  4. "They are a sign that your muscle has separated."

25. The nurse notes late decelerations on the fetal monitor of a laboring client. Which action will the nurse complete for this client?
  1. Decrease the client's intravenous rate.
  2. Insert an indwelling Foley catheter.
  3. Place the client in left side-lying position.
  4. Request an internal fetal monitor.

26. A client has given birth vaginally several minutes ago. The nurse notes blood gushing from the vagina, the umbilical cord lengthening, and a globe-shaped uterus. The nurse will monitor the client closely for which condition?
  1. Uterine involution
  2. Cervical laceration
  3. Placental separation
  4. Postpartum hemorrhage

27. While the nurse is assessing a laboring client's cervical dilation and effacement, a prolapsed cord is discovered. Which nursing intervention(s) is appropriate? Select all that apply.
  1. Administer oxytocin intravenously.
  2. Keep the client in the supine position.
  3. Position the client in the Trendelenburg position.
  4. Prepare the client for an emergency cesarean section.
  5. Move the cord back to its original location.
  6. Continuously monitor fetal heart rate.

Like my nursing instructor used to say, "Perfused tissue is happy tissue."

23. 2. During contractions, blood pressure increases and blood flow to the intervillous spaces changes, compromising the fetal blood supply. Therefore, the nurse should assess the client's blood pressure frequently to determine whether it returns to precontraction level and allows adequate fetal blood flow again. A urine output of 100 mL every 2 hours, respirations of 12 breaths/minute, and temperature changes are normal.
CN: Physiological integrity; CNS: Reduction of risk potential; CL: Analyze

24. 2. Striae are wavy, depressed streaks that may occur over the abdomen, breasts, or thighs as pregnancy progresses. They fade with time to a silvery color but will not disappear. Creams may soften the skin and reduce the appearance of striae, but they will not remove the striae completely. Separation of the rectus muscle, or diastasis recti, is a condition of pregnancy whereby the abdominal wall has difficulty stretching enough to accommodate the growing fetus, causing the muscle to separate. Striae are not an indication of this separation.
CN: Health promotion and maintenance; CNS: None; CL: Apply

25. 3. In the left side-lying position, cardiac output increases, stroke volume increases, and the pulse rate decreases, thereby promoting placental perfusion. The intravenous rate should be increased to increase placental perfusion, not decreased. A Foley catheter and internal monitor are not indicated for this client.
CN: Health promotion and maintenance; CNS: None; CL: Apply

26. 3. Placental separation causes a sudden gush or trickle of blood from the vagina, rise of the fundus in the abdomen, increased umbilical cord length at the introitus, and a globe-shaped uterus. Uterine involution causes a firmly contracted uterus, which cannot occur until the placenta is delivered. Cervical lacerations produce a steady flow of bright red blood in a client with a firmly contracted uterus. Postpartum hemorrhage results in excessive vaginal bleeding and signs of shock, such as pallor and a rapid, thready pulse.
CN: Health promotion and maintenance; CNS: None; CL: Apply

27. 3, 4, 6. A prolapsed cord necessitates an emergency cesarean section. Placing the client in the Trendelenburg position relieves pressure from the fetal head on the umbilical cord. Keeping the client supine is inappropriate. It is important to not attempt to move the cord. Monitoring fetal heart rate reveals any compromise in fetal oxygenation. Administering oxytocin is unnecessary because a cesarean, not vaginal, birth is needed.
CN: Physiological integrity; CNS: Physiological adaptation; CL: Apply

CN: Client needs category   CNS: Client needs subcategory   CL: Cognitive level

28. A client in active labor requests a holistic approach to labor and birth. Which nursing intervention best meet this client's needs during the labor and birth process?
1. A warm bath
2. A foot massage
3. Use of Reiki
4. Use of heated stones

28. 3. The use of Reiki, a gentle technique focusing on the body's energy centers by loosening blocked energy, promoting total relaxation, and establishing spiritual equilibrium and mental well-being, is the most realistic holistic approach. A warm bath or foot massage might help any client, not just those who approach their health holistically. The use of heated stones might be difficult to arrange in a labor and birth unit.
CN: Physiological integrity; CNS: Basic care and comfort; CL: Apply

29. A client comes to the labor unit reporting contractions. After assessing the client, the nurse determines the client is having Braxton Hicks contractions and provides education on the difference between true and false labor. Which statement by the client indicates effective teaching?
1. "Braxton Hicks contractions begin irregularly and become regular."
2. "Braxton Hicks contractions cause cervical dilation and effacement."
3. "Braxton Hicks contractions begin in the lower back and radiate to the abdomen."
4. "Braxton Hicks contractions begin in the abdomen and remain irregular."

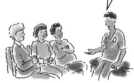

Don't be fooled by Braxton Hicks contractions; you might think they're real, but they're all in your abdomen.

29. 4. Braxton Hicks contractions begin and remain irregular. They are felt in the abdomen and remain confined to the abdomen and groin. They commonly disappear with ambulation and do not dilate the cervix. True contractions begin irregularly but become regular and predictable, causing cervical effacement and dilation. True contractions are felt initially in the lower back and radiate to the abdomen in a wavelike motion.
CN: Health promotion and maintenance; CNS: None; CL: Apply

30. A client in labor is prescribed oxytocin and asks the nurse, "What is this medication for?" The nurse will include which actions of oxytocin in the response?
1. Stimulates labor and prevents hemorrhage
2. Decreases maternal heart rate and stimulates labor
3. Slows labor progression and increases diuresis
4. Prevents hemorrhage and increases diuresis

Oxytocin is like a pair of jumper cables for a stalled labor—it helps get the contractions up and running again.

30. 1. Oxytocin is the synthetic form of the pituitary hormone used to stimulate uterine contractions, stimulate labor, and prevent hemorrhage. It may increase maternal heart rate and has an antidiuretic effect.
CN: Physiological integrity; CNS: Pharmacological and parenteral therapies; CL: Apply

31. A laboring client is having contractions every 3 to 5 minutes, lasting 45 to 55 seconds. Her cervical dilation has progressed from 4 to 7 cm. The nurse will document the client is in which phase of labor?
1. Preparatory
2. Latent
3. Active
4. Transition

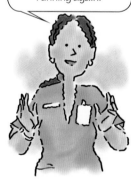

31. 3. Cervical dilation occurs more rapidly during the active phase than any of the previous phases. The active phase is characterized by cervical dilation that progresses from 4 to 7 cm, Uterine contractions occurring every 2 to 5 minutes, lasting 40 to 60 seconds. The preparatory, or latent, phase begins with the onset of regular uterine contractions and ends when rapid cervical dilation begins (1 to 3 cm). Transition is defined as cervical dilation beginning at 8 cm and lasting until 10 cm, or complete dilation.
CN: Health promotion and maintenance; CNS: None; CL: Apply

32. The nurse is reviewing information about the stages of labor with a pregnant client. The nurse determines the client has understood the information when the client states crowning occurs during which stage of labor?
1. First
2. Second
3. Third
4. Fourth

32. 2. The second stage of labor begins at full cervical dilation (10 cm) and ends when the infant is born. Crowning is present during this stage as the fetal head, pushed against the perineum, causes the vaginal introitus to open, allowing the fetal scalp to be visible. The first stage of labor begins with true labor contractions and ends with complete cervical dilation. The third stage is from the time the infant is born until the delivery of the placenta. The fourth stage is the first 4 hours following delivery of the placenta.
CN: Health promotion and maintenance; CNS: None; CL: Understand

CN: Client needs category   CNS: Client needs subcategory   CL: Cognitive level

33. During admission, a pregnant client tells the nurse that her significant other abuses her. Which nursing response is **most** appropriate?
  1. "I am going to have to contact local law enforcement."
  2. "I am so sorry you are having to deal with this while pregnant."
  3. "You have to get out of this situation for your baby's safety."
  4. "You seem upset. Let us talk about what you are experiencing."

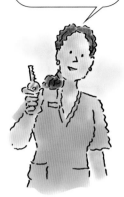

Remember—therapeutic communication is key when talking with clients.

34. For a client in active labor, the health care provider prescribes an internal electronic fetal monitoring (EFM) device. Which client finding(s) will the nurse interpret as supporting the use of an internal EFM? Select all that apply.
  1. The membranes have ruptured.
  2. The fetus is in vertex position.
  3. The cervix is 6 cm dilated.
  4. The client has an epidural.
  5. The fetal head is at 0 station.

35. The nurse is admitting a pregnant client diagnosed with gestational diabetes. A cervical assessment reveals the cervix is 3 cm dilated and 40% effaced and the fetal head is at −2 station. The client is experiencing contractions every 5 minutes that last 40 to 45 seconds. Which question is **most** important for the nurse to ask the client?
  1. "Are you planning to breastfeed or formula-feed your newborn?"
  2. "What is your current pain level on a scale of 1 to 10?"
  3. "Who do you want to be present during your birth?"
  4. "What were your blood glucose levels over the past few days?"

36. While assessing a laboring client's cervix, the nurse notes the biparietal diameter of the fetal head is 2 cm below the level of the ischial spines. Which nursing action is appropriate?
  1. Have the client void.
  2. Call the health care provider.
  3. Insert an internal fetal scalp monitor.
  4. Continue to monitor the client.

37. A laboring client is prescribed 5% dextrose in lactated Ringer's intravenously (IV) to run at 100 mL/hour. The IV tubing delivers 10 drops/mL. At which infusion rate will the nurse set the IV? Record your answer using a whole number.

_____ gtt/minute

33. 4. The most therapeutic response would be to acknowledge the client's feelings and then talk with the client to learn more about the nature of her abusive situation, such as whether the abuse is physical, mental, and/or sexual in nature. Depending on the client's response and desires, the nurse could contact law enforcement. Neither merely expressing empathy to the client nor ordering the client to get out of the situation is as appropriate or therapeutic as having the client provide more information about the abuse.
CN: Safe, effective care environment; CNS: Safety and infection control; CL: Apply

34. 1, 2, 3, 5. Internal EFM can be applied only after the client's membranes have ruptured, when the fetus is at least at −1 station and is in vertex position, and when the cervix is dilated at least 3 cm. Although the client may receive anesthesia, it is not required before application of an internal EFM device.
CN: Physiological integrity; CNS: Reduction of risk potential; CL: Analyze

35. 4. It would be most important to find out about the client's most recent blood glucose levels because this would provide information about how well her diabetes has been controlled. The nurse would also ask about feeding, pain, and birth, but these are not priorities during the latent phase of labor.
CN: Physiological integrity; CNS: Reduction of risk potential; CL: Analyze

36. 4. When the largest diameter of the presenting part (typically the biparietal diameter of the fetal head) is 2 cm (+2) below the ischial spines, this indicates normal progression of the fetus into the birth canal. The nurse would continue to monitor the client. No other interventions are needed based on the fetal station.
CN: Health promotion and maintenance; CNS: None; CL: Apply

37. 17.
Multiply the number of milliliters to be infused (100) by the drop factor (10).

$$100 \times 10 = 1,000.$$

Then divide the answer by the number of minutes to run the infusion (60).

$$1,000 \div 60 = 16.67 \,(or\, 17 \, gtt/minute)$$

CN: Physiological integrity; CNS: Pharmacological and parenteral therapies; CL: Apply

CN: Client needs category   CNS: Client needs subcategory   CL: Cognitive level

38. The nurse admits a multiparous client to the labor unit who has not received any prenatal care during this pregnancy. The client states the first day of her last menstrual period was on August 18. Using Naegele's rule, what does the nurse determine is the client's estimated date of delivery?
1. May 11
2. May 25
3. December 11
4. December 25

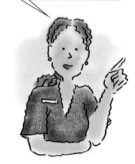

It is critical to correctly estimate the date of birth. What information do you need to do that?

38. 2. The nurse would take the first day of the last menstrual period, subtract 3 months, and then add 7 days. So, in this case, the nurse would take August and subtract 3 months to get May. Then the nurse would take 18 and add 7 to get 25, making the client's estimated date of delivery May 25.
CN: Health promotion and maintenance; CNS: None; CL: Apply

39. The registered nurse (RN) and the assistive personnel (AP) are caring for a laboring client with preeclampsia who is receiving magnesium sulfate intravenously. Which intervention is appropriate for the nurse to delegate to the AP?
1. Checking the client's deep tendon reflexes (DTRs)
2. Emptying and documenting urine output
3. Monitoring the client's blood pressure
4. Assessing the urine for the presence of protein

39. 2. The RN would delegate measuring and documenting the client's urine output to the AP. The RN would review the data to monitor for complications. Checking DTRs and urine for protein requires nursing judgment. The nurse must monitor the blood pressure to assess for changes or trends.
CN: Safe, effective care environment; CNS: Management of care; CL: Apply

40. The nurse is performing Leopold's maneuvers on a client and determines the fetus is in a frank breech presentation. Which image illustrates this position?

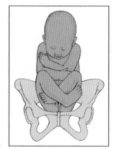
1.

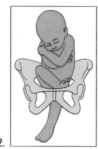
2.

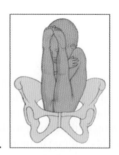
3.

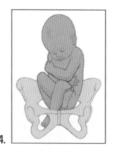
4.

40. 3. In a frank breech presentation, the buttocks are the presenting part, with the hips flexed and the knees remaining straight. In a complete breech (option 1), the knees and hips are flexed. In a footling breech (option 2), neither the hips nor the lower legs are flexed, and one or both feet may present. In an incomplete breech (option 4), one or both hips remain extended, and one or both feet or knees lie below the breech.
CN: Physiological integrity; CNS: Physiological adaptation; CL: Apply

41. A laboring client has been given an epidural anesthetic. The nurse assesses the client immediately following epidural administration. Which finding is **most** important for the nurse to report?
1. Maternal respirations decrease from 20 to 14 breaths/minute.
2. Maternal blood pressure decreases from 130/70 to 98/50 mm Hg.
3. Maternal pulse increases from 78 to 96 beats/minute.
4. Maternal temperature increases from 99°F (37.2°C) to 100°F (37.8°C).

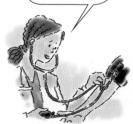

No signs of hypotensive crisis here.

41. 2. As the epidural anesthetic agent spreads through the spinal canal, it may produce hypotensive crisis, which is characterized by maternal hypotension, decreased beat-to-beat variability, and fetal bradycardia. Maternal blood pressure that decreases from 130/70 to 98/50 mm Hg is the most important finding following administration of epidural anesthesia. The respiratory rate, pulse rate, and temperature listed are within normal limits for a laboring client.
CN: Safe, effective care environment; CNS: Management of care; CL: Analyze

CN: Client needs category   CNS: Client needs subcategory   CL: Cognitive level

42. A client at 39 weeks' gestation is in labor and receiving magnesium sulfate intravenously. Which prescription will the nurse question?
1. Monitor deep tendon reflexes and vital signs.
2. Administer terbutaline subcutaneously.
3. Place calcium gluconate at the client's bedside
4. Insert a Foley catheter.

42. 2. The nurse will question administration of terbutaline. Terbutaline is a smooth muscle relaxant sometimes used to relax the uterus, especially for preterm labor and uterine hyperstimulation. The client is term and has no indication of hyperstimulation. Calcium gluconate should be kept at the bedside while a client is receiving a magnesium infusion. If magnesium toxicity occurs, administering calcium gluconate is an antidote. Monitoring vital signs, urine output, and reflexes are priority to help the nurse determine if the client is becoming toxic. All will become depressed with magnesium overdose.
CN: Physiological integrity; CNS: Pharmacological and parenteral therapies; CL: Apply

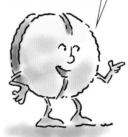

A lot of clients say that I make them sick to their stomach, but I try not to take it personally.

43. A pregnant client received dinoprostone for cervical ripening. The client tells the nurse, "I am starting to have chills." What will the nurse do **next**?
1. Check the client's temperature.
2. Notify the health care provider.
3. Document the client's statement.
4. Give acetaminophen 500 mg orally.

43. 1. The nurse should check the client's temperature to determine whether the client has a fever, which could be an adverse effect or indicate an infection. Headache, nausea, vomiting, chills, fever, and hypertension are adverse effects of dinoprostone. The nurse may then notify the health care provider and give acetaminophen if fever is present. The nurse would document the statement after assessing.
CN: Physiological integrity; CNS: Pharmacological and parenteral therapies; CL: Apply

44. A pregnant client is admitted to the labor unit. Which finding(s) indicates to the nurse the client is in the latent phase of the first stage of labor? Select all that apply.
1. Cervical dilation of 5 cm
2. Contractions occurring every 6 to 7 minutes
3. Contractions lasting about 30 to 45 seconds
4. Cervical effacement of 50%
5. Moderate contraction intensity

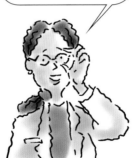

Focus on that word "latent" in question #44. It's important.

44. 2, 3. Signs indicating the latent phase of the first stage of labor include contractions occurring every 5 to 10 minutes and lasting about 30 to 45 seconds. Signs indicating the active phase of the first stage of labor include cervical dilation from 4 to 7 cm, cervical effacement from 40% to 80%, and moderate contraction intensity.
CN: Health promotion and maintenance; CNS: None; CL: Apply

45. The nurse reviews a laboring client's laboratory results, shown in the chart exhibit below. Based on the findings, the nurse will monitor the client for which complication?

Test	Result
Blood type	AB+
Hemoglobin level	10 g/dL (100 g/L)
Hematocrit	32% (0.32)
White blood cell count	18,000 mm³ (18 × 10⁹/L)
Platelet count	200,000 mm³ (200 × 10⁹/L)

1. Rh sensitization
2. Chorioamnionitis
3. Hemorrhage
4. Fetal distress

45. 4. The nurse should monitor the client for fetal distress because it is more common in women with anemia (hemoglobin level less than 11 g/dL) than in the general, nonanemic population. Rh sensitization is suspected in women with a negative rhesus factor. The white blood cell count is normal for a laboring client. No risk factors for chorioamnionitis or hemorrhage are noted.
CN: Physiological integrity; CNS: Reduction of risk potential; CL: Apply

46. An experienced nurse is determining which laboring client to assign to a new graduate nurse. Which client will be assigned to the new graduate nurse?
   1. Fetal heart rate of 145 to 155 beats/minute with 15-second accelerations to 160 beats/minute
   2. Fetal heart rate of 130 to 140 beats/minute with decreased variability
   3. Fetal heart rate of 110 to 120 beats/minute in a client whose membranes just ruptured
   4. Fetal heart rate of 165 to 175 beats/minute with late decelerations to 140 beats/minute

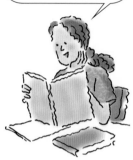

Normal fetal heart rates are way higher than those for adults, and short bursts of acceleration are nothing to be concerned about.

47. The nurse is monitoring a client who is receiving oxytocin to induce labor. The nurse will be alert for which maternal adverse reaction(s)? Select all that apply.
   1. Hypertension
   2. Jaundice
   3. Dehydration
   4. Fluid overload
   5. Uterine tetany
   6. Bradycardia

48. The nurse is educating expectant mothers about the progress of labor. Place the items below in order showing a normal progression of labor. Use all options.

1. Uncontrollable urge to push
2. Cervical dilation of 4 cm
3. 100% cervical effacement
4. Strong Braxton Hicks contractions
5. Mild contractions lasting 20 to 40 seconds

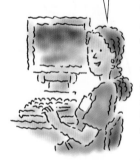

Sweet! I love these ordering questions. Now, which is most likely to occur first?

49. A client at 32 weeks' gestation is receiving terbutaline. The nurse will monitor the client for which potentially life-threatening complication?
   1. Diabetic ketoacidosis
   2. Hyperemesis gravidarum
   3. Pulmonary edema
   4. Sickle cell anemia

46. 1. The nurse should assign the new graduate nurse the least complex client. A fetal heart rate of 110 to 160 beats/minute is normal. Accelerations of up to 15 beats/minute above baseline for a duration of 15 seconds are signs of fetal well-being. The experienced nurse should care for the clients requiring complex care or with deviations. Decreased variability and late decelerations indicate fetal distress. The client with ruptured membranes needs to be assessed to determine whether any complications are present.
CN: Safe, effective care environment; CNS: Management of care; CL: Apply

47. 1, 4, 5. Maternal adverse effects of oxytocin include hypertension, fluid overload, and uterine tetany. Oxytocin's antidiuretic effect increases renal reabsorption of water, leading to fluid overload, not dehydration. Jaundice and bradycardia are adverse effects that may occur in the neonate. Tachycardia, not bradycardia, is reported as a maternal adverse effect.
CN: Physiological integrity; CNS: Pharmacological and parenteral therapies; CL: Apply

48. Ordered Response:

4. Strong Braxton Hicks contractions
5. Mild contractions lasting 20 to 40 seconds
2. Cervical dilation of 4 cm
3. 100% cervical effacement
1. Uncontrollable urge to push

Strong Braxton Hicks contractions typically occur before the onset of true labor and are considered a preliminary sign of labor. During the latent phase of the first stage of labor, contractions are mild, lasting up to 45 seconds. As the client progresses through labor, contractions increase in intensity and duration, and cervical dilation occurs. Cervical dilation of 4 cm indicates that the client has entered the active phase of the first stage of labor. Cervical effacement also occurs; effacement of 100% characterizes the transition phase of the first stage of labor. Progression into the second stage of labor is noted by the client's uncontrollable urge to push.
CN: Health promotion and maintenance; CNS: None: CL: Analyze

49. 3. Terbutaline is a tocolytic, which is a medication used to stop labor contractions. An adverse effect associated with the use of these drugs is pulmonary edema. Clients who do not have diabetes do not need to be observed for diabetic ketoacidosis. Hyperemesis gravidarum does not result from tocolytic use. Sickle cell anemia is an inherited genetic condition that does not develop spontaneously.
CN: Physiological integrity; CNS: Pharmacological and parenteral therapies; CL: Apply

50. A pregnant client in the active phase of labor states, "My head and upper abdomen are hurting. I am seeing a few spots around the room, too." What will the nurse do **next**?
1. Turn the client to her right side.
2. Have the client rate her pain.
3. Administer magnesium sulfate.
4. Check the client's blood pressure.

51. A woman is in the third stage of labor after having just given birth to a healthy newborn. Which action(s) by the nurse is **most** important during this stage? Select all that apply.
1. Assisting with skin-to-skin contact
2. Providing the woman with cool compresses
3. Encouraging the woman to breastfeed
4. Assisting the woman into a comfortable position
5. Applying a heating pad to the episiotomy site

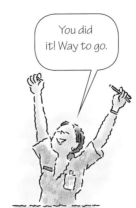

You did it! Way to go.

50. 4. The nurse should check the client's blood pressure because the client is exhibiting signs of elevated blood pressure. The nurse may reposition the client to the left side and administer magnesium sulfate if the blood pressure is significantly elevated. Having the client rate pain would be done after assessing for hypertension.
CN: Physiological integrity; CNS: Pharmacological and parenteral therapies; CL: Apply

51. 1, 3, 4. During the third stage of labor, the nurse should assist with skin-to-skin contact between the mother and the newborn, provide warm blankets to prevent shivering, encourage the woman to breastfeed if appropriate, assist the woman into a comfortable position, and apply ice to the episiotomy site.
CN: Safe, effective care environment; CNS: Management of care; CL: Apply

Chapter 23

Postpartum Care

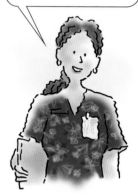

The postpartum period begins after the baby is born and lasts for 6 weeks ... but it may take the woman longer to feel like herself again.

Postpartum care refresher

Mastitis

Inflammation and infection of the breast that results from the stasis of milk; the most common infecting organism is *Staphylococcus aureus*

Key signs and symptoms

- Chills
- Localized area of redness, inflammation, and tenderness
- Temperature of 101.1°F (38.4°C) or higher

Key test results

- Culture of purulent discharge may test positive for *Staphylococcus aureus*

Key treatments

- Incision and drainage if abscess occurs
- Moist heat application
- Feed or pump breasts every 2 to 4 hours to preserve breastfeeding ability if abscess occurs
- Analgesics: acetaminophen, ibuprofen
- Antibiotics: cephalexin, cefaclor, clindamycin

Key interventions

- Administer antibiotic therapy.
- Apply moist heat.

Postpartum hemorrhage

Blood loss of 500 mL or more after a vaginal birth or 1,000 mL or more after cesarean birth; can occur within the first 24 hours (early postpartum hemorrhage) or from 24 hours to 6 weeks after birth (late postpartum hemorrhage)

Key signs and symptoms

- Blood loss greater than 500 mL within a 24-hour period; may occur up to 6 weeks after birth
- Signs of shock (tachycardia, hypotension, oliguria)
- Uterine atony

Key test results

- Hematology studies show decreased hemoglobin and hematocrit levels, low fibrinogen level, and decreased partial thromboplastin time

Key treatments

- Bimanual compression of the uterus and dilation and curettage (D&C) to remove clots
- Intravenous (IV) replacement of fluids and blood
- Parenteral administration of methylergonovine maleate
- Rapid IV infusion of dilute oxytocin

Key interventions

- Massage the fundus and express clots from the uterus.
- Perform a pad count, may weigh pads.
- Monitor the fundus for location.
- Monitor IV infusion of dilute oxytocin.

Psychological maladaptation

Changes in the mother's mood, which can range from postpartum blues (or baby blues) to postpartum depression to postpartum psychosis

Key signs and symptoms

- Inability to stop crying
- Increased anxiety about self and infant's health
- Overall feeling of sadness
- Unwillingness to be left alone
- Hallucinations/delusions with psychosis

Key treatments

- Counseling for the client and family at risk
- Psychotherapy for the client
- Antidepressants: imipramine, nortriptyline

Key interventions

- Obtain a health history during the antepartum period to determine risk of postpartum depression.

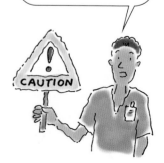

Postpartum blood loss greater than 500 mL within a 24-hour period is considered hemorrhage and should be addressed immediately.

- Evaluate client's support systems.
- Evaluate maternal–infant bonding.
- Provide emotional support and encouragement.

Puerperal infection

Fever occurring after the first 24 hours after birth, and occurring on at least 2 of the first 10 days after birth; can occur in the reproductive tract, urinary tract, or wound

Key signs and symptoms
- Abdominal pain and tenderness
- Purulent, foul-smelling lochia
- Tachycardia
- Temperature of 101.5°F (38.6°C) or higher

Key test results
- Complete blood count may show an elevated white blood cell count in the upper ranges of normal (more than 30,000/mm³ [30 × 10⁹/L]) for the postpartum period
- Cultures of the blood or the endocervical and uterine cavities may reveal the causative organism

Key treatments
- Broad-spectrum IV antibiotic therapy unless a causative organism is identified

Key interventions
- Monitor vital signs every 4 hours.
- Place client in Fowler's position.
- Maintain IV fluid administration as prescribed.
- Administer antibiotics as prescribed.

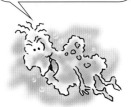

We bacteria love the postpartum period. So many opportunities to invade and multiply.

thePoint® You can download tables of drug information to help you prepare for the NCLEX®! View Generic Drug Names, Drug Classifications, Drug Actions, and Nursing Implications for the drugs discussed in this refresher at **http://thePoint.lww.com.**

Postpartum care questions, answers, and rationales

1. The nurse is assisting a postpartum client to breastfeed her newborn. The client is having difficulty in establishing an adequate supply of breast milk. The nurse understands which factor might play a role?
1. Supplemental formula feedings
2. Maternal diet high in vitamin C
3. Consumption of an alcoholic drink
4. Frequently breastfeeding the newborn

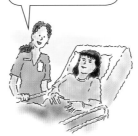

Other than being chronically sleep-deprived, having sore breasts, and hemorrhoids—I'm doing fantastic.

2. After receiving the 0700 shift report, the nurse assesses a postpartum client. The nurse notices the client's perineal pad is completely saturated with lochia rubra. What will the nurse do **next**?
1. Perform fundal massage immediately.
2. Assess the client's vital signs.
3. Determine when the client last changed the pad.
4. Administer oxytocin intravenously.

3. A G7 P5 client gave birth vaginally to a healthy neonate this morning. It is **priority** for the nurse to monitor the client for which complication?
1. Anemia
2. Uterine atony
3. Thrombophlebitis
4. Metritis

1. 1. Routine formula supplementation may interfere with establishing an adequate milk volume because decreased stimulation to the client's nipples affects hormonal levels and milk production. Vitamin C levels have not been shown to influence milk volume. One alcoholic drink has not been shown to decrease milk supply, although excessive consumption of alcohol may interfere with breastfeeding. Frequent feedings are likely to increase milk production.
CN: Health promotion and maintenance; CNS: None; CL: Apply

2. 3. First, the nurse should determine when the client last changed her perineal pad. It is possible that the client has not changed her pad in several hours. The client's lochia may have pooled during the night, resulting in a heavy flow in the morning. Fundal massage, assessing vital signs, and oxytocin may be warranted if the client has recently changed her perineal pad.
CN: Safe, effective care environment; CNS: Management of care; CL: Analyze

3. 2. Multiparous women typically experience a loss of uterine tone due to frequent distention of the uterus from previous pregnancies. As a result, this client is at higher risk for hemorrhage from uterine atony. The client does not have risk factors for anemia, thrombophlebitis, or metritis.
CN: Physiological integrity; CNS: Reduction of risk potential; CL: Apply

CN: Client needs category   CNS: Client needs subcategory   CL: Cognitive level

4. A postpartum client calls the nurse and states, "My breasts are engorged. I am giving my baby formula, not breast milk. What can I do?" Which nursing response is **most** appropriate?
   1. "You need to apply heat packs to your breasts for 10 to 15 minutes at a time."
   2. "I recommend you use a breast pump to remove some of the milk from your breasts."
   3. "The easiest thing to do is place cabbage leaves over each breast for a few days."
   4. "The best thing is to limit your oral intake of fluids to no more than 20 ounces a day."

5. The nurse is educating a postpartum client following a cesarean section. Which education will the nurse provide to the client? Select all that apply.
   1. Clean the perineum with warm water after voiding.
   2. You need to change your perineal pad once every 12 hours.
   3. Do coughing and deep-breathing exercises every hour.
   4. Perform Kegel exercises several times each day.
   5. You need to drink three or four 8-oz glasses of fluid a day.

6. A postpartum client who had a cesarean birth reports right calf pain to the nurse. Upon assessment, the nurse notes the client has nonpitting edema from her right knee to her foot. Based on this finding, the nurse expects the health care provider will order which test?
   1. Venous duplex ultrasound of the right leg
   2. Transthoracic echocardiogram
   3. Venogram of the right leg
   4. Noninvasive arterial studies of the right leg

7. A postpartum client asks the nurse how to perform Kegel exercises. Which nursing response is **most** appropriate?
   1. "You need to quickly tighten and relax your abdominal muscles."
   2. "Contract your pelvic floor muscles, hold, and then relax the muscles."
   3. "You contract and hold your abdominal muscles for 15 seconds."
   4. "To do this, bear down using your pelvic muscles, as you would for a bowel movement."

8. The nurse is caring for a postpartum client with type 1 diabetes who has developed ketoacidosis. The nurse will complete which prescription **first**?
   1. Consult an endocrinologist.
   2. Administer intravenous insulin.
   3. Apply a cardiac monitor.
   4. Monitor glucose hourly.

4. **3.** Telling the client to place cabbage leaves on each breast helps to reduce the engorgement. Cabbage leaves contain an enzyme that works to dry up a woman's milk supply. Because the client is not breastfeeding, this is an appropriate intervention. Applying heat and using a breast pump stimulate milk production, worsening the engorgement. Restricting fluids does not reduce engorgement and should not be encouraged.
CN: Physiological integrity; CNS: Basic care and comfort; CL: Apply

5. **1, 3, 4.** The nurse should encourage the woman to clean her perineum after each voiding to prevent infection, cough and perform deep-breathing exercises to prevent infection, and perform Kegel exercises to strengthen the pelvic floor following a cesarean section. The client should change her perineal pad with each voiding and bowel movement or when soiled. The client should consume at least six to eight 8-oz glasses.
CN: Physiological integrity; CNS: Reduction of risk potential; CL: Apply

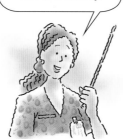

After surgery, the lungs need a good workout to stay clear and healthy.

6. **1.** Right calf pain and nonpitting edema may indicate deep vein thrombosis (DVT). Postpartum clients and clients who have had abdominal surgery are at increased risk for DVT. Venous duplex ultrasound is a noninvasive test that visualizes the veins and assesses blood flow patterns. A venogram is an invasive test that utilizes dye and radiation to create images of the veins; it would not be the first test to perform. Transthoracic echocardiography looks at cardiac structures and is not indicated at this time. Right calf pain and edema are symptoms of venous outflow obstruction, not arterial insufficiency.
CN: Safe, effective care environment; CNS: Management of care; CL: Apply

7. **2.** To perform Kegel exercises correctly, the client should tighten her pelvic muscles, hold for 8 to 10 seconds, and then relax the muscles for 10 seconds. The client should perform 10 sets three times a day. Kegel exercises do not involve the abdominal muscles.
CN: Health promotion and maintenance; CNS: None; CL: Apply

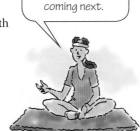

Being a nurse requires a lot of flexibility; you never know what's coming next.

8. **2.** The nurse should first administer insulin to treat the ketoacidosis. The nurse would then complete the remaining prescriptions. Clients with diabetes who become pregnant tend to become sicker and develop illnesses more quickly than pregnant clients without diabetes.
CN: Physiological integrity; CNS: Reduction of risk potential; CL: Analyze

9. The nurse will suspect a client may be experiencing a pulmonary embolus based on which assessment finding(s)? Select all that apply.
1. Sudden dyspnea
2. Hypertension
3. Chills
4. Bradycardia
5. Increased prothrombin time (PT)

10. A client had an emergency cesarean birth. Afterward, the client expresses disappointment about not being able to give birth vaginally. The nurse understands the client's feeling may be based on which concept?
1. Cesarean births cost substantially more.
2. Depression is more common after a cesarean birth.
3. The client is usually more fatigued after cesarean birth.
4. The client is not able to experience a traditional birth.

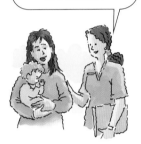

Emotional support and encouragement can be invaluable to a new mother.

11. The nurse is providing discharge instructions to a postpartum client following a vaginal birth. The nurse determines the client has understood the information when the client states which finding(s) is expected? Select all that apply.
1. Redness or swelling in the calves
2. A healed episiotomy within 3 weeks
3. Vaginal dryness after the lochial flow has ended
4. Red lochia for approximately 6 weeks after the birth
5. Strong-smelling lochia by the end of the first week

12. The nurse assesses a postpartum client and notes her fundus is deviated to the left of midline. What is the **priority** nursing action?
1. Ask the client to empty her bladder.
2. Straight catheterize the client.
3. Call the client's health care provider.
4. Massage the client's fundus.

Remember to look for the *priority* action in question #12.

13. When reviewing self-care instructions with a postpartum client, the nurse emphasizes the need for the client to report heavy or excessive bleeding. The nurse will describe heavy bleeding as saturating one sanitary pad within which time span?
1. 1 hour
2. 2 hours
3. 3 hours
4. 4 hours

9. 1. A sign of pulmonary embolus is sudden dyspnea. Other symptoms include chest pain, coughing, bloody sputum, confusion, and fainting. Chills would most likely signal an infection. An increased PT may indicate disseminated intravascular coagulation (DIC). The client with a pulmonary embolus would have tachycardia and hypotension, not bradycardia and hypertension.
CN: Physiological integrity; CNS: Reduction of risk potential; CL: Apply

10. 4. Clients occasionally feel a loss after a cesarean birth. They may feel they are inadequate because they could not give birth to their newborn vaginally. The cost of cesarean birth does not generally apply because the client usually is not directly responsible for payment. No conclusive studies support the theory that depression is more common following cesarean births. Although clients are usually more fatigued after a cesarean birth, fatigue has not been shown to cause feelings of disappointment over the method of birth.
CN: Psychosocial integrity; CNS: None; CL: Understand

11. 2, 3. An episiotomy should be healed within 2 to 3 weeks' postpartum. Vaginal dryness is a normal finding during the postpartum period due to hormonal changes. Redness or swelling in the calves is not normal and may indicate thrombophlebitis. Red lochia (indicating fresh bleeding) should last about 3 days' postpartum. Lochia at any stage should have a fleshy odor. Any other strong odor suggests an infection.
CN: Physiological integrity; CNS: Physiological adaptation; CL: Apply

12. 1. A full bladder may displace the uterine fundus to the left or right side of the abdomen. Therefore, the nurse should have the client empty her bladder and then check the fundus again. A straight catheterization is unnecessarily invasive if the client can urinate on her own. Nursing interventions should be completed before notifying the primary health care provider in a nonemergency situation. Massaging the client's fundus is performed to address atony, promote involution, alleviate pain, and prevent or stop postpartum hemorrhage.
CN: Safe, effective care environment; CNS: Management of care; CL: Apply

13. 1. Bleeding is considered heavy when a woman saturates one sanitary pad in 1 hour.
CN: Health promotion and maintenance; CNS: None; CL: Understand

14. A 7-day postpartum client is diagnosed with postpartum hemorrhage. The nurse will assess the client for which common cause(s) of delayed postpartum hemorrhage? Select all that apply.
1. Retained placental fragments
2. Endometriosis
3. Intrauterine infection
4. Uterine fibroids
5. Uterine rupture

15. The nurse is educating a postpartum client diagnosed with mastitis. The nurse determines the client understands the information when she makes which statement?
1. "Mastitis is caused when a virus is transmitted to the breasts through cracks in the nipples."
2. "I probably got mastitis from breastfeeding my baby too often during the day."
3. "The bacteria that cause mastitis can be transmitted to the breast from the baby."
4. "Mastitis happens secondary to another infection, like a sinus or ear infection."

16. The nurse is monitoring a client who gave birth vaginally 30 hours ago. The nurse determines the client is progressing as expected when the nurse assesses the client's fundus at which location?
1. Two fingerbreadths above the umbilicus
2. One fingerbreadth below the umbilicus
3. At the level of the umbilicus
4. Below the symphysis pubis

17. The nurse is educating postpartum clients on mastitis. Which information will the nurse include in the teaching?
1. The most common cause of mastitis is group A beta-hemolytic streptococci.
2. A breast abscess is a common complication of mastitis.
3. Mastitis usually develops in both breasts of a breastfeeding client.
4. Symptoms of mastitis include fever, chills, malaise, and localized breast tenderness.

18. The nurse is providing care to a G6 P5 postpartum client who had polyhydramnios during this pregnancy and had a macrosomic baby by cesarean section. Based on this, the nurse will perform which assessment **frequently** on this client?
1. Lochia flow
2. Temperature
3. Blood pressure
4. Glucose level

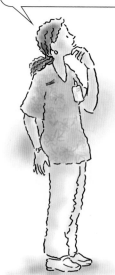

Let's see … mastitis is an infection of the breast. What symptoms do we expect to see?

14. 1, 3, 4. The most common causes of a delayed postpartum hemorrhage include retained placental fragments, intrauterine infection, and fibroids. Uterine rupture is a common cause of early, not delayed, postpartum hemorrhage. Endometriosis is not a cause of postpartum hemorrhage.
CN: Physiological integrity; CNS: Reduction of risk potential; CL: Apply

15. 3. The most common cause of mastitis is *Staphylococcus aureus*, which can be transmitted from the lining of the infant's nostrils when an opportunity such as a crack in the nipple presents itself. Mastitis is not caused by a virus, frequent feeding, or secondary to another infection.
CN: Safe, effective care environment; CNS: Safety and infection control; CL: Apply

16. 2. After a client gives birth vaginally, the height of her fundus should decrease by about one fingerbreadth (1 cm) each day. By the end of the first postpartum day, the fundus should be one fingerbreadth below the umbilicus. Immediately after birth, the fundus may be midway between the umbilicus and symphysis pubis; 6 to 12 hours after birth, it should be at the level of the umbilicus; and 10 days after birth, it should be below the symphysis pubis.
CN: Health promotion and maintenance; CNS: None; CL: Apply

17. 4. Mastitis is an infection of the breast characterized by flulike symptoms, along with redness and tenderness in the breast. The most common causative agent is *Staphylococcus aureus*. Breast abscess is rarely a complication of mastitis if the client continues to empty the affected breast. Mastitis usually occurs in one breast, not bilaterally.
CN: Physiological integrity; CNS: Physiological adaptation; CL: Apply

18. 1. The nurse should monitor the client's lochia flow closely to watch for hemorrhage. The client is at high risk for a postpartum hemorrhage from the overdistention of the uterus because of the extra amniotic fluid (polyhydramnios), the large size of the neonate (macrosomia), and high gravida. The uterus may not be able to contract as well as it would normally. The client is not at increased risk for fever, hypertension or hypotension, or diabetes mellitus.
CN: Physiological integrity; CNS: Reduction of risk potential; CL: Analyze

CN: Client needs category   CNS: Client needs subcategory   CL: Cognitive level

19. What is **priority** for the nurse to monitor on a client in the immediate postpartum period? Select all that apply.
1. Blood glucose level
2. Heart rhythm
3. Height of fundus
4. Occult stool test
5. Fluid intake

19. 3. A focused physical examination should be performed every 15 minutes for the first 1 to 2 hours' postpartum, including assessment of the fundus, lochia, perineum, blood pressure, pulse, and bladder function (urine output, not fluid intake). A blood glucose level would be obtained if the client has risk factors for an unstable blood glucose level or if she has symptoms of an altered blood glucose level. Monitoring the heart rhythm would be necessary only if the client is at risk for cardiac difficulty. A stool test for occult blood generally would not be valid during the immediate postpartum period because it is difficult to sort out lochial bleeding from rectal bleeding.
CN: Health maintenance and promotion; CNS: None; CL: Apply

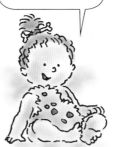

Yabba dabba doo! You're really rockin' this test.

20. During assessment of a 1-hour postpartum client, the nurse notices heavy bleeding with large clots. After initiating fundal massage, which action will the nurse perform **next**?
1. Administer oxytocin.
2. Assess the client's vital signs.
3. Give an IV fluid bolus.
4. Notify the health care provider.

20. 1. Initial management of excessive postpartum bleeding is continuous, firm massage of the fundus and administration of oxytocin. The nurse would give a fluid bolus and assess vitals if the excessive bleeding continues. The health care provider should be notified if the client does not respond to fundal massage, but other measures can be taken in the meantime.
CN: Physiological integrity; CNS: Reduction of risk potential; CL: Analyze

21. A postpartal client asks the nurse, "Why am I still having contraction pain?" Which response by the nurse is **most** appropriate?
1. "The pain you are currently experiencing is normal and is referred to as afterpains."
2. "Your uterus is still contracting to help seal off the site where your placenta was attached."
3. "I am not sure why you are still having contractions. I will call the health care provider."
4. "Do not worry about pain. I am sure the contractions will subside within a few days."

21. 2. It is most appropriate for the nurse to respond by addressing the client's concern. The pain is normal and is called afterpains, but this statement does not address the client's question. The remaining choices are not therapeutic.
CN: Health promotion and maintenance; CNS: None; CL: Apply

22. A multiparous postpartum client is being discharged 48 hours after a 16-hour vaginal birth of a 4,036-g neonate. The nurse notes the mother is rubella-immune with Rh-positive blood type. When planning to discharge the client, which intervention is **priority**?
1. The client will receive Rho(D) immune globulin intramuscularly before discharge.
2. The client will understand the need for planned rest periods.
3. The client will understand the need for and consent to a rubella vaccine before discharge.
4. The client will state the importance of reporting any change in character of lochia.

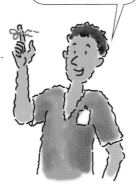

Remember to keep your priorities in order when answering question #22.

22. 4. A multiparous client who has a history of prolonged labor and birth of a large infant is at a higher risk for developing late postpartum hemorrhage. The nurse should ensure that the client understands the importance of reporting a change in lochia pattern, including increased amount, resumption of a brighter color, passage of clots, or foul odor. The client with Rh-positive blood does not require a Rho(D) immune globulin injection. Postpartum hemorrhage instruction takes precedence over planning adequate rest. A client who is rubella-immune does not require immunization.
CN: Safe, effective care environment; CNS: Management of care; CL: Analyze

23. The nurse is caring for a client who has given birth to a healthy neonate. When checking the client's fundus, which finding will the nurse expect to assess?
1. Fundus 1 cm above the umbilicus 1 hour postpartum
2. Fundus 1 cm above the umbilicus on postpartum day 3
3. Fundus palpable in the abdomen at 2 weeks' postpartum
4. Fundus slightly to the right and 2 cm above the umbilicus on postpartum day 2

24. The nurse notices an assistive personnel (AP) about to give a client with gestational diabetes her breakfast tray on her first day postpartum. Which nursing action is appropriate?
1. Ensure that the client is receiving a diabetic meal tray.
2. Obtain the client's glucose level after breakfast.
3. Have the AP obtain a fasting glucose level for the client.
4. Perform a urine dipstick test to check the urine for ketones.

25. The nurse is caring for a client with O negative blood type. The client's neonate is A positive blood type. The neonate has had a positive direct Coombs test. Which nursing intervention is appropriate?
1. Administer Rho(D) immune globulin.
2. Contact the health care provider.
3. Hold the Rho(D) immune globulin.
4. Repeat the Coombs test in 24 hours.

26. A postpartum client experiences postpartal hemorrhage. Fundal massage fails to maintain uterine contraction, and the client continues to experience hemorrhage. The nurse will anticipate which medication(s) to be prescribed? Select all that apply.
1. Oxytocin
2. Carboprost
3. Methylergonovine
4. Heparin
5. Amoxicillin

27. The nurse is caring for a postpartum client. When interacting with the client, which finding(s) concerns the nurse? Select all that apply.
1. The client does not want to hold her newborn.
2. The client refuses to feed her newborn.
3. The client cannot stop crying.
4. The client sleeps with the baby in her bed.
5. The client appears to be paranoid.

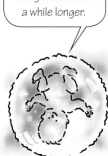

No thanks. I think I'll just hang out in here a while longer.

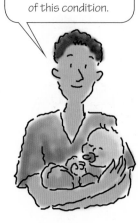

The "baby blues" might sound harmless, but it can develop into depression; monitor any client with signs of this condition.

23. 1. Within the first 12 hours' postpartum, the fundus is usually approximately 1 cm above the umbilicus. The fundus should be below the umbilicus by postpartum day 3. The fundus should not be palpated in the abdomen after day 10. A uterus that is not midline or is above the umbilicus on postpartum day 3 might be caused by a full, distended bladder or a uterine infection.
CN: Health promotion and maintenance; CNS: None; CL: Apply

24. 3. Clients with gestational diabetes need to have their fasting glucose levels assessed the morning following birth. Generally, their glucose level should now be returned to normal and no further interventions should be required. If the level is normal, a diabetic meal is not necessary. There is no need to assess urine for ketones.
CN: Safe, effective care environment; CNS: Management of care; CL: Apply

25. 3. A positive Coombs test means that the Rh-negative client is now producing antibodies to the Rh-positive blood of the neonate. Rho(D) immune globulin should not be given to a sensitized client because it will not be able to prevent antibody formation. There is no need to contact the health care provider or to repeat the Coombs test in 24 hours.
CN: Physiological integrity; CNS: Reduction of risk potential; CL: Apply

26. 1, 2, 3. If fundal massage fails to maintain uterine contraction, oxytocin, carboprost, or methylergonovine may be prescribed to maintain uterine tone and control hemorrhage. Heparin would be appropriate as treatment for deep vein thrombosis. Amoxicillin may be prescribed to treat an infection.
CN: Physiological integrity; CNS: Pharmacological and parenteral therapies; CL: Apply

27. 1, 2, 3, 4, 5. A client experiencing postpartum depression or psychosis may deny her newborn and be unable to safely care for her newborn. Signs and symptoms include refusing to care for the newborn, lack of responsiveness to the newborn, inability to stop crying, and paranoia. The client sleeping with the newborn in her bed places the newborn at risk for sudden infant death syndrome and is associated with increased infant mortality.
CN: Psychosocial integrity; CNS: None; CL: Apply

CN: Client needs category   CNS: Client needs subcategory   CL: Cognitive level

28. The nurse reviews a progress note in the client's medical record, shown below. What will the nurse do **next**?

Progress notes	
10/24	Client is 5 hours postvaginal birth with
1845	vacuum extraction. Fundus is firm;
	moderate lochia. Vital signs:
	temperature, 100.8°F (38.2°C)
	orally; heart rate, 110 beats/minute;
	respiratory rate, 22 breaths/minute; blood
	pressure, 110/78 mm Hg.
	—Elana Blain, RN

1. Notify the health care provider.
2. Reassess the client's vital signs.
3. Administer acetaminophen orally.
4. Check the client's oxygen saturation level.

29. While assessing a postpartum client's lochia, the nurse notes a continuous trickle of bright red blood from the vagina. A fundal assessment reveals her fundus is firm. The client's vital signs are as follows: blood pressure, 112/78 mm Hg; pulse rate, 68 beats/minute; oxygen saturation, 96%; respiratory rate, 20 breaths/minute. What will the nurse do **next**?
1. Prepare the client for a vaginal exam.
2. Recheck the client in 30 minutes.
3. Administer oxygen via nasal cannula at 2 L/minute.
4. Administer a normal saline bolus intravenously (IV).

30. A client is 2 days' postpartum and is experiencing bleeding. The client asks the nurse, "Will it always be like this?" Which statement by the nurse is **most** accurate?
1. "This is lochia alba and will last 4 weeks."
2. "This is lochia serosa and will last 2 days."
3. "This is lochia rubra and will last 3 to 4 days."
4. "This is your menstrual cycle and will last 6 weeks."

31. The nurse is educating a postpartum client on anticoagulant therapy. Which client statement indicates the client understands the nurse's teaching?
1. "I need to stop taking any iron supplements."
2. "I should take acetaminophen instead of aspirin."
3. "I will wear knee-high stockings when possible."
4. "Shortness of breath is a common adverse effect."

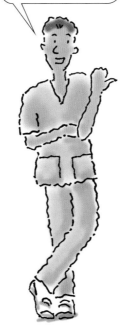

Inform your client that if heavy bleeding lasts longer than a few days, she should contact her health care provider immediately.

28. 1. The nurse should notify the health care provider of potential infection. The client's elevated temperature along with her prolonged labor and the instrumentation associated with the birth place her at risk for postpartum infection. The nurse should reassess vital signs and may administer acetaminophen after notifying the health care provider. Checking the oxygen saturation level is not needed.
CN: Physiological integrity; CNS: Reduction of risk potential; CL: Analyze

29. 1. If the uterus is firm, and thus atony is not a suspected cause of bleeding, a continuous trickle of blood may be due to cervical or vaginal lacerations, so the nurse should prepare the client for a vaginal exam. The nurse should recheck the client frequently, but preparing the client for a vaginal exam is the priority. The client does not require oxygen or an IV bolus at this time, but may if the bleeding continues.
CN: Physiological integrity; CNS: Reduction of risk potential; CL: Apply

30. 3. Lochia rubra, which is made up of blood, mucus, and tissue debris, lasts 3 to 4 days. Lochia serosa, which consists of blood, mucus, and leukocytes, lasts from day 3 to day 10 postpartum. Lochia alba, which consists largely of mucus, lasts from day 10 to day 14 postpartum. Lochia alba may last up to 6 weeks' postpartum. Postpartum bleeding is not the menstrual cycle.
CN: Physiological integrity; CNS: Physiological adaptation; CL: Apply

31. 2. Discharge education should include informing the client to avoid salicylates, such as aspirin, which may potentiate the effects of anticoagulant therapy. Iron does not affect anticoagulation therapy. Restrictive clothing such as knee-high stockings should be avoided to prevent the recurrence of thrombophlebitis. Shortness of breath is not a common adverse effect of anticoagulant therapy and should be reported immediately because it may be a symptom of pulmonary embolism.
CN: Physiological integrity; CNS: Reduction of risk potential; CL: Apply

32. Which postpartum client will the nurse see **first**?
1. A 2-day postpartum client with a fundal height 2 cm below her umbilicus.
2. A client who experienced a fetal demise 12 hours ago and is now denying the death.
3. A 3-day postpartum client with a 4-in (10-cm) stain of bright red blood on her perineal pad.
4. A client who had a cesarean section 10 hours ago occasionally passing half-inch (1.75-cm) clots.

33. The nurse obtains vital signs of a client who is 2 days postpartum and finds the temperature is 100.8°F (38.2°C). Additional assessment indicates infection is not present. The nurse will assess the client for which complication **next**?
1. Breast engorgement
2. Endometritis
3. Mastitis
4. Uterine involution

34. A Rh-positive client gives birth vaginally to a 3,007-g neonate after 17 hours of labor. It is **priority** for the nurse to monitor the client for which potential complication?
1. Infection
2. Rh antibodies
3. Mastitis
4. Uterine subinvolution

35. The nurse is caring for a client who required an episiotomy during a vaginal birth 30 hours ago. Which nursing intervention(s) is appropriate for this client? Select all that apply.
1. Apply an ice pack intermittently to the perineal area for 3 days.
2. Administer docusate 100 mg by mouth daily.
3. Provide sitz baths three to four times per day.
4. Encourage the client to do Kegel exercises.
5. Limit the number of times the perineal pad is changed.

36. A client who had an emergency cesarean birth for fetal distress 3 days ago is preparing for discharge. When reviewing the home care instructions with the nurse, the client reveals she is saddened about her cesarean and feels let down that she was not able to have a vaginal birth. When questioned further, the client states she feels "weepy about everything" and cannot stop crying. Which nursing action is **priority**?
1. Contact the health care provider.
2. Discuss the finding with the client's family.
3. Ask the client to elaborate on her feelings.
4. Document the conversation.

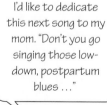

> I'd like to dedicate this next song to my mom. "Don't you go singing those low-down, postpartum blues ..."

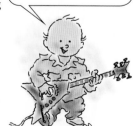

32. 2. The nurse should assess the client denying the death of her fetus first. Denial of the perinatal loss reflects dysfunctional grieving in the client and needs further assessment to ensure client safety. All other client findings are within normal range and are expected.
CN: Psychosocial integrity; CNS: None; CL: Analyze

33. 1. Breast engorgement and dehydration are noninfectious causes of postpartum fevers. Mastitis and endometritis are postpartum infections. Involution of the uterus does not cause temperature elevations.
CN: Health promotion and maintenance; CNS: None; CL: Apply

34. 1. A prolonged length of labor, such as 17 hours, places the mother at increased risk for developing an infection. A client with a positive Rhesus factor is not at risk for antibody production. There are no risk factors for mastitis or uterine subinvolution for this client.
CN: Safe, effective care environment; CNS: Safety and infection control; CL: Apply

35. 2, 3, 4. Docusate softens stool to prevent the client from straining during bowel movements. Sitz baths help decrease inflammation and promote healing in the perineal area. Kegel exercises improve circulation to the area and help reduce edema. Ice packs should be applied to the perineum for the first 24 hours only; after that time, heat should be used. The perineal pad should be changed frequently.
CN: Physiological integrity; CNS: Basic care and comfort; CL: Apply

36. 3. The client's affect is consistent with postpartum blues, a transient source of sadness experienced during the first week after birth. The nurse should offer support to the client and encourage her to elaborate on her concerns and feelings. The client's emotional state is normal, so contacting the health care provider is not indicated at this point. Discussing the client's feelings with family members is a violation of confidentiality and is not an appropriate action. Documenting the interaction is indicated but should take place after the encounter is completed and additional information is gathered.
CN: Psychosocial integrity; CNS: None; CL: Apply

CN: Client needs category CNS: Client needs subcategory CL: Cognitive level

37. A client calls the nurses' station stating she needs to void 3 hours after a vaginal birth. Which nursing action is **most** appropriate?

1. Have the assistive personnel (AP) help the client to the bathroom.
2. Instruct the client that she can get up and use the bathroom independently.
3. Inform the client that she needs to use a bedpan at this time.
4. Assess the client's vital signs before allowing the client to ambulate.

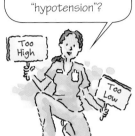

Would a sudden drop in blood pressure be "hypertension" or "hypotension"?

37. 1. The rapid decrease in intra-abdominal pressure occurring after birth causes splanchnic engorgement. The client is at risk for orthostatic hypotension when standing due to the blood pooling in this area; therefore, the nurse should have the AP assist the client when standing immediately after birth. The client should not ambulate alone the first time due to the risk of falling. The client does not require a bedpan or a vital sign assessment prior to ambulation.

CN: Safe, effective care environment; CNS: Safety and infection control; CL: Apply

38. The nurse is caring for a client who gave birth by cesarean section 3 days ago. The client plans to formula feed her infant. The nurse completes an assessment, the findings of which are noted in the chart exhibit below. Which nursing action is **most** appropriate?

Progress notes	
11/15	The client is sitting in the chair bottle
1745	feeding her newborn. Vital signs:
	temperature, 99.1°F (37.3°C); blood
	pressure, 110/72 mm Hg; heart rate,
	64 beats/minute; respiratory rate,
	16 breaths/minute. The fundus is
	4 fingerbreadths below the umbilicus; a small
	amount of lochia rubra is on the perineal
	pad. The client reports discomfort in her
	breasts, which are hard and warm to the
	touch.

1. Tell the client to wear a supportive bra.
2. Have the client stand in a warm shower.
3. Reassess the client in one hour.
4. Recommend the client use a breast pump.

38. 1. These assessment findings are normal for the third postpartum day. Hard, warm breasts indicate engorgement, which occurs about three days after birth. The client should be encouraged to wear a supportive bra to help minimize engorgement and decrease nipple stimulation. The nurse should do something at this time to help the client instead of waiting to reassess. Showering in warm water and using a breast pump stimulate milk production, which would be inappropriate for this client because she is planning to formula feed her infant.

CN: Physiological integrity; CNS: Basic care and comfort; CL: Apply

39. A postpartum client who has developed mastitis is being discharged. What recommendation is **most** appropriate for the nurse to make when the client voices concern about breastfeeding her neonate?

1. "Stop breastfeeding until you complete the antibiotic."
2. "Supplement feedings with formula until the infection resolves."
3. "Do not use analgesics because they are not safe with breastfeeding."
4. "It is okay to continue breastfeeding; mastitis will not infect the neonate."

39. 4. The client with mastitis should be encouraged to continue breastfeeding while taking antibiotics for the infection. Mastitis will not infect the neonate. No supplemental feedings are necessary because breastfeeding does not need to be altered and actually encourages resolution of the infection. Analgesics are safe and should be administered as needed.

CN: Safe, effective care environment; CNS: Safety and infection control; CL: Apply

40. The nurse is assessing a client at 6 weeks' post-partum. The nurse notes her uterus is enlarged and soft and that she is experiencing vaginal bleeding. Based on the findings, which condition does the nurse suspect?
1. Cervical laceration
2. Clotting deficiency
3. Perineal laceration
4. Uterine subinvolution

40. 4. Late postpartum bleeding is usually the result of subinvolution of the uterus. Retained products of conception or infection commonly cause subinvolution. Cervical or perineal lacerations can cause an immediate postpartum hemorrhage. A client with a clotting deficiency may have an immediate postpartum hemorrhage if the deficiency is not corrected at the time of birth.
CN: Physiological integrity; CNS: Physiological adaptation; CL: Apply

41. A 3-week-postpartum client is brought to the emergency department by her husband after he noticed she was acting strangely. The husband reports the client has been having trouble sleeping, experiencing extreme fatigue, and crying all the time. The nurse suspects the client may be experiencing postpartal psychosis based on which additional finding(s)? Select all that apply.
1. Euphoria
2. Preoccupation with guilt
3. Statements about being worthless
4. Thoughts of hurting herself
5. Hallucinations

41. 2, 3, 4, 5. Signs and symptoms associated with postpartum psychosis include: sleep disturbances, fatigue, depression, tearfulness, confusion, and preoccupation with feelings of guilt and worthlessness that may escalate to delirium, hallucinations, anger toward herself or her infant, bizarre behavior, mania, and thoughts of hurting herself or her infant. There may be a loss of touch with reality and a high risk for suicide or infanticide. Euphoria is not associated with postpartum psychosis.
CN: Psychosocial integrity; CNS: None; CL: Apply

42. A client, who gave birth vaginally 16 hours ago, states she does not need to void at this time. The nurse reviews the documentation and finds the client has not voided for 7 hours. Which response by the nurse is indicated?
1. "If you do not attempt to use the bathroom, I will need to catheterize you."
2. "It is common for you to have a full bladder even though you cannot sense it."
3. "I will need to contact your health care provider right away for instructions."
4. "I will come back and check on you in a few hours to see if you can go."

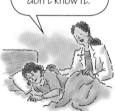
Sometimes you "gotta go" even when you don't know it.

42. 2. After a vaginal birth, the client should be encouraged to void every 4 to 6 hours. As a result of anesthesia and trauma, the client may be unable to sense the filling bladder. It is premature to catheterize the client without allowing her to attempt to void first. Additionally, the statement is threatening to the client. There is no need to contact the health care provider at this time, as the client is demonstrating common adaptations in the early postpartum period. Allowing the client's bladder to fill for another 2 to 3 hours may cause overdistention.
CN: Physiological integrity; CNS: Physiological adaptation; CL: Apply

43. The nurse is preparing to administer a routine injection of insulin to a client with type 1 diabetes who has just given birth vaginally to a newborn. The client asks the nurse, "Why are you giving me less insulin than I took yesterday?" Which nursing response is **most** appropriate?
1. "You need less insulin now because you no longer have a fetus using your insulin too."
2. "Your body needs less insulin after birth because of hormone changes."
3. "The health care provider may have made an error. Let me go check on the dosage."
4. "Your insulin need changes after birth and you may not need any insulin after a few days."

Birth significantly changes the insulin needs of clients with type 1 diabetes. Note any dosage changes and monitor blood glucose levels closely.

43. 2. The placenta produces the hormone human placental lactogen, an insulin antagonist. After birth, the placenta, the major source of insulin resistance, is gone. Insulin needs decrease, and women with type 1 diabetes may need only one half to two thirds of the prenatal insulin dose during the first few postpartum days, though these clients will still need insulin. Blood glucose levels should be monitored and insulin dosages adjusted as needed. The remaining statements are not accurate.
CN: Physiological integrity; CNS: Physiological adaptation; CL: Apply

44. The nurse is providing discharge education to a postpartum client who is rubella nonimmune. Which statement by the client indicates the need for further education?
1. "I can continue to breastfeed my baby after taking the rubella vaccine."
2. "There may be some soreness or tenderness at the injection site for a few days."
3. "The immunization will be given at my 6 weeks' postpartum examination."
4. "Although I have had a tubal ligation, I still need the rubella vaccine."

45. The nurse is caring for a client following a cesarean birth. The client received magnesium sulfate for management of gestational hypertension prior to the cesarean section. It is **priority** for the nurse to perform which assessment?
1. Check the fundus.
2. Monitor heart rate.
3. Measure urine output.
4. Assess gag reflex.

46. A health care provider has prescribed continuation of magnesium sulfate for a 1-hour postpartum client with preeclampsia. During assessment the nurse notes a respiratory rate of 13 breaths/minute and urine output of 30 mL/hour. The client's magnesium sulfate serum level is 6 mg/dL (3 mmol/L). The client reports feeling warm and flushed. Which action by the nurse is appropriate?
1. Reduce the dosage of magnesium sulfate by half.
2. Discontinue the magnesium sulfate immediately.
3. Document the findings.
4. Notify the health care provider.

47. A postpartum client with type 1 diabetes desires to breastfeed. She asks the nurse whether she needs to make any changes to her regular treatment regimen while breastfeeding. Which nursing response is appropriate?
1. "You will need to increase your daily insulin dosage."
2. "You will not need to take insulin while breastfeeding."
3. "You will need to take metformin in addition to insulin while breastfeeding."
4. "You will probably need less insulin while you are breastfeeding."

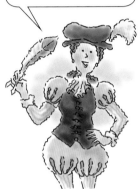

Methinks thou shalt be well prepared to smite that formidable foe, the NCLEX-RN.

44. 3. The rubella vaccine is administered at the time of discharge, not at the 6 weeks' postpartum examination. It is safe for both bottle-feeding and breastfeeding mothers. The medication is given as an intramuscular injection; there may be some localized tenderness, which will subside. To promote community health and wellness, the vaccine is administered to women who have had a tubal ligation.

CN: Health promotion and maintenance; CNS: None; CL: Apply

45. 1. Magnesium sulfate has properties that act as a smooth-muscle relaxant; therefore, the uterus may fail to adequately contract after administration. The nurse should monitor the consistency of the fundus. Failure of the uterus to contract may result in excessive blood loss. Urine output should be monitored closely for signs of magnesium toxicity in clients receiving magnesium sulfate. However, priority would be to monitor for hemorrhage. The heart rate and gag reflex are not affected by the administration of magnesium sulfate.

CN: Physiological integrity; CNS: Pharmacological and parenteral therapies; CL: Apply

46. 3. Magnesium sulfate is associated with feelings of warmth and flushing; these symptoms do not indicate toxicity or complications. A respiratory rate of 13 breaths/minute is considered normal. Urine output should be at least 30 mL/hour. Serum levels of magnesium sulfate should be 4 to 8 mg/dL (2 to 4 mmol/L) to promote a therapeutic response.

CN: Physiological integrity; CNS: Pharmacological and parenteral therapies; CL: Analyze

47. 4. Breastfeeding has an antidiabetic effect. Insulin needs are decreased, but not eliminated, because carbohydrates are used in milk production. Breastfeeding clients are at a higher risk for hypoglycemia in the first postpartum days after birth because glucose levels are lower. Clients with type 1 diabetes do not require oral diabetic medications while breastfeeding.

CN: Physiological integrity; CNS: Pharmacological and parenteral therapies; CL: Apply

CN: Client needs category   CNS: Client needs subcategory   CL: Cognitive level

48. The nurse is assisting a postpartum woman with breastfeeding her newborn. Which action(s) will the nurse recommend to help the new mother breastfeed? Select all that apply.
  1. Suggest the mother cuddle and caress the infant while feeding.
  2. Remind her that breastfeeding is a natural skill.
  3. Encourage her to breastfeed when the infant is alert and hungry.
  4. Show her the different positions for holding the infant for feeding.
  5. Remind her to limit feedings to 10 minutes each time.

49. The nurse is caring for a postpartum client who just had an uncomplicated vaginal birth of an 8 lb, 2 oz (3,693 g) neonate. The client has an intact perineum, equivocal rubella status, and desires to breastfeed. While planning care for this client, which nursing intervention is **priority**?
  1. Encourage high-fiber foods.
  2. Assist the client with breastfeeding.
  3. Administer a rubella vaccination.
  4. Provide an initial sitz bath.

50. While examining a client who gave birth 6 hours ago, the nurse notes the client has saturated a perineal pad in the past 30 minutes and the client's fundus is boggy, 1 cm above the umbilicus. Which nursing action(s) is appropriate? Select all that apply.
  1. Give an intravenous (IV) infusion of lactated Ringer's.
  2. Assess the client's vital signs.
  3. Continue to massage the client's fundus.
  4. Place the client in high Fowler's position.
  5. Administer oxytocin IV.

51. The nurse is assessing a postpartum client's fundus. Which nursing action is appropriate?
  1. Place the client in the supine position with arms overhead.
  2. Have the client empty her bladder before the examination.
  3. Wear sterile gloves when assessing the pad and perineum.
  4. Perform the examination as quickly as possible.

52. On the first postpartum day, a client requests the nurse show her how to change the newborn's diaper. The nurse identifies the client is most likely in which phase?
  1. Depression phase
  2. Letting-go phase
  3. Taking-hold phase
  4. Taking-in phase

Watch out for a boggy uterus. This is a common cause of postpartum hemorrhage.

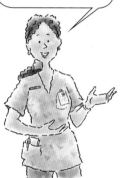

48. 1, 3, 4. Breastfeeding is a learned skill, and some newborns are able to adapt immediately while others take more time. The nurse should suggest that the mother cuddle and caress the infant during feedings, making sure that the infant is alert, awake, and showing signs of hunger. In addition, the nurse should show the mother different positions that can be used for feeding and encourage her to allow sufficient time for her and her baby to enjoy each other in an unhurried atmosphere.
CN: Health promotion and maintenance; CNS: None; CL: Apply

49. 2. With an uncomplicated vaginal birth, the average client is hospitalized for 48 hours or less. It is priority to assist the client with breastfeeding to facilitate the process, provide education, and encourage success. The rubella vaccine is given on the day of discharge. This client has an intact perineum, so fiber and a sitz bath are not priority.
CN: Safe, effective care environment; CNS: Management of care; CL: Analyze

50. 1, 2, 3, 5. Assessing vital signs provides information about the client's circulatory status and identifies significant changes to report to the health care provider. The nurse should continue to massage the client's fundus and give oxytocin to promote uterine contractions. Administering an IV infusion replenishes fluid volume. Placing the client in high Fowler's position may lower blood pressure and harm the client.
CN: Physiological integrity; CNS: Reduction of risk potential; CL: Apply

51. 2. An empty bladder facilitates the examination of the fundus. The client should be in a supine position with her arms at her sides and her knees bent. Clean gloves should be used when assessing the perineum; sterile gloves are not necessary. The postpartum examination should not be done quickly. The nurse can take this time to review information with the client about the changes in her body after birth.
CN: Health promotion and maintenance; CNS: None; CL: Apply

52. 4. The taking-in phase occurs in the first 24 hours after birth. The taking-hold phase occurs when the client is ready to take responsibility for her care as well as her neonate's care, such as in changing the newborn's diaper. During this phase, the client is concerned with her own needs and requires support from others. The letting-go phase begins several weeks later, when the client incorporates the new infant into the family unit. The depression phase is not a postpartum phase.
CN: Health promotion and maintenance; CNS: None; CL: Apply

CN: Client needs category   CNS: Client needs subcategory   CL: Cognitive level

53. The nurse observes several interactions between a new mother and her neonate. Which behavior(s) by the mother concerns the nurse? Select all that apply.

1. Talks and coos to her baby
2. Cuddles her baby close to her
3. Does not make eye contact with her baby
4. Never feeds or changes the baby
5. Encourages the father to hold the baby
6. Takes a nap when the baby is sleeping

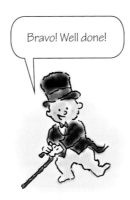

Bravo! Well done!

53. 3, 4. Avoiding eye contact and not providing care are signs that the mother is not bonding with her baby. Eye contact, touching, and speaking are important to establish attachment with an infant. Talking to, cooing to, and cuddling are positive signs that the mother is adapting to her new role. Encouraging the dad to hold the baby facilitates attachment between the neonate and the father. Resting while the infant is sleeping conserves needed energy and allows the mother to be alert and awake when her infant is awake.

CN: Psychosocial integrity; CNS: None; CL: Apply

Chapter 24

Neonatal Care

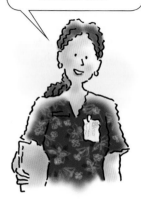

Neonates depend on you for everything. Let's show 'em you've got what it takes for neonatal care!

Neonatal care refresher

Fetal alcohol spectrum disorder

Spectrum of birth defects and behavioral and neurocognitive disabilities resulting from maternal use of alcohol during pregnancy

Key signs and symptoms
- Difficulty establishing respirations
- Lethargy
- Opisthotonos
- Seizures
- Slow pre- and postnatal growth
- Distinctive facial features
- Microcephaly

Key test results
- Chest x-ray may reveal congenital heart defect

Key treatments
- Swaddling
- IV phenobarbital

Key interventions
- Provide a stimulus-free environment for the neonate; darken the room, if necessary.
- Provide gavage feedings, if necessary.
- Early diagnosis improves outcome of birth defects and cognitive development.

Human immunodeficiency virus (HIV)

Infection with HIV virus can be transmitted to the fetus in utero or during the birth process or through breast milk; incidence can be reduced if the HIV-positive pregnant woman receives treatment with antiretroviral therapy

Key signs and symptoms
- Produces no symptoms at birth

Key test results
- Test interpretation is problematic because most neonates with an HIV-positive mother test positive at birth
- Uninfected neonates lose this maternal antibody between 8 and 15 months, and infected neonates remain seropositive
- Testing should be repeated at age 15 months

Key treatments
- Antimicrobial therapy to treat opportunistic infections
- Zidovudine administration based on neonate's lymphocyte count

Key interventions
- Monitor cardiovascular and respiratory status.
- Keep umbilical stump meticulously clean.
- Maintain standard precautions.

Hypothermia

Neonates are at risk for hypothermia due to their immature temperature regulating system

Key signs and symptoms
- Kicking and crying (a mechanism used to increase the metabolic rate to produce body heat)
- Core body temperature lower than 97.7°F (36.5°C)
- Weak suck
- Tachypnea, grunting
- Hypotonia

Key test results
- Arterial blood gas (ABG) analysis shows hypoxemia
- Blood glucose level reveals hypoglycemia

Key treatments
- Radiant warmer

Key interventions
- Dry the neonate immediately after birth.
- Allow mother to hold the neonate skin to skin.
- Monitor vital signs every 15 to 30 minutes.
- Provide a knitted cap for the neonate.
- Wrap the neonate in warmed blankets.
- Place the neonate in a radiant warmer.

Neonatal drug dependency

Dependency caused by exposure to an addictive drug while in the womb

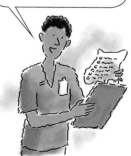

Neonates are especially at risk for hypothermia.

Key signs and symptoms

- Neonatal abstinence syndrome (including seizures, hyperactive reflexes, poor feeding, respiratory disturbances)
- High-pitched cry
- Irritability
- Jitteriness
- Poor sleeping pattern
- Tremors

Key test results

- Urine toxicology screen determines drug exposure
- Meconium screening reveals drug exposure

Key treatments

- Gavage feedings, if necessary

Opioid withdrawal
- Methadone, morphine

Nonopioid withdrawal
- Phenobarbital, chlorpromazine, diazepam

Key interventions

- Monitor cardiovascular status.
- Use tight swaddling for comfort.
- Place the neonate in a dark, quiet environment.
- Encourage use of a pacifier.
- Be prepared to administer gavage feedings (in cases of methadone withdrawal).
- Maintain fluid and electrolyte balance.

Neonatal infections

Neonates are at risk for infections due to their need to rely on maternal antibodies for protection; with birth, the neonate is no longer protected by the intrauterine environment and must develop its own defenses against the environment

Key signs and symptoms

- Feeding pattern changes, such as poor sucking or decreased intake
- Sternal retractions
- Subtle, nonspecific behavioral changes, such as lethargy or hypotonia
- Temperature instability

Key test results

- Blood and urine cultures positive for the causative organism, most commonly gram-positive beta-hemolytic streptococci and the gram-negative *Escherichia coli, Aerobacter, Proteus,* and *Klebsiella*
- Complete blood count shows an increased white blood cell count

Key treatments

- IV therapy to provide adequate hydration

- Antibiotic therapy: broad-spectrum until causative organism is identified and then specific antibiotic

Key interventions

- Monitor cardiovascular and respiratory status.
- Administer broad-spectrum antibiotics before culture results are received.
- Administer specific antibiotic therapy after culture results are received.

Neonatal jaundice

Yellowing of the skin caused by the accumulation of bilirubin in the blood and deposited in the skin and mucous membranes; in the newborn, the rate of bilirubin production must balance the rate of excretion; if production exceeds excretion, hyperbilirubinemia and jaundice result

Key signs and symptoms

- Jaundice
- Lethargy

Key test results

- Bilirubin levels exceed 12 mg/dL in premature or term neonates

Key treatments

- Increased fluid intake
- Phototherapy

Key interventions

- Monitor neurologic status.
- Monitor serum bilirubin levels.
- Initiate and maintain phototherapy
  - provide eye protection while under phototherapy lights
  - remove eye shields promptly when removed from the phototherapy lights.

Respiratory distress syndrome

Respiratory disorder commonly seen in premature neonates that results from lung immaturity and a lack of surfactant in the alveoli

Key signs and symptoms

- Cyanosis and pallor
- Expiratory grunting
- Fine crackles and diminished breath sounds
- Seesaw respirations
- Sternal, substernal, and intracostal retractions
- Tachypnea (more than 60 breaths/minute)

Key test results

- ABG analysis reveals respiratory acidosis
- Chest x-ray reveals bilateral diffuse reticulogranular density

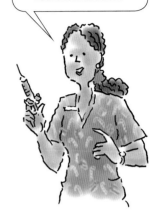

What type of antibiotic therapy is called for initially to treat a neonatal infection?

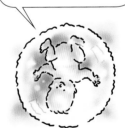

Some infections can be transmitted to the fetus in utero.

Key treatments

- Oxygenation and continuous positive airway pressure (CPAP)
- Endotracheal (ET) intubation and mechanical ventilation
- Nutrition supplements (total parenteral nutrition [TPN] or enteral feedings if possible)
- Surfactant replacement by way of ET tube
- Temperature regulation with a radiant warmer

Key interventions

- Monitor cardiovascular, respiratory, and neurologic status.
- Monitor vital signs.
- Maintain ventilator support status.
- Administer medications, including ET surfactant as prescribed.
- Provide adequate nutrition through enteral feedings, if possible, or TPN.

Tracheoesophageal fistula

Abnormal opening between the trachea and the esophagus; during embryonic development, the esophagus and trachea do not separate as they normally should

Key signs and symptoms

- Difficulty feeding, such as choking or aspiration; cyanosis during feeding
- Signs of respiratory distress

Key test results

- Abdominal x-ray shows the fistula and a gas-free abdomen

Key treatments

- Emergency surgical intervention to prevent pneumonia, dehydration, and fluid and electrolyte imbalances
- Maintenance of patent airway

Key interventions

- Monitor cardiovascular, respiratory, and GI status.
- Place neonate in high Fowler's position.
- Keep a laryngoscope and ET tube at bedside.
- Provide neonate with a pacifier.
- Provide gastrostomy tube feedings postoperatively.

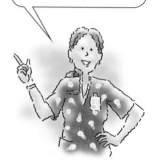

A neonate you are caring for chokes, aspirates, and turns blue during feeding. What condition should you suspect?

thePoint® You can download tables of drug information to help you prepare for the NCLEX®! View Generic Drug Names, Drug Classifications, Drug Actions, and Nursing Implications for the drugs discussed in this refresher at **http://thePoint.lww.com**

Neonatal care questions, answers, and rationales

1. The nurse is providing teaching to a new mother of a premature neonate about the benefits of breast milk for her child. The nurse knows additional teaching is needed if the mother makes which statement?
1. "My baby will be less likely to have ear infections if I breastfeed for the first 6 months."
2. "Breastfed babies tend to have less allergies compared to formula-fed babies."
3. "Preterm neonates that are breastfed have a higher incidence of necrotizing enterocolitis."
4. "Breast milk contains antibodies that help babies fight of bacteria and viruses."

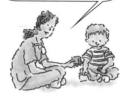

No worries. This chapter is child's play.

2. The nurse is providing education to a new mother on the purpose of administering surfactant to her neonate. The nurse knows the client understands the teaching when she makes which statement?
1. "My baby received surfactant to help regulate her breathing pattern."
2. "Surfactant will help clear out any amniotic fluid still in my baby's lungs."
3. "Giving my baby surfactant will finish developing her airway and lungs."
4. "Surfactant helps keep my baby's lungs from collapsing when she breathes."

1. 3. Components specific to breast milk have been shown to lower, not increase, the incidence of necrotizing enterocolitis in premature neonates. All other statements are true regarding breastfeeding. When exclusively breastfed (no formula given) for at least the first 6 months of life, infants have fewer cases of otitis media, bouts of diarrhea, and respiratory illnesses.

CN: Safe, effective care environment; CNS: Management of care; CL: Apply

2. 4. Surfactant works by reducing surface tension in the lung, which allows the lung to remain slightly expanded, preventing it from collapsing with exhalation and decreasing the amount of work required for inspiration. Surfactant has not been shown to influence upper airway maturation, clear the respiratory tract, or regulate the neonate's breathing pattern.

CN: Physiological integrity; CNS: Pharmacological and parenteral therapies; CL: Apply

CN: Client needs category   CNS: Client needs subcategory   CL: Cognitive level

3. While assessing a 2-hour-old neonate, the nurse notes acrocyanosis. Which action will the nurse complete?

1. Immediately activate the rapid response team.
2. Document the finding in the medical record.
3. Assess the neonate's axillary temperature.
4. Apply an oxygen saturation monitor to the neonate.

4. The nurse is teaching a group of parents about infant cardiopulmonary resuscitation (CPR) prior to discharge of their newborns. Place the steps of single-rescuer infant CPR in the sequence in which the nurse will instruct the parents to complete them for a witnessed collapse. Use all answer choices once.

| 1. Activate emergency response system. |
| 2. Begin cycles of 30 compressions and 2 breaths. |
| 3. Check a brachial pulse and for breathing. |
| 4. Ensure the scene is safe. |
| 5. Analyze heart rhythm with an automated external defibrillator (AED). |

5. The nursery nurse is caring for healthy neonates. Which action is important for the nurse to complete to prevent infection?

1. Check the neonates' temperatures frequently.
2. Use sterile technique when changing diapers.
3. Always practice meticulous hand washing.
4. Wear gloves when providing any care or holding.

6. The nurse is assessing a neonate. The nurse determines the neonate is adequately hydrated based on which assessment finding?

1. The neonate has desquamation of the hands.
2. The neonate's anterior fontanel is flat.
3. The mother reports excessive spitting up.
4. No urine output in the first 24 hours of life.

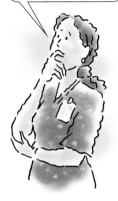

Acrocyanosis is just a bluish discoloration of the hands and feet—a very common finding in newborns.

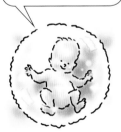

With all that's waiting for me out there— cold, infections, diseases—I think I'll just stay put.

3. 2. Acrocyanosis, or a bluish discoloration of the hands and feet of the neonate (also called peripheral cyanosis), is a normal finding and should not last more than 48 hours after birth. Activating the rapid response team, taking the neonate's temperature, and applying an oxygen saturation monitor are inappropriate because this is a normal finding.
CN: Physiological integrity; CNS: Physiological adaptation; CL: Apply

4. Ordered Response:

| 4. Ensure the scene is safe. |
| 3. Check a brachial pulse and for breathing. |
| 1. Activate emergency response system. |
| 2. Begin cycles of 30 compressions and 2 breaths. |
| 5. Analyze heart rhythm with an AED. |

CN: Health promotion and maintenance; CNS: None; CL: Apply

5. 3. To prevent and control infection, the nurse should practice meticulous hand washing, scrubbing for 3 minutes before entering the nursery, washing frequently during caregiving activities, and scrubbing for 1 minute after providing care. Checking for signs of infection can detect, not prevent, infection. The nurse should use sterile technique for invasive procedures, not when changing diapers. The nurse should wear gloves whenever contact with blood or body fluids is possible.
CN: Safe, effective care environment; CNS: Safety and infection control; CL: Apply

6. 2. A flat fontanel best indicates adequate hydration. Desquamation, or peeling, of the hands may be a normal finding, but this does not indicate adequate hydration. A sunken fontanel and no urine output in the first 24 hours of life are signs of poor hydration. In the case of no urine output, kidney dysfunction would also be a concern. Frequent spitting up is normal in neonates. Excessive spitting up, however, may result in poor hydration.
CN: Physiological integrity; CNS: Basic care and comfort; CL: Apply

7. The nurse is providing care to a 10 lb (4,536 g) neonate whose mother has diabetes. Which nursing intervention is **most** appropriate for the neonate?
1. Perform glucose checks.
2. Check the hemoglobin A1C level.
3. Monitor urine output.
4. Assess for jitteriness and weight loss.

7. 1. Macrosomic neonates of mothers with diabetes are at risk for hypoglycemia due to increased insulin levels. During gestation, an increased amount of glucose is transferred to the fetus through the placenta. The neonate's liver cannot initially adjust to the changing glucose levels after birth. This inability may result in an overabundance of insulin in the neonate, causing hypoglycemia. It is not appropriate to check hemoglobin A1C in a neonate. Serum glucose checks provide better insight into the neonate condition than monitoring for late symptoms such as alterations in urine output, jitteriness, and weight loss.
CN: Safe, effective care environment; CNS: Management of care; CL: Analyze

8. When collecting data on a neonate born at 39 weeks' gestation which finding(s) will the nurse identify as expected? Select all that apply.
1. Distended abdomen
2. "Sunset" eyes
3. Positive Babinski sign
4. Non-reactive pupils
5. Flaccid extremities

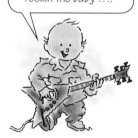

This next song goes out to Nurse Joy: "Keep on a rockin' me baby. Keep on a rockin' me baby …."

8. 3. A positive Babinski sign is present in infants until approximately age 1 year and is normal in neonates, though abnormal in adults. The abdomen should be slightly protuberant, soft, and symmetrical, not distended. The appearance of "sunset" eyes, in which the sclera is visible above the iris, results from cranial nerve palsies and may indicate increased intracranial pressure. A neonate's pupils normally react to light as an adult's would. Flaccid extremities are not expected and could indicate a neurological complication.
CN: Health promotion and maintenance; CNS: None; CL: Apply

9. When bathing a 1-hour-old neonate, which nursing action is **most** appropriate?
1. Feed the neonate immediately after bathing is complete.
2. Place the neonate in a tub of warm water to bathe.
3. Sponge bathe the neonate while under a radiant warmer.
4. Continuously monitor the neonate's temperature while bathing.

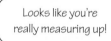
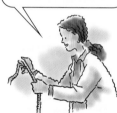

Looks like you're really measuring up!

9. 3. During the first several hours after birth, a neonate's thermal regulatory system is adapting to extrauterine life. When bathing a neonate under a radiant warmer, the external heat decreases the chances for cold stress by decreasing the number of internal mechanisms the neonate must use to stay warm. The neonate should not be placed in a tub until the umbilical cord comes off. Feeding immediately after bathing and continuous monitoring are not necessary. The neonate should be fed on demand. The temperature should be assessed before bathing.
CN: Safe, effective care environment; CNS: Management of care; CL: Apply

10. The nurse is providing care to a neonate who has received prolonged mechanical ventilation following birth. The nurse will carefully monitor the neonate for the development of which condition?
1. Bronchopulmonary dysplasia
2. Esophageal atresia
3. Hydrocephalus
4. Renal failure

10. 1. Bronchopulmonary dysplasia commonly results from the high pressures that must sometimes be used to maintain adequate oxygenation. Esophageal atresia, a structural defect in which the esophagus and trachea do not communicate with each other, does not relate to mechanical ventilation. Hydrocephalus and renal failure do not typically occur in neonates who received prolonged mechanical ventilation following birth.
CN: Physiological integrity; CNS: Reduction of risk potential; CL: Apply

11. The parents of a neonate born 20 minutes ago state, "We do not understand why our baby needs so many shots. Maybe we should not let our baby get a vitamin K shot." Which nursing response is **most** appropriate?
1. "It is painful for your baby so I see why you would not want your baby to get another injection."
2. "Although any injection does cause discomfort, vitamin K helps blood to clot and prevent serious bleeding."
3. "If you would prefer, you can defer the vitamin K injection until your baby's follow-up appointment."
4. "I highly recommend that your baby receives a vitamin K injection within one hour of being born."

11. **2.** The nurse should address the parents' concern and educate them as they state a lack of understanding of the purpose of the vitamin K injection. Vitamin K, deficient in the neonate, is needed to activate clotting factors II, VII, IX, and X. In the event of trauma, the neonate would be at risk for excessive bleeding. Stating that injections are painful and giving the nurse's personal recommendation do not address the lack of knowledge. Vitamin K cannot be deferred; it should be given within 1 hour of birth.
CN: Physiological integrity; CNS: Pharmacological and parenteral therapies; CL: Apply

12. The nurse is caring for a neonate birthed by a mother who tested positive for hepatitis B surface antigen (HBsAg) during pregnancy. Which intervention(s) will the nurse perform for this neonate? Select all that apply.
1. Giving hepatitis B immune globulin (HBIG) within 12 hours after birth
2. Administering recombinant hepatitis B vaccine prior to discharge
3. Drawing up both the HBIG and hepatitis B vaccine in the same syringe
4. Telling the parents the neonate will need two more doses of the hepatitis B vaccine
5. Injecting HBIG and hepatitis B vaccine at the same site

Read the answers to question #12 carefully—it's all about medication administration.

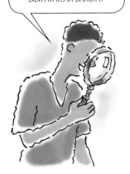

12. **1, 2, 4.** It is recommended that neonates birthed by mothers positive for HBsAg receive HBIG 0.5 mL intramuscularly (IM) once they are physiologically stable, optimally within 12 hours after birth. Hepatitis B vaccine, derived or recombinant, should be given IM in three doses of 0.5 mL each. HBIG and hepatitis B vaccine cannot be mixed or given at the same site. Each injection should be given independently at a different site.
CN: Health promotion and maintenance; CNS: None; CL: Apply

13. The nurse is preparing to give a hepatitis B vaccine to a neonate. Which action(s) will the nurse perform? Select all that apply.
1. Administer the injection to the neonate intramuscularly (IM).
2. Place a 5/8″ long needle on the syringe for administration.
3. Administer the injection in the neonate's deltoid muscle.
4. Insert the needle at a 90-degree angle.
5. Explain to the neonate's mother that the child will require one more dose.

13. **1, 2, 4.** Hepatitis B vaccine injections for neonates should be given IM in the vastus lateralis. The deltoid may be used for certain IM injections once the child is a toddler. The hepatitis B vaccine should be given in three doses of 0.5 mL each. It is correct to use a 5/8-in needle on the syringe and to insert the needle at a 90-degree angle.
CN: Physiological integrity; CNS: Basic care and comfort; CL: Apply

14. The amniotic fluid of a neonate, who is about to be born, is stained with meconium. Which nursing action is **priority** following birth of the neonate?
1. Help the mother to breastfeed the neonate.
2. Assess the umbilical cord and placenta.
3. Auscultate the abdomen for bowel sounds.
4. Monitor the neonate's respiratory effort.

14. **4.** The nurse's priority is to monitor for respiratory distress such as grunting, retractions, tachycardia, poor muscle tone, and cyanosis. The nurse will help the mother with feeding, assess the cord and placenta, and auscultate the abdomen; however, these actions are not priority over monitoring for respiratory distress. Early intervention is vital to achieving positive outcomes for the neonate.
CN: Safe, effective care environment; CNS: Management of care; CL: Analyze

CN: Client needs category   CNS: Client needs subcategory   CL: Cognitive level

15. The nurse is caring for several neonates, all born vaginally. Which neonate will the nurse monitor for the development of respiratory distress syndrome (RDS)?
1. The neonate born at 32 weeks' gestation
2. The neonate born at 41 weeks' gestation
3. The neonate with a pH level of 7.37
4. The neonate with 54 respirations per minute

15. 1. Prematurity is the single most important risk factor for developing RDS. The second born of twins and neonates born by cesarean birth are also at increased risk for RDS. Surfactant deficiency, which commonly results in RDS, is not a problem for postdate neonates. A pH of 7.35 to 7.45 and 54 breaths/minute are normal findings.
CN: Physiological integrity; CNS: Reduction of risk potential; CL: Analyze

16. Which neonate will the nurse assess **first**?
1. A 3-hour-old neonate who occasionally sneezes
2. A 10-hour-old neonate with yellowing sclera
3. A 15-hour-old neonate with acrocyanosis
4. A 23-hour-old neonate with a negative direct Coombs test

16. 2. A neonate with yellowing sclera within the first 24 hours of life is indicative of pathologic jaundice. Causes include blood incompatibility, liver disease, sepsis, toxoplasmosis, rubella, and erythroblastosis fetalis. Occasional sneezing is common initially following birth to aid in clearing the airway. Acrocyanosis is an expected finding during the first 48 hours after birth. A negative direct Coombs test indicates that no antibodies are present in the neonate's blood, so no treatment is needed.
CN: Safe, effective care environment; CNS: Management of care; CL: Analyze

17. The nurse is caring for a neonate and is preparing to administer erythromycin ointment. The parents ask the nurse why this medication is given. Which nursing response is appropriate?
1. "It is given to prevent the development of cataracts later in life."
2. "This medication is given to prevent ophthalmia neonatorum."
3. "Erythromycin is the best treatment for retinopathy of prematurity."
4. "The ointment is great at inhibiting the progress of strabismus."

Hint: Erythromycin is an antibiotic.

17. 2. Eye prophylaxis is administered to the neonate immediately or soon after birth to prevent ophthalmia neonatorum (conjunctivitis contracted during birth from passage through the birth canal). Erythromycin ointment is not given to prevent or treat cataracts, retinopathy of prematurity (ROP), or strabismus. Cataracts are opacities of the lens of the eye in children with congenital rubella, galactosemia, or cortisone therapy. ROP is caused by abnormal growth of retinal blood vessels in premature infants and can lead to blindness. Strabismus is neuromuscular incoordination of the eye alignment.
CN: Health promotion and maintenance; CNS: None; CL: Apply

18. The nurse caring for a male neonate notes a yellow-white exudate around the circumcision site 2 days after the procedure. Which action by the nurse is **most** appropriate?
1. Document the finding in the medical record.
2. Report the exudate to the health care provider.
3. Take the neonate's axillary temperature.
4. Remove the exudate with a warm cloth.

18. 1. The yellow-white exudate is part of the granulating process and a normal finding for a healing penis after circumcision. There is no need to act; the nurse would document the findings. Therefore, notifying the health care provider is not necessary. There is no indication of an infection that would necessitate taking the neonate's temperature. The exudate should not be removed.
CN: Health promotion and maintenance; CNS: None; CL: Apply

19. A client has just given birth at 42 weeks' gestation. When assessing the neonate, which finding does the nurse expect?
1. A sleepy and lethargic neonate
2. Abundant lanugo covering the neonate's body
3. Desquamation of the neonate's epidermis
4. Vernix caseosa covering the neonate's body

19. 3. Postdate neonates lose the vernix caseosa, and the epidermis may become desquamated. A neonate at 42 weeks' gestation is usually very alert and missing lanugo.
CN: Health promotion and maintenance; CNS: None; CL: Apply

20. After assessing a 3-day-old neonate, the nurse suspects the neonate may have an infection based on which finding?
  1. Flushed facial cheeks
  2. Heart rate of 150 beats/minute
  3. Temperature of 96.8°F (36.0°C)
  4. Increased activity level

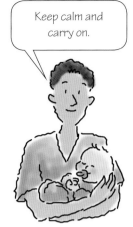

Keep calm and carry on.

20. 3. A decreased temperature in the neonate, such as 96.8°F (36.0°C), may be a sign of infection. The neonate's color commonly changes with an infectious process but generally becomes ashen or mottled, not flushed. The neonate with an infection usually shows a decrease in activity level or lethargy. A heart rate of 150 beats/minute is considered normal.
CN: Physiological integrity; CNS: Reduction of risk potential; CL: Analyze

21. The nurse is providing care to a small-for-gestational-age neonate who is in the transitional period. The nurse will monitor the neonate for the development of which complication?
  1. Anemia
  2. Hyperthermia
  3. Hyperglycemia
  4. Polycythemia

21. 4. The small-for-gestational-age neonate is at risk for developing polycythemia, not anemia, during the transitional period in an attempt to decrease hypoxia. This neonate is also at increased risk for developing hypoglycemia and hypothermia due to decreased glycogen stores.
CN: Physiological integrity; CNS: Reduction of risk potential; CL: Apply

22. Which neonate will the registered nurse (RN) assign to the licensed practical nurse (LPN)?
  1. The neonate exhibiting mild nasal flaring
  2. The neonate with light, audible grunting
  3. The neonate with a respiratory rate of 54 breaths/minute
  4. The neonate with a heart rate of 167 beats/minute

22. 3. The neonate with a respiratory rate of 54 breaths/minute is the most stable because this rate is normal for a neonate during the transitional period. The RN would assign this client to the LPN because the client is stable. Nasal flaring and audible grunting are signs of respiratory distress. A heart rate of 167 beats/minute is elevated; 110 to 160 beats/minute is a normal range.
CN: Safe, effective care environment; CNS: Management of care; CL: Analyze

23. The nurse is caring for a neonate whose mother received magnesium sulfate during labor. The nurse will closely monitor the neonate for which potential problem(s)? Select all that apply.
  1. Hypoglycemia
  2. Twitching
  3. Respiratory depression
  4. Tachycardia
  5. Bradycardia

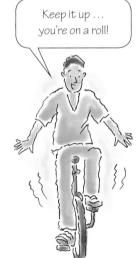

Keep it up . . . you're on a roll!

23. 3, 5. Magnesium sulfate crosses the placenta, and adverse neonatal effects include respiratory depression, hypotonia, and bradycardia. The serum blood glucose level is not affected by magnesium sulfate. The neonate would experience hypotonia, not twitching.
CN: Physiological integrity; CNS: Pharmacological and parenteral therapies; CL: Apply

24. The nurse is caring for a neonate whose mother abused opioids during pregnancy. Which nursing intervention is **priority**?
  1. Place the incubator in a quiet area of the nursery.
  2. Administer intravenous (IV) fluids.
  3. Monitor for the development of seizures.
  4. Request a prescription for methadone.

24. 1. Neonates experiencing opioid withdrawal need a supportive environment, which includes decreasing environmental stimuli, swaddling, skin-to-skin contact, and pacifier use. IV fluids may be needed if the neonate becomes dehydrated or has severe vomiting or diarrhea. The nurse should monitor for the development of seizures; however, this is not priority as it is only a potential problem at this time. Medications such as phenobarbital, methadone, and diazepam should be given only if supportive measures are not sufficient.
CN: Physiological integrity; CNS: Reduction of risk potential; CL: Analyze

25. The nurse is caring for the neonate of a mother with diabetes. The nurse will monitor the neonate for the development of which complication(s)? Select all that apply.

1. Respiratory distress syndrome
2. Atelectasis
3. Microcephaly
4. Pneumothorax
5. Congenital anomalies
6. Hyperbilirubinemia

25. 1, 5, 6. Neonates of mothers with diabetes are at increased risk for respiratory distress syndrome, hypoglycemia, hypocalcemia, hyperbilirubinemia, and congenital anomalies. They are not at greater risk for atelectasis or pneumothorax. Microcephaly is usually the result of cytomegalovirus or rubella virus infection.

CN: Health promotion and maintenance; CNS: None; CL: Apply

26. The nurse is administering erythromycin ointment to a neonate. Place the actions in the sequence in which the nurse will complete them. Use all options.

1.	Obtain a single-dose application tube.
2.	Close the eye for several seconds.
3.	Gently pull the lower eyelid downward.
4.	Place a line of ointment into the lower conjunctival sac.
5.	Wipe away any excess ointment after about 1 minute.

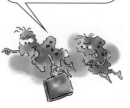

Go for the eyes and pray they forget the erythromycin.

26. Ordered Response:

1.	Obtain a single-dose application tube.
3.	Gently pull the lower eyelid downward.
4.	Place a line of ointment into the lower conjunctival sac.
2.	Close the eye for several seconds.
5.	Wipe away any excess ointment after about 1 minute.

CN: Physiological integrity; CNS: Pharmacological and parenteral therapies; CL: Apply

27. The nurse suspects a 3-hour-old neonate is experiencing newborn distress based on which finding(s)? Select all that apply.

1. Respiratory rate of 15 breaths/minute
2. Sternal retractions
3. Acrocyanosis
4. Grunting
5. Nasal flaring

27. 1, 2, 4, 5. Bradypnea, sternal retractions, and the use of accessory chest muscles all indicate distress. Grunting and nasal flaring also indicate the infant is working very hard to breathe. Acrocyanosis is normal cyanosis, as indicated by discoloring of the hands and feet.

CN: Physiological integrity; CNS: Physiological adaptation; CL: Apply

28. The nurse is maintaining a neutral thermal environment for a neonate by quickly drying the neonate following a bath. The nurse's action reflects prevention of heat loss by which mechanism?

1. Conduction
2. Convection
3. Evaporation
4. Radiation

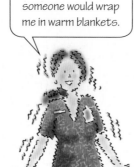

Ugh. I can't stand hypothermia. I wish someone would wrap me in warm blankets.

28. 3. Evaporation is the loss of heat that occurs when a liquid is converted to a vapor. Drying neonates quickly and applying caps to the dried hair help to reduce this type of heat loss. Convection heat loss is the flow of heat from the body surface to cooler air. Keeping the nursery temperature warm and wrapping the neonate in blankets help to prevent this type of heat loss. Conduction is the loss of heat from the body surface to cooler surfaces in direct contact. Covering the surfaces of the neonate's body with warmed blankets helps to prevent this type of heat loss. Radiation is the loss of heat from the body surface to cooler, solid surfaces that are not in direct contact but are in relative proximity. Keeping neonates away from cooler surfaces helps to prevent this type of heat loss.

CN: Health promotion and maintenance; CNS: None; CL: Understand

CN: Client needs category   CNS: Client needs subcategory   CL: Cognitive level

29. The nurse is caring for a 36-hour-old neonate and notices the skin and sclera appear yellow. What will the nurse do **first**?
1. Encourage frequent feedings.
2. Assess the bilirubin level.
3. Provide phototherapy.
4. Document the findings.

30. A 3-day-old neonate is ordered to undergo phototherapy. Which nursing intervention will the nurse complete?
1. Administration of tube feedings to the neonate
2. Feeding the neonate while under phototherapy lights
3. Use of eye patches to prevent retinal damage
4. Temperature monitoring every 6 hours

31. The nurse is teaching a new parent about the changes in a neonate's stools. After describing meconium as the first stool, which description of the stool by the parent demonstrates understanding?
1. Soft, pale yellow
2. Hard, pale brown
3. Sticky, greenish black
4. Loose, golden yellow

32. A neonate has been diagnosed with caput succedaneum. Which nursing action is appropriate?
1. Measure the head circumference every 12 hours.
2. Mark the borders of the edematous tissue hourly.
3. Monitor hemoglobin and hematocrit levels daily.
4. Document the findings in the electronic medical record.

33. The nurse is caring for a neonate and suspects the development of early-onset sepsis. Which finding(s) indicates to the nurse this is occurring? Select all that apply.
1. Tachypnea
2. Hypoglycemia
3. Lethargy
4. Constipation
5. Exaggerated sucking reflex

29. 2. The nurse should first assess the neonate's bilirubin level using a transcutaneous bilirubinometry device or with a serum test to determine what type of treatment the neonate needs. Physiologic hyperbilirubinemia, or jaundice, in full-term neonates first appears after 24 hours. Neonates with this condition are otherwise healthy and have no medical problems. The nurse would encourage frequent feeding to facilitate removal of bilirubin from the body and document the findings after assessing the level. Phototherapy may be needed depending on the bilirubin level.
CN: Physiological integrity; CNS: Reduction of risk potential; CL: Analyze

30. 3. The neonate's eyes must be covered with eye patches to prevent damage. The neonate can be removed from the lights and held for feedings. Tube feedings are not indicated. The neonate's temperature should be monitored every 2 to 4 hours because of the risk of hyperthermia with phototherapy.
CN: Physiological integrity; CNS: Reduction of risk potential; CL: Apply

31. 3. Meconium collects in the gastrointestinal tract during gestation and is initially sterile. Meconium is viscous and greenish black because of occult blood. The stools of formula-fed babies are typically soft and pale yellow after feeding is well established. The stools of breastfed neonates are loose and golden yellow after the transition to extrauterine life. Neonate stools typically are not hard or pale brown.
CN: Health promotion and maintenance; CNS: None; CL: Understand

32. 4. Caput succedaneum is the swelling of tissue over the presenting part of the fetal scalp due to sustained pressure. This boggy, edematous swelling is present at birth, crosses the suture line, and most commonly occurs in the occipital area. The nurse should document the findings in the medical record; no treatment is needed. Caput succedaneum resolves within 3 to 4 days. The nurse may monitor hemoglobin and hematocrit levels for cephalohematoma, a collection of blood between the skull and periosteum that does not cross cranial suture lines and resolves in 3 to 6 weeks.
CN: Health promotion and maintenance; CNS: None; CL: Apply

33. 1, 2, 3. Signs and symptoms of early-onset neonatal sepsis include respiratory distress such as tachypnea, hypoglycemia, lethargy, and diarrhea, not constipation. The sucking reflex is usually diminished, not exaggerated.
CN: Physiological integrity; CNS: Physiological adaptation; CL: Apply

---

---

34. The nurse is assigned to care for four neonates. The nurse will monitor which neonate for hyperbilirubinemia?

1. Neonate birthed by a mother with poorly controlled gestational diabetes
2. Neonate whose birth weight was 3,685 g 36 hours ago
3. Neonate with A positive blood birthed by a mother with O negative blood
4. Neonate born 12 hours ago with Apgar scores of 7 and 9 at 1 and 5 minutes, respectively

34. 3. Neonates of Rh-negative mothers tend to have hyperbilirubinemia. The mother's blood type, which is different from the neonate's, impacts the neonate's bilirubin level due to the antigen-antibody reaction. Therefore, a neonate with ABO and Rhesus incompatibilities would be at highest risk for developing hyperbilirubinemia. Gestational diabetes and normal weight are not associated with hyperbilirubinemia. Low Apgar scores, not high ones such as 7 and 9, may indicate a risk for hyperbilirubinemia.

CN: Safe, effective care environment; CNS: Management of care; CL: Analyze

35. A neonate develops significant respiratory distress 14 hours after birth. After reviewing the neonate's medical record, the nurse finds the mother's membranes were ruptured for 23 hours before birth. Which additional finding will the nurse expect to note in the neonate's medical record?

1. Neonate's initial heart rate 166 beats/minute and respirations 52 breaths/minute.
2. Neonate's 1-minute Apgar was 8 and 5-minute Apgar was 9.
3. Mother received an epidural for pain management during labor.
4. Mother tested positive for group B beta-hemolytic streptococci.

35. 4. Transmission of group B beta-hemolytic streptococci to the fetus results in respiratory distress that can rapidly lead to septic shock. This organism is a major cause of infection in the neonate, especially with prolonged ruptured membranes. A heart rate of 166 beats/minute and respiratory rate of 52 breaths/minute are both within normal range for the neonate. Apgar scores of 7 or higher indicate successful transition to the extrauterine environment. The mother receiving an epidural would not lead to neonate infection.

CN: Physiological integrity; CNS: Physiological adaptation; CL: Analyze

36. The nurse cares for a neonate who was born at 28 weeks' gestation. Which finding(s) will the nurse expect to assess? Select all that apply.

1. The skin is pale and no vessels show through it.
2. Creases appear on the interior two-thirds of the sole.
3. The pinna of the ear is soft, flat, and stays folded.
4. The neonate has 5 to 6 mm of breast tissue.
5. The neonate shows little extremity recoil.

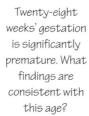

Twenty-eight weeks' gestation is significantly premature. What findings are consistent with this age?

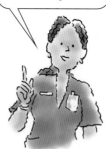

36. 3, 5. In a preterm neonate, the ear has a soft pinna that is flat and stays folded, and the infant exhibits minimal to no extremity recoil. Pale skin with no vessels showing through, and 5 to 6 mm of breast tissue, are characteristic of a neonate at 40 weeks' gestation. Creases on the anterior two-thirds of the sole are characteristic of a neonate at 36 weeks' gestation.

CN: Physiological integrity; CNS: Physiological adaptation; CL: Apply

37. The nurse is attempting to interact with a neonate experiencing drug withdrawal. The nurse determines the neonate is willing to interact based on which behavior?

1. Quiet, alert state
2. Gaze aversion
3. Hiccups
4. Yawning

37. 1. When caring for neonates experiencing drug withdrawal, the nurse must be alert for distress signals from the infant. Stimuli should be introduced one at a time when the neonate is in a quiet, alert state. Gaze aversion, yawning, sneezing, hiccups, and body arching are distress signals that indicate the neonate cannot handle stimuli at that time.

CN: Psychosocial integrity; CNS: None; CL: Apply

38. When caring for a neonate of a mother with diabetes, the nurse will suspect the neonate is experiencing hypoglycemia based on which finding(s)? Select all that apply.

1. Hyper-alert state
2. Jitteriness
3. Excessive crying
4. Serum glucose level of 60 mg/dL (3.3 mmol/L)
5. Diaphoresis

38. 2, 5. Hypoglycemia in a neonate is expressed as jitteriness, lethargy, diaphoresis, and a serum glucose level below 40 mg/dL (2.2 mmol/L). A hyper-alert state in a neonate is more suggestive of neuralgic irritability and has no correlation to blood glucose levels. Excessive crying is not found in hypoglycemia.

CN: Physiological integrity; CNS: Reduction of risk potential; CL: Apply

39. The nurse is caring for a neonate born 30 minutes ago to a mother who was treated for *Chlamydia trachomatis* at 20 weeks' gestation. Which action will the nurse complete **next**?
1. Give erythromycin ophthalmic ointment.
2. Monitor the neonate's eyes hourly.
3. Administer oral azithromycin for 3 days.
4. Assess the neonate's rectal temperature.

40. The nurse is educating new parents on umbilical cord care. The nurse determines the parents understand the information when they make which statement(s)? Select all that apply.
1. "The cord should fall off in 7 to 10 days."
2. "We need to apply alcohol to the cord daily."
3. "We can pull the stump once it is about to fall off."
4. "If the stump bleeds, we need to put gauze over it."
5. "We should fold the diaper below the cord."

41. The nurse is assessing a 38 weeks' gestation neonate immediately following birth. The nurse notes a thick, white, cheesy coating on the neonate's skin. What will the nurse do **next**?
1. Continue to assess the neonate.
2. Bathe the neonate under the radiant warmer.
3. Obtain a specimen of the substance.
4. Assess the neonate's temperature.

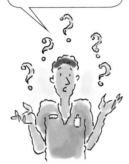

White, cheesy coating? I'm guessing mozzarella is out.

42. The nurse is preparing to administer vitamin K to a neonate. The parent states, "I do not want my baby to get that shot." Which action will the nurse take **next**?
1. Explain that vitamin K is mandatory.
2. Consult with the ethics committee.
3. Explain the purpose of giving vitamin K.
4. Hold the administration of vitamin K.

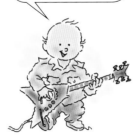

A healthy baby is the goal; any other accomplishment is a bonus!

43. The nurse is caring for a healthy neonate born at 39 weeks' gestation. Which finding(s) will the nurse expect to assess? Select all that apply.
1. Simian crease
2. Rooting reflex
3. Cystic hygroma
4. Bulging fontanel
5. Head circumference of 14 in (35.5 cm)

39. 1. Erythromycin ophthalmic ointment is given for prophylactic treatment of ophthalmia neonatorum (ON), usually within 1 hour after birth. The most common cause of ON is *Chlamydia*, which the mother was treated for during pregnancy. A history of sexually transmitted infections (STIs) places a client at high risk for future STIs due to lifestyle choices. The nurse should monitor the neonate's eyes and a rectal temperate as needed, unless already assessed for rectal patency, but these are not priority. Azithromycin may be given for ON caused by *Neisseria gonorrhoeae*.
CN: Physiological integrity; CNS: Pharmacological and parenteral therapies; CL: Analyze

40. 1, 5. The umbilical stump deteriorates over the first 7 to 10 days' postpartum due to dry gangrene and usually falls off by day 10. The diaper should be folded below the level of the stump to prevent irritation. It is no longer recommended to apply alcohol to the stump. The stump should never be pulled on; it should be allowed to fall off on its own to prevent infection. If bleeding occurs, the parents should notify the health care provider.
CN: Health promotion and maintenance; CNS: None; CL: Apply

41. 1. Vernix, a normal finding at 38 weeks' gestation, is the white, cheesy material present on the neonate's skin at birth. Vernix serves to protect the skin in utero, while surrounded by amniotic fluid. The nurse should wait until the neonate is stable before bathing. Vernix will not harm the extrauterine neonate's skin. Vernix does not require testing, nor does it indicate infection.
CN: Health promotion and maintenance; CNS: None; CL: Analyze

42. 4. The nurse will hold the medication at this time. Medications are not mandatory and can be refused by the neonate's caregivers. The nurse may explain the purpose of administering vitamin K to the parents and answer any questions they may have to ensure an informed decision is being made. This would not qualify as an ethical issue.
CN: Physiological integrity; CNS: Pharmacologic and parenteral therapies; CL: Apply

43. 2, 5. Rooting is a reflex seen in neonates that disappears from 3 to 6 months of age. When the neonate's cheek is brushed or stroked near the corner of the mouth, the neonate turns its head to that side. Another normal finding is the head circumference, which normally ranges from 13 to 15 in (32 to 38 cm). A simian crease is present in 40% of neonates with trisomy 21 (Down syndrome). Cystic hygroma is a neck mass that can obstruct the airway. Bulging fontanels are a sign of intracranial pressure.
CN: Health promotion and maintenance; CNS: None; CL: Apply

44. The nurse is caring for a neonate immediately after birth. Which nursing intervention is **priority**?
1. Obtain a glucose reading.
2. Give the initial bath.
3. Assess Apgar scores.
4. Cover the neonate's head with a cap.

44. 3. The Apgar scores should be assessed at 1 and 5 minutes following birth to determine whether the neonate is transitioning well to extrauterine life. A glucose reading, appropriate for neonates with risk factors for hyperglycemia, is obtained at 30 minutes to 1 hour of age. The initial bath is not given until the neonate's temperature is stable. The neonate's head should not be covered until the hair is dried under a radiant warmer.

CN: Safe, effective care environment; CNS: Management of care; CL: Analyze

45. The nurse notes small, white papules surrounded by erythematous dermatitis on a neonate's skin during assessment. Which action will the nurse take?
1. Inform the parents that the spots will resolve.
2. Apply erythromycin cream to the spots.
3. Cover the areas with sterile gauze.
4. Monitor the neonate's immunoglobulin E level.

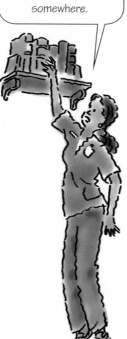

Erythema toxicum—hmm … I remember reading about that somewhere.

45. 1. The nurse should educate the parents on erythema toxicum. Erythema toxicum progresses from papules to erythema and then disappears. The papules occur sporadically on the face, trunk, and limbs. They occur when the immature immune system reacts to the environment. No treatment is needed.

CN: Health promotion and maintenance; CNS: None; CL: Apply

46. The nurse is reviewing the medical record of a neonate. Which data from the record will the nurse identify as the **best** indicator of fetal lung maturity?
1. Meconium in the amniotic fluid
2. Glucocorticoid treatment just before birth
3. Lecithin-sphingomyelin ratio of more than 2:1
4. Absence of phosphatidylglycerol in amniotic fluid

46. 3. Lecithin and sphingomyelin are phospholipids that help compose surfactant in the lungs; lecithin peaks at 36 weeks, and sphingomyelin concentrations remain stable. Meconium is released due to fetal stress before birth, but it is chronic fetal stress that matures lungs. Glucocorticoids must be given at least 48 hours before birth. The presence of phosphatidylglycerol indicates lung maturity.

CN: Physiological integrity; CNS: Physiological adaptation; CL: Apply

47. The nurse is preparing to give a neonate the initial bath. Which nursing action is **priority**?
1. Assess the neonate's temperature.
2. Use warm water and mild soap.
3. Allow the parents to assist.
4. Thoroughly wash the neonate.

47. 1. It is priority for the nurse to assess the neonate's temperature prior to initiating the bath to ensure it is stable. If the neonate's temperate is not stable, cold stress could occur. The other actions, though correct, are of lower priority than assessing the neonate's temperature. The nurse would use warm water and mild soap on a neonate to prevent drying out the skin. Parents can assist if they desire and the neonate is stable. The neonate should be thoroughly washed to remove bacteria from the birth canal.

CN: Health promotion and maintenance; CNS: None; CL: Analyze

48. While caring for a neonate at risk for cold stress, which nursing intervention(s) is appropriate? Select all that apply.
1. Immediately dry the neonate after bathing.
2. Swaddle the neonate in warm blankets.
3. Place the neonate skin-to-skin with the mother.
4. Pre-warm the radiant warmer before using.
5. Keep the neonate away from windows.

48. 1, 2, 3, 4, 5. Immediately drying the neonate decreases evaporative heat loss from the neonate's moist body from birth. Swaddling in warn blankets and placing skin-to-skin decreases heat loss from conduction. Pre-warming equipment decreases heat loss from convection. Keeping the neonate away from cold areas or equipment not in direct contact with the neonate decreases heat loss from radiation.

CN: Health promotion and maintenance; CNS: None; CL: Apply

CN: Client needs category   CNS: Client needs subcategory   CL: Cognitive level

49. A male neonate has just been circumcised. Following this procedure, which intervention will the nurse perform?
1. Apply alcohol to the site daily.
2. Change the diaper every 10 minutes.
3. Keep the neonate in the prone position.
4. Apply petroleum gauze to the site.

50. The nurse is caring for several neonates in a busy nursery. When weighing a neonate, which action will the nurse take?
1. Leave the diaper on the neonate.
2. Place a sterile paper on the scale.
3. Keep a hand on the neonate's abdomen.
4. Weigh neonates daily at the same time.

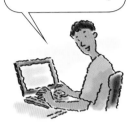

When it comes to measurement, there's a lot to be said for consistency.

51. The nurse is administering the initial bath to a neonate who is 4 hours old and weighs 3,235 g. The pre-bath vital signs were: pulse rate, 126 beats/minute; respiratory rate, 42 breaths/minute; and rectal temperature, 98.4°F (36.9°C). The neonate cries lustily throughout the bath. While drying the neonate, the nurse notes the neonate's color becomes slightly dusky, cry is weak, and vigorous movement stops. Which action will the nurse do **first**?
1. Obtain a pulse oximetry reading and administer oxygen.
2. Immediately place the neonate under the radiant warmer.
3. Use a bulb syringe to suction the neonate's nose and oropharynx.
4. Use a bag and mask device to provide two rescue breaths.

52. The nurse will suspect a neonate is experiencing a metabolic response to cold stress based on which finding?
1. Dysrhythmia
2. Hypoglycemia
3. Elevated liver function tests
4. Hypertension

Hooray! You're doing awesome! Keep it up.

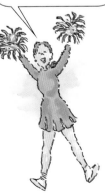

53. The nurse is caring for a full-term neonate who is receiving phototherapy for hyperbilirubinemia. Which finding(s) will the nurse report **immediately**? Select all that apply.
1. Seizure activity
2. Maculopapular rash
3. Absent Moro reflex
4. Greenish stool
5. Bronze-colored skin
6. Lethargy

49. 4. The nurse should apply petroleum gauze to the site to prevent the skin edges from sticking to the diaper. Alcohol is contraindicated for circumcision care. The nurse should change diapers more frequently to inspect the site, but not every 10 minutes. Neonates are initially kept in the supine position.
CN: Health promotion and maintenance; CNS: None; CL: Apply

50. 4. A neonate of any age should be weighed at the same time each day, using the same technique. A neonate should be weighed while undressed. Clean scale paper should be used when weighing the neonate; sterile scale paper is unnecessary. The nurse should keep a hand near or above, not on, the abdomen when weighing the neonate.
CN: Health promotion and maintenance; CNS: None; CL: Apply

51. 2. Because this neonate is receiving a bath, the neonate is at risk for becoming cold and metabolizing brown fat. Immediately placing the neonate under the warmer helps restore body temperature and stops the acidosis that occurs with the metabolism of brown fat. After placing the neonate under the warmer, the nurse can continue collecting data. If the neonate continues to deteriorate, the other actions may be necessary and should be performed under the warmer. There is no initial evidence that the neonate's respirations are compromised; the neonate continues to cry, although weakly. The dusky color is not respiratory in origin but is due to metabolic acidosis. Based on the findings, there is no need to suction or give rescue breaths.
CN: Physiological integrity; CNS: Reduction of risk potential; CL: Analyze

52. 2. Hypoglycemia occurs as the consumption of glucose increases with the increase in metabolic rate. Dysrhythmia and increases in blood pressure occur due to cardiorespiratory manifestations. Liver function declines in cold stress.
CN: Health promotion and maintenance; CNS: None; CL: Apply

53. 1, 3, 6. An absent Moro reflex, lethargy, and seizures are symptoms of bilirubin encephalopathy, which can be life threatening. A maculopapular rash, greenish stools, and bronze-colored skin are minor adverse effects of phototherapy that should be monitored but do not require immediate intervention.
CN: Safe, effective care environment; CNS: Management of care; CL: Apply

54. How will the nurse monitor a preterm neonate who is receiving phototherapy treatment for insensible water loss? Select all that apply.
  1. Monitor the sodium level.
  2. Weigh the neonate daily.
  3. Monitor urine output.
  4. Check bilirubin levels daily.
  5. Assess heart rate every 2 hours.

54. 1, 2, 3. Increased insensible water loss occurs from evaporation through the skin from the lights. Assessing daily weights, sodium level, and urine output helps the nurse determine whether the neonate is experiencing insensible water loss associated with the use of phototherapy. Bilirubin levels may be checked daily, but the level is not associated with insensible water loss. There is no need to monitor the heart rate every 2 hours, as it is not associated with insensible water loss.
CN: Physiological integrity; CNS: Reduction of risk potential; CL: Apply

55. The nurse assesses a neonate's temperate in the mother's room. The neonate's temperate is 97.6° F (36.4°C) while lying in the bassinette without a cap. Which nursing action is **priority**?
  1. Immediately place the neonate skin-to-skin with the mother.
  2. Recheck the neonate's axillary temperature in 30 minutes.
  3. Educate the mother on the importance of keeping a cap on the neonate's head.
  4. Take the neonate to the nursery and place under a radiant warmer.

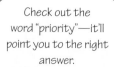

Check out the word "priority"—it'll point you to the right answer.

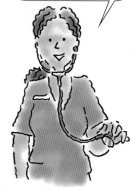

55. 1. The nurse needs to increase the neonate's temperature while preventing the temperature from further decreasing. Placing the neonate skin-to-skin is priority over providing education. The nurse should recheck the temperature, but an intervention is needed first. The temperature does not warrant removing the neonate from the mother at this time. Normal temperature range for a neonate is 97.7°F (36.5°C) to 99°F (37.2°C).
CN: Safe, effective care environment; CNS: Management of care; CL: Analyze

56. Which neonatal assessment finding will the nurse flag as priority for the health care provider to review?
  1. Icteric sclera in a 15-day-old neonate
  2. Bilirubin level of 15 mg/dL (256.5 µmol/L) in a 10-hour-old neonate
  3. Yellowing skin and sclera in a neonate born 48 hours ago
  4. Bilirubin level increasing by 5 mg/dL (85.5 µmol/L) a day

56. 2. Increased bilirubin levels in the liver usually do not cause blood bilirubin levels of 15 mg/dL (256.5 µmol/L) until the third day of life; such a rise within the first 24 hours of life indicates pathological jaundice. This rise results from the impaired conjugation and excretion of bilirubin and difficulty clearing bilirubin from plasma. The other findings suggest physiological jaundice, which is a lower priority than pathological jaundice.
CN: Physiological integrity; CNS: Reduction of risk potential; CL: Analyze

57. The nurse is caring for a neonate receiving phototherapy. Which action is important for the nurse to complete?
  1. Decrease the amount of formula given.
  2. Dress the neonate warmly.
  3. Massage the neonate's skin with lotion.
  4. Reposition the neonate frequently.

57. 4. Phototherapy works by the chemical interaction between a light source and the bilirubin in the neonate's skin. Therefore, the larger the skin area exposed to light, the more effective the treatment. Changing the neonate's position frequently ensures maximum exposure. Because the neonate loses water through the skin as a result of evaporation, the amount of formula or water may need to be increased. The neonate is typically undressed to ensure maximum skin exposure. The eyes are covered to protect them from light, and an abbreviated diaper is used to prevent soiling. The skin should be clean and patted dry. Use of lotions interferes with phototherapy.
CN: Physiological integrity; CNS: Reduction of risk potential; CL: Apply

58. A 2-day-old male is scheduled for a circumcision. Which nursing action is important following the procedure?
1. Monitoring the neonate for voiding
2. Keeping the neonate's penis exposed to air
3. Feeding the neonate clear fluids for the first 12 hours
4. Placing a small ice cap on the neonate's penis

58. 1. After a circumcision, urine retention may occur. Therefore, the nurse should monitor and document the time of the neonate's voiding. Although the penis should be inspected for swelling and bleeding, further care is unnecessary. A petroleum dressing is commonly applied to the penis; then the neonate is diapered. Feeding restrictions are unnecessary, as anesthetics are not generally used. Ice should not be used on a neonate.
CN: Safe, effective care environment; CNS: Safety and infection control; CL: Apply

59. The nurse will suspect a neonate is experiencing breast milk jaundice based on which finding?
1. History of poor sucking and latching
2. Decreased bilirubin level on day 3 of life
3. Yellowing skin and sclera 7 days after birth
4. Increased bilirubin level 12 hours after birth

59. 3. Breast milk jaundice is an elevation of indirect bilirubin in a breastfed neonate that develops 7 days after birth and peaks during weeks 2 to 3 of life. It is caused by insufficient production or intake of breast milk. A history of poor sucking and latching is indicative of breastfeeding jaundice, not breast milk jaundice. Increased bilirubin levels before 24 hours indicate pathological jaundice.
CN: Health promotion and maintenance; CNS: None; CL: Apply

60. Which assessment finding will the nurse **immediately** report to the health care provider?
1. A 2-hour-old neonate with bilateral crackles
2. A 15-hour-old neonate with bluish hands and feet
3. A neonate with a respiratory rate of 70 breaths/minute
4. A neonate who last nursed 3 hours ago and is refusing to nurse now

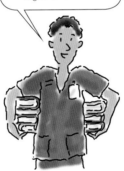

I get tachypnea every time I run up a flight of stairs.

60. 3. Tachypnea and expiratory grunting occur early in respiratory distress syndrome to help improve oxygenation. This neonate needs support, such as oxygen administration. Bilateral crackles and acrocyanosis are expected findings based on the neonate's age. Neonates should breastfeed every 2 to 4 hours.
CN: Safe, effective care environment; CNS: Management of care; CL: Analyze

61. The nurse is providing discharge education to a 48-hour-postpartum client. The client voices concern because her neonate's birth weight has declined by 2 oz. She states, "I will continue to breastfeed but will supplement after each breastfeeding with 4 oz of formula." Which response by the nurse is **best**?
1. "Good idea. It is difficult to determine if your breastfed baby is getting enough to eat."
2. "To see if your baby is eating enough, you can weigh the baby before and after each feeding."
3. "It is normal for babies to lose weight. Supplementing may cause a drop in your milk supply."
4. "Supplementing with formula is never recommended for breastfed infants."

61. 3. Normal neonatal weight loss can range from 5% to 10% of birth weight. The normal neonate's stomach holds about 3 oz (90 mL), and supplementing may lead to the neonate nursing less often, which may result in decreased milk production. A breastfed neonate's continued weight gain indicates the neonate is eating a sufficient amount. It can be concerning to the client to not know exactly how much the breastfed neonate is consuming, but this statement does not address the client's concern. While the premature or low-birth-weight neonate is weighed before and after eating in the clinical setting, this is not an action that is ordinarily taken for the normal neonate at home. Supplementation is not recommended for all breastfeeding clients but may be recommended if milk supply is low and cannot be increased.
CN: Health promotion and maintenance; CNS: None; CL: Apply

62. A neonate develops a mild respiratory disorder shortly after birth. After evaluation, the nurse believes the neonate is experiencing transient tachypnea of the newborn (TTN). Which nursing action is **most** appropriate?

1. Auscultate the neonate's heart.
2. Notify the health care provider.
3. Monitor the neonate's output.
4. Transfer the neonate to the intensive care unit.

62. 2. Transient tachypnea is a mild respiratory disorder that is self-limiting. It has an invariably favorable outcome after several hours to several days, but generally lasts less than 24 hours. The nurse should notify the health care provider to determine if additional prescriptions are needed (chest x-ray, complete blood count, oxygen therapy). The nurse will assess the heart and monitor output; however, treatment for TTN is priority. The health care provider will determine if the neonate should be transferred.
CN: Safe, effective care environment; CNS: Management of care; CL: Apply

63. The nurse is providing education to a new mother. The client asks the nurse, "Did my baby receive all the immune protection needed from me?" Which nursing response is **most** appropriate?

1. "Your baby did receive passive immunity from you but is still susceptible to bacteria and viruses."
2. "Your neonate only received immunity from you against viruses you received immunizations for during pregnancy."
3. "I wish babies received immunity from mothers. They have no immunity against any bacteria or virus."
4. "Babies receive some immunity while in utero, but this protection only lasts for about 30 days after birth."

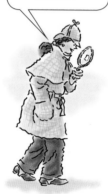

IgG crosses the placenta and provides passive immunity. Which one is it?

63. 1. Neonates do receive passive immunity in utero from the mother. However, they are still susceptible to bacteria and viruses found in their environment and need protection, such as meticulous hand washing by caregivers. The other statements are not accurate.
CN: Health promotion and maintenance; CNS: None; CL: Apply

64. A 10-hour-old neonate appears exceptionally irritable, cries easily, and startles when touched. The results of a meconium drug test indicate the neonate is positive for cocaine. Which nursing action will **most** help soothe the neonate?

1. Leave a light on beside the bassinet at night.
2. Wrap the neonate snugly in a blanket.
3. Provide multisensory stimulation while awake.
4. Give the neonate a warm bath.

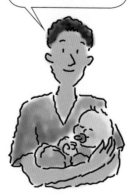

It's a wrap! Swaddling can help soothe both healthy and struggling neonates.

64. 2. The practice of tightly wrapping, or swaddling, a cocaine-addicted neonate provides a safe, secure environment and maintains body warmth, both of which are soothing. A cocaine-addicted neonate typically experiences withdrawal 8 to 10 hours after birth; signs and symptoms include constant crying, jitteriness, poor feeding, emesis, respiratory distress, and seizures. To minimize or prevent these signs and symptoms, the nurse should keep sensory stimulation to a minimum and the neonate in a quiet, dimly lit environment. A bath would necessitate the removal of clothing and exposure to changes in temperature, both of which are too stimulating for the cocaine-addicted neonate.
CN: Physiological integrity; CNS: Basic care and comfort; CL: Apply

65. A neonate of a mother with diabetes was born full-term and weighs 4,600 g. While caring for this neonate, the nurse checks the clavicles for which reason?

1. Neonates of mothers with diabetes have brittle bones.
2. Clavicles are commonly absent in neonates of mothers with diabetes.
3. One of the neonate's clavicles may have been broken during birth.
4. Large-for-gestational-age (LGA) neonates have glucose deposits on their clavicles.

65. 3. Clavicular fractures are common during birth in LGA neonates. The nurse should assess all LGA neonates for this occurrence. Neonates of mothers with diabetes do not have brittle bones or glucose deposits, nor are their clavicles absent.
CN: Physiological integrity; CNS: Reduction of risk potential; CL: Apply

CN: Client needs category   CNS: Client needs subcategory   CL: Cognitive level

66. The nurse is caring for a neonate diagnosed with fetal alcohol syndrome (FAS). When assessing this neonate, which finding(s) will the nurse expect? Select all that apply.
1. Microphthalmia
2. Microcephaly
3. Wide palpebral fissures
4. Well-developed philtrum
5. Difficulty hearing

67. A neonate born at 36 weeks' gestation weighs 1,800 g. The neonate also has microcephaly and microphthalmia. When reviewing the maternal history, the nurse will expect which finding?
1. Alcohol abuse
2. Use of marijuana
3. Gestational diabetes
4. Group B streptococci infection

68. The nurse is caring for a 4-hour-old neonate. The heel stick hematocrit test result is 48% (0.48). What will the nurse do **next**?
1. Notify the health care provider.
2. Document the level in the medical record.
3. Reassess the level in 12 hours.
4. Check the respiratory rate.

69. Which neonate will the registered nurse (RN) assign to the licensed practical nurse (LPN)?
1. The neonate with a temperature of 100.9°F (38.3°C), heart rate of 112 beats/minute, and blood pressure of 92/50 mm Hg
2. The neonate with a temperature 98.4°F (36.9°C), respiratory rate of 68 breaths/minute, and blood pressure of 70/48 mm Hg
3. The neonate with a chest circumference of 12 in (30.5 cm) and weight of 4,600 g
4. The neonate with a head circumference of 13 in (33 cm) and length of 19 in (48.3 cm)

70. The nurse is providing discharge teaching to the parents of a 2-day-old neonate. The neonate was circumcised earlier today and is breastfed. Which statement(s) by the parents indicates to the nurse teaching was effective? Select all that apply.
1. "My newborn should breastfeed every 2 to 4 hours once we get home."
2. "We will apply petroleum gauze to the end of the penis with each diaper change."
3. "My newborn's stools will begin to transition to a greenish color tomorrow."
4. "We should give our baby acetaminophen orally every 4 hours for pain for a few days."
5. "We can give our baby a tub bath once the umbilical stump falls off."

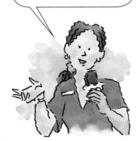

Hang in there— you're almost done. Then you can have a treat.

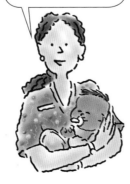

Remember to "select all that apply" in question #70.

66. 1, 2, 5. Distinctive facial dysmorphology of children with FAS most commonly involves the eyes (microphthalmia). Microcephaly is generally seen with FAS, as are short palpebral fissures and a poorly developed philtrum. Hearing and vision problems are common with FAS.
CN: Physiological integrity; CNS: Physiological adaptation; CL: Apply

67. 1. The most common sign of the effects of alcohol on fetal development is retarded growth in weight, length, and head circumference (microcephaly). Intrauterine growth retardation is not characteristic of marijuana use. Gestational diabetes usually produces large-for-gestational-age neonates. Infection with group B streptococci is not a relevant risk factor.
CN: Physiological integrity; CNS: Reduction of risk potential; CL: Apply

68. 1. Hematocrit of 52% (0.52) to 58% (0.58) is normal in a neonate because of increased blood supply during intrauterine life. Hematocrit of 48% (0.48) indicates a complication such as anemia, and the health care provider needs to be notified first. Then the nurse may complete the other actions.
CN: Health promotion and maintenance; CNS: None; CL: Analyze

69. 4. The RN will delegate this neonate to the LPN because all findings are within normal range. Normal ranges are: temperature, 97.7°F (36.5°C) to 99°F (37.2°C); heart rate, 120 to 160 beats/minute; average blood pressure, 65/41 mm Hg; respiratory rate, 30 to 60 breaths/minute; head circumference, 13 to 14 in (33 to 35.6 cm); chest circumference, 12 to 13 in (30.5 to 33 cm); length, 19 to 21 in (48.3 to 53.3 cm); and weight, 2,500 g to 4,000 g. The other neonates listed have findings that are not normal and thus should be monitored by the RN for potential complications.
CN: Safe, effective care environment; CNS: Management of care; CL: Analyze

70. 1, 2, 3, 5. Breastfed neonates should eat every 2 to 4 hours, as that is the approximate stomach emptying time. Petroleum jelly should be applied to the glans with each diaper change until the site is healed, which is typically in 2 to 4 days. Breastfed neonate stools begin transitioning around day 3 to a greenish color. Tub baths are appropriate once the stump falls off and the circumcision heals, to prevent infection. If the neonate appears to be in pain, the health care provider should be notified to assess for complications.
CN: Health promotion and maintenance; CNS: None; CL: Apply

71. The nurse is eliciting reflexes in a neonate during the initial assessment. Identify the area the nurse will touch to elicit a plantar grasp reflex.

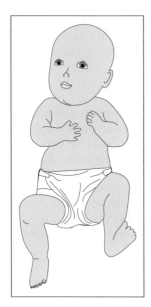

71. Touching the sole near the base of the digits elicits a plantar grasp reflex and causes flexion or grasping. This reflex disappears around age 9 months.

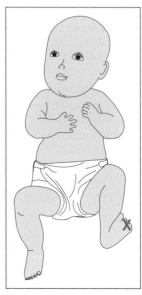

cn: Health promotion and maintenance; cns: None; cl: Apply

72. The nurse notes a neonate is pink with acrocyanosis at 5 minutes after birth; the knees are flexed, fists are clinched, a whimpering cry is present, and the heart rate is 128 beats/minute. The neonate withdraws the foot in response to a slap on the sole. What 5-minute Apgar score will the nurse record for this neonate?

Apgar Scoring Chart			
	Score		
Sign	0	1	2
Heart rate	Absent	Slow (<100)	>100
Breathing	Absent	Slow, irregular; weak cry	Good; strong cry
Muscle tone	Flaccid	Some flexion of extremities	Well flexed
Reflex response			
Response to catheter in nostril	No response	Grimace	Cough or sneeze
or			
Slap of sole of foot	No response	Grimace	Cry and with-drawal of foot
Color	Blue, pale	Body pink, extremities blue	Completely pink

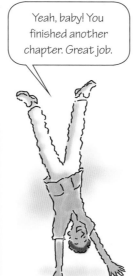

Yeah, baby! You finished another chapter. Great job.

72. **8.** The Apgar score quantifies neonatal heart rate, respiratory effort, muscle tone, reflexes, and color. Each category is assessed 1 minute after birth and again 5 minutes after birth. Scores in each category range from 0 to 2. This neonate has a heart rate above 100 beats/minute, which equals 2; is pink in color with acrocyanosis, which equals 1; is well-flexed, which equals 2; has a weak cry, which equals 1; and has a good response to slapping the soles, which equals 2. Therefore, the nurse should record a total Apgar score of 8 for this neonate.

cn: Physiological integrity; cns: Physiological adaptation; cl: Analyze

Part V

Care of the Child

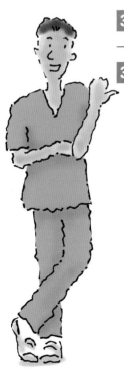

Chapter 25

Growth & Development

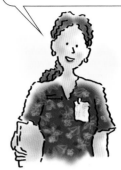

Here's a short but important chapter that covers the growth and development of children. Enjoy!

Growth & development refresher

Infant (birth to age 1)

Neonatal period
- All behavior is under reflex control; extremities are flexed
- Normal pulse rate ranges from 110 to 160 beats/minute
- Normal blood pressure is 65/41 mm Hg
- Normal respiratory rate is 30 to 60 breaths/minute. Respirations are irregular and from the abdomen; the neonate is an obligate nose breather
- Temperature regulation is poor

1 to 4 months
- Posterior fontanel closes
- Begins to hold up the head
- Cries to express needs
- Thumb opposition at fourth month

5 to 6 months
- Rolls over from stomach to back
- Cries when caregiver leaves

7 to 9 months
- Fear of strangers appears to peak during the eighth month
- Sits unsupported
- Crawls on hands and knees with belly off floor
- Verbalizes all vowels and most consonants but speaks no intelligible words

10 to 12 months
- Holds onto furniture while walking (cruising) at age 10 months, walks with support at age 11 months, and stands alone and takes first steps at age 12 months
- Says "mama" and "dada" and responds to own name
- Can say about five words but understands many more

Toddler (ages 1 to 3)
- Normal pulse rate is 70 to 110 beats/minute
- Normal blood pressure range is 90 to 105/55 to 70 mm Hg

- Normal respiratory rate is 20 to 30 breaths/minute
- Separation anxiety arises
- Toilet-trained; day dryness is achieved between ages 18 months and 3 years and night dryness between ages 2 and 5
- Speaks 2- to 4-word sentences

Preschool child (ages 3 to 6)
- Normal pulse rate ranges from 65 to 110 beats/minute
- Normal blood pressure ranges from 95 to 110/60 to 75 mm Hg
- Normal respiratory rate is 20 to 25 breaths/minute
- May express fear of animal noises, new experiences, and the dark

School-age child (ages 6 to 12)
- Normal pulse rate ranges from 85 to 95 beats/minute
- Normal blood pressure ranges from 95 to 120/55 to 76 mm Hg
- Normal respiratory rate ranges from 17 to 25 breaths/minute
- Accidents are a major cause of death and disability during this period
- Plays with peers, develops a first true friendship, and develops a sense of belonging, cooperation, and compromise
- Learns to read and spell

Adolescent (ages 12 to 18)
- Experiences puberty-related changes in body structure and psychosocial adjustment
- Vital signs approach adult values
- Normal pulse rate ranges from 65 to 85 beats/minute
- Normal blood pressure ranges from 118 to 120/70 to 80 mm Hg
- Normal respiratory rate ranges from 15 to 20 breaths/minute
- Peers influence behavior and values

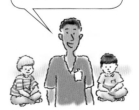

I bet this chapter will grow on you. I've developed quite a fondness for it.

Infants and nutrition

Primary nutrition guidelines for first year of life

- Begin with formula or breast milk; give no more than 30 oz (887 mL) of formula each day; breastfeed on demand (every 2 to 4 hours)
- Iron supplements may be necessary by 6 months
- No solid foods should be given for the first 4 to 6 months
- Provide rice cereal as the first solid food, followed by any other cereal except wheat
- Single ingredient vegetables and fruits may be given at 6 months
- Give junior foods or soft table foods after 9 months

Growth & development questions, answers, and rationales

1. A parent of a 2-year-old child states "I think my child may have attention deficit hyperactivity disorder (ADHD) because my child has so much energy, does not pay attention for long, and is always getting into things." Which response by the nurse is **best**?
1. "This behavior is normal. The child is exploring and learning about the world."
2. "You should talk to your child's health care provider. You have definite concerns."
3. "You need to keep your child's intake of sugar and sugary treats to a minimum."
4. "I recommend requesting a referral for a child psychologist for evaluation."

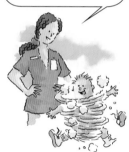

Two year olds can be quite energetic.

1. **1.** It is normal for a 2-year-old child to eagerly explore the environment for new sensory experiences. Talking to the health care provider is inappropriate because the nurse is assuming a corrective, parental role toward the parent without addressing concerns. Restricting the child's intake of sugar and sugary treats is incorrect because the nurse is making assumptions and recommendations that do not relate to the parent's concerns. Suggesting evaluation by a psychologist reinforces the parent's fear that something is wrong with the child.
CN: Health promotion and maintenance; CNS: None; CL: Apply

2. The nurse is planning to administer immunizations to children during their well-child appointments. To which child(ren) will the nurse question administering the prescribed vaccination? Select all that apply.
1. Influenza to a child who is allergic to gelatin and penicillin.
2. Rotavirus (RV) to a child with a history of Celiac disease.
3. Inactivated polio vaccine (IPV) to a child with a temperature of 100.6°F (38.1°C).
4. *Haemophilus influenzae* Type B (Hib) to a child with a history of chronic otitis media.
5. Pneumococcal conjugate vaccine (PCV) to a child whose mother is pregnant.
6. Diphtheria, tetanus, and pertussis (DTaP) to a child who has had seizures in the past.

2. **2, 3.** The nurse would question giving RV to a child with a history of a gastrointestinal disorder, such as Celiac disease and any vaccination to a child who is acutely ill. Varicella and measles, mumps, rubella (MMR) are contraindicated if the client is allergic to gelatin or neomycin. No vaccinations are contraindicated for an allergy to penicillin. Vaccines are safe to administer to children of pregnant mothers. DTaP, in rare cases, has led to seizure activity; however, it is safe to give to clients with a history of seizures that are now controlled.
CN: Health promotion and maintenance; CNS: None; CL: Analyze

3. Which developmental milestone(s) will the nurse expect to assess in a 10-month-old infant? Select all that apply.
1. Holding the head erect
2. Self-feeding
3. Have good bowel and bladder control
4. Sitting on a firm surface without support
5. Walking while holding on to furniture
6. Walking alone

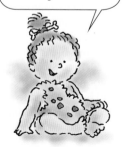

"All by myself!" Infants and toddlers are constantly learning new skills.

3. **1, 4, 5.** By age 10 months, an infant should be able to hold the head erect, a developmental milestone achieved by age 3 months. The infant should also be able to sit on a firm surface without support and bear the majority of his or her weight on the legs (for example, walking while holding on to furniture). Self-feeding and bowel and bladder control are developmental milestones of toddlers. By age 12 months, the infant should be able to stand alone and may take first steps.
CN: Health promotion and maintenance; CNS: None; CL: Apply

4. A parent brings a 2-year-old child to the clinic for a routine wellness check. During assessment, the nurse notes: blood pressure, 90/70 mm Hg; pulse, 94 beats/minute; and respirations, 20 breaths/minute. What will the nurse do **next**?
1. Notify the health care provider.
2. Document the findings.
3. Give oxygen via a nasal cannula.
4. Measure urine output.

5. A 14-month-old is admitted to the pediatric floor with a diagnosis of croup. The nurse will expect the client to exhibit which developmental milestone(s)? Select all that apply.
1. Strong hand grasp
2. Hold one object while looking for another
3. Smile in recognition of familiar voices
4. Presence of Moro reflex
5. Weight that is triple the birth weight
6. Closed anterior fontanel

6. The nurse assessing an adolescent male documents his sexual maturity as Tanner stage 3. Which image depicts this stage?

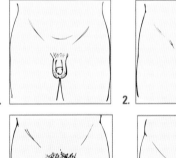
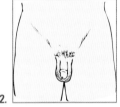
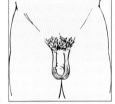
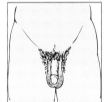

1.   2.

3.   4.

7. When discussing death and dying with 10- and 11-year-old children which guides will the nurse incorporate? Select all that apply.
1. Logical explanations are not appropriate for this age.
2. The children will be curious about the physical aspects of death.
3. The children will know that death is inevitable and irreversible.
4. The children will be influenced by the attitudes of the adults in their lives.
5. Educating children about death and dying should not start before age 11.
6. Telling children that death is the same as going to sleep is appropriate.

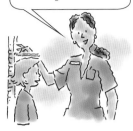

Looks like you really measure up. Keep up the good work.

4. 2. The nurse would document the assessment findings. Normal vital signs for toddlers are pulse rate is 70 to 110 beats/minute, blood pressure range is 90 to 105/55 to 70 mm Hg, and respiratory rate is 20 to 30 breaths/minute.
CN: Health promotion and maintenance: CNS: None; CL: Apply

5. 1, 2, 3, 5. A strong hand grasp is demonstrated within the first month of life. Holding one object while looking for another is accomplished by the 20th week. Within the first year of life, the toddler masters smiling at familiar faces and voices, birth weight triples, and the Moro reflex disappears. The anterior fontanel closes by approximately 18 months of age.
CN: Health promotion and maintenance; CNS: None; CL: Apply

6. 2. In Tanner stage 3, pubic hair extends across the pubis. Testes and scrotum begin to enlarge, and the penis increases in length. Option 1 depicts Tanner stage 2, option 3 shows Tanner stage 4, and option 4 depicts Tanner stage 5.
CN: Physiological integrity; CNS: Physiological adaptation; CL: Apply

7. 2, 3, 4. School-age children are curious about the physical aspects of death and may wonder what happens to the body. By age 9 or 10, most children know that death is universal, inevitable, and irreversible. Their cognitive abilities are advanced, and they respond well to logical explanations. They should be encouraged to ask questions. Because adults influence children's attitudes toward death, they should be encouraged to include children in the family rituals and be prepared to answer questions that may seem shocking. Educating children about death should begin early in childhood. Comparing death to sleep can be frightening for children and cause them to fear falling asleep.
CN: Psychosocial integrity; CNS: None; CL: Apply

CN: Client needs category   CNS: Client needs subcategory   CL: Cognitive level

Chapter 26

Cardiovascular Disorders

Pediatric cardiovascular refresher

Increased pulmonary blood flow defects and obstructions to blood flow from the ventricles

Key signs and symptoms
- Congested cough
- Diaphoresis
- Fatigue
- Machine-like heart murmur (in patent ductus arteriosus)
- Mild cyanosis (if the condition leads to right-sided heart failure)
- Respiratory distress
- Tachycardia
- Tachypnea

Key test results
- Chest x-ray, echocardiography, and cardiac catheterization confirm type of heart defect

Key treatments
- Surgical repair
- Digoxin
- Diuretic (e.g., furosemide)

Key interventions
- Monitor vital signs, pulse oximetry, and intake and output.
- Monitor cardiovascular and respiratory status.
- Take apical pulse for 1 minute before giving digoxin (bradycardia is considered to be a pulse below 100 beats/minute in infants).
- Monitor fluid status.

Decreased pulmonary blood flow and mixed blood flow defects

Key signs and symptoms
- Clubbing
- Crouching position assumed frequently

- Cyanosis
- History of inadequate feeding
- Irritability
- Tachycardia
- Tachypnea

Key test results
- Arterial blood gas analysis shows diminished arterial oxygen saturation
- Complete blood count shows polycythemia

Key treatments
- Corrective surgery to redirect blood flow for transposition of the great vessels or arteries
- Complete repair or palliative treatment for tetralogy of Fallot
- Surgery to restructure the heart or heart transplantation for hypoplastic left-heart syndrome
- Surgery to recreate the pulmonary trunk and repair the ventricular septal defect for truncus arteriosus

Key interventions
- Monitor cardiovascular and respiratory status.
- Monitor vital signs, pulse oximetry, and intake and output.
- Administer prophylactic antibiotics.

Rheumatic fever

Inflammatory condition that may result as a complication after experiencing a group A streptococcus infection; may cause chronic cardiac complications

Key signs and symptoms
- Carditis
- Chorea
- Erythema marginatum (temporary, disk-shaped, nonpruritic, reddened macules

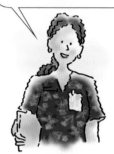

Ah, there you are. You've reached our test on cardiovascular disorders in children. Before starting these practice questions, why not bolster yourself with a heart-healthy snack of celery and low-fat cream cheese? Yum!

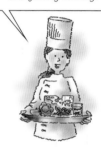

This pump keeps everything flowing!

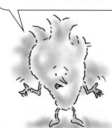

When I'm defective, not enough oxygen gets to the rest of the body, which is bad news.

that fade in the center, leaving raised margins)
- Polyarthritis
- Subcutaneous nodules

Key test results
- Erythrocyte sedimentation rate is increased
- Electrocardiogram shows prolonged PR interval
- Echocardiography shows damage to heart structures

Key treatments
- Bed rest until the sedimentation rate normalizes
- Penicillin to prevent additional damage from future attacks
- Anti-inflammatory drug to reduce pain and inflammation

Key interventions
- Monitor vital signs and intake and output.

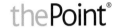 You can download tables of drug information to help you prepare for the NCLEX®! View Generic Drug Names, Drug Classifications, Drug Actions, and Nursing Implications for the drugs discussed in this refresher at **http://thePoint.lww.com**

Cardiovascular questions, answers, and rationales

1. When auscultating heart sounds on a 2-year-old child, where will the nurse place the stethoscope to hear the first heart sound **best**?
1. Third or fourth intercostal space
2. The apex with the stethoscope bell
3. Second intercostal space, midclavicular line
4. Fifth intercostal space, left midclavicular line

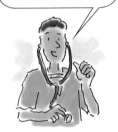

1. 4. The first heart sound can best be heard at the fifth intercostal space, left midclavicular line. The second heart sound is heard at the second intercostal space. The third heart sound is heard with the stethoscope bell at the apex of the heart. The fourth heart sound can be heard at the third or fourth intercostal space.
CN: Health promotion and maintenance; CNS: None; CL: Understand

2. The nurse has auscultated the second heart sound. When does the nurse determine this sound is occurring?
1. Late in diastole
2. Early in diastole
3. With closure of the mitral and tricuspid valves
4. With closure of the aortic and pulmonic valves

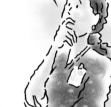

2. 4. The second heart sound occurs during diastole with closure of the aortic and pulmonic valves. The first heart sound occurs during systole with closure of the mitral and tricuspid valves. The third heart sound is heard early in diastole. The fourth heart sound is heard late in diastole and may be a normal finding in children.
CN: Health promotion and maintenance; CNS: None; CL: Understand

3. During assessment, a child's parent states the child has a grade 1 heart murmur. Which finding will the nurse expect with auscultation?
1. A sound equal in volume to the heart sounds
2. A sound softer than the heart sounds
3. A sound that can be heard with the naked ear
4. A sound associated with a precordial thrill

3. 2. A grade 1 heart murmur is usually difficult to hear and softer than the heart sounds. A grade 2 murmur is usually equal in volume to the heart sounds. A grade 4 murmur can be associated with a precordial thrill. A thrill is a palpable manifestation associated with a loud murmur. A grade 6 murmur can be heard with the naked ear or with the stethoscope off the chest.
CN: Health promotion and maintenance; CNS: None; CL: Apply

CN: Client needs category   CNS: Client needs subcategory   CL: Cognitive level

4. A 17-year-old client is diagnosed with cardiogenic shock. Which finding(s) will the nurse expect to note during assessment? Select all that apply.
1. Blood pressure of 70/40 mm Hg
2. Respiratory rate of 41 breaths/minute
3. Oxygen saturation of 96%
4. Urine output of 95 mL in 3 hours
5. Pale skin with cool extremities

5. The nurse suspects a neonate has a patent ductus arteriosus (PDA). Which assessment finding(s) will the nurse expect this client to exhibit? Select all that apply.
1. Poor feeding pattern
2. Bounding heart rate of 150 beats/minute
3. Acrocyanosis
4. Icteric sclera
5. Respiratory rate of 75 breaths/minute

6. The nurse is caring for a 4-year-old child in a shock state. Which finding **most** concerns the nurse?
1. Heart rate of 114 beats/minute
2. Blood pressure of 75/46 mm Hg
3. Capillary refill of 4 seconds
4. Pale, cool, mottled hands

7. The nurse is assessing a 1-month-old infant. Which finding will the nurse report to the health care provider **immediately**?
1. The infant is lethargic and uninterested in drinking formula from a bottle.
2. The infant's current weight is 8 lb (3,629 g) and birth weight was 7 lb (3,175 g).
3. The caregiver states the infant refuses to take naps during the day.
4. The infant's blood pressure is 62/40 mm Hg and heart rate is 150 beats/minute.

8. A 2-year-old child is showing signs of shock. A 10 mL/kg bolus of normal saline is prescribed. The child weighs 55 lb (25 kg). How many milliliters will the nurse administer? Record your answer using a whole number.

_____ mL

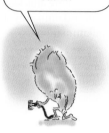

Speaking of "cardiogenic shock," check this out ...

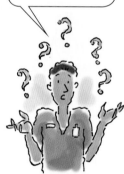

That word "most" in question #6 looks important. Which finding is most concerning?

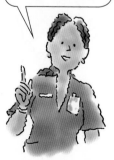

Try not to overthink question #8. As math problems go, it's pretty easy.

4. 1, 2, 5. Cardiogenic shock occurs when cardiac output is suddenly decreased, and tissue oxygen needs are not adequately met. Signs and symptoms include hypotension; severe shortness of breath; rapid breathing; oliguria; weak pulses; and pale, cool skin. Decreased, not normal, oxygen saturation and urine output levels would be expected in this client.
CN: Physiological integrity; CNS: Physiological adaptation; CL: Analyze

5. 1, 2, 5. A PDA results when the ductus arteriosus does not close at birth. This usually results within 15 hours of life. Symptoms are consistent with the condition include a full, bounding pulse; dyspnea; poor feeding; tiring easily; and tachypnea. Acrocyanosis refers to a blue discoloration in the extremities. This is commonly seen in the first hours after birth and is not associated with PDA. Icteric sclera indicates jaundice, which is not associated with PDA.
CN: Physiological integrity; CNS: Physiological adaptation; CL: Apply

6. 2. Hypotension is considered a late sign of shock in children. This represents a decompensated state and impending cardiopulmonary arrest. Tachycardia, delayed capillary refill, and pale, cool, mottled skin are earlier indicators of shock that may show compensation.
CN: Physiological integrity; CNS: Physiological adaptation; CL: Analyze

7. 1. Infants and children with heart defects tend to have poor nutritional intake and weight loss, indicating poor cardiac output, heart failure, or hypoxemia. The child appears lethargic or tired because of the heart failure or hypoxia. Gray, pale, or mottled skin may indicate hypoxia or poor cardiac output. Some infants do not nap well, which does not indicate a cardiac condition. The listed vital signs and weight gain are normal for an infant.
CN: Health promotion and maintenance; CNS: None; CL: Analyze

8. 250. To determine the dose, multiply the dose prescribed, by the child's weight in kilograms:

$$10 \, mL/kg \times 25 \, kg = 250 \, mL$$

CN: Physiological integrity; CNS: Pharmacological and parenteral therapies; CL: Apply

9. Which client will the nurse monitor **most** closely for the development of an arrhythmia?
1. A 3-day-old exposed to toxoplasmosis in utero
2. A 6-month-old receiving indomethacin for a patent ductus arteriosus
3. A 1-year-old returning from surgery to correct a ventricular septal defect
4. A 6-year-old with a blood pressure of 95/55 mm Hg and heart rate of 85 beats/minute

10. The nurse is caring for a neonate recently diagnosed with tetralogy of Fallot. The neonate's parents do not seem to be accepting of the diagnosis and the changes the diagnosis will make in their lives. Which nursing action is **most** therapeutic?
1. Encourage the parents to have genetic testing before future pregnancies.
2. Listen as the parents discuss their feelings about the loss of their baby's health.
3. Ensure the parents understand the diagnosis and treatment plan requirements.
4. Consult with case management to get the parents a referral for counseling.

11. The nurse is talking with the parent of a 3-year-old child who has coarctation of the aorta. The parent reports feeling concern the child does not seem to be maturing at the same rate as the two older children in the family. Which response by the nurse is **most** appropriate?
1. "All children mature at different rates so comparisons are not really appropriate."
2. "Children who have chronic health issues may experience developmental delays."
3. "The immature actions may just be your child's way of coping with being different."
4. "You will need to lower your expectations for your child's level of maturity."

12. A neonate with a patent ductus arteriosus (PDA) was born 6 hours ago and is currently being held by his mother. As the nurse enters the room to assess the neonate's vital signs, the mother says, "The health care provider says my baby has a heart murmur. Does that mean my baby has a bad heart?" Which response(s) by the nurse is appropriate? Select all that apply.
1. "We need to do more tests on your baby to determine if he has a bad heart."
2. "Your baby will need to be placed on oxygen therapy for a few weeks."
3. "Do not worry, many babies have transient murmurs right after they are born."
4. "The murmur is caused by a natural opening that may take a day or two to close."
5. "Many newborns experience murmurs while transitioning to life outside the womb."

9. **3.** Arrhythmia development in children is most common in the early postoperative period following surgery for congenital heart disorders. Toxoplasmosis can cause cardiac anomalies in utero, not arrhythmia after birth. Indomethacin is administered intravenously, and if successful, the client will not require surgery. The vital signs listed are within normal range for a school-age client.
CN: Safe, effective care environment; CNS: Management of care; CL: Analyze

10. **2.** Grief and feelings of loss by the parents are expected phenomena when a baby receives a diagnosis of a chronic health concern. Parents will need to work through the feelings about the anticipated future of their baby being modified. Genetic counseling may be needed if the disorder is hereditary, but in this case it is premature and the focus needs to be on assisting the family to navigate through their feelings and focus on the care of their child. Education about the diagnosis and treatment plan is needed but does not address the parents' concerns. Counseling may be of benefit but the nurse must first promote communication with the parents.
CN: Psychosocial integrity; CNS: None; CL: Apply

11. **2.** Chronic illnesses can impact a child's growth and development both emotionally and cognitively. The child with a cardiac disorder may experience delays as a result of hypoxic episodes or because of repeated hospitalizations. Educating parents about these possibilities helps initiate the discussion about the child's level of maturity. Although children mature at different rates, this is not the best response. Children may act out in response to illness or other factors but there is no information that supports this reason for the child's behavior. Encouraging parents to lower their expectations is not therapeutic.
CN: Psychosocial integrity; CNS: None; CL: Apply

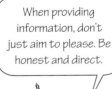

When providing information, don't just aim to please. Be honest and direct.

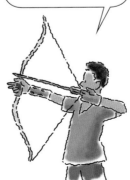

12. **4, 5.** Although the nurse may want to tell the mother not to worry, the most appropriate response would be to explain the neonate's present condition to relieve her fears, and to acknowledge an awareness of the condition. A neonate's vascular system changes with birth; certain factors help to reverse the flow of blood through the PDA and ultimately favor its closure. This closure typically begins within the first 24 hours after birth and ends within a few days after birth. There is no indication that the neonate needs additional testing or oxygen at this time.
CN: Health promotion and maintenance; CNS: None; CL: Apply

CN: Client needs category   CNS: Client needs subcategory   CL: Cognitive level

13. A school-age client is scheduled to have a cardiac catheterization and reports increasing anxiety as the day of the procedure approaches. Which nursing action(s) is appropriate for the client prior to the procedure? Select all that apply.
 1. Provide the client with a map of the entire hospital.
 2. Restrict the client's visitors to immediate family members only.
 3. Give a tour of the hospital and catheterization laboratory.
 4. Let the client touch the equipment used for the procedure.
 5. Explain what will happen before, during, and after the procedure.

13. **3, 4, 5.** A tour of the facility will help minimize fears and allay anxieties for the child. It gives the opportunity for questions and education. Having familiarity with appropriate equipment required for the procedure will be of assistance. It will also allow a time for questions to be asked. The nurse should explain to the client what to expect before, during, and after the procedure to help alleviate anxiety. A map of the hospital will not reduce concerns about the procedure. Restricting visitors may cause more stress and anxiety for the client.
CN: Physiological integrity; CNS: Physiological adaptation; CL: Apply

14. A 15-year-old client is scheduled to have a cardiac catheterization. Which statement(s) by the client indicates to the nurse further instruction is needed? Select all that apply.
 1. "A consent form will need to be signed by my parents for this procedure."
 2. "My health care provider will put me to sleep for the catheterization."
 3. "The sound waves will let the health care provider see how my heart moves."
 4. "It provides visualization of the heart and great vessels with radiopaque dye."
 5. "They will pass a small catheter through an artery in my leg to look at my heart."

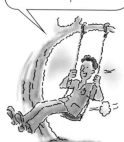

Now you've got the swing of things. Keep it up!

14. **2, 3.** Cardiac catheterization provides visualization of the heart and great vessels. It is an invasive procedure in which a thin catheter is passed into the chambers of the heart through a peripheral vein or artery. A signed consent form will be required. Conscious sedation is usually given before cardiac catheterization. General anesthesia is not generally done. High-frequency sound waves are used during ultrasound and echocardiography, not cardiac catheterization.
CN: Health promotion and maintenance; CNS: None; CL: Apply

15. The nurse is caring for a child who underwent a cardiac catheterization 1 hour ago. Which nursing intervention(s) is appropriate while caring for this child? Select all that apply.
 1. Keep the television off in the child's room.
 2. Encourage the child to remain flat in bed.
 3. Assess the child's vital signs every 15 minutes until awake and stable.
 4. Replace the dressing if bleeding occurs at the insertion site.
 5. Do not let the child eat for 24 hours after the procedure.

15. **2, 3.** During recovery, the child should remain flat in bed, keeping the punctured leg straight for the prescribed time. The child should avoid raising the head, sitting, straining the abdomen, or coughing. Vital signs are taken every 15 minutes until the child is awake and stable, then every half hour, and then hourly as prescribed. If bleeding occurs at the insertion site, the nurse should reinforce the dressing and monitor for changes, not replace it. There is no reason for the child not to watch television or to be NPO after the procedure.
CN: Physiological integrity; CNS: Physiological adaptation; CL: Analyze

16. The nurse is providing discharge education to a teenager following a cardiac catheterization. Which statement(s) made by the client indicates the need for further instruction? Select all that apply.
 1. "I can follow my normal diet at home."
 2. "I need to drink extra water for a few days."
 3. "I will be able to go to school tomorrow."
 4. "It will be at least 2 weeks before I can play basketball."
 5. "I will be able to take a shower or bath in a few days."

16. **3, 4.** After a cardiac catheterization a regular diet may be resumed. Increased fluid intake is recommended as it will help to flush the dye from the system. The client can normally return to school in 3 to 5 days. Most regular activities including exercise will be permissible after 3 to 5 days. Taking a bath or shower is permissible after a few days.
CN: Physiological integrity; CNS: Physiological adaptation; CL: Apply

17. A 2-year-old child is being monitored after cardiac surgery. Which finding(s) will the nurse flag for the health care provider? Select all that apply.
1. Blood pressure of 80/45 mm Hg
2. Urinary output of 45 mL in 2 hours
3. Weak peripheral pulses
4. Capillary refill of less than 2 seconds
5. Heart rate of 100 beats/minute

18. A 3-year-old child is experiencing distress after having cardiac surgery. The nurse suspects cardiac tamponade based on which finding(s)? Select all that apply.
1. Blood pressure of 120/85 mm Hg
2. Muffled heart sounds
3. Pulse pressure of 65 mm Hg
4. Increased chest tube drainage
5. Respiratory rate of 44 breaths/minute

19. The nurse is reviewing laboratory results for a 17-year-old client scheduled for a cardiac procedure. Which finding(s) will the nurse report to the health care provider? Select all that apply.
1. Potassium 3.1 mEq/L (3.1 mmol/L)
2. Sodium 151 mEq/L (151 mmol/L)
3. Calcium 9 mg/dL (2.25 mmol/L)
4. Chloride 100 mEq/L (100 mmol/L)
5. Magnesium 2.0 mEq/L (1 mmol/L)

20. The nurse is providing education on wound and skin care to a pediatric client's parents following cardiac surgery. Which information will the nurse include in the education? Select all that apply.
1. "Avoid using powders near the incision location."
2. "Your child will be able to begin taking tub baths tomorrow."
3. "Your child may feel tingling, itching, and numbness at the wound site."
4. "If you notice foul-smelling drainage from the incision, call the health care provider."
5. "If the sterile adhesive strips over the incision fall off, call the health care provider."

21. The nurse is caring for a child following cardiac surgery. While preparing for discharge, the child's parents ask the nurse, "Do we need to limit our child's activity level?" Which nursing response is **best**?
1. "There are no activity limitations for your child."
2. "Your child will be able to return to school in 3 days."
3. "Your child needs to maintain a balance of rest and activity."
4. "Your child can't climb or participate in contact sports for 1 week."

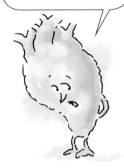

When my blood pressure is down, I just can't pump out the red stuff like usual.

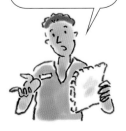

As my grandpa always says, "Everything in moderation."

17. 1, 2, 3. Signs of decreased cardiac output include weak peripheral pulses, low urine output, delayed capillary refill, hypotension, and cool extremities. These should be reported to the health care provider. The normal blood pressure for a child of this age may range from 90/55 to 105/70 mm Hg. The blood pressure presented is well below this value. Urinary output of less than 30 mL/hour signals reduced cardiac output. A heart rate of 100 beats per minute is within normal limits (70 to 110 beats/minute) for a 2-year-old child.
CN: Physiological integrity; CNS: Physiological adaptation; CL: Analyze

18. 2, 5. Symptoms of cardiac tamponade include muffled heart sounds, hypotension, sudden cessation of chest tube drainage, rapid respirations, and a narrowing pulse pressure. Cardiac tamponade occurs when a large volume of fluid interferes with ventricular filling and pumping and collects in the pericardial sac, decreasing cardiac output.
CN: Physiological integrity; CNS: Physiological adaptation; CL: Analyze

19. 1, 2. The normal range for serum potassium is 3.5 to 5.5 mEq/L. Serum sodium levels should range from 135 to 145 mEq/L. The values found for both sodium and potassium are not within normal limits and require notification. The calcium, chloride, and magnesium levels are within normal limits.
CN: Health promotion and maintenance; CNS: None; CL: Analyze

20. 1, 3, 4. Lotions and powders should be avoided during the first 2 weeks after surgery. As the area heals, tingling, itching, and numbness are normal sensations that will eventually go away. Foul-smelling drainage or a fever could indicate infection. A complete bath should be delayed for the first week. Adhesive strips may loosen or fall off on their own, which is a common and normal occurrence.
CN: Physiological integrity; CNS: Physiological adaptation; CL: Apply

21. 3. Activity should be increased gradually each day, allowing for a sensible balance of rest and activity. School and large crowds should be avoided for at least 2 weeks to prevent exposure to people with active infections. Sports and contact activities should be restricted for about 6 weeks, giving the sternum enough time to heal.
CN: Physiological integrity; CNS: Physiological adaptation; CL: Apply

CN: Client needs category   CNS: Client needs subcategory   CL: Cognitive level

22. Which discharge education is appropriate for the nurse to provide to a child after surgery to correct a cardiac anomaly?
1. "You must take all medications as prescribed."
2. "Do not eat any foods that contain sodium."
3. "You can keep your dental appointment for next month."
4. "You should not receive any more vaccines in the future."

23. The nurse is caring for a pediatric client who has a chest tube not connected to suction. Which finding will the nurse expect when assessing the client?
1. The water level rises with inhalation.
2. Bubbling is seen in the suction chamber.
3. Bubbling is seen in the water seal chamber.
4. Water seal is obtained by clamping the tube.

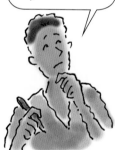

Make sure your priorities are in order in question #24.

24. During assessment, the nurse notes a client's chest tube is dislodged. Which action will the nurse perform **first**?
1. Place a dry gauze dressing over the insertion site.
2. Place a petroleum gauze dressing over the insertion site.
3. Wipe the tube with alcohol and reinsert it.
4. Call the health care provider immediately.

25. The nurse is caring for 5-year-old pediatric client diagnosed with heart failure. Based on the assessment findings noted in the chart exhibit below, what will the nurse do **next**?

Progress notes	
3/28	Client is supine in bed at this time. Vital signs:
1429	temperature, 98.6°F (37°C); blood pressure,
	105/72 mm Hg; heart rate, 112 beats/minute;
	respiratory rate, 30 breaths/minute; oxygen
	saturation, 96%. Gallop heart rhythm and mild
	peripheral edema noted during auscultation.

1. Reassess the respiratory rate in 15 minutes.
2. Put the child in semi-Fowler's position.
3. Prepare the child for an echocardiography.
4. Notify the child's health care provider.

22. 1. Drugs such as digoxin and furosemide should not be stopped abruptly. There are no diet restrictions, so the child may resume a regular diet. Routine dental care is usually delayed 4 to 5 months after surgery. Immunizations may be delayed 6 to 8 weeks after surgery.
CN: Physiological integrity; CNS: Physiological adaptation; CL: Apply

23. 1. The water seal chamber is functioning appropriately when the water level rises in the chamber with inhalation and falls with expiration. This shows that negative pressure required in the lung is being maintained. Bubbling in the suction chamber should only be seen when suction is being used. Bubbling in the water seal chamber generally indicates the presence of an air leak. The chest tube should never be clamped; a tension pneumothorax may occur. Water seal is activated when the suction is disconnected.
CN: Physiological integrity; CNS: Physiological adaptation; CL: Apply

24. 2. Petroleum gauze should immediately be placed over the insertion site to prevent a pneumothorax. The health care provider should be notified after this step. A dry gauze dressing would allow air to escape, leading to a pneumothorax. The tube may only be reinserted by a primary health care provider using a sterile thoracotomy tray.
CN: Safe, effective care environment; CNS: Management of care; CL: Apply

25. 2. The nurse would first change the client's position to facilitate breathing. The child is showing signs of respiratory compromise. A gallop heart rhythm, tachycardia, and peripheral edema are expected findings in a child with heart failure. When the heart stretches beyond efficiency, an extra heart sound or S3 gallop murmur may be audible. This is related to excessive preload and ventricular dilation. Tachycardia occurs as a compensatory mechanism to the decrease in cardiac output. It also attempts to increase the force and rate of myocardial contraction and increase oxygen consumption of the heart. The nurse should reassess the client after changing positions. An echocardiogram is not indicated at this time. The nurse should perform interventions before notifying the health care provider.
CN: Safe, effective care environment; CNS: Management of care; CL: Analyze

26. The nurse is assessing a child with left-sided heart failure. Which finding(s) will the nurse expect to assess? Select all that apply.
1. Weight gain
2. Peripheral edema
3. Jugular vein distention
4. Tachypnea
5. Dyspnea

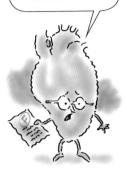

What do you mean I'm a failure? I'm pumping as hard as I can!

26. 1, 2, 3, 4, 5. Unlike adults, children with heart failure do not show separate left- and right-sided signs and symptoms. Failure of one side of the heart leads to reciprocal change in the opposite chamber in children. Therefore, the nurse would expect to see a combination of signs and symptoms associated with left- and right-sided heart failure. Respiratory symptoms, such as tachypnea and dyspnea, are seen due to pulmonary congestion. Weight gain, peripheral edema, and jugular vein distention are seen due to systemic venous congestion. Fluid accumulates in the interstitial spaces due to blood pooling in the venous circulation.
CN: Physiological integrity; CNS: Physiological adaptation; CL: Apply

27. The nurse receives 0700 shift report on an infant diagnosed with heart failure and begins to plan care. The nurse notes it will be time to reassess the client's vital signs at 0730. At 0800, it will be time for the client to receive a bottle. Which nursing action is **most** appropriate?
1. Have the assistive personnel (AP) obtain the client's vital signs now.
2. Visually assess the client, but wait until 0800 to obtain vitals and feed the client together.
3. Assess the client at 0700 and allow the client to rest until time to feed at 0800.
4. Obtain the client's vital signs and feed the client ahead of schedule at 0700.

27. 2. Energy expenditures need to be limited to reduce metabolic and oxygen needs of the infant. Nursing care should be clustered, followed by long periods of undisturbed rest. Visually assessing the client, without disturbing the client, allows the nurse to determine whether the client is safe and stable. The nurse would return at 0800 to obtain vitals and feed the client. Feeding the client an hour early could result in decreased caloric intake.
CN: Safe, effective care environment; CNS: Management of care; CL: Apply

28. The nurse is educating parents of a 3-week-old infant diagnosed with heart failure. Which teaching is **priority** for the nurse to include?
1. Feed your baby a 22-kcal/oz formula.
2. Weigh your baby each day at the same time.
3. Once your baby is eating solids, sodium may be restricted.
4. You need to feed your baby every 4 hours during the day.

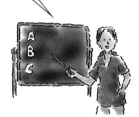

Teach parents that kids with heart failure need calories, calories, calories.

28. 1. Formulas with increased caloric content are given to meet the greater caloric requirements from the overworked heart and labored breathing. Daily weights at the same time of day on the same scale before feedings are recommended to follow trends in nutritional stability and diuresis but are not priority. Discussing sodium requirements for once the infant is consuming solids is not priority. Infants often are hungry every 2 to 4 hours; the infant should be fed when exhibiting hunger signs.
CN: Physiological integrity; CNS: Basic care and comfort; CL: Analyze

29. The nurse is caring for a child with heart failure. The child's parent ask why the child needs oxygen. Which nursing response is appropriate?
1. "Oxygen helps your child rest well."
2. "Oxygen facilitates healing of the heart."
3. "Oxygen is a pulmonary bed constrictor."
4. "Oxygen decreases the work of breathing."

29. 4. Oxygen decreases the work of breathing and increases arterial oxygen levels, so it is indicated in this situation. Oxygen usually is administered at low levels with humidification. While decreasing the workload of the body will facilitate resting and healing, these are not primary reasons for administering oxygen. Oxygen is a pulmonary bed dilator, not constrictor, and can exacerbate any condition in which the lungs are overloaded.
CN: Physiological integrity; CNS: Physiological adaptation; CL: Apply

30. The nurse is caring for a 2-year-old client receiving digoxin. Which finding(s) will cause the nurse to withhold the upcoming dose of digoxin and notify the health care provider? Select all that apply.
1. Weight gain
2. Respiratory rate of 25 breaths/minute
3. Nausea and vomiting
4. Blood pressure of 100/70 mm Hg
5. Apical heart rate of 55 beats/minute

31. A teenage client diagnosed with heart failure is taking digoxin. The client asks the nurse, "What will this drug do for my heart?" What is the **best** response by the nurse?
1. "It will cause vasodilation and help with chest pain."
2. "It will decrease the workload of the heart."
3. "It will help your body excrete sodium."
4. "It will increase your resting heart rate."

32. An 11-month-old infant with heart failure weighs 30.9 lbs (14 kg). Digoxin is prescribed as 0.01 mg/kg in divided doses every 12 hours. How many milligrams will the nurse give the infant with each dose? Record your answer using two decimal places.

_____ mg/dose

33. The nurse is caring for adolescents with congestive heart failure, each prescribed captopril. To which client will the nurse question administering captopril?
1. An adolescent stating she is 10 weeks' gestation with her first baby.
2. An adolescent who does not like having the blood pressure checked.
3. An adolescent whose blood pressure is 140/90 mm Hg and heart rate is 90 beats/minute.
4. An adolescent who took 500 mg of acetaminophen this morning for a headache.

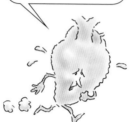

Phew! I sure could use a hit of digoxin. I'm feeling beat after all this beating.

30. 3, 5. Digoxin toxicity in infants and children may present with nausea, vomiting, anorexia, or a slow, irregular apical heart rate. Weight gain is not seen in digoxin toxicity. A respiratory rate of 25 breaths/minute and blood pressure of 100/70 mm Hg are normal findings in a 2-year-old.
CN: Physiological integrity; CNS: Pharmacological and parenteral therapies; CL: Analyze

31. 2. Digoxin is a cardiac glycoside. It decreases the workload of the heart and improves myocardial function. It will not cause vasodilation or increase sodium excretion. Diuretics help remove excess fluid. Digoxin is not a vasodilator and will slow the heart rate, not increase it.
CN: Physiological integrity; CNS: Pharmacological and parenteral therapies; CL: Apply

32. 0.07.
Use the following equations:

$$weight \times dose = mg\ prescribed\ per\ day$$
$$14\ kg \times 0.01\ mg/kg = 0.14\ mg$$
$$Hours\ per\ day \div dosage\ frequency = number\ of\ doses\ prescribed\ per\ day$$
$$24\ hours/12\ hours/dose = 2\ doses$$
$$mg\ prescribed\ per\ day \div doses\ prescribed\ per\ day = mg\ prescribed\ per\ dose$$
$$0.14\ mg/2\ doses = 0.07\ mg/dose$$

CN: Physiological integrity; CNS: Pharmacological and parenteral therapies; CL: Analyze

33. 1. Angiotensin-converting enzyme inhibitors, such as captopril, block the conversion of angiotensin I to angiotensin II in the kidneys. This causes decreased aldosterone levels, vasodilation, and increased sodium excretion. As a vasodilator, it also acts to reduce vascular resistance by the manipulation of afterload. Captopril should not be administered to pregnant clients because it is associated with fetal and neonatal morbidity and death. The nurse must work with the client who does not like having blood pressure assessed because this will be necessary for care. Captopril will assist in lowering hypertension. This medication is safe to take with acetaminophen.
CN: Physiological integrity; CNS: Pharmacological and parenteral therapies; CL: Analyze

34. The nurse is assessing a neonate and notes the following: a systolic murmur with a continuous machinery sound, blood pressure of 70/22 mm Hg, bounding pulses, and capillary refill greater than 5 seconds. Based on these findings, which prescription will the nurse expect when notifying the health care provider?
1. Administer intravenous indomethacin.
2. Prepare the client for surgery.
3. Give prostaglandin E intravenously.
4. Give acetylsalicylic acid.

35. A 10-year-old who is hospitalized with a diagnosis of rheumatic heart disease reports feeling "trapped in a diseased body." Which action by the nurse is **most** appropriate?
1. Provide the client with information on the diagnosis.
2. Allow the client to participate in planning each day.
3. Ask the client to invite friends to visit while in the hospital.
4. Encourage the client's parents to bring familiar items from home.

36. The nurse is caring for an infant immediately following a cardiac catheterization. Which nursing action is appropriate?
1. Keep the operative leg flexed.
2. Change the catheterization dressing.
3. Monitor for oozing or bleeding.
4. Keep the infant uncovered.

37. The nurse has observed that the mother of a 6-month-old child diagnosed with aortic stenosis seems to be uninterested in her child's daily routine. Which action by the nurse is **most** appropriate?
1. Request that a case manager assess the mother.
2. Give the mother information on local support groups.
3. Invite the mother to assist with performing the infant's care.
4. Provide education to the mother on aortic stenosis.

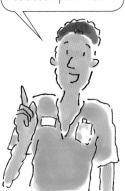

Sounds like the client would like a little more control. What's the best way to accomplish that?

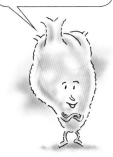

Wow! You're really pumping out the answers—impressive output.

34. 1. The nurse should suspect that the client has a patent ductus arteriosus (PDA) based on the assessment findings (wide pulse pressure, bounding pulses, machinery-sounding murmur, delayed capillary refill). Treatment for PDA includes administration of prostaglandin inhibitors, such as indomethacin, to promote closure of the PDA. If the PDA does not respond to pharmacological treatment, surgery may be required. Prostaglandins are given to keep the ductus arteriosus open with other cardiac anomalies. Acetylsalicylic acid may be given for rheumatic heart disease and Kawasaki's disease.
CN: Physiological integrity; CNS: Physiological adaptation; CL: Analyze

35. 2. All of the interventions listed may be considered in the client's plan of care. The most appropriate would be allowing the child to become more involved in the plan of treatment to promote feelings of control. Providing information on the diagnosis does not address the child's feelings. Involvement of friends is most appropriate for a teenage client. Comfort items are most appropriate for young children.
CN: Psychosocial integrity; CNS: None; CL: Analyze

36. 3. Monitoring the operative site for oozing or bleeding is appropriate. The operative leg should be kept straight and immobile to prevent trauma and bleeding. The pressure dressing should not be changed, but it may be reinforced if bleeding occurs. Keeping the infant uncovered would result in decreased temperature, which would lead to increased stress on the infant's body and should be avoided.
CN: Physiological integrity; CNS: Reduction of risk potential; CL: Apply

37. 3. Caring for an infant with a cardiac disorder may be overwhelming for the mother. She may fear harming the child and may have a sense of powerlessness. The focus should be to increase the mother's involvement in the infant's care. This may be a gradual process. There is no indication that a case management referral is needed. A support group and education on the diagnosis may be of benefit but they are not the initial intervention needed.
CN: Psychosocial integrity; CNS: None; CL: Apply

38. Which finding will the nurse expect when assessing a child with an acyanotic heart defect?
1. Excess weight gain
2. Hepatomegaly
3. Bradycardia
4. Decreased respiratory rate

38. 2. Hepatomegaly may result from blood backing up into the liver due to increased resistance in the right side of the heart. Poor growth and development, not excess weight gain, may be seen because of the increased energy required for breathing. The increase in blood flow to the lungs may cause tachycardia (not bradycardia) and an increased respiratory rate to compensate.
CN: Physiological integrity; CNS: Physiological adaptation; CL: Apply

39. A child hospitalized with right-sided heart failure is tearful and states, "My parents do not want me to be active and say I always need to rest." Which action by the nurse is **most** appropriate?
1. Explain to the child that becoming tired is a concern with this condition.
2. Explain to the child that the parents are just showing love and care.
3. Ask if the child would like assistance sharing these concerns with the parents.
4. Determine whether the child would like to visit the unit's playroom.

39. 3. Fatigue is a concern in a child with heart failure. Efforts should be made to ensure adequate periods of rest. Activity and play are normal needs for a child. Parents of chronically ill children may at times be overprotective. Encouraging a meeting with the parents and child may be of benefit to highlight the child's concerns. Explaining that fatigue is a concern and that the parents love the child, while true, does not address the child's concerns. Visiting the playroom also does not address the child's concerns.
CN: Safe, effective care environment; CNS: Management of care; CL: Apply

40. The nurse is caring for an 8-week-old infant diagnosed with a ventricular septal defect. Which finding(s) will the nurse report to the health care provider immediately? Select all that apply.
1. Weight gain of 4.9 lbs (2.2 kg) since birth
2. Loud, harsh murmur
3. Heart rate of 170 beats/minute
4. Diminished carotid pulses
5. Blood pressure of 42/26 mm Hg

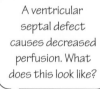

A ventricular septal defect causes decreased perfusion. What does this look like?

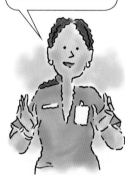

40. 4, 5. Diminished carotid pulses and hypotension are associated with aortic stenosis. They are not expected in this infant and should be reported immediately. A ventricular septal defect is an abnormal opening in the wall of the heart. The clinical manifestations vary depending on the size and location and generally present at 4 to 8 weeks of age. Expected findings include symptoms of heart failure; a loud, harsh murmur; poor growth and development; failure to thrive; and tachycardia.
CN: Safe, effective care environment; CNS: Management of care; CL: Analyze

41. When caring for a neonate suspected to have a ventricular septal defect, which prescription will the nurse question?
1. Prepare the client for an echocardiogram.
2. Monitor intake and output.
3. Furosemide 1 mg/kg/day intravenously.
4. Indomethacin 0.2 mg/kg for three doses.

41. 4. Failure of a septum to develop between the ventricles results in a left-to-right shunt, which is noted as a ventricular septal defect (VSD). Clients with VSDs may present with cyanosis, poor feeding, edema, systolic murmur, fatigue, and tachycardia. The nurse would question administering indomethacin, as this is given to close a patent ductus arteriosus (PDA). An echocardiogram or chest x-ray is used to confirm the diagnosis and determine severity. Intake and output need to be monitored to ensure adequate intake (poor feeding) and output (edema). Diuretics (furosemide) may be given for edema. ACE inhibitors may also be given to relax blood vessels and lower blood pressure.
CN: Physiological integrity; CNS: Physiological adaptation; CL: Analyze

42. A 6-month-old infant with uncorrected tetralogy of Fallot suddenly becomes increasingly cyanotic and diaphoretic, with weak peripheral pulses and a respiratory rate of 64 breaths/minute. What is the **priority** action by the nurse?
1. Administer oxygen.
2. Administer morphine sulfate.
3. Place the infant in a knee–chest position.
4. Notify the health care provider.

42. 3. The knee–chest position reduces the workload of the heart by increasing the blood return to the heart and keeping the blood flow more centralized. Oxygen should be administered quickly but only after placing the infant in the knee–chest position. Morphine should be administered after positioning and oxygen administration are completed. The health care provider would be notified after completing these actions.
CN: Safe, effective care environment; CNS: Management of care; CL: Analyze

43. A child with a ventricular septal defect is receiving digoxin. Which statement(s) will the nurse include when educating the child's parents on digoxin administration? Select all that apply.
1. "Give digoxin to your child at the same time each day."
2. "Keep administering digoxin even if your child seems better."
3. "If you miss giving your child a dose, it is okay to double the next dose."
4. "You need to ensure that your child drinks plenty of fluids."
5. "Notify the health care provider immediately if your child's heart rate is low."

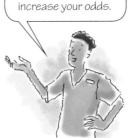

If you're having trouble finding the right answer, try eliminating a few wrong ones; it will increase your odds.

43. 1, 2, 4, 5. Digoxin is given before corrective surgery to prevent heart failure. It helps the heart beat stronger and with regular rhythm. Digoxin should be given at approximately the same time each day. Suddenly halting digoxin could lead to worsening symptoms. If a dose is missed and the next dose is due in less than 12 hours, the missed dose cannot be taken. Staying hydrated is important because risk of toxicity is increased in the dehydrated client. Sinus bradycardia is the earliest and most frequent manifestation of digoxin toxicity in children and should be reported immediately.
CN: Physiological integrity; CNS: Pharmacological and parenteral therapies; CL: Apply

44. A child returns to the unit after a cardiac catheterization. The nurse will include which statement when providing education to the child and parents?
1. "You may sit in a chair with the affected extremity immobilized."
2. "You must stay in the bed with no further activity restrictions."
3. "You need to stay in the bed with the affected extremity immobilized."
4. "You are permitted to get out of bed to go to the bathroom as needed."

44. 3. Following cardiac catheterization, the child should be maintained on bed rest with the affected extremity immobilized to prevent hemorrhage. Allowing the child to sit in a chair with the affected extremity immobilized, to move the affected extremity while on bed rest, or to have bathroom privileges places the child at risk for hemorrhage.
CN: Physiological integrity; CNS: Reduction of risk potential; CL: Apply

45. The nurse is teaching a mother to administer digoxin to her 6-month-old infant prior to discharge. Which statement by the parent indicates the need for additional education?
1. "I will count the baby's pulse before every dose."
2. "I will make sure the pulse is regular before every dose."
3. "I will measure the dose using the dosing syringe provided."
4. "I will withhold the medication if the pulse is below 60."

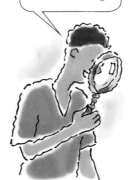

Remember— "need for additional education" is code for "wrong."

45. 4. A pulse rate under 60 beats/minute is an indication for withholding digoxin from an *adult*. Withholding digoxin from an infant is appropriate if the infant's pulse is under 90 beats/minute. The pulse rate must be counted before each dose of digoxin is given to an infant. An irregular pulse may be a sign of digoxin toxicity; if this occurs, the health care provider should be consulted before the drug is given. The dose must be measured carefully to decrease the risk of toxicity.
CN: Physiological integrity; CNS: Pharmacological and parenteral therapies; CL: Apply

46. The nurse is caring for an infant following a left femoral cardiac catheterization. During assessment, the nurse notes a weak left dorsalis pedis pulse. What will the nurse do **next**?
1. Recheck both pedis pulses in 15 minutes.
2. Notify the health care provider.
3. Elevate the left leg above the level of the heart.
4. Monitor the client's urine output.

46. 2. The nurse should notify the health care provider. The pulse below the catheterization site should be strong and equal to the unaffected extremity. A weakened pulse may indicate vessel obstruction or perfusion problems. The nurse should recheck the site and monitor urine output, but notification to the health care provider is priority. Elevating the leg would cause increased tissue perfusion compromise and should be avoided.
CN: Physiological integrity; CNS: Reduction of risk potential; CL: Apply

47. Propranolol has been prescribed for a teen diagnosed with hypertension. When the nurse is providing education on propranolol to the teen, which statement by the teen indicates the need for additional education?
1. "I should take this medication daily on an empty stomach."
2. "It is best to take this medication at the same time each day."
3. "I may experience dizziness while taking this medication."
4. "I will call my health care provider if I experience weight gain."

47. 1. Propranolol is used in the management of hypertension. The drug should be taken with food and at the same time daily. Side effects include changes in sleep pattern, dizziness, and light headedness. Side effects such as skin afflictions, weight gain, and difficulty breathing should be reported promptly to the health care provider.
CN: Physiological integrity; CNS: Pharmacological and parenteral therapies; CL: Apply

48. The nurse is caring for a child who underwent atrial septal repair 2 days ago. Which nursing intervention(s) is appropriate for this child? Select all that apply.
1. Give the child nothing by mouth.
2. Maintain strict bed rest.
3. Take vital signs at least every 4 hours.
4. Administer an analgesic as needed.
5. Monitor intake and output.

Remember: kids with heart conditions are still kids. Encourage them to play, as appropriate.

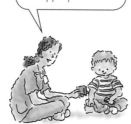

48. 3, 4, 5. Vital signs should be monitored every 4 hours, minimum. Pain management is a concern and should be given on an as-needed basis. By day 3, the child should be advancing to a regular diet. Monitoring intake and output to ensure there is no fluid overload or deficits should be included in the plan of care. Bed rest is not indicated 2 days after surgery. Activity should be allowed as the child is able, with coughing and deep-breathing exercises.
CN: Physiological integrity; CNS: Physiological adaptation; CL: Apply

49. The parents of a 14-year-old child who underwent an atrial septal repair 6 days ago have asked whether a few family members can visit. Which response by the nurse is **most** appropriate?
1. "Your child is extremely fragile right now, and visitations are not recommended."
2. "Your child can call friends and family on the phone instead of having visitors."
3. "It would be best if your child did not have visitors for another few days."
4. "A few visitors would not be a problem at this stage of your child's recovery."

49. 4. Prevention of infection after any surgical procedure is important. After 5 days the child's risk for infection, while still present, is lessened. If all visitors are free of infection, a visit would be fine.
CN: Safe, effective care environment; CNS: Safety and infection control; CL: Apply

50. When educating the pediatric client's family regarding coarctation of the aorta, which statement will the nurse include?
1. "Your child will need to be monitored for low blood pressure."
2. "Your child will be prescribed a prostaglandin."
3. "Your child may experience cramping in the arms and legs."
4. "Chest pain is common with this condition in older children."

51. The nurse is assessing a neonate an hour after birth. The nurse's findings are noted in the chart exhibit below. Which prescription(s) will the nurse anticipate from the health care provider for this client? Select all that apply.

Progress notes	
7/19	The neonate is lying under the radiant
1845	warmer with extremities flexed and pink
	upper extremities and pale lower extremities
	present. Vital signs: temperature, 98.4°F
	(36.9°C); blood pressure, 86/54 mm Hg in the
	left arm and 70/40 mm Hg in the left leg;
	heart rate, 175 beats/minute; respiratory rate,
	68 breaths/minute. Mild nasal flaring and
	bounding brachial pulses are noted.

1. Administer digoxin 20 mcg/kg.
2. Apply warm, humidified oxygen.
3. Give prostaglandin intravenously.
4. Administer furosemide 1 mg/kg.
5. Weigh diapers.

52. The nursery nurse suspects an infant has a cardiac anomaly. Which nursing intervention is **priority** to perform on the infant?
1. Assess skin turgor.
2. Check blood pressure in each extremity.
3. Measure chest circumference.
4. Measure pupil size and reaction to light.

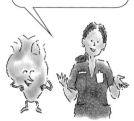

Watch out for those cardiac anomalies. I suspect they adore nursing interventions

53. A child with coarctation of the aorta experiences a postsurgical recoarctation. Which treatment will the nurse expect the health care provider to prescribe?
1. Bypass graft repair
2. Balloon angioplasty
3. Patch aortoplasty
4. Left subclavian flap angioplasty

50. 3. Coarctation of the aorta consists of a localized constriction or narrowing of the aortic wall. Symptoms include claudication (cramping of the extremities), hypertension (not hypotension), and decreased femoral pulses. Medications, such as prostaglandins, are not effective in treating coarctation of the aorta, only surgical procedures are used. Chest pain is noted in clients with aortic stenosis.
CN: Health promotion and maintenance; CNS: None; CL: Apply

51. 1, 2, 3, 4, 5. The neonate is exhibiting signs and symptoms of coarctation of the aorta, which include dyspnea, hypertension in the upper body, pulmonary edema, pink upper extremities and cyanotic lower extremities, bounding pulses in the arms, and absent or diminished femoral pulses. The nurse should anticipate digoxin and diuretics to prevent heart failure. Oxygen is given to facilitate breathing and limit effort expended by the neonate. Prostaglandin is given to maintain a patent ductus arteriosus. Weighing diapers is part of maintaining an accurate intake and output.
CN: Physiological integrity; CNS: Physiological adaptation; CL: Analyze

52. 2. Measuring blood pressure in all four extremities in a child with a possible cardiac anomaly is necessary to document hypertension and the blood pressure gradient between the upper and lower extremities. Skin turgor, chest circumference, and pupillary assessment are also important, but they are not as specific for cardiac assessment as blood pressure.
CN: Safe, effective care environment; CNS: Management of care; CL: Analyze

53. 2. Balloon angioplasty is the treatment of choice for postsurgical recoarctation. Bypass graft repair, patch aortoplasty, and left subclavian flap angioplasty are surgical options to treat the original coarctation.
CN: Physiological integrity; CNS: Physiological adaptation; CL: Apply

54. Which nursing intervention is appropriate postoperatively for a child with repair of a coarctation of the aorta?
1. Give a vasoconstrictor.
2. Maintain hypothermia.
3. Give a bolus of intravenous fluids.
4. Maintain a low blood pressure.

54. 4. Blood pressure should be closely managed and kept low, so there is no excessive pressure on the fresh suture lines. Vasoconstrictors would be contraindicated. Normal body temperature is maintained, and diuretics may be given to decrease fluid volume.
CN: Physiological integrity; CNS: Physiological adaptation; CL: Apply

55. The nurse will notify the health care provider **immediately** if which finding is noted in a 10-year-old with tetralogy of Fallot?
1. Clubbing of the fingers and toes
2. Prominent inferior sternum
3. Cyanotic spell with bowel movements
4. Higher pressure in the upper extremities than in the lower extremities

55. 4. Higher pressures in the upper extremities are characteristic of coarctation of the aorta and not associated with tetralogy of Fallot. This unexpected finding should be reported immediately. Expected findings do not require immediate notification. Clubbing is seen in older children as a result of chronic hypoxia. A prominent inferior sternum is associated with right ventricular hypertrophy. A child with tetralogy of Fallot is mildly cyanotic at rest and has increasing cyanosis with crying, activity, or straining, as with a bowel movement.
CN: Physiological integrity; CNS: Physiological adaptation; CL: Apply

56. The nurse notices a 12-year-old child with tetralogy of Fallot has clubbing of the fingers and toes. Which nursing action is appropriate?
1. Apply a continuous oxygen saturation monitor.
2. Document the finding in the medical record.
3. Check hemoglobin and hematocrit levels.
4. Prepare the child for a cardiac catheterization.

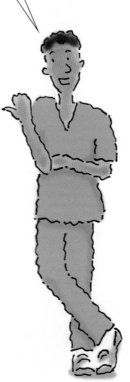

No, not *that* kind of clubbing. We're talking about fingers and toes swelling due to a lack of oxygen, not nightlife.

56. 2. Clubbing of the fingers and toes is an expected finding in an older child with untreated tetralogy of Fallot. Clubbing results from chronic hypoxia. The nurse should document the expected finding. Applying a continuous oxygen saturation monitor and assessing laboratory findings are not necessary, as they would not alter the finding. A cardiac catheterization provides visualization of the cardiac defects.
CN: Physiological integrity; CNS: Physiological adaptation; CL: Apply

57. The nurse notices a child with tetralogy of Fallot squat after running around the unit. What will the nurse do **next**?
1. Assess the client's respiratory rate.
2. Notify the health care provider.
3. Have the child sit and rest for a while.
4. Administer propranolol now.

57. 3. The nurse needs to have the client rest. A child may squat or assume a knee–chest position to reduce venous blood flow from the lower extremities and to increase systemic vascular resistance, which diverts more blood flow into the pulmonary artery during activity. The nurse would then check the client's respiratory status and notify the health care provider, if necessary. Propranolol is given to prevent the spells and would not be appropriate in this situation.
CN: Safe, effective care environment; CNS: Management of care; CL: Analyze

58. The nurse is caring for a newborn recently diagnosed with tetralogy of Fallot. Which test will the nurse expect to prepare the newborn for initially?
1. Chest radiography
2. Echocardiography
3. Electrocardiography
4. Cardiac catheterization

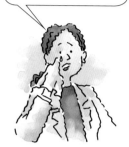

Don't get upset if you can't figure out a question—just move on to the next one.

58. 4. Cardiac catheterization provides specific information about the direction and amount of shunting, coronary anatomy, and each portion of the heart defect. This test assists the health care provider in determining what method of treatment will be best for this client. The remaining tests are used to diagnose tetralogy of Fallot but not to determine what treatment is needed. Chest radiographs show right ventricular hypertrophy pushing the heart apex upward, resulting in a boot-shaped silhouette. Echocardiogram scans define such defects as large ventricular septal defects, pulmonary stenosis, and malposition of the aorta. Electrocardiograms show right ventricular hypertrophy with tall R waves.
CN: Physiological integrity; CNS: Physiological adaptation; CL: Apply

59. The parents of a 3-year-old with congenital heart disease tell the nurse they are concerned about their child receiving the flu vaccine. Which nursing response is **most** appropriate?
1. "Because the vaccine can cause complications for your child, I recommend the rest of the family be immunized instead."
2. "The flu vaccine is both safe and recommended to children who have chronic illnesses such as heart disease."
3. "You are right to be concerned because this vaccine should be administered to children who are older than 3 years of age."
4. "As long as you are careful who your child is exposed to during flu season, it should be fine to not vaccinate your child."

59. 2. Children who have heart disease or another chronic illness are more vulnerable to the flu. Immunization is recommended for the child. Any possible side effects are of lesser concern than contracting the flu. Children ages 6 months and older may receive the flu vaccine. It is important to avoid exposing a vulnerable child to at-risk populations, but this is not an acceptable substitute for vaccinating the child.
CN: Safe, effective care environment; CNS: Safety and infection control; CL: Apply

60. The nurse is educating parents of a fetus diagnosed with tricuspid atresia. Which statement(s) indicates the parents understand the education? Select all that apply.
1. "Our baby's tricuspid valve failed to develop."
2. "Our baby will receive prostaglandin E after birth."
3. "Our baby will need to have surgery soon after birth."
4. "The nurses will closely monitor our baby's kidney function."
5. "Our baby will need to receive antibiotics for endocarditis."

60. 1, 2, 3, 4. Tricuspid atresia is failure of the tricuspid valve to develop, leaving no communication between the right atrium and the right ventricle. A continuous prostaglandin E infusion is given to maintain a patent ductus until surgery is performed. Kidney function should be closely monitored to assess for complications such as fluid overload and renal anomalies. The child is not at greater risk for developing endocarditis.
CN: Physiological integrity; CNS: Physiological adaptation; CL: Apply

61. Which finding will the nurse expect to assess when caring for a child diagnosed with tricuspid atresia?
1. Cyanosis
2. Machinery murmur
3. Decreased respiratory rate
4. Capillary refill less than 3 seconds

61. 1. Cyanosis is the most consistent clinical sign of tricuspid atresia. A machinery (Gibson) murmur is characteristic of a patent ductus arteriosus. Tricuspid atresia does not have a characteristic murmur. Tachypnea and dyspnea are typically present because of the pulmonary blood flow and right-to-left shunting. Decreased oxygenation increases capillary refill time.
CN: Physiological integrity; CNS: Physiological adaptation; CL: Apply

62. When assessing laboratory results of a child diagnosed with tricuspid atresia, which finding will the nurse expect?
1. Acidosis
2. Alkalosis
3. Normal red blood cell (RBC) count
4. Normal arterial oxygen saturation level

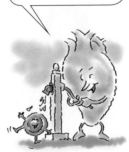

Hearts are the most important pumps in the world. Keep us healthy so we can do our job.

62. 1. In tricuspid atresia, the tricuspid valve is completely closed so that no blood flows from the right atrium to the right ventricle. Therefore, no oxygenation of blood occurs. The child has chronic hypoxemia and acidosis, not alkalosis, due to decreased atrial oxygenation. This chronic hypoxemia leads to polycythemia, so a normal RBC count would not result. Arterial oxygenation is not normal, as the blood bypasses the lungs and the step of oxygenation.
CN: Physiological integrity; CNS: Physiological adaptation; CL: Apply

63. Which action is **priority** for the nurse to perform before administering digoxin to an infant?
1. Educate the parent's about digoxin.
2. Check the apical heart rate.
3. Weigh the infant daily.
4. Monitor for peripheral edema.

63. 2. Digoxin is used to decrease heart rate and prevent heart failure secondary to structural defects, such as congenital heart defects. The apical pulse must be carefully monitored to detect a severe reduction. Administering digoxin to an infant with a heart rate less than 90 beats/minute could further reduce the rate and compromise cardiac output. The nurse would educate the parents and monitor for signs and symptoms of heart failure, but those actions are not priority over assessing the heart rate.
CN: Physiological integrity; CNS: Pharmacological and parenteral therapies; CL: Apply

64. The nurse is assigned four pediatric clients. Which client will the nurse see **first**?
1. A 13-year-old child hospitalized with suspected cardiomyopathy scheduled for a cardiac catheterization tomorrow.
2. An 8-year-old child who had a cardiac catheterization 3 hours ago and has a 2-cm spot of drainage on the dressing.
3. A 9-year-old child who had cardiac surgery 1 day ago and is reporting pain rated a level 5 on a 10-point scale.
4. A 14-year-old child who had cardiac surgery 2 days ago and who has had 200 mL of urinary output over the past 8 hours.

64. 4. A urinary output of 200 mL over 8 hours is an average of 25 mL each hour. This signals potential renal complications. This child should be seen first. The other children are considered stable compared to this child.
CN: Safe, effective care environment; CNS: Management of care; CL: Analyze

65. The nurse is caring for a child who is experiencing a hypercyanotic episode. Which nursing action(s) is appropriate? Select all that apply.
1. Encourage the child to take deep breaths.
2. Assist the child to a semi-Fowler's position.
3. Provide the child supplemental oxygen.
4. Assist the child into a knee–chest position.
5. Use a soothing tone of voice when talking.

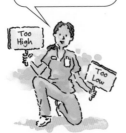

Hyper-cyanosis means hypo-oxygen; so, what interventions are needed here?

65. 1, 3, 4, 5. Cyanosis has resulted from a lack of oxygenation. Activities should focus on relieving anxiety and promoting oxygenation and perfusion to the body's tissues. Deep breaths and supplemental oxygen provide increased oxygen intake. Knee–chest positioning improves pulmonary oxygenation. A soothing tone of voice enhances relaxation and calms the child. The use of a semi-Fowler's position would not improve oxygenation.
CN: Physiological integrity; CNS: Basic care and comfort; CL: Apply

66. The nurse is admitting a child with a total anomalous pulmonary venous return defect and notes recurrent respiratory infections in the child's medical record. Which nursing action is **most** appropriate?
1. Educate the family on proper handwashing.
2. Continue with the admission process.
3. Ask if the child is up to date on immunizations.
4. Assess the child's temperature.

66. 2. Children with total anomalous pulmonary venous return defects are prone to repeated respiratory infections due to increased pulmonary blood flow. There is no indication the family does not understand proper handwashing or that the child is not up to date on vaccinations. The nurse would assess the child's temperature as part of the admission process, not due to the finding.
CN: Safe, effective care environment; CNS: Management of care; CL: Apply

67. An infant has undergone a repair of total anomalous pulmonary venous return and develops pulmonary hypertension postoperatively. Which finding indicates to the nurse the infant may be experiencing a complication?
1. Respiratory rate of 82 breaths/minute
2. Heart rate of 160 beats/minute
3. Oxygen saturation level of 95%
4. Blood pressure of 78/50 mm Hg

67. 1. Pulmonary hypertension may result as a postoperative complication of this procedure, which can cause hypoxia. Symptoms of hypoxia include tachypnea, cyanosis, chest retractions, and fatigue. The respiratory rate listed represents tachypnea. The other findings are within normal range for an infant.
CN: Physiological integrity; CNS: Physiological adaptation; CL: Analyze

68. The nurse is reviewing a prescription from the health care provider for a child scheduled for cardiac surgery the following day. Which prescription(s) will the nurse question? Select all that apply.
1. Complete blood count
2. Electrolyte levels
3. Urinalysis
4. 2-step tuberculosis (TB) test
5. Partial prothrombin time (PTT)

68. 4. The nurse should question a 2-step TB test, as this is not needed for a client scheduled for a cardiac procedure. Tests that are commonly prescribed during the preoperative period include a complete blood count, electrolyte levels, urinalysis, and bleeding time studies such as a PTT.
CN: Health promotion and maintenance; CNS: None; CL: Apply

69. Which finding will the nurse expect to observe in an infant diagnosed with pulmonary stenosis?
1. Diminished carotid pulses
2. Hypotension
3. Dull, gray mucous membranes
4. Harsh systolic ejection murmur

69. 3. Pulmonary stenosis is a narrowing or fusing of the pulmonic valve leaflets that interferes with right ventricular outflow to the lungs. This leads to mild or moderate cyanosis, so mucous membranes may appear dull or gray. Diminished carotid pulses and hypotension are associated with aortic stenosis. A harsh systolic ejection murmur heard along the left sternal border, usually accompanied by a thrill, is associated with truncus arteriosus.
CN: Physiological integrity; CNS: Physiological adaptation; CL: Apply

70. The health care provider has prescribed digoxin and a diuretic for an infant. How will the nurse administer these medications to the child?
1. Use a measuring spoon.
2. Use a graduated dropper.
3. Mix the medications with baby food.
4. Add the medications to a full bottle.

When administering digoxin, it's important for the dosage to be exact.

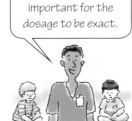

70. 2. Using a graduated dropper allows the exact dosage to be given. A measuring spoon is not as exact as a graduated dropper, and exact measures are necessary. Mixing medications in a bottle or in food is problematic because, if the child does not completely finish the meal, the nurse cannot determine the exact amount ingested. In addition, this may prevent the child from drinking or eating in the future for fear of tasting the medications.
CN: Physiological integrity; CNS: Pharmacological and parenteral therapies; CL: Apply

71. The nurse is caring for a newborn with transposition of the great arteries. When reviewing the neonate's medical record, which finding(s) related to the mother's health history does the nurse expect? Select all that apply.
1. Diabetes
2. Bacterial pneumonia during the pregnancy
3. Excessive alcohol use during the pregnancy
4. Chronic hypertension
5. Use of combination oral contraceptives at time of conception

71. 1, 3. Although the exact cause of transposition of the great arteries is unknown, maternal risk factors include diabetes, excessive alcohol intake in pregnancy, and viral, not bacterial, infections during pregnancy. Maternal hypertension and use of oral contraceptives at the time of conception are not tied to the condition.
CN: Physiological integrity; CNS: Reduction of risk potential; CL: Apply

72. The nurse is caring for a gravid woman whose health care provider is concerned the fetus may have transposition of the great arteries. The nurse will expect to prepare the client for which procedure?
1. Amniocentesis
2. Fetal echocardiography
3. Percutaneous umbilical cord sampling
4. Nuchal translucency measurement

72. 2. An echocardiogram can be used to diagnose transposition of the great arteries in a fetus in utero. Amniocentesis is used to collect a sample of amniotic fluid to screen for genetic disorders. Percutaneous umbilical cord sampling is used to collect a fetal blood sample to screen for genetic disorders. Nuchal translucency is used to assess for the presence of Down's syndrome.
CN: Health promotion and maintenance; CNS: None; CL: Apply

73. Which change will the nurse expect to assess after applying oxygen to an infant with uncorrected tetralogy of Fallot?
1. Disappearance of the murmur
2. No evidence of cyanosis
3. Improvement of finger clubbing
4. Decreased agitation

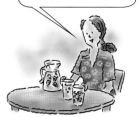

Feeling weary? Take a short break and refresh yourself.

73. 4. Supplemental oxygen helps the infant breathe more easily and feel less anxious or agitated. None of the other findings occurs as the result of supplemental oxygen administration.
CN: Physiological integrity; CNS: Basic care and comfort; CL: Apply

74. The nurse is caring for a child with transposition of the great arteries. Which associated defect will the nurse assess this client for?
1. Mitral atresia
2. Tricuspid atresia
3. Patent foramen ovale
4. Hypoplasia of the left ventricle

74. 3. A patent foramen ovale, patent ductus arteriosus, and ventricular septal defect are defects associated with transposition of the great arteries. A patent foramen ovale is the most common atrial septal defect and is necessary to provide adequate mixing of blood between the two circulations. Tricuspid atresia is failure of the tricuspid valve to develop, leaving no communication between the right atrium and the right ventricle; this defect is not associated with transposition of the great arteries. Hypoplasia of the left ventricle and mitral atresia are two defects associated with hypoplastic left heart syndrome.
CN: Physiological integrity; CNS: Physiological adaptation; CL: Apply

75. A 9-year-old child had cardiac surgery 2 days ago. The child tells the nurse he is sore and does not want to move much today. Which action by the nurse is **most** appropriate?
1. Agree to allow the child to rest today after promising to get up tomorrow.
2. Medicate the child for discomfort and then begin activities related to ambulation.
3. Tell the child he will not be allowed to watch television if he does not get up.
4. Ask the parents to encourage the child to get up and walk around the unit.

75. 2. Postoperative pain is an anticipated occurrence. Despite the discomfort the client must ambulate. Prolonging ambulation for a day may promote complications. Medicating the child allows him to achieve an increased level of comfort prior to the activity. The child should not be threatened with an ultimatum of ambulation or television. The parents should be involved in the care being delivered but should not be used to threaten the child; this again does not alleviate the issue, which is pain.
CN: Health promotion and maintenance; CNS: None; CL: Apply

CN: Client needs category   CNS: Client needs subcategory   CL: Cognitive level

76. Balloon dilation valvuloplasty treatment is planned for an adolescent with valvular pulmonic stenosis. When educating the teen, which statement(s) by the client indicates the need for further instruction? Select all that apply.
1. "I will be prescribed diuretic therapy for an indefinite period after my procedure."
2. "The outcomes for this procedure are positive for the majority of clients."
3. "This procedure may need to be repeated in about 10 years."
4. "I will likely need to have open heart surgery within 6 to 12 months of this procedure."
5. "I will not be able to participate in sporting activities after my recovery."

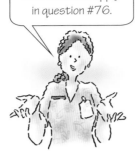

Remember to "select all that apply" in question #76.

76. 1, 4, 5. The narrowing in the vessels for the client with valvular pulmonic stenosis is often successfully managed with balloon dilation valvuloplasty. This procedure has a positive outcome rating for adolescents and may have to be repeated in approximately 10 years. This procedure is usually all that is needed, and, if successful, open heart surgery will not be necessary. Diuretic therapy is not indicated in the management of this condition. Participation in sports is not prohibited for those with this condition.
CN: Health promotion and maintenance; CNS: None; CL: Apply

77. The parents of a 3-week-old infant diagnosed with tricuspid atresia are discussing the planned courses of therapy with the nurse. Which statement(s) indicates an understanding of the education provided by the nurse? Select all that apply.
1. "My child will likely need a series of corrective procedures."
2. "It will be difficult, but the surgical repairs will be completed by my child's first birthday."
3. "The initial procedures will be performed to increase blood flow."
4. "Children with this disorder often have a significantly reduced life expectancy."
5. "The final procedures will be completed once my child is a teen and has stopped growing."

77. 1, 3. In tricuspid atresia, one of the tricuspid valves has not developed and is instead a solid band of tissue. Management of the condition traditionally includes a series of surgical corrections. The first procedure can be done between 3 and 6 months of age. The final procedure can usually be completed once the child reaches 2 years of age. Procedures performed initially are to increase blood flow. The children who have this condition usually have corrective procedures and then are able to live a relatively normal life into adulthood.
CN: Physiological integrity; CNS: Reduction of risk potential; CL: Apply

78. Which finding does the nurse expect during cardiac catheterization of a child with pulmonic stenosis?
1. Right-to-left shunting
2. Right ventricular hypertrophy
3. Decreased pressure in the right side of the heart
4. Increased oxygenation in the left side of the heart

78. 1. In pulmonic stenosis, right-to-left shunting develops through a patent foramen ovale due to right ventricular failure and an increase in pressure in the right side of the heart. Right ventricular hypertrophy and decreased pressure in the right side of the heart are not associated with pulmonic stenosis. Decreased oxygenation in the left side of the heart is noted due to the right-to-left shunt.
CN: Physiological integrity; CNS: Physiological adaptation; CL: Understand

79. The nurse is caring for a child diagnosed with aortic stenosis. The child tells the nurse, "My chest hurts sometimes when I am riding my bicycle." Which question by the nurse is **most** appropriate?
1. "How old were you when you first experienced chest pain?"
2. "Does the pain subside when you stop riding your bike and rest?"
3. "Have either of your parents suffered a myocardial infarction (MI)?"
4. "What would you rate your chest pain on a 0 to 10 pain scale?"

79. 2. Children with aortic stenosis may develop chest pain similar to angina when they are active. The nurse would expect the pain to subside with rest, indicating a normal response to aortic stenosis. How old the client was at the onset of chest pain and the pain rating are irrelevant. This pain is an expected finding and not indicative of an MI.
CN: Physiological integrity; CNS: Physiological adaptation; CL: Apply

80. The nurse is educating parents of a child with congenital aortic stenosis. Which statement will the nurse include in the education?
   1. "It can result from rheumatic fever."
   2. "It is the most common congenital defect."
   3. "It causes an increase in cardiac output."
   4. "It causes increased pulmonary blood flow."

81. The nurse is educating the mother of a newborn diagnosed with hypoplastic left heart syndrome about nutritional needs. What statement(s) will the nurse include in the education? Select all that apply.
   1. "Feedings should be limited to 15-minute sessions."
   2. "High-calorie formulas may be added to the baby's diet."
   3. "Frequent weighing of the baby will be needed."
   4. "Tube feedings may be instituted."
   5. "Bottle feeding is recommended for your child."

82. Which statement by the nurse is **most** appropriate for parents of a child with symptomatic aortic stenosis?
   1. "You need to restrict your child's exercise."
   2. "Only give prostaglandin E1 for a week."
   3. "You may give digoxin in water."
   4. "Assess your child daily for a murmur."

83. The nurse is educating the parent of a 5-year-old child. The parent reports having recently read an article about rheumatic fever and heart disease and questions how to prevent this from happening to the child. What is the **best** response by the nurse?
   1. "Prompt treatment of strep infections is a key to preventing this condition."
   2. "Getting your child an annual influenza vaccine is the best thing you can do."
   3. "Your child is not susceptible because there is no history of cardiac problems."
   4. "Giving your child a low-dose salicylate daily will prevent rheumatic fever."

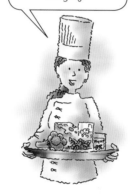

Make sure your neonatal clients are plumping up—especially after surgery.

Why is rheumatic fever in a cardiovascular chapter? What's the connection?

80. 1. Aortic stenosis can result from rheumatic fever (infection with group A streptococci), which can damage the aortic valve in the first 8 weeks of pregnancy. It accounts for only about 5% of all congenital heart defects and is not the most common congenital defect. It causes a decrease in cardiac output. It is classified as an acyanotic defect with obstructed flow from the ventricles and does not increase pulmonary blood flow.
CN: Physiological integrity; CNS: Physiological adaptation; CL: Understand

81. 2, 3, 4. The infant with hypoplastic left heart syndrome may experience difficulty with feeding. Feeding may be tiring. This may result in inadequate weight gain or weight loss. High-caloric formulas maybe prescribed. Frequent weighing will be needed to assess weight gain. Tube feedings may be instituted if weight loss becomes a concern. Limiting the duration of feedings may be necessary, but not to 15 minutes or less. Bottle feeding is not encouraged over breastfeeding.
CN: Physiological integrity; CNS: Basic care and comfort; CL: Apply

82. 1. In a child with symptomatic aortic stenosis, exercise should be restricted due to low cardiac output and left ventricular failure. Prostaglandin E1 is recommended to maintain the patency of the ductus arteriosus to allow for improved systemic blood flow, but should not be limited to just 1 week. Digoxin may be required for critically ill children experiencing heart failure as a result of severe aortic stenosis but should not be added to food or drink. It is expected for the child to have a rough, systolic murmur; however, the parents do not need to assess for the murmur at home.
CN: Physiological integrity; CNS: Physiological adaptation; CL: Apply

83. 1. Rheumatic fever is often caused by a strep infection in children. Seeking prompt care and following treatment recommendations is key in prevention of complications. Although the influenza vaccine is recommended for a 5-year-old child, it does not reduce the risk of rheumatic fever or rheumatic heart disease. A history of cardiac disease is not associated with contracting rheumatic fever. Salicylates may be given to treat rheumatic fever but do not prevent acquiring rheumatic fever.
CN: Safe, effective care environment; CNS: Safety and infection control; CL: Apply

84. A 3-year-old child with tetralogy of Fallot is experiencing polycythemia. Which nursing action is **priority**?
1. Promote adequate fluid intake.
2. Ensure appropriate daily caloric intake.
3. Administer ferrous sulfate as prescribed.
4. Encourage a daily period of exercise.

85. A child is taking prednisone following a heart transplantation. The nurse will notify the health care provider if which adverse reaction is assessed?
1. Weight gain of 2.5 lbs (1.1 kg) over 3 weeks
2. Temperature of 99.0°F (37.2°C)
3. Increased appetite
4. Arm wound with purulent drainage

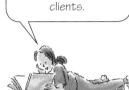

Wow—prednisone has a lot of adverse effects. I should mention these to my clients.

86. A child is prescribed 0.5 mg/kg/day of prednisone divided into two doses. The child weighs 30.9 lbs (14 kg). How many milligrams will the nurse give the child with each dose? Record your answer using one decimal place.

_____ mg

87. The clinic nurse is educating the father of a teenager diagnosed with bacterial endocarditis. Which statement(s) by the father indicates understanding of the condition? Select all that apply.
1. "It is caused by bacteria invading only tissues of the heart."
2. "My child will have to be hospitalized to receive antibiotics intravenously."
3. "Tender, raised, subcutaneous lesions may appear on my child's fingers or toes."
4. "Hemorrhagic areas with white centers may appear on my child's retina."
5. "My child needs to be monitored very closely for signs of heart failure."

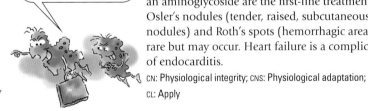

Ooh, look! It's the heart—my favorite organ to infect. We can do some real damage there.

88. A child receives prednisone after undergoing a heart transplantation. The nurse understands which outcome indicates the prednisone is effective?
1. The client's appetite is increased.
2. The white blood cell count is low.
3. Wound healing is improved.
4. Fluid retention does not occur.

84. 1. Dehydration is a concern with polycythemia. Adequate fluid intake helps prevent complications. The other items may be included in the plan of care but are not of the highest priority.
CN: Health promotion and maintenance; CNS: None; CL: Analyze

85. 4. The nurse should notify the health care provider of poor wound healing with purulent drainage. This could indicate infection and should be treated immediately to prevent more severe complications. The other findings are common adverse reactions to prednisone, which include weight gain, delayed temperature response, increased appetite, delayed sexual maturation, growth impairment, and a Cushingoid appearance. The school-aged child who has received prednisone is usually overweight and has a moon-shaped face.
CN: Physiological integrity; CNS: Pharmacological and parenteral therapies; CL: Apply

86. 3.5
First, determine the dose per day:

dose prescribed × client weight = dose per day

$$0.5 \ mg / kg \times 14 \ kg = 7 \ mg / day$$

Then, because the child is to receive the drug in two doses, divide the daily amount in half.

$$7 \ mg / 2 \ doses = 3.5 \ mg / dose$$

CN: Physiological integrity; CNS: Pharmacological and parenteral therapies; CL: Analyze

87. 2, 3, 4, 5. Bacterial/infective endocarditis is an infection of the valves and inner lining of the heart. It is usually caused by the bacterium *Streptococcus viridans* and frequently affects children with acquired or congenital anomalies of the heart or great vessels. Intravenous penicillin and an aminoglycoside are the first-line treatments. Osler's nodules (tender, raised, subcutaneous nodules) and Roth's spots (hemorrhagic areas) are rare but may occur. Heart failure is a complication of endocarditis.
CN: Physiological integrity; CNS: Physiological adaptation; CL: Apply

88. 2. The goal of prednisone for this client is to suppress the immune system, thereby preventing organ rejection. Prednisone is often used in combination with other immunosuppressant medications to prevent rejection. Although corticosteroids do stimulate the appetite, that is not the desired effect for this child. Prednisone and other corticosteroids decrease wound healing; fluid retention is one of their side effects.
CN: Physiological integrity; CNS: Physiological adaptation; CL: Apply

89. A child with suspected bacterial endocarditis arrives at the emergency department. Which prescription will the nurse complete **first**?
1. Obtain blood cultures.
2. Administer penicillin.
3. Assess for Janeway lesions.
4. Monitor urine output.

90. The nurse is assessing a child with suspected bacterial endocarditis. The child also has aortic stenosis. Which finding indicates to the nurse this child is at risk for this disease?
1. History of a cold for 3 days
2. Dental work pretreated with antibiotics
3. Peripheral intravenous (IV) catheter in place for 1 day
4. Currently being treated for a urinary tract infection

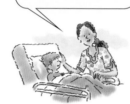

Routes for infection abound in the hospital. Become an expert at identifying them and taking preventive measures.

91. Erythromycin is given to a 6-year-old child before dental work to prevent endocarditis. The child weighs 50 lb (22.7 kg). The prescription is for 20 mg/kg by mouth 2 hours before the procedure. How many milligrams will the nurse tell the parents to give to this child? Record your answer using a whole number.

_____ mg

92. A pediatric client is prescribed enteric-coated erythromycin. The nurse educates the parents on common adverse effects. Which adverse effect(s) will the nurse include in the education? Select all that apply.
1. Abdominal pain
2. Anorexia
3. Diarrhea
4. Weight gain
5. Nausea
6. Vomiting

93. Which finding will the nurse expect to assess in a child in the acute phase of Kawasaki's disease?
1. Polymorphous rash and cervical lymphadenopathy
2. Normal blood values and swollen hands and feet
3. Strawberry tongue and increased irritability
4. Desquamation of the hands and feet and a red throat

89. 1. The nurse should first obtain blood cultures, and then administer antibiotics. Cultures are needed to determine the causative organism. Blood cultures should be obtained from three different sites, with an hour between each stick. Urine output would be monitored to assess for complications such as heart failure. Janeway lesions, purplish macules on the palms or soles, are rare findings.
CN: Safe, effective care environment; CNS: Management of care; CL: Analyze

90. 4. Bacterial organisms can enter the bloodstream from any site of infection, such as a urinary tract infection. Gram-negative bacilli are common causative agents. A peripheral IV catheter is a potential entry site for bacteria but would not be an indication of increased risk for bacterial endocarditis unless the signs and symptoms of infection were present at the site. Moreover, long-term indwelling catheters pose a higher risk of infection than do those that are in place for only 1 day. Colds are usually viral, not bacterial. Dental work is a common portal of entry if not pretreated with antibiotics. Heart surgery is also a common cause of endocarditis, especially if synthetic material is used.
CN: Physiological integrity; CNS: Physiological adaptation; CL: Apply

91. 454.
To determine the dose, multiply the dose prescribed, by the child's weight in kilograms
$$20 \ mg \ / \ kg \times 22.7 \ kg = 454 \ mg$$
CN: Physiological integrity; CNS: Pharmacological and parenteral therapies; CL: Analyze

92. 1, 2, 3, 5, 6. Erythromycin is an antibacterial antibiotic. Common adverse effects include nausea, vomiting, anorexia, diarrhea, and abdominal pain. Weight gain is not an adverse effect associated with erythromycin. It should be given with a full glass (8 oz) of water after meals or with food to lessen gastrointestinal symptoms.
CN: Physiological integrity; CNS: Pharmacological and parenteral therapies; CL: Apply

93. 1. Findings of the acute phase include polymorphous rash, cervical lymphadenopathy, red throat, swollen hands and feet, fever, and irritability. Findings of the subacute phase include desquamation of the hands and feet, strawberry tongue, joint pain, and thrombocytosis. Blood values return to normal at the end of the convalescent phase.
CN: Physiological integrity; CNS: Physiological adaptation; CL: Apply

94. The nurse is providing discharge education to the parents of a client diagnosed with endocarditis. Which symptom(s) will the nurse inform the parents could indicate a potential cardiac complication? Select all that apply.
1. Skin rash
2. Diarrhea
3. Increasing fatigue
4. Lower extremities swelling
5. Poor appetite

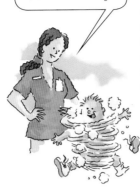

No problem with fatigue here. His mother, however, is a different story.

95. A child presents with a strawberry tongue. The parents tell the nurse the child has had a temperature of 103°F (39.4°C) for several days that does not respond to acetaminophen or ibuprofen. Which prescription(s) will the nurse anticipate from the health care provider? Select all that apply.
1. Intravenous immunoglobulin (IVIG)
2. Acetylsalicylic acid
3. Influenza vaccination prior to discharge
4. Corticosteroids
5. Penicillin intravenously

96. The nurse is educating the parents of a child with Kawasaki's disease. Which statement(s) will the nurse include in the education provided to the parents? Select all that apply.
1. "It is an acute systemic vasculitis of unknown cause."
2. "It mostly occurs in the fall and winter months."
3. "Diagnosis can be made by laboratory testing."
4. "It manifests in three stages: acute, subacute, and convalescent."
5. "Your other children need to be treated prophylactically."

97. Which finding in a child with Kawasaki's disease will the nurse report to the health care provider **immediately**?
1. Desquamation of the skin of the hands and feet
2. Sudden abdominal pain with vomiting
3. Pain in the joints rated an 8 on a 0 to 10 pain scale
4. Erythrocyte sedimentation rate of 20 mm/ hour (20 mm/hour)

94. 3, 4, 5. The client with endocarditis is at risk for the development of further cardiac complications. Increasing fatigue may signal cardiac insufficiency. Swelling and poor appetite are associated with heart failure. The client with endocarditis will be discharged to home with continued antibiotic therapy. A skin rash and diarrhea signal possible reactions to the antibiotic therapy and are not likely cardiac in nature.
CN: Heath promotion and maintenance; CNS: None; CL: Apply

95. 1, 2. Inflammation of the pharynx and oral mucosa develops in Kawasaki's disease, causing red, cracked lips and a "strawberry" tongue, in which the normal coating of the tongue sloughs off. Having a high fever for 5 or more days that is unresponsive to antibiotics and antipyretics is also part of the diagnostic criteria. Treatment for Kawasaki's disease includes IVIG to reduce the immune response and acetylsalicylic acid to control the fever and symptoms of inflammation and for antiplatelet action. Influenza vaccine is recommended to prevent Reye's syndrome but should not be given for 5 months following IVIG administration. Corticosteroids and penicillin are given for rheumatic fever.
CN: Physiological integrity; CNS: Physiological adaptation; CL: Apply

96. 1, 4. Kawasaki's disease can best be described as an acute systemic vasculitis of unknown cause with three stages: acute, subacute, and convalescent. Most cases are geographic and seasonal, occurring in the late winter and early spring. Diagnosis is based on clinical findings of five of the six diagnostic criteria and associated laboratory results. There is no specific laboratory test for diagnosis. Family members cannot be treated prophylactically.
CN: Physiological integrity; CNS: Physiological adaptation; CL: Apply

97. 2. The most serious complication of Kawasaki's disease is cardiac involvement. Abdominal pain, vomiting, and restlessness are the main symptoms of an acute myocardial infarction in children. Desquamation and joint pain are expected and occur in the subacute phase. An increased erythrocyte sedimentation rate is a reflection of the inflammatory process and may be seen for 2 to 4 weeks after the onset of symptoms.
CN: Safe, effective care environment; CNS: Management of care; CL: Apply

CN: Client needs category   CNS: Client needs subcategory   CL: Cognitive level

98. The nurse is caring for a child in the subacute phase of Kawasaki's disease. Which finding(s) will the nurse expect in this stage of the illness? Select all that apply.
1. Diarrhea
2. Abdominal pain
3. Joint pain
4. Swollen, reddened palms
5. Peeling skin

99. A child diagnosed with Kawasaki's disease is prescribed intravenous gamma globulin 400 mg/kg/day for 4 days. The child weighs 39.7 lb (18 kg). How many milligrams will the nurse administer with each dose? Record your answer using a whole number.

_____ mg

100. A 2-month-old infant arrives in the emergency department with a heart rate of 180 beats/minute and a rectal temperature of 103.1°F (39.5°C). Which nursing intervention is **most** appropriate?
1. Give acetaminophen.
2. Encourage fluid intake.
3. Apply carotid massage.
4. Place the infant's feet in cold water.

101. A child is prescribed aspirin for Kawasaki's disease. The prescription is for 80 mg/kg/day orally in four divided doses until the child is afebrile. The child weighs 22.1 lb (10 kg). How many milligrams will the nurse administer with each dose? Record your answer using a whole number.

_____ mg

102. The nurse is providing discharge education to parents of a child with Kawasaki's disease. Which statement by the parents indicates an understanding of the educational information?
1. "We need to get our child a soft-bristled toothbrush."
2. "Our child can eat regular foods once at home."
3. "Our child may have black, tarry stools on and off."
4. "Our child can participate in physical education next week."

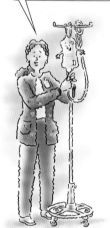

My little friend here is not that great at math. Can you calculate his dose in question #99?

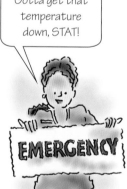

Gotta get that temperature down, STAT!

98. 1, 2, 3, 5. Kawasaki's disease is characterized by inflammation of the walls of the body's arteries, including those of the heart. The condition has three phases. In the subacute phase, symptoms include gastrointestinal problems, such as abdominal pain and diarrhea, joint pain, and skin peeling on the hands and feet. Red, swollen palms are seen in the acute phase of the disease.
CN: Physiological integrity; CNS: Physiological adaptation; CL: Apply

99. 7,200
To determine the dose per day:

dose prescribed × client weight = dose per day

$$400\ mg / kg \times 18\ kg = 7,200\ mg$$

CN: Physiological integrity; CNS: Pharmacological and parenteral therapies; CL: Analyze

100. 1. Acetaminophen should be given first to decrease the infant's temperature. A heart rate of 180 beats/minute is normal in an infant with a fever. Fluid intake is encouraged after the acetaminophen is given to help replace insensible fluid losses. Carotid massage is an attempt to decrease the heart rate as a vagal maneuver; it will not work in this infant because the source of the increased heart rate is fever. A tepid sponge bath may be given to help decrease the temperature and calm the infant.
CN: Safe, effective care environment; CNS: Management of care; CL: Apply

101. 200
First, determine the dose per day:

dose prescribed × client weight = dose per day
$$80\ mg / kg \times 10\ kg = 800\ mg$$

Then, because the child is to receive the drug in four doses, divide the daily amount by 4.

$$800\ mg / 4\ doses = 200\ mg / dose$$

CN: Physiological integrity; CNS: Pharmacological and parenteral therapies; CL: Analyze

102. 1. Because of the anticoagulant effects of aspirin therapy, the child should use a soft-bristled toothbrush to prevent bleeding of the gums. A low-cholesterol diet should be followed until coronary artery involvement resolves, usually within 6 to 8 weeks. Black, tarry stools are abnormal and are signs of bleeding that should be reported to the health care provider immediately. Contact sports should be avoided because of the cardiac involvement and excessive bruising that may occur due to aspirin therapy.
CN: Physiological integrity; CNS: Physiological adaptation; CL: Apply

103. The nurse is providing discharge teaching to the caregiver of a child with Kawasaki's disease. Which instruction is **priority** for the nurse to include?
   1. Continue aspirin as prescribed.
   2. Erythrocyte sedimentation rate may be elevated for a few weeks.
   3. Your child is at increased risk for acquired heart disease.
   4. Frequent echocardiography will be needed.

103. 1. Aspirin therapy may be continued for weeks after the onset of symptoms. The caregiver should be instructed to continue treatment as prescribed to prevent cardiac complications. All other instructions are appropriate, but not priority over continuing treatment.
CN: Physiological integrity; CNS: Physiological adaptation; CL: Analyze

104. The mother of a 10-year-old diagnosed with an upper respiratory infection questions the nurse about the potential development of rheumatic heart disease. Which information is appropriate for the nurse to include in the response? Select all that apply.
   1. The condition is genetically more likely to occur in some individuals.
   2. The condition is more likely to occur if there is a family history of heart disease.
   3. Not all strains of streptococcus bacteria result in rheumatic heart disease.
   4. Antiviral therapy administered at the onset of the infection can prevent the condition.
   5. The acute phase of the condition lasts for up to 2 weeks.

Yo. The name's strep. Let's just say I'm a real heartbreaker.

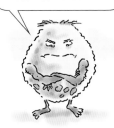

104. 1, 3, 5. Rheumatic heart disease may result in individuals who have been experiencing group A streptococcus infections. The acute phase of the condition lasts about 10 to 14 days. The condition is more likely to occur in individuals with certain genetic makeups. Not all strains of the bacteria cause the infection. A family history of heart disease does not increase the occurrence of this complication. Antiviral therapy is not used in the prevention of the complication.
CN: Health promotion and maintenance; CNS: None; CL: Apply

105. The nurse is caring for a child with acute rheumatic fever. Which finding will the nurse anticipate observing in this child?
   1. Leukocytosis
   2. Normal electrocardiogram
   3. High fever for 5 or more days
   4. Erythrocyte sedimentation rate of 10 mm/h

Ugh. I feel a little warm. Maybe I should have my white blood cells checked out.

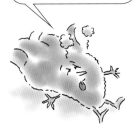

105. 1. Leukocytosis can be seen as an immune response triggered by colonization of the pharynx with group A streptococci. The electrocardiogram shows a prolonged PR interval as a result of carditis. A low-grade fever is a minor manifestation. A high fever for 5 or more days may indicate Kawasaki's disease. The inflammatory response causes an elevated erythrocyte sedimentation rate.
CN: Physiological integrity; CNS: Physiological adaptation; CL: Apply

106. The nurse is assessing a child admitted with suspected rheumatic fever. Which finding will the nurse expect in this child?
   1. Abnormal laboratory test results
   2. Fever and the presence of four Jones criteria
   3. Positive blood cultures for *Staphylococcus* organisms
   4. Presence of multiple Jones criteria and a streptococcal infection

106. 4. Two major (or one major and two minor) manifestations from Jones criteria, and the presence of a streptococcal infection, indicate the diagnosis of rheumatic fever. There is no single laboratory test for diagnosis. Fever and four diagnostic criteria are required to diagnose Kawasaki's disease. Blood cultures would be positive for *Streptococcus*, not *Staphylococcus*, organisms.

Jones criteria for diagnosing rheumatic fever

Major criteria	Minor criteria
Carditis	Fever
Migratory polyarthritis	Arthralgia
Sydenham chorea	Elevated acute phase reactants
Subcutaneous nodules	Prolonged PR interval
Erythema marginatum	

CN: Physiological integrity; CNS: Physiological adaptation; CL: Apply

107. The nurse is providing discharge education to a 17-year-old client who received care for rheumatic fever with cardiac inflammation. Which statement by the teenage client indicates the need for further instruction?
  1. "I will be able to go back to school in just a few days."
  2. "By taking my medications, I have a good chance of avoiding more complications."
  3. "I may have an extended need for bed rest."
  4. "We may not know the extent of damage to my heart for a while."

108. The nurse is discussing criteria for rheumatic fever with a child's parents. The nurse realizes the parents understand chorea when they make which statement?
  1. "My child may not be able to walk."
  2. "Long movies may help for relaxation."
  3. "My child might have difficulty in school."
  4. "Many activities and visitors are recommended."

109. The nurse is caring for a 9-year-old child with a positive culture for *Streptococcus* organisms. Which nursing intervention is **most** appropriate?
  1. Administer aspirin.
  2. Give penicillin.
  3. Start corticosteroids.
  4. Monitor fluid intake.

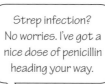

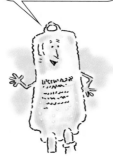

110. A nurse is educating parents of a child diagnosed with rheumatic fever without carditis. Which information will the nurse include?
  1. "Administer aspirin for signs of chorea."
  2. "Your child will need to take penicillin for a month."
  3. "Notify the health care provider if you see a macular rash."
  4. "Your child does not need penicillin before dental procedures."

111. The nurse is caring for a child with rheumatic fever. Which is the **greatest** area of concern for the nurse?
  1. Nutrition
  2. Anxiety management
  3. Cognitive delays
  4. Prevention of falls

107. **1.** After rheumatic fever, rest is needed. The cardiac involvement requires an extended period of rest and relaxation. The remaining statements indicate an accurate understanding of the condition.
CN: Health promotion and maintenance; CNS: None; CL: Apply

108. **3.** Chorea may last 1 to 6 months. Central nervous system involvement contributes to a shortened attention span, so children might have difficulty learning in school or even sustaining interest in long movies. Muscle incoordination may cause the child to be more clumsy than usual when walking, but the child should be able to walk. A quiet environment is required for treatment.
CN: Physiological integrity; CNS: Physiological adaptation; CL: Apply

109. **2.** Infection caused by *Streptococcus* organisms is treated with antibiotics, mainly penicillin. This will ensure the organism is destroyed, and prevent rheumatic fever. Antipyretics, such as acetaminophen, may be given for fever. Aspirin is not recommended. Corticosteroids are not indicated. Fluid intake is encouraged to prevent dehydration from decreased oral intake due to a sore throat, or to replace fluids lost due to possible diarrhea from the antibiotics.
CN: Physiological integrity; CNS: Physiological adaptation; CL: Analyze

110. **4.** Children who might benefit from prophylactic penicillin include those with unrepaired congenital heart defects, those with heart defects repaired with synthetic material, those with prior infective endocarditis, and some children with heart transplants. Because this child does not have carditis, prophylactic treatment with penicillin is not needed. A macular rash found predominately on the trunk, erythema marginatum, is an expected finding and does not require notifying the health care provider. Aspirin is not indicated for signs of chorea.
CN: Physiological integrity; CNS: Pharmacological and parenteral therapies; CL: Apply

111. **4.** The child with rheumatic fever has a risk for chorea. This can lead to falls. In addition, the child may experience weakness, which can also increase the risk for falls. The remaining items are not typical concerns for rheumatic fever.
CN: Safe, effective care environment; CNS: Safety and infection control; CL: Apply

112. An exercise stress test has been prescribed for a 12-year-old child. Which statement by the child indicates to the nurse the need for additional education?
1. "I will be allowed to eat whatever I want after the test is finished."
2. "I will eat the breakfast my mom prepares for me before I take the test."
3. "If I have any pain or trouble breathing during the test I will let you know."
4. "The test should take only about 30 to 45 minutes to complete."

113. A child with sinus bradycardia is prescribed atropine 0.02 mg/kg/dose. The child weighs 70.6 lb (32 kg). How many milligrams will the nurse administer the child per dose? Record your answer using one decimal place.

_____ mg

114. The nurse is assigned four pediatric clients. The nurse understands that which client may exhibit asymptomatic sinus bradycardia?
1. Preterm neonate
2. Term neonate
3. Growth-delayed adolescent
4. Physically conditioned adolescent

115. The nurse is administering atropine to a 9-year-old child with sinus bradycardia. Which finding will the nurse expect following administration?
1. The heart rate changes from 72 to 85 beats/minute.
2. The blood pressure changes from 130/86 to 115/74 mm Hg.
3. The respiratory rate changes from 12 to 18 breaths/minute.
4. The oxygen saturation level changes from 90% to 96%.

116. The nurse is caring for an 11-month-old infant taking atropine. During assessment, the nurse notes the infant does not cry tears when upset. Which nursing action is **most** appropriate?
1. Hold the next dose of atropine.
2. Begin weighing the client's diapers.
3. Administer an intravenous bolus.
4. Document the finding in the medical record.

117. When assessing a child, the nurse notes sinus tachycardia. Which condition in the child's health history places the client at risk for sinus tachycardia?
1. Febrile illness
2. Hypothermia
3. Hypothyroidism
4. Hypoxia

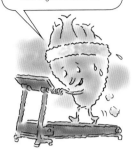

Speaking of "stress test," how's your practice test going? Don't sweat it. I'm sure you'll ace it.

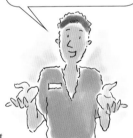

If the whole point of atropine is to treat bradycardia, then what effect should it have?

112. 2. The exercise stress test monitors the heart rate, blood pressure, and oxygen consumption during a period of activity. The child should be NPO for at least 4 hours prior to the test. The remaining statements are correct.
CN: Health promotion and maintenance; CNS: None; CL: Apply

113. 0.64
To determine the dose per day:

$$dose\ prescribed \times client\ weight = dose\ per\ day$$

$$0.02\ mg\ /\ kg \times 32\ kg = 0.64\ mg$$

CN: Physiological integrity; CNS: Pharmacological and parenteral therapies; CL: Analyze

114. 4. A physically conditioned adolescent might have a lower-than-normal heart rate, which is of no significance. Growth-delayed adolescents do not have bradycardia as a normal finding. Neonates have characteristic elevated heart rates.
CN: Physiological integrity; CNS: Physiological adaptation; CL: Apply

115. 1. Atropine blocks vagal impulses to the myocardium and stimulates the cardio-inhibitory center in the medulla, thereby increasing heart rate and cardiac output. Atropine is not given to directly increase blood pressure or dilate the bronchial tubes.
CN: Physiological integrity; CNS: Pharmacological and parenteral therapies; CL: Analyze

116. 4. Atropine dries up secretions and also lessens the response of ciliary and iris sphincter muscles in the eye, causing mydriasis. The finding should be documented in the medical record. The nurse should not hold the medication due to an expected reaction. No other interventions are needed at this time.
CN: Physiological integrity; CNS: Pharmacological and parenteral therapies; CL: Apply

117. 1. Sinus tachycardia is commonly seen in children with a fever. It is usually a result of a non-cardiac cause. Hypothermia, hypothyroidism, and hypoxia all result in sinus bradycardia.
CN: Physiological integrity; CNS: Physiological adaptation; CL: Understand

CN: Client needs category   CNS: Client needs subcategory   CL: Cognitive level

118. The nurse is educating parents of a child who had surgery for tetralogy of Fallot. Which statement(s) by the parents demonstrate an understanding of the condition? Select all that apply.
  1. "My son will not be able to play any sports when he gets older."
  2. "My son's life expectancy has been diminished by this diagnosis."
  3. "My son will need to be seen throughout his life by a cardiologist."
  4. "My son's heart may at times have irregular rhythm patterns."
  5. "Repeated surgical procedures will likely be needed to manage my son's condition."

118. 3, 4. Tetralogy of Fallot is a congenital cardiac condition in which there are four primary defects of the heart's structure and function. These include a large ventricular septal defect, pulmonary stenosis, right ventricular hypertrophy, and an overriding aorta. The condition is typically managed with surgical intervention in infancy. This procedure is usually all that is needed to manage the condition. The ability to live a full life with few restrictions is possible for these clients. There is not a significant loss of life years with the condition. The child with this condition will need lifelong monitoring by a cardiologist. Individuals with this condition have an increased risk for the development of cardiac dysrhythmias.
CN: Physiological integrity; CNS: Physiological adaptation; CL: Apply

119. The health care provider prescribes digoxin 0.1 mg orally every morning for a 6-month-old infant with heart failure. Digoxin is available in a 400 mcg/mL concentration. How many milliliters of digoxin will the nurse administer? Record your answer using two decimal places.

_____ mL

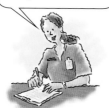

Oh look, another math problem—my favorite. Don't forget to convert.

119. 0.25
First, convert milligrams to micrograms:
$$1{,}000\ mcg\ /\ 1\ mg = X\ mcg\ /\ 0.1\ mg$$
$$X = 100\ mcg$$

Then, calculate drug dose:
$$Dose\ on\ hand\ /\ Quantity\ on\ hand = Dose\ desired\ /\ X.$$
$$400\ mcg\ /\ mL = 100\ mcg\ /\ X$$
$$X = 0.25\ mL$$

CN: Physiological integrity; CNS: Pharmacological and parenteral therapies; CL: Analyze

120. The nurse is caring for a female adolescent diagnosed with Wolff-Parkinson-White syndrome. When asking the teen how she is feeling, which response is **most** consistent with this condition?
  1. "I feel like my heart has episodes of beating very slowly."
  2. "I feel an aching feeling in my left arm and shoulder."
  3. "My breathing seems to be slow today."
  4. "There were times today when my heart seemed to beat very fast."

120. 4. Wolff-Parkinson-White syndrome is a condition in which electrical impulses arrive at the ventricles prematurely. It is often termed a "pre-excitation syndrome." Manifestations of the condition include tachycardia, dizziness or fainting, and heart palpitations.
CN: Physiological integrity; CNS: Physiological adaptation; CL: Apply

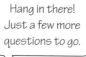

Hang in there! Just a few more questions to go.

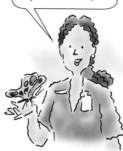

121. An infant who weighs 17.7 lb (8 kg) is to receive ampicillin 25 mg/kg intravenously every 6 hours. How many milligrams will the nurse administer per dose? Record your answer using a whole number.

_____ mg

121. 200
To determine the dose per day:
$$dose\ prescribed \times client\ weight = dose\ per\ day$$
$$25\ mg/kg \times 8\ kg = 200\ mg$$

CN: Physiological integrity; CNS: Pharmacological and parenteral therapies; CL: Analyze

122. The nurse is providing preoperative education to the parents of a 9-month-old infant who is having surgery to repair a ventricular septal defect. Identify the area of the heart where the defect is located.

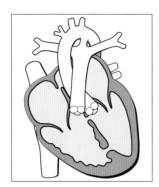

122. A ventricular septal defect is a hole in the septum between the ventricles. The defect can be anywhere along the septum but is most commonly located in the middle of the septum.

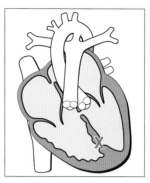

CN: Physiological integrity; CNS: Physiological adaptation; CL: Apply

123. A 6-year-old arrives in the emergency department reporting dizziness and collapses in the waiting room. Prioritize in ascending chronologic order the steps the nurse will take during initial intervention. Use all options.

1. Provide 30 chest compressions.
2. Tilt the child's head back to open up the airway.
3. Check the carotid pulse.
4. Give two rescue breaths.
5. Establish unresponsiveness and call for help.

All done? Super! Time for a nap.

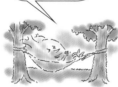

123. Ordered Response:

5. Establish unresponsiveness and call for help.
3. Check the carotid pulse.
1. Provide 30 chest compressions.
2. Tilt the child's head back to open up the airway.
4. Give two rescue breaths.

The first step is to establish unresponsiveness and call for help. Then check the carotid pulse for no more than 10 seconds. If there is no pulse, begin chest compressions (30 compressions:2 breaths for a single rescuer). Then tilt the child's head back to open the airway and give two breaths.

CN: Safe, effective care environment; CNS: Management of care; CL: Apply

Chapter 27

Hematologic & Immune Disorders

Pediatric hematologic & immune refresher

Acquired immunodeficiency syndrome (AIDS)

Grouping of symptoms that signal a loss of immune response in one who is positive for human immunodeficiency virus (HIV)

Key signs and symptoms
- Failure to thrive
- Mononucleosis-like prodromal symptoms
- Night sweats
- Recurring diarrhea
- Weight loss

Key test results
- CD4+ T-cell count measures the severity of immunosuppression
- Enzyme-linked immunosorbent assay and Western blot are positive for HIV antibody
- Viral culture or p24 antigen test reveals presence of HIV in children younger than age 18 months

Key treatments
- Antibiotic therapy according to sensitivity of infecting organisms
- Antiviral agents such as zidovudine
- Monthly gamma globulin administration

Key interventions
- Monitor vital signs, intake and output, and growth and development.
- Monitor respiratory and neurologic status.
- Maintain standard precautions.

Hemophilia

Deficiency of clotting factors, in which the absence of these clotting factors results in abnormal bleeding times

Key signs and symptoms
- Multiple bruises without petechiae
- Prolonged bleeding after circumcision, immunizations, or minor injuries

Key test results
- Prolonged partial thromboplastin time (PTT)

Key treatments
- Cryoprecipitate (frozen factor VIII) administration to maintain an acceptable serum level of the clotting factor; usually done by the family at home
- Fresh frozen plasma

Key interventions
- Monitor vital signs, intake, and output.
- When bleeding occurs:
  - elevate the affected extremity above the heart
  - immobilize the site
  - apply pressure to the site for 10 to 15 minutes
  - decrease the child's anxiety.

Iron deficiency anemia

Deficiency of red blood cells, which are responsible for carrying oxygen in the body

Key signs and symptoms
- Fatigue, listlessness
- Increased susceptibility to infection
- Pallor
- Tachycardia
- Numbness and tingling of the extremities
- Vasomotor disturbances

Key test results
- Hemoglobin (Hb), hematocrit, and serum ferritin levels are low
- Serum iron levels are low, with high binding capacity

Key treatments
- Oral preparation of iron or a combination of iron and ascorbic acid (which enhances iron absorption)

Key interventions
- Administer iron before meals with citrus juice.
- Give liquid iron through a straw; for infants, administer by oral syringe toward the back of the mouth.
- Do not give iron with milk products.

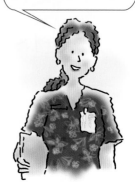

This chapter covers sickle cell disease, varicella, Rocky Mountain spotted fever, leukemia, and many other blood and immune system disorders in kids. It's a whopper of a chapter on a critical area. If you're ready, let's begin!

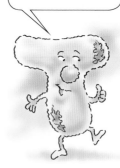

No immunosuppression here. I'm feeling T-rrific.

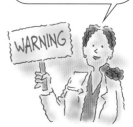

Iron and milk products don't mix. Serve iron with a citrus juice and have your client sip it through a straw.

WARNING

Leukemia

Cancer of the blood-forming cells of the body

Key signs and symptoms

- Fatigue
- History of infections
- Low-grade fever
- Lymphadenopathy
- Pallor
- Petechiae and ecchymosis
- Poor wound healing and oral lesions

Key test results

- Blast cells appear in the peripheral blood
- Blast cells may be as high as 95% in the bone marrow
- Initial white blood cell count may be 10,000/µL (10×10^9/L) at time of diagnosis in a child between 3 and 7 years of age with acute lymphocytic leukemia (ALL)

Key treatments

- Bone marrow transplantation
- Radiation therapy
- Chemotherapy

Key interventions

- Provide pain relief.
- Monitor vital signs, intake, and output.
- Inspect the skin frequently.
- Provide nursing measures to ease adverse effects of radiation and chemotherapy.

Reye's syndrome

Serious condition impacting all organs and tissues of the body, but acts most severely on the brain and liver, where it is associated with swelling; many affected will experience a viral infection prior to syndrome development

Key signs and symptoms

- Stage I: persistent vomiting (may be diarrhea in infant), signs of brain dysfunction, listlessness, liver dysfunction
- Stage II: restlessness, combativeness, hyperventilation, hyperreflexia, delirium, lethargy
- Stage III: disorientation, confusion, irrational behavior, combativeness, decorticate rigidity

- Stage IV: decerebrate rigidity, seizures, coma, fixed pupils
- Stage V: seizures, deep coma, flaccid paralysis, absent reflexes, respiratory arrest (death is usually a result of cerebral edema or cardiac arrest)

Key test results

- Blood test results show elevated serum ammonia, serum fatty acid, and lactate levels
- Coagulation studies reveal prolonged prothrombin time (PT) and partial thromboplastin time (PTT)
- Liver biopsy shows fatty droplets distributed through cells
- Liver function studies show aspartate aminotransferase (AST) and alanine aminotransferase (ALT) elevated to twice normal levels

Key treatments

- Endotracheal intubation and mechanical ventilation
- Exchange transfusion
- Induced hypothermia

Key interventions

- Monitor vital signs and pulse oximetry.
- Monitor cardiac, respiratory, and neurologic status.
- Monitor fluid intake and output.
- Monitor blood glucose levels.
- Maintain seizure precautions.
- Keep head of bed at 30-degree angle.
- Maintain oxygen therapy, which may include intubation and mechanical ventilation.
- Administer blood products as necessary.
- Administer medications and monitor for adverse effects.
- Maintain hypothermia blanket as needed and monitor temperature every 15 to 30 minutes while in use.
- Check for loss of reflexes and signs of flaccidity.

Sickle cell anemia

Autosomal recessive condition in which the red blood cells are sickle shaped, resulting in ineffective ability to carry oxygen to the body's tissues; the cells become lodged in the body's organs and vessels

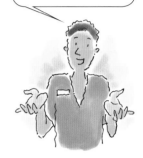

A client is suspected of having leukemia. What tests should you expect to be prescribed?

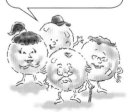

Leukemia mutates white blood cells, turning them from heroes to villains.

Key signs and symptoms

- In infants, signs and symptoms usually do not develop until 4 to 6 months of age due to the presence of fetal hemoglobin
- Swollen hands and feet (may be the first sign noted in infants)
- Periodic episodes of pain (sickle cell crisis)
- Chronic fatigue
- Delayed growth
- Frequent infections
- Splenomegaly

Key test results

- More than 50% Hb S indicates sickle cell disease; a lower level of Hb S indicates sickle cell trait

Key treatments

- Hydration with IV fluid administration
- Transfusion therapy as necessary
- Treatment for acidosis
- Analgesics: morphine or hydromorphone
- Oral penicillin prophylactically until 5 years of age
- Daily folic acid supplementation

Key interventions

- Monitor vital signs, intake, and output.
- Administer pain medications and note effectiveness.

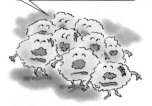

Time for a head count! Elevated white blood cell count can be an indicator of a problematic immune response.

thePoint® You can download tables of drug information to help you prepare for the NCLEX®! View Generic Drug Names, Drug Classifications, Drug Actions, and Nursing Implications for the drugs discussed in this refresher at **http://thePoint.lww.com**

Hematologic & immune questions, answers, and rationales

1. The parents of a child with continuous vomiting, extreme drowsiness, and confusion state the child recently took salicylates for a cold. The child begins to have a seizure while the nurse is assessing the child. Which nursing intervention is **priority**?

1. Place the child in a side-lying position.
2. Attempt to arouse the child.
3. Notify the health care provider of Reye's syndrome.
4. Determine which stage of the illness the child is in.

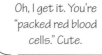

Oh, I get it. You're "packed red blood cells." Cute.

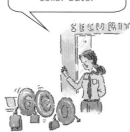

2. A child with Reye's syndrome is in stage I of the illness. Which intervention will the nurse expect to for the health care provider to prescribe?

1. Invasive monitoring
2. Endotracheal intubation
3. Hypertonic glucose solution
4. Pancuronium

1. 1. The nurse should first ensure the child is safe during the seizure. Placing the child side-lying would help keep the child's airway clear. The nurse should not attempt to arouse the child during a seizure; clients are unresponsive during a seizure. The health care provider should be notified quickly, as early diagnosis and therapy are essential because of the rapid, clinical course of Reye's syndrome and its high mortality. Staging, although important to therapy, occurs after a differential diagnosis is made.

CN: Safe, effective care environment; CNS: Management of care; CL: Analyze

2. 3. For children in stage I of Reye's syndrome, treatment is primarily supportive and directed toward restoring blood glucose levels and correcting acid–base imbalances. Intravenous administration of dextrose solutions with added insulin helps to replace glycogen stores and may help prevent progression of the syndrome. Noninvasive monitoring is adequate to assess the status at this stage. Endotracheal intubation may be necessary later. Pancuronium is used as an adjunct to endotracheal intubation and would not be used in stage I of Reye's syndrome.

CN: Physiological integrity; CNS: Reduction of risk potential; CL: Analyze

3. The nurse is caring for a 9-month-old with Reye's syndrome. Which intervention will the nurse include when caring for this infant?
1. Assess the skin every shift.
2. Perform range-of-motion (ROM) exercises.
3. Monitor the child's intake and output.
4. Place the child in protective isolation.

4. A child with Reye's syndrome is exhibiting signs of increased intracranial pressure (ICP). Which nursing intervention is **most** appropriate for this child?
1. Position the child with head elevated and neck in a neutral position.
2. Prepare the child and caregivers for mechanical ventilation.
3. Space apart interventions that may induce stress.
4. Assess the child's pupils and level of consciousness.

5. The nurse is comforting an adolescent upset at the loss of hair related to the administration of chemotherapy. Which statement(s) will the nurse include when talking with the adolescent? Select all that apply.
1. "Options to cover your hair loss include a cap, scarf, or wig."
2. "You should not stress about this; hair loss is completely temporary."
3. "You should begin to interact with your friends as soon as possible."
4. "Please share your feelings about this change with your parents."
5. "You do not have to wear a head cover unless it is for protection from the sun or cold."

6. A child with pauciarticular juvenile rheumatoid arthritis (JRA) is being seen for an annual physical examination. The child's parent reports not understanding why the child will need to have an annual eye examination if there are no visual problems. Which statement by the nurse is **most** appropriate?
1. "The common complication is painless, so your child will not have symptoms."
2. "An annual examination is just easier for everyone to remember."
3. "You need to ask the health care provider why your child needs to be checked yearly."
4. "If your child is not reporting any pain or vision changes, a yearly checkup is not needed."

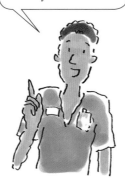
Heads up! Finding the most appropriate intervention is critical in question #4.

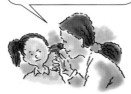
No, I can't see your thoughts—just some ear wax.

3. 3. Monitoring intake and output alerts the nurse to the development of dehydration and cerebral edema, complications of Reye's syndrome. Although checking the skin for signs of breakdown is important because the child may not be as active as normal, it is not as critical as monitoring the infant's intake and output. Active ROM exercises may not be needed and are not as important as monitoring the child's intake and output. Placing the child in protective isolation is not necessary.
CN: Physiological integrity; CNS: Reduction of risk potential; CL: Apply

4. 1. Positioning the child with Reye's syndrome with the head elevated and the neck in neutral position helps decrease ICP. Spacing interventions is appropriate; however, a more immediate effect would result from an immediate intervention. The nurse should monitor the child's pupils to monitor for ICP. Mechanical ventilation is not required at this time.
CN: Safe, effective care environment; CNS: Management of care; CL: Analyze

5. 1, 3, 4, 5. The loss of hair is a common reaction to chemotherapy. This loss is temporary, but it is not therapeutic to tell the client not to stress. New hair growth begins in 3 to 6 months. The new hair may be a different color or texture than the hair that was lost. Children may choose to cover their scalps with wigs, hats, or scarves. Covering should be done to protect from elements such as cold and sun when present. Sharing feelings is important so that support may be received from those closest to the child. Remaining in contact with peers is helpful and important for psychosocial development among adolescents.
CN: Psychosocial integrity; CNS: None; CL: Apply

6. 1. Painless iritis may be found in up to 75% of children with pauciarticular JRA. If left untreated, permanent scarring in the anterior chamber of the eye may occur, with loss of vision. Children should have annual slit-lamp examinations by an ophthalmologist for early detection. The nurse should not tell the parents the question to the health care provider; if the nurse does not know, the nurse should seek the information to answer a client or family's questions.
CN: Health promotion and maintenance; CNS: None; CL: Apply

CN: Client needs category   CNS: Client needs subcategory   CL: Cognitive level

7. An 8-year-old child is brought to the clinic during the summer with watery eyes, clear nasal drainage that has lasted more than 10 days, and an absence of fever. The nurse notes dark circles under the child's eyes and a crease above the tip of the nose. Which intervention is the nurse's **priority**?

1. Assess for potential environmental allergy triggers.
2. Administer amoxicillin 25 mg/kg PO every 12 hours.
3. Give the influenza vaccine intramuscularly.
4. Prepare the child and caregivers for sinus x-rays.

8. The nurse is caring for a child with juvenile arthritis prescribed oral prednisone. The parents ask whether their child will always have to take prednisone. Which response by the nurse is **most** appropriate?

1. "Prednisone is given for the shortest duration possible to promote normal growth and limit the risk of infections."
2. "The only effective treatment for juvenile arthritis is prednisone, so yes, your child will always need this medicine."
3. "How long a medication is needed really depends on how your child responds to the particular medication."
4. "We will monitor your child's blood for antinuclear antibodies. This test will determine how long prednisone is needed."

9. The nurse is providing education to the parent of a 12-year-old child recently diagnosed with systemic juvenile arthritis. Which statement(s) by the parent **best** indicates the nurse's education was effective? Select all that apply.

1. "Maintaining an appropriate, regular exercise program is very important."
2. "Joint stiffness, pain, swelling, and tenderness are common symptoms."
3. "We will come to the emergency room if my child starts limping."
4. "It is important that my child's diet include 1,300 mg of calcium daily."
5. "Warm showers in the morning may help ease my child's morning discomforts."

10. The nurse is assessing an infant scheduled to receive the first dose of the rotavirus vaccine today. Which finding(s) will the nurse highlight for the health care provider? Select all that apply.

1. Temperature 102°F (38.9°C)
2. Blood pressure 75/50 mm Hg
3. History of intussusception
4. Allergy to penicillin
5. Maternal history of diabetes

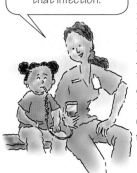

All normal. Looks like your body did a great job fighting off that infection.

7. 1. Cold symptoms that last longer than 10 days without fever, dark circles under the eyes (from increased blood flow near the sinuses), and a crease near the tip of the nose (from upward nose wiping) are all signs and symptoms of perennial allergic rhinitis. The nurse's priority is to collect data about potential indoor and outdoor environmental allergen triggers. Amoxicillin is used to treat bacterial infections, not allergies. Influenza vaccination is indicated annually during flu season (fall and winter). Sinus x-rays may be necessary to check for structural abnormalities, but they are not the priority at this time.

CN: Safe, effective care environment; CNS: Safety and infection control; CL: Apply

8. 1. Prednisone should be prescribed for the shortest possible duration. Long-term prednisone use is associated with poor growth and immunosuppression; it may aggravate or mask serious infections. Prednisone is not the only treatment; nonsteroidal anti-inflammatory drugs and disease-modifying antirheumatic drugs are given to relieve joint pain and swelling and slow the progression. Antinuclear antibodies are proteins produced by the immune system in clients with autoimmune disorders and indicate an increased risk for eye inflammation.

CN: Physiological integrity; CNS: Pharmacological and parenteral therapies; CL: Apply

9. 1, 2, 4, 5. Maintaining a regular, appropriate exercise program is important to maintain muscle strength and joint flexibility. Joint stiffness (especially in the mornings), pain, swelling, limping, persistent fever, rash, weight loss, fatigue, and tenderness are common symptoms. It is important for a 12-year-old child to consume 1,300 mg of calcium daily to maintain bone health. Morning pain and stiffness are concerns of the child with juvenile arthritis. The longer a joint has been inactive, the more discomfort may be experienced. Heat-related treatments are often effective in managing these concerns. Because limping is a common finding, there is no need to come to the ER.

CN: Health promotion and maintenance; CNS: None; CL: Apply

10. 1,3. The nurse will highlight a fever and a history of gastrointestinal disorders for the health care provider to review. Both are potential contraindications to the infant receiving the vaccine. The blood pressure is within normal range. An allergy to penicillin and a maternal history of diabetes are not significant factors on whether the infant should receive the rotavirus vaccine.

CN: Safe, effective care environment; CNS: Safety and infection control; CL: Apply

CN: Client needs category   CNS: Client needs subcategory   CL: Cognitive level

11. The nurse is caring for a child newly diagnosed with leukemia. Which action will the nurse include to help the parents cope with the diagnosis?
1. Not accepting aggressive behavior from parents
2. Minimizing the expression of feelings and concerns
3. Letting parents interpret the child's behaviors and responses
4. Encouraging the parents to talk about their feelings

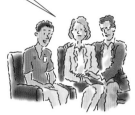

Leukemia is a scary diagnosis. Help parents to verbalize their emotions about it.

11. 4. As the parents are encouraged to talk about their feelings, stress is reduced. Aggressive behavior should not be tolerated, but instead recognized as a symptom of poor coping skills, indicating their need for greater emotional support; however, this action would not help parents cope with the diagnosis. It is critical to not minimize the feelings and concerns of the parents because this may increase their stress. It is important for the nurse to explain the child's behavior to the parents so they do not misinterpret the meaning.
CN: Psychosocial integrity; CNS: None; CL: Apply

12. The nurse is preparing to administer an immunization to a 2-month-old child. The child's parent states, "I am going to put off the immunization because I hate to see my child hurt." Which response by the nurse is **most** appropriate?
1. "I personally believe the pain your child will endure is worth it in the long run."
2. "Do not worry, your baby will not even remember this little shot."
3. "Although your baby will feel discomfort now, it will be short lived."
4. "Deciding to forgo the planned immunization is not in the baby's best interests."

12. 3. Parents often experience anxiety when care that causes discomfort or stress is administered to a child. The nurse should acknowledge the parent's stress or anxiety. The nurse should not provide personal believes or opinions. While the child will not recall the shot in the future, this does not address the parent's current concerns. Immunizations are recommended but telling the parent the decision is not in the baby's best interest is inappropriate.
CN: Health promotion and maintenance; CNS: None; CL: Apply

13. The nurse will question administering which pediatric client the prescribed vaccination?
1. Hepatitis B (Hep B) vaccine to an infant whose mother's hepatitis B surface antigen (HbsAg) is positive.
2. Diphtheria, tetanus, and pertussis (DTaP) vaccine to a child who experienced increased irritability after the previous dose.
3. *Haemophilus influenzae* type B (Hib) vaccine to a child with a history of otitis media, conjunctivitis, and sinusitis.
4. Measles, mumps, and rubella (MMR) vaccine to a child who is allergic to neomycin and penicillin.

13. 4. The nurse will question administering MMR to a child allergic to neomycin or gelatin. An infant whose mother is positive for HbsAg should receive the Hep B vaccine along with hepatitis B immune globulin (HBIG). It is common for children to experience irritability, loss of appetite, or swelling or tenderness at the injection site following DTaP. Hib is given to limit the occurrence of otitis media, conjunctivitis, and sinusitis in children.
CN: Safe, effective care environment; CNS: Safety and infection control; CL: Apply

14. Which child will the nurse assess **first**?
1. A 6-month-old waiting to receive an influenza vaccine before going home
2. A 12-year-old with juvenile arthritis (JA) reporting right knee pain
3. A 2-year-old with Reye's syndrome whose parent states the child is seizing
4. An 8-year-old diagnosed with HIV who has a CD4+ level of 175 cells/μL

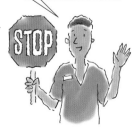

A nurse is always thinking about safety.

14. 3. The nurse should first assess the child actively seizing to ensure the child's safety during the seizure. Discharge of a client is not priority over safety. Joint pain is expected in a child with JA and is not life threatening. A CD4+ level below 200 cells/μL indicates that the client's HIV is progressing to acquired immune deficiency syndrome. This is not priority over the immediate safety and assessment of a seizing client.
CN: Safe, effective care environment; CNS: Safety and infection control; CL: Analyze

15. The nurse is educating the parents of a child diagnosed with HIV regarding immunizations. Which information will the nurse include in the teaching? Select all that apply.
   1. The immunization schedule should be followed as usual.
   2. Immunizations may be delayed for this child.
   3. The child will be put on an accelerated immunization schedule.
   4. The child will receive no further immunizations.
   5. The child may receive fewer vaccines given in a single visit.

16. The parents of an infant report they are concerned about giving their child immunizations due to their association with autism. Which response by the nurse is **most** appropriate?
   1. "Studies do not support a link between autism and immunizations."
   2. "There are limited risks of autism with the use of 'live' vaccines."
   3. "Getting more than one vaccine at a time has shown a slight increase in autism."
   4. "Inactivated vaccines have been linked to the development of autism in populations at risk."

17. A child is admitted to the hospital for asthma exacerbation. The history reveals this client was exposed to varicella 2 weeks ago. Which nursing intervention is **priority**?
   1. Administer the varicella vaccine.
   2. Place the child on airborne precautions.
   3. Administer diphenhydramine.
   4. Notify the health care provider.

18. The nurse is preparing to administer the second dose of measles, mumps, and rubella (MMR) vaccine to a 6-year-old child. Which action(s) will the nurse perform? Select all that apply.
   1. Use a 5/8-inch needle to administer the vaccine.
   2. Inject the vaccine into the deltoid muscle.
   3. Explain to the caregiver the immunization will be given intravenously.
   4. Ensure the caregiver understands risks and benefits of the vaccine.
   5. Explain to the caregiver that a third dose will need to be administered in 2 weeks.

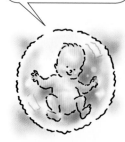

Vaccinations are like a protective bubble. Remind my parents to get them for me.

15. 2, 5. Immunizations should be delayed until the health care provider has determined the child is ready. The particular type and number of immunizations given at one time may vary for this child. The child may be put on a schedule to catch up eventually, but that would not be the first response. The child would not typically be excluded from immunizations in the future.
CN: Health promotion and maintenance; CNS: None; CL: Apply

16. 1. There has been a great deal of discussion about the risk of autism being increased with the administration of immunizations. Studies do not presently show a correlation, regardless of whether they are live or inactivated vaccines.
CN: Safe, effective care environment; CNS: Management of care; CL: Understand

17. 2. The child should immediately be placed on airborne precautions to limit exposing others to the virus. The incubation period for varicella is 2 to 3 weeks, with an average of 13 to 17 days. A person is infectious from 1 day before eruption of lesions until after the vesicles have formed crusts. The vaccine would not protect the child from the virus because the child has already been exposed to the virus. Diphenhydramine may help control pruritus; however, limiting exposure is priority. The health care provider should be notified after placing the child on precautions.
CN: Safe, effective care environment; CNS: Safety and infection control; CL: Analyze

18. 1, 4. The MMR vaccine is administered subcutaneously into the anterolateral aspect of the thigh in smaller children or into the posterior triceps aspect of the upper arm in older children and adolescents. A 3/8- to 5/8-inch needle should be used for subcutaneous injections. The vaccine should not be injected intramuscularly or intravenously. The nurse should ensure the caregiver receives appropriate vaccine information according to the Centers for Disease Control and Prevention (CDC) or the Public Health Agency of Canada prior to administering a vaccine. According to the CDC and Public Health Agency of Canada, only two doses of the MMR vaccine are required, not three, and these doses should be separated by a minimum interval of 4 weeks.
CN: Health promotion and maintenance; CNS: None; CL: Apply

19. The nurse is caring for an adolescent receiving steroid therapy as a part of the cancer treatment plan. The adolescent tearfully asks the nurse, "Why does my face look so fat?" Which response by the nurse is appropriate?
1. "The facial tissues are retaining fluid as a result of your cancer."
2. "An activity plan to promote calorie use will be helpful for you."
3. "Drinking more fluids will help flush toxins and will reduce this look."
4. "This change is temporary and will subside once the steroid medication is not needed."

20. While assessing a child's skin integrity, the nurse notes a pruritic rash with some macules, papules, and vesicles. The rash is profuse on the trunk and sparse on the distal limbs. Which personal protective equipment (PPE) will the nurse apply when caring for this client? Select all that apply.
1. Gloves
2. Surgical mask
3. N95 respirator
4. Gown
5. Face shield

21. Which response is appropriate for the nurse to provide to a parent asking, "When can my child with chickenpox return to school?"
1. "When the child is afebrile."
2. "When all vesicles have dried."
3. "When vesicles begin to crust over."
4. "When lesions and vesicles are gone."

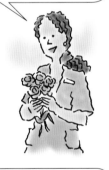

I'd much rather have roses than roseola.

22. A parent reports her child has roseola. Which clinical manifestations will the nurse expect to find during assessment?
1. Apparent sickness, fever, and rash
2. Rash, without history of fever or illness
3. Fever for 3 to 4 days, followed by rash
4. Rash for 3 to 4 days, followed by high fever

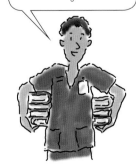

Your client with hemophilia has sudden hematuria, bruising, and joint pain. What should you do?

23. A pediatric client with hemophilia presents with hematuria, bruising, and joint pain that started suddenly after falling at home. The child's prothrombin time (PT) level is 19 seconds. Which nursing action is **priority**?
1. Give a desmopressin injection.
2. Assess the child's pain level.
3. Administer fresh frozen plasma.
4. Reassess the PT in an hour.

19. 4. Steroid therapy is associated with an increased roundness of the face. This may be a source of distress to the child and parents. It is important to explain this is the result of the medication therapy and will subside.
CN: Physiologic integrity; CNS: Pharmacological and parenteral therapies; CL: Apply

20. 1, 3, 4. The nurse should suspect that the child has varicella, which begins with a macule, rapidly progresses to a highly pruritic papule, and then becomes a vesicle. All three stages are present in varying degrees at one time. The child should be placed on airborne precautions immediately. The PPE required for airborne precautions are gloves, gown, and a respirator. A surgical mask or face shield would not be sufficient protection.
CN: Safe, effective care environment; CNS: Safety and infection control; CL: Analyze

21. 2. Chickenpox is contagious. It is transmitted through direct contact, droplet spread, and contact with contaminated objects. Vesicles break open; therefore, the child is considered contagious until all vesicles have dried. A child may be fever-free but continue to have vesicles and remain contagious. Some vesicles may be crusted over, but new ones may have formed so the child remains contagious. It is not necessary to wait until dried lesions have disappeared. Isolation is usually necessary only for about 1 week after the onset of the disease.
CN: Safe, effective care environment; CNS: Safety and infection control; CL: Apply

22. 3. Roseola is manifested by persistent high fever for 3 to 4 days followed by a rash. When the rash appears, a precipitous drop in fever occurs and the temperature returns to normal.
CN: Health promotion and maintenance; CNS: None; CL: Understand

23. 3. The nurse should administer fresh frozen plasma first to facilitate clotting. Desmopressin is given to stimulate the body to release more clotting factors but does not have an immediate effect. Assessing pain is not priority. The nurse should monitor the client's PT level, but this is not priority over controlling blood loss. A normal PT is 9 to 12 seconds.
CN: Safe, effective care environment; CNS: Management of care; CL: Analyze

24. The nurse expects the health care provider to prescribe which medication for a child who presents with a strawberry tongue; fine, red rash with the texture of sandpaper in the groin and behind the knees; fever; and a sore throat?
1. Acyclovir
2. Amphotericin B
3. Ibuprofen
4. Penicillin

24. 4. The nurse should suspect the child has scarlet fever. The causative agent of scarlet fever is group A beta-hemolytic streptococci, which are susceptible to penicillin. Erythromycin is used for penicillin-sensitive children. Acyclovir is used in the treatment of herpes infections. Amphotericin B is used to treat fungal infections. Anti-inflammatory drugs, such as ibuprofen, are not indicated for children with scarlet fever.

CN: Physiological integrity; CNS: Pharmacological and parenteral therapies; CL: Analyze

25. The nurse is caring for a 4-month-old infant who has recently tested positive for HIV. Which intervention(s) will the nurse include in the infant's care? Select all that apply.
1. Administer prophylactic sulfamethoxazole–trimethoprim for the first year of life.
2. Administer sulfamethoxazole–trimethoprim for the first 6 months after diagnosis.
3. Follow the recommended vaccination schedule in the absence of severe immunosuppression.
4. Place the infant on droplet precautions for the first year of life.
5. Initiate antiretroviral medications immediately upon diagnosis with HIV.

Remember, certain conditions affect children's vaccination schedules.

25. 1, 3, 5. The HIV-positive infant should begin antiretroviral medications at the time of diagnosis. These medications are used to delay the onset of illness and to strengthen the body's response in the event of infection. *Pneumocystis carinii* pneumonia is a common infection encountered by HIV-positive children. Health care providers should initiate prophylactic sulfamethoxazole–trimethoprim for the first year of life. Children should be scheduled to receive immunizations in the first year per the recommended schedule as long as there is no evidence of severe immunosuppression. The infant would not need to be placed on any precautions beyond contact.

CN: Physiological integrity; CNS: Pharmacological and parenteral therapies; CL: Apply

26. The nurse is educating the caregiver of a child diagnosed with rubella. Which information will the nurse include in the teaching?
1. This disorder is caused by exposure to a virus.
2. The child will be on droplet precautions for 7 days after the onset of the rash.
3. The rash starts on the face and spreads down the body.
4. The child should not be around pregnant women while contagious.

26. 4. Rubella (German measles) has a teratogenic effect on the fetus; therefore, children with rubella should avoid contact with pregnant women. All other information is correct regarding rubella.

CN: Safe, effective care environment; CNS: Safety and infection control; CL: Apply

27. A 2-year-old child presents to the clinic with rose-pink macules that blanch when mild pressure is applied. The parent states the child had a temperature of 103°F to 104°F (39.4°C to 40°C) a few days ago. Which prescription(s) does the nurse anticipate? Select all that apply.
1. Administer amoxicillin orally.
2. Alternate acetaminophen and ibuprofen for fever.
3. Give oatmeal baths with tepid water.
4. Apply hydrocortisone cream to macules.
5. Encourage increased fluid intake.

27. 2, 5. The nurse should suspect that the child has roseola. The rash associated with roseola is discrete, features rose-pink macules or maculopapules that blanch on pressure, and usually lasts 1 to 2 days. Treatment is symptomatic as roseola is viral. Acetaminophen and ibuprofen would be prescribed to prevent a febrile seizure. Fluid replacement is needed due to the history of a high fever to prevent dehydration. Antibiotics are given for viral illnesses. Oatmeal baths and hydrocortisone are not needed, as pruritus is not generally associated with roseola.

CN: Health promotion and maintenance; CNS: None; CL: Apply

28. A 2-year-old hospitalized child is HIV positive and has severe thrush. The child's anxious grandparents are at the bedside, continually calling the nurse with various concerns. The staff speaks disparagingly about them because they are tired of responding to the frequent call lights. When working with the unit's staff, which response by the nurse manager is **most** appropriate?
  1. "This situation will improve as you respond to the call light more promptly."
  2. "This couple is demanding, but we need to handle things in a professional manner."
  3. "It might be best to have the child transferred to a facility that is better staffed."
  4. "If we stop by the room before the light goes on, they may be less anxious."

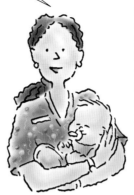

This is the part of the job I love.

28. 4. Although the situation may improve with more prompt responses to the call light, stopping by the room before the light goes on addresses the needs of the family. This response encourages the staff to be proactive and compassionate and provide prompt nursing intervention. The staff should handle the situation more professionally, providing individualized care based on the needs of the family. Transferring the child to a better-staffed facility is not a therapeutic solution.
CN: Safe, effective care environment; CNS: Management of care; CL: Apply

29. Which instruction will the nurse include when providing education to the parents of a child diagnosed with chickenpox?
  1. Administer penicillin as prescribed.
  2. Apply hydrocortisone cream to the lesions.
  3. Provide peer interaction as a distraction.
  4. The child can return to school in 2 days.

29. 2. Chickenpox is highly pruritic. Preventing the child from scratching is necessary to prevent scarring and secondary infection caused by irritation of lesions. Antibiotics are not used to treat chickenpox. Interaction with other children would be contraindicated due to the risk of disease transmission, unless the other children have previously had chickenpox or have been immunized. The child cannot return to school until all lesions have crusted.
CN: Safe, effective care environment; CNS: Safety and infection control; CL: Apply

30. The nurse is caring for a toddler diagnosed with scarlet fever. The parent asks when the child can return to day care. Which response by the nurse is appropriate?
  1. "The child can return once the diaper rash disappears."
  2. "The child cannot return until antibiotic therapy is complete."
  3. "The child can return once fever-free for 24 hours."
  4. "The child can return 24 hours after initiation of treatment."

30. 4. A child requires respiratory isolation until 24 hours after initiation of treatment. The rash may persist for 3 weeks. It is not necessary to wait until the end of treatment. The child usually becomes afebrile 24 hours after therapy has begun. It is not necessary to maintain isolation for an additional 24 hours.
CN: Safe, effective environment; CNS: Safety and infection control; CL: Apply

31. A pregnant woman recently found out she is HIV positive. When discussing the impact of the condition and care of the infant, what information will the nurse provide? Select all that apply.
  1. Definitively diagnosing a newborn with HIV is challenging during the first year of life.
  2. HIV symptoms typically develop in an infant beginning around 6 months of age.
  3. Taking antiviral medications during pregnancy will significantly lower the risk of HIV transmission to the baby.
  4. Vaginal birth will be permissible if the woman has been compliant with prescribed antiviral therapies.
  5. Breastfeeding is permissible in the first few weeks of life if the fetus is taking antiviral medication.

31. 1, 3. A confirmed diagnosis is difficult during the first 15 months because of the presence of maternal antibody. Symptoms are unlikely to present prior to 1 year of age in an infected newborn. The use of antiviral therapies in a pregnant woman who is HIV-positive can reduce the chance of transmission to the newborn to less than 1%. The recommended method of birth is cesarean section. Breastfeeding is not recommended for women who are HIV positive.
CN: Health promotion and maintenance; CNS: None; CL: Apply

32. A mother infected with human immunodeficiency virus (HIV) asks about breastfeeding her infant. Which response by the nurse is **best**?
1. "It is not advisable to breastfeed if you have HIV."
2. "Breastfeeding is safe for your infant if you have HIV."
3. "You can breastfeed your infant if you are taking zidovudine."
4. "It is best for you to supplement breastfeeding with formula."

33. The nurse is caring for a teen who was recently sexually assaulted and has concerns about becoming infected with HIV. Which symptom(s) associated with early infection will the nurse inform the client to report? Select all that apply.
1. Night sweats
2. Diarrhea
3. Enlarged lymph nodes in the groin region
4. Fatigue
5. Weight loss
6. Fever
7. Headache

34. The nurse working in a public health clinic is talking with a teen about having HIV testing. The teen is concerned about people finding out the results. Which statement will the nurse include when teaching the teen?
1. "When you are tested for HIV, the only people who will be told are your parents."
2. "HIV test results must be released to the local health department."
3. "You may choose to have confidential testing so only you can access your results."
4. "Anonymous testing will allow you to use a private ID number to retrieve your test results."

35. A child with sickle cell anemia is being treated for a vaso-occlusive crisis and reports significant discomfort. Which nursing action(s) is appropriate for this child? Select all that apply.
1. Cluster care interventions.
2. Encourage fluid intake.
3. Perform passive range-of-motion exercises.
4. Administer oxygen therapy as prescribed.
5. Assist the child into knee-chest position.

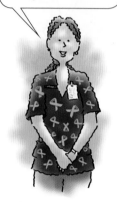

Keep an eye on that word "early" in question #33. It will point you to the right answers.

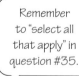

Remember to "select all that apply" in question #35.

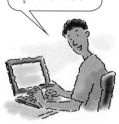

32. 1. Mothers infected with HIV should not breastfeed because the virus has been isolated in breast milk and can be transmitted to the infant. Taking zidovudine does not prevent transmission of the virus in breast milk, and supplementing breastfeeding with formula would not reduce exposure of the infant to the HIV virus in breast milk.
CN: Safe, effective care environment; CNS: Safety and infection control; CL: Apply

33. 3, 4, 6, 7. Early HIV infection has few clinical symptoms. These symptoms may be attributed to other factors or overlooked. Symptoms seen in the first weeks after infection include fever, headache, fatigue, and swollen lymph nodes in the neck or groin regions. Later symptoms seen in HIV infection include weight loss, night sweats, and diarrhea.
CN: Physiological integrity; CNS: Physiological adaptation; CL: Apply

34. 4. HIV testing is recommended for every individual ages 13 to 64 years at least once as a part of routine care. HIV testing may be performed either confidentially or anonymously. The confidential test allows the results to be tied to the individual. These results then become a part of the individual's permanent medical record. This makes the results available to insurance companies and health care providers who are involved with the individual. Anonymous testing assigns a personal identification number to the individual to retrieve the results and no other individuals or agencies will be privy to the results.
CN: Safe, effective care environment; CNS: Management of care; CL: Understand

35. 1, 2, 4. Sickle cell anemia is a condition characterized by red blood cells that are crescent or "sickle" in shape. At times these cells may become clumped in the blood vessels, resulting in what is referred to as a vaso-occlusive crisis. Interventions to promote increased comfort for this client include clustering of care activities. Clustering of care allows the child to have periods of rest and periods of organized activity. This reduces fatigue and discomfort for the child. Hydration is important in managing and preventing further facilitation of the crisis. Oxygen is often prescribed for the child in crisis. Range-of-motion exercises, although beneficial to promote joint mobility, do not improve comfort to the individual who is experiencing pain related to a vaso-occlusive crisis. Knee-chest positioning would not be of benefit to this client.
CN: Physiological integrity; CNS: Basic care and comfort; CL: Apply

36. The nurse is assessing a child with sickle cell anemia. The nurse will assess the child for which bone-related complication?
1. Arthritis
2. Osteoporosis
3. Osteogenic sarcoma
4. Spontaneous fractures

37. The nurse caring for a child with sickle cell anemia who is experiencing a vaso-occlusive crisis avoids palpating the child's abdomen. The nurse knows this action could lead to which result?
1. Splenic rupture
2. Vomiting
3. Increased abdominal pain
4. Blood cell destruction

38. A child tests positive for the sickle cell trait and the parents ask the nurse what this means. Which response by the nurse is **most** appropriate?
1. "This means your child has sickle cell anemia."
2. "Your child is a carrier but does not have the disease."
3. "Your child is a carrier and will pass the disease to any offspring."
4. "Your child does not have the disease now but may develop the disease."

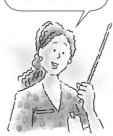

Great job! You really know how to stick to it.

39. When caring for a child with sickle cell anemia in vaso-occlusive crisis, which nursing intervention is **priority**?
1. Manage pain.
2. Provide a cool environment.
3. Immobilize the affected part.
4. Restrict fluids.

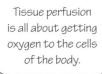

Tissue perfusion is all about getting oxygen to the cells of the body.

40. Which nursing intervention is **most** effective in maximizing tissue perfusion for a child in vaso-occlusive crisis?
1. Administer analgesics.
2. Monitor intravenous fluids.
3. Encourage activity as tolerated.
4. Administer oxygen as prescribed.

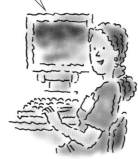

36. 2. Sickle cell anemia causes hyperplasia and congestion of the bone marrow, resulting in osteoporosis. Arthritis does not occur secondary to sickle cell anemia; however, a crisis can cause localized swelling over joints, resulting in arthralgia. Bones do weaken, but spontaneous fractures do not occur as a result. Osteogenic sarcoma is bone cancer; sickle cell anemia does not cause bone cancer.
CN: Physiological integrity; CNS: Physiological adaptation; CL: Apply

37. 1. Palpating a child's abdomen in a vaso-occlusive crisis should be avoided because sequestered red blood cells may precipitate splenic rupture. Abdominal pain alone is not a reason to avoid palpation. Vomiting or blood cell destruction does not occur from palpation of the abdomen.
CN: Physiological integrity; CNS: Reduction of risk potential; CL: Analyze

38. 2. A child with sickle cell trait is only a carrier and may never show any symptoms, except under special hypoxic conditions. A child with sickle cell trait does not have the disease and will never test positive for sickle cell anemia. Sickle cell anemia would be transmitted to offspring only as the result of a union between two individuals who are positive for the trait.
CN: Health promotion and maintenance; CNS: None; CL: Apply

39. 1. Pain management is an important aspect in the care of a child with sickle cell anemia in vaso-occlusive crisis. The goal is to prevent sickling. This can be accomplished by promoting tissue oxygenation, adequate hydration, and rest, which minimize energy expenditure and oxygen utilization. A cool environment can cause vasoconstriction and thus more sickling and pain. Immobilization can promote stasis and increase sickling.
CN: Physiological integrity; CNS: Basic care and comfort; CL: Apply

40. 4. Administering oxygen is the most effective way to maximize tissue perfusion. Short-term oxygen therapy helps to prevent hypoxia, which leads to metabolic acidosis, causing sickling. Long-term oxygen therapy depresses erythropoiesis. Analgesics are used to control pain. Hydration is essential to promote hemodilution and maintain electrolyte balance. Bed rest should be promoted to reduce oxygen utilization.
CN: Safe, effective care environment; CNS: Management of care; CL: Analyze

41. Which nursing action is **most** important to decrease the risk of postoperative complications in a child with sickle cell anemia?
 1. Increasing fluids
 2. Preparing the child psychologically
 3. Discouraging coughing
 4. Limiting the use of analgesics

41. **1.** The main surgical risk from anesthesia is hypoxia; however, emotional stress, demands of wound healing, and the potential for infection can each increase the sickling phenomenon. Increased fluids are encouraged because keeping the child well-hydrated is most important for hemodilution to prevent sickling. Preparing the child psychologically to decrease fear minimizes undue emotional stress. Deep coughing is encouraged to promote pulmonary hygiene and prevent respiratory tract infection. Analgesics are used to control wound pain and to prevent abdominal splinting and decreased ventilation.
CN: Safe, effective care environment; CNS: Management of care; CL: Apply

42. Which instruction is **priority** for the clinic nurse to include when educating the parents about prevention of infection in their child with sickle cell anemia?
 1. Perform adequate handwashing.
 2. Avoid emotional stress.
 3. Visit the health care provider when sick.
 4. Avoid strenuous physical exertion.

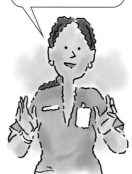

The two biggest problems in a sickle cell crisis are dehydration and pain. What interventions are best at addressing these issues?

42. **1.** The nurse must emphasize the importance of adequate handwashing as the priority to prevent infection in children with sickle cell anemia. Frequent medical supervision can prevent infection, often a predisposing factor toward development of a crisis. Avoiding stress and strenuous physical exertion helps prevent sickling, but adequate handwashing remains priority.
CN: Safe, effective care environment; CNS: Management of care; CL: Analyze

43. The nurse is working in the emergency department when a child is admitted in sickle cell crisis. Which intervention(s) will the nurse expect to perform? Select all that apply.
 1. Give blood transfusions.
 2. Administer antibiotics.
 3. Increase fluid intake.
 4. Administered morphine.
 5. Prepare the child for a splenectomy.
 6. Apply oxygen via a nasal cannula.

43. **3, 4, 6.** The primary therapy for sickle cell crisis is to increase fluid intake (according to age), give analgesics, and administer oxygen. Blood transfusions are given conservatively to avoid iron overload. Antibiotics are given to children with fever. Routine splenectomy is not recommended. Splenectomy in a child with sickle cell anemia is controversial.
CN: Physiological integrity; CNS: Physiological adaptation; CL: Apply

44. The health care provider has prescribed diagnostic testing for a client suspected of having thalassemia. When reviewing this client's laboratory results, which finding(s) does the nurse determine are consistent with the disorder? Select all that apply.
 1. Hemoglobin 8.8 g/dL (88 g/L)
 2. Platelet 200,000 mm^3
 3. Hematocrit 36% (0.36)
 4. Red blood cell count $2.9 \times 10^6/\mu L$ ($2.9 \times 10^{12}/L$)
 5. White blood cell count $5.2 /\mu L$ ($5.2 \times 10^9/L$)

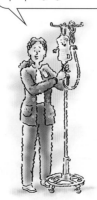

Remember to keep clients who are having a vaso-occlusive crisis properly hydrated.

44. **1, 4.** A complete blood cell count can be anticipated in the client suspected of having thalassemia. In thalassemia the number of red blood cells and hemoglobin level are reduced. A normal hemoglobin level for the client in this age group would be 12.5 to 16.1 g/dL (125 to 161 g/L). The normal range for red blood cell count for a client in this age range would be 4.1 to $5.3 \times 10^6/\mu L$ (4.1 to $5.3 \times 10^{12}/L$). The hematocrit level, white blood cell count, and platelet count are within normal range.
CN: Physiological integrity; CNS: Physiological adaptation; CL: Analyze

45. When assessing a child with sickle cell anemia, which finding will **most** concern the nurse?
 1. Pain upon urination
 2. Pain with ambulation
 3. Reports of throat pain
 4. Fever with associated rash

45. **2.** Bone pain, such as may occur with ambulation, is one of the major symptoms of vaso-occlusive crisis. Painful urination and throat pain could indicate subsequent infections. Fever is one of the major symptoms of vaso-occlusive crisis but is not associated with rash. All findings are concerning; however, treating a vaso-occlusive crisis is priority.
CN: Safe, effective care environment; CNS: Management of care; CL: Analyze

46. The nurse is caring for a child who has just been diagnosed with sickle cell anemia. Which initial nursing action is **most** therapeutic for this client?
1. Discuss plans for contraception with the parents.
2. Refer the parents for genetic counseling.
3. Offer emotional support to the child and parents.
4. Ensure that the parents understand that illness is easy to treat.

46. 3. The nurse can be instrumental in providing support, encouragement, and correct information to the parents of a child newly diagnosed with sickle cell anemia. Offering emotional support to the child and parents is the most therapeutic initial action. Selective birth control methods, such as in vitro fertilization of an embryo without markers for sickle cell disease, should be discussed, but after the nurse has provided emotional support and when the parents are ready. All heterozygous, or trait-positive, parents should be referred for genetic counseling, but offering emotional support would be more appropriate initially. Sickle cell disorder requires complex care.
CN: Psychological integrity; CNS: None; CL: Apply

47. A 14-year-old client is admitted for sickle cell crisis. Which nursing intervention is **most** important?
1. Allow the child's friends to visit the child in the hospital.
2. Monitor the child's temperature every 2 hours.
3. Provide adequate oxygenation, hydration, and pain management.
4. Make sure the family is involved in every step of the child's care.

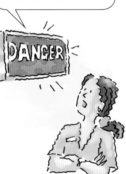

Be on the lookout for these symptoms of a transfusion reaction—it's serious business.

47. 3. The most critical need of a child in sickle cell crisis is to provide adequate oxygenation, hydration, and pain management until the crisis passes. Obtaining a temperature every 2 hours is not the priority intervention. Although allowing friends to visit an adolescent and involving the family in the child's care are important, they are not the priority interventions during a sickle cell crisis.
CN: Safe, effective care environment; CNS: Management of care; CL: Analyze

48. The nurse is administering a blood transfusion to a child with sickle cell anemia. The nurse notes urticaria, flushing, and wheezing while assessing the child. Which nursing intervention is **priority**?
1. Assess the oxygen saturation level.
2. Administer normal saline.
3. Notify the health care provider.
4. Stop the blood transfusion.

48. 4. The nurse should recognize these as signs of an allergic reaction and stop the transfusion immediately. The nurse should administer normal saline intravenously, check the oxygen saturation level, and notify the health care provider after stopping the transfusion.
CN: Physiological integrity; CNS: Reduction of risk potential; CL: Analyze

49. A parent of a toddler asks the clinic nurse how often the influenza vaccine should be given to the child. Which response is **most** accurate?
1. "The vaccine is usually given annually to children with certain risk factors."
2. "I would not worry about influenza; your child does not need the vaccine."
3. "The vaccine is given every other year to children at their yearly examination."
4. "It is given annually to kids 6 months of age and older during fall and winter months."

49. 4. The influenza virus vaccine is recommended to be administered annually to all children 6 months and older during the fall and winter months, not just to children with certain risk factors or every other year.
CN: Health promotion and maintenance; CNS: None; CL: Apply

50. A 3-year-old sibling of a neonate is diagnosed with pertussis. Which information will the clinic nurse include when educating the parent about possible infection of the neonate?
1. The neonate will inevitably contract pertussis
2. Immune globulin is effective in protecting the neonate
3. The risk to the neonate depends on the parent's immune status
4. Erythromycin will be administered prophylactically to the neonate

50. 4. In exposed, high-risk clients, such as neonates, erythromycin may be effective in preventing or lessening the severity of pertussis if administered during the pre-paroxysmal stage. Immune globulin is not indicated; it is used as an immunization against hepatitis A. Neonates exposed to pertussis are at considerable risk, regardless of the parent's immune status; however, infection is not inevitable.
CN: Health promotion and maintenance; CNS: None; CL: Apply

CN: Client needs category   CNS: Client needs subcategory   CL: Cognitive level

51. A child has recently been admitted to the pediatric unit with a hemoglobin A2 level of 6% (0.06). Based on this finding, the nurse plans care for which complication?
1. Beta-thalassemia trait
2. Iron deficiency
3. Lead poisoning
4. Sickle cell anemia

52. A 4-year-old is asymptomatic but has a petechial rash. The client's platelet count is 20,000 μL (20 × 10⁹/L), and the hemoglobin level and white blood cell (WBC) count are normal. Which diagnosis does the nurse **most** likely suspect?
1. Acute lymphocytic leukemia (ALL)
2. Disseminated intravascular coagulation (DIC)
3. Idiopathic thrombocytopenic purpura (ITP)
4. Systemic lupus erythematosus (SLE)

53. A child has been diagnosed with leukemia. Which finding **most** concerns the nurse?
1. Presence of a mediastinal mass
2. Late central nervous system leukemia
3. White blood cell (WBC) count of 11,000/μL (5 × 10⁹/L)
4. The child being 4 years of age

54. Which action is **most** important for the nurse to incorporate when providing education to the parents of a neonate diagnosed with sickle cell anemia?
1. Stress the importance of folic acid supplementation.
2. Show how to give monthly vitamin B$_{12}$ injections.
3. Teach how to take an accurate temperature.
4. Emphasize the importance of getting immunizations.

55. The nurse is providing education to the parents of an adolescent newly diagnosed with Hodgkin's lymphoma. Which statement(s) will the nurse include? Select all that apply.
1. "Bring your child in for evaluation if the child has a temperature above 100.4°F (38°C)."
2. "Your child may experience severe itching, leading to excoriated skin."
3. "Recent advances in medicine have greatly improved the outcome of this disease."
4. "Secondary malignancies are a severe complication of Hodgkin's lymphoma."
5. "Your child will receive multiple chemotherapeutic agents during treatment."

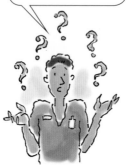

Confused by all the data in question #52? Try focusing on the words "petechial rash."

51. 1. The concentration of hemoglobin A2 is increased with the beta-thalassemia trait. In severe iron deficiency, hemoglobin A2 may be decreased. The hemoglobin A2 level is normal in lead poisoning and sickle cell anemia.
CN: Physiological integrity; CNS: Reduction of risk potential; CL: Apply

52. 3. The onset of ITP typically occurs between ages 1 and 6. Children with ITP are asymptomatic, except for a petechial rash and a low platelet count. ALL is associated with a low platelet count, as well, but an abnormal hemoglobin level and WBC count. DIC is secondary to a severe underlying disease. SLE is rare in a 4-year-old child.
CN: Safe, effective care environment; CNS: Management of care; CL: Analyze

53. 1. The presence of a mediastinal mass indicates a poor prognosis for children with leukemia and would be very concerning. Early central nervous system leukemia and a WBC count of 100,000/μL or higher indicate a poor prognosis for a child with leukemia. The prognosis is poorer if age at onset is less than 2 years or greater than 10 years.
CN: Safe, effective care environment; CNS: Management of care; CL: Analyze

54. 3. Parents should be able to take an accurate temperature. A temperature of 101.3°F to 102.2°F (38.5°C to 39°C) calls for emergency evaluation, even if the neonate appears well. Folic acid requirement is increased in sickle cell anemia; therefore, supplementation is prudent. However, it is not as important as taking accurate temperature readings. Vitamin B$_{12}$ supplementation is not necessary. Parents should be encouraged to keep the immunizations up to date, but this is not as important as taking accurate temperature readings.
CN: Safe, effective care environment; CNS: Management of care; CL: Analyze

55. 1, 2, 3, 4, 5. Children with Hodgkin's lymphoma should be evaluated for secondary symptoms, including fevers, night sweats, unexplained weight loss, and severe pruritus. The outcome for these clients has improved, with more than 90% living more than 5 years with treatment. Secondary malignancies are one of the most severe long-term complications. Effective treatment does include administration of multiple chemotherapeutic agents and possible radiation.
CN: Physiological integrity; CNS: Physiological adaptation; CL: Apply

56. A 1-year-old infant is pale, but the assessment is otherwise normal. Blood studies reveal a hematocrit of 24% (0.24). Which question by the nurse to the parents will be **most** useful in helping to establish a diagnosis of anemia?
1. "Is the infant on any medications?"
2. "What is the infant's usual daily diet?"
3. "Did the infant receive phototherapy for jaundice?"
4. "What is the pattern and appearance of bowel movements?"

57. The nurse assesses a child and notes the following: temperature of 101.1°F (38.4°C), pruritus, and a generalized rash with macules, papules, vesicles, and crusts. The caregiver reports the child is immunocompromised. Which health care provider prescription(s) will the nurse question? Select all that apply.
1. Complete blood count
2. Acetylsalicylic acid orally
3. Acyclovir liquid suspension
4. Topical diphenhydramine cream
5. Placement in a negative pressure room

58. A 14-year-old is seen at the clinic with a history of a mild sore throat, low-grade fever, and diffuse maculopapular rash and reports swelling of the wrists and redness in the eyes. The nurse will interpret these findings as indications of which condition?
1. Rubella
2. Rubeola
3. Roseola
4. Varicella

59. The nurse is caring for a toddler diagnosed with iron deficiency anemia. The child's current hemoglobin level is 9 g/dL (90 g/L). The nurse will anticipate educating the child and parents on which treatment option?
1. Blood transfusion
2. Oral ferrous sulfate
3. An iron-fortified cereal
4. Intramuscular iron dextran

60. The nurse will assess which client diagnosed with hemophilia **first**?
1. The client reporting a "bad headache"
2. The client with bruises in various stages
3. The client experiencing mild epistaxis
4. The client whose left knee is swollen and red

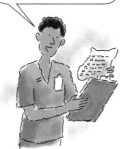

What's the most likely cause of anemia in a 1-year-old?

56. 2. Iron deficiency anemia is the most common nutritional deficiency in infants 9 to 15 months old. Anemia in a 1-year-old is mostly nutritional in origin, and its cause would be suggested by a detailed nutrition history. The other questions would not be helpful in diagnosing anemia.
CN: Safe, effective care environment; CNS: Management of care; CL: Apply

57. 2. The nurse should question administering acetylsalicylic acid to a child with varicella, and this child is showing signs of varicella. Administering salicylate products to a pediatric client during afebrile illness places the client at risk for Reye's syndrome. All other prescriptions are appropriate for an immunocompromised client with varicella.
CN: Safe, effective care environment; CNS: Management of care; CL: Apply

58. 1. Rubella presents with a diffuse maculopapular rash, mild sore throat, low-grade fever, and, occasionally, conjunctivitis, arthralgia, or arthritis. Rubeola is associated with high fever, which reaches its peak at the height of a generalized macular rash and typically lasts for 5 days. Roseola involves high fever and is abruptly followed by a rash. Varicella presents with fever; small erythematous macules on the trunk or scalp, which progress to papules; and clear vesicles on an erythematous base.
CN: Physiological integrity; CNS: Physiological adaptation; CL: Analyze

59. 2. A prompt rise in hemoglobin level and hematocrit follows the administration of oral ferrous sulfate. The hemoglobin level is low but not critical. Blood transfusion is rarely indicated unless a child becomes symptomatic or is further compromised by a superimposed infection. Dietary modifications are appropriate long-term measures, but these modifications will not make enough iron quickly available to replenish iron stores. Intramuscular iron dextran is reserved for use when compliance cannot be achieved; it is expensive, painful, and no more effective than oral iron.
CN: Physiological integrity; CNS: Pharmacological and parenteral therapies; CL: Analyze

60. 1. The nurse should assess the client reporting a "bad headache" first, as this is a sign of increased intracranial pressure from intracranial hemorrhage. Bruises in various stages, epistaxis, and swollen joints are expected findings in a client with hemophilia.
CN: Safe, effective care environment; CNS: Management of care; CL: Analyze

61. Which statement by a caregiver indicates to the nurse a 10-month-old infant is at **high** risk for iron deficiency anemia?
1. "The baby is sleeping through the night without a bottle."
2. "The baby drinks about five 8 oz bottles of milk per day."
3. "The baby likes to eat egg yolk for breakfast several times a week."
4. "The baby likes all vegetables except carrots and most fruits."

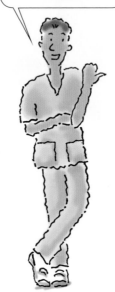

Drinking too much milk means not eating enough solid food. Those little tummies can only hold so much, after all.

62. An iron dextran injection has been prescribed for an 8-month-old baby with iron deficiency anemia. When providing information about the medication to the parents, which statement by the parents indicates to the nurse the need for further instruction?
1. "Most side effects of this medication will be noted within 12 hours of administration."
2. "If my child experiences any side effects, they should subside within 3 to 4 days."
3. "This medication will work to increase my baby's red blood cell count."
4. "Our child will need to have serum blood testing in the future."

63. When providing education to parents about preventing nutritional iron deficiency, the nurse will emphasize including which food(s) in the child's diet? Select all that apply.
1. Peas
2. Fish
3. Beans
4. Milk products
5. Dried fruits

64. Which instruction will the nurse include when teaching the parents about proper administration of oral iron supplements to a preschool-age child? Select all that apply.
1. Give the supplements with food or mixed in a small amount of food.
2. Stop the medication if the child experiences vomiting.
3. Follow the medication's administration with a glass of milk.
4. Allow the child to drink the medicine through a straw.
5. Increase dietary intake of fruits, vegetables, and fiber to prevent constipation.

61. 2. The recommended intake of milk, which does not contain iron, is 24 oz/day; 40 oz/day exceeds the recommended allotment and may reduce iron intake from solid food sources, risking iron deficiency anemia. Sleeping through the night without a bottle is an anticipated behavior at this age. Egg yolk is a good source of iron and would minimize any risk factor related to nutritional anemia. Because only dark-green vegetables are good sources of iron, a dislike of carrots would not be significant for this client.
CN: Physiological integrity; CNS: Basic care and comfort; CL: Analyze

62. 1. When iron dextran injection is administered to clients with anemia, the majority of side effects manifest within about 24 hours of administration. The remaining statements are correct.
CN: Physiological integrity; CNS: Pharmacological and parenteral therapies; CL: Apply

63. 1, 3, 5. Good dietary sources of iron include red meat, peas, beans, leafy green vegetables, and dried fruits such as apricots and raisins. Fish is not a good source of dietary iron. Milk is deficient in iron and should be limited in cases of nutritional anemia.
CN: Physiological integrity; CNS: Basic care and comfort; CL: Apply

64. 4, 5. Liquid iron preparations may temporarily stain the teeth; therefore, the drug should be given by dropper or through a straw, depending on the age of the child. Constipation can be decreased by increasing intake of fiber. Supplements should be given between meals, when the presence of free hydrochloric acid is greatest. If vomiting occurs, supplementation should not be stopped; instead, it should be administered with food.
CN: Physiological integrity; CNS: Pharmacological and parenteral therapies; CL: Apply

65. While assessing a child, the nurse recognizes which finding as the primary clinical manifestation of hemophilia?
1. Petechiae on the face
2. Prolonged bleeding time
3. Decreased clotting time
4. Decreased white blood cell (WBC) count

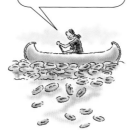

Looks like there's no absence of clotting factors here.

66. The nurse is providing discharge education for the parents of a child with hemophilia. The nurse will prepare them to initiate which **immediate** treatment(s) if the child experiences external bleeding? Select all that apply.
1. Apply an ice pack to the affected area.
2. Withhold factor replacement.
3. Apply pressure for at least 10 minutes.
4. Immobilize the affected area.
5. Elevate the affected area.

67. A child with hemophilia is hospitalized with internal bleeding at the right knee. Which action will the nurse take **first**?
1. Administer a whole blood transfusion.
2. Provide a plasma transfusion.
3. Perform range-of-motion (ROM) exercises.
4. Elevate the affected extremity.

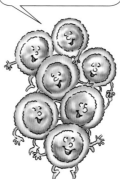

Look, guys—there's the laceration. Now clump together and chant, "Hemostasis."

68. Which information will the nurse discuss with the parents of a child with hemophilia to limit joint degeneration?
1. Avoiding the use of analgesics
2. Using aspirin for pain relief
3. Administering replacement factor
4. Using active range-of-motion (ROM) exercises

69. A pediatric client is diagnosed with von Willebrand disease. The nurse will monitor which area **most** closely for bleeding?
1. Brain tissue
2. Gastrointestinal (GI) tract
3. Mucous membranes
4. Spinal cord

65. 2. The effect of hemophilia is prolonged bleeding, anywhere from or within the body. With severe deficiencies, hemorrhage can occur as a result of minor trauma. Petechiae are uncommon in persons with hemophilia because repair of small hemorrhages depends on platelet function, not on blood clotting mechanisms. Clotting time is increased in a client with hemophilia. A decrease in WBCs is not indicative of hemophilia.
CN: Physiological integrity; CNS: Physiological adaptation; CL: Understand

66. 1, 3, 4, 5. Immobilizing and elevating the area above the level of the heart decreases blood flow. Application of cold promotes vasoconstriction and decreases bleeding. Pressure should be applied to the area for at least 10 to 15 minutes to allow clot formation. Factor replacement should not be delayed.
CN: Safe, effective care environment; CNS: Safety and infection control; CL: Apply

67. 4. Bleeding into the joints is the most common type of bleeding episode in the more severe hemophilia forms. Elevating the affected part and applying pressure and cold are indicated. The nurse should anticipate transfusing the missing clotting factor, not whole blood or plasma, which would not stop the bleeding promptly and might pose a risk of fluid overload. Active ROM exercises are contraindicated because they may cause more bleeding, injury, and pain.
CN: Safe, effective care environment; CNS: Management of care; CL: Apply

68. 3. Prevention of bleeding is the ideal goal and is achieved by factor replacement therapy. Analgesics should be administered before physical therapy to control pain and provide the maximum benefit. Acetaminophen should be used for pain relief because aspirin has anticoagulant effects and has been linked to Reye's syndrome. Passive ROM exercises are usually instituted after the acute phase.
CN: Physiological integrity; CNS: Physiological adaptation; CL: Apply

69. 3. The most characteristic clinical feature of von Willebrand disease is an increased tendency to bleed from mucous membranes, which may be seen as frequent nosebleeds or menorrhagia. In hemophilia, the joint cavities are the most common site of internal bleeding. Bleeding into the GI tract, spinal cord, and brain tissue can occur, but these are not the most common sites for bleeding.
CN: Safe, effective care environment; CNS: Management of care; CL: Apply

70. Which nursing action(s) will be appropriate for the child with von Willebrand disease (VWD) experiencing epistaxis? Select all that apply.
1. Lay the client in a supine position.
2. Pack the nostrils with sterile gauze.
3. Pinch the end of the child's nose.
4. Apply pressure to the nose.
5. Have the child sit leaning forward.

70. 2, 4, 5. Applying pressure to the nose may stop bleeding because most bleeds occur in the anterior part of the nasal septum. The child should be instructed to sit up and lean forward to avoid aspiration of blood. Pressure should then be maintained for at least 10 minutes, just above the nostrils, to allow clotting to occur. Packing with tissue or cotton may be used to help stop bleeding, although care must be taken in removing packing to avoid dislodging the clot.
CN: Physiological integrity; CNS: Physiological adaptation; CL: Apply

71. The nurse is assessing a child diagnosed with acute lymphocytic leukemia (ALL) in the hospital. Which nursing action is **priority**?
1. Check the intravenous site.
2. Monitor blood work.
3. Assess the pain rating.
4. Palpate cervical lymph nodes.

Ready for some adventures in assessment? Make sure you're equipped with all the right gear.

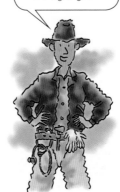

71. 1. It is priority for the nurse to assess the child with ALL for infection, such as at the intravenous site. The nurse should monitor the child's laboratory values and notify the health care provider as needed. The nurse would also assess the child for pain and intervene as needed. Painless swelling of cervical lymph nodes is expected in children with ALL.
CN: Safe, effective care environment; CNS: Management of care; CL: Analyze

72. The nurse is educating the parents of a child with leukemia about complications to monitor for at home. Which complication(s) will the nurse include in the teaching? Select all that apply.
1. Bone deformities
2. Spherocytosis
3. Anemia
4. Infection
5. Delayed growth
6. Decreased clotting time
7. Bleeding tendencies

72. 3, 4, 7. The three main complications of leukemia are anemia, caused by decreased erythrocyte production; infection secondary to neutropenia; and bleeding tendencies from decreased platelet production. Bone deformities do not occur with leukemia. Spherocytosis refers to erythrocytes taking on a spheroid shape and is not a feature of leukemia. Growth delay can be a result of large doses of steroids but is not common in leukemia. Clotting times would be prolonged.
CN: Physiological integrity; CNS: Physiological adaptation; CL: Apply

73. The nurse is assessing a child reporting bone and joint pain. Which additional finding(s) will lead the nurse to suspect the child has leukemia? Select all that apply.
1. Fever
2. Pallor
3. Abdominal pain
4. Unexplained weight gain
5. Diarrhea
6. Petechiae
7. Fatigue

73. 1, 2, 3, 6, 7. Signs and symptoms of leukemia result from infiltration of the bone marrow. These include petechiae, fever, pallor, abdominal pain, fatigue, weight loss (not gain), anorexia, and joint pain with decreased activity level. Diarrhea is not a finding associated with ALL.
CN: Physiological integrity; CNS: Physiological adaptation; CL: Apply

74. The nurse is preparing a child newly diagnosed with leukemia for a spinal tap. The parents state, "Why is the health care provider doing this?" What is the **best** response by the nurse?
1. "It will rule out bacterial meningitis."
2. "It will decrease intracranial pressure (ICP)."
3. "It will aid in classification of the leukemia."
4. "It will assess for central nervous system infiltration."

74. 4. A spinal tap is performed to assess for central nervous system infiltration. A spinal tap can be done to rule out meningitis, but this is not the reason for the test on a child with leukemia. A spinal tap does not decrease ICP or aid in the classification of the leukemia.
CN: Safe, effective care environment; CNS: Management of care; CL: Apply

75. Which finding(s) in a child with leukemia will the nurse determine indicates the cancer has metastasized to the brain? Select all that apply.
1. Headache
2. Vomiting
3. Restlessness
4. Tachycardia
5. Hypervigilance
6. Anxious behavior
7. Hypotension

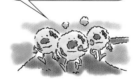

Remember to select all that apply in question #75.

75. 1, 2. The usual effect of leukemic infiltration of the brain is increased intracranial pressure. The proliferation of cells interferes with the flow of cerebrospinal fluid in the subarachnoid space and at the base of the brain. The increased fluid pressure causes dilation of the ventricles, which creates symptoms of severe headache, vomiting, irritability, lethargy, increased blood pressure, decreased heart rate, and, eventually, coma. Children with a variety of illnesses are typically hypervigilant and anxious when hospitalized.
CN: Physiological integrity; CNS: Physiological adaptation; CL: Analyze

76. The nurse is caring for an adolescent diagnosed with acute lymphocytic leukemia. A review of the laboratory report indicates a platelet count of 125,500/µL (125 × 10^9/L). Which assessment finding is **most** consistent with this laboratory result?
1. Abdominal swelling
2. Joint swelling
3. Bruising
4. Swollen axillary lymph nodes

76. 3. Platelet production may be impaired in the client with leukemia. A platelet count of 125,000/µL (125 × 10^9/L) is less than normal. This may be accompanied by bruising or reports of nosebleeds. The child with leukemia may experience abdominal swelling resulting from an accumulation of leukemia cells in the abdomen. Joint swelling may result from an accumulation of leukemia cells in the joint. Swollen lymph nodes are often seen in leukemia and result from the body attempting to fight the illness.
CN: Safe, effective care environment; CNS: Management of care; CL: Apply.

77. Before the initiation of chemotherapy, the nurse will prepare a pediatric client with leukemia for which test?
1. Lumbar puncture
2. Liver function studies
3. Complete blood count (CBC)
4. Peripheral blood smear

Never fear! The white blood cells are here. Now where's that pesky invader?

77. 2. Liver and kidney function studies are done before initiation of chemotherapy to evaluate the child's ability to metabolize the chemotherapeutic agents. A lumbar puncture is performed to assess for central nervous system infiltration. A CBC is performed to assess for anemia. A peripheral blood smear is done to assess the level of immature white blood cells (blastocytes).
CN: Physiological integrity; CNS: Pharmacological and parenteral therapies; CL: Apply

78. When providing education for an adolescent with iron deficiency anemia about diet choices, which menu selection by the adolescent indicates to the nurse more teaching is needed?
1. Caesar salad, pretzels, and 2% milk
2. Cheeseburger, carrot sticks, and milkshake
3. Red beans, rice with sausage, and juice
4. Egg sandwich, peanuts, and water

78. 1. Caesar salad, milk, and pretzels are not foods high in iron and protein. Meats (especially organ meats), eggs, beans, and nuts have high protein and iron.
CN: Physiological integrity; CNS: Basic care and comfort; CL: Apply

79. The nurse is providing discharge education to a parent of a child on methotrexate. The parent asks the nurse how the drug works. Which statement by the nurse is **most** accurate?
1. "The drug interferes with the use of folic acid by cancer cells."
2. "The drug keeps the cancer cell wall from forming."
3. "The drug makes the cancer cells ineffective by massing them together."
4. "The drug interferes with mitochondrial activity."

79. 1. Methotrexate is an antimetabolite and antifolate. It prevents folic acid from being used to create nucleic acid. As a result, it interferes with mitosis, which prevents the cancer cells from multiplying. It does not interfere with the cell wall, cause massing of the cells, or interfere with mitochondrial activity.
CN: Physiological integrity; CNS: Pharmacological and parenteral therapies; CL: Understand

CN: Client needs category   CNS: Client needs subcategory   CL: Cognitive level

80. A 4-year-old child is diagnosed as having acute lymphocytic leukemia. The white blood cell (WBC) count is 3,000 µ/L (3 × 10⁹/L) and platelet count is 180,000 × 10³/L (80 × 10⁹/L). Which education is **priority** for the nurse to teach the parents?

1. Protect the child from falls because of the increased risk of bleeding.
2. Protect the child from infections because the resistance to infection is decreased.
3. Provide the child with frequent rest periods throughout the day.
4. Treat constipation, which frequently accompanies a decrease in WBCs.

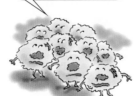

Immune cells of the body unite! And get ready to fight.

80. 2. One of the complications of both acute lymphocytic leukemia and its treatment is a decreased WBC count, specifically a decreased absolute neutrophil count. Because neutrophils are the body's first line of defense against infection, the child must be protected from infection. Bleeding is a risk factor if platelets or other coagulation factors are decreased. A decreased hemoglobin level, hematocrit, or both would reduce the oxygen-carrying capacity of the child's blood and cause the child to need more frequent rest periods throughout the day. Constipation is not related to the WBC count.
CN: Safe, effective care environment; CNS: Safety and infection control; CL: Apply

81. Which medication, administered as prophylaxis against pneumocystis pneumonia, does the nurse anticipate providing education on for a child diagnosed with leukemia?

1. Sulfamethoxazole–trimethoprim
2. Oral nystatin suspension
3. Prednisone
4. Vincristine sulfate

81. 1. The most common cause of death from leukemia is overwhelming infection. Pneumocystis pneumonia infection is lethal to a child with leukemia. As prophylaxis against pneumocystis pneumonia, continuous low dosages of sulfamethoxazole–trimethoprim are usually prescribed. Oral nystatin suspension would be indicated for the treatment of thrush. Prednisone is not an antibiotic and increases susceptibility to infection. Vincristine sulfate is an antineoplastic agent.
CN: Physiological integrity; CNS: Pharmacological and parenteral therapies; CL: Apply

82. A child is admitted to the pediatric unit with an unknown mass in the lower left abdomen. Which nursing action is **priority**?

1. Obtain the history of the illness from the caregivers.
2. Place a "Do Not Palpate Abdomen" sign over the bed.
3. Obtain a complete set of vital signs from the child.
4. Schedule a hemoglobin and hematocrit test for early morning.

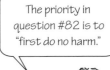

The priority in question #82 is to "first do no harm."

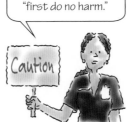

Caution

82. 2. The nurse must take measures to prevent palpation of the mass, if possible. If the mass is a malignant tumor, a do-not-palpate warning would help prevent trauma and rupture of the suspected tumor capsule. Rupture of the tumor capsule may cause seeding of cancer cells throughout the abdomen. Obtaining the history and vital signs and scheduling laboratory work are important but not the priority.
CN: Safe, effective care environment; CNS: Management of care; CL: Analyze

83. The nurse is caring for a client who has painful mouth ulcers that have resulted from chemotherapy treatments. Which nursing action(s) will be beneficial in promoting comfort for this client? Select all that apply.

1. Use lemon glycerin swabs.
2. Administer milk of magnesia.
3. Provide a bland, moist, soft diet.
4. Use alcohol-based mouthwash.
5. Provide a straw with drinks.

83. 3, 5. Oral ulcers are red, eroded, and painful. Providing a bland, moist, soft diet would make chewing and swallowing less painful. Drinking from a straw would prevent liquids from irritating the ulcerated areas. The use of lemon glycerin swabs and milk of magnesia should be avoided. Glycerin, a trihydric alcohol, absorbs water and dries the membranes. Milk of magnesia also has a drying effect because unabsorbed magnesium salts exert an osmotic pressure on tissue fluids. Frequent mouthwashes consisting of a half-teaspoon tsp of salt plus a half-teaspoon of baking soda dissolved in an 8-oz glass of water are recommended. Alcohol-based mouthwashes should be avoided because they would irritate the ulcers and dry the membranes.
CN: Physiological integrity; CNS: Basic care and comfort; CL: Apply

84. A pediatric client undergoing radiation and chemotherapy is experiencing nausea and vomiting. When is the **best** time for the nurse to begin administering antiemetics?

1. 30 minutes before initiation of therapy
2. With the administration of therapy
3. Immediately after nausea begins
4. When therapy is completed

85. The nurse is educating the parent of a child receiving procarbazine on dietary needs. Which statement by the parent indicates to the nurse teaching was successful?

1. "I will decrease my child's spicy food intake."
2. "I will decrease my child's fluid intake between meals."
3. "I will include foods such as liver in my child's meals."
4. "I will keep my child away from cheese and pepperoni pizza."

86. The nurse is providing education to a client who has hemorrhagic cystitis caused by bladder irritation from chemotherapeutic medications. Which recommendation will the nurse provide to prevent future occurrences?

1. Stop chemotherapy.
2. Take prophylactic antibiotics.
3. Increase intake of cranberry juice.
4. Aggressively increase oral fluid intake.

87. Which action by the nurse will assist in preparing the parents and child receiving chemotherapy for alopecia?

1. Provide the child with several wigs to try on and play with prior to any hair loss.
2. Encourage the child's family to shave their heads when the child begins to lose hair.
3. Stress that hair loss during a second treatment with the same medication will be more severe.
4. Explain as hair thins that keeping it clean, short, and fluffy may camouflage partial baldness.

88. The nurse is caring for a child diagnosed with influenza. Which personal protective equipment will the nurse apply when entering the child's room? Select all that apply.

1. Gloves
2. Gown
3. Facemask
4. Shoe covers
5. Goggles

84. 1. Antiemetics are most beneficial if given before the onset of nausea and vomiting. The first dose is given 30 minutes to 1 hour before nausea is expected, and then every 2, 4, or 6 hours for approximately 24 hours after chemotherapy. If the antiemetic were given with the medication or after the medication, it could lose its maximum effectiveness when needed.

CN: Physiological integrity; CNS: Pharmacological and parenteral therapies; CL: Apply

85. 4. Procarbazine has monoamine oxidase inhibitory activity. Foods high in tyramine, such as cheese and pepperoni, should be avoided. There is no chemotherapeutic or physiologic reason to restrict spicy foods. Increased fluid intake is essential to prevent calculi formation. Liver should be avoided because it contains tyramine, which can cause tremors, palpitations, and increased blood pressure.

CN: Physiological integrity; CNS: Pharmacological and parenteral therapies; CL: Apply

86. 4. Sterile hemorrhagic cystitis is an adverse effect of chemical irritation of the bladder from cyclophosphamide. It can be prevented by liberal fluid intake (at least 1½ times the recommended daily fluid requirement). Stopping chemotherapy, prophylactic antibiotics, and consuming cranberry juice are not appropriate recommendations.

CN: Physiological integrity; CNS: Reduction of risk potential; CL: Apply

87. 4. The nurse must prepare parents and children for possible hair loss. Cutting the hair short lessens the impact of seeing large quantities of hair on bed linens and clothing. Sometimes, keeping the hair short and fuller can make a wig unnecessary. A child should be encouraged to pick out a wig similar to their own hair style and color before the hair falls out, to foster adjustment to hair loss. Providing wigs to play with, encouraging family to shave their heads, and stressing that hair loss during a second treatment will be worse are not therapeutic in preparing for actual hair loss by the child.

CN: Psychosocial integrity; CNS: None; CL: Apply

88. 1, 2, 3. Influenza clients will be placed on droplet precautions. When caring for a client on droplet precaution, the nurse should apply gloves, gown, and mask before entering the client's room. Shoe covers and goggles are not necessary.

CN: Safe, effective care environment; CNS: Safety and infection control; CL: Apply

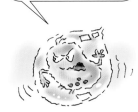

That's right—keep on sneezing. Droplets are my favorite way to get around.

89. The nurse is preparing a school-age child for a bone marrow biopsy to rule out leukemia. The nurse explains the sample will be taken from the anterior iliac crest. Identify this area.

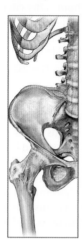

89. A bone marrow biopsy may be taken from the anterior or posterior iliac crest, as shown. A bone marrow biopsy may also be taken from the sternum, vertebral spinous process, rib, or tibia.

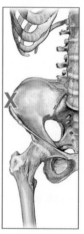

CN: Physiological integrity; CNS: Physiological adaptation; CL: Apply

90. The parents of a child diagnosed with leukemia have stated they will give aspirin to their child for pain relief. Which statement by the nurse about aspirin is **most** accurate?
1. "It is okay for you to give your child aspirin for pain relief."
2. "It is contraindicated because it promotes bleeding tendencies."
3. "Aspirin is not a strong enough analgesic for your child."
4. "It decreases the effects of methotrexate and should be avoided."

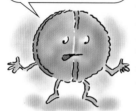

If bleeding is an issue for you, then you'd better steer clear of me.

90. 2. Aspirin would be contraindicated because it promotes bleeding. Aspirin use has also been associated with Reye's syndrome in children. For home use, acetaminophen is recommended for mild-to-moderate pain. Aspirin enhances the effects of methotrexate. Nonopioid analgesia has been effective for mild-to-moderate pain in children with leukemia.

CN: Physiological integrity; CNS: Pharmacological and parenteral therapies; CL: Apply

91. Which action(s) by the nurse represents use of proper precautions to prevent the spread of communicable diseases? Select all that apply.
1. Donning a mask, gown, and gloves when caring for a child with erythema infectiosum
2. Wearing a face shield when assessing the pain level of a child with hand–foot–mouth disease
3. Donning a gown, gloves, and respirator when helping a child with rubeola to the bathroom
4. Putting on gloves, gown, and mask before entering the room of a child with mumps
5. Wearing a mask, gown, and gloves when taking the vital signs of a child with tuberculosis

91. 1, 3, 4. Erythema infectiosum (fifth disease) and mumps (parotitis) require droplet precautions (mask, gown, gloves). Rubeola (measles) and tuberculosis require airborne precautions (gown, gloves, respirator). The nurse should follow contact precautions (gloves and gown) when caring for a child with hand–foot–mouth disease.

CN: Safe, effective care environment; CNS: Safety and infection control; CL: Analyze

92. While caring for a 6-year-old client diagnosed with sickle cell, the nurse documents the chart exhibit seen below. Which primary health care provider prescription will the nurse question?

> **Progress notes**
>
> Client is in bed resting at this time. Vital signs: blood pressure 100/70 mm Hg, pulse 100 beats/minute, respiratory rate 25 breaths/minute, O₂ 89% on RA, and temperature 101.3°F (38.5°C). Pain rated at an 8 using 10-point pain scale.
>
> —G. Lopez, RN

1. Give morphine sulfate IV for pain.
2. Administer influenza vaccine.
3. Apply oxygen via a facemask.
4. Give acetaminophen orally.

93. The nurse is meeting with a 17-year-old client who recently tested positive for human immuno-deficiency virus (HIV). The client asks, "What information will be told to others?" Which response by the nurse is appropriate?
1. "You will need to disclose information to your school."
2. "Your employers have a legal right to know your HIV status."
3. "In some jurisdictions, laws require you to tell future sexual partners."
4. "You are legally required to tell all past sexual partners."

94. The health care provider has prescribed hydroxyurea for a pediatric client with sickle cell anemia. When providing education to this client and family, which information will the nurse include? Select all that apply.
1. "This medication may initially cause nausea and vomiting."
2. "If you forget to take a dose, take it as soon as you remember."
3. "Do not take two doses of this medication at the same time."
4. "If you feel excessively weak, contact your health care provider."
5. "Report any darkening of your skin or fingernails."

95. The health care provider has recommended a diet high in folic acid for an adolescent with sickle cell anemia. Which food(s) will the nurse recommend to the child and caregivers? Select all that apply.
1. Legumes
2. String cheese
3. Grapefruit
4. Bananas
5. Kale

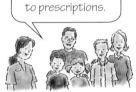

Be sure to assess clients for contraindications to prescriptions.

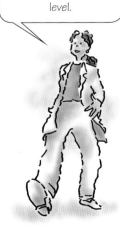

You sure are a smart one. Time to step up to the next level.

92. 2. The nurse would question administering a vaccine to this child due to the presence of a fever. Pain medication is needed to control pain and limit a vaso-occlusive crisis. Oxygen is also needed to limit a vaso-occlusive crisis. Acetaminophen is appropriate to decrease the child's temperature.
CN: Safe, effective care environment; CNS: Management of care; CL: Analyze

93. 3. Most jurisdictions have laws requiring HIV-positive people to share their status with future contacts prior to sexual activity. Sharing a positive HIV status is an obvious area of concern for a client. Studies have shown that those who disclose their status to friends and family experience a greater source of support and benefit from it. Disclosures to teachers, employers, friends, and family are voluntary and not a requirement. Disclosures of a positive HIV status to past contacts are a courtesy and, although recommended, are not legally required.
CN: Safe, effective care environment; CNS: Management of care; CL: Apply

94. 1, 2, 3, 4. Hydroxyurea may be prescribed for the client with sickle cell anemia. This medication is used to prevent the frequency of crisis episodes. The medication is administered orally. It may initially cause nausea and vomiting. If a dose is missed it should be taken when realized. If the dose is recalled at the time the next is due, do not double up on the dosage. The medication may have adverse effects that require immediate notification of the health care provider, such as excessive weakness or fatigue. Darkening of the skin and fingernails is a side effect of the medication and does not require notification of the health care provider.
CN: Physiological integrity; CNS: Pharmacological and parenteral therapies, CL: Apply

95. 1, 3, 5. Folic acid is associated with red blood cell production. Folic acid is encouraged in the diet for individuals with sickle cell anemia. Sources of folic acid include peas, legumes, citrus fruits (such as grapefruit), and leafy green vegetables (such as kale). String cheese and bananas are not considered good sources of folic acid.
CN: Physiological integrity; CNS: Basic care and comfort; CL: Apply

Chapter 28

Respiratory Disorders

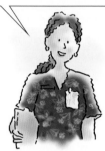

From the simple otitis media to the uncommon and dangerous epiglottitis, this chapter covers a wide variety of respiratory disorders in children. So, take a deep breath and go for it!

Pediatric respiratory refresher

Asthma

Lung disease that inflames and narrows the airways

Key signs and symptoms

- Diaphoresis
- Dyspnea
- Prolonged expiration with an expiratory wheeze; in severe distress, inspiratory wheeze
- Unequal or decreased breath sounds
- Use of accessory muscles

Key test results

- Oxygen saturation via pulse oximetry may show decreased oxygen saturation
- Arterial blood gas measurement may show increased partial pressure of arterial carbon dioxide from respiratory acidosis

Key treatments

- Short-acting bronchodilator: albuterol
- Chromone derivative: cromolyn
- Long-acting bronchodilator: salmeterol, formoterol
- Leukotriene modifiers: montelukast, zafirlukast
- Inhaled glucocorticoids: fluticasone, budesonide, flunisolide

Key interventions

- Monitor respiratory and cardiovascular status.
- Monitor vital signs during an acute attack.
- Allow the child to sit upright to ease breathing; provide moist oxygen, if necessary.
- Monitor for alterations in vital signs (especially cardiac stimulation and hypotension).

Bronchiolitis

Infection of the bronchioles usually caused by a viral infection and usually found in children under 2 years of age

Key signs and symptoms

- Retractions
- Tachypnea

Key test results

- Bronchial mucus culture shows respiratory syncytial virus (RSV)

Key treatments

- Humidified oxygen
- IV fluids

Key interventions

- Monitor vital signs and pulse oximetry.
- Monitor respiratory and cardiovascular status.
- Administer humidified oxygen therapy.

Bronchopulmonary dysplasia

Chronic bronchial tube and lung disease that affects infants who have been on a ventilator

Key signs and symptoms

- Crackles, rhonchi, wheezes
- Dyspnea
- Retractions

Key test results

- Chest x-ray reveals pulmonary changes (bronchiolar metaplasia and interstitial fibrosis)

Key treatments

- Chest physiotherapy
- Continued ventilatory support and oxygen
- Bronchodilators: albuterol

Key interventions

- Monitor respiratory and cardiovascular status.
- Monitor vital signs, pulse oximetry, and intake and output.

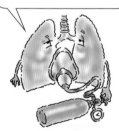

Some respiratory disorders are treated with oxygen therapy.

Croup

Upper respiratory tract viral infection that causes a barking cough

Key signs and symptoms

- Barking, brassy cough or hoarseness
- Inspiratory stridor with varying degrees of respiratory distress
- Fever may be low grade or up to 104°F (40°C)

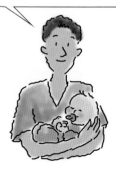

Bronchiolitis is usually found in children of what age?

Key test results
- Laryngoscopy may reveal inflammation and obstruction in epiglottis and laryngeal areas
- Neck x-ray shows areas of upper airway narrowing and edema in subglottic folds

Key treatments
- Cool humidification during sleep with a cool mist tent or room humidifier
- Inhaled racemic epinephrine and corticosteroids: methylprednisolone sodium succinate
- Tracheostomy, oxygen administration

Key interventions
- Monitor vital signs and pulse oximetry.
- Administer oxygen therapy and maintain the child in a cool environment, if needed.
- Allow parent to hold the child.

Cystic fibrosis

Inherited disease that causes thick, sticky mucus to form in the lungs, pancreas, and other organs

Key signs and symptoms
- History of a chronic, productive cough and recurrent respiratory infections, often due to *Pseudomonas* infections
- Parents report salty taste on the child's skin
- History of poor weight gain and growth; intestinal blockage; foul-smelling, greasy stools

Key test results
- Sweat test using pilocarpine iontophoresis is positive
- Newborn screening test may reveal cystic fibrosis
- Sputum cystic fibrosis respiratory screen reveals bacterial or fungal lung infection

Key treatments
- Chest physiotherapy
- Oral pancreatic enzyme replacement
- Antibiotics: tobramycin, azithromycin
- Bronchodilators
- Mucolytics: dornase alfa

Key interventions
- Monitor respiratory and cardiovascular status.
- Administer pancreatic enzymes with meals and snacks.

- Encourage breathing exercises and perform chest physiotherapy two to four times a day.

Epiglottitis

Acute inflammation of the epiglottis; an emergency that may result in death if not treated quickly

Key signs and symptoms
- Difficult and painful swallowing
- Increased drooling
- Restlessness
- Stridor

Key test results
- Lateral neck x-ray shows enlarged epiglottis

Key treatments
- Emergency endotracheal intubation or tracheotomy
- Oxygen therapy
- 10-day course of parenteral antibiotics

Key interventions
- Have emergency tracheotomy and intubation equipment at the bedside.
- Monitor vital signs and pulse oximetry.
- Monitor respiratory and cardiovascular status.
- Defer inspection of the throat until the arrival of emergency personnel and supplies.

Sudden infant death syndrome (SIDS)

Sudden and unexpected death of an infant younger than 1 year of age

Key signs and symptoms
- Death takes place during sleep without noise or struggle

Key test results
- Autopsy is the only way to diagnose SIDS

Key treatments
- Emotional and other support for the parents

Key interventions
- Let parents touch, hold, and rock the infant.
- Reinforce the fact that the death was not the parents' fault.

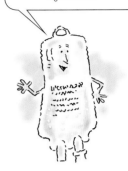

Don't forget to keep your clients with bronchiolitis well hydrated.

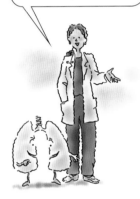

Your client has a history of chronic, productive cough and thick, sticky mucus in the lungs. What condition should you suspect?

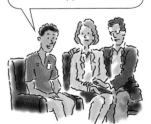

Parents who have lost a child to SIDS will likely need a lot of emotional support.

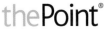

Respiratory questions, answers, and rationales

1. The nurse is educating a parent on sudden infant death syndrome (SIDS) prevention. Which statement made by the parent indicates a correct understanding of SIDS?

1. "I will place my infant on the stomach to sleep."
2. "I will breastfeed my infant for at least 6 months."
3. "I will cover my infant with a warm blanket while sleeping."
4. "I will put my infant in my bed while we are napping."

1. 2. SIDS can best be defined as the sudden death of an infant (a child younger than 1 year) that remains unexplained after autopsy. Ways to lower an infant's risk of SIDS include breastfeeding for at least 6 months, sleeping on the back, no blankets on the infant while sleeping (sleep sacks are recommended), no stuffed animals in the crib, using a firm crib mattress, and not placing the infant in the parent's bed to sleep (should be on a firm crib mattress or in a bassinet).

CN: Physiological integrity; CNS: Physiological adaptation; CL: Apply

2. While teaching a class to new parents, the nurse will identify which child as having an increased risk of sudden infant death syndrome (SIDS)?

1. A male born at 32 weeks' gestation, weighing 3.1 lb (14,000 g)
2. A 2-year-old female with a history of asthma
3. A 8-month-old male with a temperature of 102.2°F (39°C)
4. A 3-year-old male whose father has cystic fibrosis

2. 1. Premature infants, especially those with low birth weight, have an increased risk for SIDS. Males are also slightly more likely to die from SIDS. Infants with apnea, central nervous system disorders, or respiratory disorders also have a higher risk of SIDS. The peak age for SIDS is between 2 and 4 months, and by definition SIDS only occurs in infants (children 0 to 12 months of age), not in toddlers. A fever or family history of cystic fibrosis does not increase a child's risk for SIDS.

CN: Physiological integrity; CNS: Reduction of risk potential; CL: Analyze

3. A 3-month-old who is not breathing is brought to the emergency department. A preliminary diagnosis of sudden infant death syndrome (SIDS) is made. Which action will the nurse complete **first**?

1. Ask the parents if they want to hold their infant.
2. Document what the parents state happened at home.
3. Complete required forms for an autopsy.
4. Gather the infant's clothing for the parents.

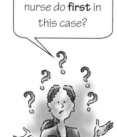

What will the nurse do **first** in this case?

3. 1. The parents need time with their infant to assist with the grieving process. The nurse should complete each of the other actions; however, they are not priority.

CN: Psychosocial integrity; CNS: None; CL: Analyze

4. A client who just birthed a full-term newborn tells the nurse sudden infant death syndrome (SIDS) is a big fear. When educating the mother about SIDS, which factor(s) will the nurse identify as being associated with SIDS? Select all that apply.

1. Breastfeeding
2. Gestational age of 42 weeks
3. Immunizations
4. Low birth weight
5. Smoking in the home
6. Recent respiratory infection

4. 4, 5, 6. Prematurity, low birth weight, secondhand smoke, male sex, recent respiratory infection, brain defects, overheating, sleeping in a prone position, race, and family history are all risk factors for SIDS. Breastfeeding and term and post-term gestational age are not related to SIDS. Immunizations have been disproved to be associated with the disorder.

CN: Physiological integrity; CNS: Reduction of risk potential; CL: Apply

5. The parents of an infant suspected to have just died from sudden infant death syndrome (SIDS) are crying and shouting, "Why did this happen to our beautiful baby?" Which response by the nurse is **most** appropriate?
1. "Did the infant have a blanket or pillow in the crib?"
2. "You seem upset. I am going to sit with you a while."
3. "What position did the infant usually sleep in?"
4. "I know this is a terrible experience and it is not fair."

5. 2. It is most appropriate for the nurse to acknowledge the parents' feelings and provide emotional support. During the initial history in the emergency department, only factual questions should be asked of the parents whose child has died of SIDS. The questions listed imply blame, guilt, or neglect. Expressing an opinion about the situation is not therapeutic.

CN: Psychosocial integrity; CNS: None; CL: Apply

6. Which intervention will the nurse include when caring for an infant with an increased risk of sudden infant death syndrome (SIDS)?
1. Perform pulmonary function testing at regular intervals.
2. Consult case management for home apnea monitoring.
3. Assess the infant's pulse oximetry hourly while sleeping.
4. Schedule the infant for a chest x-ray at age 1 month.

6. 2. A home apnea monitor is recommended for infants with an increased risk of SIDS. Diagnostic tests, such as pulmonary function tests, pulse oximetry, and chest x-rays, cannot diagnose the risk of surviving or dying from SIDS.

CN: Physiological integrity; CNS: Reduction of risk potential; CL: Apply

7. The nurse will anticipate the family of an infant who has just died from sudden infant death syndrome (SIDS) to exhibit which action?
1. Having feelings of blame or guilt
2. Being accepting of the loss of their infant
3. Requesting to have the infant's belongings
4. Beginning planning to become pregnant again

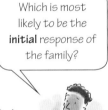

Which is most likely to be the **initial** response of the family?

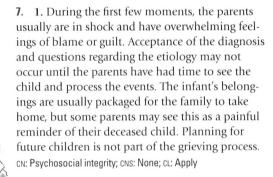

7. 1. During the first few moments, the parents usually are in shock and have overwhelming feelings of blame or guilt. Acceptance of the diagnosis and questions regarding the etiology may not occur until the parents have had time to see the child and process the events. The infant's belongings are usually packaged for the family to take home, but some parents may see this as a painful reminder of their deceased child. Planning for future children is not part of the grieving process.

CN: Psychosocial integrity; CNS: None; CL: Apply

8. The parents of an infant who just died from sudden infant death syndrome (SIDS) are angry at God and refuse to see any members of the clergy. Which process **best** defines this situation?
1. Ineffective coping
2. Spiritual distress
3. Complicated grieving
4. Chronic sorrow

8. 2. The defining characteristics of spiritual distress include anger and refusal to interact with spiritual leaders. Although anger is part of the grieving process, there is no indication that the parents are not coping effectively or are experiencing complicated grieving. Chronic sorrow, as the name implies, occurs over a period of time and may be cyclical. These are not nursing diagnoses but appropriate feelings that parents experience after such a horrible event.

CN: Psychosocial integrity; CNS: None; CL: Apply

9. The nurse is assessing a toddler with suspected acute otitis media. Which finding(s) will the nurse expect to assess? Select all that apply.
1. Pulling at the affected ear(s)
2. Anorexia
3. Increased crying
4. Intermittent vomiting
5. Nasal congestion

9. 1, 2, 3, 5. Expected symptoms of acute otitis media in children include: pain (pulling/tugging at the affected ear), fever, loss of appetite, vertigo, crying, irritability, and nasal congestion or a recent history of a respiratory infection. Vomiting is not associated with otitis media.

CN: Health promotion and maintenance; CNS: None; CL: Apply

CN: Client needs category   CNS: Client needs subcategory   CL: Cognitive level

10. The nurse is providing discharge education to the mother of an infant at increased risk for sudden infant death syndrome (SIDS). Which statement(s) will the nurse include in the teaching? Select all that apply.
   1. "Your infant can have a blanket in the crib at 6 months of age."
   2. "You must breastfeed the infant until 4 months of age."
   3. "You should always place your infant on the back to sleep."
   4. "The infant should always be on a firm surface when sleeping."
   5. "Be sure to keep your infant's room very warm when sleeping."
   6. "Your infant should not sleep in the bed with you."

10. 3, 4, 6. To help prevent SIDS, the nurse should recommend always placing the infant supine, on a firm mattress/surface, in the crib/bassinet when sleeping. It is not recommended to give infants blankets or pillows in cribs. Breastfeeding does decrease the chance of SIDS, but the nurse cannot demand that the mother breastfeed. Overheating may be a risk factor for SIDS. The nurse should caution parents to never sleep with their infant in bed with them.
CN: Physiological integrity; CNS: Reduction of risk potential; Apply

11. A few days after the death of an infant from sudden infant death syndrome (SIDS), the nurse making a home visit notices the parents are disorganized in their thought patterns. What is the **best** action for the nurse?
   1. Realize this is a normal process for the impact phase of crisis.
   2. Instruct the parents they need to try to accept the loss of their infant.
   3. Inform the parents that many parents go through this and they will be okay.
   4. Tell the parents they need to focus on other aspects of their lives.

11. 1. Within a day or two of the infant's death, the parents enter the impact phase of crisis, which consists of disorganized thoughts in which they cannot deal with the crisis in concrete terms. This is a normal reaction at this time. Telling them to accept the loss, that they will be okay, and to go on with their lives would only add to the parents' distress and is not compassionate or therapeutic.
CN: Psychosocial integrity; CNS: None; CL: Apply

12. When providing discharge education for a parent of a newborn, which statement made by the parent indicates a need for further instruction?
   1. "I will make sure the crib mattress is firm before using the crib."
   2. "I will place my infant on the stomach position when napping."
   3. "I will not put any stuffed animals in the crib or bassinet."
   4. "I will allow tummy-time only while I am playing with my infant."

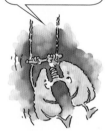

Now you've got the swing of things.

12. 2. Research indicates to place infants supine only when sleeping as a way to reduce the risk of sudden infant death syndrome. It is, however, acceptable to place the infant prone while awake and playing, with supervision. The infant should sleep on a firm mattress, and nothing should be placed in the crib, to prevent external airway obstruction.
CN: Health promotion and maintenance; CNS: None; CL: Apply

13. The nurse is admitting a 4-year-old child to the hospital for a tonsillectomy. The child appears anxious. Which nursing intervention(s) is appropriate for this child? Select all that apply.
   1. Allow the child to hold a stethoscope before using it on the child.
   2. Have the parents bring the child's favorite blanket from home.
   3. Show the child how the procedure will be done using a doll.
   4. Inform the parents that one of them needs to stay with the child.
   5. When asking admission questions, allow the child to sit on a parent's lap.

13. 1, 2, 3, 4, 5. It is important to help a child cope with new and strange surroundings. This can be accomplished by having a parent present, allowing the child to have a favorite blanket, explaining procedures in simple terms using models when possible, allowing the child to touch medical equipment when appropriate, and allowing the child to be in a comfortable, safe place (such as a parent's lap).
CN: Psychosocial integrity; CNS: None; CL: Apply

14. A child presents with inspiratory stridor and a seal-like barking cough. Which nursing action is **priority**?
1. Provide oxygen via a face mask.
2. Establish and maintain the airway.
3. Administer intravenous antibiotics.
4. Assess the oxygen saturation rate.

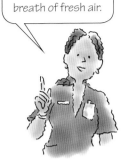

Let's take a breath of fresh air.

14. 2. The initial priority is to establish and maintain the airway. Edema and accumulation of secretions may contribute to airway obstruction. It is not clear that antibiotics are indicated at this time, as the cause of the child's dyspnea is unknown; moreover, even if antibiotics were indicated, establishing and maintaining the airway would still be the priority. Oxygen should be administered as soon as the airway is established to decrease the child's distress. The nurse would assess the oxygen saturation to determine the effectiveness of interventions to maintain the airway and oxygen administration. This is not priority, however, because the child is in distress.
CN: Safe, effective care environment; CNS: Management of care; CL: Apply

15. The nurse is educating the parents of a 5-year-old child diagnosed with croup. Which intervention will the nurse include to help alleviate worsening symptoms during the night?
1. Give warm liquids.
2. Raise the heat setting on the thermostat.
3. Place the child in a tub of cool water.
4. Provide humidified air with cool mist.

15. 4. High humidity with cool mist, such as from a cool mist humidifier, provides the most (and safest form of) relief. Providing cool, not warm, liquids for the child to drink would be best for the child. If unable to take liquid, the child needs emergency care. Raising the heat on the thermostat would result in dry, warm air, which might cause secretions to adhere to the airway wall. A warm, running shower provides a mist that may be helpful to moisten and decrease the viscosity of airway secretions and may also decrease laryngeal spasm. Placing the child in a tub of cool water might result in hypothermia and would not necessarily improve respirations, as the water would not be in a mist.
CN: Physiological integrity; CNS: Physiological adaptation; CL: Apply

16. A 5-year-old child is admitted with a diagnosis of croup. Which characteristic sign(s) will the nurse expect to assess in this client? Select all that apply.
1. Barking cough
2. Temperature of 100.8°F (38.2°C)
3. Blood pressure of 105/60 mm Hg
4. Respiratory rate of 25 breaths/minute
5. Heart rate of 140 beats/minute

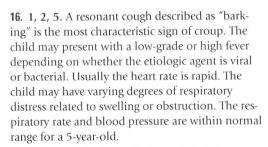

Croup may have a low or high fever, depending on the etiology.

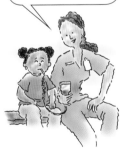

16. 1, 2, 5. A resonant cough described as "barking" is the most characteristic sign of croup. The child may present with a low-grade or high fever depending on whether the etiologic agent is viral or bacterial. Usually the heart rate is rapid. The child may have varying degrees of respiratory distress related to swelling or obstruction. The respiratory rate and blood pressure are within normal range for a 5-year-old.
CN: Physiological integrity; CNS: Physiological adaptation; CL: Apply

17. Which finding warrants **immediate** nursing intervention in a child diagnosed with croup?
1. A barking cough
2. Intercostal retractions
3. Clubbing of the fingers
4. Temperature of 99.6°F (37.6°C)

17. 2. Intercostal retractions occur as the child's breathing becomes more labored and the use of other muscles is necessary to draw air into the lungs. A barking cough occurs in a child with croup and in itself is not a sign that the condition is worsening. Clubbing of the fingers is expected with chronic, not acute, respiratory conditions. A low-grade fever is an expected finding in a child with croup. Facilitating breathing is priority over a low-grade fever.
CN: Physiological integrity; CNS: Physiological adaptation; CL: Apply

CN: Client needs category   CNS: Client needs subcategory   CL: Cognitive level

18. Which nursing intervention is **priority** when caring for a child with croup experiencing spasmodic episodes?
1. Reduce the child's environmental stimuli.
2. Have intubation equipment at the bedside.
3. Administer humidified oxygen.
4. Give albuterol to the child as prescribed.

18. 2. The priority nursing intervention is to maintain the child's airway by having intubation equipment at the bedside. The danger of glottal obstruction due to inflammation is very real. Only after making preparations to ensure that the airway can be established and maintained should the nurse administer albuterol and then oxygen to facilitate breathing. The nurse should reduce stimuli to provide a calming environment, but only after performing the other interventions listed.
CN: Safe, effective care environment; CNS: Management of care; CL: Analyze

19. The nurse is assessing a 2-year-old child with croup. Which finding requires **immediate** action from the nurse?
1. Capillary refill less than 3 seconds
2. Temperature of 100.2°F (37.9°C)
3. Grunting and head bobbing
4. Respiratory rate of 28 breaths/minute

19. 3. Grunting and head bobbing is seen in a child in respiratory distress. Capillary refill time of less than 3 seconds and a respiratory rate of 28 breaths/minute are normal findings. An elevated temperature does not indicate respiratory distress; rather, this indicates infection.
CN: Safe, effective care environment; CNS: Management of care; CL: Apply

20. The nurse is caring for a child with congenital laryngomalacia. Which precaution is **most** appropriate for the nurse to use when caring for this child?
1. Apply an N95 mask.
2. Perform proper hand washing.
3. Place the child in isolation.
4. Wear goggles and a mask.

Protect yourself and your clients from infection by washing your hands frequently, observing your facility's protocols.

20. 2. Congenital laryngomalacia is a congenital laryngeal cartilage abnormality. Hand washing would help prevent the spread of infections to this child. An N95 respirator mask is used to protect against airborne illnesses, such as tuberculosis. Isolation, goggles, and a mask are not required, as this is a congenital abnormality.
CN: Health promotion and maintenance; CNS: None; CL: Apply

21. The parent of a child who is receiving nebulizer treatments at home asks the nurse, "When is the best time of day to administer a nebulizer treatment to my child?" Which response by the nurse is **most** appropriate?
1. "Giving the treatments to your child after eating meals is best."
2. "You should administer the treatments to your child at naptime."
3. "I recommend incorporating treatments into your child's playtime."
4. "Any time of the day is fine to give your child a nebulizer treatment."

21. 2. The nurse should recommend administering nebulizer treatments at prescribed intervals at certain times of the day. Administering treatment at naptime allows for as little disruption as possible. A child should be given a treatment before, not after, eating so that the airway is open, and the work of eating is decreased. Administering the treatment during playtime would disrupt the child's daily pattern.
CN: Physiological integrity; CNS: Pharmacological and parenteral therapies; CL: Apply

22. The parents brings their child to the emergency department reporting difficulty swallowing, increased drooling, restlessness, and stridor. The nurse observes the child in a tripod sitting position. Which condition will the nurse suspect this child is experiencing?
1. Asthma
2. Epiglottitis
3. Bronchiolitis
4. Croup

22. 2. Epiglottitis is associated with difficult swallowing, increased drooling, restlessness, stridor, and a tripod sitting position. Asthma is accompanied dyspnea, fatigue, wheezing, decreased breath sounds, and the use of accessory muscles. Bronchiolitis normally is diagnosed by a cough, sternal retractions, thick mucus, and an elevated temperature. Croup is identified by the presence of a barking cough, crackles, and/or decreased breath sounds, increased dyspnea, and inspiratory stridor.
CN: Physiological integrity; CNS: Physiological adaptation; CL: Apply

23. Which education is **most** important for the nurse to provide to the parents of a child in the recovery stage of croup?
1. Limit the child's oral fluid intake.
2. Recognize signs of respiratory distress.
3. Provide three nutritious meals per day.
4. Allow the child to go to the playground.

23. 2. Although most children with croup recover without complications, the parents should be able to recognize signs and symptoms of respiratory distress and know how to access emergency services. Oral fluids should be encouraged because fluids help to thin secretions. Although nutrition is important, frequent small, nutritious snacks are usually more appealing than an entire meal. Children should have optimal rest and engage in quiet play. A comfortable environment free of noxious stimuli lessens respiratory distress.
CN: Safe, effective care environment; CNS: Management of care; CL: Apply

24. The nurse is assessing a child with suspected epiglottitis. Which finding(s) will the nurse expect to observe in this child? Select all that apply.
1. Restlessness
2. Drooling
3. High fever
4. Spontaneous cough
5. Tripod position

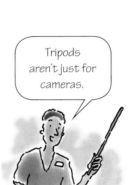

Tripods aren't just for cameras.

24. 1, 2, 3, 5. Restlessness indicates respiratory distress, which is associated with epiglottitis. Drooling is common due to the pain of swallowing, excessive secretions, and sore throat. The child usually has a high fever and the absence of a spontaneous cough. The classic clinical picture of this condition is the child in a tripod position with mouth open and tongue protruding.
CN: Physiological integrity; CNS: Physiological adaptation; CL: Apply

25. Which nursing intervention is **priority** when caring for a child with acute epiglottitis?
1. Keep the child calm.
2. Put the child in semi-Fowler's position.
3. Give intravenous (IV) antibiotics.
4. Place the child in respiratory isolation for 48 hours.

25. 1. Airway support is priority for this child; therefore, it is imperative to keep the child calm to minimize agitation and distress, which could lead to respiratory distress. The etiologic agent for epiglottitis is usually bacterial, and IV antibiotic therapy is needed; however, avoiding respiratory distress is the priority. The child should be placed in Fowler's position or any position that provides the most comfort and security. Respiratory isolation is not required.
CN: Safe, effective care environment; CNS: Management of care; CL: Apply

26. The nurse finds a 6-month-old client unresponsive and not breathing in the crib. Which action will the nurse take **next**?
1. Assess for a brachial pulse.
2. Begin chest compressions.
3. Start mouth-to-mouth resuscitation.
4. Call a code and get the automated external defibrillator (AED).

26. 1. Initially, the nurse will check the infant for a brachial pulse. If no pulse is detected, perform chest compressions (30 as a single rescuer). Next, open the airway and give two rescue breaths. This nurse should determine whether the infant has a pulse before calling a code or requesting an AED.
CN: Safe, effective care environment; CNS: Management of care; CL: Analyze

27. The nurse is caring for a child with a diagnosis of croup. Which response will the nurse provide to the caregiver when concern is expressed about the child waking at night coughing?
1. Immediately call 911 for assistance.
2. Transport the child to an ambulatory care center.
3. Take the child in a bathroom, shut the door, and turn on a hot shower.
4. Administer a home nebulizer treatment to the child.

27. 3. Steam from the shower would decrease laryngeal spasms, so taking the child to the bathroom and turning on a hot shower should help. It is not necessary to call 911 each time a child has a coughing episode with croup. Driving the child to a patient care center would be dangerous if the child's condition worsened on the way. While having a spasmodic coughing episode, the child would not be able to do a breathing treatment successfully.
CN: Physiological integrity; CNS: Physiological adaptation; CL: Apply

CN: Client needs category   CNS: Client needs subcategory   CL: Cognitive level

28. A 5-year-old client is found in respiratory arrest and cardiopulmonary resuscitation is started. Which site will the nurse use to assess for the client's pulse?

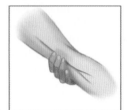

1.

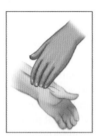

2.

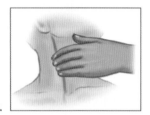

3.

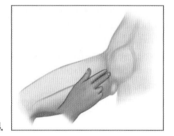

4.

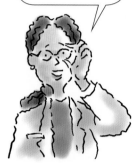

Arm yourself with knowledge and I'm sure you'll be able to answer question #28.

28. 3. Palpation of the carotid artery is recommended starting at age 1 year. The brachial is used on infants. The femoral and radial pulses are not recommended for indicating central artery perfusion during cardiopulmonary resuscitation.
CN: Physiological integrity; CNS: Physiological adaptation; CL: Apply

29. The nurse is teaching parents how to perform infant cardiopulmonary resuscitation (CPR). The nurse knows the parents understand the correct infant CPR procedure if the parents state they will perform which action to open the infant's airway when providing ventilation?
1. Head-tilt-chin-lift
2. Chin tuck
3. Hyperextend the head
4. Jaw thrust

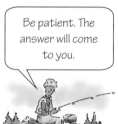

Be patient. The answer will come to you.

29. 1. The head-tilt-chin-lift maneuver would be used to correctly open the infant's airway. The nurse must not tilt the infant's head too far back or the airway will become obstructed. The other positions would not open the airway.
CN: Physiological integrity; CNS: Physiological adaptation; CL: Understand

30. Which chest compression to ventilation ratio will the nurse use when performing cardiopulmonary resuscitation on a 3-year-old client alone?
1. 15 compressions to one ventilation
2. 15 compressions to two ventilations
3. 30 compressions to one ventilation
4. 30 compressions to two ventilations

30. 4. The single rescuer should use a ratio of 30 chest compressions to two ventilations (30:2) for children ages 1 year to the onset of adolescence. A ratio of 15:2 is indicated if there are two rescuers. Ratios of 15:1 and 30:1 would not provide optimal compression and ventilation.
CN: Physiological integrity; CNS: Physiological adaptation; CL: Understand

31. Which intervention(s) will the nurse perform when providing care for a child with suspected epiglottitis? Select all that apply.
1. Place the child on NPO status.
2. Maintain the child on bed rest.
3. Prepare to insert an intravenous line.
4. Place intubation equipment at the bedside.
5. Establish the child's airway.

32. The nurse finds a 7-year-old child in the room coughing as a result of choking. Which action will the nurse take **first**?
1. Look inside the child's mouth for the object.
2. Encourage the child to continue coughing.
3. Attempt a blind finger sweep on the child.
4. Notify the child's health care provider.

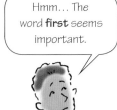

Hmm… The word **first** seems important.

33. The nurse enters the room of a 3-year-old child and notes a seal-like barking cough and nasal flaring. Which action will the nurse complete **first**?
1. Give the child humidified oxygen.
2. Auscultate the lungs bilaterally.
3. Assess an oxygen saturation level.
4. Administer albuterol as prescribed.

34. The parents bring their 2-year-old child to urgent care stating the child swallowed a toy. The nurse notes the child is cyanotic and not able to cough or speak. Which nursing action is **priority**?
1. Give oxygen via a face mask.
2. Administer five back blows.
3. Determine the type of toy swallowed.
4. Provide upward abdominal thrusts.

35. A 3-year-old child is receiving ampicillin for acute epiglottitis. Which finding leads the nurse to suspect the child is experiencing a common adverse effect of this drug?
1. The child has not had a bowel movement in several days.
2. A generalized rash is noted on the child's torso and extremities.
3. The child has been eating more food with meals and asking for snacks.
4. The child's temporal temperature is 99.8°F (37.7°C).

31. 1, 2, 4, 5. The nurse should establish the child's airway and place intubation equipment at the bedside in case it is needed to maintain the airway. The child with epiglottitis should be kept calm by being placed on bed rest and should be NPO to maintain the airway. Inserting an IV line would cause distress in the child and could lead to a lost airway. Before inserting an IV, the nurse must ensure the airway is safe.
CN: Physiological integrity; CNS: Physiological adaptation; CL: Apply

32. 2. The nurse should encourage a client who is coughing while choking to continue coughing. Coughing indicates the client can move air and is the most efficient way to dislodge the object. If the client becomes unconscious, the nurse should begin cardiopulmonary resuscitation while looking for the object when opening the airway. If the object is visible, the nurse should remove it. A blind finger sweep should never be performed as this may further lodge the object. Notifying the health care provider is not necessary at this time.
CN: Safe, effective care environment; CNS: Management of care; CL: Apply

33. 4. First, the nurse would administer albuterol via a nebulizer to open the child's airway. The child is exhibiting signs of respiratory distress. The nurse would give oxygen once the airway was open. A respiratory assessment, including auscultation of the lungs and assessment of oxygen saturation level, would be completed once the child was stable.
CN: Safe, effective care environment; CNS: Management of care; CL: Analyze

34. 4. A child 1 to 8 years old should receive upward abdominal thrusts to help dislodge the object. Administering oxygen would not help if the airway is occluded. Infants (children younger than age 1 year) should receive back blows before chest thrusts. It is not priority to determine the type of toy.
CN: Safe, effective care environment; CNS: Management of care; CL: Apply

35. 2. Some children with epiglottitis may develop an erythematous or maculopapular rash after 3 to 14 days of therapy; however, this complication does not necessitate discontinuing the drug. Nausea, vomiting, epigastric pain, diarrhea, and respiratory symptoms of anaphylaxis are adverse effects that may necessitate discontinuation of the drug. Constipation, increased appetite, and fever are not common adverse effects of this drug.
CN: Physiological integrity; CNS: Pharmacological and parenteral therapies; CL: Apply

36. A health care provider prescribes amoxicillin 40 mg/kg/day to be given in three divided doses for an 8-month-old infant with otitis media. The child weighs 26.5 lb (12 kg). How many milligrams will the nurse administer to the child per dose? Record your answer using a whole number.

_____ mg

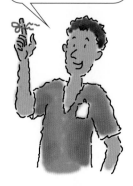

Remember—you are looking for the number of milligrams **per dose**.

36. 160.
The child should receive 160 mg per dose. First, calculate the total daily dose.

milligrams per dose × child's weight in kilograms
= total dose per day

40 mg × 12 kg = 480 mg/day

Then, divide the total daily dose by the number of doses.

480 mg/3 doses = 160 mg/dose

CN: Physiological integrity; CNS: Pharmacological and parenteral therapies; CL: Analyze

37. A 3-year-old child diagnosed with epiglottitis is prescribed ampicillin 50 mg/kg/day to be administered in six divided doses. The client weighs 32 lb (14.5 kg). How many milligrams of ampicillin will the nurse administer per dose? Record your answer using a whole number.

_____ mg

37. 121.
The child should receive 121 mg per dose. First, calculate the total daily dose.

milligrams per dose × child's weight in kilograms
= total dose per day

50 mg × 14.5 kg = 725 mg/day

Then, divide the total daily dose by the number of doses.

725 mg/6 doses = 121 mg/dose

CN: Physiological integrity; CNS: Pharmacological and parenteral therapies; CL: Analyze

38. A 3-year-old child is given a preliminary diagnosis of acute epiglottitis. Which nursing action is **most** important?
1. Obtain a throat culture immediately.
2. Place the child in a side-lying position.
3. Do not attempt to visualize the epiglottis.
4. Use a tongue depressor to look inside the throat.

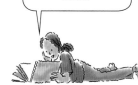

Sometimes the best intervention is to do nothing at all.

38. 3. The nurse should not attempt to visualize the epiglottis. The use of tongue blades or throat culture swabs may cause the epiglottis to spasm and totally occlude the airway. Throat inspection should be attempted only when immediate intubation or tracheostomy can be performed, in the event of further or complete obstruction. The child should always remain in the position that provides the most comfort, security, and ease of breathing.
CN: Safe, effective care environment; CNS: Management of care; CL: Apply

39. The parents of a 7-year-old child ask the nurse how they can decrease the chance of their child contracting epiglottitis. Which response by the nurse is **most** appropriate?
1. "Limit taking your child to public locations around lots of children."
2. "Ensure your child receives the haemophilus influenzae type B (Hib) vaccine."
3. "Have your child wash the hands after using public restrooms."
4. "Do not worry; epiglottitis only effects children 3 years of age and younger."

39. 2. Epiglottitis is caused by the bacterial agent _H. influenzae_. It is recommended children receive the Hib conjugate vaccine. A decline in the incidence of epiglottitis has been seen as a result of this vaccination regimen. A school-age child cannot avoid exposure to other children. It is important for a child to wash the hands after using the restroom; however, this is not most appropriate to prevent epiglottitis. Epiglottitis can affect clients of all ages, including adults.
CN: Safe, effective care environment; CNS: Management of care; CL: Apply

40. Which finding(s) in a 3-year-old child with acute epiglottitis indicates to the nurse the child is beginning to experience respiratory distress? Select all that apply.
1. Progressive, barking cough
2. Acute anorexia
3. Increasing heart rate
4. Productive cough
5. Tachypnea

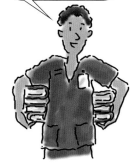

Which answer is an early sign of hypoxia?

40. 3, 5. Increasing heart rate and tachypnea are early signs of hypoxia. A progressive, barking cough is characteristic of spasmodic croup. Acute anorexia may be noted in ill children; however, it is not a sign of respiratory distress. A productive cough shows secretions are moving, and the child can effectively clear them.
CN: Physiological integrity; CNS: Physiological adaptation; CL: Apply

41. Before examining a child with acute epiglottitis, it is **priority** for the nurse to have which item(s) at the bedside? Select all that apply.
1. Cool, humidified oxygen
2. Endotracheal tube
3. Oxygen saturation monitor
4. The child's security blanket
5. Laryngoscope with blade
6. Stylet or bougie

41. 2, 5, 6. Emergency intubation equipment (appropriately sized endotracheal tube, laryngoscope with blade, and a stylet or bougie) should be at the bedside to secure the airway if the examination precipitates further or complete obstruction. All other items are needed, but not priority.
CN: Safe, effective care environment; CNS: Safety and infection control; CL: Analyze

42. The nurse notes a child is drooling, sitting upright, and leaning forward with the chin thrusting out, mouth open, and tongue protruding. Which nursing action is **most** appropriate?
1. Check the child's gag reflex with a tongue blade.
2. Allow the child to cry to keep the lungs expanded.
3. Check the airway for a foreign body obstruction.
4. Support the child in an upright position on the parent's lap.

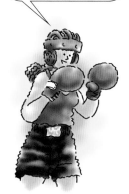

Float like a butterfly, sting like a bee. Hang in there!

42. 4. The classic signs of epiglottitis are drooling, sitting upright, and leaning forward with the chin thrust out, mouth open, and tongue protruding. The child should be kept in an upright position to ease the work of breathing, to avoid aspiration of secretions, and to help prevent obstruction of the airway by the swollen epiglottis. Placing the child on the lap of a parent may help reduce the child's anxiety. The gag reflex of a child with epiglottitis should never be checked unless emergency personnel and equipment are immediately available to perform a tracheotomy (in the event that the airway becomes obstructed by the swollen epiglottis). Allowing the child to cry and inspecting the airway for a foreign body may also cause complete airway obstruction.
CN: Physiological integrity; CNS: Reduction of risk potential; CL: Apply

43. The nurse is caring for a 3-year-old child with right lower lobe pneumonia. Which position will the nurse place the child in after completing an assessment?
1. Supine
2. Prone
3. Right side-lying
4. Left side-lying

43. 4. The child with right lower lobe pneumonia should be placed on the left side. This places the unaffected left lung in a position to allow gravity to promote blood flow through the healthy lung tissue and improve gas exchange. Placing the child on the right side, back, or stomach would not promote circulation to the unaffected lung.
CN: Physiological integrity; CNS: Physiological adaptation; CL: Apply

44. The arterial blood gas analysis of a child with asthma shows a pH level of 7.30, $PaCO_2$ level of 56 mm Hg, and HCO_3^- level of 25 mEq/L. The nurse determines the child has which condition?
1. Metabolic acidosis
2. Metabolic alkalosis
3. Respiratory acidosis
4. Respiratory alkalosis

44. 3. Respiratory acidosis is an acid–base disturbance characterized by excess CO_2 in the blood, indicated by a $PaCO_2$ level greater than 45 mm Hg. The pH level is usually below the normal range of 7.35 to 7.45. The HCO_3 level is normal in the acute stage and elevated in the chronic stage.
CN: Physiological integrity; CNS: Physiological adaptation; CL: Apply

45. Which action will the nurse take for a 2-year-old child with laryngotracheobronchitis who is lethargic, tachypneic, and has labored breathing?
1. Stimulate the child to maintain alertness.
2. Provide an atmosphere of cool mist, high humidity.
3. Offer frequent, oral feedings.
4. Administer acetaminophen as prescribed.

Looks like a trip to the rainforest might be in order.

46. When caring for a child with increased laryngotracheal edema, the nurse will closely monitor the child for which early sign of hypoxia?
1. Decreased heart and respiratory rates and a high peak flow rate
2. Increased heart rate, retractions, and restlessness
3. Decreased blood pressure, lethargy, and tripod positioning
4. Increased temperature, blood pressure, and respiratory rate

47. Which action will the nurse complete when caring for an infant with bronchopulmonary dysplasia?
1. Provide frequent, playful stimuli.
2. Decrease oxygen during feedings.
3. Place the infant on a set schedule.
4. Place the infant in an open crib.

Great job! You've taken a great step forward.

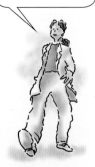

48. Which finding does the nurse identify as **priority** for an infant with bronchopulmonary dysplasia?
1. Imbalanced nutrition
2. Effective breastfeeding
3. Impaired gas exchange
4. Imbalanced fluid volume

45. 2. An atmosphere of cool mist and high humidity reduces mucosal edema and prevents drying of secretions, thus helping to maintain an open airway in a child exhibiting signs of respiratory distress. Keeping the child calm, not stimulated, helps to reduce oxygen need. Oral feedings may need to be withheld in a child experiencing respiratory distress because eating may interfere with the ability to breathe. Acetaminophen is not indicated for respiratory distress.
CN: Physiological integrity; CNS: Physiological adaptation; CL: Analyze

46. 2. Increased heart and respiratory rates, retractions, and restlessness are classic indicators of hypoxia. The heart and respiratory rates increase to enable increased oxygenation. Accessory breathing muscles are used, causing retractions in substernal, suprasternal, and intercostal areas. Reduced oxygen to the brain causes restlessness initially and altered level of consciousness later. A decrease in heart and respiratory rates would be a late, ominous sign of decompensation. Peak flow rate is a test used in asthma. A decrease, not increase, in peak flow is diagnostic of disease. Decreased blood pressure would be a late sign of hypoxia. An increase in temperature is more indicative of infection or inflammation than respiratory distress.
CN: Physiological integrity; CNS: Physiological adaptation; CL: Apply

47. 3. Timing care activities with rest periods to avoid fatigue and to decrease respiratory effort is essential. Early stimulation activities are recommended, but the infant would have limited tolerance for them because of the illness. Oxygen is usually increased during feedings to help decrease respiratory and energy requirements. Thermoregulation is important because both hypothermia and hyperthermia would increase oxygen consumption and might increase oxygen requirements. These infants are usually maintained on warmer beds or in isolettes.
CN: Safe, effective care environment; CNS: Management of care; CL: Apply

48. 3. The infant would have impaired gas exchange related to retention of carbon dioxide and borderline oxygenation secondary to fibrosis of the lungs. Although the infant may require increased caloric intake and may have excess fluid volume, the other nursing diagnoses are not the priority.
CN: Safe, effective care environment; CNS: Management of care; CL: Apply

49. Which intervention is **most** appropriate for the nurse to recommend to the parents of a child newly diagnosed with bronchopulmonary dysplasia to assist with coping?
1. Educate the parents on cardiopulmonary resuscitation.
2. Provide the parents pamphlets on local support groups.
3. Help the parents identify necessary lifestyle changes.
4. Evaluate the parents' current stress and anxiety levels.

50. Which action is **most** appropriate for the nurse to include when caring for an infant with bronchopulmonary dysplasia?
1. Provide chest physiotherapy.
2. Administer enteral feedings.
3. Offer age-appropriate activities.
4. Promote parent and infant bonding.

51. Theophylline 24 mg/kg/day given in four divided doses is prescribed for a 20-month-old child with bronchopulmonary dysplasia. The child weighs 33.1 lb (15 kg). How many milligrams will the nurse administer per dose? Record your answer using a whole number.

_____ mg

52. The nurse is caring for an infant with bronchopulmonary dysplasia. The nurse will provide more rest periods if which finding(s) is noted in the infant? Select all that apply.
1. Diaphoresis
2. Poor eye contact
3. Cyanosis
4. Sternal retractions
5. Falling asleep during care
6. Increased irritability

53. Before discharge, the nurse will ensure the parents of a child with bronchopulmonary dysplasia have met which goal?
1. They have increased levels of stress regarding home care
2. They can make safe decisions with help from the nurse
3. They assist in routine, but not complex, caretaking activities
4. They verbalize how to perform care for their infant at home

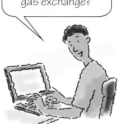
Which intervention will best improve gas exchange?

49. 4. The emotional impact of bronchopulmonary dysplasia is clearly a crisis situation. The parents are experiencing grief and sorrow over the loss of a "healthy" child. The other strategies are more appropriate for long-term intervention.
CN: Psychosocial integrity; CNS: None; CL: Apply

50. 1. All of these activities are appropriate to include in the care of a child with bronchopulmonary dysplasia; however, providing chest physiotherapy is the nursing action that addresses impairment of gas exchange and thus is the priority.
CN: Safe, effective care environment; CNS: Management of care; CL: Analyze

51. 90.
The child should receive 90 mg/dose. First, calculate the total daily dose.

$$\textit{milligrams per dose} \times \textit{child's weight in kilograms} = \textit{total dose per day}$$

$$24\ mg \times 15\ kg = 360\ mg/dose$$

Then, divide the total daily dose by the number of doses.

$$60\ mg/4\ doses = 90\ mg/dose$$

CN: Physiological integrity; CNS: Pharmacological and parenteral therapies; CL: Analyze

52. 1, 2, 3, 4, 5, 6. Signs of overstimulation in an infant with chronic respiratory dysfunction include cyanosis, avoidance of eye contact, vomiting, diaphoresis, irritability, signs of respiratory distress (such as sternal retractions), and falling asleep during care.
CN: Psychosocial integrity; CNS: None; CL: Apply

53. 4. The parents should understand the care requirements of their infant by the time of discharge. Asking the parents to verbalize this information is the only way to assess their understanding. The parents should report decreased levels of stress, be capable of making decisions independently, and participate in routine and complex care prior to discharge.
CN: Physiological integrity; CNS: Basic care and comfort; CL: Apply

CN: Client needs category   CNS: Client needs subcategory   CL: Cognitive level

54. The nurse is caring for a child with broncho-pulmonary dysplasia. Which characteristic will the nurse expect the child to exhibit during the early stage of this disease?
1. Clubbing of the fingers
2. Barrel chest
3. Cyanosis
4. Dyspnea upon exertion

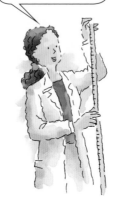

Impressive. Your performance is off the scale.

54. 4. The early stage is characterized by early interstitial changes and resembles respiratory distress syndrome (including dyspnea with exertion). As the disease progresses, signs of chronic disease appear, including interstitial edema, signs of emphysema, and pulmonary hypertension. Clubbing of the fingers, barrel chest, and cyanosis would be observed in the later stage of the disease. CN: Physiological integrity; CNS: Physiological adaptation; CL: Apply

55. The nurse is caring for a child with broncho-pulmonary dysplasia prescribed furosemide. The nurse will monitor this child for which adverse effect?
1. Hypercalcemia
2. Hyperkalemia
3. Hypernatremia
4. Irregular heart rhythm

55. 4. An irregular heart rhythm and muscle cramps are adverse effects associated with hypokalemia and hypocalcemia, which can be caused by taking furosemide. Diuretics cause volume depletion by inhibiting reabsorption of sodium and chloride. Hypocalcemia is related to the urinary excretion of calcium. Hypokalemia can occur with excessive fluid loss or as part of contraction alkalosis. CN: Physiological integrity; CNS: Pharmacological and parenteral therapies; CL: Apply

56. The nurse is caring for a child prescribed furosemide 4 mg/kg/day. The child weighs 40 lb (18 kg). How many milligrams will the nurse administer in each dose? Record your answer using a whole number.

_____ mg

56. 72.
The child will receive 72 mg per dose. To calculate the milligrams per dose:

$$milligrams\ per\ dose \times child's\ weight\ in\ kilograms = milligrams\ per\ dose$$

$$4\ mg \times 18\ kg = 72\ mg/day$$

CN: Physiological integrity; CNS: Pharmacological and parenteral therapies; CL: Apply

57. A 2-year-old child with bronchopulmonary dysplasia is prescribed furosemide daily. Which food(s) will the nurse recommend the parents include in the child's diet? Select all that apply.
1. Figs
2. Apples
3. Oranges
4. Peaches
5. Raisins

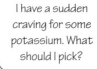

I have a sudden craving for some potassium. What should I pick?

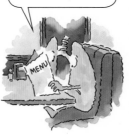

57. 1, 5. The nurse should recommend foods high in potassium to prevent hypokalemia from furosemide. Raisins, dates, figs, and prunes are among the most potassium-rich foods. They average 17 to 20 mEq (17 to 20 mmol/L) of potassium. Apples, oranges, and peaches have very low amounts of potassium. Each averages 3 to 4 mEq (3 to 4 mmol/L). CN: Physiological integrity; CNS: Pharmacological and parenteral therapies; CL: Apply

58. The nurse is caring for an infant with broncho-pulmonary dysplasia. Several attempts to wean the infant from the ventilator have been unsuccessful. Which action will the nurse complete?
1. Prepare the infant for possible tracheostomy tube placement.
2. Teach the parents how to use a continuous positive airway pressure (CPAP) machine.
3. Discuss end-of-life care measures with the infant's parents.
4. Continue to monitor the infant for signs of increasing respiratory distress.

58. 1. Tracheostomy may be required after a child has been dependent on a ventilator and cannot wean from it. The child would not need CPAP or monitoring for increasing respiratory distress at this time. The nurse would not discuss end-of-life care at this time. CN: Physiological integrity; CNS: Physiological adaptation; CL: Apply

59. A 3-year-old child with bronchopulmonary dysplasia has just returned from surgery for a tracheostomy. Which nursing intervention(s) is appropriate? Select all that apply.
1. Keep extra tracheostomy tubes at the bedside.
2. Secure ties at the back of the child's neck.
3. Change the tracheostomy tube 1 day after surgery.
4. Secure the tracheostomy ties tightly.
5. Monitor the child for respiratory distress.

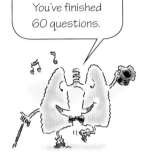

Happy day! You've finished 60 questions.

60. Based on the nurse's note in the chart shown below, which nursing intervention is **priority** for an 11-month-old infant with bronchopulmonary dysplasia?

Progress notes	
11/15	The infant is lying in the bassinet and
1730	appears restless. Tracheostomy is in place.
	Vital signs: temperature, 98°F (36.7°C);
	blood pressure, 80/50 mm Hg; heart rate,
	180 beats/minute; respiratory rate,
	66 breaths/minute; oxygen saturation rate, 88%.
	—G. Tremblay, RN

1. Auscultate breath sounds.
2. Suction the tracheostomy tube.
3. Notify the health care provider.
4. Administer humidified oxygen.

61. Which nursing intervention is **most** appropriate when suctioning thick secretions through a tracheostomy tube from a 2-year-old child?
1. Hyperventilate the child after suctioning.
2. Repeat the suctioning process for two intervals.
3. Insert the catheter 1 to 2 cm below the tracheostomy tube.
4. Inject a small amount of normal saline into the tube before suctioning.

62. A child comes to the clinic with consistent sneezing and itching of the eyes and nose. Which prescription will the nurse anticipate from the primary health care provider?
1. Amoxicillin
2. Cetirizine
3. Cefdinir
4. Albuterol

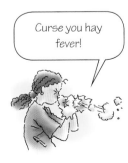

Curse you hay fever!

59. 1, 2, 5. Extra tracheostomy tubes should be kept at the bedside in case of an emergency, including one size smaller in case the appropriate size does not fit due to edema. The ties should be placed securely but should allow some space (the width of a pinky finger) to prevent excessive pressure or skin breakdown. The first tracheostomy tube change is usually performed by the health care provider after 7 days. Ties are placed at the back of the neck. The nurse would monitor for complications such as respiratory distress.
CN: Physiological integrity; CNS: Physiological adaptation; CL: Apply

60. 2. Tracheostomy tubes, particularly in small children, require frequent suctioning to remove mucous plugs and excessive secretions. The tracheostomy tube can be changed if suctioning is unsuccessful. Auscultating breath sounds and notifying the health care provider is not necessary at this time. Humidified oxygen would only help if the airway were patent.
CN: Safe, effective care environment; CNS: Management of care; CL: Apply

61. 4. Injecting a small amount of normal saline solution helps to loosen secretions for easier aspiration but should not be done routinely. Preservative-free normal saline solution should be used. The child should be hyperventilated *before* and *after* suctioning to prevent hypoxia. The suctioning process should be repeated until the trachea is clear. The catheter should be inserted 0.5 cm beyond the tracheostomy tube. If the catheter is inserted too far, it will irritate the carina and may cause blood-tinged secretions.
CN: Safe, effective care environment; CNS: Management of care; CL: Apply

62. 2. The nurse would suspect the client has seasonal allergies. Allergies elicit consistent bouts of sneezing, are seldom accompanied by fever, and tend to cause itching of the eyes and nose. Common antihistamine medications used to treat seasonal allergies in children include cetirizine, fexofenadine, and loratadine. Amoxicillin and cefdinir are antibiotics used to treat bacterial infections. Albuterol is a bronchodilator used to treat respiratory conditions such as asthma.
CN: Safe, effective care environment; CNS: Management of care; CL: Apply

CN: Client needs category   CNS: Client needs subcategory   CL: Cognitive level

63. The nurse is caring for a 10-year-old child with asthma. Which finding **most** concerns the nurse?
1. Exercise intolerance
2. Respiratory rate of 24 breaths/minute
3. Recurrent cough
4. Diminished breath sounds

63. 4. Diminished breath sounds are an indication that the child is in distress and not exchanging air adequately; this is an immediate concern. The nurse would anticipate the child with asthma to have exercise intolerance. The respiratory rate is normal for a 10-year-old child. Cough is not a concern at this time because the child is still able to clear the airway.
CN: Safe, effective care environment; CNS: Management of care; CL: Apply

64. A 2-year-old child is diagnosed with asthma. The parents ask the nurse about asthma triggers. Which potential trigger(s) will the nurse include in the education? Select all that apply.
1. Weather
2. Air quality
3. Peanut butter
4. Exercise
5. Sulfites

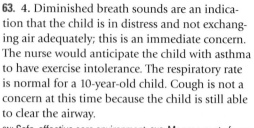

Uh oh. Trigger alert!

64. 1, 2, 4, 5. Excessively cold air, wet or humid weather, and changes in seasons; air pollution; exercise; and food additives (sulfites) are common asthma triggers. Peanut butter can be a food allergen and can lead to anaphylactic reactions but is not an asthma trigger.
CN: Physiological integrity; CNS: Physiological adaptation; CL: Apply

65. A child is seen in the emergency department with severe chest tightness and wheezing. The parents inform the nurse these symptoms have been constant, and bronchodilators have not helped. Which primary health care provider prescription will the nurse question for this client?
1. High-dose albuterol
2. Ipratropium bromide
3. Theophylline
4. Montelukast

65. 4. Severe asthma, or status asthmaticus, can best be described as constant attacks unrelieved by bronchodilators. Current treatments include higher dosage of albuterol, ipratropium bromide, and theophylline (bronchodilators). Montelukast is a leukotriene modifier used for the prevention of bronchospasms.
CN: Safe, effective care environment; CNS: Management of care; CL: Analyze

66. When assessing a child with asthma, which finding **most** concerns the nurse?
1. Expiratory stridor
2. Tachycardia
3. Coughing
4. Wheezing

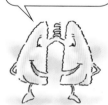

You really know your stuff. That helps me breathe a little easier.

66. 1. The nurse would be most concerned if stridor were assessed in a child with asthma. Expiratory stridor is not associated with asthma and indicates the child is experiencing a disrupted airflow, usually from a blockage in the trachea. Asthma frequently occurs with wheezing and coughing due to increased mucus production, as well as tachycardia.
CN: Safe, effective care environment; CNS: Management of care; CL: Apply

67. An adolescent with asthma comes to the school nurse to use the peak flow meter. It measures in the red zone. Which response by the school nurse is **most** appropriate?
1. "When was the last time you used albuterol inhaler?"
2. "I am calling your parents to take you to your health care provider."
3. "You need to use your albuterol inhaler promptly."
4. "I need to give you a dose of your montelukast now."

67. 2. Peak flow meters provide clients with a color scale (green, yellow, and red). The different color zones help determine a management plan for the client. The red zone indicates airway narrowing, a medical emergency. The client needs to use a bronchodilator and may need an oral corticosteroid or to seek emergency care. It is not priority to know when the child last used the inhaler. The child's parents should be notified and the child may need additional medical care. Montelukast is a leukotriene modifier used for prevention of bronchospasms, not to treat airway narrowing.
CN: Physiological integrity; CNS: Reduction of risk potential; CL: Apply

68. A 2-year-old child with severe asthma is admitted and begins to receive continuous albuterol nebulizers. The nurse will observe the client for which adverse reaction(s)? Select all that apply.
1. Tachycardia
2. Nervousness
3. Tremors
4. Tachypnea
5. Irritability

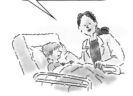

This question should get your heart rate up.

69. A 10-year-old child admitted with asthma is prescribed an aminophylline infusion. A loading dose of 6 mg/kg is prescribed. The client weighs 66 lb (30 kg). How many milligrams of aminophylline will the nurse administer to the client in the loading dose? Record your answer using a whole number.

_____ mg

70. Which complication will the nurse monitor for in a child receiving mechanical ventilation?
1. Pneumothorax
2. High cardiac output
3. Polycythemia
4. Hypovolemia

71. The nurse is reviewing diagnostic test results for a child admitted with severe asthma. The chest x-ray results indicate hyperexpansion and atelectasis. Which action will the nurse take?
1. Continue to monitor the client as prescribed.
2. Assess the client's oxygen saturation level.
3. Have the client use the peak flow meter.
4. Administer formoterol to the client.

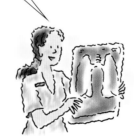

Hmm… Looks a little deflated. Do you remember the medical term for that?

72. The nurse is caring for a child with atelectasis as a result of severe asthma. Which nursing action is **priority** for this child?
1. Increase intravenous (IV) fluids.
2. Perform chest physiotherapy.
3. Administer humidified oxygen.
4. Get arterial blood gas (ABG) levels.

68. **1, 2, 3, 5.** Albuterol is a rapid-acting bronchodilator. Common adverse effects include tachycardia, nervousness, tremors, insomnia, irritability, nausea and vomiting, and headache. Tachypnea is not a common adverse effect of this drug.
CN: Physiological integrity; CNS: Pharmacological and parenteral therapies; CL: Apply

69. **180.**
The child will receive 180 mg for the loading dose. To calculate the loading dose:

$$milligrams\ per\ dose \times child's\ weight\ in\ kilograms = total\ dose$$

$$6\ mg \times 30 = 180\ mg$$

CN: Physiological integrity; CNS: Pharmacological and parenteral therapies; CL: Apply

70. **1.** Mechanical ventilation can cause barotrauma, as occurs with pneumothorax. A child receiving mechanical ventilation must be carefully monitored. Mechanical ventilation decreases, not increases, cardiac output. Polycythemia is the result of chronic hypoxia, not mechanical ventilation. Mechanical ventilation can cause fluid overload, not hypovolemia.
CN: Physiological integrity; CNS: Physiological adaptation; CL: Apply

71. **1.** Hyperexpansion, atelectasis, and a flattened diaphragm are typical x-ray findings for a child with asthma. Air becomes trapped behind the narrowed airways and the residual capacity rises, leading to hyperinflation. Hypoxemia results from areas of the lung not being well perfused. The nurse would continue to monitor the client as prescribed. Since the findings are typical, there is no indication of a need to assess an oxygen saturation, use a peak flow meter, or administer formoterol (bronchodilator).
CN: Physiological integrity; CNS: Physiological adaptation; CL: Analyze

72. **2.** Chest physiotherapy and incentive spirometry help to enhance the clearance of mucus and open the alveoli. Although not the most important intervention, giving IV and oral fluids is recommended to help liquefy and thin secretions. Administration of oxygen would not provide enough pressure to open the alveoli. Obtaining ABG levels is not necessary unless the client has signs of hypoxemia.
CN: Safe, effective care environment; CNS: Management of care; CL: Analyze

73. The parents of a 10-year-old child diagnosed with asthma ask the nurse if their child can continue to play soccer. Which nursing response is **most** appropriate?
  1. "Absolutely, because physical activity does not lead to asthma attacks."
  2. "It is best to limit your child's physical activities to reduce asthma attacks."
  3. "As long as your child does not have a respiratory illness at the time, it is okay."
  4. "A peak flow meter will help us see how your child tolerates physical activity."

74. A child with a thoracic water-seal drainage system is on the elevator. The assistive personnel (AP) placed the drainage system on the stretcher. Which action will the registered nurse (RN) take **first**?
  1. Assist the AP in placing the drainage system lower than the child's chest.
  2. Report the incident to the nurse administrator upon return to the unit.
  3. Immediately auscultate to assess the child's respiratory and heart rates.
  4. Inform the AP to no longer provide care for clients with a drainage system.

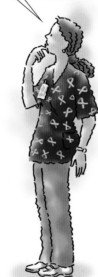

Which action will the RN take **first** in question #74?

75. Which nursing intervention is **most** appropriate for a 2-year-old child with asthma based on the chart exhibit below?

Progress notes	
5/21	Child was crying during assessment, no tears
1135	noted. Child's current weight is 22.1 lb (10 kg).
	Vital signs are as follows: Heart rate, 140
	beats/minute; respiratory rate, 38 breaths/
	minute; blood pressure, 82/44 mm Hg. Dry
	mucous membranes are noted. Urine output was
	30 mL over the past 4 hours.
	— Quinton Macdonald, RN

  1. Have the child drink warm liquids.
  2. Provide the child an ice pop.
  3. Give the child an electrolyte drink.
  4. Administer intravenous (IV) fluids.

76. The nurse is educating parents of a child being discharged with asthma. Which information will the nurse include in the teaching?
  1. Cover floors with carpet or area rugs.
  2. Allow the child to play in the basement.
  3. Dust the home thoroughly twice a month.
  4. Use foam rubber pillows and synthetic blankets.

73. 4. Participation in sports is encouraged but should be evaluated on an individual basis using a peak flow meter as long as the asthma is under control. Exercise-induced asthma is an example of the airway hyperactivity common to asthmatics. Exclusion from sports or activities may hamper peer interaction. Respiratory illnesses do place children more at risk for an asthma attack, but this does not address the parent's overall concern.
CN: Safe, effective care environment; CNS: Management of care; CL: Apply

74. 1. The drainage device must be kept below the level of the chest to maintain straight gravity drainage. Placing it on the stretcher may cause a backflow of drainage into the thoracic cavity, which could collapse the partially expanded lung. Reporting the incident is indicated, but the immediate safety of the child takes priority. After the drainage system has been properly repositioned, the child's respiratory and heart rates may be taken. The nurse administrator would decide whether disciplinary action is needed, not the staff RN.
CN: Safe, effective care environment; CNS: Management of care; CL: Apply

75. 4. The assessment reveals that the child is severely dehydrated and needs to have fluids replaced intravenously. The heart and respiratory rates are increased, blood pressure is decreased, and expected urine output for a toddler is 1 to 2 mL/kg/hour. Liquids are best tolerated if they are warm and can be given in conjunction with IV fluids, but not in place of IV fluids. Cold liquids may cause bronchospasm and should be avoided. A warmed electrolyte drink may be provided.
CN: Safe, effective care environment; CNS: Management of care; CL: Apply

76. 4. Bedding should be free from allergens and have nonallergenic covers. Unnecessary rugs and carpets should be removed, and floors should be mopped a few times per week to reduce dust. Basements or cellars should be avoided to lessen the child's exposure to molds and mildew. Dusting and cleaning should occur daily or at least weekly.
CN: Physiological integrity; CNS: Physiological adaptation; CL: Apply

CN: Client needs category   CNS: Client needs subcategory   CL: Cognitive level

77. The nurse on the pediatric unit is caring for a child with asthma. Which complication will the nurse expect to address in this child?
1. Overeating at meal times
2. Edema related to fluid overload
3. Inability to play due to fatigue
4. Straining to pass hard stools

77. 3. Ineffective oxygen supply and demand may lead to activity intolerance. The nurse should promote rest and encourage developmentally appropriate activities. Nutrition may be decreased, not increased, due to respiratory distress and gastrointestinal upset. Dehydration is common due to diaphoresis, insensible water loss, and hyperventilation. Medications given to treat asthma may cause nausea, vomiting, and diarrhea, not constipation.
CN: Physiological integrity; CNS: Physiological adaptation; CL: Analyze

78. The clinic nurse is providing education to the caregivers of a 1-year-old diagnosed with bronchiolitis. Which statement made by the parents demonstrates an understanding of the nurse's education?
1. "We can give our child ibuprofen every 3 to 4 hours."
2. "The nebulizer medication should be given daily at bedtime."
3. "It is safe for our child to return to day care tomorrow."
4. "We will place a cool-mist humidifier in the child's room."

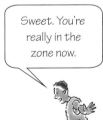

I love causing inflammation. You could say I get a real rise out of it.

78. 4. Bronchiolitis is an infection of the bronchioles, causing the mucosa to become edematous, inflamed, and full of mucus. A cool-mist humidifier will help ease congestion and coughing by moistening the air. Ibuprofen can be given for pain, inflammation, or fever to children over 6 months of age; however, it should be given every 6 to 8 hours to prevent overdosing. Nebulizers may be given several times a day as needed for respiratory distress. Children may return to day care once they do not have signs of respiratory distress.
CN: Physiological integrity; CNS: Physiological adaptation; CL: Apply

79. A 5-month-old infant is diagnosed with bronchiolitis from respiratory syncytial virus (RSV). Which symptom warrants **immediate** nursing intervention?
1. Mild wheezing
2. Poor appetite
3. Nasal flaring
4. Paroxysmal coughing

79. 4. In bronchiolitis, the bronchioles become narrowed and edematous. These infants typically have a 2- to 3-day history of an upper respiratory infection and feeding difficulties with loss of appetite due to nasal congestion and increased work of breathing. This combination leads to respiratory distress. Paroxysmal coughing is violent, frequent coughing that compromises the infant's respiratory status. The nurse must maintain the child's airway and facilitate breathing first, and then address the other findings.
CN: Safe, effective care environment; CNS: Management of care; CL: Analyze

80. The nurse is caring for a child diagnosed with bronchiolitis. Which symptom **most** concerns the nurse?
1. Multiple sternal retractions
2. Presence of thick mucus
3. Temperature of 100.6°F (38.1°C)
4. Oxygenation saturation level of 95%

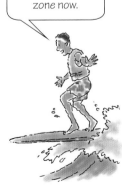

Sweet. You're really in the zone now.

80. 1. Bronchiolitis is a lower respiratory infection and is characterized by possible air trapping, tachypnea, thick mucus, and sternal retraction. A child with multiple sternal retractions has more difficulty breathing; therefore, not enough air is getting into the lungs. This needs to be a high priority and needs to be monitored closely. The other findings are expected in a child with this condition.
CN: Safe, effective care environment; CNS: Management of care; CL: Apply

81. A child comes to the emergency department with symptoms of asthma, and the health care provider prescribes a sputum culture. Which explanation for this test is **best** for the nurse to provide the parents?
1. "It will identify the causative agent of the asthma attack."
2. "It will rule out a respiratory infection in your child."
3. "It will complete the protocol for asthma treatment."
4. "It will identify any risk factors associated with asthma."

82. Which personal protective equipment (PPE) will the nurse caring for a 2-month-old infant with respiratory syncytial virus (RSV) don before entering the room? Select all that apply.
1. Gloves
2. Gown
3. Mask
4. Eye shield
5. N95 respirator

83. The nurse will anticipate administering palivizumab to which client?
1. A 2-month-old born at 37 weeks' gestation with a cleft lip and palate
2. A 3-month-old born at 32 weeks' gestation with tetralogy of Fallot
3. A 6-month-old born at 42 weeks' gestation with Hirschsprung's disease
4. A 3-year-old born at 39 weeks' gestation recently diagnosed with asthma

84. The nurse is caring for a 6-year-old client with cystic fibrosis prescribed azithromycin 12 mg/kg 2 days ago. The nurse will report which finding to the primary health care provider?
1. Presence of loose, watery stools
2. History of jaundice 1 week after birth
3. Client reports intermittent nausea, lasting 10 minutes
4. Aspartate aminotransferase (AST) level 20 U/L (0.33 µkat/L)

85. A child is diagnosed with respiratory syncytial virus (RSV). Which medication will the nurse anticipate administering?
1. Albuterol
2. Aminophylline
3. Cromolyn sodium
4. Ribavirin

81. 2. When a client has asthma, it is appropriate to do a sputum analysis to rule out a respiratory infection. It is not part of the protocol for asthma treatment and it would not identify risk factors for asthma or agents that precipitated an asthma attack.
CN: Physiological integrity; CNS: Physiological adaptation; CL: Apply

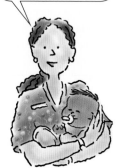

Remember to gear up when your client has RSV—it's highly contagious.

82. 1, 2, 3. RSV is highly contagious and is spread through direct contact with infectious secretions via hands, droplets, and fomites. A gown, gloves, and mask should be worn for care of the infant to prevent the spread of infection, in addition to practicing proper hand washing between clients. An eye shield and N95 respirator are not required PPE for RSV.
CN: Safe, effective care environment; CNS: Safety and infection control; CL: Apply

83. 2. Clients at highest risk for respiratory syncytial virus (RSV) include preterm infants with cardiac or pulmonary conditions. Palivizumab is a synthetic antibody to RSV given to high-risk clients for 5 consecutive months from November to April. Gastrointestinal disorders do not place an infant at high risk for RSV. Children 2 years and younger are at greatest risk for RSV.
CN: Physiological integrity; CNS: Reduction of risk potential; CL: Analyze

Don't let question #84 make you anxious. You'll figure it out.

84. 1. Azithromycin is an antibiotic given to treat bacterial infections. The nurse will report loose, watery (or bloody) stools after the use of azithromycin. This could indicate *Clostridium difficile*–associated diarrhea. Jaundice while taking azithromycin, not a previous history of, should be reported as this could indicate liver damage. Nausea is a common side effect in clients taking azithromycin. The AST level is in the normal range of 10 to 40 U/L (0.17 to 0.67 µkat/L).
CN: Safe, effective care environment; CNS: Management of care; CL: Apply

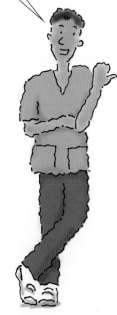

85. 4. Ribavirin is an antiviral agent sometimes used to reduce the severity of bronchiolitis caused by RSV in high-risk clients. It is used rarely due to its potential for teratogenic effects. Aminophylline and albuterol are bronchodilators and have not been proven effective in treating viral bronchiolitis. Cromolyn sodium is an inhaled anti-inflammatory agent.
CN: Physiological integrity; CNS: Pharmacological and parenteral therapies; CL: Apply

CN: Client needs category   CNS: Client needs subcategory   CL: Cognitive level

86. The registered nurse (RN) and assistive personnel (AP) are caring for a 1-year-old client with bronchiolitis. Which task will the RN delegate to the AP?
   1. Obtain the child's respiratory rate.
   2. Decrease the oxygen flow rate as prescribed.
   3. Show the parents how to give acetaminophen.
   4. Help the mother with breastfeeding.

86. 1. The nurse can delegate obtaining a respiratory rate to the AP, as this is a consistent, unchanging procedure. The AP cannot titrate oxygen, administer medications, or provide education on administering medications. The nurse needs to assist with breastfeeding to assess the infant's ability to breathe while feeding and determine what guidance the mother may need.
CN: Safe, effective care environment; CNS: Management of care; CL: Analyze

87. When developing a care plan for an 8-month-old infant with bronchiolitis, which finding will the nurse determine is **priority**?
   1. 2 lb (1 kg) weight loss over 1 week
   2. Oxygen saturation rate 89% (0.89) on room air
   3. Infant appears uninterested in toys
   4. Caregiver infrequently holds infant

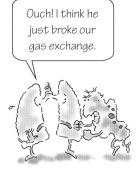

Ouch! I think he just broke our gas exchange.

87. 2. Infants with bronchiolitis have impaired gas exchange related to bronchiolar obstruction, atelectasis, and hyperinflation. Nutrition may be seen as less than body requirements but is not as important as gas exchange. If respiratory distress is present, these infants should have nothing by mouth and fluids given intravenously only. These infants may be too uncomfortable and fatigued to be interested in toys. A lack of bonding should be addressed but is not priority at this time.
CN: Safe, effective care environment; CNS: Management of care; CL: Apply

88. The nurse is providing discharge education to the parents of an infant being treated for bronchiolitis. Which information will the nurse include in the teaching?
   1. Place the child in a prone position for sleeping.
   2. Bring the child back to the hospital if the infant does not sleep.
   3. Notify the health care provider for grunting or nasal flaring.
   4. Provide the infant several activities throughout the day.

88. 3. It is essential for parents to be able to recognize signs of increasing respiratory distress and to notify the health care provider. The child should be positioned with the head of the bed elevated to facilitate removal of secretions and ease the work of breathing. Infants may not sleep well while sick, but this is not a reason to come to the hospital. Quiet play activities are required only as the child's energy level permits.
CN: Physiological integrity; CNS: Physiological adaptation; CL: Apply

89. The nurse is caring for a child diagnosed with pneumonia. What prescription will the nurse complete **first**?
   1. Increase oral fluid intake.
   2. Administer oxygen as needed.
   3. Perform chest physiotherapy.
   4. Give acetaminophen for fever.

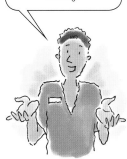

Sometimes a little percussion to the back is just the thing to clear the airway.

89. 3. Pneumonia is an inflammation of the pulmonary parenchyma, and ventilation decreases as secretions thicken. The most effective treatment to promote a clear airway is chest physiotherapy, including postural drainage, coughing, and deep breathing, as well as incentive spirometry. Dietary changes, especially forcing fluids, would help, but chest physiotherapy, coughing, and deep breathing are more effective. Oxygen therapy would help to increase oxygen saturation but does not work well if the bronchioles are blocked with mucus or constricted. Antipyretics would decrease a fever, but opening the airways is priority.
CN: Safe, effective care environment; CNS: Management of care; CL: Analyze

90. The nurse is caring for a 15-year-old client with bacterial pneumonia. The health care provider prescribes a sputum culture. Place the steps in the chronological order the nurse will correctly complete them for the procedure. Use all options.

1. Provide a container and instruct the client not to touch the inside of the container.
2. Securely apply the lid to the container and label with appropriate information.
3. Inform the client to expectorate sputum directly into the provided container.
4. Explain the procedure to the client.
5. Have the client repeat coughing until a sufficient amount is collected.
6. Instruct the client to take a slow, deep breath and cough after full inhalation.

90. Ordered Response:

4. Explain the procedure to the client.
1. Provide a container and instruct the client not to touch the inside of the container.
6. Instruct the client to take a slow, deep breath and cough after full inhalation.
3. Inform the client to expectorate sputum directly into the provided container.
5. Have the client repeat coughing until a sufficient amount is collected.
2. Securely apply the lid to the container and label with appropriate information.

CN: Safe, effective care environment; CNS: Safety and infection control; CL: Apply

91. A 2-year-old client is diagnosed with bacterial otitis media. Which education is **priority** for the nurse to include?
1. How to perform proper hand washing in a public setting
2. The importance of completing prescribed antibiotics
3. Signs and symptoms of hearing loss from otitis media
4. About myringotomy and tympanostomy tube insertion

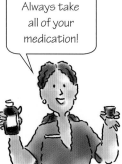

Always take all of your medication!

91. 2. The nurse should first educate the caregiver on proper antibiotic administration to ensure complete healing. The nurse would also educate the caregiver on proper hand washing to decrease future infections. Hearing loss and tube insertion would be discussed if the child has had multiple diagnoses of otitis media.

CN: Health promotion and maintenance; CNS: None; CL: Analyze

92. The nurse is caring for a 1-year-old client diagnosed with pertussis. Which assessment finding will the nurse flag for the primary health care provider?
1. The child resting after coughing
2. The presence of a whooping cough
3. Temperature of 100.6°F (38.1°C)
4. Blood pressure of 75/40 mm Hg

92. 4. The nurse should flag the low blood pressure, as this is an unexpected finding in a child with pertussis. Resting is expected as the child is fatigued from coughing. Pertussis is characterized by consistent short, rapid coughs followed by a sudden inspiration with a high-pitched whooping sound. Pertussis usually is accompanied by a low-grade fever.

CN: Safe, effective care environment; CNS: Management of care; CL: Apply

93. A homeless teenager comes to the clinic with a history of a chronic cough with blood in the sputum, anorexia, night sweats, and a temperature 102.6°F (39.2°C). Which test does the nurse expect to perform on this client?
1. Chest x-ray
2. Sputum culture
3. Tuberculin skin test
4. Tuberculin blood test

93. 2. A sputum culture is the definitive test for tuberculosis (TB) in children. The tuberculin skin test and blood test would only indicate the child has been exposed to TB but would not confirm active infection. A chest x-ray may be helpful, but a sputum culture is preferred.

CN: Physiological integrity; CNS: Physiological adaptation; CL: Analyze

94. After a coin was removed from a preschool child's trachea, which action(s) will the nurse recommend to the parents before discharge?
1. "Cut hot dogs and sausages into small pieces."
2. "Chop up raisins before giving to your child."
3. "Cut cherry tomatoes in half when eating."
4. "Supervise your child while eating hard candy."

CN: Client needs category   CNS: Client needs subcategory   CL: Cognitive level

94. 1. Cherry tomatoes, hot dogs, and sausage should be cut into many small pieces (not just in half). Hard candy, raisins, popcorn, and peanuts should be avoided for children aged 4 years and younger.

CN: Physiological integrity; CNS: Reduction of risk potential; CL: Apply

95. A child is diagnosed with tuberculosis (TB). When educating the parents about care of the child, which statement made by the parent indicates to the nurse a need for further instruction?
1. "As long as I keep a surgical mask on I will not get TB."
2. "I understand that tuberculosis is highly contagious."
3. "I am willing to follow the rigid medication regimen."
4. "Increasing my child's calories is important at this time."

Cheers! You're doing great.

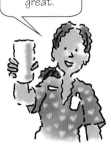

95. 1. Tuberculosis is highly contagious. To prevent the spread of infection, a negative pressure room is needed, and the caregivers must wear N95 medical respirators when around the child while contagious. A regular surgical mask is not effective. A rigid medication regimen is required. Increasing calories, including carbohydrates and proteins, as well as vitamins, is important during care for TB.
CN: Physiological integrity; CNS: Physiological adaptation; CL: Apply

96. The nurse is teaching the parents of a toddler about foreign body aspiration prevention. Which statement will the nurse include in the education?
1. "Provide finger foods for your child to eat while playing."
2. "Encourage your child to take bites off of large pieces of food."
3. "Your child can eat whole popcorn and peanuts while supervised."
4. "Buckle your child into a highchair while eating meals and snacks."

96. 4. Children should remain seated while eating. The risk of aspiration increases if children are running, jumping, or talking with food in their mouths. Food should be cut into small pieces before given to the child. Toys are a dangerous distraction to toddlers and young children and should be avoided while eating. Children need constant supervision and should be monitored while eating; however, whole popcorn and peanuts should not be given to children under 5 regardless of whether they are supervised or not.
CN: Safe, effective care environment; CNS: Safety and infection control; CL: Apply

97. A child is admitted for possible foreign body aspiration. Which assessment finding(s) indicates to the nurse this has occurred? Select all that apply.
1. Inspiratory stridor
2. Coughing
3. Expiratory wheezing
4. Drooling
5. Cyanosis

97. 1, 2, 3, 4, 5. All listed findings are symptoms of foreign body aspiration in children.
CN: Physiological integrity; CNS: Physiological adaptation; CL: Apply

98. The parent of a 2-year-old child taking rifampin after testing positive for tuberculosis calls the nurse and states, "My child's urine is orange." What response by the nurse is **most** appropriate?
1. "How long has your child been taking rifampin?"
2. "This is actually a normal side effect to rifampin."
3. "Your child needs to be seen today at the clinic."
4. "Have your child's tears or feces been orange, too?"

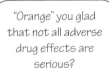

"Orange" you glad that not all adverse drug effects are serious?

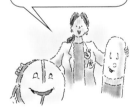

98. 2. Rifampin and its metabolites turn urine, feces, sputum, tears, and sweat an orange color. This is not a serious adverse effect. Rifampin may also cause gastrointestinal upset, headache, drowsiness, dizziness, vision disturbances, and fever. It is not important to ask how long the child has been taking the medication or whether other products are orange in color as well. The child does not need to be seen as this is an expected reaction.
CN: Physiological integrity; CNS: Pharmacological and parenteral therapies; CL: Apply

99. A 2-year-old child comes to the clinic with a cough, stridor, drooling, and mild cyanosis. The nurse will prepare the child for which procedure?
1. Chest x-ray
2. Laparotomy
3. Lateral neck x-ray
4. Bronchoscopy

99. 4. The nurse should suspect foreign body aspiration and prepare the child for a bronchoscopy. Bronchoscopy can give a definitive diagnosis of the presence of foreign bodies and is also the best choice for removal of the object with direct visualization. Chest x-ray and lateral neck x-ray may also be used but findings vary. Some films may appear normal or show changes such as inflammation related to the presence of the foreign body. A laparotomy is a surgical procedure of the abdominal cavity.
CN: Physiological integrity; CNS: Physiological adaptation; CL: Analyze

CN: Client needs category   CNS: Client needs subcategory   CL: Cognitive level

100. The nurse will complete which prescription **first** for a child with cystic fibrosis who is having difficulty clearing secretions?
1. Perform chest physiotherapy.
2. Give pancreatic enzymes.
3. Administer oxygen via nasal cannula.
4. Provide a high-calorie, high-protein meal.

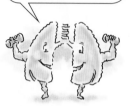

I just love chest PT. It makes me feel so strong and healthy.

100. 1. Chest physiotherapy should be performed to mobilize secretions so that they can be more easily cleared. Pancreatic enzymes should be administered with meals to aid in digestion, but this is lower priority than mobilizing secretions. Administering oxygen may improve oxygenation but will not help clear secretions. A high-calorie, high-protein diet is important for normal growth and development, but it will not aid in clearing secretions.
CN: Physiological integrity; CNS: Reduction of risk potential; CL: Analyze

101. Which statement by the parent of an 18-month-old child with cystic fibrosis **most** concerns the nurse?
1. "My child is finally starting to pull up on furniture."
2. "My child is saying a few words and short phrases."
3. "My child does not want to play with other children."
4. "My child always cries when I leave the room."

101. 1. A toddler should be walking by 15 months. A child should be able to hold onto furniture while walking around 10 months of age, walk with support around 11 months of age, and take the first steps around 12 months of age. By 12 months, a child should be able to say a few words, with more words and short phrases being added each month. A child at 16 months typically engages in solitary play and has little interaction with other children. Separation anxiety is common in toddlers.
CN: Health promotion and maintenance; CNS: None; CL: Apply

102. The nurse is assessing a newborn being tested for cystic fibrosis. Which finding will the nurse recognize as an early indicator of the disease?
1. Constipation
2. Decreased appetite
3. Hyperalbuminemia
4. Meconium ileus

102. 4. Meconium ileus is a common early sign of cystic fibrosis. Thick, mucilaginous meconium blocks the lumen of the small intestine, causing intestinal obstruction, abdominal distention, and vomiting. Large-volume, loose, frequent, foul-smelling stools are common. The undigested food is excreted, increasing the bulk of feces. These infants may have an increased appetite related to poor absorption from the intestine. Hypoalbuminemia is a common result from the decreased absorption of protein.
CN: Physiological integrity; CNS: Physiological adaptation; CL: Understand

103. The parents of a child with cystic fibrosis ask the nurse about proper nutrition for their child. Which recommendation will the nurse include when providing dietary education?
1. Fat-restricted, high-protein diet
2. High-calorie, high protein diet
3. Low-protein, fat-restricted diet
4. Sodium-restricted, high calorie diet

103. 2. A well-balanced, high-calorie, high-protein diet is recommended for a child with cystic fibrosis due to impaired intestinal absorption. Fat restriction is not required because digestion and absorption of fat in the intestine are impaired. The child usually increases enzyme intake when high-fat foods are eaten. Low-sodium foods can lead to hyponatremia; therefore, high-salt foods are recommended, especially during hot weather or when the child has a fever.
CN: Physiological integrity; CNS: Basic care and comfort; CL: Apply

Cystic fibrosis is all in the genes.

104. A newborn has been diagnosed with cystic fibrosis. The parents ask the nurse, "Which of us passed on the gene that caused this disorder?" How will the nurse respond?
1. "The father passed on the gene."
2. "Either parent could have passed on the gene."
3. "Both parents had to pass on the gene."
4. "The mother probably passed on the gene."

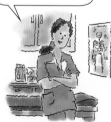

104. 3. Cystic fibrosis is an autosomal recessive disease. Therefore, both parents have to pass the gene to the fetus.
CN: Health promotion and maintenance; CNS: None; CL: Apply

CN: Client needs category   CNS: Client needs subcategory   CL: Cognitive level

105. The nurse is providing educating on the administration of pancreatic enzymes to the parents of a toddler with cystic fibrosis. Which statement by the parents indicates the education was effective?
1. "We will not open the medication capsules when administered."
2. "We can crush the microcapsules and mix in food."
3. "We will administer the enzymes with a glass of water."
4. "The enzymes should be given with meals and snacks."

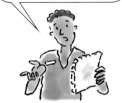

Enzymes help promote digestion. So, when would be a logical time to take them?

105. 4. Enzymes are administered with each feeding, meal, and snack to optimize absorption of the nutrients consumed. Microcapsules should not be crushed due to the enteric coating. Regular capsules may be opened, and the contents mixed with a small amount of applesauce or other nonalkaline food.
CN: Physiological integrity; CNS: Physiological adaptation; CL: Apply

106. The nurse is caring for a child with cystic fibrosis. Ranitidine 4 mg/kg/day every 12 hours is prescribed. The child weighs 33.1 lb (15 kg). How many milligrams per dose will the nurse give the child? Record your answer using a whole number.

_____ mg

106. 30.
The child will receive 30 mg per dose. First, calculate the total daily dose.

milligrams per dose × child's weight in kilograms = total dose per day

4 mg × 15 kg = 60 mg

Then, calculate the number of doses to give per day.

24 hours/12 hours = 2 doses

Then, divide the total daily dose by the number of doses.

60 mg/2 doses = 30 mg/dose

CN: Physiological integrity; CNS: Pharmacological and parenteral therapies; CL: Apply

107. Which nursing intervention(s) is appropriate when caring for a school-age child with cystic fibrosis? Select all that apply.
1. Encourage appropriate exercise and physical activity.
2. Administer cough suppressants and antihistamines.
3. Educate the child and family on proper hand washing.
4. Provide chest physiotherapy two to four times per day.
5. Give bronchodilator treatments prior to chest physiotherapy.

107. 1, 3, 4, 5. Chest physiotherapy is recommended two to four times per day to help loosen and move secretions to facilitate expectoration. Exercise and physical activity are recommended to stimulate mucus secretion and to establish a good habitual breathing pattern. Cough suppressants and antihistamines are contraindicated. Proper hand washing is essential to prevent pulmonary infections. The goal is for the child to be able to cough and expectorate mucus secretions. Bronchodilator or nebulizer treatments are given before chest physiotherapy to help open the bronchi for easier expectoration.
CN: Safe, effective care environment; CNS: Management of care; CL: Apply

108. The nurse is caring for a 9-year-old client admitted with pneumonia and a history of cystic fibrosis. Which finding will the nurse report to the health care provider **first**?
1. Temperature 101.6°F (38.7°C)
2. Respiratory rate 24 breaths/minute
3. Child has a productive cough
4. Nasal flaring noted with respirations

108. 4. The nurse would first report nasal flaring as this is a sign of respiratory distress. The child's temperature would need to be reported; however, this is not priority over respiratory distress. The respiratory rate is on the high end of normal and should be monitored. A productive cough is expected with pneumonia.
CN: Safe, effective care environment; CNS: Management of care; CL: Apply

109. A 3-year-old child is admitted with pneumonia and exhibits a productive cough and difficulty breathing. The parents inform the nurse of the child's poor appetite and inactivity. Which intervention(s) will the nurse include while caring for the child? Select all that apply.
1. Restrict fluid intake.
2. Perform chest physiotherapy as prescribed.
3. Encourage coughing and deep breathing.
4. Keep the head of the bed flat.
5. Perform postural drainage.
6. Use a cool mist humidifier.

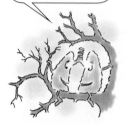

You're almost done. Hang in there!

110. The nurse is caring for a 5-year-old client admitted to the pediatric unit with cystic fibrosis. The caregiver states the child has been having foul-smelling, fatty stools at home. Which nursing action is appropriate?
1. Assess the child's next bowel movement.
2. Notify the primary health care provider.
3. Ask what medications the child takes at home.
4. Palpate the child's abdomen.

111. Ceftazidime is prescribed for a child with cystic fibrosis. The prescription states to give 40 mg/kg every 8 hours. The child is 3 years old and weighs 40.6 lb (18.4 kg). How many milligrams will the nurse administer in each dose? Record your answer using a whole number.

_____ mg

Put on your math cap. Time to crunch some numbers.

112. The nurse is caring for a 15-year-old female with cystic fibrosis. The client has questions about her future and the consequences of her disease. Which nursing statement(s) about cystic fibrosis is accurate? Select all that apply.
1. Breast development is frequently delayed
2. The adolescent is at risk for developing diabetes
3. Pregnancy and birth are not affected
4. Normal sexual relationships can be expected
5. Only females carry the gene for the disease
6. Current life expectancy is about 37 years

109. 2, 3, 5, 6. Chest physiotherapy and postural drainage work together to break up congestion and drain secretions. Coughing and deep breathing are also effective to remove congestion. A cool mist humidifier helps loosen thick mucus and relax airway passages. Fluids should be encouraged, not restricted. The child should be placed in semi-Fowler's or high-Fowler's position (not supine) to facilitate breathing and promote optimal lung expansion.
CN: Physiological integrity; CNS: Physiological adaptation; CL: Apply

110. 1. The nurse would assess the child's bowel movement. Children with cystic fibrosis have an abnormal electrolyte transport system in the cells that eventually blocks the pancreas, preventing the secretion of enzymes that digest certain foods such as protein and fats. This results in foul-smelling, fatty stool. The health care provider does not need to be notified of an expected finding. The nurse does not need to ask about medications because this is not a result of medication administration. There is no indication the child's abdomen needs to be palpated at this time.
CN: Physiological integrity; CNS: Physiological adaptation; CL: Apply

111. 245.
The child will receive 245 mg per dose. First, calculate the total daily dose.

$$milligrams\ per\ dose \times child's\ weight\ in\ kilograms = total\ dose\ per\ day$$

$$40\ mg \times 18.4\ kg = 736\ mg$$

Then, calculate the number of doses to give per day.

$$24\ hours/8\ hours = 3\ doses$$

Then, divide the total daily dose by the number of doses.

$$736\ mg/3\ doses = 245\ mg/dose$$

CN: Physiological integrity; CNS: Pharmacological and parenteral therapies; CL: Apply

112. 1, 2, 4, 6. Cystic fibrosis delays growth and the onset of puberty. Children with cystic fibrosis tend to be smaller-than-average size and develop secondary sexual characteristics later in life. In addition, clients with cystic fibrosis are at risk for developing diabetes because the pancreatic duct becomes obstructed as pancreatic tissue is damaged. Adolescents with cystic fibrosis can expect to have normal sexual relationships, but fertility may be affected because of changes in mucous membranes. Both males and females carry the gene for cystic fibrosis. The current life expectancy for people with cystic fibrosis is about 37 years.
CN: Physiological integrity; CNS: Physiological adaptation; CL: Apply

CN: Client needs category   CNS: Client needs subcategory   CL: Cognitive level

113. The nurse is preparing to administer tobramycin to an adolescent with cystic fibrosis. The prescription is for 3 mg/kg intravenously daily in three divided doses. The client weighs 99 lb (45 kg). How many milligrams will the nurse administer per dose? Record your answer using a whole number.

_____ mg

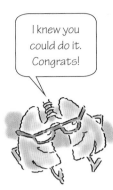

I knew you could do it. Congrats!

113. 45. The adolescent will receive 45 mg per dose. First, calculate the total daily dose.

milligrams per dose × child's weight in kilograms
= total dose per day

3 mg × 45 kg = 135 mg

Then, divide the total daily dose by the number of doses.

135 mg/3 doses = 45 mg/dose

CN: Physiological integrity; CNS: Pharmacological and parenteral therapies; CL: Analyze

Chapter 29

Neurosensory Disorders

Pediatric neurosensory refresher

Attention deficit hyperactivity disorder

Displaying signs of inattentiveness, hyperactivity, and impulsivity; often, difficulty staying on task or concentrating for long periods of time

Key signs and symptoms
- Decreased attention span
- Hyperactivity
- Impulsivity
- Difficulty organizing tasks and activities
- Easily distracted

Key test results
- Complete psychological, medical, and neurologic evaluations rule out other problems

Key treatments
- Behavioral modification and psychological therapy
- Amphetamines: methylphenidate, dextroamphetamine sulfate, amphetamine sulfate, and amphetamine aspartate

Key interventions
- Give one simple instruction at a time.
- Provide consistency in child's daily routine.
- Reduce environmental stimuli.
- Promote self-esteem.
- Monitor nutrition.
- Praise child for accomplishments.

Cerebral palsy

Nonprogressive brain disorder that is often associated with spasticity and difficulty with posture; usually occurs due to some type of brain injury during pregnancy or early childhood; symptoms can range from mild to severe, and may or may not be associated with intellectual disorders

Key signs and symptoms
- Abnormal muscle tone and coordination (most common associated problem)
- Difficulty sucking or keeping a nipple or food in mouth
- Involuntary movements

- Exaggerated reflexes
- Difficulty walking (scissor gait)

Key test results
- Neuroimaging studies determine site of brain impairment
- Cytogenic studies (genetic evaluation of the child and other family members) rule out other potential causes
- Metabolic studies rule out other causes

Key treatments
- Braces or splints and special appliances (such as adapted eating utensils and a low toilet seat with arms) to help child perform activities independently
- Range-of-motion (ROM) exercises to minimize contractures
- Muscle relaxants or neurosurgery to decrease spasticity, if appropriate

Key interventions
- Assist with locomotion, communication, and educational opportunities.
- Divide tasks into small steps.
- Perform ROM exercises if child is spastic.

Down's syndrome

Genetic disorder, trisomy 21, in which there are distinct physical manifestations, as well as some degree of cognitive disorder; the severity of the disorder is often not known until the child stops meeting developmental milestones

Key signs and symptoms
- Flat, broad forehead
- Mild to moderate retardation
- Short stature with pudgy hands
- Small head with slow brain growth
- Small jaw
- Upward slanting eyes
- Transverse palmar creases

Key test results
- Amniocentesis allows prenatal diagnosis

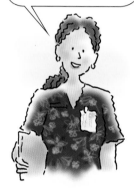

Here are three Web sites for more information about neurosensory disorders in children: *www.chadd.org* (Children and Adults with Attention-Deficit Hyperactivity Disorder), *www.ndss.org* (National Down's Syndrome Society), and *www.spinabifidaassociation.org* (Spina Bifida Association of America).

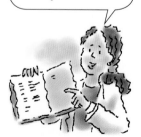

Can you remember the key signs and symptoms of Down's syndrome?

Key treatments

- Treatment for coexisting conditions such as congenital heart problems, visual defects, or hypothyroidism

Key interventions

- Provide activities appropriate for the child's mental rather than chronological age.
- Set realistic, reachable, short-term goals; break tasks into small steps.
- Provide stimulation and communicate at a level appropriate to the child's mental age rather than chronologic age.

Hydrocephalus

Dysfunction between cerebrospinal fluid production and absorption, resulting in increased fluid within the ventricles of the brain, which leads to increased intracranial pressure; may be fatal if not treated promptly; may be congenital or acquired

Key signs and symptoms

- High-pitched cry
- Rapid increase in head circumference and full, tense, bulging fontanels (before cranial sutures close)

Key test results

- Skull x-ray shows thinning of the skull with separation of the sutures and widening of fontanels

Key treatments

- Ventriculoperitoneal shunt insertion to allow cerebrospinal fluid (CSF) to drain from the lateral ventricle in the brain
- Anticonvulsants: carbamazepine, phenobarbital, diazepam, phenytoin

Key interventions

- Monitor vital signs, intake, and output.
- Monitor neurologic status.
- After shunt is inserted, do not lay child on the side of the body where it is located.
- Lay the child flat.
- If the caudal end of the shunt must be externalized because of infection, keep the bag at ear level.

Meningitis

Infection and inflammation of the meninges surrounding the brain and spinal cord; may be caused by viruses, bacteria, and other organisms; bacterial meningitis is highly contagious; viral meningitis is not

Key signs and symptoms

- Nuchal rigidity that may progress to opisthotonos (severe posturing with arched back and head thrown backwards)
- Positive Brudzinski's sign (flexion of the knees and hips in response to passive neck flexion)
- Positive Kernig's sign (inability to extend leg when hip and knee are flexed)
- Bulging anterior fontanel (before cranial sutures close)

Key test results

- Lumbar puncture shows increased CSF pressure, cloudy color, increased white blood cell count and protein level, and decreased glucose level if the meningitis is caused by bacteria

Key treatments

- Airborne precautions should be maintained until at least 24 hours of effective antibiotic therapy have elapsed; continued precautions recommended for meningitis caused by *Haemophilus influenzae or Neisseria meningitidis*
- Seizure precautions
- Analgesics to treat pain of meningeal irritation
- Corticosteroids: dexamethasone
- Parenteral antibiotics: ceftazidime, ceftriaxone; possibly intraventricular administration of antibiotics

Key interventions

- Monitor vital signs, intake, and output.
- Monitor child's neurologic status frequently.
- Examine young infant for bulging fontanels and measure head circumference.

Otitis media

Infection of the middle part of the ear that causes pain; repeated ear infections may lead to hearing loss

Key signs and symptoms

Acute suppurative otitis media
- Fever (mild to very high)
- Severe, deep, throbbing pain (from pressure behind the tympanic membrane)
- Pain that suddenly stops (if tympanic membrane ruptures)
- Signs of upper respiratory tract infection (sneezing, coughing)

Acute secretory otitis media
- Popping, crackling, or clicking sounds on swallowing or with jaw movement
- Sensation of fullness in the ear

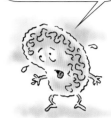

What are the possible causes of brain inflammation?

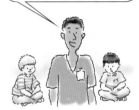

Remember—bacterial meningitis is highly contagious. Observe airborne precautions for 24 hours after starting antibiotics.

Chronic otitis media
- Cholesteatoma (cystlike mass in the middle ear)
- Decreased or absent tympanic membrane mobility
- Painless, purulent discharge in chronic suppurative otitis media

Key test results

Acute suppurative otitis media
- Otoscopy reveals obscured or distorted bony landmarks of the tympanic membrane

Acute secretory otitis media
- Otoscopy reveals clear or amber fluid behind the tympanic membrane and tympanic membrane retraction, which causes the bony landmarks to appear more prominent; if hemorrhage into the middle ear has occurred, as in barotrauma, the tympanic membrane appears blue-black

Chronic otitis media
- Otoscopy shows thickening, sometimes scarring, and decreased mobility of the tympanic membrane

Key treatments

Acute suppurative otitis media
- Myringotomy for children with severe, painful bulging of the tympanic membrane
- Antibiotic therapy, usually amoxicillin

Acute secretory otitis media
- Inflation of the eustachian tube by performing Valsalva maneuver several times a day, which may be the only treatment required
- Nasopharyngeal decongestant therapy

Chronic otitis media
- Elimination of eustachian tube obstruction
- Excision of cholesteatoma
- Mastoidectomy
- Antibiotic therapy: amoxicillin

Key interventions
- Watch for and report headache, fever, severe pain, or disorientation.
- Instruct parents not to feed their infant in a supine position or put to bed with a bottle.
- After myringotomy, maintain drainage flow; place sterile cotton loosely in the external ear and change cotton frequently.
- After tympanoplasty, reinforce dressings and observe for excessive bleeding from the ear canal.
- Warn the child against blowing his or her nose or getting the ear wet when bathing.

Seizure disorders

Abnormal movements or behaviors, resulting from unusual electrical activity in the brain; there are many different types of seizures; all can produce unusual symptoms

Key signs and symptoms
- Aura just before the seizure's onset (reports of unusual tastes, feelings, or odors)
- Eyes deviating to a particular side or blinking
- Usually unresponsive during tonic-clonic muscular contractions; may experience incontinence
- Irregular breathing with spasms

Key test results
- Electroencephalogram (EEG) results help differentiate epileptic from non-epileptic seizures; each seizure has a characteristic EEG tracing

Key treatments
- IV diazepam or lorazepam
- Anticonvulsants: phenobarbital, diazepam, fosphenytoin
- Anticonvulsants: phenytoin or carbamazepine to keep neuron excitability below the seizure threshold

Key interventions
- Monitor neurologic status.
- Stay with the child during a seizure.
- Move the child to a flat surface.
- Place the child on his or her side to allow saliva to drain out.
- Do not try to interrupt the seizure.

Spina bifida

Neural tube defect that occurs at the time of brain and neural tube formation. It can range from mild, such as spina bifida occulta, to a myelomeningocele with permanent neurological dysfunction

Key signs and symptoms

Spina bifida occulta
- Dimple on the skin over the spinal defect
- No neurologic dysfunction (usually), except occasional foot weakness or bowel and bladder disturbances

Meningocele
- No neurologic dysfunction (usually)
- Saclike structure protruding over the spine

Myelomeningocele
- Permanent neurologic dysfunction (paralysis below the spinal defect, bowel and bladder incontinence)

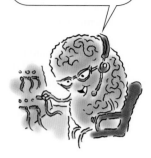

I'm sorry—we're having an electrical disturbance; I can't make your connection at the moment.

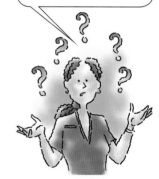

A pediatric client is diagnosed with otitis media. Which interventions should you perform?

Key test results

- Elevated alpha-fetoprotein levels in mother's blood or amniotic fluid may indicate the presence of a neural tube defect
- Acetylcholinesterase measurement can be used to confirm diagnosis
- Ultrasound may detect spina bifida prenatally

Key interventions

- Teach parents how to cope with their infant's physical problems.
- Teach parents how to recognize early signs of complications, such as hydrocephalus, pressure ulcers, and urinary tract infections.
- Before surgery:
  - watch for signs of hydrocephalus; measure head circumference daily; be sure to mark the spot where the measurement was made.
  - watch for signs of meningeal irritation, such as fever and nuchal rigidity.
- After surgery:
  - watch for hydrocephalus, which commonly follows surgery; measure the infant's head circumference as prescribed.

Reye's syndrome

Complication that occurs when recovering from a viral illness with concurrent aspirin use to reduce fever/body aches; starts with an accumulation of fat in the liver and other organs, and increased pressure in the brain; syndrome goes through several phases and is considered a medical emergency

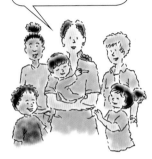

Teach parents and family members how to recognize signs of complications.

Key signs and symptoms

- Vomiting, listlessness
- Disorientation, confusion
- Convulsions
- Coma

Key test results

- Elevated aspartate aminotransferase (AST, also known as SGOT) and alanine aminotransferase (ALT, also known as SGPT) in the absence of jaundice

Key interventions

- Recognize the problem early.
- Maintain airway and brain oxygenation.
- Provide ICU placement with intubation.

thePoint® You can download tables of drug information to help you prepare for the NCLEX®! View Generic Drug Names, Drug Classifications, Drug Actions, and Nursing Implications for the drugs discussed in this refresher at **http://thePoint.lww.com**

Neurosensory questions, answers, and rationales

1. A 12-year-old child presents to the clinic for a follow-up after starting methylphenidate for attention deficit hyperactivity disorder (ADHD). Which finding will the nurse highlight for the health care provider?
   1. Apical heart rate of 100 beats/minute
   2. Able to concentrate for longer periods of time
   3. Improved performance on tests in school
   4. One-pound weight gain over 2 months

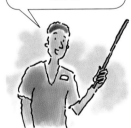

I'm sure you'll have no problem staying focused on these disorders. Let's dive in.

1. 1. A side effect of methylphenidate is tachycardia and should be reported to the health care provider. A normal heart rate for a 12-year-old is 65 to 85 beats/minute. The purpose of the medication is to increase the ability of the child to concentrate; consequently, improved grades may occur. A change in weight of 1 lb (0.5 kg) over 2 months is not significant; however, the nurse should monitor weight at the next checkup. Weight loss is a complication from the medication.
CN: Physiological integrity; CNS: Pharmacological and parenteral therapies; CL: Apply

2. Following birth, the nurse will be concerned regarding which finding in a neonate with a myelomeningocele?
   1. Apgar score of 8 at 5 minutes
   2. Greasy covering over the body
   3. Dark green, thick stool
   4. Temperature of 101°F (38.3°C)

2. 4. During the first hours of life, the most life-threatening event in a child with a myelomeningocele would be an infection. The other findings are expected. An Apgar of 8 indicates the neonate is transitioning to extrauterine life successfully. Vernix is a greasy covering over the body and meconium stool is dark green and thick.
CN: Physiological integrity; CNS: Reduction of risk potential; CL: Apply

CN: Client needs category   CNS: Client needs subcategory   CL: Cognitive level

3. Which finding(s) will the nurse expect to assess when caring for a neonate diagnosed with hydrocephalus? Select all that apply.
1. Bulging anterior fontanel
2. Difficulty consoling
3. Eyes rotated downward
4. High-pitched cry
5. Increased interest in feeding
6. Head circumference of 14 inches (35.6 cm)

3. **1, 2, 3, 4.** Hydrocephalus is caused by an alteration in circulation of the cerebrospinal fluid (CSF). As CSF volume increases, it causes the fontanel to bulge. This also causes an enlarged head circumference and an increase in intracranial pressure. This increase in pressure causes the neonate's eyes to deviate downward (the "setting sun sign"), the neonate's cry becomes high-pitched, and irritability is increased (difficulty consoling). Increased interest in feeding would not be expected. The head circumference listed here is in the normal range.
CN: Physiological integrity; CNS: Physiological adaptation; CL: Apply

4. A 13-year-old diagnosed with attention deficit hyperactivity disorder (ADHD) is taking methylphenidate. Which finding **most** concerns the nurse?
1. Pulse of 65 beats/minute and respiratory rate of 15 breaths/minute
2. A weight loss of 13.2 lb (6 kg) over the past month
3. The child is lying in bed watching television
4. Blood pressure of 120/70 mm Hg and oxygen saturation level of 95%

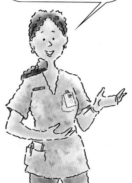

Knowing what to expect and what to be concerned about is important!

4. **2.** A weight loss of 13.2 lb (6 kg) over 1 month is significant and indicates a complication from the medication. Lying quietly indicates that the medication effects are successful. All other findings are in normal range for an adolescent.
CN: Physiological integrity; CNS: Pharmacological and parenteral therapies; CL: Apply

5. The registered nurse (RN) is caring for a child immediately following shunt insertion on the left side of the head to relieve hydrocephalus. The RN observes the licensed practical nurse (LPN) place the child in the left side-lying position. Which action by the RN is **priority**?
1. Teach the LPN the proper position for this procedure.
2. Immediately place the child in the supine position.
3. Document the child's position in the medical record.
4. Inform the child's parents regarding proper positioning.

5. **2.** The child should be placed flat in bed to avoid rapid decompression of cerebrospinal fluid (CSF) and supine or on the unaffected side—in this case, the right side— to avoid occlusion of the shunt and blockage of the drainage of CSF. Placing the child on the affected side (the left side, in this case) is incorrect. The RN should teach the LPN and parents proper positioning for this child and document; however, positioning the child is priority.
CN: Safe, effective care environment; CNS: Management of care; CL: Analyze

6. The nurse is caring for a child with a seizure disorder. Which nursing action is appropriate during a seizure?
1. Administer rectal diazepam.
2. Monitor the child's respiratory status.
3. Gently restrain the child's extremities.
4. Insert a padded tongue blade into the mouth.

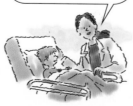

The hospital can be a scary place, especially for kids. Take time to comfort your clients and calm their fears.

6. **2.** When a child has a seizure, the most important aspect of care is airway maintenance. Monitoring for signs of an obstructed airway is important to ensure patency. The nurse may administer diazepam for a prolonged seizure, after ensuring airway patency. It is not recommended to restrain the child, as this can cause extremity damage; or to put anything into the child's mouth, as this can cause airway obstruction and possible injury to the oral cavity.
CN: Physiological integrity; CNS: Reduction of risk potential; CL: Apply

7. The parents bring their infant to the urgent clinic stating the infant had a seizure at home. Which laboratory result from the chart exhibit below will the nurse report to the health care provider?

Laboratory results	
Parameter	*Results*
Blood glucose	*120 mg/dL (6.7 mmol/L)*
Chloride	*104 mEq/L (104 mmol/L)*
Potassium	*4 mEq/L (4 mmol/L)*
Sodium	*125 mEq/L (125 mmol/L)*
Casts	*None*

  1. Blood glucose
  2. Chloride
  3. Potassium
  4. Sodium

7. 4. The nurse should report the sodium level to the health care provider. Normal serum sodium level for an infant is 135 to 145 mEq/L (135 to 145 mmol/L). Hyponatremia is one of the causes of seizures in infants and can be caused by diluting formula. The other laboratory values are all within normal limits.

CN: Safe, effective care environment; CNS: Management of care; CL: Analyze

8. A neonate is admitted with suspected bacterial meningitis. Which finding(s) will the nurse expect to assess in this neonate? Select all that apply.
  1. Crying and agitation
  2. Temperature of 96.2°F (35.7°C)
  3. Nuchal rigidity
  4. Sunken fontanel
  5. Poor feeding

8. 1, 2, 5. The clinical appearance of a neonate with meningitis is different from that of a child or an adult. The neonate may be either hypothermic or hyperthermic. The irritation to the meninges causes the neonate to be irritable and to have a decreased appetite. The neonate may be pale and mottled with a bulging, full fontanel. Older children and adults with meningitis have headaches, nuchal rigidity, and hyperthermia as clinical manifestations. Sunken fontanels are associated with dehydration.

CN: Physiological integrity; CNS: Physiological adaptation; CL: Apply

9. The nurse will be **most** concerned if which behavior is exhibited by a 9-year-old client diagnosed with attention deficit hyperactivity disorder (ADHD)?
  1. The child reacts impulsively
  2. The child reports fighting at school
  3. The child reverses words while reading
  4. The child is unable to sit still during the exam

9. 3. Children who reverse letters and words while reading have dyslexia, which is not associated with ADHD. Two of the most common characteristics of children with ADHD include inattention and impulsiveness. Although it is not a characteristic that aids in the diagnosis of this disorder, aggressiveness is common in children with ADHD.

CN: Health promotion and maintenance; CNS: None; CL: Apply

10. Which statement by the parent of a child with cerebral palsy indicates the nurse's teaching is successful?
  1. "My child's muscles will get stronger with therapy."
  2. "My child's condition will progressively get worse."
  3. "My child will have a low intelligence level."
  4. "My child will need lifelong therapy."

In other words, which statement is *true* in question #10?

10. 4. The child with cerebral palsy needs continual treatment and therapy to maintain or improve functioning. Without therapy, muscles get progressively weaker and more spastic. Although some children with cerebral palsy have an intellectual disability, many have normal intelligence. Even with therapy, the child's muscles will not get stronger.

CN: Health promotion and maintenance; CNS: None; CL: Apply

11. A toddler is diagnosed with acute otitis media. Which finding(s) will the nurse expect to assess? Select all that apply.
  1. Acute anorexia
  2. Tugging on the ear(s)
  3. A mild respiratory infection
  4. Temperature of 101.3°F (38.5°C)
  5. Bulging tympanic membrane

11. 1, 2, 3, 4, 5. All are common findings in a child with otitis media. A child with otitis media usually exhibits a bulging and/or discolored tympanic membrane (bright red or dull gray), acute anorexia, tugging on the ears, a mild respiratory infection, and fever.

CN: Physiological integrity; CNS: Physiological adaptation; CL: Apply

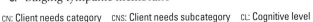

CN: Client needs category   CNS: Client needs subcategory   CL: Cognitive level

12. A child is prescribed methylphenidate 20 mg QD for attention deficit hyperactivity disorder (ADHD). The nurse has methylphenidate 10 mg/tablets. How many tablets will the nurse administer to the child per dose? Record your answer using one decimal place.

_____ tablet(s)

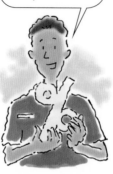

Get ready to crunch some numbers—it's another math question.

13. The nurse is educating the caregivers of a toddler diagnosed with otitis media about the prescribed amoxicillin. Which statement by the caregivers indicates the nurse's education was effective?
1. "We can mix the dosage of amoxicillin in our child's milk."
2. "If our child has diarrhea, we will let the health care provider know."
3. "When our child stops pulling at her ears, we can stop giving this medication."
4. "If our child has a rash, we should put hydrocortisone cream on the bumps."

14. The nurse is educating the parents of a 1-year-old client on the correct method for instilling eardrops for a middle ear infection. Place the steps in the chronological order the nurse will instruct the parents to follow. Use each option once.
1. Have the child remaining side-lying for a few minutes while gently massaging the tragus.
2. Place the child side-lying with the affected ear upward.
3. Gently pull the pinna down and back.
4. Wipe away any excess medication with a clean tissue.
5. Stabilize the child's head.
6. Hold the dropper above the ear canal and instill the prescribed number of drops.

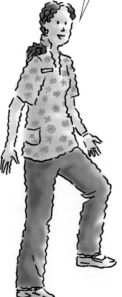

You're making great strides. Keep on going.

15. After a child returns from surgery for a left myringotomy, which nursing intervention is **priority**?
1. Apply gauze to the left ear.
2. Position the child left side-lying.
3. Assess the child's hearing.
4. Apply warm compresses to the left ear.

12. 2.
The correct formula to calculate a drug dose is:

$$\frac{Dose\ on\ hand}{Quantity\ on\ hand} = \frac{Dose\ desired}{X}$$

The child is taking 20 mg, which is the dose desired. The pharmacy has available 10-mg tablets, which is the dose on hand.

$$\frac{10\ mg}{1\ tablet} = \frac{20\ mg}{X}$$

X = 2 tablets

CN: Physiological integrity; CNS: Pharmacological and parenteral therapies; CL: Analyze

13. 2. Diarrhea is a common adverse effect of amoxicillin and indicates a new infection may be present. Medications should not be added to large amounts of drink or food because the caregiver cannot determine how much is consumed unless the child drinks or eats it all. The full prescribed dosage of antibiotics should be taken. If a rash appears, the parents should notify the health care provider, as this could indicate an allergic reaction.
CN: Physiological integrity; CNS: Pharmacological and parenteral therapies; CL: Apply

14. Ordered Response:
2. Place the child side-lying with the affected ear upward.
5. Stabilize the child's head.
3. Gently pull the pinna down and back.
6. Hold the dropper above the ear canal and instill the prescribed number of drops.
1. Have the child remaining side-lying for a few minutes while gently massaging the tragus.
4. Wipe away any excess medication with a clean tissue.

CN: Physiological integrity; CNS: Pharmacological and parenteral therapies; CL: Apply

15. 2. The child should be positioned on the left side to facilitate drainage. Gauze dressings are not necessary after surgery. Assessing hearing and applying warm compresses (which may help to facilitate drainage) are not priority over positioning.
CN: Safe, effective care environment; CNS: Management of care; CL: Apply

16. A child is diagnosed with chronic otitis media. Which information will the nurse include when educating the child's parents? Select all that apply.
1. Administer acetaminophen or ibuprofen for pain.
2. Provide soft foods and liquids for eating.
3. Avoid exposing the child to tobacco smoke.
4. Position the child on the unaffected side.
5. Clean the child's ear with a cotton swab daily.

17. The nurse is using an otoscope to assess a child's tympanic membrane. Which finding(s) will the nurse report to the health care provider? Select all that apply.
1. A pearl-gray tympanic membrane
2. Presence of a cone of light
3. Lateral process of malleus
4. Bright red, bulging tympanic membrane
5. A dull-gray tympanic membrane

18. Which statement by the parent of a child with otitis media indicates to the nurse additional teaching is needed?
1. "I will give my child the full course of prescribed antibiotics."
2. "My child may experience muffled or temporary hearing loss."
3. "Ear infections usually develop after a viral respiratory illness."
4. "I will know my child has another ear infection because he will pull his ears."

19. A child with a history of otitis media presents to the clinic crying and holding the left ear. Upon assessment, the nurse notes a ruptured tympanic membrane. Which prescription from the health care provider will the nurse anticipate?
1. Admit to the hospital for surgical repair.
2. Administer amoxicillin 90 mg/kg twice a day.
3. Administer morphine sulfate 3 mg IM.
4. Pack the ear canal with sterile cotton.

20. The parents of a child diagnosed with otitis media ask the nurse, "Why do kids get so many ear infections?" Which statement made by the nurse is **most** appropriate?
1. "The ear cartilage lining is underdeveloped in children."
2. "Kids get more ear infections because they have more respiratory illnesses."
3. "Immature humoral defense mechanisms place children at risk of infection."
4. "Eustachian tubes in children are short, wide, and straight and lie in a horizontal plane."

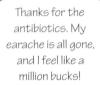
Thanks for the antibiotics. My earache is all gone, and I feel like a million bucks!

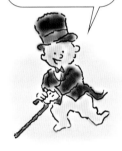

16. **1, 2, 3.** Analgesics, such as acetaminophen or ibuprofen, can be given for pain as needed. Soft foods and liquids help decrease pain from chewing. Eliminating tobacco smoke and other allergens from the environment can help prevent otitis media. The child should be placed on the affected side to promote drainage. It is not recommended to insert cotton swabs into the ear canal.
CN: Health promotion and maintenance; CNS: None; CL: Apply

17. **4, 5.** A bright red, bulging tympanic membrane indicates acute otitis media. A dull-gray membrane with fluid is consistent with subacute or chronic otitis media. A pearl-gray tympanic membrane, cone of light, and lateral process of malleus are normal findings.
CN: Safe, effective care environment; CNS: Management of care; CL: Apply

18. **4.** Not all children pull at their ears with otitis media. Some children may exhibit anorexia, elevated temperature, otorrhea, increased irritability, or decreased activity with otitis media. All other statements are correct regarding otitis media in children.
CN: Physiological integrity; CNS: Physiological adaptation; CL: Apply

19. **2.** A ruptured tympanic membrane is the most common complication of acute otitis media as the exudate accumulates and pressure increases. Antibiotic therapy is the recommended treatment to treat the infection. Surgical repair is not needed as the membrane self-heals in hours to days. Pain is not generally associated with rupturing; clients often experience relief because the pressure is released. Nothing should be inserted into the ear canal.
CN: Safe, effective care environment; CNS: Management of care; CL: Apply

20. **4.** The eustachian tubes in children are short, wide, and straight and lie in a horizontal plane, allowing them to be more easily blocked by conditions such as large adenoids and infections. Until the eustachian tubes change in size and angle, children are more susceptible to otitis media. Cartilage lining is underdeveloped, making the tubes more distensible and more likely to open inappropriately, but this does not make children more susceptible to ear infections. Children do acquire more respiratory illnesses than adults, but this does not fully answer the parent's question. Immature humoral defense mechanisms increase the risk of infection in general, but this does not fully answer the question.
CN: Physiological integrity; CNS: Physiological adaptation; CL: Apply

21. A parent states their 9-year-old child is having increased difficulty concentrating, completing tasks, and sitting still in school. Which intervention will the nurse complete for this child?
1. Assess the child's hearing bilaterally.
2. Refer for a learning disability assessment.
3. Administer dextroamphetamine as prescribed.
4. Prepare for an electroencephalogram (EEG).

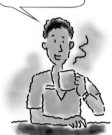

Relax. You're doing fine.

21. 3. The child is exhibiting symptoms of attention deficit hyperactivity disorder (ADHD). Dextroamphetamine is used to treat ADHD symptoms. A mild hearing problem usually is exhibited as leaning forward, talking louder, listening to louder TV and music than usual, and a repetitive "what?" from the child. The symptoms do not indicate a learning disability or seizures (for which an EEG would be indicated).
CN: Physiological integrity; CNS: Physiological adaptation; CL: Analyze

22. The nurse is admitting a preschooler to the hospital with a diagnosis of bacterial meningitis. Which action will the nurse perform **first**?
1. Obtain an axillary temperature.
2. Place the child on droplet precautions.
3. Assess for a Brudzinski's sign.
4. Monitor the level of consciousness.

22. 2. First, the nurse should take necessary precautions to protect the nurse and others from possible infection from the bacterial organism causing meningitis. The affected child should immediately be placed on droplet precautions. The nurse should then monitor the level of consciousness. Obtaining a temperature and assessing for a Brudzinski's sign would also be done, but after placing the child on droplet precautions.
CN: Safe, effective care environment; CNS: Safety and infection control; CL: Analyze

23. A toddler diagnosed with bacterial meningitis began taking ceftazidime 36 hours ago. Which nursing action is appropriate at this time?
1. Discontinue droplet precautions and initiate standard precautions.
2. Begin flexing the toddler's neck at least every 4 hours.
3. Take the toddler to a treatment room to administer the medication.
4. Assess the toddler's white blood cell (WBC) level daily.

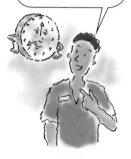

Focus on the time frame given in #23, it is important!

23. 1. With bacterial meningitis, respiratory isolation must be maintained for at least 24 hours after beginning antibiotic therapy; therefore, this client can now be placed on standard precautions. Moving the toddler's head to maintain range of motion would cause pain because the meninges are inflamed. Children are generally administered medications in their room and taken to a treatment room for procedures. Assessing a WBC level daily is not necessary.
CN: Safe, effective care environment; CNS: Safety and infection control; CL: Apply

24. A 2-month-old infant is being seen for a well-baby checkup. The registered nurse (RN) notes the assistive personnel (AP) documented the infant's head circumference at the 95th percentile. Which action will the RN take **first**?
1. Have the AP obtain vital signs.
2. Remeasure the infant's head.
3. Assess for sun-setting eyes.
4. Notify the health care provider.

24. 2. Whenever there is a question about vital signs or assessment data, the first logical step is to reassess and determine whether an error has been made initially. In this case, remeasuring the head would be the priority. Notifying the health care provider and assessing neurologic and vital signs are important and would follow the head reassessment, if warranted.
CN: Safe, effective care environment; CNS: Management of care; CL: Analyze

25. A preschool-age child is admitted to the pediatric unit with a diagnosis of bacterial meningitis. Which nursing intervention is appropriate to include in the plan of care?
1. Provide movies for the child to watch.
2. Obtain a temperature each shift.
3. Limit visitors in the child's room.
4. Encourage the parents to hold the child.

Our brains need a break, too. Remember to get up and walk around occasionally.

25. 3. A child with the diagnosis of meningitis is much more comfortable with decreased environmental stimuli. Visitors, noise, television, and bright lights stimulate the child and can be irritating, causing the child to cry, in turn increasing intracranial pressure. Vital signs would be taken initially every hour and temperature monitored every 2 hours. Children with bacterial meningitis are usually much more comfortable if allowed to lie flat because this position does not cause increased meningeal irritation.
CN: Physiological integrity; CNS: Physiological adaptation; CL: Apply

26. The nurse is caring for a school-age client who had a ventriculoperitoneal shunt placed a few weeks ago for hydrocephalus. The client complains of a headache upon arrival to the urgent care clinic. Which nursing intervention is **priority**?
1. Obtain the client's vital signs.
2. Assess the shunt surgical suture site.
3. Notify the client's health care provider.
4. Measure the client's head circumference.

27. A 17-month-old child with a history of febrile seizures is being seen in the clinic for a wellness check. Which statement by the parent indicates to the nurse additional teaching is needed?
1. "I keep ibuprofen on hand at all times."
2. "I hope my child outgrows these seizures."
3. "I always keep phenobarbital with me in case of a fever."
4. "The most likely time for a seizure is when the fever is rising."

28. When assessing a 6-month-old infant, which finding will the nurse highlight for the health care provider to review?
1. Absent grasp reflex
2. Rolls from back to side
3. Balances head when sitting
4. Presence of Moro embrace reflex

29. An adolescent is started on valproic acid to treat seizures. Which statement will the nurse include when educating the adolescent?
1. "This medication has no adverse effects."
2. "A common adverse effect is weight loss."
3. "Drowsiness and irritability commonly occur."
4. "Your liver enzymes will be monitored."

30. The nurse is caring for a child newly diagnosed with cerebral palsy who is experiencing excessive drooling. Which primary health care provider prescription will the nurse question?
1. Consult physical and occupational therapies.
2. Give baclofen PRN for muscle spasms.
3. Administer diazepam every 8 hours.
4. Apply scopolamine transdermal patch.

31. Which nursing action will be included in the care plan to promote comfort in a preschool-age child hospitalized with bacterial meningitis?
1. Rock the child at night to assist with sleeping.
2. Let the child's siblings stay in the room.
3. Keep the overhead lights on in the room.
4. Avoid making noise when in the child's room.

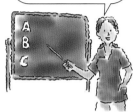

Make sure the parents of pediatric clients understand the purpose of their medications.

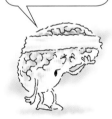

Whew! This test is giving me quite a workout. I think I need a break.

26. 4. The nurse would first assess the child's head circumference to determine whether the shunt is functioning properly. The nurse would assess vital signs and the surgical site after measuring the head. The health care provider should be notified, if needed, based on assessment findings.
CN: Safe, effective care environment; CNS: Management of care; CL: Analyze

27. 3. Antiepileptics, such as phenobarbital, are administered to children with prolonged seizures or neurologic abnormalities. Ibuprofen or acetaminophen, not phenobarbital, are given for fever. Febrile seizures usually occur after age 6 months and are unusual after age 5 years. Treatment is to decrease the temperature because seizures occur as the temperature rises.
CN: Health promotion and maintenance; CNS: None; CL: Apply

28. 4. Moro embrace reflex should be absent at 4 months. Grasp reflex begins to fade at 2 months and should be absent at 3 months. A 4-month-old infant should be able to roll from back to side and balance the head when sitting.
CN: Health promotion and maintenance; CNS: None; CL: Apply

29. 4. Valproic acid can cause liver failure. Weight gain, not loss, is a common adverse effect of valproic acid. Drowsiness and irritability are adverse effects more commonly associated with phenobarbital.
CN: Physiological integrity; CNS: Pharmacological and parenteral therapies; CL: Apply

30. 3. The nurse would question administering diazepam, an anxiolytic and sedative, to treat muscle spasms. However, routine, long-term use is not recommended due to the risk of dependence and incidence of increased drooling. Administering every 8 hours could oversedate the child. Physical and occupational therapies are a few of the many referrals the family will receive. Baclofen is used to treat muscle spasms. Scopolamine is given to decrease drooling.
CN: Safe, effective care environment; CNS: Management of care; CL: Apply

31. 4. Meningeal irritation may cause seizures and heightens a child's sensitivity to all stimuli, including noise, lights, movement, and touch. Frequent rocking, presence of siblings, and bright lights would increase stimulation.
CN: Physiological integrity; CNS: Basic care and comfort; CL: Apply

CN: Client needs category   CNS: Client needs subcategory   CL: Cognitive level

32. A 6-month-old infant is admitted with a diagnosis of bacterial meningitis. The nurse will assign the infant to which room?
1. A private room near the nurses' station
2. A negative pressure room on the unit
3. A room shared with a child with a urinary tract infection
4. A shared room with an infant with failure to thrive

33. When caring for a school-age child immediately after a head injury, the nurse notes a blood pressure of 110/60 mm Hg, a heart rate of 82 beats/minute, dilated and nonreactive pupils, minimal response to pain, and slow response to name. Which finding causes the nurse the **most** concern?
1. Vital signs
2. Nonreactive pupils
3. Slow response to name
4. Minimal response to pain

34. An older child is scheduled for a craniotomy to remove a brain tumor. Which statement made by the parents indicates to the nurse that additional teaching is needed?
1. "Our child will be monitored closely for infection after surgery."
2. "We know our child will have a lengthy recovery process."
3. "We are so thankful our child's tumor is benign."
4. "Part of our child's skull will be removed during the surgery."

35. Which developmental milestone(s) will the nurse expect an 11-month-old infant to exhibit? Select all that apply.
1. Thumb opposition
2. Sitting independently
3. Walking independently
4. Building a tower with four blocks
5. Playing pat-a-cake

36. Which prescription is **priority** for the nurse to complete when caring for a 10-month-old infant with bacterial meningitis?
1. Administer ceftriaxone.
2. Assist with breastfeeding.
3. Monitor for seizures.
4. Assess temperature hourly.

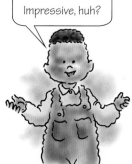

Sometimes symptoms are hidden and have to be discovered.

Check out what I can do. Impressive, huh?

32. 1. A child who has the diagnosis of bacterial meningitis is considered contagious and should be placed in a private room until he or she has received intravenous antibiotics for 24 hours. Additionally, bacterial meningitis can be quite serious; therefore, the child should be placed near the nurses' station for close monitoring and easier access in case of a crisis. A negative pressure room is not required for a child with bacterial meningitis.
CN: Safe, effective care environment; CNS: Safety and infection control; CL: Apply

33. 2. Dilated and nonreactive pupils indicate that anoxia or ischemia of the brain has occurred. If the pupils are also fixed (do not move), then herniation of the brain through the tentorium has occurred. The vital signs are normal. Slow response to name can be normal after a head injury. Minimal response to pain is an indication of the child's level of consciousness.
CN: Physiological integrity; CNS: Basic care and comfort; CL: Apply

34. 3. Final pathology results for a brain tumor typically are not available for several days after a craniotomy, so it is premature to state that the tumor is benign or malignant. The child is at high risk for infection following surgery and should be closely monitored. Usually after a craniotomy, it takes several weeks or longer before the child is back to normal. In a craniotomy, part of the skull, termed a bone flap, is removed and replaced.
CN: Psychosocial integrity; CNS: None; CL: Apply

35. 1, 2, 5. Thumb opposition is noted in infants who are about 4 months of age. Infants typically sit independently, without support, by age 8 months. Walking independently may be accomplished as late as age 15 months and still be within the normal range. Building a tower of three or four blocks is a milestone of an 18-month-old. Playing pat-a-cake is a milestone accomplished by 9 months of age.
CN: Health promotion and maintenance; CNS: None; CL: Apply

36. 1. Beginning antibiotic therapy is priority to limit effects of the disease and prevent spreading the disease. The child must be on precautions until 24 hours after the antibiotic is given. Maintaining nutrition and monitoring for seizures and hyperthermia are also important, but antibiotic therapy is priority.
CN: Physiological integrity; CNS: Reduction of risk potential; CL: Analyze

37. The nurse is educating the parents of a 1-year-old with spastic cerebral palsy on interventions to prevent a scissoring position. Which intervention(s) will the nurse include? Select all that apply.
  1. Remove leg braces for bathing only.
  2. Allow the child to periodically ride in a stroller.
  3. Encourage the child to keep the legs touching.
  4. Try to keep the child as quiet as possible.
  5. Carry the child by placing on the hip.

37. 5. To interrupt the scissoring position, flex the knees and hips. Placing the child with spastic cerebral palsy on the hip is an easy way to stop this common spastic positioning. This child needs stimulation and movement to reach the goal of development to the fullest potential. Wearing leg braces the majority of the day is inappropriate and does not allow the child to move freely. Trying to keep the child quiet, in a stroller, and with legs touching are inappropriate measures.
CN: Physiological integrity; CNS: Basic care and comfort; CL: Apply

38. A 4-year-old child with a ventriculoperitoneal shunt presents to the emergency room with a temperature of 101.2°F (38.4°C), blood pressure of 108/68 mm Hg, pulse of 110 beats/minute, lethargy, and vomiting. Which nursing intervention will the nurse complete **next**?
  1. Administer acetaminophen as prescribed.
  2. Place the child on contact precautions.
  3. Consult the health care provider.
  4. Reassess the pulse in 30 minutes.

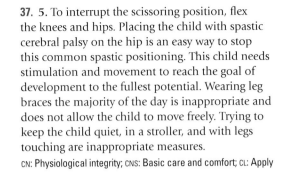

Lots of data to analyze here. What do they all add up to?

38. 3. The nurse should consult the health care provider. The child is exhibiting symptoms of infection and may need antibiotic therapy. One of the complications of a ventriculoperitoneal shunt is a shunt infection. The nurse would give acetaminophen after notifying the health care provider. Contact precautions are not warranted. The nurse would continue to monitor for changes in the child's condition.
CN: Physiological integrity; CNS: Basic care and comfort; CL: Apply

39. The parents of a 10-year-old child with attention deficit hyperactivity disorder (ADHD) state they do not want their child to take the prescribed methylphenidate. Which response by the nurse is **most** appropriate?
  1. "You should give your child the medication anyway."
  2. "Why do you not try the medicine and see how your child does?"
  3. "Do you not want your child to behave better in school and at home?"
  4. "Can you tell me what concerns you about this medicine?"

39. 4. The nurse should be therapeutic when communicating and determine what concerns the parents have regarding the medication. Telling the parents to give the medication and to see what happens are not therapeutic, nor do they address the parent's concerns. Asking the parents about better behavior is confrontational.
CN: Physiological integrity; CNS: Pharmacological and parenteral therapies; CL: Apply

40. A child is prescribed 240 mg of acetaminophen for fever control. The pharmacy sends acetaminophen 160 mg per 5 mL. How many milliliters will the nurse administer the client for each dose? Record your answer using one decimal place.

_____ mL

40. 7.5.
Use the following equations:

$$\frac{Dose\ on\ hand}{Quantity\ on\ hand} = \frac{Dose\ desired}{X}$$

$$\frac{160\ mg}{5\ mL} = \frac{240\ mg}{X}$$

$$X = 7.5\ mL$$

CN: Physiological integrity; CNS: Pharmacological and parenteral therapies; CL: Apply

41. The nurse is caring for an infant with suspected bacterial meningitis. Which findings will the nurse anticipate?
  1. Flat fontanel, fever, and drowsiness
  2. Irritability, fever, and vomiting
  3. Jaundice, drowsiness, and refusal to eat
  4. Negative Kernig's and Brudzinski's signs

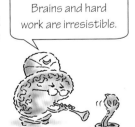

Brains and hard work are irresistible.

41. 2. Findings associated with acute bacterial meningitis may include irritability, fever, vomiting, and seizure activity. Fontanels would be bulging as intracranial pressure rises, and Kernig's and Brudzinski's signs would be present due to meningeal irritation. Jaundice, drowsiness, and refusal to eat indicate a gastrointestinal disturbance rather than meningitis.
CN: Physiological integrity; CNS: Physiological adaptation; CL: Apply

42. The nurse reviews the chart shown below while caring for a school-age child who had a brain tumor removed. Which action will the nurse perform **next**?

Progress notes	
6/9 0952	Pupils are equal and reactive to light; motor strength is equal; client is aware of name and date but not location. Client is reporting headache.
	—Q. Hart, RN

1. Measure the child's head circumference.
2. Determine the child's prior level of consciousness.
3. Administer acetaminophen 240 mg orally.
4. Notify the child's health care provider.

43. The nurse is assisting the health care provider performing a lumbar puncture (LP) on a child. The health care provider tells the nurse to place the child side-lying, with the back curved. Which action by the nurse is appropriate?
1. Stop the procedure and notify the charge nurse.
2. Ask the health care provider to repeat the prescription.
3. Place the child in the stated position.
4. Position the child supine with the head turned to the side.

44. The nurse is assessing a 10-month-old client and notes the anterior and posterior fontanels are open. What will the nurse do **first**?
1. Obtain vital signs.
2. Notify the health care provider.
3. Measure head circumference.
4. Assess the level of consciousness.

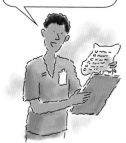

In other words, what's the priority intervention in question #44?

45. A 10-year-old child with a concussion is admitted to the pediatric unit. The nurse will assign this client to which room?
1. A room with a 6-year-old child with hydrocephalus
2. A room with an 8-year-old child with Down's syndrome
3. A room with a 10-year-old child with viral meningitis
4. A room with a 12-year-old child with Reye's syndrome

42. 2. When there is an abnormality in current assessment data, it is vital to determine what the client's previous status was to determine whether the status has changed or remained the same. Providing medication for the headache would be done after ascertaining the previous level of consciousness. The head circumference is generally only measured if the child is under 2 years of age. Contacting the health care provider is not necessary before a final assessment has been made.
CN: Safe, effective care environment; CNS: Management of care; CL: Apply

43. 3. Lumbar puncture involves placing a needle between the lumbar vertebrae into the subarachnoid space. For this procedure, the nurse should position the client on one side with the back curved; curving the back maximizes the space between the lumbar vertebrae, facilitating needle insertion. A prone position does not achieve maximum separation of the vertebrae. There is no reason to stop the procedure or have the prescription repeated.
CN: Safe, effective care environment; CNS: Management of care; CL: Apply

44. 3. The nurse should first measure the child's head circumference to see whether the head is abnormally large, indicating a complication. By age 18 months, the child's anterior and posterior fontanels should be closed. The diamond-shaped anterior fontanel normally closes between ages 9 and 18 months. The triangular posterior fontanel normally closes between ages 2 and 3 months. The nurse would then assess level of consciousness and vital signs before notifying the health care provider.
CN: Safe, effective care environment; CNS: Management of care; CL: Analyze

45. 2. A child with a concussion should be placed with a roommate who is free from infection, stable, and close to the child's age. The children with hydrocephalus, viral meningitis, and Reye's syndrome would benefit from a quiet environment due to the potential for increased intracranial pressure.
CN: Safe, effective care environment; CNS: Safety and infection control; CL: Analyze

CN: Client needs category   CNS: Client needs subcategory   CL: Cognitive level

46. The nurse is caring for a child with spina bifida. The child's mother asks the nurse what she did to cause the birth defect. Which response by the nurse is **best**?
1. "Older age at conception is one of the major causes of spina bifida."
2. "It is a common complication when you have an amniocentesis."
3. "Spina bifida has been linked to maternal alcohol consumption during pregnancy."
4. "This was not caused by one certain thing. The cause is actually unknown."

47. The parent of a 14-year-old child with a head injury asks the nurse, "Why is my child occasionally making inappropriate statements, being combative, and having violent outbursts?" Which nursing response is **best**?
1. "This shows your child's brain is going through the healing process."
2. "If you let your child know this behavior is inappropriate, the child will stop."
3. "This is a normal finding among teenagers and is not related to the brain injury."
4. "Let me refer your child to therapy that can help with aggressive behavior."

48. A child hospitalized for increased intracranial pressure (ICP) reports a severe headache. The parents ask the nurse, "Does this mean our child is getting worse?" Which response by the nurse is **most** appropriate?
1. "There is no way to know if your child is getting worse."
2. "We need to decrease your child's environmental stimuli."
3. "I will check with the health care provider for an update."
4. "Headaches are expected with increased intracranial pressure."

49. The nurse is assessing a child newly diagnosed with petit mal seizures. Which observation will the nurse report to the health care provider to review?
1. A loss of consciousness followed by muscle convulsions
2. Appearing to stare into space for a few seconds
3. Brief periods of lip smacking and eyelid fluttering
4. No alteration in muscle tone, with a brief loss of consciousness

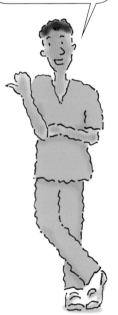

If you concentrate hard enough on question #47, I'm sure you'll get it right.

46. **4.** There is no one known cause of spina bifida, but scientists believe it is linked to hereditary and environmental factors. Neural tube defects, including spina bifida, have been strongly linked to low dietary intake of folic acid. Maternal age does not impact spina bifida. An amniocentesis is performed to help diagnose spina bifida in utero but does not cause the disorder. Maternal alcohol intake during pregnancy has been linked to intellectual disability, craniofacial defects, and cardiac abnormalities but not spina bifida.
CN: Physiological integrity; CNS: Physiological adaptation; CL: Apply

47. **1.** Clients with head injuries may pass through eight stages during their recovery. Stage 1, marked by unresponsiveness, is the worst stage. Stage 8, characterized by purposeful, appropriate behavior, is the final stage of healing. This child is somewhere between stage 4 (confused, agitated behavior) and stage 6 (confused, appropriate behavior) because sometimes the child can answer appropriately but at other times becomes confused and angry, resorting to violent behavior. The other responses are inappropriate and do not answer the parent's question.
CN: Health promotion and maintenance; CNS: None; CL: Apply

48. **4.** Headaches are an expected finding with increased ICP. The mechanism producing the headache that accompanies increased ICP may be the stretching of the meninges and pain fibers associated with blood vessels. The child's stimuli should be decreased, but this statement does not address the parents' concern. The other responses are not accurate or appropriate.
CN: Safe, effective care environment; CNS: Management of care; CL: Apply

49. **1.** A loss of consciousness followed by muscle contractions is indicative of a grand mal seizure (tonic-clonic seizure). The nurse would report this observation as it is not expected with petit mal seizures. Petit mal seizures, or absence seizures, consist of a brief loss of responsiveness with minimal or no alteration in muscle tone. They may go unrecognized because the child's behavior changes very little. Children appear to stare into space for a few seconds during the seizures and may exhibit lip smacking, eyelid fluttering, or chewing motions.
CN: Safe, effective care environment; CNS: Management of care; CL: Apply

50. The nurse is assessing a 12-month-old client. Which finding will the nurse highlight for the health care provider to review?
1. The child does not search for objects the child sees the caregiver hide.
2. The child is pulling up and cruising around furniture, but is not walking yet.
3. The child can say about five words and understand simple commands.
4. The child does not attempt to copy actions the caregiver performs.

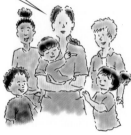

Nurses need to know expected milestones for kids of all ages.

50. 1. By 12 months of age, children should search for items hidden while they are watching. At 12 months, most children understand the word "no" and other simple commands and can say approximately five words, including "mama" and "dada." By this age, children are usually pulling up and cruising; they may or may not be standing alone, taking steps, or walking. Walking should occur by 18 months of age. The nurse would be concerned if an 18-month-old client did not attempt to copy actions of others.
CN: Health promotion and maintenance; CNS: None; CL: Apply

51. The nurse is assessing a 3-year-old child with nuchal rigidity and notes a positive Kernig's sign. Which nursing action(s) is appropriate based on these findings? Select all that apply.
1. Administer dexamethasone.
2. Document the finding.
3. Assess for a Brudzinski's sign.
4. Call the rapid response team.
5. Prepare the child for magnetic resonance imaging (MRI).

51. 1, 2, 3. Dexamethasone, a corticosteroid, is used to treat meningitis. A positive Kernig's sign indicates nuchal rigidity, caused by an irritative lesion of the subarachnoid space. A positive Brudzinski's sign also is indicative of the condition. The nurse would document these expected findings in the medical record. Calling the rapid response team and preparing the child for an MRI are not necessary.
CN: Physiological integrity; CNS: Physiological adaptation; CL: Apply

52. A child with a diagnosis of meningococcal meningitis develops sudden signs of sepsis and a purpuric rash on the lower extremities. The nurse will suspect the child is experiencing which complication?
1. A severe allergic reaction to the antibiotic prescribed
2. Syndrome of inappropriate antidiuretic hormone (SIADH)
3. Fulminant meningococcemia (Waterhouse-Friderichsen syndrome)
4. Adhesive arachnoiditis

52. 3. Meningococcemia is a serious complication usually associated with meningococcal infection. When onset is severe, sudden, and rapid (fulminant), it is known as Waterhouse-Friderichsen syndrome. Allergic reactions do not present as sepsis. SIADH can be an acute complication but would not be accompanied by the purpuric rash. Adhesive arachnoiditis occurs in the chronic phase of the disease and leads to obstruction of the flow of cerebrospinal fluid.
CN: Physiological integrity; CNS: Reduction of risk potential; CL: Apply

53. The nurse is planning care for a 12-year-old client with Down's syndrome. Which nursing action is **most** appropriate?
1. Treat the child the same way the nurse would any other 12-year-old.
2. Allow the child to decide whether the parents will be involved in the care.
3. Communicate with the child on a preschool level.
4. Determine the child's current developmental level.

Which intervention in question #54 would be most effective in alleviating fear?

53. 4. Before developing a care plan, the nurse should assess the child's developmental level and plan care at that level. The nurse should not plan care geared toward the child's chronologic age without first assessing the child. The nurse should not assume that the child is at a lower developmental level without assessment. The parents would need to be involved in the child's care to maintain consistency based on the home schedule and upon discharge.
CN: Health promotion and maintenance; CNS: None; CL: Apply

54. Which nursing intervention is appropriate to calm a preschool-age child prior to an electroencephalogram (EEG) procedure?
1. Administer intravenous fentanyl to the child.
2. Allow the child to hold a security blanket.
3. Have the child sit on the bed with the nurse.
4. Give the child a handout about the procedure.

54. 2. Allowing the child to hold a security item assists in calming the child at this age. Fentanyl is not necessary for an EEG procedure and may interfere with the results. Having the child sit with a parent would be appropriate. A handout is not age-appropriate. The nurse could demonstrate the procedure using dolls and allow the child to see and touch the equipment to be used, if able.
CN: Physiological integrity; CNS: Basic care and comfort; CL: Apply

55. The nurse is caring for a child suspected to have meningitis. The nurse will complete which prescription **first**?
1. Reduce the child's environmental stimuli.
2. Obtain intravenous access.
3. Administer ceftriaxone intravenously.
4. Collect cerebrospinal fluid (CSF) and blood for culture.

56. The nurse will monitor which client **most** closely for the development of a complication of meningitis?
1. A 1-month-old with bacterial meningitis and increased head circumference
2. A 6-month-old diagnosed with meningococcal meningitis
3. A 1-year-old with bacterial meningitis and a temperature of 102.4°F (39.1°C)
4. A 6-year-old with bacterial meningitis and positive Brudzinski's sign

57. A 3-month-old infant is admitted to the pediatric unit and diagnosed with bacterial meningitis. Which finding(s) by the nurse supports the diagnosis? Select all that apply.
1. Change in feeding pattern
2. Diarrhea
3. Fever
4. Vomiting
5. Sun-setting eyes

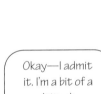

Okay—I admit it. I'm a bit of a multitasker.

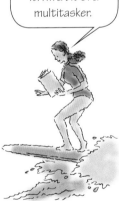

58. The nurse is caring for a child with meningitis. Which goal will the nurse recognize as **most** difficult to achieve?
1. Protecting self and others from possible infection
2. Avoiding actions that increase discomfort
3. Keeping environmental stimuli to a minimum
4. Maintaining intravenous (IV) access

59. The nurse is assessing an infant during a routine examination. Which method will the nurse use to test for Babinski's sign?
1. Raise the child's leg with the knee flexed and then extend the child's leg at the knee to determine whether resistance is noted.
2. With the infant's knee flexed, dorsiflex the foot to determine whether pain is present in the calf of the leg.
3. Flex the child's head while the child is in a supine position to determine whether the knees or hips flex involuntarily.
4. Stroke the bottom of the infant's foot to determine whether there is fanning and dorsiflexion of the big toe.

55. 4. Antibiotic therapy should always begin immediately *after* the collection of CSF and blood cultures. After the specific organism is identified, bacteria-specific antibiotics can be administered if the initial choice of antibiotic therapy is not appropriate. The nurse would obtain IV access, start antibiotics, and reduce stimuli after assisting with the collection of specimens.
CN: Safe, effective care environment; CNS: Management of care; CL: Analyze

56. 1. Infants younger than age 2 months with bacterial meningitis commonly have complications such as hearing loss, impaired vision, seizures, and cardiac and renal abnormalities. Increased head circumference indicates hydrocephalus, which is a complication of meningitis. Complications are seen less commonly among children diagnosed with meningococcal meningitis. Fever and positive Brudzinski's sign are expected with bacterial meningitis.
CN: Physiological integrity; CNS: Physiological adaptation; CL: Analyze

57. 1, 2, 3, 4. Fever, change in feeding patterns, vomiting, and diarrhea are commonly observed in infants and young children with bacterial meningitis. Sun-setting eyes are a common manifestation of hydrocephalus.
CN: Physiological integrity; CNS: Physiological adaptation; CL: Apply

58. 4. One of the most difficult problems in the nursing care of children with meningitis is maintaining the IV infusion for the length of time needed to provide adequate therapy. All of the other options are important aspects in the provision of care for the child with meningitis, but are less difficult than maintaining an IV infusion for antimicrobial therapy.
CN: Physiological integrity; CNS: Basic care and comfort; CL: Apply

59. 4. To test for Babinski's sign, stroke the bottom of the foot to determine whether there is fanning and dorsiflexion of the big toe. Raising the child's leg with the knee flexed and then extending the leg at the knee to determine whether resistance is noted tests for Kernig's sign. Dorsiflexion of the foot with the knee flexed to determine whether there is pain in the calf of the leg tests for Homans' sign. Flexing the child's head while the child is in a supine position to determine whether the knees or hips flex involuntarily tests for Brudzinski's sign.
CN: Physiological integrity; CNS: Physiological adaptation; CL: Understand

CN: Client needs category   CNS: Client needs subcategory   CL: Cognitive level

60. The nurse is teaching the parents of a child who had a febrile seizure about methods to reduce the child's body temperature. Which statement(s) made by the parents indicates to the nurse teaching was effective? Select all that apply.
1. "We can sponge our child off with ice water."
2. "We can alternate giving our child acetaminophen and ibuprofen."
3. "We will not cover our child with a quilt while the child has a fever."
4. "We will remove all our child's clothing except the underwear."
5. "We can rub our child's body with a water and alcohol solution."

60. 2, 3, 4. Appropriate measures to decrease a child's temperature include sponging with tepid water, alternating medications, and limiting clothing and blankets that would hold in heat. It is not comfortable to sponge the child with cold water or safe to apply a water and alcohol solution to the child's body.

CN: Health promotion and maintenance; CNS: None; CL: Apply

61. The parent of a child with a history of a closed-head injury asks the nurse why the child would begin having seizures now. Which response by the nurse is the **most** appropriate?
1. "Clonic seizure activity is usually interpreted as falling."
2. "It is not unusual to develop seizures after a head injury because of brain trauma."
3. "Focal discharge in the brain may lead to absence seizures that go unnoticed."
4. "The brain needs multiple stimuli before it manifests as a seizure."

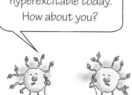

I'm feeling a little hyperexcitable today. How about you?

61. 2. Stimuli from an earlier injury may eventually elicit seizure activity, a process known as kindling. Atonic seizures, not clonic seizures, are commonly accompanied by falling. Focal seizures are partial seizures; absence seizures are generalized seizures. Focal seizures do not lead to absence seizures. The epileptogenic focus consists of a group of hyperexcitable neurons responsible for initiating synchronous, high-frequency discharges that lead to a seizure and do not need multiple stimuli.

CN: Safe, effective care environment; CNS: Management of care; CL: Apply

62. The nurse is caring for a child with tubercular meningitis. Which finding **most** concerns the nurse?
1. Temperature of 101.8°F (38.8°C)
2. Presence of nuchal rigidity
3. New onset of urinary incontinence
4. Intracranial pressure (ICP) at 30 mm Hg

62. 4. Assessment of fever and evaluation of nuchal rigidity are important aspects of care, but assessment for signs of increasing ICP should be the highest priority due to the life-threatening implications. Increased ICP is defined as pressure at 20 mm Hg or higher. Urinary incontinence can occur in a child who is ill from nearly any cause but does not pose a great danger to life.

CN: Physiological integrity; CNS: Reduction of risk potential; CL: Analyze

63. The nurse is educating the parents of a child with hydrocephalus who has been prescribed phenytoin. Which statement made by the parents indicates a need for additional teaching?
1. "It is okay for us to switch between tablets and capsules."
2. "This medicine will help stop our child's seizures."
3. "We will not abruptly stop administering phenytoin."
4. "Our child will need to have blood work every 6 months."

63. 1. Differences in bioavailability of phenytoin exist among different formulations (tablets and capsules) and among the same formulations produced by different manufacturers. Children should not be switched from one formulation to another or from one brand to another without approval from the health care provider. All other statements are correct.

CN: Physiological integrity; CNS: Pharmacological and parenteral therapies; CL: Apply

64. Which behavioral response(s) to pain will the nurse expect in a 7-month-old client? Select all that apply.
1. Localized withdrawal
2. Facial grimacing
3. Reflex withdrawal to stimulus
4. Clenching fists
5. Low frustration level
6. Striking out physically

64. 2, 3. Infants younger than age 1 year become irritable and exhibit reflex withdrawal to the painful stimulus. Facial grimacing also occurs. Localized withdrawal is experienced by toddlers (ages 1 to 3), not infants, in response to pain. The nurse would observe clenching fists in school-age children. Preschoolers show a low frustration level and strike out physically.

CN: Physiological integrity; CNS: Physiological adaptation; CL: Apply

CN: Client needs category   CNS: Client needs subcategory   CL: Cognitive level

65. The parents of a child who takes phenytoin ask the nurse why it is difficult to maintain therapeutic plasma levels of this medication. Which statement by the nurse is **most** appropriate?
1. "A drop in the plasma drug level leads to a toxic state."
2. "The capacity to metabolize the drug becomes overwhelmed over time."
3. "Small increments in dosage lead to sharp increases in plasma drug levels."
4. "Large increments in dosage lead to a more rapid, stabilizing therapeutic effect."

66. A child is newly diagnosed with a seizure disorder and is started on carbamazepine. Which education is **priority** for the nurse to include in the discharge teaching?
1. Blood work will be monitored while taking this medication.
2. Drug dosage may be adjusted depending on seizure activity.
3. Notify the primary health care provider if seizures continue.
4. Monitor the child closely for any changes in behavior.

67. The nurse will closely monitor a child with meningitis receiving intravenous (IV) fluids for which condition?
1. Cerebral edema
2. Renal failure
3. Left-sided heart failure
4. Cardiogenic shock

68. The nurse will include which instruction(s) when educating the parents of a child prescribed phenytoin? Select all that apply.
1. Obtain a medical identification bracelet for the child.
2. Maintain a seizure frequency chart.
3. Avoid potentially hazardous activities.
4. Discontinue the drug immediately for adverse effects.
5. Limit physical activity for the first month.

69. A couple wants their fetus tested for neural tube defects. The nurse will anticipate preparing the couple for which procedure?
1. Abdominal x-ray
2. Serum alpha-fetoprotein screening
3. Amniocentesis
4. Non-stress test

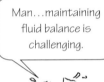

Monitor clients when they first start taking me.

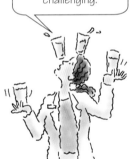

Man…maintaining fluid balance is challenging.

65. 3. Within the therapeutic range for phenytoin, small increments in dosage produce sharp increases in plasma drug levels. The capacity of the liver to metabolize phenytoin is affected by slight changes in the dosage of the drug, not necessarily the length of time the client has been taking the drug. Large increments in dosage greatly increase plasma levels, leading to drug toxicity.
CN: Physiological integrity; CNS: Pharmacological and parenteral therapies; CL: Understand

66. 4. When anticonvulsants are initially started, clients should be monitored for behavior changes, as these could indicate depression or suicidal thoughts or behaviors. All other statements are important too; however, client safety is priority.
CN: Physiological integrity; CNS: Pharmacological and parenteral therapies; CL: Analyze

67. 1. The child with meningitis is already at increased risk for cerebral edema and increased intracranial pressure due to inflammation of the meningeal membranes; therefore, the nurse should carefully monitor fluid intake and output to avoid fluid volume overload. Renal failure and cardiogenic shock are not complications of IV therapy. The child with a healthy heart would not be expected to develop left-sided heart failure.
CN: Physiological integrity; CNS: Pharmacological and parenteral therapies; CL: Apply

68. 1, 2, 3. Ongoing evaluation of therapeutic effects can be accomplished by maintaining a frequency chart that indicates the date, time, and nature of the child's seizure activity. These data may be helpful in making dosage alterations and specific drug selection. Wearing a medical identification bracelet and avoiding hazardous activities are ways to minimize danger related to seizure activity. Anticonvulsant drugs should never be discontinued abruptly due to the potential for development of status epilepticus. Physical activity should not be limited.
CN: Physiological integrity; CNS: Pharmacological and parenteral therapies; CL: Apply

69. 2. Screening for significant levels of alpha-fetoprotein is 90% effective in detecting neural tube defects. Prenatal screening begins with maternal serum screening. If levels are abnormal, amniotic fluid levels may be tested via amniocentesis. X-rays of the abdomen and non-stress tests are not diagnostic for neural tube defect.
CN: Health promotion and maintenance; CNS: None; CL: Apply

70. A 13-year-old with structural scoliosis had Cotrel-Dubousset rods inserted. The registered nurse (RN) observes the licensed practical nurse (LPN) place the child supine in bed. Which action by the RN is appropriate?
1. Place the child in semi-Fowler's position.
2. Continue to monitor the child.
3. Show the LPN the correct position for this child.
4. Notify the unit nurse manager.

71. The parents of a child newly diagnosed with seizures ask the nurse, "What time of day is seizure activity most likely to occur?" Which response by the nurse is **most** accurate?
1. "During the rapid eye movement (REM) stage of sleep."
2. "During long periods of excitement."
3. "While falling asleep and on awakening."
4. "While eating, particularly if the child is hurried."

72. The family of a child with seizures asks the nurse when they should activate the emergency medical services. Which nursing response is **best**?
1. "Activate if your child continues to vomit for 15 minutes after a seizure."
2. "Activate if stereotypic or automatous body movements occur during the onset."
3. "Activate if your child has a lack of facial expressions during the seizure."
4. "Activate if bilateral posturing of one or more extremities occurs during the onset."

73. The nurse educates a child's parents on factors that may trigger seizure activity. Which factor(s) will the nurse include in the teaching? Select all that apply.
1. Striped wallpaper
2. Ceiling fans
3. Sleep interruption during the night
4. Periods of intense physical activity
5. Caffeinated beverages
6. Missed medication

74. Which nursing intervention will be included to support the goals of avoiding injury, respiratory distress, and aspiration during a seizure for a child?
1. Position the child with the head hyperextended.
2. Place a hand under the child's head for support.
3. Use pillows to prop the child into the sitting position.
4. Work a small plastic airway between the teeth.

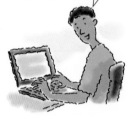

What position would you want to be in after having rods put in your back?

You're almost done. Cheers!

70. 2. The RN should continue to monitor this child, as the supine position is appropriate and should be maintained. Other positions, such as the side-lying, semi-Fowler's, and high Fowler's positions, could prove damaging because the rods will not be able to maintain the spine in a straight position. Other options are inappropriate.
CN: Safe, effective care environment; CNS: Management of care; CL: Apply

71. 3. Falling asleep or awakening from sleep are periods of functional instability of the brain; seizure activity is more likely to occur during these times. Eating quickly, excitement without undo fatigue, and REM sleep have not been identified as contributing factors.
CN: Physiological integrity; CNS: Physiological adaptation; CL: Understand

72. 1. Continuous vomiting after a seizure has ended can be a sign of an acute problem and indicates that the child requires an immediate medical evaluation. All of the other body responses to seizure are normally present in various types of seizure activity and do not require immediate medical evaluation.
CN: Physiological integrity; CNS: Reduction of risk potential; CL: Apply

73. 1, 2, 4, 5, 6. Striped wallpaper and ceiling fans can be triggers for seizure activity if the child is photosensitive. Avoidance of fatigue can reduce seizure activity; therefore, intense physical activity for extended periods of time should be avoided. Restricting caffeine intake by using caffeine-free soda is a dietary modification that may prevent seizures. Missing medication dosages can lead to seizure activity. Sleep interruption has not been identified as a triggering factor.
CN: Physiological integrity; CNS: Physiological adaptation; CL: Apply

74. 2. Placing a hand, small cushion, or blanket under the child's head can help prevent injury. Position the child with the head in midline, not hyperextended, to promote a good airway and adequate ventilation. Do not attempt to prop the child up into a sitting position but ease the child to the floor to prevent falling and possible injury. Do not put anything in the child's mouth because it could cause infection or obstruct the airway.
CN: Physiological integrity; CNS: Reduction of risk potential; CL: Apply

75. The nurse is caring for an adolescent client prescribed carbamazepine. Which finding(s) will the nurse highlight for the health care provider? Select all that apply.
1. Blood urea nitrogen (BUN) level 18 mg/dL (6.43 mmol/L)
2. Platelet count 300,000/mm³ (300 × 10⁹/L)
3. Reticulocyte count 15 × 10³/µL (15 × 10⁹/L)
4. Alanine aminotransferase (ALT) level 22 U/L (0.37 µkat/L)
5. Sodium level 139 mEq/L (139 mmol/L)

75. 3. Carbamazepine is an anticonvulsant. The nurse would highlight a low reticulocyte count for review. Carbamazepine use can cause aplastic anemia, which will significantly lower a client's reticulocyte count. Normal reticulocyte count is 25 to 75 × 10³/L (25 to 75 × 10⁹/L). All other levels are within range for an adolescent client.
CN: Safe, effective care environment; CNS: Management of care; CL: Analyze

76. The nurse is caring for an infant recently born with spina bifida. The nurse will monitor the neonate for which complication?
1. Clubfoot
2. Hip extension
3. Ankylosis of the knee
4. Abduction and external rotation of the hip

76. 1. The type and extent of deformity in the lower extremities of a child with spina bifida depend on the muscles that are active or inactive. Passive positioning in utero may result in deformities of the feet, such as equinovarus (clubfoot), knee flexion and extension contractures, and hip flexion with adduction and internal rotation leading to subluxation or dislocation of the hip.
CN: Physiological integrity; CNS: Physiological adaptation; CL: Apply

77. The nurse notes a 4-year-old child with cerebral palsy has a weight at the 30th percentile and a height at the 60th percentile. Which teaching information is appropriate for this child's parents?
1. The child should eat more carbohydrates and fats
2. The child's weight and height are within the normal range
3. The child needs to increase the daily caloric intake
4. The child is small and will remain so through adolescence

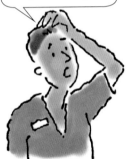

What's the normal percentile range for weight and height?

77. 2. The weight and height are between the 25th and 75th percentiles, so the child is considered within normal range. The other options are incorrect.
CN: Health promotion and maintenance; CNS: None; CL: Apply

78. An 8-month-old infant is diagnosed with an ear infection. The parent asks the nurse, "Why do children have more ear infections than adults?" The nurse shows the parent a diagram of the ear and explains the differences in anatomy. Identify the portion of the infant's ear that allows fluid to stagnate and act as a medium for bacteria.

78. The eustachian tube in an infant is shorter and wider than in an adult or older child. It also slants horizontally. Because of these anatomical features, nasopharyngeal secretions can enter the middle ear more easily, stagnate, and cause infections.

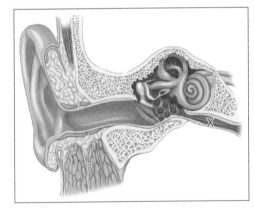

CN: Health promotion and maintenance; CNS: None; CL: Understand

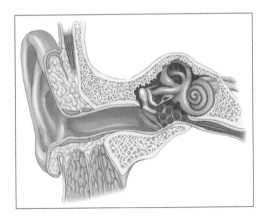

CN: Client needs category   CNS: Client needs subcategory   CL: Cognitive level

79. Which finding(s) indicates to the nurse an infant with a myelomeningocele has an Arnold-Chiari malformation? Select all that apply.
1. Rapidly progressing scoliosis
2. Changes in urologic functioning
3. Back pain below the site of the sac closure
4. Respiratory stridor
5. Apneic periods
6. Difficulty swallowing

79. 4, 5, 6. Children with a myelomeningocele have a 90% chance of being born with an Arnold-Chiari malformation, in which brain tissue extends into the spinal canal. This may lead to respiratory function problems, such as respiratory stridor associated with paralysis of the vocal cords, apneic episodes of unknown cause, difficulty swallowing, and an abnormal gag reflex. Scoliosis and urologic function changes occur with myelomeningocele, but these complications are not specifically related to an Arnold-Chiari malformation. Lower back pain does not occur because the infant has a loss of sensory function below the level of the cord defect.
CN: Physiological integrity; CNS: Reduction of risk potential; CL: Apply

80. The clinic nurse is assessing a child with a recent history of a viral illness. The parent states the child was given aspirin to control the fever. The child is now vomiting, lethargic, confused, and has hyperactive reflexes. What will the nurse do **first**?
1. Assess the child's temperature.
2. Notify the health care provider.
3. Draw blood to assess electrolyte levels.
4. Prepare the child for a liver biopsy.

80. 2. The nurse should notify the health care provider as this child is exhibiting signs of cerebral edema associated with Reye's syndrome. The child needs to be admitted to the hospital for treatment. The other actions may be done for this child, but priority is stabilizing the child, which may include assisted ventilation and intracranial pressure monitoring.
CN: Safe, effective care environment; CNS: Management of care; CL: Analyze

81. The nurse is caring for a 10-year-old client who fell off his bike and hit his head without a helmet on. Which finding(s) indicates to the nurse the client is experiencing increased intracranial pressure (ICP)? Select all that apply.
1. Decreased responsiveness
2. Increased pulse rate
3. Double vision
4. Headache
5. Vomiting

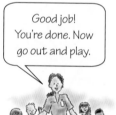

Good job! You're done. Now go out and play.

81. 1, 3, 4, 5. Signs and symptoms of increased ICP in a child include behavior changes, decreased alertness, headache, lethargy, seizures, vomiting, and vision alterations. With increased ICP, blood pressure rises while the pulse rate falls.
CN: Physiological integrity; CNS: Physiological adaptation; CL: Apply

Chapter 30

Musculoskeletal Disorders

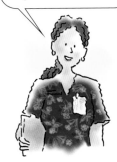

Challenge yourself with these questions on musculoskeletal system disorders in children. I'm betting you'll have a blast!

Pediatric musculoskeletal refresher

Clubfoot

Abnormality of the foot, which is usually congenital, in which the tendons are shorter than normal

Key signs and symptoms
- Cannot be corrected manually (distinguishes true clubfoot from apparent clubfoot)

Key test results
- X-rays show superimposition of the talus and calcaneus and a ladder-like appearance of the metatarsals

Key treatments
- Correcting deformity with a series of casts or surgical correction
- Maintaining correction until foot gains normal muscle balance
- Observing foot closely for several years to prevent foot deformity from recurring

Key interventions
- Ensure that shoes fit correctly.
- Prepare for surgery, if necessary.

Developmental hip dysplasia

Dislocation or instability of the hip at birth, which may result in hip dysplasia

Key signs and symptoms
- Affected side exhibits an increased number of folds on posterior thigh when child is supine with knees bent
- Appearance of shortened limb on affected side when child is supine
- Restricted abduction of hips

Key test results
- Barlow's sign: A click is felt when the infant is placed supine with hips flexed 90 degrees and when the knees are fully flexed and the hip is brought into midabduction
- Ortolani click: Can be felt by the health care provider's fingers at the hip area as the femur head snaps out of and back into the acetabulum; it is also palpable during examination with the child's legs flexed and abducted

- Positive Trendelenburg test: When child stands on the affected leg, the opposite pelvis dips to maintain erect posture.

Key treatments
- Hip spica cast or corrective surgery for older children
- Bryant traction
- Casting or a Pavlik harness to keep the hips and knees flexed and the hips abducted for at least 3 months

Key interventions
- Give reassurance that early, prompt treatment will probably result in complete correction.
- Assure parents that the child will adjust to restricted movement and return to normal sleeping, eating, and playing in a few days.

Duchenne muscular dystrophy

Incurable inherited disorder that involves muscle weakness and wasting, which progresses rapidly

Key signs and symptoms
- Eventual muscle weakness and wasting
- Gowers sign (use of hands to push self up from floor)
- Pelvic girdle weakness, indicated by waddling gait and falling

Key test results
- Electromyography typically demonstrates short, weak bursts of electrical activity in affected muscles
- Muscle biopsy shows variation in the size of muscle fibers and, in later stages, shows fat and connective tissue deposits, with no dystrophin

Key treatments
- Physical therapy
- Surgery to correct contractures
- Use of such devices as splints, braces, trapeze bars, overhead slings, and a wheelchair to help preserve mobility

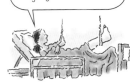

Be sure to use appropriate precautions when moving a client who is being treated for a musculoskeletal injury or disorder.

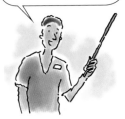

What key signs and symptoms would you expect to see in Duchenne muscular dystrophy?

573

Key interventions

- Perform range-of-motion exercises.
- If respiratory involvement occurs, encourage:
  - coughing
  - deep-breathing exercises
  - diaphragmatic breathing.
- Encourage adequate fluid intake.
- Increase dietary fiber.
- Obtain a prescription for a stool softener.

Fractures

Complete or incomplete break of a bone

Key signs and symptoms

- Loss of motor function
- Muscle spasm
- Pain or tenderness
- Skeletal deformity
- Swelling

Key test results

- X-rays may be used to confirm location and extent of fracture

Key treatments

- Casting
- Reduction and immobilization of the fracture
- Surgery: open reduction and external fixation of the fracture

Key interventions

- Keep child in proper body alignment.
- Provide support above and below fracture site when moving the child.
- Elevate the fracture above the level of the heart.
- Apply ice to the fracture to promote vasoconstriction.
- Monitor pulses distal to the fracture every 2 to 4 hours.
- Monitor color, temperature, and capillary refill.

Juvenile rheumatoid arthritis

Most common form of arthritis in children; long-term (chronic) disease resulting in joint pain and swelling which may or may not resolve in adulthood

Key signs and symptoms

- Inflammation around joints
- Stiffness, pain, and guarding of affected joints

Key test results

- Hematology studies reveal:
  - elevated erythrocyte sedimentation rate
  - positive antinuclear antibody test
  - presence of rheumatoid factor

Key treatments

- Heat therapy: warm compresses, baths
- Splint application

Key interventions

- Monitor joints for deformity.

Scoliosis

Abnormal lateral curvature of the spine

Key signs and symptoms

- Disappearance of the curve in the spinal column
- Nonstructural scoliosis
- When child bends at the waist to touch the toes, the curve in the spinal column disappears

Structural scoliosis

- Failure of the spinal curve to straighten; asymmetry of the hips, ribs, shoulders, and shoulder blades when the child bends forward with the knees straight and the arms hanging down toward the feet

Key test results

- X-rays may aid in diagnosing

Key treatments

- Nonstructural scoliosis: postural exercises, shoe lifts
- Structural scoliosis: steel rods, prolonged bracing, spinal fusion

Key interventions

- After spinal fusion and insertion of rods:
  - turn the child by logrolling only
  - maintain the child in correct body alignment
  - maintain the bed in a flat position.

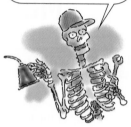

Fractured ulna? No problem. You just need to gather the right tools for the job.

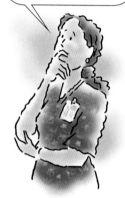

Your client with juvenile rheumatoid arthritis complains of joint pain and swelling. What's a good treatment?

thePoint® You can download tables of drug information to help you prepare for the NCLEX®! View Generic Drug Names, Drug Classifications, Drug Actions, and Nursing Implications for the drugs discussed in this refresher at **http://thePoint.lww.com**

Musculoskeletal questions, answers, and rationales

1. The nurse is caring for a neonate newly diagnosed with clubfoot. Which primary health care provider prescription(s) will the nurse question? Select all that apply.
  1. Gather supplies for Ponseti method.
  2. Prepare neonate for surgery.
  3. Give acetaminophen for pain Q 6 hr.
  4. Monitor for cardiac anomaly.
  5. Consult pediatric orthopedist.

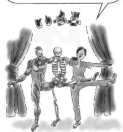

Get out there and break a leg—or at least sprain an ankle.

1. **2, 3, 4.** Talipes equinovarus, or clubfoot, is a birth defect which causes the foot to be turned inward. Initial treatment includes either the Ponseti method (stretching and casting) or the French method (stretching and taping), If the selected method is not successful, surgery may be needed as the neonate grows. Clubfoot is not painful in infancy; therefore, pain medication is not necessary. The neonate does not need to be monitored for cardiac anomalies, as these are not associated with clubfoot. A pediatric orthopedist would be consulted for treatment.
CN: Safe, effective care environment; CNS: Management of care; CL: Apply

2. The nurse observes an assistive personnel (AP) place an 18-month-old in Bryant traction with the hips resting on the bed. Which action will the nurse complete **first**?
  1. Slightly elevate the toddler's hips off the bed.
  2. Take the AP in the room and explain correct positioning.
  3. Immediately notify the health care provider.
  4. Notify the nurse educator of the incident.

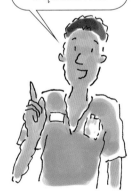

Remember— more than one answer may be right in question #3.

2. **1.** In Bryant traction, the child's hips should be slightly elevated off the bed at a 15-degree angle. The nurse should first correct the toddler's positioning. The nurse should explain correct positioning to the AP, but not in the client's room. There is not a need to notify the health care provider. If the AP needed additional training, the nurse educator could be notified.
CN: Safe, effective care environment; CNS: Management of care; CL: Analyze

3. The nurse is providing education to the caregivers of a child prescribed corticosteroid therapy for juvenile rheumatoid arthritis. Which statement(s) will the nurse include in the education? Select all that apply.
  1. "This medication can be taken orally."
  2. "This medication is given subcutaneously."
  3. "This medication is injected into the joint."
  4. "This medication is given intermuscularly."
  5. "This medication is applied as a topical cream."

3. **1, 3.** This medication can be given orally or by injection directly into the joint to control symptoms of juvenile rheumatoid arthritis. The other routes of administration do not apply to this medication.
CN: Physiological integrity; CNS: Pharmacological and parenteral therapies; CL: Apply

4. The nurse is providing education to the parent of a neonate with clubfoot. Which information will the nurse include?
  1. Clubfoot is a hereditary disorder.
  2. This condition causes intermediate pain.
  3. This will be treated over a few months.
  4. Surgery is required at 6 months of age.

4. **3.** Clubfoot is treated with serial casting or taping of the affected foot for a few months. If these methods are not successful or adhered to, surgery may be required. The cause of clubfoot is unknown, and it does not cause pain.
CN: Physiological integrity; CNS: Physiological adaptation; CL: Apply

5. A 9-month-old infant has torticollis with the head rotated to the left and bent to the right side. The nurse will place the infant in which position?
  1. Prone
  2. Supine
  3. Left side-lying
  4. Right side-lying

5. **3.** The left side-lying position assists with lengthening of the shortened muscles associated with torticollis because this position makes it easier to stretch the sternocleidomastoid and upper trapezius. No other positions would assist in increasing muscle length.
CN: Physiological integrity; CNS: Reduction of risk potential; CL: Apply

6. The nurse is preparing to give an intramuscular injection into the left leg of a 2-year-old client. Place an "X" on the area where the nurse will administer the injection.

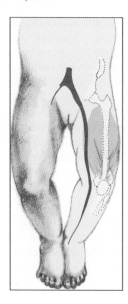

6. The nurse should administer intramuscular injections in the vastus lateralis, located in the child's thigh. To give the injection, the nurse should first divide the distance between the greater trochanter and the knee joints into quadrants and then inject in the center of the upper quadrant.

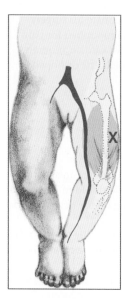

CN: Physiological integrity; CNS: Pharmacological and parenteral therapies; CL: Apply

7. The nurse is educating parents of a 3-month-old infant who has severe torticollis, with the head rotated to the left and bent to the right side. Which statement by the parents indicates the education has been effective?
1. "It involves shortening of the left upper trapezius."
2. "It involves shortening of the right middle trapezius."
3. "It involves shortening of the left sternocleidomastoid."
4. "It involves shortening of the right sternocleidomastoid."

7. 4. The right sternocleidomastoid is shortened when the head rotates left. The left upper trapezius is not shortened. The middle trapezius is not affected, and the left sternocleidomastoid is lengthened.

CN: Physiological integrity; CNS: Physiological adaptation; CL: Apply

8. The nurse is assessing an 11-year-old client. The nurse notes the client leans to one side and the waist appears uneven in height. Which action will the nurse complete **first**?
1. Have the client rate and describe the pain.
2. Have the client lean forward.
3. Prepare the client for an x-ray.
4. Notify the primary health care provider.

8. 2. The nurse would suspect the client has scoliosis, which is defined as "S" curves along the longitudinal axis of the body. The nurse would first assess the client's spine for scoliosis by having the client lean forward with knees straight and arms hanging down. After assessing, the nurse will determine if the health care provider needs to be notified and if an x-ray is needed. Pain is not associated with scoliosis in early development.

CN: Safe, effective care environment; CNS: Management of care; CL: Analyze

9. The nurse is caring for an infant who received a hip spica cast 24 hours ago for hip dysplasia. Which assessment finding will the nurse highlight for the health care provider?
1. Oxygen saturation level of 96%
2. Absent pedal pulses
3. Capillary refill time of less than 3 seconds
4. Urinary output of 35 mL/hr

10. A child with scoliosis is prescribed a Milwaukee brace. The child states, "This brace is uncomfortable, and I feel confined." Which response by the nurse is **most** appropriate?
1. "By the looks of that brace, I see what you are saying."
2. "You have the right to refuse to wear this brace."
3. "I am sorry, but you have to wear this for 23 hours a day."
4. "It is common to feel that way when you first wear this brace."

11. A child with juvenile rheumatoid arthritis comes to the outpatient infusion clinic to receive the first infusion of etanercept. The child's caregiver asks about dangerous adverse effects of the medication. Which response(s) by the nurse is appropriate? Select all that apply.
1. "The child may develop an infection."
2. "The child may experience chills."
3. "It is possible to develop malignant tumors."
4. "The child may have a sore throat."
5. "The child may experience nausea."

12. The nurse expects which finding while assessing a child for scoliosis?
1. Scapula winging
2. Forward head posture
3. Raised right iliac crest
4. Forward flexion of the cervical spine

13. The nurse is educating the parents of a neonate with talipes equinovarus. The nurse knows additional education is needed if the parents make which statement?
1. "Our baby's foot is mostly cartilage, making it moldable."
2. "Casting slowly stretches the tissue to correct the deformity."
3. "We will sponge bathe our baby while the casts are worn."
4. "Our baby cannot ride in a normal car seat with casts on."

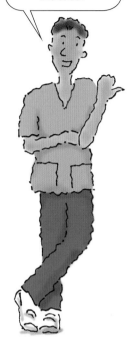

Which data indicate neurovascular compromise due to the cast?

9. 2. Neurovascular compromise is an assessment finding that would need to be reported immediately due to swelling within the confined space of the cast. All the other assessment data are within normal limits.
CN: Safe, effective care environment; CNS: Management of care; CL: Analyze

10. 4. This is a common feeling described by children when they start wearing this brace. Telling the child that he or she can refuse the brace is not the most appropriate response as the child may not be mentally mature enough to make the best decision and the child does need to allow time to get used to the brace. The other options are not therapeutic.
CN: Physiological integrity; CNS: Reduction of risk potential; CL: Apply

11. 1, 3. Clients who are treated with etanercept are at an increased risk of serious infection and malignancies, specifically lymphoma. Chills, nausea, and sore throat are common side effects of etanercept, but are not dangerous.
CN: Physiological integrity; CNS: Pharmacological and parenteral therapies; CL: Apply

12. 3. A raised iliac crest may be a warning sign of some curvature secondary to the attachment of the pelvis to the spine. Scapula winging could be caused by muscle paralysis. Forward head posture is not a result of scoliosis. Forward flexion is not indicative of lateral curves in the spine.
CN: Physiological integrity; CNS: Physiological adaptation; CL: Apply

13. 4. The casting process does not affect how infants are placed in a car seat. All other statements are correct concerning clubfoot.
CN: Physiological integrity; CNS: Reduction of risk potential; CL: Apply

14. The nurse is caring for an adolescent who sustained a left femur fracture yesterday in a motor vehicle accident. A cast was applied following surgery. Which finding will **most** concern the nurse?
1. Pain rated a 5 out of 10 on a pain scale
2. Left toes that are cool and mottled
3. Local swelling of the left toes
4. Respiratory rate of 15 breaths/minute

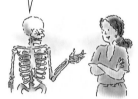

14. 2. The client with a cast is at risk for compartment syndrome. The nurse should monitor the client for severe pain, pallor, paresthesia, pulselessness, and paralysis. Cool, pale, mottled extremities indicate decreased blood flow and require immediate intervention. Moderate pain, local swelling, and loss of function are all typical findings after a fracture. The respiratory rate is normal for an adolescent.
CN: Physiological integrity; CNS: Reduction of risk potential; CL: Analyze

15. Which statement made by an adolescent with scoliosis indicates the education provided by the nurse was successful?
1. "I will wear the brace at night and during the day."
2. "I cannot do any exercising until my spine is fixed."
3. "I will have to wear a brace for several months."
4. "Surgery is required when I am done wearing the brace."

15. 1. The child must wear the brace all day, even during school and sleep. A brace worn to correct scoliosis must be worn for several years to correct the spinal deformity. Exercises are commonly prescribed to be performed several times per day to stretch and strengthen back muscles. Surgery may be needed if the brace is not effective.
CN: Physiological integrity; CNS: Basic care and comfort; CL: Apply

16. A child has just returned to the hospital room following surgical repair of a fractured femur. The nurse notes a scant amount of blood on the child's cast. Which action will the nurse take **next**?
1. Obtain the child's pulse rate and blood pressure.
2. Outline the bloody drainage and monitor it frequently.
3. Assess the child's level of consciousness (LOC).
4. Document the size and color of the drainage.

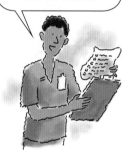

16. 1. The most appropriate action for the nurse is to assess the child's vital signs for evidence of hemorrhage, such as tachycardia and hypotension. The nurse should also assess the LOC and outline the drainage to accurately visualize for continued bleeding, but these should be done after taking the child's vital signs. The nurse would document the findings last.
CN: Physiological integrity; CNS: Reduction of risk potential; CL: Analyze

17. The nurse is providing crutch training to an adolescent. Which finding indicates to the nurse the crutches are a proper fit for the adolescent?
1. The crutches fit snugly under the axilla.
2. The crutches end 3 in (7.5 cm) below the axilla.
3. The elbow is flexed 25 degrees.
4. The client reports the crutches are comfortable.

17. 3. The client's elbow should be flexed 20 to 30 degrees, and the crutches should end 2 in (5 cm) below the axilla. The client stating the crutches are comfortable is not a proper indication.
CN: Physiological integrity; CNS: Basic care and comfort; CL: Apply

18. Which nursing intervention is appropriate for a 3-month-old client diagnosed with torticollis?
1. Administer morphine sulfate.
2. Only place the infant supine.
3. Offer a bottle on the unaffected side.
4. Perform passive neck exercises.

18. 4. Performing neck stretching exercises may help loosen the tight muscles and strengthen weaker ones. Severe pain is not generally associated with torticollis. The bottle or breast should be offered in a manner that causes the infant to turn to the affected side. The infant should also be positioned to encourage turning the affected side.
CN: Health promotion and maintenance; CNS: None; CL: Apply

19. The nurse is assigned to care for an infant with torticollis prescribed stretches. The nurse feels uncomfortable performing stretching techniques on the infant. Which nursing action is appropriate?
1. Omit the infant's stretches for this shift.
2. Switch assignments with another nurse on the unit.
3. Ask the assistive personnel (AP) to do the stretches.
4. Notify the charge nurse of the feelings.

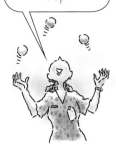

You're juggling these questions like a pro. Keep it up!

19. 4. The nurse should notify the charge nurse to discuss the feelings and determine a solution. The only cure for the torticollis is exercise or surgery, so the stretches cannot be omitted. The nurse should not switch assignments without consulting the charge nurse, as assignments are based on client acuity and a nurse's skill set. Having the AP perform the stretches is not appropriate, as the nurse should assess the client's response to and the effectiveness of the exercise while performing it.
CN: Safe, effective care environment; CNS: Management of care; CL: Apply

20. The nurse will monitor a child with severe scoliosis for which complication?
1. Adventitious breath sounds
2. Increased oxygen uptake
3. Diminished vital capacity
4. Decreased residual volume

20. 3. Scoliosis of greater than 60 degrees can shift organs and decrease the ability of the ribs to expand, thus decreasing vital capacity. Adventitious breath sounds and increased oxygen uptake would not occur secondary to a decrease in chest expansion. Residual volume would increase secondary to decreased ability of the lungs to expel air.
CN: Physiological integrity; CNS: Physiological adaptation; CL: Apply

21. An infant has developed right torticollis, with the head bent to the right side and rotated to the left. Which exercise is **most** beneficial for the nurse to perform for this infant?
1. Rotation exercises to the right
2. Rotation exercises to the left
3. Cervical extension exercises
4. Cervical flexion exercises

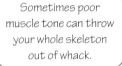

Sometimes poor muscle tone can throw your whole skeleton out of whack.

21. 1. Performing rotation exercises to the right helps increase the length of the shortened right sternocleidomastoid. Rotation to the left would exacerbate the torticollis, as the head is already rotated in that direction. Cervical extension exercises would not lengthen tightened muscles. Cervical flexion would shorten the muscles further.
CN: Physiological integrity; CNS: Reduction of risk potential; CL: Apply

22. A preschool-age child is diagnosed with thoracic scoliosis secondary to cerebral palsy. Which finding will the nurse expect contributed to the child's scoliosis?
1. Hyperreflexia
2. Hypotonia
3. Intellectual disability
4. Involuntary extremity movement

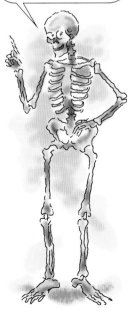

22. 2. Cerebral palsy is usually associated with some degree of hypotonia or hypertonia. Poor muscle tone may result in scoliosis. All other findings are associated with cerebral palsy but not scoliosis.
CN: Physiological integrity; CNS: Physiological adaptation; CL: Analyze

23. During a scoliosis screening, the school nurse examines a child and notes a raised right iliac crest. Which action by the nurse is **most** appropriate?
1. Have someone take the child to the urgent care clinic.
2. Notify the child's parents and provide a referral.
3. Document the findings in the child's medical record.
4. Assess the child for difficulty walking up stairs.

23. 2. A raised iliac crest may be indicative of a leg length discrepancy or a curvature in the lumbar spine. The nurse should notify the child's parents and suggest they have the child further evaluated by a health care provider. The nurse would document the findings after notifying the parents. The other options are not appropriate for this child.
CN: Health promotion and maintenance; CNS: None; CL: Apply

CN: Client needs category   CNS: Client needs subcategory   CL: Cognitive level

24. A child with muscular dystrophy is admitted to the hospital with reports of chest pain. The electrocardiogram shows cardiac muscle damage. Which medication(s) will the nurse anticipate administering? Select all that apply.
1. Benazepril
2. Enalapril
3. Metoprolol
4. Amlodipine
5. Nifedipine

25. A school nurse is performing a scoliosis screening on a group of students. Which student does the nurse recognize as being at **greatest** risk for developing scoliosis?
1. A 7-year-old with asthma
2. A 10-year-old with Down syndrome
3. A 12-year-old whose mom has scoliosis
4. A 13-year-old born with spina bifida

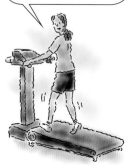

Nursing is an endurance sport. Pace yourself!

26. The nurse is caring for a 12-year-old who had a Harrington rod placed 2 days ago. Which finding **most** concerns the nurse?
1. Temperature of 101.8° F (38.8° C)
2. Reports of pain along the incision
3. Urine output of 38 mL/hr
4. Hypoactive bowel sounds

27. When assessing a child suspected of having scoliosis, which structure(s) will the nurse focus on during the screening process? Select all that apply.
1. Thoracic spine
2. Lumbar spine
3. Acromion processes
4. Posterior superior iliac spines
5. Cervical spine

28. The nurse is caring for an infant just diagnosed with talipes equinovarus. What action will the nurse complete **next**?
1. Educate the parents on the condition.
2. Prepare the infant for serial casting.
3. Measure the infant for leg braces.
4. Assess the infant for primitive reflexes.

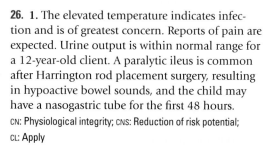

When come it comes to prioritizing, think quick! Your client will thank you.

29. A 6-year-old is crying after having surgical repair and a short cast applied for a fracture of the left radius. The nurse notes the client's fingers on the left hand are cool to the touch. Which nursing action is **priority**?
1. Ask the child to wiggle the fingers.
2. Elevate the child's arm on a pillow.
3. Administer prescribed pain medication.
4. Assess the brachial pulses bilaterally.

24. 1, 2, 3. When cardiac muscle damage in relation to muscular dystrophy has occurred, the health care provider would likely prescribe angiotensin-converting enzyme inhibitors (benazepril, enalapril) or beta blockers (metoprolol). Calcium channel blockers (amlodipine, nifedipine) would not be prescribed as first-line treatment for cardiac muscle damage.
CN: Physiological integrity; CNS: Pharmacological and parenteral therapies; CL: Apply

25. 3. Scoliosis typically develops during the growth spurt prior to puberty. There is an increased risk with family history of scoliosis. Asthma, Down syndrome, and spina bifida are not risk factors for scoliosis.
CN: Physiological integrity; CNS: Physiological adaptation; CL: Analyze

26. 1. The elevated temperature indicates infection and is of greatest concern. Reports of pain are expected. Urine output is within normal range for a 12-year-old client. A paralytic ileus is common after Harrington rod placement surgery, resulting in hypoactive bowel sounds, and the child may have a nasogastric tube for the first 48 hours.
CN: Physiological integrity; CNS: Reduction of risk potential; CL: Apply

27. 1, 2, 5. Thoracic, lumbar, and cervical areas of the spine are the best bony landmarks to identify when attempting to screen for scoliosis because they show lateral deviation of the column. Abnormalities in the acromion processes and posterior superior iliac spines are not indicative of scoliosis.
CN: Physiological integrity; CNS: Physiological adaptation; CL: Apply

28. 1. The nurse should first help educate the parents on talipes equinovarus (clubfoot) and discuss treatment options. The nurse should anticipate then preparing the infant for serial casting. Corrective shoes are used instead of short leg braces. It is not priority to assess the infant's primitive reflexes.
CN: Physiological integrity; CNS: Reduction of risk potential; CL: Analyze

29. 1. The nurse should first determine whether the child has paralysis, indicating compartment syndrome. The pulse would be assessed below the cast to determine whether blood flow is appropriate. The other options are appropriate if the nurse determines the child is stable.
CN: Physiological integrity; CNS: Reduction of risk potential; CL: Analyze

30. The primary health care provider has prescribed oral prednisone for a client diagnosed with Duchenne muscular dystrophy. The parents ask the nurse why this medication is prescribed. Which response(s) by the nurse is appropriate? Select all that apply.
1. "Prednisone can strengthen the bones."
2. "Prednisone can improve muscle strength."
3. "Prednisone can stop the progression of the disease."
4. "Prednisone can delay the progression of the disease."
5. "Prednisone can decrease depression."

31. While assessing an infant, the nurse notes asymmetrical skin folds, a Galeazzi sign, and a positive Barlow test. The nurse will anticipate preparing the infant for which diagnostic test?
1. X-ray
2. Ortolani's test
3. Computed tomography (CT) scan
4. Magnetic resonance imaging (MRI)

32. The primary health care provider has prescribed a child with juvenile rheumatoid arthritis to receive an intravenous infusion of methylprednisolone. The child weighs 49.6 lb (22.5 kg). The prescription reads to administer 10 mg/kg over 1 hour. The vial comes in 100 mg/mL. How many milliliters will the nurse infuse? Record your answer using two decimal places.

_____ mL

33. The registered nurse (RN) is caring for a child newly diagnosed with Duchenne muscular dystrophy. Which task will the nurse delegate to the assistive personnel (AP)?
1. Document intake and output.
2. Assist the child with ambulation.
3. Monitor muscle movement.
4. Teach the family how to prevent obesity.

34. Which finding indicates to the nurse the parent of an infant with developmental hip dysplasia correctly understands the discharge education?
1. A folded towel is placed between the infant's legs.
2. The infant is wearing three diapers.
3. The infant is tightly swaddled in a blanket.
4. The infant is placed in the prone position to sleep.

30. 2, 4. Prednisone's benefits to the client with Duchenne muscular dystrophy are that it can delay the progression of the disease and improve muscle strength. Prednisone would not stop the progression of the disease nor would it strengthen the bones; in fact, it weakens the bones. Prednisone has been shown to possibly increase depression, not decrease it.
CN: Physiological integrity; CNS: Pharmacological and parenteral therapies; CL: Apply

31. 1. An x-ray can confirm the diagnosis of developmental dysplasia of the hip (DDH). Based on the assessment findings, the nurse should suspect that the infant has DDH. A positive finding on Ortolani's test is common in clients with DDH but would not be diagnostic. The CT scan and MRI are inappropriate tests for this client.
CN: Physiological integrity; CNS: Physiological adaptation; CL: Apply

32. 2.25.

$$dose\ prescribed \times weight = total\ dose$$
$$10\ mg/kg\ (22.5\ kg) = 225\ mg$$
$$total\ dose \div dose\ on\ hand \times mL = dose\ to\ infuse$$
$$225\ mg\ /\ 100\ mg = 2.25 \times 1\ mL = 2.25\ mL$$

CN: Physiological integrity; CNS: Pharmacological and parenteral therapies; CL: Analyze

33. 1. The RN should delegate to the AP documenting intake and output for this client. Muscular dystrophy usually affects muscles of the upper arms, legs, and trunk first, causing the child to have difficulty walking and requiring assessment of functional level and assistance from the RN. The RN should not delegate assessments or education.
CN: Safe, effective care environment; CNS: Management of care; CL: Analyze

34. 2. Placing several diapers on the infant keeps the hips abducted. A towel placed between the legs is not enough to abduct the hips. Swaddling the infant tightly straightens the legs and does not allow the hips to abduct. Placing the infant in a prone position will not keep the hips abducted and is not recommended due to the increased risk of sudden infant death syndrome.
CN: Physiologic integrity; CNS: Basic care and comfort; CL: Apply

35. The clinic nurse is trying to weigh a 5-year-old child with Duchenne muscular dystrophy who has difficulty standing. What is the **best** way for the nurse to obtain an accurate weight?
1. Ask the parent to approximate the child's current weight.
2. Ask the parent to hold the child and record the combined weight.
3. Weigh the parent and child and subtract the parent's weight from the combined weight.
4. Determine what the child weighted at the last visit and add 2 ounces per day.

35. 3. Subtracting the parent's weight from the combined weight yields the child's weight. Weight is an important parameter used in calculating drug dosages based on kilograms per body weight. It also provides the most accurate information about the child's fluid balance. For these reasons, weight should never be approximated. Adding a couple of ounces per day to the admission weight would be inaccurate.
CN: Health promotion and maintenance; CNS: None; CL: Apply

36. The nurse is caring for a child who sustained a dislocated hip and a subcapital fracture a few weeks ago. The client states the pain has gotten much worse since the accident occurred. Which complication will the nurse suspect?
1. Avascular necrosis
2. Osteomyelitis
3. Internal hemorrhage
4. Poor postoperative ambulation

36. 1. Avascular necrosis is common with fractures to the subcapital region secondary to possible compromise of blood supply to the femoral head. Postoperative infection is always a concern but not a priority at first. Hemorrhage should not occur. Poor postoperative ambulation is of concern but not as much as the possibility of avascular necrosis.
CN: Physiological integrity; CNS: Reduction of risk potential; CL: Apply

37. When assessing a child for developmental dysplasia of the hip, how will the nurse perform Ortolani's test?
1. Abduct the thigh to the table midline while lifting up the greater trochanter.
2. Adduct the thigh toward midline while trying to displace the femoral head posteriorly.
3. Assess the hips while having the child alternate standing on each leg.
4. Monitor for a limp while having the child walk down a hallway.

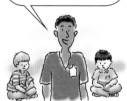
So many tests to learn. Can you remember what they all indicate?

37. 1. Ortolani's test involves abducting the thigh to the table midline while lifting up the greater trochanter with the finger and feeling for a click or clunk. Adducting the thigh is done with the Barlow test. Assessing the hips is done with a Trendelenburg test. A limp while walking is referred to as a Trendelenburg gait.
CN: Physiological integrity; CNS: Physiological adaptation; CL: Understand

38. The nurse is educating the parents of a child newly diagnosed with Duchenne muscular dystrophy. Which information will the nurse include in the teaching? Select all that apply.
1. It is an inherited, progressive disease.
2. It leads to muscle weakness and atrophy.
3. The child will have difficulty learning to crawl.
4. It involves degeneration of muscle fibers.
5. It is equally common in girls and boys.

38. 1, 2, 4. Degeneration of muscle fibers with progressive weakness and wasting best describes Duchenne muscular dystrophy. It is an X-linked recessive disorder and affects mostly males. Symptoms generally present between the ages of 2 and 5 years; therefore, crawling would not be delayed.
CN: Physiological integrity; CNS: Physiological adaptation; CL: Apply

39. When a 2-year-old child is suspected of having muscular dystrophy, the nurse will expect which muscle(s) to be affected **first**? Select all that apply.
1. Upper arm muscles
2. Leg muscles
3. Hand and feet muscles
4. Lung and heart muscles
5. Trunk muscles
6. Pelvic muscles

39. 1, 2. 5. Muscles of the upper arms, legs, and trunk are affected first. Progression later advances to muscles of the foot, hand, and pelvis. Involuntary muscles, such as the muscles of respiration and cardiac, are affected last.
CN: Physiological integrity; CNS: Physiological adaptation; CL: Apply

CN: Client needs category   CNS: Client needs subcategory   CL: Cognitive level

40. The nurse will prepare a child with suspected muscular dystrophy for which diagnostic test?
1. X-ray of the femurs
2. Muscle biopsy
3. Electrocardiogram (EKG)
4. Lumbar puncture

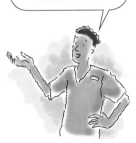

Which diagnostic test will reveal the degeneration of muscle fibers?

40. 2. A muscle biopsy shows the degeneration of muscle fibers and infiltration of fatty tissue. It is used for diagnostic confirmation of muscular dystrophy. X-ray is best for identifying an osseous deformity. An EKG would be done later in the disease process as the cardiac and respiratory systems become involved. A lumbar puncture is not indicated for muscular dystrophy.
CN: Health promotion and maintenance; CNS: None;
CL: Apply

41. The nurse is reviewing the laboratory test results of a child diagnosed with muscular dystrophy. Which result **most** concerns the nurse?
1. Total bilirubin level of 0.8 mg/dL (13.68 µmol/L)
2. Creatinine level of 1.6 mg/dL (144.4 µmol/L)
3. Potassium level of 2.1 mEq/L (2.1 mmol/L)
4. Sodium level of 145 mEq/L (145 mmol/L)

41. 3. The potassium level is critically low and warrants immediate intervention. Bilirubin is a by-product of liver function and should remain normal. Creatinine is a by-product of muscle metabolism as the muscle hypertrophies; the creatinine level is expected to be elevated in a client with muscular dystrophy. The sodium level is within normal range.
CN: Health promotion and maintenance; CNS: None;
CL: Analyze

42. Which client will the registered nurse (RN) assign to the licensed practical nurse (LPN)?
1. A 5-month-old admitted for suspected developmental dysplasia of the hip (DDH)
2. A 6-year-old who had a cast applied 3 days ago and is now reporting itching under the cast
3. A 9-year-old with Duchenne muscular dystrophy whose respiratory rate is 32 breaths/minute
4. A 14-year-old diagnosed with scoliosis who is being fitted for a Milwaukee brace

42. 2. The RN should assign the most stable client to the LPN. Itching under a cast applied 3 days ago is an expected finding. The infant with suspected DDH would require testing. A respiratory rate of 32 is elevated, indicating difficulty breathing. The child being fitted for a brace would need education.
CN: Safe, effective care environment; CNS: Management of care;
CL: Analyze

43. Which finding(s) are **most** concerning to the nurse caring for a school-age child with muscular dystrophy? Select all that apply.
1. Heart rate of 140 beats/minute
2. Respiratory rate of 40 breaths/minute
3. Increased lumbar lordosis
4. Gowers' sign
5. Shortness of breath
6. Difficulty sitting

43. 1, 2, 5. The nurse should be most concerned regarding symptoms indicating respiratory distress, such as tachycardia, tachypnea, and dyspnea. Increased lumbar lordosis, Gowers' sign, and difficulty sitting are expected findings with muscular dystrophy.
CN: Physiological integrity; CNS: Physiological adaptation;
CL: Analyze

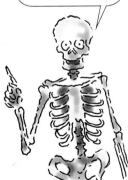

No bones about it—you're doing great!

44. The health care provider has prescribed a child with an open femur fracture morphine sulfate 10 mg PO. The elixir on hand is 100 mg/5 mL. How many milliliters will the nurse administer to the child? Record your answer using one decimal place.

_____ mL

44. 0.5.

$$\frac{Dose\ on\ hand}{Quantity\ on\ hand} = \frac{Dose\ desired}{X}$$
$$10\ mg/100\ mg = 0.1$$
$$0.1\ mg \times 5\ mL = 0.5\ mL$$

CN: Physiological integrity; CNS: Pharmacological and parenteral therapies; CL: Apply

45. A child with muscular dystrophy has lost complete control of the lower extremities. There is some strength bilaterally in the upper extremities but poor trunk control. Which mechanism is **most** important for the nurse to apply to the child's wheelchair?
1. Anti-tip device
2. Extended brakes
3. Headrest support
4. Wheelchair belt

46. When assessing a 4-year-old client with a history of muscular dystrophy, the nurse notes the child's legs appear to be held together and the knees are touching. The nurse suspects contraction of which muscles?
1. Hip abductors
2. Hip adductors
3. Hip extensors
4. Hip flexors

47. A child diagnosed with muscular dystrophy is hospitalized secondary to a fall and is scheduled for surgery and skeletal traction. The nurse is preparing to administer meperidine to the child. Which nursing assessment is **priority** following the administration of meperidine?
1. Check level of consciousness (LOC).
2. Monitor respiratory rate.
3. Measure urine output.
4. Assess pain level.

48. The nurse anticipates which complication in an adolescent female diagnosed with severe scoliosis?
1. Respiratory distress
2. Low self-worth
3. Decreased appetite
4. Poor compliance

49. The nurse is caring for an adolescent with bilateral femur fractures in bilateral leg skeletal traction. Which nursing action(s) is appropriate while caring for this client? Select all that apply.
1. Teach the client how to perform Kegel exercises.
2. Provide the client with a high-fiber diet.
3. Ensure the client maintains adequate fluid intake.
4. Perform range-of-motion (ROM) exercises several times a day.
5. Have the client perform coughing and deep breathing exercises.

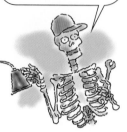
What are some devices in the health care provider's "toolbox" that might be used to treat musculoskeletal disorders?

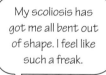
My scoliosis has got me all bent out of shape. I feel like such a freak.

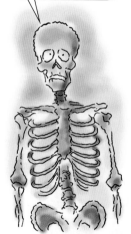

45. 4. Because the child has poor trunk control, a belt would prevent the child from falling out of the wheelchair. Anti-tip devices, headrest supports, and extended brakes are all important options but are not the most important mechanisms in this situation.
CN: Safe, effective care environment; CNS: Safety and infection control; CL: Apply

46. 2. The child's hip adductors are in a shortened position. The abductors are in a lengthened position. This position is not indicative of hip flexor or hip extensor shortening.
CN: Physiological integrity; CNS: Physiological adaptation; CL: Understand

47. 2. Respiratory depression is the life-threatening side effect the nurse should monitor for when administering opioids. It is important for the nurse to assess LOC, urine output, and pain, but respiratory status is priority.
CN: Physiological integrity; CNS: Pharmacological and parenteral therapies; CL: Analyze

48. 2. Low self-worth is a major issue with many adolescents, but the use of orthopedic appliances such as those used to treat scoliosis make this issue much more significant for teens with scoliosis. Although respiratory distress, poor compliance, and decreased appetite may surface with scoliosis, they are not as common as self-esteem problems in adolescent females with this condition.
CN: Health promotion and maintenance; CNS: None; CL: Apply

49. 1, 2, 3, 4, 5. To limit complications of immobility, the nurse would have the client perform Kegel exercises to keep the child from becoming incontinent. A high-fiber diet and adequate fluid intake will limit constipation. ROM exercises help limit muscle atrophy. Respiratory hygiene helps prevent respiratory complications such as pneumonia.
CN: Physiological integrity; CNS: Basic care and comfort; CL: Apply

50. A child has developed difficulty ambulating, and the nurse notes the child walking on the toes. Which nursing action is **priority**?
1. Continue to monitor the client during ambulation.
2. Document the findings in the medical record.
3. Prepare the client for surgery.
4. Notify the health care provider.

51. It is **priority** for the nurse to include which information when providing discharge education to the parents of a child with Legg-Calvé Perthes disease?
1. Activity restrictions
2. Pain control techniques
3. Appropriate diet
4. Physical therapy needs

52. The nurse is assessing the lower extremity strength of a child diagnosed with muscular dystrophy. Which muscle group is **most** important for the nurse to assess?
1. Gastrocnemius
2. Gluteus maximus
3. Hamstrings
4. Quadriceps

53. A child is newly diagnosed with muscular dystrophy. The child is noted to have mild muscle weakness but has not lost movement at this time. The nurse will anticipate educating the family on which equipment?
1. Long leg braces
2. Motorized wheelchair
3. Manual wheelchair
4. Walker

54. A child with muscular dystrophy is having increased difficulty getting out of the chair at school. The nurse will recommend the child use which equipment?
1. A seat cushion
2. Long leg braces
3. Powered wheelchair
4. Removable armrests on a wheelchair

55. Which assessment finding will the nurse expect while palpating the muscles of a child with muscular dystrophy?
1. Soft on palpation
2. Firm or woody on palpation
3. Extremely hard on palpation
4. No muscle consistency on palpation

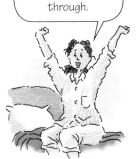

Wake up! We still have a lot of questions to get through.

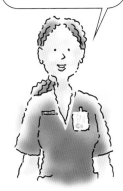

Muscular dystrophy involves infiltration of connective tissue and fatty tissue into the muscle. So, on palpation, how would the muscles feel?

50. 4. A shortened Achilles tendon may cause a child to walk on the toes. The nurse would notify the health care provider to determine if the client needs surgery for a release of the tendon. The nurse will continue to monitor and document after notifying the health care provider.
CN: Physiological integrity; CNS: Reduction of risk potential; CL: Apply

51. 1. It is most important for the nurse to teach the parents and child about activity restrictions to preserve the head of the femur. Pain control, diet, and physical therapy are also important; however, preventing permanent deformity is priority.
CN: Safe, effective care environment; CNS: Management of care; CL: Analyze

52. 2. The gluteus maximus is the strongest muscle in the body and is important for standing as well as for transfers. All of the named muscles are important, but the maintenance of the gluteus maximus would enable maximum function.
CN: Health promotion and maintenance; CNS: None; CL: Apply

53. 1. Long leg braces are functional assistive devices that provide increased independence and increased use of upper and lower body strength. Wheelchairs, both motorized and manual, provide less independence and less use of upper and lower body strength. Walkers are functional assistive devices that provide less independence than braces.
CN: Physiological integrity; CNS: Basic care and comfort; CL: Apply

54. 1. A seat cushion would put the hip extensors at an advantage and make it somewhat easier to get up. Long leg braces would not be the first choice. A powered wheelchair would not assist with the transfer. Removable armrests have no bearing on assisting the client.
CN: Physiological integrity; CNS: Basic care and comfort; CL: Apply

55. 2. Muscles in a child with muscular dystrophy are usually firm on palpation secondary to the infiltration of fatty tissue and connective tissue into the muscle. The muscles would not be soft secondary to the infiltration or extremely hard upon palpation. There is some consistency to the muscle, although in advanced stages atrophy is present.
CN: Physiological integrity; CNS: Physiological adaptation; CL: Apply

56. The nurse will teach a child with muscular dystrophy who uses a wheelchair how to perform which exercise to **best** prevent skin breakdown?
1. Wheelchair pushups
2. Leaning side-to-side
3. Sloping forward
4. Gluteal sets

57. The nurse observes a child diagnosed with muscular dystrophy displaying Gowers' sign. Which nursing action is **most** appropriate?
1. Document the observation in the medical record.
2. Assess the client for muscle weakness.
3. Consult physical therapy for additional sessions.
4. Request an increase in the client's prednisone dosage.

58. Which statement made by a parent of a child with osteogenesis imperfecta indicates to the nurse additional teaching is needed?
1. "Kids with osteogenesis imperfecta have thick bones."
2. "We will increase our child's calcium daily intake."
3. "My child may develop scoliosis secondary to this disease."
4. "The white of my child's eye may become bluish tinged."

59. A toddler is hospitalized for treatment of multiple injuries. The parents state the injuries occurred when their child fell down the stairs. However, inconsistencies between the history and physical findings suggest child abuse. What will the nurse do **next**?
1. Refer the parents to a "parents anonymous" group.
2. Prepare the child for foster care placement.
3. Prevent the parents from seeing their child.
4. Report the incident to proper authorities.

60. A child with bilateral fractured femurs is scheduled for a double hip spica cast and says to the nurse, "Only 3 more months and I can go home." Which nursing response is **most** appropriate?
1. "I know you will be super excited to finally get to go home."
2. "You will be able to go home 2 to 4 days after casting."
3. "It is hard to say when the health care provider will discharge you."
4. "I think you will be able to go home in another month or so."

56. 1. Wheelchair pushups would alleviate the most pressure to the buttocks. Leaning side-to-side would help, but not as much as wheelchair pushups. Sloping forward and gluteal sets would not help with pressure relief.
CN: Health promotion and maintenance; CNS: None; CL: Apply

57. 1. Gowers' sign is an expected finding in clients with muscular dystrophy; therefore, the nurse would document the finding. It indicates weakness of the proximal muscles. Muscle weakness is already being assessed in a client with muscular dystrophy. The client does not need additional physical therapy sessions or an increase in prednisone.
CN: Physiological integrity; CNS: Physiological adaptation; CL: Apply

58. 1. Osteogenesis imperfecta is also known as brittle bone disease. These clients have fragile bones that break easily. Calcium can aid in bone healing. Scoliosis and bow legs can develop. The bluish tinge is related to poor connective tissue formation.
CN: Physiological integrity; CNS: Physiological adaptation; CL: Apply

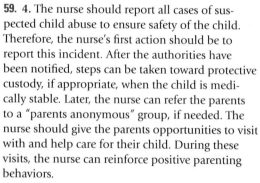
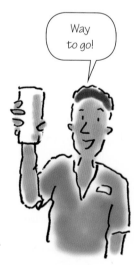

Way to go!

59. 4. The nurse should report all cases of suspected child abuse to ensure safety of the child. Therefore, the nurse's first action should be to report this incident. After the authorities have been notified, steps can be taken toward protective custody, if appropriate, when the child is medically stable. Later, the nurse can refer the parents to a "parents anonymous" group, if needed. The nurse should give the parents opportunities to visit with and help care for their child. During these visits, the nurse can reinforce positive parenting behaviors.
CN: Safe, effective care environment; CNS: Safety and infection control; CL: Analyze

60. 2. The double hip spica cast dries fairly rapidly with the use of fiberglass casting material. The time spent in the hospital after casting, typically 2 to 4 days, would be for educating the child and family about home care and for evaluating the child's skin integrity and neurovascular status before discharge. The time frames in the other options given are inaccurate for application of a double hip spica cast.
CN: Health promotion and maintenance; CNS: None; CL: Apply

CN: Client needs category   CNS: Client needs subcategory   CL: Cognitive level

61. An adolescent with a repaired fractured femur is currently in traction. The adolescent asks the nurse, "What would happen if the hospital caught on fire?" Which response by the nurse is **best**?
1. "You really should not worry about crazy things like that."
2. "The hospital has protocols for fires and emergencies."
3. "You seem concerned. Let us talk for a little while."
4. "The fire department would be in very quickly."

61. 3. Something prompted the client to ask such a question, and the nurse needs to take advantage of this opportunity to further explore the client's concerns and fears. Telling the client not to worry discounts the client's feelings and may actually increase anxiety. Telling the client about hospital protocols or the fire department does not explore the client's feelings.
CN: Psychosocial integrity; CNS: None; CL: Apply

62. The nurse receives report on a child admitted with severe muscular dystrophy receiving corticosteroids. The nurse will monitor the child for which potential side effect(s)? Select all that apply.
1. Weight gain
2. Blurred vision
3. Weakened bones
4. Restlessness
5. Loss of peripheral vision

62. 1, 2, 3, 4. Weight gain, blurred vision, weakened bones, and restlessness are all possible side effects. Loss of peripheral vision is not a possible side effect.
CN: Physiological integrity; CNS: Pharmacological and parenteral therapies; CL: Apply

63. Which finding in a client with a cast following fracture of the radius **most** concern the nurse?
1. Pain at the site of the break
2. Fingers that are pink and warm
3. Mild swelling of the fingers
4. Discomfort over a bony prominence

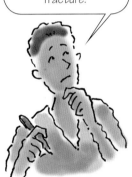

You're looking for something that would be unusual, not typical signs and symptoms of a fracture.

63. 4. Pain over a bony prominence, such as in the wrist or elbows, signals an impending pressure ulcer and requires prompt attention. Pain or discomfort at the site of the fracture is expected and is relieved by analgesics. Warm and pink fingers are an expected finding. Swelling may be relieved by elevation of the extremity. Swelling that is not relieved by elevation of the affected limb should be reported to the health care provider.
CN: Physiological integrity; CNS: Reduction of risk potential; CL: Analyze

64. The parents of a child diagnosed with osteogenesis imperfecta are crying and withdrawn. Which nursing statement is **most** appropriate?
1. "Why are you crying? You have a beautiful child and should be thankful."
2. "Would you like the hospital chaplain to come talk to you?"
3. "A support group will let you talk with others experiencing these emotions."
4. "Let's talk about what this condition means for your child."

64. 4. The nurse should talk to the parents about their concerns and feelings, and about the disease. Asking "why" is not therapeutic and may make the parents become defensive. The nurse should address the parents first, not refer them to someone else. This may be done after the nurse talks with the parents.
CN: Psychosocial integrity; CNS: None; CL: Apply

65. The nurse notes an infant has asymmetrical thigh folds. Which nursing action is **priority**?
1. Prepare the infant for a spica cast.
2. Determine the infant's fetal position at birth.
3. Attempt to abduct the infant's hips.
4. Notify the health care provider.

65. 3. The nurse would suspect the infant may have developmental dysplasia of the hip (DDH) and should further assess the infant before notifying the health care provider. Breech positioning is a risk factor for DDH, but determining the infant's fetal position at birth is not priority over assessing the infant's current state. The infant may need a spica cast if diagnosed with DDH.
CN: Safe, effective care environment; CNS: Management of care; CL: Analyze

CN: Client needs category   CNS: Client needs subcategory   CL: Cognitive level

66. Which pediatric client will the registered nurse (RN) appropriately assign to the licensed practical nurse (LPN)?
1. A 4-year-old who had a Harrington rod inserted yesterday and is receiving IV antibiotics
2. A 6-year-old newly diagnosed with Legg-Calvé Perthes disease requesting pain medication
3. A 10-year-old with Blount's disease who had surgery 2 days ago and needs help ambulating
4. A 14-year-old with scoliosis who had halo traction applied and is being discharged today

66. 3. The LPN can best care for the stable child needing help with ambulation. The LPN cannot administer intravenous medications or provide education for a new diagnosis or at discharge.
CN: Safe, effective care environment; CNS: Management of care; CL: Analyze

67. The nurse is caring for a child with a hip spica cast. The nurse notes the cast is soiled. Which nursing action is appropriate?
1. Clean the cast with a damp cloth.
2. Clean the cast with soap and water.
3. Allow the cast to absorb the spill.
4. Remove the cast and apply a clean cast.

67. 1. A damp cloth is best for cleaning the cast. Water would break down the cast. Changing the cast is not practical. The cast would give off a foul odor if the spill is allowed to absorb into the material.
CN: Physiological integrity; CNS: Basic care and comfort; CL: Apply

68. The nurse is providing care to a child in a hip spica cast who states, "I need to use the potty." The nurse will perform which intervention?
1. Elevate the child's head and shoulders and have the child use a bedpan.
2. Place the child supine with a bedpan under the child.
3. Lift the child from the bed and place the child on a toilet chair.
4. Position the child supine and apply a diaper.

68. 1. The head and shoulders need to be elevated to toilet the child on a bedpan to prevent the cast from becoming soiled. Supine positioning would soil the cast. The child cannot use a toilet chair while in a hip spica cast. The toilet-trained child should not be forced to use a diaper.
CN: Physiological integrity; CNS: Basic care and comfort; CL: Apply

69. The parents of a child with a fractured femur who has been prescribed Buck's traction ask the nurse about the purpose of traction. Which nursing response is **most** appropriate?
1. "Traction will ensure that your child's leg heals straight."
2. "Buck's traction helps to decrease pain and maintain length."
3. "Buck's traction limits the risk of complications after surgery."
4. "Traction allows the bone to heal quickly without surgery."

69. 2. Buck's traction is used preoperatively to decrease pain and maintain fracture length. Traction decreases pain by limiting movement and reducing the fracture while maintaining straight alignment and length of the bone. The other statements are not correct.
CN: Physiological integrity; CNS: Basic care and comfort; CL: Apply

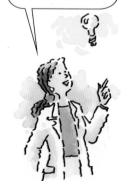

Read the question again. I'm sure the light bulb will come on.

70. The registered nurse (RN) and assistive personnel (AP) are caring for a child with developmental hip dysplasia. The RN observes the AP internally rotating the client's affected hip while changing the bed linen. Which action by the RN is **priority**?
1. Tell the AP to externally rotate the hip next time.
2. Immediately correct the client's positioning.
3. Ask the AP to come to the nurse's station.
4. Assess the client's affected hip for dislocation.

70. 2. Internal rotation increases the risk of hip dislocation; therefore, the RN would immediately correct the client's positioning. It would be appropriate to tell the AP to externally rotate the hip next time; however, this is not priority over safety. The nurse would educate the AP outside of the client's room and assess the client's hip after placement correction.
CN: Safe, effective care environment; CNS: Management of care; CL: Analyze

71. The health care provider has prescribed sulfasalazine for a child with juvenile rheumatoid arthritis. The nurse questions the prescription when reading the client has an allergy to which medication?
1. Alprazolam
2. Naproxen
3. Sulfamethoxazole-trimethoprim
4. Penicillin

72. A toddler is immobilized with traction to the legs. Which play activity will the nurse include in this child's plan of care?
1. Pounding boards
2. Tinker toys
3. Pull toy
4. Board games

73. The nurse expects to see which activity level prescribed for a client immediately after a spinal fusion?
1. Supine bed rest
2. No weight bearing
3. No restrictions
4. Limited weight bearing

74. Which intervention is appropriate for the nurse to use to prevent venous stasis for an adolescent in skeletal traction?
1. Bed rest with bathroom privileges
2. Convoluted foam mattress
3. Vigorous pulmonary care
4. Antiembolism stockings

75. The school nurse suspects a 13-year-old has structural scoliosis. How will the nurse assess the child for this condition?
1. Ask the child to bend over and touch toes while the nurse observes from behind.
2. Ask the child to stand sideways while the nurse observes the profile.
3. Ask the child to assume a knee-chest position on the examination table.
4. Ask the child to arch the back while the nurse observes from behind.

76. Which nursing intervention is **priority** for a child with a suspected fracture at the scene of a motor vehicle accident?
1. Assess level of consciousness.
2. Monitor blood loss.
3. Move the child to a safe place.
4. Immobilize the extremity.

Working with pediatric clients comes with its own set of challenges.

71. 3. Sulfamethoxazole-trimethoprim is a sulfa drug, as is sulfasalazine. If a person has a reaction to one sulfa drug, it is highly probable the person would have a reaction to another. Alprazolam, naproxen, and penicillin should not make the nurse question the prescription.
CN: Physiological integrity; CNS: Pharmacological and parenteral therapies; CL: Apply

72. 1. A pounding board is appropriate for an immobilized toddler because it promotes physical development and provides an acceptable energy outlet. Toys with small parts, such as tinker toys, are not suitable because a toddler may swallow the parts. A pull toy is suitable for most toddlers but not for one who is immobilized. Board games are too advanced for the developmental skills of most toddlers.
CN: Health promotion and maintenance; CNS: None; CL: Apply

73. 1. After a spinal fusion, the child is usually placed on bed rest and prescribed to lie flat. In 2 to 4 days, the child is allowed to sit up in and get out of bed. Other activities are gradually reintroduced.
CN: Physiological integrity; CNS: Basic care and comfort; CL: Apply

74. 4. To prevent venous stasis after skeletal traction application, antiembolism stockings or an intermittent compression device are used on the unaffected leg. Convoluted foam mattresses and pulmonary care do not prevent venous stasis. Bed rest can cause venous stasis.
CN: Health promotion and maintenance; CNS: None; CL: Apply

75. 1. As the child bends over, the curvature of the spine is more apparent. The scapula on one side becomes more prominent, and the one on the opposite side hollows. Scoliosis cannot be properly assessed from the side or with the back arched. The knee-chest position is used for lumbar puncture, not assessment of scoliosis.
CN: Health promotion and maintenance; CNS: None; CL: Understand

76. 4. At the scene of a trauma, the nurse should immobilize the extremity of a child with a suspected fracture and then move the child to safety. The nurse should assess the child once safety is achieved.
CN: Safe, effective care environment; CNS: Safety and infection control; CL: Apply

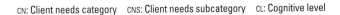

CN: Client needs category   CNS: Client needs subcategory   CL: Cognitive level

77. Which statement will the nurse include in the education plan for the parents of a child about to undergo a closed fracture reduction?
1. "Closed reductions have a high infection rate."
2. "Fracture reduction restores alignment."
3. "Undisplaced fractures may be reduced."
4. "Fracture reduction usually has minimal discomfort."

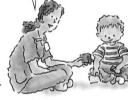

You're making this test look like child's play.

77. 2. Fracture reduction restores alignment. Closed reductions have a lower infection rate. Some fractures, such as undisplaced fractures, cannot be reduced. Fracture reduction is usually painful.
CN: Physiological integrity; CNS: Reduction of risk potential; CL: Apply

78. A child in skeletal traction for a fracture of the right femur reports new and constant left calf pain. The nurse notes the child's left calf is 1 in (2.54 cm) larger than the right and with nonpitting edema below the left knee. The nurse knows these signs are **most** consistent with which condition?
1. A fat embolus
2. An infection
3. A pulmonary embolism
4. Deep vein thrombosis (DVT)

78. 4. Constant unilateral leg pain and significant edema should lead the nurse to suspect DVT. Symptoms of fat emboli include restlessness, tachypnea, and tachycardia and are more common in long bone injuries. It is unlikely that an infection would occur on the side opposite the fracture without cause. Tachycardia, chest pain, and shortness of breath may be symptoms of a pulmonary embolism.
CN: Physiological integrity; CNS: Reduction of risk potential; CL: Apply

79. The nurse is providing care for a child in traction. Which nursing intervention is **priority**?
1. Assessing pin sites at least every shift
2. Ensuring that the rope knots do not catch on the pulley
3. Adding and removing weights as prescribed
4. Placing unaffected joints through range of motion every shift

79. 1. If the child has pins, it is priority to assess the pins to monitor for complications such as infection. The nurse would complete the other interventions after assessing the pins.
CN: Physiological integrity; CNS: Basic care and comfort; CL: Analyze

80. After assisting the health care provider to apply a cast, the nurse will include which intervention in **immediate** cast care?
1. Rest the cast on the bedside table.
2. Dispose of the plaster water in the sink.
3. Support the cast with the palms of the hand.
4. Wait until the cast dries before cleaning surrounding skin.

80. 3. After a cast has been applied, it should be immediately supported with the palms of the nurse's hands. Later, the nurse should dispose of the plaster water in a sink with a plaster trap or in a garbage bag. Then the nurse should clean the surrounding skin before the cast dries and make sure that the cast is not resting on a hard or sharp surface.
CN: Safe, effective care environment; CNS: Management of care; CL: Apply

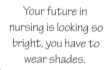

Your future in nursing is looking so bright, you have to wear shades.

81. The parents of a child who just had a synthetic cast applied ask the clinic nurse how long before they can go home. Which response by the nurse is accurate?
1. "You and your child can go home now."
2. "It will be about 20 minutes before you can leave."
3. "We need to monitor your child for the next hour."
4. "You can go but will need to come back tomorrow."

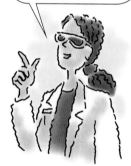

81. 2. The client will be able to go home after the cast is dry/set. Synthetic casts take about 20 minutes to set. After that time, if there are no complications, the client and parents will be able to leave the clinic. There is no need for continued monitoring for an hour after the cast is applied or to return the following day.
CN: Safe, effective care environment; CNS: Management of care; CL: Apply

82. Which nursing intervention can **best** prevent foot drop in a client with a casted leg?
1. Encourage frequent bed rest.
2. Elevate the foot on multiple pillows.
3. Support the foot with 90 degrees of flexion.
4. Place a stocking on the foot.

82. 3. To prevent foot drop in a casted leg, the foot should be supported with 90 degrees of flexion. Bed rest can cause foot drop. Keeping the extremity warm or elevated would not prevent foot drop.
CN: Health promotion and maintenance; CNS: None; CL: Understand

83. While the child's cast is drying, the child states, "My leg feels hot under this cast." Which nursing intervention is appropriate?
1. Remove the cast immediately.
2. Notify the health care provider.
3. Assess the child for signs of infection.
4. Explain that this is a normal sensation.

84. The nurse suspects a child with juvenile rheumatoid arthritis has presented with ibuprofen toxicity. Which laboratory test(s) will the nurse expect the health care provider to prescribe? Select all that apply.
1. Liver function panel
2. Blood urea nitrogen (BUN)
3. Creatinine
4. Blood cultures
5. Cerebrospinal fluid (CSF) cultures

85. The nurse determines an adolescent with a fractured left femur correctly understands the instructions to perform touch-down weight bearing when making what statement?
1. "I will place only a small portion of my weight on my left leg."
2. "I will allow my left leg to touch the floor without placing weight on it."
3. "I will place full weight on my left leg when ambulating."
4. "I will keep my left leg completely off the floor when walking."

86. The nurse notes a 90-degree curvature of the spine in a pediatric client. Which statement is appropriate for the nurse to tell the child and the parents?
1. "Your child will have to be in traction for 23 hours a day."
2. "This curvature will require chiropractic treatment."
3. "Your child will need to use a brace and traction."
4. "This curvature will require surgical intervention."

87. The nurse will order which meal for an adolescent with Duchenne muscular dystrophy?
1. Baked chicken, strawberry spinach salad with low-fat vinaigrette, orange slices, and 1% milk
2. Fried fish sandwich, green bean casserole, chocolate pudding, and orange juice
3. Baked spaghetti with cheese, side salad with ranch dressing, vanilla cake, and water
4. Pepperoni pizza, corn on the cob, mixed fruit cup, and a carbonated beverage

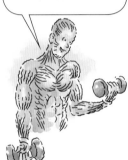

Tell your client to take it easy with the weight bearing after a fracture.

83. 4. It is normal for the child to report heat from the cast as it is drying. The nurse should offer reassurance that this is a normal sensation. Notifying the health care provider or removing the cast is unnecessary. Heat from a newly applied cast is not a sign of infection.
CN: Safe, effective care environment; CNS: Management of care; CL: Apply

84. 1, 2, 3. The health care provider would prescribe a liver function panel, BUN level, and creatinine level in addition to the other tests to determine ibuprofen toxicity. There is no need to prescribe blood cultures or CSF cultures because there is no evidence of infection.
CN: Physiological integrity; CNS: Pharmacological and parenteral therapies; CL: Apply

85. 2. Touch-down weight bearing allows the child to put no weight on the extremity, but the child may touch the floor with the affected extremity. Full weight bearing allows the child to bear all of the weight on the affected extremity. Partial weight bearing allows for only 30% to 50% weight bearing on the affected extremity. Non–weight bearing means bearing no weight on the extremity, and it must remain elevated.
CN: Physiological integrity; CNS: Basic care and comfort; CL: Understand

86. 1. A child with a curvature of the spine greater than 80 degrees requires traction, which must be worn for 23 hours a day. The other statements are not correct for this client.
CN: Health promotion and maintenance; CNS: None; CL: Apply

87. 1. A child with Duchenne muscular dystrophy is prone to constipation and obesity, so dietary intake should include a diet low in calories, high in protein, and high in fiber.
CN: Physiological integrity; CNS: Basic care and comfort; CL: Analyze

88. Which pediatric client will the nurse assign the lowest priority when making rounds?
1. A child with an ulna fracture reporting cool, pale fingers
2. A child newly diagnosed with Legg-Calvé-Perthes disease prescribed traction
3. An infant with clubfoot scheduled for surgery today
4. A child with scoliosis requesting help with bathing

89. Which is the **best** strategy for the nurse to include when educating an adolescent about preventing sports-related injuries?
1. Perform warm-up exercises before participating in the sport.
2. Pace the rate of activity during the sport.
3. Include weight lifting while training to build strength.
4. When playing the sport, maintain moderate activity intensity.

90. Which activity is **best** for the nurse to recommend for a child prescribed full activity after repair of a clubfoot?
1. Playing catch at the park
2. Standing when feasible
3. Swimming laps in the pool
4. Walking around a track

91. An adolescent sustains a broken leg as a result of a motor vehicle accident and is taken to the emergency department. A plaster cast is applied. Before discharge, the nurse provides the child with instructions regarding cast care. Which instruction(s) is appropriate for the nurse to include? Select all that apply.
1. Elevate the cast intermittently.
2. Avoid getting the cast soiled.
3. Move the toes on the affected side often.
4. Apply powder to the inside of the cast after it dries.
5. Notify the health care provider if itching occurs under the cast.
6. Avoid putting straws or hangers inside the cast.

92. A client is taking high doses of methotrexate for juvenile rheumatoid arthritis. The nurse will question which new prescription(s)? Select all that apply.
1. Ibuprofen
2. Aspirin
3. Prednisone
4. Acetaminophen
5. Multivitamin

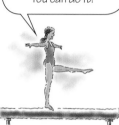

Stay focused and nail your dismount. You can do it!

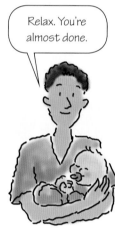

Relax. You're almost done.

88. 4. The nurse should assign the most stable client the lowest priority when making rounds. The child with scoliosis requesting help with bathing is stable. Cool, pale extremities indicate decreased tissue perfusion and require assessment. A new diagnosis requires intense education. The child going to surgery would require frequent assessment for complications after surgery.
CN: Safe, effective care environment; CNS: Management of care; CL: Analyze

89. 1. To prevent sports-related injuries, the nurse should teach the adolescent that the best prevention is warming up. Pacing activity, building strength, and using moderate intensity are other helpful injury-prevention measures.
CN: Health promotion and maintenance; CNS: None; CL: Apply

90. 4. Walking stimulates all of the involved muscles and helps with strengthening. All of the other activities are good exercises, but walking is the best choice.
CN: Physiological integrity; CNS: Physiological adaptation; CL: Apply

91. 1, 2, 3, 6. The nurse should instruct the child to elevate the affected extremity to limit edema, avoid getting the cast soiled to limit unpleasant odors, move the toes to prevent stiffness, and not place anything inside of the cast to avoid the risk of impairing the skin and causing infection. Powder should not be used because it can cake under the cast. Itching is a common occurrence with casts because the skin cells cannot slough as they normally would and the dry skin causes itching. The health care provider is not usually called for this problem.
CN: Physiological integrity; CNS: Basic care and comfort; CL: Apply

92. 1, 2. Nonsteroidal anti-inflammatory drugs, such as ibuprofen, and salicylates such as aspirin are contraindicated because methotrexate decreases platelet levels, and adding these would possibly cause hematologic toxicity. All other listed medications would not cause adverse effects to the client if used with methotrexate.
CN: Physiological integrity; CNS: Pharmacological and parenteral therapies; CL: Apply

93. The nurse is observing the chest of a child who has been diagnosed with pectus excavatum. Which graphic depicts this abnormality?

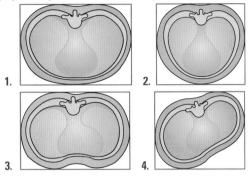

1.   2.

3.   4.

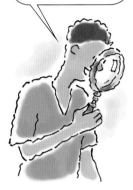

Pectus excavatum—do you remember what that condition looks like?

94. The health care provider prescribes methylprednisolone 1.5 mg/kg for a child weighing 112.4 lb (51 kg). Methylprednisolone is available as 125 mg/2 mL. How many milliliters will the nurse administer? Record your answer using two decimal places.

_____ mL

95. A child has a fractured femur. The health care provider prescribes morphine sulfate 0.15 mg/kg/dose intravenously every 4 hours PRN pain. The child weighs 110.2 lb (50 kg). Morphine sulfate is supplied at 2 mg/mL. How many milligrams may the nurse administer to the child in 24 hours? Record your answer using a whole number.

_____ mg

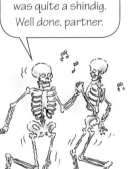

Yee-haw! That was quite a shindig. Well done, partner.

93. 3. Pectus excavatum, as shown in option 3, is an indentation of the lower portion of the sternum. Option 1 shows a normal chest. Option 2 shows a barrel chest contour. Option 4 shows a thoracic scoliosis chest contour.

CN: Physiological integrity; CNS: Physiological adaptation; CL: Apply

94. **1.22.**

$$dose\ prescribed \times kilogram\ weight = total\ dose$$
$$1.5\ mg \times 51\ kg = 76.5\ mg$$
$$total\ dose \div dose\ on\ hand = does\ to\ infuse$$
$$76.5\ mg \div 125\ mg/2\ mL = 1.224\ mL$$

In pediatric doses, it is rounded to the nearest hundredth, which would make the answer 1.22 mL.

CN: Physiological integrity; CNS: Pharmacological and parenteral therapies; CL: Apply

95. **45.**

$$dose\ prescribed \times kilogram\ weight = amount\ per\ dose$$
$$0.15\ mg/kg/dose \times 50\ kg = 7.5\ mg/dose$$
$$amount\ per\ dose \times$$
$$number\ of\ \frac{doses}{day} = total\ administered\ per\ day$$

$$7.5\ mg/dose \times 6\ doses/day = 45\ mg/day.$$

CN: Physiological integrity; CNS: Pharmacological and parenteral therapies; CL: Analyze

CN: Client needs category   CNS: Client needs subcategory   CL: Cognitive level

Chapter 31

Gastrointestinal Disorders

Pediatric gastrointestinal refresher

Accidental poisoning

Ingestion of a toxic substance, which overwhelms the body's ability to clear or detoxify the substance

Key treatments
- Prevention:
  - educating parents and those who care for children about poisoning hazards
  - keeping child safety locks on cabinets
  - keeping hazardous chemicals and medications out of the reach of children
  - teaching parents or those who care for children to place the number for Poison Control near the phones for ease of access.
- Always treat the child first by stopping further exposure to the substance and stabilizing the child

Acetaminophen poisoning

Ingestion of a toxic amount of acetaminophen, which occurs in an 8-hour period or less

Key signs and symptoms
- Diaphoresis, pallor, and hypothermia (2 to 4 hours)
- Slow, weak pulse (24 to 36 hours)
- Nausea and vomiting (2 to 4 hours)
- Right upper quadrant pain (48 hours)

Key test results
- Serum aspartate aminotransferase (AST) and serum alanine aminotransferase (ALT) levels (liver necrosis occurs in 2 to 5 days) become elevated soon after ingestion; BUN and creatinine
- Acetaminophen levels are greatly elevated

Key treatments
- Gastric lavage and induced vomiting
- *N*-acetylcysteine antidote: most effective in 8 to 10 hours; must be given within 24 hours; administer orally every 4 hours × 72 hours or IV × 3 doses

Key interventions
- Monitor cardiovascular, respiratory, renal, and GI status.
- Monitor vital signs, intake, and output, and maintain hydration status.
- Monitor lab results for liver and kidney function.

Corrosive agent poisoning

Ingestion of substances containing hydrocarbon (e.g., drain or oven cleaner, bleach, or battery acid) that adversely affect the body's systems

Key signs and symptoms
- Burning in the mouth and throat
- White, swollen mucous membranes
- Vomiting

Key test results
- Inspection of the face, mouth, and oropharynx
- Urine and serum blood analysis
- Chest x-ray

Key treatments
- Gastric lavage and activated charcoal
- IV fluids

Key interventions
- Monitor respiratory, cardiovascular, neurologic, GI, and renal status.
- Assess vital signs, face, mouth, and oropharynx.
- Do not induce vomiting.
- Administer IV fluids and oral fluids when indicated.
- Provide comfort measures for the child and supportive measures for the parents.

Hydrocarbon poisoning

Ingestion of substances containing hydrocarbon (e.g., kerosene, turpentine, or gasoline) that adversely affect the body's systems

Key signs and symptoms
- Burning in the mouth and throat
- Choking and gagging
- CNS depression

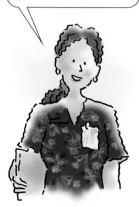

I'll bet when you started nursing school, you had no idea kids could be subject to so many GI disorders. This chapter tests you on the most common ones. Good luck!

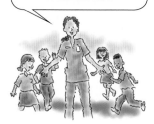

Poisoning is preventable. Encourage parents to keep all medications in a high, locked cabinet.

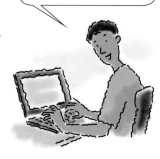

Which interventions will you make for a client who consumed drain cleaner?

Key test results

- Urine and serum blood analysis
- Chest x-ray and EEG, if indicated

Key treatments

- Gastric lavage and activated charcoal
- IV fluids

Key interventions

- Monitor respiratory, cardiovascular, neurologic, GI, and renal status.
- Assess vital signs.
- Administer IV fluids and oral fluids when indicated.
- Provide comfort measures for the child and supportive measures for the parents.

Lead poisoning

Ingestion of lead or lead-containing products that build up in the body over a period of time

Key signs and symptoms

- Impaired growth and clumsiness
- Developmental regression and irritability
- Neurologic involvement

Key test results

- Blood lead levels above 9 mcg/dL (0.43 µmol/L) are considered elevated
- Erythrocyte protoporphyrin (EP) level
- Complete blood count (CBC) and long bone x-rays (may reveal radiopaque material "lead lines")

Key treatments

- Chelation therapy (dimercaprol, calcium disodium edetate, succimer, and deferoxamine)
- IV fluids and hydration

Key interventions

- Conduct neurologic assessment, physical examination, biophysical measurements (height, weight, head circumference if indicated).
- Provide for hydration (IV or oral) and a diet high in calcium and iron.
- Rotate injection sites for chelation therapy.
- Educate parents to wash the child's hands and toys, and to frequently remove lead dust.
- Teach parents about sources of lead (flaking paint, crumbling plaster, pottery with lead glaze, lead solder in pipes, and other sources).
- Teach parents about reading labels on toy packaging for possible lead contents.

- Screen and monitor young children who place objects in their mouth (toddlers) for lead exposure/poisoning.
- Remove lead from the child's environment.

Salicylate poisoning

Ingestion of a toxic amount of salicylate that builds up in the system over a period of time

Key signs and symptoms

- High fever from the stimulation of carbohydrate metabolism
- Petechiae and bleeding tendency

Key test results

- Prothrombin time (PT) is prolonged
- Serum salicylate levels are elevated

Key treatments

- Gastric lavage and activated charcoal
- IV fluids
- Sodium bicarbonate and vitamin K
- Peritoneal dialysis for severe cases

Key interventions

- Monitor respiratory, cardiovascular, GI, renal, and neurologic status.
- Assess vital signs and urine pH.
- Administer oral and IV fluids.
- Provide comfort measures.

Appendicitis

Inflammation of the appendix that results from a blockage of the organ and causes infection and pus accumulation

Key signs and symptoms

- Periumbilical pain that radiates to the right lower abdomen (McBurney's point) and rebound tenderness
- Low-grade fever and elevated WBC count
- Nausea and vomiting
- Sudden cessation of pain (indicates rupture)

Key test results

- Hematology shows moderately elevated white blood cell count
- Ultrasound or CT of the abdomen shows a distended or enlarged appendix

Key treatments

- Appendectomy

Key interventions

- Assess and monitor vital signs, abdomen, GI status, and pain.

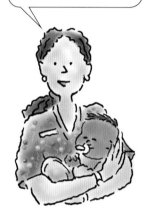

Be sure parents understand the sources of lead poisoning, such as flaking paint, and how to address them.

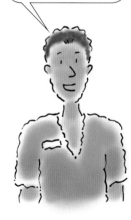

A client is suspected of having acute appendicitis. What signs will you look for?

- Avoid laxatives and applying heat to the area.
- Perform preoperative care and teaching appropriate for child's developmental level
  - involve the parents as appropriate
  - assess parents' and child's understanding.
- Provide postoperative care by assessing vital signs and cardiac, respiratory, and abdominal status
  - position right side-lying or semi-Fowler's if surgery is post-rupture
  - provide pain relief
  - encourage deep breathing, coughing, and use of incentive spirometer or other age-appropriate devices, as indicated
  - teach incisional splinting, change positions slowly, and promote early ambulation
  - maintain nothing-by-mouth (NPO) status until bowel sounds return postoperatively and then advance diet as tolerated.
- Monitor for postoperative complications:
  - atelectasis (dyspnea, cyanosis)
  - bleeding/hemorrhage (decreased blood pressure; increased pulse rate; cool, clammy skin)
  - peritonitis (rigid abdomen and guarding)
  - fluid and electrolyte disturbances
  - paralytic ileus (absence of bowel sounds, inability to pass gas or stool, and abdominal distention)
  - infection (redness, swelling, or abnormal drainage from the incision).

Celiac disease

Intolerance to gluten (protein found in wheat, rye, and barley)

Key signs and symptoms
- Generalized malnutrition and failure to thrive due to protein and carbohydrate malabsorption
- Steatorrhea and chronic diarrhea due to fat malabsorption
- Weight and height below normal for age group

Key test results
- Immunologic assay screen is positive for celiac disease
- Bowel biopsy

Key treatments
- Gluten-free diet (avoid wheat, rye, and barley)

- Vitamin supplementation (fat-soluble vitamins A, D, E, and K)

Key interventions
- Monitor and plot growth and development using appropriate forms such as growth charts.
- Give small, frequent meals avoiding wheat, rye, and barley; substitute corn, oats, and rice.
- Teach parents to read labels to identify foods containing hidden gluten.

Cleft lip and palate

Congenital malformation, which causes fissure(s) that involve any of these facial or mouth structures: lip, nasal septum, anterior maxilla, and soft and hard palates

Key signs and symptoms
- Cleft lip is obvious at birth (with or without cleft palate): ranges from simple notch on upper lip to complete cleft from lip edge to floor of the nostril, on either side of the midline but rarely along the midline itself
- Cleft palate without cleft lip may not be detected until mouth examination or observation of feeding difficulties

Key test results
- Prenatal ultrasound may indicate severe defects
- Physical examination of the face, lips, and palate (soft and hard) reveals the deformity

Key treatments
- Cheiloplasty performed between 2 and 3 months of age to unite lip and gum edges in anticipation of teeth eruption
- Cleft palate repair surgery
  - scheduled between 12 and 18 months to allow for growth of palate and to be done before infant develops speech patterns
  - infant must be free from ear and respiratory infections

Key interventions
- Visualize the face, lips, nose, and gums, and palpate the soft and hard palates for deformities at birth.
- Use interventions that encourage a positive view of the child and that facilitate parent-infant bonding.
- Assess infant's ability to suck and swallow at birth
  - keep suction equipment and bulb syringe at bedside.

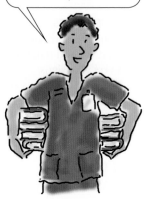

You have a client who has diarrhea after eating wheat or rye bread or oatmeal. Which condition will you suspect?

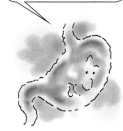

Dietary intolerances can be managed with ingredient substitutions and vitamin supplementation.

- Monitor intake and output and weigh daily.
- Before cleft lip repair surgery
  - assess for signs and symptoms of ear or respiratory infection
  - be alert for respiratory distress while feeding and hold the infant when feeding
  - maintain adequate nutrition by feeding small amounts in an upright position; feed utilizing special nipples and feeders, burp frequently, and promote sucking between meals
  - provide information to the parents and allow time for verbalization of feelings.
- After cleft lip repair surgery
  - maintain airway, observe for distress, and position infant to prevent aspiration
  - keep infant's hands away from the mouth by using restraints or pinning the sleeves to the shirt; use adhesive strips to hold the suture line in place
  - clean the suture line after each feeding as prescribed
  - provide soothing measures (rocking, cuddling), age-appropriate activities, and minimize crying
  - administer pain medications and antibiotics as prescribed.
- After cleft palate repair surgery
  - place a suction setup and endotracheal tray at the bedside and position the toddler on the abdomen or side
  - anticipate edema and a reduction in airway clearance from palate closure and assess for signs of altered oxygenation
  - teach parents to keep hard or pointed objects (utensils, straws, frozen dessert sticks) away from the mouth and to monitor for signs of infection (infection increases the chance of scarring)
  - provide referrals to speech therapy and orthodontists as needed.

Esophageal atresia and tracheoesophageal fistula

Malformation of the esophagus that results in a blind pouch or an opening between the esophagus and trachea

Key signs and symptoms
Esophageal atresia
- Excessive salivation and drooling due to inability to pass food through the esophagus

Tracheoesophageal fistula
- Choking, coughing, and intermittent cyanosis caused by secretions, or during feeding due to secretions, or food that goes through the fistula into the trachea

Key test results
- Abdominal x-ray reveals a stomach filled with air
- NG tube insertion does not yield gastric aspirate when verifying placement
- Radiologic visualization of the tube does not reveal it in the stomach (curls in the blind pouch)
- Neonates are fed first with a few sips of sterile water to detect these anomalies and to prevent aspiration of formula or breast milk into the lungs

Key treatments
- Surgical correction by ligating the tracheoesophageal fistula and reanastomosing the esophageal ends; in many cases, done in stages
- Transport to neonatal intensive care (NICU) when possible
- Antibiotic therapy started early because of aspiration

Key interventions
- Before surgery
  - monitor respiratory status and cardiac and GI systems; monitor vital signs
  - manage secretions with nasal and oral suctioning; position to promote airway drainage and to prevent aspiration
  - administer antibiotics and other medications as prescribed
  - manage the gastrostomy tube and facilitate drainage; weigh daily and monitor intake and output.
- After surgery
  - monitor respiratory, cardiac, and GI status; position to prevent aspiration; and manage secretions with suctioning
  - provide care of the incision; maintain total parenteral nutrition (TPN) until gastrostomy or oral feedings are tolerated (check for cloudy fluid color, agitate the bag periodically, use a 10-micron filter, is greater than 10% glucose concentration administered only through a central line); weigh daily and monitor intake and output
  - monitor for postoperative complications (respiratory difficulty, aspiration, bleeding, infection, and fluid balance and electrolyte disturbances)

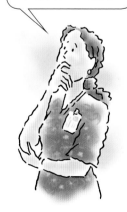

Esophageal atresia … tracheoesophageal fistula—what do these terms mean?

○ teach parents soothing techniques, positioning, CPR, care of the incision, signs and symptoms to report, and when to follow up postoperatively.

Failure to thrive

When a child's current weight or rate of weight gain is much lower than that of other children of similar age and gender

Key signs and symptoms
- Altered body posture (child is stiff or floppy and does not cuddle)
- Avoids eye contact
- Disparities between chronologic age and height, weight, and head circumference
- History of insufficient stimulation and inadequate parental knowledge of child development

Key test results
- Growth chart analysis and Denver Developmental Screening (Ages and Stages)
- Complete blood count (CBC), chemistry panel, and hormone studies in older children

Key treatments
- High-calorie diet
- Parental counseling
- Vitamin and mineral supplements

Key interventions
- Assign care to the same team of caregivers when possible.
- Provide adequate food and fluid intake and interact appropriately with the child.
- Provide the child with visual and auditory stimulation.
- When caring for child in parent's presence, act as role model for effective parenting skills.
- Demonstrate comfort measures and show the mother how to hold infant in the en-face position.

Gastroenteritis

Increase in the frequency of liquid stool expulsion and vomiting

Key signs and symptoms
- Increase in fluid content, frequency, and volume of stool
- Frequent nausea and vomiting
- Abdominal cramping
- Weight loss (1 g of weight equals 1 mL of body fluid)

Key test results
- Serum electrolytes, complete blood count, blood cultures, and stool cultures
- History becomes important because antibiotic use, diet (lactose intolerance), travel, and exposure to contagious illnesses can also cause diarrhea

Key treatments
- IV therapy to correct fluid and electrolyte imbalances and antidiarrheal medications
- Correction of the underlying problem, as indicated

Key interventions
- Assess vital signs, weight, and skin, and for signs of dehydration (poor skin turgor [tenting of skin when pinched], sunken eye sockets, sunken fontanels, absence of tears, dry mouth, decreased urine output).
- Administer IV rehydration therapy as prescribed, weigh daily, and maintain strict intake and output measurements.
- Monitor laboratory results and observe for signs of electrolyte imbalance (deep breathing, listlessness, and other changes in level of consciousness).
- Maintain nothing by mouth (NPO) status until reintroduction of oral food is prescribed.
- Introduce clear liquids slowly and frequently in small amounts using over-the-counter oral rehydration fluid; avoid apple juice or juices high in sugar.
- Administer antidiarrheal medications as prescribed.
- Report bloody stools, continued weight loss, physiologic changes in condition, decreased urinary output, bloody stool, persistent diarrhea or vomiting, or changes in level of consciousness.

Intestinal obstruction

Partial or complete obstruction of the small or large intestine resulting from intussusception, Hirschsprung's disease, other mechanical blockage by a foreign object, or a volvulus

Key signs and symptoms
- Complete small-bowel obstruction:
  ○ bowel contents are propelled toward mouth (instead of rectum) by vigorous peristaltic waves causing vomiting
  ○ persistent epigastric or periumbilical pain

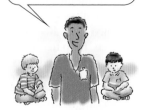

Don't be alarmed by the term "failure to thrive"—it usually just means a child is not gaining as much weight as needed.

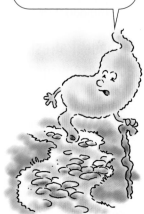

Ugh. I'm feeling a little ... obstructed. What should I do?

- Partial large-bowel obstruction:
  - leakage of liquid stool around the obstruction (common) resulting in soiling or reports of diarrhea
- Hirschsprung's disease:
  - abdominal distention is common in all age groups
  - neonate signs and symptoms: failure to pass first meconium stool within 24 to 48 hours, refusal to eat, and vomiting bile
  - infant signs and symptoms: failure to thrive, constipation, vomiting, and diarrhea
  - older children signs and symptoms: ribbon-like stool, palpable fecal mass, visible peristalsis, and malnourished appearance
- Intussusception:
  - sudden onset of acute abdominal pain
  - stools with mucus and blood that resemble currant jelly
  - palpable "sausage" mass in the right upper quadrant of the abdomen and/or a tender distended abdomen

Key test results

- With large-bowel obstruction, barium enema reveals a distended, air-filled colon
- With sigmoid volvulus, barium enema reveals a closed loop of sigmoid with extreme distention or the presence of an intussusception
- X-rays confirm the diagnosis
- Abdominal films show the presence and location of intestinal gas or fluid
- Abdominal ultrasound to determine presence of intussusception (telescoping of the intestine into itself)
- Full thickness and/or rectal biopsies to determine presence of Hirschsprung's disease, which is an absence of ganglion (nerve) cells in the colon

Key treatments

- IV therapy to correct fluid and electrolyte imbalances
- Laparoscopic surgery or open abdominal surgery to correct the underlying problem
- Surgical reduction (if inflating the bowel with air or administering a barium enema is not successful)
- Proton pump inhibitors (omeprazole) and histamine-2 (H_2) receptor antagonist (ranitidine) for intussusception
- Analgesics and antibiotics for Hirschsprung's disease

Key interventions

- Monitor vital signs and respiratory and cardiovascular status.
- Observe child closely for signs of shock (pallor, rapid pulse, and hypotension).
- Monitor for fluid and electrolyte disturbances.
- Maintain strict intake and output measurements.
- Weigh daily.
- Position child side lying with head elevated to prevent aspiration during vomiting episodes.
- Stay alert for signs and symptoms of:
  - metabolic alkalosis (changes in sensorium; slow, shallow respirations; hypertonic muscles; tetany)
  - metabolic acidosis (dyspnea on exertion; disorientation; deep, rapid breathing; weakness; malaise).
- Document characteristics, amount of emesis, and behaviors during vomiting episodes.
- Provide meticulous oral care after vomiting.
- Watch for signs and symptoms of secondary infection.
- Provide preoperative and postoperative care as indicated.

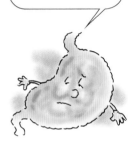

I've clearly ingested something I shouldn't.

Pyloric stenosis

Narrowing of the pylorus, the opening from the stomach into the small intestine

Key signs and symptoms

- Projectile vomiting during or shortly after feedings
- Hunger immediately after vomiting and possible olive shaped mass in the right upper quadrant of the abdomen
- Peristaltic wave moves from right to left when lying flat
- Failure to gain weight
- Signs of dehydration

Key test results

- Ultrasound of the abdomen reveals hypertrophied sphincter

Key treatments

- Pyloromyotomy performed by laparoscopy

Key interventions

- Provide small, frequent, thickened feedings with the head of the bed elevated.
- Burp frequently.

- Position child on the right side or with head slightly elevated to prevent aspiration.
- Weigh daily and monitor intake and output.
- Maintain NPO status and document amount and characteristics of emesis along with the behaviors observed.

- Maintain IV fluid replacement and monitor for fluid and electrolyte disturbances.
- Perform preoperative teaching and encourage parents to verbalize feelings.
- Provide postoperative care, maintain NG tube placement and patency, and maintain NPO status until bowel sounds return.

thePoint® You can download tables of drug information to help you prepare for the NCLEX®! View Generic Drug Names, Drug Classifications, Drug Actions, and Nursing Implications for the drugs discussed in this refresher at **http://thePoint.lww.com**

Gastrointestinal questions, answers, and rationales

1. Which intervention(s) will the nurse perform when caring for a child receiving total parenteral nutrition (TPN)? Select all that apply.
1. Inspect the central line insertion site.
2. Monitor the child's vital signs.
3. Agitate the IV bag frequently.
4. Monitor the child's visitors.
5. Assess blood glucose levels.
6. Observe the fluid's clarity.

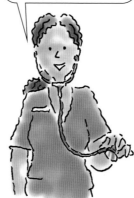

No, "total parenteral nutrition" doesn't mean that the parents are the only ones feeding the client.

1. **1, 2, 3, 5, 6.** The high sugar content of TPN solutions increases the possibility of bacteria growth in the bag and tubing and can raise the blood glucose levels. This increases the client's risk for infection. Crystallization of the mixture can occur in the bag. The nurse should assess for elevated temperature, inspect the central line insertion site for signs of infection, inspect the TPN mixture for clarity, and assess blood glucose levels. TPN should not be stopped abruptly or infused rapidly. Special tubing is used that contains an in-line filter to remove bacteria and particulate material. Monitoring visitors does not apply to the care for TPN but for clients with compromised immune functioning.
CN: Physiological integrity; CNS: Pharmacological and parenteral therapies; CL: Apply

2. The nurse is caring for a child with celiac disease. Which finding **most** indicates the child's treatment plan is successful?
1. The child's growth is appropriate for both height and weight.
2. The child only has erythematous lesions on the buttocks.
3. The child's extremities appear thin, but face has a normal appearance.
4. The child's parents report flatulence and steatorrhea are present.

2. **1.** Because celiac disease is a disease that involves protein and carbohydrate malabsorption, the child is at risk for failure to thrive. The main goal of care is to promote a normal growth pattern for the child. Following the prescribed diet is a way to reach the goal of maintaining the child's growth. Erythematous lesions (dermatitis herpetiformis), thin extremities with a normal face, flatulence, and steatorrhea are all findings associated with celiac disease.
CN: Physiological integrity; CNS: Reduction of risk potential; CL: Apply

3. Which food item(s) selected by a child with celiac disease will cause the nurse to intervene? Select all that apply.
1. Yogurt with granola, skim milk, and a banana
2. A bologna, lettuce, and tomato pita sandwich
3. Sliced cheese, sausage and vegetable pizza
4. A wheat tortilla with southwestern chicken and rice
5. Steamed broccoli florets with a grilled pork chop
6. Sliced strawberries with a tossed green salad

3. **1, 2, 3, 4.** Sources of gluten found in wheat, rye, and barley should be avoided. Rice, corn, and oats are suitable substitutes because they do not contain gluten. Pizza crust, granola, some cereals, noodles, baked goods, some sauces and gravies, and breads contain gluten and, when broken down, cannot be digested by people with celiac disease. Processed lunch meats may contain gluten. The remaining dietary choices do not contain gluten.
CN: Physiological integrity; CNS: Reduction of risk potential; CL: Apply

CN: Client needs category   CNS: Client needs subcategory   CL: Cognitive level

4. The nurse interviewing the parents of a child diagnosed with celiac disease will expect them to make which statement?
1. "Our child's behavior has not changed."
2. "There are no problems with weight gain."
3. "Playing is our child's favorite way to pass the time."
4. "Our child has 5 to 6 oily looking stools a day."

5. To help promote a normal life for a school-age child with celiac disease, which intervention will the nurse recommend to the child's parents?
1. Give the child special treatment over siblings.
2. Focus on restrictions that make them feel different.
3. Introduce the child to a peer with celiac disease.
4. Do not allow the child to express doubt about following dietary restrictions.

6. The nurse will review which data to **best** evaluate the effectiveness of nutritional therapy for a child with celiac disease?
1. Daily vital signs
2. Stool characteristics
3. Serum creatinine levels
4. Intake and output

7. Which finding(s) concern the nurse evaluating a child with celiac disease who started the prescribed diet 1 week ago? Select all that apply.
1. Increased diarrhea
2. Foul-smelling stools
3. Improved appetite
4. Weight gain
5. Abdominal cramping

8. The nurse is caring for an infant immediately following cheiloplasty. The nurse will incorporate which intervention(s) while caring for this infant? Select all that apply.
1. Clean the sutures after feedings.
2. Pin the infant's arms to the shirt.
3. Place the infant supine after feeding.
4. Remove the lip device from the infant after surgery.
5. Monitor vital signs.

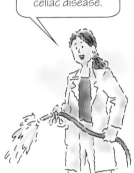

Bulky stool may be a sign of celiac disease.

4. 4. Diarrhea is common due to the child's inability to absorb the protein gluten and fat. Profuse watery diarrhea is usually a sign of celiac crisis. Behavior changes such as irritability, uncooperativeness, and apathy are common, and they usually are not pleasant. Poor weight gain would be a symptom of celiac disease because impaired absorption leads to malnutrition.
CN: Physiological integrity; CNS: Physiological adaptation; CL: Apply

5. 3. Introducing the child to a peer with celiac disease will let this child know he or she is not alone. It will show the child how other people live a normal life with similar restrictions. Instead of focusing on restrictions that make the child feel different, the parents should focus on ways the child can be normal. They should treat the child no differently than other siblings but set appropriate limits. Allow the child with celiac disease to express feelings about dietary restrictions.
CN: Psychosocial integrity; CNS: None; CL: Apply

6. 2. The fat, bulky, foul-smelling stools should be gone when a child with celiac disease follows a gluten-free diet. Vital signs, serum creatinine levels, and intake and output are not affected by a gluten-free diet.
CN: Physiological integrity; CNS: Basic care and comfort; CL: Analyze

7. 1, 2, 5. The nurse would be concerned about findings indicating no improvement, such as increased diarrhea, continued steatorrhea, and cramping. Within a day or two of starting the diet, most children show improved appetite and reduction or disappearance of diarrhea. Steatorrhea (fatty, oily, foul-smelling stool) disappearance and weight gain are good indicators that the child's ability to absorb nutrients is improving.
CN: Physiological integrity; CNS: Physiological adaptation; CL: Apply

8. 1, 2, 5. The nurse would clean the sutures following repair of the cleft lip after feedings to prevent bacterial growth from milk accumulation. The infant's arms should be restrained to prevent the infant from rubbing the sutures. It is imperative to monitor vital signs to ensure an airway is maintained. The infant would be placed on the right side to prevent aspiration and promote digestion. The lip device should not be removed by the nurse.
CN: Physiological integrity; CNS: Reduction of risk potential; CL: Apply

9. Which intervention will the nurse use to prevent tissue infection after cleft palate and lip repair?
1. Cover the suture line with sterile gauze.
2. Allow the infant to suck on a pacifier.
3. Rinse the infant's mouth after each feeding.
4. Feed the infant with a syringe or cup.

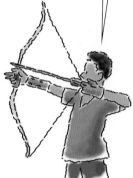

If you aim at nothing, you'll hit it every time. Keep your sights set on the best answer.

10. Which health care provider prescription will the nurse question when caring for an adolescent diagnosed with failure to thrive?
1. Assess hormone levels.
2. Administer daily multivitamin.
3. Obtain weight BID.
4. Monitor thyroid function.

11. Which nursing intervention is **priority** when caring for a toddler during the first 24 hours after palatoplasty surgery?
1. Clean the suture line after feedings using sterile technique.
2. Position the infant in the side-lying position after feedings.
3. Use a syringe or cup to feed the toddler.
4. Start the child on clear liquids and progress to a soft diet.

12. The nurse is educating the parents of an infant following cleft lip repair. Which instruction(s) will the nurse provide the parents? Select all that apply.
1. Offer a pacifier as needed.
2. Lay the infant on the back to sleep.
3. Sit the infant up for each feeding.
4. Loosen the arm restraints every 4 hours.
5. Clean the suture line after each feeding.
6. Give the infant extra care and support.

9. **3.** To prevent milk buildup around the suture line, the infant's mouth is usually rinsed. The sutures should be kept clean, dry, and uncovered (to prevent aspiration and suffocation). Placing objects in the mouth is generally avoided after surgery. Infants are fed by mouth using a catheter-tipped, plunger-type syringe or a cup; however, this prevents damage to the suture line, not infection.
CN: Physiological integrity; CNS: Physiological adaptation;
CL: Apply

10. **3.** Adolescents with failure to thrive are 20% underweight for their height. Obtaining weights BID is not necessary. Daily weight assessment is commonly prescribed. These adolescents often experience delayed pubertal changes; therefore, testing hormone and thyroid levels is appropriate. These adolescents need a multivitamin to help restore imbalances.
CN: Safe, effective care environment; CNS: Management of care;
CL: Apply

11. **2.** Palatoplasty is repair of the cleft palate. Priority is maintaining the toddler's airway by placing the toddler side-lying to prevent aspiration. The suture line must be cleaned after each feeding to reduce the risk of infection, which could adversely affect the healing and cosmetic results; however, airway is priority. A syringe or cup would be used to feed the child to prevent injury to the suture line, and the diet would begin with clear liquids and progress as feedings resumed, but airway is priority.
CN: Physiological integrity; CNS: Reduction of risk potential;
CL: Analyze

12. **2, 3, 5, 6.** An infant with a repaired cleft lip should be put to sleep on the back to prevent trauma to the surgery site. The infant should be fed in the upright position with a syringe and attached tubing to prevent stress to the suture line from sucking. To prevent infection, the suture line should be cleaned after each feeding by dabbing it with half-strength hydrogen peroxide or saline solution. The infant should receive extra care and support because the emotional needs cannot be met by sucking. Extra care and support may also prevent crying, which stresses the suture line. Pacifiers should not be used during the healing process because they stress the suture line. Arm restraints are used to keep the infant's hands away from the mouth and should be loosened every 2 hours to allow for muscle movement.
CN: Physiological integrity; CNS: Reduction of risk potential;
CL: Apply

13. Which nursing intervention is essential in the care of an infant with cleft lip and palate?
1. Discourage breastfeeding.
2. Hold the infant flat while feeding.
3. Involve the parents in the infant's care.
4. Use a normal bottle nipple for feedings.

14. The parents of an infant born with cleft lip and palate are seeing their child for the first time. Which nursing action will **best** assist with facilitating parent–infant bonding?
1. Point out the infant's positive features when providing care.
2. Discuss the parent's feelings of frustration with the situation.
3. Recognize the parent's ambivalence toward the infant.
4. Allow the parents to share their feeling of dissatisfaction.

15. The nurse will educate the parents of a child who had a cheiloplasty on which potential long-term complication?
1. Deviated septum
2. Recurring tonsillitis
3. Tooth decay
4. Hearing loss

16. The parent of a neonate born with a cleft lip and palate prepares to feed the child for the first time. Which education is **priority** for the nurse to provide prior to the parent attempting the first feeding?
1. How to lay the neonate down
2. Methods of burping the neonate
3. How to clean the neonate's mouth
4. Proper positioning of the neonate

17. The nurse prepares to provide discharge education to the parents of a child who had surgical repair of a cleft palate. Which instruction will the nurse include in the teaching?
1. Provide the child a normal diet.
2. Continue using arm restraints at home.
3. Avoid allowing the child to drink from a cup.
4. The proper method to brush the child's teeth.

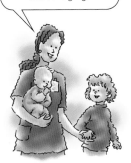

Congenital defects in infants, such as cleft palate, can be upsetting to the family. Stay optimistic and be encouraging.

13. 3. The sooner the parents become involved, the quicker they can determine the method of feeding best suited for them and the infant. Breastfeeding, like bottle feeding, may be difficult but can be facilitated if the mother intends to breastfeed. Sometimes, especially if the cleft is not severe, breastfeeding may be easier because the human nipple conforms to the shape of the infant's mouth. Feedings are usually given in the upright position to prevent aspiration. Various special nipples have been devised for infants with cleft lip or palate; a normal nipple is not effective.
CN: Physiological integrity; CNS: Physiological adaptation; CL: Apply

14. 1. To relieve the parents' anxiety, positive aspects of the infant's physical appearance need to be emphasized. Showing optimism toward surgical correction and showing a photograph of possible cosmetic improvements may be helpful. The other nursing responses are inappropriate to facilitate bonding. These items may be discussed later or with a support group.
CN: Psychosocial integrity; CNS: None; CL: Apply

15. 4. Improper draining of the middle ear, caused by repair of the cleft lip, causes recurrent otitis media and scarring of the tympanic membrane, which lead to varying degrees of hearing loss. The septum remains intact with cleft palate repair. Cleft palate does not cause problems with the tonsils. Improper tooth alignment, not tooth decay, is common.
CN: Physiological adaptation; CNS: Reduction of risk potential; CL: Analyze

16. 4. When neonates are held in the upright position, the formula or breast milk is less likely to leak out the nose or mouth. Neonates need to be burped frequently during the feeding, but positioning to prevent aspiration is priority. The nurse can educate on cleaning the mouth and properly laying the neonate after the feeding session.
CN: Safe, effective care environment; CNS: Management of care; CL: Analyze

17. 2. Arm restraints are also used at home to keep the child's hands away from the mouth until the palate is healed. A soft diet is recommended. No food harder than mashed potatoes can be eaten. Fluids are best taken from a cup. Proper teeth brushing is resumed about 1 to 2 weeks following surgery.
CN: Physiological integrity; CNS: Physiological adaptation; CL: Apply

CN: Client needs category   CNS: Client needs subcategory   CL: Cognitive level

18. Which toddler, following repair of a cleft palate, will the nurse assess **first**?
1. The toddler sucking on a pacifier
2. The toddler lying on the left side
3. The toddler whose respiratory rate is 45 breaths/minute
4. The toddler with a soiled diaper

18. 1. The nurse will first assess the toddler sucking on a pacifier because the pacifier needs to be taken away. Pacifiers are not recommended during the immediate postoperative period to prevent damage to the suture lines. The infant should be positioned on the side to allow oral secretions to drain from the mouth, so suctioning is not necessary. The respiratory rate is within normal range for a toddler. The soiled diaper needs to be changed to prevent damage to the skin, after removing the pacifier.
CN: Physiological integrity; CNS: Reduction of risk potential; CL: Analyze

19. The registered nurse (RN) and assistive personnel (AP) are caring for a toddler following a palatoplasty. Which action(s) by the AP warrants immediate intervention by the RN? Select all that apply.
1. Providing a popsicle for the toddler to eat
2. Allowing the toddler to walk in the hall
3. Providing the toddler water in a cup
4. Obtaining the toddler's temperature orally
5. Giving the child a whistle to play with

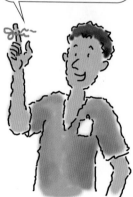

Keep hard and pointed objects out of the child's mouth following a cheiloplasty or a palatoplasty.

19. 1, 4, 5. Nothing hard or pointed should be placed in the child's mouth to prevent injury to the sutures. A popsicle has a hard stick and a portion of the whistle would be placed in the mouth. Tympanic or axillary methods should be used for obtaining the temperature. It is appropriate for the child to ambulate in the hall; this will assist in expending energy. The toddler can drink from a cup.
CN: Safe, effective care environment; CNS: Management of care; CL: Analyze

20. After an infant with a cleft lip has surgical repair and heals, the nurse will educate the parents on which expected finding?
1. Misaligned teeth
2. A larger upper lip
3. Distortion of the jaw
4. Minimal scarring

20. 4. If there is no trauma or infection to the site, healing occurs with little scar formation. There may be some inflammation right after surgery, but after healing the lip is a normal size. No jaw malformation occurs with cleft lip repair.
CN: Physiological integrity; CNS: Physiological adaptation; CL: Understand

21. Which assessment finding in a neonate born with esophageal atresia is **most** concerning to the nurse?
1. Blowing bubbles
2. Sucking on hands
3. Increased irritability
4. Distended abdomen

21. 1. The neonate blowing bubbles indicates excessive mucus in mouth and required suctioning to prevent aspiration. Sucking on the hands indicates hunger. Increased irritability and distended abdomen are expected findings.
CN: Safe, effective care environment; CNS: Management of care; CL: Analyze

22. The nurse assesses a 1-day-old neonate with esophageal atresia. Which finding will the nurse highlight for the health care provider?
1. Passing meconium
2. A sunken anterior fontanel
3. Weight loss of 2 oz (0.6 g)
4. Brisk return of the skin when pinched

You're doing udderly awesome! Seriously, you must be dairy smart. Okay—I think I've milked this joke for all it's worth.

22. 2. A sunken anterior fontanel is a sign of dehydration in the neonate. Mild weight loss is expected in all neonates following birth due to normal fluid loss. Skin that returns quickly when pinched is a sign of adequate hydration.
CN: Physiological integrity; CNS: Reduction of risk potential; CL: Apply

23. The nurse is caring for a neonate suspected of having esophageal atresia. Which assessment finding will the nurse expect in this neonate?
1. Decreased breath sounds
2. Absent bowel sounds
3. Inability to pass meconium
4. Inability to aspirate gastric contents

23. 4. In a neonate suspected of having esophageal atresia, a catheter will meet resistance and not reach the stomach because the esophagus is blocked. The neonate will not be able to aspirate gastric contents. If the esophagus is patent, the catheter will pass unobstructed to the stomach. Breath sounds and bowel sounds are not affected in esophageal atresia. The neonate would be able to pass meconium as this is already in the bowel.
CN: Physiological integrity; CNS: Physiological adaptation; CL: Apply

24. Which intervention will the nurse expect the health care provider to prescribe for a neonate diagnosed with a tracheoesophageal fistula?
1. Antibiotic therapy
2. Continuous supine position
3. Limited oral feedings
4. Remove esophageal catheter

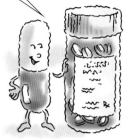

When aspiration pneumonia is a threat, I'm your guy.

25. Which intervention will the nurse perform **first** when caring for a neonate suspected of having tracheoesophageal fistula and esophageal atresia?
1. Administer oxygen.
2. Notify the health care provider.
3. Prepare the neonate for surgery.
4. Suction the neonate.

26. A nurse is assigned to care for a neonate immediately following surgical repair of a tracheoesophageal fistula. It is **priority** for the nurse to monitor the neonate for which complication?
1. Aspiration
2. Aversion to sucking
3. Stomach distention
4. Infection

27. Which initial finding will the nurse anticipate in a neonate suspected of having esophageal atresia with a distal tracheoesophageal fistula?
1. Decreased oral secretions
2. Normal respiratory effort
3. Bulky stools
4. Abdominal distention

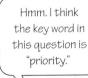

Hmm. I think the key word in this question is "priority."

28. A neonate returns from the operating room after surgical repair of a tracheoesophageal fistula and esophageal atresia. Which nursing intervention is **priority**?
1. Monitor respirations.
2. Give the neonate a pacifier.
3. Begin parent–infant bonding.
4. Monitor chest tube drainage.

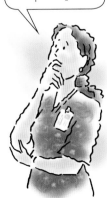

24. 1. Antibiotic therapy is started for the neonate with a tracheoesophageal fistula because aspiration pneumonia is inevitable and appears early. The neonate's head is usually kept in an upright position to prevent aspiration. IV fluids are started, and the neonate is not allowed any oral intake. The catheter is left in the upper esophageal pouch to easily remove fluid that collects there.
CN: Safe, effective care environment; CNS: Management of care; CL: Apply

25. 4. Suctioning is priority to prevent aspiration when tracheoesophageal fistula or esophageal atresia is suspected. Oxygen should be given after suctioning if needed. The nurse would notify the health care provider and prepare the neonate for surgery as prescribed.
CN: Safe and effective care environment; CNS: Management of care; CL: Analyze

26. 1. Respiratory complications are a threat to the neonate's life preoperatively and postoperatively due to the continual risk of aspiration. Stomach distention is more likely to occur preoperatively due to air filling the stomach cavity. An aversion to sucking generally does not develop after being NPO for a short time. Careful attention is paid postoperatively when neonates begin to eat to make sure they can swallow appropriately. Infection would not be an immediate complication and is not priority over airway. The neonate is generally given antibiotics preoperatively to prevent infection.
CN: Safe, effective care environment; CNS: Management of care; CL: Analyze

27. 4. Crying may force air into the stomach, causing distention. Secretions in a client with this condition may be more visible, though normal in quantity, due to the client's inability to swallow effectively. Respiratory effort is usually more difficult. Bulky stools are noted with other disorders such as celiac disease and cystic fibrosis.
CN: Physiological integrity; CNS: Physiological adaptation; CL: Apply

28. 1. Maintaining a patent airway is essential after surgery for repair of a tracheoesophageal fistula and esophageal atresia until sedation wears off. Monitoring respirations will indicate distress. A pacifier can be given to promote comfort and facilitate the sucking reflex. Bonding should begin as soon as possible. Chest tube drainage should be monitored. However, these interventions do not have priority over monitoring for respiratory distress.
CN: Safe, effective care environment; CNS: Management of care; CL: Analyze

29. Before discharging a neonate with a repaired tracheoesophageal fistula and esophageal atresia, which teaching is **priority** for the nurse to provide to the caregivers?
1. Antibiotic administration
2. Proper handwashing techniques
3. Signs of esophageal constriction
4. Appropriate diet progression

29. 3. It is priority for the nurse to educate the caregivers on recognizing and reporting signs of respiratory distress and esophageal constriction, such as drooling and difficulty swallowing. It is important for the nurse to educate the client on antibiotic administration (if prescribed), proper handwashing to limit infection, and diet progression. However, ensuring the airway is maintained is priority.
CN: Physiological integrity; CNS: Basic care and comfort; CL: Analyze

30. The nurse is reviewing the chart exhibit noted below from a neonate's chart and suspects the neonate has which structural defect?

Progress notes	
5/22 1300	4-day-old neonate admitted with coughing, choking, and sneezing following feedings. Neonate's mother states, "My baby seems to have a lot of saliva and drools quite a bit." —Emma Bean, RN

1. Cleft lip
2. Pyloric stenosis
3. Gastroschisis
4. Tracheoesophageal fistula

30. 4. Because of an ineffective swallow, saliva and secretions appear in the mouth and around the lips of the neonate with a tracheoesophageal fistula and esophageal atresia. Coughing, choking, and sneezing occur for the same reason and usually after an attempt at eating. Cleft lip does not produce excessive salivation. None of these symptoms occurs with pyloric stenosis or gastroschisis.
CN: Physiological integrity; CNS: Physiological adaptation; CL: Analyze

31. The nurse is caring for an infant diagnosed with Hirschsprung's disease. Which information will the nurse include when providing education to the parents?
1. "The affected section of your baby's bowel will be surgically removed."
2. "Your baby will need to maintain a gluten-free diet in the future."
3. "Your baby needs to have a surgical procedure for a permanent colostomy."
4. "Your baby will need to have the bowel irrigated at least twice a week."

31. 1. With Hirschsprung's disease, there is an absence of ganglionic innervation of the muscle of a section of the large intestine. Treatment involves removing the affected section of the bowel. A gluten-free diet is maintained with celiac disease. This disease does not normally result in a permanent colostomy. A temporary colostomy may be needed following surgery to allow for healing. The bowel will not need to be irrigated.
CN: Safe, effective care environment; CNS: Management of care; CL: Apply

32. Which nursing action helps verify that a nasogastric (NG) tube is properly positioned in a child's stomach?
1. Invert the tube into a glass of water and observe for bubbling.
2. Aspirate contents from the NG tube and examine it with a pH test strip.
3. Clamp the tube for 10 minutes and auscultate for increased peristalsis.
4. Instill 30 mL of normal saline solution and observe the child's response.

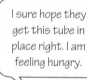

I sure hope they get this tube in place right. I am feeling hungry.

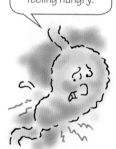

32. 2. To verify positioning of an NG tube, the gastric aspirate should be tested with a pH test strip. Probability of gastric placement is increased if the aspirate has a typical gastric fluid appearance (grassy green, clear and colorless with mucus shreds, or brown) and the pH is ≤7.0. Inverting the tube into a glass of water and observing for bubbling would be done to verify that an NG tube is in the respiratory tract. Clamping the tube and listening for increased peristalsis provides no information on the location of the tube. If the tube is in the respiratory tract, instilling normal saline causes respiratory distress.
CN: Safe, effective care environment; CNS: Safety and infection control; CL: Understand

33. The nurse is caring for an infant with suspected pyloric stenosis. Which finding will the nurse expect to assess?
  1. Anorexia
  2. Chronic diarrhea
  3. Projectile vomiting
  4. Excessive drooling

34. The parent of an infant with pyloric stenosis expresses feelings of guilt and fear of having caused the child's condition. Which response by the nurse is **most** appropriate?
  1. "The actual cause of pyloric stenosis is not known."
  2. "I understand since the cause of pyloric stenosis is believed to be hereditary."
  3. "Pyloric stenosis is typically caused by poor nutrition in pregnancy."
  4. "You should not blame yourself for things beyond your control."

35. When assessing a neonate, the nurse notes visible peristaltic waves across the epigastrium. Which condition will the nurse suspect in this neonate?
  1. Hypertrophic pyloric stenosis
  2. Imperforate anus
  3. Intussusception
  4. Hirschsprung's disease

36. The nurse admits an infant diagnosed with pyloric stenosis. Which nursing intervention will the nurse complete **first**?
  1. Weigh the infant.
  2. Check urine specific gravity.
  3. Place an IV catheter.
  4. Monitor output.

37. The nurse is caring for an infant diagnosed with pyloric stenosis. The nurse notes: respiratory rate, 50 breath/min; pulse, 150 beats/min; O₂ saturation, 96% on room air. Which nursing action is appropriate for this infant?
  1. Monitor intake and output.
  2. Provide humidified oxygen.
  3. Administer intravenous fluids.
  4. Insert a 6 French feeding tube.

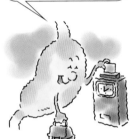

Your gastrointestinal system works hard for you 'round the clock. Be sure to give it high-quality fuel.

33. 3. The obstruction seen in pyloric stenosis does not allow food to pass through to the duodenum. The classic sign of projectile vomiting occurs when the stomach becomes full and the infant vomits for relief. Drooling would not be a finding in a child with pyloric stenosis, but rather in a child with tracheoesophageal fistula. Chronic hunger is commonly seen. There is no diarrhea because food does not pass through the stomach.
CN: Physiological integrity; CNS: Physiological adaptation; CL: Apply

34. 1. The cause of the narrowing of the pyloric musculature is unknown. A hereditary link has not been established. Poor nutrition in pregnancy and poor muscle development in the stomach may relate to this defect, but neither has been established as a definitive cause.
CN: Safe, effective care environment; CNS: Management of care; CL: Apply

35. 1. The diagnosis of pyloric stenosis can be established from a finding of hypertrophic pyloric stenosis. Imperforate anus, intussusception, and Hirschsprung's disease are diagnosed by other symptoms.
CN: Physiological integrity; CNS: Physiological adaptation; CL: Apply

36. 1. Weighing the infant diagnosed with pyloric stenosis would be done first so that a baseline weight can be established and weight changes can be assessed. After a baseline weight is obtained, an IV catheter can be placed to maintain hydration because oral feedings generally are not given. These infants are usually dehydrated, so while checking output and specific gravity are important tools to help assess client status, these actions are not the first priority.
CN: Safe, effective care environment; CNS: Management of care; CL: Analyze

37. 3. The nurse's findings indicate the infant is stable. The nurse would focus on replacing hydration due to excessive vomiting associated with pyloric stenosis. The nurse would monitor intake and output after starting intravenous therapy. Oxygen and a feeding tube are not indicated.
CN: Physiological integrity; CNS: Physiological adaptation; CL: Apply

38. When preparing to feed an infant following pyloric stenosis repair, which nursing intervention(s) is appropriate? Select all that apply.
   1. Begin with small amounts.
   2. Burp the infant frequently.
   3. Discourage parental participation.
   4. Hold the infant side-lying while feeding.
   5. Provide a pacifier between feedings.

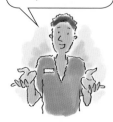

After a big meal, belching is one of my highest priorities.

39. The nurse is caring for an infant following a pyloromyotomy. The nurse notes occasional vomiting. Which nursing action is **most** appropriate?
   1. Hold the next feeding.
   2. Notify the health care provider.
   3. Continue feeding the infant.
   4. Document the emesis characteristics.

40. Which intervention will the nurse perform to help prevent vomiting in an infant diagnosed with pyloric stenosis?
   1. Hold the infant for 1 hour after feeding.
   2. Handle the infant minimally after feedings.
   3. Space out feedings and give large amounts.
   4. Lay the infant prone with the head of the bed elevated.

41. Which nursing intervention provides the **best** support to the parents of an infant diagnosed with pyloric stenosis?
   1. Keep the parents informed of the infant's progress.
   2. Provide all care for the infant, even when the parents visit.
   3. Tell the parents to minimize handling of the infant.
   4. Ask the health care provider to keep the parents informed.

42. Which nursing intervention is **priority** when caring for a child suffering from accidental poisoning?
   1. Stabilize the child.
   2. Notify the parents.
   3. Identify the poison.
   4. Determine when it occurred.

38. 1, 2, 5. Following repair of pyloric stenosis the nurse will begin feedings with small amounts and increase as tolerated to a normal diet. The infant should be burped often to limit distention. A pacifier may be offered to satisfy the sucking instinct. Parents should be involved. The infant should be held upright while feeding to prevent aspiration.
CN: Physiological integrity; CNS: Physiological adaptation; CL: Apply

39. 2. A pyloromyotomy is the surgical procedure done to correct pyloric stenosis. If the nurse notes vomiting, the health care provider should be notified as this could indicate a complication. The nurse would document the emesis characteristics after notifying the health care provider. Additional interventions will be based on any new prescriptions received.
CN: Safe, effective care environment; CNS: Management of care; CL: Apply

40. 2. Minimal handling, especially after a feeding, will help prevent vomiting. Holding the infant would provide too much stimulation, increasing the risk of vomiting. Feedings are given frequently and slowly in small amounts. An infant should be positioned in semi-Fowler's position and slightly on the right side after a feeding.
CN: Physiological integrity; CNS: Physiological adaptation; CL: Apply

41. 1. Keeping the parents informed of their child's progress will decrease their anxiety. The nurse should encourage the parents to be involved with the infant's care. Telling the parents to minimize handling of the infant is not appropriate because parent–child contact is important. The health care provider is responsible for updating the parents on the infant's medical condition, and the nurse is responsible for updating the parents on the day-to-day activities of the infant and his improvement with the day's activities.
CN: Psychosocial integrity; CNS: None; CL: Apply

42. 1. Stabilization and the initial emergency treatment of the child (such as respiratory assistance, circulatory support, or control of seizures) will prevent further damage to the body from the poison. If the parents did not bring the child, they can be notified as soon as the child is stabilized or treated. Although identification of the poison is crucial and should begin at the same time as the stabilization of the child, the assessment of airway, breathing, and circulation should occur first. Determining when the poisoning took place is an important consideration, but emergency stabilization and treatment are most important.
CN: Safe, effective care environment; CNS: Management of care; CL: Analyze

43. Which symptom(s) will the nurse likely find in an infant diagnosed with pyloric stenosis? Select all that apply.
1. Slow response to stimuli
2. Sunken anterior fontanel
3. Irregular heart rate
4. Dryness of the lips
5. Low body temperature

43. 2, 4. Dry lips and sunken anterior fontanel are signs of dehydration, which is common in infants with pyloric stenosis. These infants are constantly hungry due to their inability to retain feedings. A slow response to stimuli, dysrhythmias, and hypothermia are not clinical findings with pyloric stenosis.
CN: Physiological integrity; CNS: Physiological adaptation; CL: Apply

44. The nurse is caring for an infant diagnosed with intussusception. Which health care provider prescription will the nurse question?
1. Omeprazole
2. Vitamin K
3. Ranitidine
4. Lactated Ringer's

44. 2. Intussusception is invagination of the intestine. Vitamin K is given to promote clotting, which is not a symptom of intussusception. Treatment for intussusception includes omeprazole (proton pump inhibitor), ranitidine (histamine₂ receptor antagonist), and intravenous fluids to correct hydration and electrolyte imbalances.
CN: Safe, effective care environment; CNS: Management of care; CL: Apply

45. The nurse admits a child who has a suspected bowel obstruction. Which assessment finding(s) will the nurse anticipate in this child? Select all that apply.
1. Abdominal distention
2. Hyperactive bowel sounds
3. Temperature 99° F (37.2° C)
4. Abdominal pain
5. Vomiting

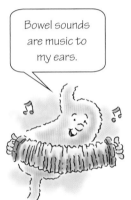

Bowel sounds are music to my ears.

45. 1, 4, 5. Children with a bowel obstruction may have various symptoms depending on the cause of the obstruction. General assessment findings include abdominal pain, abdominal distention, diarrheal stool leakage around the obstruction, soiling, nausea, and vomiting. A low-grade fever may or may not be present depending on symptoms of dehydration. Bowel sounds are usually hypoactive.
CN: Physiological integrity; CNS: Physiological adaptation; CL: Apply

46. A preschooler is brought to the emergency department after ingesting a large amount of liquid acetaminophen. Which assessment finding(s) will the nurse anticipate in this child? Select all that apply.
1. Bradycardia
2. Diaphoresis
3. Pallor
4. Hypertension
5. Tachypnea
6. Tinnitus
7. Hypothermia

46. 1, 2, 3, 7. A weak-slow pulse (bradycardia), diaphoresis, pallor, hypothermia, nausea and vomiting, and right upper quadrant pain are all signs of acetaminophen poisoning. The other conditions are not associated with acetaminophen ingestion.
CN: Physiological integrity; CNS: Physiological adaptation; CL: Apply

47. The nurse admits a child who ingested drain cleaner. Which intervention(s) will the nurse include in this child's plan of care? Select all that apply.
1. Evaluate vital signs.
2. Assess the child's ability to speak.
3. Monitor for fluid balance disturbances.
4. Assess for swelling of the tongue.
5. Position the child semi-Fowler's in bed.

47. 1, 2, 4, 5. Subtle changes in vital signs can indicate changes in oxygenation in children. Assessing the ability to speak and for tongue swelling helps to determine airway compromise and patency. The child should be positioned semi-Fowler's or high-Fowler's to maintain airway patency and to prevent aspiration if the child is vomiting. Fluid balance disturbances do not commonly occur after drain cleaner ingestion.
CN: Physiological integrity; CNS: Physiological adaptation; CL: Apply

CN: Client needs category   CNS: Client needs subcategory   CL: Cognitive level

48. A parent brings their child to the clinic after ingestion of an unknown poisonous substance. Which nursing action is **priority**?
1. Induce vomiting with syrup of ipecac.
2. Notify the health care provider.
3. Give large amounts of water to drink.
4. Assess the child for additional symptoms.

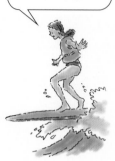

You're doing great. Keep riding that wave!

48. 2. Notify the health care provider first so that appropriate care is initiated. Inducing vomiting is important but is contraindicated with some poisons. Only small amounts of water are recommended so the poison is confined to the smallest volume. Large amounts of water will let the poison pass the pylorus. The small intestine absorbs fluid rapidly, increasing the risk of toxicity. The nurse will continue to monitor the child after notifying the health care provider.
CN: Safe, effective care environment; CNS: Management of care; CL: Analyze

49. A parent brings a child to the emergency department after ingesting a poisonous hydrocarbon. What is the **priority** nursing action?
1. Administer IV fluids.
2. Keep the child calm and relaxed.
3. Auscultate bowel sounds.
4. Educate on preventing poisoning.

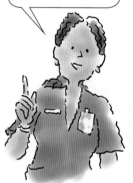

Only one of these interventions will actually help *prevent* poisoning.

49. 2. Keeping the child calm and relaxed will help prevent vomiting in a child who has ingested poisonous hydrocarbons. If vomiting occurs, there is a great chance the esophagus will be damaged from regurgitation of the gastric poison. Additionally, the risk of chemical pneumonitis exists if vomiting occurs. The nurse would perform a head-to-toe assessment and provide education once the child is stabilized. IV fluids are not indicated at this time.
CN: Safe, effective care environment; CNS: Management of care; CL: Analyze

50. The nurse is providing education about salicylate poisoning to a parent. Which information is **most** important for the nurse to include in the teaching?
1. Characteristics a child will exhibit if salicylate overdose occurs
2. How to educate children on the hazards of ingesting nonfood items
3. Allowing children to hold medication bottles to decrease curiosity
4. To keep large amounts of drugs on hand but out of reach of children

50. 2. Educating children on the hazards of ingesting nonfood items will help prevent ingestion of poisonous substances. Identifying the overdose level will not prevent it from occurring. Aspirin and drugs should be kept out of the sight and reach of children. Parents should be warned about keeping large amounts of drugs on hand.
CN: Safe, effective care environment; CNS: Safety and infection control; CL: Apply

51. The nurse caring for a conscious child diagnosed with salicylate poisoning will prepare the child for which treatment?
1. Activated charcoal
2. Hypothermia blankets
3. Hemodialysis
4. Vitamin K injection

51. 1. The nurse would anticipate preparing the conscious child for administration of activated charcoal as soon as possible. This can be repeated Q4H if bowel sounds are present, until charcoal is noted in the child's stool. Hemodialysis is reserved for children experiencing severe neurologic impairment, renal or respiratory insufficiency, and unresolved acidemia. Hypothermia blankets may be used to reduce the possibility of seizures. Vitamin K may be used to decrease bleeding tendencies but only if evidence of this exists.
CN: Physiological integrity; CNS: Physiological adaptation; CL: Apply

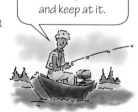

Fishing for the right answer takes time. Be patient and keep at it.

52. A child is diagnosed with acetaminophen poisoning. Which sign(s) will the nurse expect when assessing the client 18 hours after ingestion? Select all that apply.
1. Hypothermia
2. Decreased urine output
3. Profuse sweating
4. Rapid pulse
5. Right upper quadrant pain

52. 1, 2, 3, 5. During the first 12 to 24 hours, profuse sweating, hypothermia, decreased urine output, and right upper quadrant pain are signs of acetaminophen poisoning. Weak pulse is also a common finding.
CN: Physiological integrity; CNS: Physiological adaptation; CL: Apply

CN: Client needs category   CNS: Client needs subcategory   CL: Cognitive level

53. The nurse is caring for a child with suspected accidental poisoning. Which action will help the nurse determine which poison was ingested?
1. Call poison control center.
2. Ask the child.
3. Ask the parents.
4. Save all evidence of poison.

54. It is **priority** for the nurse to monitor which laboratory result(s) following an acute overdose of acetaminophen? Select all that apply.
1. Alanine transaminase (ALT)
2. Acetaminophen level
3. Aspartate transaminase (AST)
4. Hemoglobin
5. White blood cell count (WBC)
6. Erythrocyte sedimentation rate (ESR)

55. The nurse is evaluating the effectiveness of therapy with acetylcysteine in a child with acetaminophen poisoning. Which laboratory value is **most** important for the nurse to monitor?
1. Serum alanine aminotransferase (ALT)
2. Serum calcium levels
3. Prothrombin time (PT)
4. Serum glucose levels

56. The nurse is providing community education on lead poisoning in children. Which risk factor(s) will the nurse include in the teaching? Select all that apply.
1. Age
2. Gender
3. Ethnicity
4. Living environment
5. Anemia

57. Which finding will the nurse expect to assess **first** in a child just diagnosed with lead poisoning?
1. Anemia
2. Diarrhea
3. Overeating
4. Paralysis

53. 4. Saving all evidence of poison (container, vomitus, urine) will help determine which drug was ingested and how much. Calling the local poison control center may help get information on specific poisons or determine if a certain household placed a call; rarely can the poison control center determine which poison has been ingested. Asking the child may help, but the child may fear punishment and may not be honest about the incident. The parent may be helpful in some instances, but not if the parent was not present when the ingestion occurred.
CN: Physiological integrity; CNS: Reduction of risk potential;
CL: Apply

54. 1, 2, 3. It is priority for the nurse to monitor liver function tests and serum acetaminophen levels. The damage to the hepatic system is not from acetaminophen but from one of its metabolites. This metabolite binds to liver cells in large quantities. Brain damage, heart failure, and kidney damage may develop later but not initially. Hemoglobin, WBCs, and ESR are not needed at this time.
CN: Physiological integrity; CNS: Physiological adaptation;
CL: Apply

55. 1. Acetaminophen poisoning damages the liver, leading to elevated ALT and AST levels. After therapy with acetylcysteine is started, these liver enzyme levels should begin to decrease. Serum calcium levels may fall following chelation therapy in children with lead poisoning. Because PT is elevated and blood glucose levels are reduced with salicylate poisoning, the nurse should observe that the PT and blood glucose levels return to normal after treatment is initiated.
CN: Physiological integrity; CNS: Reduction of risk potential;
CL: Analyze

56. 1, 3, 4, 5. Risk factors for lead poisoning include age (young children tend to put things in their mouths), ethnicity (African-Americans have a higher incidence of lead poisoning), living environments (older homes may contain lead-based paint and paint chips may be eaten directly by the child, or they may cling to toys or hands that are then put into the child's mouth), and anemia (children with iron deficiency anemia absorb lead more readily). Poisoning is not gender-related.
CN: Health promotion and maintenance; CNS: None; CL: Apply

57. 1. Lead is dangerously toxic to the biosynthesis of heme. The reduced heme molecule in red blood cells causes anemia. Constipation (not diarrhea), poor appetite, and vomiting (not overeating) are signs of lead poisoning. Paralysis may occur as toxic damage to the brain progresses, but it is not an initial sign.
CN: Safe, effective care environment; CNS: Management of care;
CL: Apply

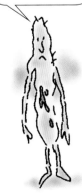

Lead poisoning really does a number on the body.

58. An infant is admitted to the hospital with gastroenteritis. Which nursing action is **priority**?
1. Observe for signs of pain.
2. Introduce oral feedings as indicated.
3. Monitor for decreased urine output.
4. Assess the infant's skin turgor.

58. 3. Monitoring for decreased urinary output is a priority. If urinary output decreases while the child is receiving treatment for gastroenteritis, it should be reported to the health care provider. Young children with gastroenteritis are at high risk for developing a fluid volume deficit. Their intestinal mucosa allows for more fluid and electrolytes to be lost when they have gastroenteritis. The main goal should be to rehydrate the infant. The other nursing actions are important, but decreased urine output (indicates deficient fluid volume) is the most life threatening.
CN: Safe, effective care environment; CNS: Management of care; CL: Analyze

59. The nurse explains to the parent of a child with lead poisoning x-rays are necessary. What is the **best** response by the nurse when the parent questions the necessity of the x-ray?
1. "The x-ray will show how much lead has been absorbed by your child's bones."
2. "The x-ray is a routine procedure for children experiencing lead poisoning."
3. "You should trust the health care provider to prescribe only what is needed."
4. "Performing x-rays will help us determine what to do next."

59. 1. Ingested lead is initially absorbed by bone. The other statements do not adequately address the parent's concern.
CN: Safe, effective care environment; CNS: Management of care; CL: Analyze

60. The nurse is gathering data from a child suspected of ingesting paint chips from an old home. Which system will the nurse closely monitor for serious effects?
1. Central nervous system (CNS)
2. Hematologic system
3. Renal system
4. Respiratory system

60. 1. Damage that occurs to the CNS after lead poisoning is difficult to repair. Damage to the renal and hematologic systems can be reversed if treated early. The respiratory system is not affected until coma and death occur.
CN: Physiological integrity; CNS: Physiological adaptation; CL: Understand

61. The nurse will prepare a child with lead poisoning scheduled for chelation therapy for which intervention(s)? Select all that apply.
1. Limited activity
2. Insertion of an IV catheter
3. Being in the hospital
4. Serum laboratory testing
5. Burning at the administration site

61. 1, 2, 3, 4, 5. The nurse will prepare the child for each listed intervention. Chelation therapy involves receiving a medication several times via an IV or in pill format. The child will be hospitalized and in bed while receiving IV therapy, which will limit activity. Laboratory testing will be used to determine the effectiveness and monitor for potential damage from the ingested lead. Burning at the site, nausea, fever, vomiting, and headaches are potential complications of chelation therapy.
CN: Physiological integrity; CNS: Physiological adaptation; CL: Apply

62. The nurse is caring for a 5-year-old child whose parents think the child has been exposed to lead. The nurse will assess the child for which sign(s) of lead poisoning? Select all that apply.
1. Jaundice
2. Coagulation abnormalities
3. Difficulty concentrating
4. Tremors
5. Headache

62. 3, 4, 5. Signs and symptoms of lead poisoning depend on the degree of toxicity. General fatigue, difficulty concentrating, tremors, and headache indicate moderate toxicity. Jaundice and coagulation abnormalities are observed in acetaminophen poisoning.
CN: Physiological integrity; CNS: Physiological adaptation; CL: Apply

CN: Client needs category   CNS: Client needs subcategory   CL: Cognitive level

63. A child is admitted to the unit after being treated in the emergency department with gastric lavage for ingestion of a bottle of acetaminophen. The nurse has a prescription to administer *N*-acetylcysteine 140 mg/kg stat. The child weighs 15 lb (6.8 kg). The package label reads 2 g/40 mL. How many milliliters will the nurse administer? Record your answer using one decimal place.

_____ mL

64. During a well-child visit, a child's parents ask the nurse, "How can we prevent lead poisoning in our child?" Which response by the nursing is **best**?
1. "You need to put child locks on cabinets in your home."
2. "Inspect painted toys to determine if lead is in the paint."
3. "Your child does not have risk factors, so do not worry."
4. "Do not let your child play in any dirt outside."

65. The nurse is monitoring a child with lead poisoning during chelation therapy. For which condition is this monitoring the **priority**?
1. Hypercalcemia
2. Hypokalemia
3. Hypernatremia
4. Hypoglycemia

66. Which symptom(s) will the nurse expect to assess for in a child suspected of having acute appendicitis? Select all that apply.
1. Reports pain in epigastric area
2. Decreased heart rate
3. Abdominal pain
4. Pain descending to the lower left quadrant
5. Temperature 102.2° F (39° C)

67. Which recommendation will the nurse give over the phone to the parent of a 7-year-old child with right lower abdominal pain, fever, and vomiting?
1. "Give prune juice to relieve constipation."
2. "Test for rebound tenderness in the left lower abdominal quadrant."
3. "Encourage fluids to prevent dehydration."
4. "Bring your child to the emergency room."

In question #64, look for the **best** response.

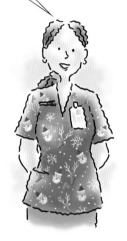

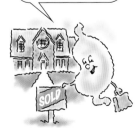

Keeping your gastrointestinal system healthy is always a good investment.

63. **38.1.**
Multiply child's weight in kilograms × 140 mg/kg

$$6.8 \; kilograms \times 140 \frac{mg}{kg} = 952 \; mg \; of \; N\text{-}acetylcysteine$$

Convert 2 grams to mg by multiplying by 1,000 (1 gram = 1,000 mg)

$$2 \; grams \times 1{,}000 \; mg/gram = 2{,}000 \; mg$$

Use the formula Dose desired/Dose on hand × Form of the drug

$$952 \; mg/2{,}000 \; mg \times 40 \; mL = 38.1 \; mL \; administered$$

CN: Physiological integrity; CNS: Pharmacological and parenteral therapies; CL: Apply

64. **2.** Reading toy labels and visually inspecting the age of toys will help to identify toys that may contain lead and may help reduce lead exposure. Locked cabinets prevent poisoning from cleaners and medications. Telling parents not to worry is not therapeutic and does not address their concern. It is not appropriate to state the child cannot play in any dirt. If the soil is thought to be contaminated, it should be tested.

CN: Safe, effective care environment; CNS: Safety and infection control; CL: Apply

65. **2.** A calcium chelating agent is used for the treatment of lead poisoning, so calcium is removed from the body with the lead, resulting in hypocalcemia. Hypokalemia, hypernatremia, and hypoglycemia do not occur as a result of chelation therapy.

CN: Safe, effective care environment; CNS: Management of care; CL: Analyze

66. **3, 5.** Elevated temperature (fever), abdominal pain, and tenderness are the first symptoms of appendicitis. Tachycardia, not bradycardia, is seen. Pain can be generalized or periumbilical. It usually descends to the lower right quadrant, not to the left.

CN: Physiological integrity; CNS: Physiological adaptation; CL: Apply

67. **4.** The parent of a child with abdominal pain, fever, and vomiting (the cardinal signs of appendicitis) should be urged to seek immediate emergency care to reduce the risk of complications from potential appendix rupture. Prune juice has laxative effects and should not be given because laxatives increase the risk of rupture of the appendix. Testing for rebound tenderness may elicit McBurney's sign in the right lower quadrant (an indication of appendicitis); however, the nurse should not rely on the parent's findings. The child should be given nothing by mouth in case surgery is needed.

CN: Physiological integrity; CNS: Reduction of risk potential; CL: Analyze

CN: Client needs category   CNS: Client needs subcategory   CL: Cognitive level

68. Which intervention will the nurse perform preoperatively for a child with appendicitis?
1. Give clear fluids.
2. Apply heat to the abdomen.
3. Maintain complete bed rest.
4. Administer an enema, if prescribed.

68. 3. Bed rest will prevent aggravating the condition. Clients scheduled for surgery are not allowed anything by mouth. Cold applications are placed on the abdomen, as heat would increase blood flow to the area and possibly spread infection. Enemas may aggravate appendicitis.
CN: Physiological integrity; CNS: Physiological adaptation; CL: Apply

69. Which nursing intervention is **priority** for a child with peritonitis from a ruptured appendix following an appendectomy?
1. Slowly advance diet.
2. Monitor pain level.
3. Assess the temperature.
4. Give parenteral antibiotics.

69. 4. Parenteral antibiotics are used for 7 to 10 days' postoperatively to help prevent the spread of peritonitis infection. The nurse will slowly advance the diet following abdominal surgery, monitor pain, and assess temperature; however, these are not priority over administering antibiotics.
CN: Safe, effective care environment; CNS: Management of care; CL: Analyze

70. After surgical repair of a ruptured appendix, which position is **most** appropriate for the nurse to place the child?
1. High-Fowler's position
2. Left side-lying
3. Semi-Fowler's position
4. Supine with knees flexed

70. 3. Semi-Fowler's or right side-lying position after surgery for a ruptured appendix will facilitate drainage from the peritoneal cavity and prevent the formation of a subdiaphragmatic abscess. High Fowler's, left side-lying, and supine positions will not facilitate drainage from the peritoneal cavity.
CN: Safe, effective care environment; CNS: Management of care; CL: Apply

71. The nurse assesses the laboratory results for a 9-year-old child hospitalized with severe vomiting and diarrhea. The child's potassium level is 3.1 mEq/L (3.1 mmol/L). Which nursing action is **priority**?
1. Document the finding.
2. Notify the health care provider.
3. Monitor apical heart rate.
4. Transfer the child to intensive care unit.

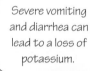

Severe vomiting and diarrhea can lead to a loss of potassium.

71. 2. The nurse would notify the health care provider. Potassium is lost through diarrhea and is expected to be low normal or low. The normal potassium level in children ranges from 3.5 to 5.8 mEq/L (3.5 to 5.8 mmol/L). Low levels of potassium can lead to serious complications. The child may need parenteral replacement. The nurse will document the findings and monitor the heart rate and rhythm. The child may be transferred, depending on emergence of additional symptoms.
CN: Physiological integrity; CNS: Reduction of risk potential; CL: Apply

72. A neonate is suspected of having a tracheoesophageal fistula. Which finding will the nurse expect to see during the initial assessment?
1. Excessive drooling
2. Distended abdomen
3. Mottling of the skin
4. Slow respiratory rate

72. 1. In tracheoesophageal fistulas, saliva will pool in this pouch and cause the child to drool. The other findings are not expected initially.
CN: Physiological integrity; CNS: Physiological adaptation; CL: Apply

73. When assessing a client suspected of having pyloric stenosis, which finding will the nurse expect?
1. An "olive" mass in the right upper quadrant
2. Passing ribbon-like stools
3. A "sausage" mass in the right upper quadrant
4. Aching during and after feedings

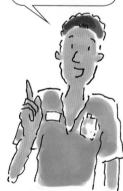

Yuck! I never did like olives.

73. 1. Pyloric stenosis involves hypertrophy of the circular muscle fibers of the pylorus. This hypertrophy is palpable as an "olive" mass in the right upper quadrant of the abdomen. Ribbon-like stool is noted in children with Hirschsprung's disease. A "sausage" mass is palpable in the right upper quadrant in children with intussusception. Arching is noted in children with reflux.
CN: Physiological integrity; CNS: Physiological adaptation; CL: Apply

74. A 5-year-old child is admitted with diarrhea and vomiting for the past 2 days. Vital signs are: temperature, 98.8° F (37.1° C); pulse, 132 beats/minute; respirations, 28 breaths/minute; and blood pressure, 88/56 mm Hg. The nurse notes poor skin turgor, dry mucous membranes, and tearless crying. Which intervention will the nurse perform **next**?
1. Obtain a stool specimen, complete blood count (CBC), and blood chemistries.
2. Implement nothing-by-mouth (NPO) status and start an IV.
3. Begin offering an oral electrolyte solution.
4. Obtain a blood culture and sensitivity test.

74. 2. This child shows signs of severe dehydration and should be put on NPO status to rest the bowel. An IV should be started immediately to begin the rehydration process. A stool specimen; hematocrit (HCT), CBC, and chemistries; and IV antibiotics may be prescribed, but they are not the priority intervention. There is no reason to suspect that the child will need a blood culture at this time because the temperature is not elevated.
CN: Physiological integrity; CNS: Basic care and comfort; CL: Analyze

75. The nurse caring for an infant with pyloric stenosis will expect which laboratory values?
1. pH, 7.30; chloride, 120 mEq/L (120 mmol/L)
2. pH, 7.38; chloride, 110 mEq/L (110 mmol/L)
3. pH, 7.43; chloride, 100 mEq/L (100 mmol/L)
4. pH, 7.49; chloride, 90 mEq/L (90 mmol/L)

75. 4. Infants with pyloric stenosis vomit hydrochloric acid. This causes them to become alkalotic and hypochloremic. Normal serum pH is 7.35 to 7.45; levels above 7.45 represent alkalosis. The normal serum chloride level is 99 to 111 mEq/L (99 to 111 mmol/L); levels below 99 mEq/L (99 mmol/L) represent hypochloremia.
CN: Physiological integrity; CNS: Physiological adaptation; CL: Analyze

76. A 13-month-old is admitted to the pediatric unit with a diagnosis of gastroenteritis. The toddler has experienced vomiting and diarrhea for the past 3 days, and laboratory tests reveal the child is dehydrated. Which nursing intervention(s) is appropriate? Select all that apply.
1. Provide the child a balanced diet.
2. Give clear liquids in small amounts.
3. Give milk as the child requests.
4. Provide the child non-salty soups and broths.
5. Monitor the IV solution per the health care provider's prescription.
6. Withhold all solid food and liquids until the symptoms pass.

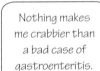

Nothing makes me crabbier than a bad case of gastroenteritis.

76. 2, 4, 5. A child experiencing nausea and vomiting will not be able to tolerate a regular diet. The child should be given sips of clear liquids, and the diet should be advanced as tolerated. Unsalted soups and broths are appropriate clear liquids. IV fluids should be monitored to maintain the fluid status and help to rehydrate the child. Milk should not be given because it can worsen the child's diarrhea. Solid foods may be withheld throughout the acute phase, but clear fluids should be encouraged in small amounts (3 to 4 tablespoons every half-hour).
CN: Physiological integrity; CNS: Basic care and comfort; CL: Apply

77. Which nursing intervention is **priority** when caring for a 1-month-old infant admitted with projectile vomiting after feeding?
1. Providing small, frequent, thickened feedings
2. Positioning child on the right side
3. Promoting breastfeeding
4. Weighing the infant daily

77. 2. Projectile vomiting in infants is a sign of pyloric stenosis, a condition that requires surgical correction. Positioning aspiration is a priority before and after surgical intervention. This is accomplished by positioning the infant on the right side or by elevating the head of the bassinette or crib slightly. Providing thickened and small, frequent feedings is a correct action but is not a priority over airway clearance. Promoting breastfeeding is also a correct action but is not a priority in this situation. Fluid and electrolyte imbalances can occur because of the vomiting, and the nurse should monitor for this by weighing the infant and monitoring for signs and symptoms of electrolyte imbalance; however, maintaining a patent airway takes priority.
CN: Physiological integrity; CNS: Reduction of risk potential; CL: Apply

78. The nurse is assigned to care for a child prescribed activated charcoal dosing 1 gram/kg orally via nasogastric tube once. The child weighs 51 lb (23.13 kg). The package insert reads: dilute 20 to 30 grams in 240 mL of water. How many grams of activated charcoal will the nurse administer to the child? Record your answer using a whole number.

_____ g

79. Which medication will the nurse prepare to administer to a child with confirmed ingestion of a toxic amount of acetaminophen?
1. Sodium bicarbonate
2. Dimercaprol
3. Acetylcysteine
4. Syrup of ipecac

80. Which intervention(s) will the nurse perform when assessing a child for a suspected ingestion of household bleach? Select all that apply.
1. Obtain a complete set of vital signs.
2. Inspect the mouth and oropharynx.
3. Monitor respiratory status.
4. Offer oral fluids.
5. Induce vomiting.

> Congrats—you finished the chapter! You're on top of the world.

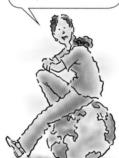

78. 23.
Multiply child's weight in kilograms by the dose:

$$23.13\ kg \times 1\ gram/kg = 23.13\ grams\ of\ activated\ charcoal$$

CN: Physiological integrity; CNS: Pharmacological and parenteral therapies; CL: Apply

79. 3. *N*-acetylcysteine is the antidote for acetaminophen overdose. Sodium bicarbonate is given for salicylate poisoning to correct the metabolic acidosis. Dimercaprol and deferoxamine are given for lead poisoning.

CN: Physiological integrity; CNS: Pharmacological and parenteral therapies; CL: Understand

80. 1, 2, 3. Inspection of the face, mouth, and oropharynx gathers assessment data to support a suspected ingestion of bleach. The mucous membranes, lips, and oropharynx will have a white appearance. Obtaining a complete set of vital signs provides additional data for the assessment. Monitoring respiratory status is important as the child is at risk for respiratory compromise if bleach was consumed. The nurse will not offer fluids until a diagnosis is made to see if fluids are appropriate. Inducing vomiting is an incorrect treatment for the ingestion of a corrosive agent.

CN: Physiological integrity; CNS: Physiological adaptation; CL: Apply

Chapter 32

Endocrine Disorders

Pediatric endocrine refresher

Diabetes mellitus type 1

Chronic metabolic syndrome that is auto-immune in origin. Destruction of the beta cells of the pancreas results in lack of insulin production.

Key signs and symptoms

- Polydipsia
- Polyphagia
- Polyuria
- Insidious onset with lethargy, weakness, and weight loss
- If left untreated, ketoacidosis will develop

Key test results

- Fasting plasma glucose level (no calorie intake for at least 8 hours) is greater than or equal to 126 mg/dL (6.99 mmol/L)
- Plasma glucose value in the 2-hour sample of the oral glucose tolerance test is greater than or equal to 200 mg/dL (11.1 mmol/L); this test should be performed after a loading dose of 75 g of anhydrous glucose
- A random plasma glucose value (obtained without regard to the time of the child's last food intake) greater than or equal to 200 mg/dL (11.1 mmol/L) accompanied by symptoms of diabetes indicates diabetes
- Glycosylated hemoglobin (HbA1c): 6%–9% (0.06–0.09) represents good control, values greater than 12% (0.12) indicate poor control

Key treatments

- Well-balanced diet that meets growth and development needs while distributing food intake so that the diet aids metabolic control; should be individualized in accordance with the child's ethnicity, age, sex, weight, activity level, family economics, and personal preference
- Precise insulin administration
- Regular exercise

Key interventions

- Monitor vital signs, intake, output, and blood glucose.

- Provide appropriate treatment for hyperglycemia and hypoglycemia.
- Teach the child and parents about:
  - complying with the prescribed treatment program
  - monitoring blood glucose levels at home
  - rotating injection sites
  - preventing, recognizing, and treating hypoglycemia and hyperglycemia at home.

Hypothyroidism

Deficiency in hormone secretions of the thyroid gland. It may be congenital or acquired (autoimmune/Hashimoto's thyroiditis).

Key signs and symptoms

Untreated hypothyroidism in infants
- Hoarse crying
- Poor feeding
- Persistent jaundice
- Large fontanelles
- Puffy face and swollen tongue
- Sluggish, sleeps a lot, floppy when handled
- If left untreated, irreversible mental retardation and physical disabilities result

Untreated hypothyroidism in older children
- Growth retardation (short stature)
- Delayed puberty
- Delayed skeletal maturation
- Cognitive impairment
- Weight gain
- Fatigue
- Constipation
- Coarse, dry hair

Key test results

- Thyroid function studies confirm hypothyroidism with low thyroxine levels (T_4), elevated thyroid stimulating hormone (TSH), and normal triiodothyronine (T_3) levels
- Screening test for hypothyroidism is routinely performed at birth in the United States and Canada

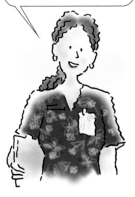

Caring for a child with an endocrine system disorder can be overwhelming. To get started on the right track, check out the website of the Juvenile Diabetes Research Foundation at www.jdrf.org. Go for it!

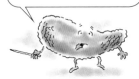

When it comes to diabetes mellitus type 1, remember the three polys: -dipsia, -phagia, and –uria.

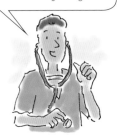

Hypothyroidism means low (hypo) hormone secretions from the thyroid gland.

617

Key treatments

- Oral thyroid hormone: levothyroxine
- Supplemental vitamin D: calcitriol (to prevent rickets from rapid bone growth)

Key interventions

- During early management of infantile hypothyroidism, monitor blood pressure and pulse rate and report hypertension and tachycardia immediately.
- Check axillary temperature every 2 to 4 hours; keep infant warm and skin moist.
- If the infant's tongue is unusually large, position side-lying and observe frequently.
- Teach child and parents to recognize signs of supplemental thyroid hormone overdose (rapid pulse rate, irritability, insomnia, fever, sweating, weight loss).

Hyperthyroidism (Graves' disease)

Overproduction in hormone secretions of the thyroid gland

Key signs and symptoms

Hyperthyroidism in infants
- Tachycardia
- Hypertension
- Goiter
- Irritability
- Difficulty feeding

Hyperthyroidism in older children
- Weight loss
- Heat intolerance
- Hyperactivity
- Goiter
- Tachycardia
- Hypertension
- Emotional lability
- Exophthalmos
- Growth acceleration
- Delayed puberty
- Advanced bone age

Key test results

- Thyroid function studies confirm hyperthyroidism with elevated thyroxine levels (T_4) and triiodothyronine (T_3) levels and decreased, possibly undetectable thyroid stimulating hormone (TSH) levels
- Thyroid ultrasound

Key treatments

- Oral antithyroid medication: methimazole
- Beta-blocking agents: propranolol, atenolol
- Radioactive iodine
- Thyroidectomy

Key interventions

- Monitor for thyroid storm if untreated for a long period of time.
- Monitor blood pressure and pulse.
- Accurately measure and document weight.
- Provide family teaching regarding medication administration and side effects.

Diabetes insipidus

Insufficient antidiuretic hormone (ADH) secreted by the pituitary gland, resulting in excretion of copious volumes of urine. Diabetes insipidus can be central, caused by damage to the pituitary gland, or nephrogenic, caused by a defect in the tubules of the kidneys.

Key signs and symptoms

- Polydipsia (consumption of 4 to 40 L/day)
- Polyuria (greater than 5 L/day of dilute urine)
- Dehydration
- Infant: Irritability, poor feeding, failure to grow, high fevers

Key test results

- Urine chemistry shows:
  - urine specific gravity less than 1.005
  - osmolality 50 to 200 mOsm/kg (50 to 200 mmol/L)
  - decreased urine pH
  - decreased sodium and potassium levels.

Key treatments

- IV therapy: hydration (when first diagnosed, intake and output must be matched milliliter to milliliter to prevent dehydration), electrolyte replacement
- Synthetic drugs with ADH activity that reduce urine output: desmopressin acetate, vasopressin, or lypressin

Key interventions

- Monitor fluid balance and daily weight.
- Monitor and record vital signs, intake, output (urine output should be measured every hour when first diagnosed), urine specific gravity (check every 1 to 2 hours when first diagnosed), and laboratory studies.
- Maintain IV fluid.
- Teach family about medication: signs and symptoms of disorder which indicate a need for desmopressin acetate, and signs and symptoms of over-dosage (decreased urine output, headache, fluid retention, weight gain).

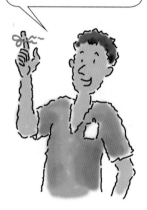

Remember—polyuria means "much urine"; that is, you have to pee a lot.

Growth hormone deficiency (idiopathic hypopituitarism or idiopathic growth hormone failure)

Diminished secretion of growth hormone by the pituitary gland

Key signs and symptoms
- Short stature but proportional height and weight
- Delayed epiphyseal closure

Key test results
- Decreased growth hormone levels (peak < 10 ng/mL [<10 µg/L] on stimulation test)
- Insulin-like growth factor 1 (IGF-1)
- Bone-age radiographs of the hand

Key treatments
- Somatropin (human growth hormone) subcutaneous injection given at bedtime
- Growth hormone therapy lasts until the conclusion of growth during late puberty

Key interventions
- Accurate measurement, documentation, and interpretation of height.
- Family teaching regarding medication administration (technique for administration, site selection and rotation, administer at bedtime).
- Child 10 years of age or older can learn to self-administer the drug.
- Promote positive body image.

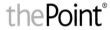 **the Point**® You can download tables of drug information to help you prepare for the NCLEX®! View Generic Drug Names, Drug Classifications, Drug Actions, and Nursing Implications for the drugs discussed in this refresher at **http://thePoint.lww.com**

Endocrine questions, answers, and rationales

1. The nurse explains the causes of hypothyroidism to the parents of a newly diagnosed infant. The nurse recognizes further education is needed when the parents ask which question(s)? Select all that apply.
1. "So, hypothyroidism can be only temporary, right?"
2. "Are you saying this is caused by a problem in the way the thyroid gland developed?"
3. "Do you mean this may be caused by a problem in the way the body makes thyroxine?"
4. "So, this is a condition that will require thyroid replacement therapy for life?"
5. "Hypothyroidism can be treated by exposing our baby to a special light, right?"

In question #1, you're looking for incorrect statements from the parents.

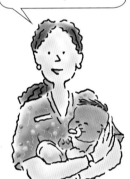

2. An infant with hypothyroidism is receiving oral thyroid hormone. Which assessment finding(s) will the nurse **immediately** report to the health care provider? Select all that apply.
1. Tachycardia
2. Excessive sleepiness
3. Irritability
4. Diaphoresis
5. Bradycardia
6. Dry, scaly skin
7. Cool extremities

3. The nurse is caring for a child with hyperthyroidism and notes exophthalmos. Which nursing action is **most** appropriate?
1. Notify the health care provider.
2. Hold the next dose of methimazole.
3. Assess the thyroxine (T₄) level.
4. Document the finding.

1. 4, 5. Congenital hypothyroidism can be permanent or transient and may result from a defective thyroid gland or an enzymatic defect in thyroxine synthesis. Phototherapy is not used to treat physiologic jaundice and indicates that the parents need more information. Thyroid replacement therapy can be a lifelong treatment. However, because some congenital hypothyroidism is transient, the child is reevaluated at age 3 for continued need for thyroid replacement.
CN: Health promotion and maintenance; CNS: None; CL: Apply

2. 1, 3, 4. Clinical manifestations of thyroid hormone overdose in an infant include tachycardia, irritability, and diaphoresis. The nurse would first report finding of overdose to the health care provider. Bradycardia; excessive sleepiness; dry, scaly skin; and cool extremities are expected manifestations of hypothyroidism or inadequate hormone replacement (underdosage).
CN: Physiological integrity; CNS: Pharmacological and parenteral therapies; CL: Apply

3. 4. Exophthalmos occurs when there is an overproduction of thyroid hormone and is an expected finding in clients with hyperthyroidism. The nurse would document the findings. The other actions are not appropriate. Methimazole is an antithyroid medication given to limit symptoms.
CN: Health promotion and maintenance; CNS: None; CL: Analyze

CN: Client needs category   CNS: Client needs subcategory   CL: Cognitive level

4. The nurse is educating parents of a neonate newly diagnosed with hypothyroidism. Which statement will the nurse include in the teaching?
1. "A goiter in a neonate does not present a problem."
2. "Preterm neonates usually are not affected by hypothyroidism."
3. "Hypothyroidism does not require medication treatment."
4. "The severity of the disorder depends on the amount of thyroid tissue present."

5. When assessing an infant, which finding(s) will cause the nurse to suspect hypothyroidism? Select all that apply.
1. Diarrhea
2. Lethargy
3. Severe jaundice
4. Poor feeding
5. Tachycardia
6. Hypotonia

6. Which result(s) of a male child will the nurse report to the health care provider? Select all that apply.
1. Thyroxine (T$_4$) level 1.1 µg/dL (14.16 nmol/L)
2. Triiodothyronine (T$_3$) 200 ng/dL (3.08 nmol/L)
3. TSH level 10 mU/L
4. Calcitonin 15 pg/mL (4.38 pmol/L)
5. Testosterone 500 ng/dL (17.35 nmol/L)

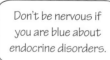
Don't be nervous if you are blue about endocrine disorders.

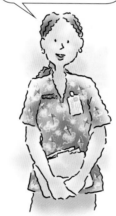

7. When assessing a neonate with congenital hypothyroidism, which finding requires **immediate** intervention by the nurse?
1. Anemia
2. Cyanosis
3. Retarded bone age
4. Delayed central nervous system (CNS) development

8. When caring for an 11-month-old infant with congenital hypothyroidism, which finding **most** concerns the nurse?
1. The infant began treatment at 9 months of age.
2. The infant's thyroxine (T$_4$) level is 6 µg/dL (77.23 nmol/L).
3. The infant is currently taking levothyroxine daily.
4. The infant has gained 10 lb (4.5 kg) since birth.

4. 4. The severity of hypothyroidism depends on the amount of thyroid tissue present. The more thyroid tissue present, the less severe the disorder. Usually, the neonate does not exhibit obvious signs of the disorder because of maternal circulation. A large goiter in a neonate could possibly occlude the airway and lead to obstruction. Hyperthyroidism treatment includes administration of levothyroxine.
CN: Physiological integrity; CNS: Physiological adaptation; CL: Apply

5. 2, 4, 6. Signs of hypothyroidism that may be seen shortly after birth include lethargy, poor feeding, prolonged jaundice, respiratory difficulty, cyanosis, hypotonia, constipation, and bradycardia. Diarrhea and severe jaundice are not normal signs of hypothyroidism. Tachycardia typically occurs in hyperthyroidism, not hypothyroidism.
CN: Physiological integrity; CNS: Physiological adaptation; CL: Apply

6. 1, 3. The nurse will report abnormal values to the health care provider. Screening results that show a low T$_4$ level (normal range is 4 to 12.3 µg/dL [51.48 to 158.31 nmol/L]) and a high TSH level (normal range is 0.35 to 5.5 mU/L) indicate congenital hypothyroidism and the need for further testing to determine the cause of the disease. T$_3$ (normal range is 60 to 171 ng/dL [0.92 to 2.63 nmol/L]) and testosterone (normal range is 300 to 1200 ng/dL [10.41 to 41.64 nmol/L]) are in normal range, which is expected with congenital hypothyroidism. Calcitonin level (3 to 26 pg/mL [0.88 to 7.59 pmol/L]) may be decreased.
CN: Physiological integrity; CNS: Reduction of risk potential; CL: Analyze

7. 2. The nurse would be most concerned if cyanosis is noted as this indicates airway compromise. This could be a result of an enlarged tongue, cognitive damage, or lethargy. The other findings are concerning, but airway is priority.
CN: Safe, effective care environment; CNS: Management of care; CL: Analyze

8. 1. The severity of the intellectual deficit is related to the degree of hypothyroidism and the duration of the condition before treatment. The nurse would be concerned about potential cognitive impairment with delayed treatment. The T$_4$ level is within normal range. The infant should be taking levothyroxine daily and this will continue throughout life. The infant has gained an appropriate amount of weight since birth for the age.
CN: Safe, effective care environment; CNS: Management of care; CL: Analyze

9. The nurse is caring for an adolescent diagnosed with Graves' disease prescribed methimazole. Which laboratory finding will the nurse flag for the health care provider to review?
1. White blood cell (WBC) count 9,000 mm³ (9.0 ×10⁹/L)
2. Thyroxine (T₄) level 10.5 μg/dL (135.15 nmol/L)
3. Prothrombin time (PT) level 19 seconds
4. Triiodothyronine (T₃) 150 ng/dL (2.31 nmol/L)

10. The nurse is providing education on therapeutic management to parents of a neonate diagnosed with congenital hyperthyroidism. Which response by a parent indicates the need for further education?
1. "My baby will need regular measurements of thyroxine levels."
2. "Treatment involves lifelong thyroid hormone replacement therapy."
3. "Treatment should begin as soon as possible after diagnosis is made."
4. "As my baby grows, the thyroid gland will mature and medication will not be needed."

11. Which comment made by the parent of a neonate at a 2-week office visit will cause the nurse to suspect congenital hypothyroidism?
1. "My baby is unusually quiet and good."
2. "My baby seems to study my face during feeding time."
3. "After feedings, my baby pulls the legs up and cries."
4. "My baby seems to be a yellowish color."

12. Which statement(s) will the nurse include when providing education to a parent about giving levothyroxine to the neonate diagnosed with hypothyroidism? Select all that apply.
1. "Administer in the morning, at the same time each day."
2. "The drug has a bitter taste."
3. "The pill should not be crushed."
4. "Never put the medication in formula or juice."
5. "Give levothyroxine on an empty stomach."

13. The nurse is providing education to parents about signs that indicate levothyroxine overdose. Which comment by a parent indicates the need for further education?
1. "Irritability is a sign of overdose."
2. "If my baby's heartbeat is fast, I should count it."
3. "If my baby loses weight, I should be concerned."
4. "I should not worry if my baby does not sleep very much."

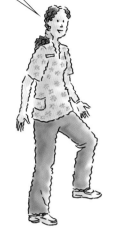

One step at a time … you can do it!

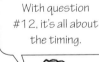

With question #12, it's all about the timing.

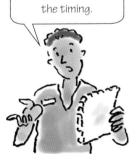

9. 3. The nurse would be most concerned about the client's PT level. Normal PT is 9.5 to 12 seconds. Methimazole can lower WBC and alter the body's ability to clot. All other levels are within normal range.
CN: Health promotion and maintenance; CNS: None; CL: Apply

10. 4. Treatment involves lifelong thyroid hormone replacement therapy that begins as soon as possible after diagnosis. The goal of treatment is to abolish all signs of hypothyroidism and to reestablish normal physical and mental development. The drug of choice is synthetic levothyroxine. Regular measurements of thyroxine levels are important in ensuring optimal treatment.
CN: Physiological integrity; CNS: Physiological adaptation; CL: Apply

11. 1. Parental remarks about an unusually "quiet and good" neonate, together with any of the early physical manifestations, should lead to a suspicion of hypothyroidism, which requires a referral for specific tests. The normal neonate likes looking at the human face and should show this interest at age 2 weeks. If the neonate is pulling the legs up and crying after feedings, he or she might be showing signs of colic. If a neonate begins to look yellow in color, hyperbilirubinemia may be the cause.
CN: Health promotion and maintenance; CNS: None; CL: Analyze

12. 1, 5. Levothyroxine should be administered daily at a consistent time. Morning is the ideal time. The medication is best absorbed on an empty stomach, given 1 hour before or 2 hours after meals. The importance of compliance with the drug regimen must be emphasized for the neonate to achieve normal growth and development. Because the drug is flavorless, it can be crushed and added to formula or breast milk.
CN: Physiological integrity; CNS: Pharmacological and parenteral therapies; CL: Apply

13. 4. Parents need to be aware of signs indicating overdose, such as insomnia, rapid pulse, dyspnea, irritability, fever, sweating, and weight loss. The parents are given acceptable parameters for the heart rate and weight loss or gain. If the baby is experiencing a heart rate or weight loss outside of the acceptable parameters, the health care provider should be called.
CN: Physiological integrity; CNS: Pharmacological and parenteral therapies; CL: Apply

CN: Client needs category   CNS: Client needs subcategory   CL: Cognitive level

14. The nurse is assessing a child with juvenile hypothyroidism. Which common clinical finding(s) will the nurse likely observe? Select all that apply.
1. Accelerated growth
2. Constipation
3. Dry skin
4. Fatigue
5. Insomnia

15. The nurse is caring for a preschool-age child with Hashimoto's thyroiditis. Which finding(s) will the nurse report to the health care provider? Select all that apply.
1. Fatigue
2. Reports of feeling cool
3. Pale appearance
4. Heart rate 130 bpm
5. Mild enlargement of the tongue
6. Hair loss
7. Dry skin

16. When counseling parents of a neonate with congenital hypothyroidism desiring to have another baby, the nurse will encourage which action?
1. Seek professional genetic counseling.
2. Retrace the family tree for others born with this condition.
3. Talk to relatives who have gone through a similar experience.
4. Consider adoption to prevent having another affected baby.

17. Which symptom(s) will lead the nurse to suspect a child is experiencing hypoglycemia? Select all that apply.
1. Irritability
2. Drowsiness
3. Headache
4. Abdominal pain
5. Nausea and vomiting
6. Hunger
7. Jitteriness

18. The parents of a child with diabetes mellitus type 1 ask the nurse if their child can continue to play soccer. Which response by the nurse is **most** appropriate?
1. "Your child will need to increase food intake on days the child plays soccer."
2. "We need to wait and see how your child responds to insulin before making a decision."
3. "It is not recommended for children with diabetes to participate in strenuous activities."
4. "It will increase the risk of hypoglycemia, so you may not want your child to play soccer."

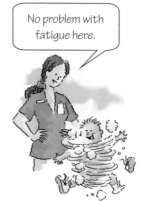

No problem with fatigue here.

Uh oh. Looks like another breakdown in insulin production.

14. 2, 3, 4. Children with hypothyroidism have dry skin, fatigue, constipation, and dry, brittle hair. The other clinical findings are not evident in children with juvenile hypothyroidism.
CN: Health promotion and maintenance; CNS: None; CL: Apply

15. 4. Hashimoto's thyroiditis (autoimmune hypothyroidism) results in inadequate thyroid production to meet a child's needs. The nurse would report tachycardia because it is not an expected finding in Hashimoto's thyroiditis. Clinical signs include fatigue; sensitivity to cold; pale, dry skin; bradycardia; enlarged tongue (would be reported if the client was having respiratory distress); hair loss; brittle nails; and constipation.
CN: Safe, effective care environment; CNS: Management of care; CL: Apply

16. 1. Seeking professional genetic counseling is the best option for parents who have a neonate with a genetic disorder and are desiring to have another baby. Retracing the family tree and talking to relatives will not help the parents understand the chance of having another baby with a genetic disorder. Telling the couple to consider adoption is not appropriate.
CN: Health promotion and maintenance; CNS: None; CL: Apply

17. 1, 3, 6, 7. Signs of hypoglycemia include irritability, shaky feeling, hunger, headache, and dizziness. Drowsiness, abdominal pain, nausea, and vomiting are signs of hyperglycemia.
CN: Physiological integrity; CNS: Physiological adaptation; CL: Apply

18. 1. If a child is more active at one time of the day than another, food or insulin should be altered to meet the child's activity pattern. Food intake should be increased when a child with diabetes mellitus type 1 is more physically active. Children with diabetes mellitus type 1 are encouraged to continue physical activity. Hypoglycemia is a risk but should not deter the child from continuing normal activities. Interventions should be taken to prevent hypoglycemia.
CN: Physiological integrity; CNS: Reduction of risk potential; CL: Apply

19. An adolescent with diabetes tells the nurse, "I recently started drinking alcohol on the weekends." Which action is **most** appropriate for the nurse to take?
1. Refer the adolescent to counseling.
2. Make the adolescent promise to stop drinking.
3. Discuss with the adolescent reasons for drinking.
4. Educate the adolescent about the effects of alcohol on diabetes.

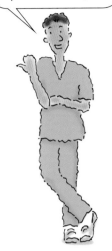

The words "**most appropriate**" are the key to getting question #19 right.

20. The nurse is providing education to an adolescent diagnosed with diabetes mellitus type 1. Which instruction by the nurse about preventing hypoglycemia is **most** appropriate?
1. "Limit participation in planned exercise activities that involve competition."
2. "Carry crackers or fruit to eat before or during periods of increased activity."
3. "Increase the insulin dosage before planned or unplanned strenuous exercise."
4. "Check blood glucose level before exercising, and eat a protein snack if elevated."

21. The nurse is caring for a 2-year-old child admitted for new onset diabetes mellitus type 1. Which finding(s) concerns the nurse? Select all that apply.
1. Increased appetite
2. Seizure
3. Decreased fluid intake
4. Weight loss
5. Frequent urination

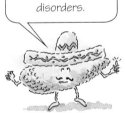

Muy bueno! You really know your endocrine disorders.

22. At 1130 the nurse is admitting a pediatric client diagnosed with diabetic ketoacidosis. Which prescription will the nurse complete **first**?
1. Order a diabetic lunch tray for the client.
2. Obtain intravenous (IV) access.
3. Consult diabetes center to see client.
4. Obtain urine specimen for a urinalysis.

19. 4. The adolescent must be taught the effects of alcohol on diabetes mellitus. Ingestion of alcohol inhibits the release of glycogen from the liver, resulting in hypoglycemia. Teens who drink alcohol may become hypoglycemic, manifesting behaviors that are similar to intoxication including shakiness, combativeness, slurred speech, and loss of consciousness. Recommending that the teen see a counselor is a good option, but the adolescent should first be taught about the effects of alcohol consumption. The nurse cannot stop an adolescent from doing something if the teen does not understand why it is wrong. Discussing the reason for the adolescent's drinking should be left up to the counselor.

CN: Health promotion and maintenance; CNS: None; CL: Apply

20. 2. Hypoglycemia can usually be prevented if an adolescent with diabetes mellitus type 1 eats more food before or during exercise. Because exercise with adolescents is not commonly planned, carrying additional carbohydrate foods such as crackers or fruit is a good preventive measure.

CN: Health promotion and maintenance; CNS: None; CL: Apply

21. 2, 3. The nurse would be most concerned about seizures and decreased fluid intake as these are not expected findings in a child with diabetes mellitus type 1. Polyphagia, polyuria, polydipsia, and weight loss are cardinal signs of diabetes mellitus type 1. Other signs include irritability, shortened attention span, lowered frustration tolerance, fatigue, dry skin, blurred vision, sores that are slow to heal, and flushed skin. If on initial presentation the child was in diabetic ketoacidosis, signs and symptoms would include fruity odor to the breath, Kussmaul respirations, and stupor.

CN: Health promotion and maintenance; CNS: None; CL: Apply

22. 2. Diabetic ketoacidosis, the most complete state of insulin deficiency, is a life-threatening situation. The child should be admitted to an intensive care facility for management, which consists of rapid assessment, adequate insulin to reduce the elevated blood glucose level, fluids to overcome dehydration, and electrolyte replacement (especially potassium). The nurse would first obtain IV access to administer IV fluids, IV insulin, and IV electrolytes. The nurse would then obtain a urine specimen, order the client a lunch tray, and complete the consult.

CN: Safe, effective care environment; CNS: Management of care; CL: Analyze

23. The nurse is caring for an adolescent client recently diagnosed with diabetes mellitus type 1. Which adolescent consideration(s) will the nurse consider when planning care for this client? Select all that apply.
   1. Desire to be an individual
   2. Desire to be like peers
   3. Preoccupation with future plans
   4. Ability to educate peers about the disease
   5. Desire to become independent of parents

24. While educating the parents of an infant diagnosed with diabetes insipidus, the nurse will include which treatment?
   1. Blood product administration
   2. Antihypertensive medications
   3. Hormone replacement
   4. Fluid restrictions

25. The nurse is preparing a mixed insulin injection of 15 units of humulin N and 5 units of humulin R for a child with diabetes mellitus type 1. Place the steps in the order the nurse will perform them. Use all options.

   1. Wipe the stoppers of both vials of insulin with alcohol.

   2. Inject 5 units of air into the humulin R vial.

   3. Draw up 5 units of humulin R.

   4. Draw up 15 units of humulin N.

   5. Inject 15 units of air into the vial of humulin N.

   6. Gently roll the bottle of humulin N in the hands.

   7. Draw up 20 units of air into the insulin syringe.

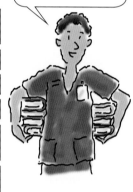

Question #25 is about putting the steps in the right order.

23. **2, 5.** Adolescents appear to have the most difficulty adjusting to diabetes mellitus type 1. Adolescence is a time when being "perfect" and being like one's peers are emphasized, and having diabetes mellitus means the adolescent is different. One of the tasks of adolescents is to become independent from their parents and develop decision-making skills.
CN: Safe, effective care environment; CNS: Management of care; CL: Apply

24. **3.** The usual treatment for diabetes insipidus is hormone replacement with vasopressin or desmopressin (DDAVP). Blood products should not be needed. Hypertension is not associated with this condition, and fluids should not be restricted.
CN: Physiological integrity; CNS: Pharmacological and parenteral therapies; CL: Apply

25. Ordered Response:

   6. Gently roll the bottle of humulin N in the hands.

   1. Wipe the stoppers of both vials of insulin with alcohol.

   7. Draw up 20 units of air into the insulin syringe.

   5. Inject 15 units of air into the vial of humulin N.

   2. Inject 5 units of air into the humulin R vial.

   3. Draw up 5 units of humulin R.

   4. Draw up 15 units of humulin N.

Mixing insulins begins with washing the hands, followed by gently rolling the vial of humulin N (cloudy insulin). The intermediate acing insulin can precipitate; therefore, it must be mixed well before drawing up. Wipe the stoppers of both vials of insulin with alcohol. Twenty units of air is drawn into the insulin syringe—first 15 units of air are injected into the humulin N vial and then 5 units of air are injected into the humulin R vial. Without removing the needle from the humulin R vial, it is inverted and 5 units of humulin R are drawn up. The needle is then inserted in the topper of the humulin N vial, the vial is inverted, and 15 units of humulin N are drawn up. The regular insulin (humulin R) is drawn up first to prevent contamination of the regular insulin vial with the intermediate acting insulin (humulin N). The mnemonic "clear to cloudy" helps to remember to draw up the regular insulin first. The humulin N is drawn up to the 20-unit marking, as the 15 units are added to 5 units of humulin R drawn up initially.
CN: Physiological integrity; CNS: Pharmacological and parenteral therapies; CL: Apply

26. A child has experienced symptoms of hypoglycemia and has eaten sugar cubes. Which nursing action is **most** appropriate?
1. Give the child apple juice.
2. Recheck the child in 30 minutes.
3. Request a fasting glucose level for the morning.
4. Give the child crackers with peanut butter.

26. 4. When a child exhibits signs of hypoglycemia, most cases can be treated with a simple concentrated sugar, such as honey or sugar cubes, that can be held in the mouth for a short time. This will elevate the blood glucose level and alleviate the symptoms. The simpler the carbohydrate, the more rapidly it will be absorbed. A complex carbohydrate and protein, such as a slice of bread or a cracker spread with peanut butter, should follow the rapid-releasing sugar, or the child may become hypoglycemic again. The nurse will reassess the child, but immediate intervention is needed. A fasting glucose is not needed.
CN: Health promotion and maintenance; CNS: None; CL: Apply

27. The nurse is educating an 11-year-old child recently diagnosed with diabetes mellitus about insulin injections. On which consideration will the nurse base the teaching?
1. The parents do not need to be involved in learning this procedure.
2. Self-injection techniques are not usually taught until the child reaches age 16.
3. At age 11, the child should be old enough to give injections independently.
4. Self-injection techniques should be taught only when the child can reach all injection sites.

27. 3. The parents must supervise and manage the child's therapeutic program, but the child should assume responsibility for self-management as soon as possible. Children can learn to collect their own blood for glucose testing at a relatively young age (4 to 5 years), and most can check their blood glucose level and administer insulin at all injection sites by about age 9. Some children can do it earlier.
CN: Health promotion and maintenance; CNS: None; CL: Apply

28. A child with diabetes mellitus type 1 tells the nurse, "I feel shaky." The nurse notes the child's skin is pale and sweaty. Which action will nurse initiate **immediately**?
1. Hold the next dose of insulin.
2. Give a 4 mg dextrose tablet to the child.
3. Administer glucagon subcutaneously.
4. Offer the child peanut butter and milk.

28. 2. Shakiness and pale, sweaty skin are symptoms of hypoglycemia. Rapid treatment involves giving the alert child a glucose tablet or, if unavailable, a glass of glucose-containing liquid. Either would be followed by a complex carbohydrate snack and protein. Holding the next dose of insulin would be determined based on the glucose level at the time the dose is due. Glucagon would be given only if there were a risk of aspiration with oral glucose, such as if the child was semiconscious.
CN: Safe, effective care environment; CNS: Management of care; CL: Analyze

29. The parents of a child diagnosed with diabetes mellitus ask the nurse about maintaining metabolic control during a minor illness with loss of appetite. Which nursing response is **most** appropriate?
1. "Decrease your child's insulin by one-half of the usual dose when sick."
2. "Your child will probably have to be hospitalized to manage glucose levels when sick."
3. "Give your child increased amounts of clear liquids to prevent dehydration during illness."
4. "Substitute calorie-containing liquids for uneaten solid food during sickness."

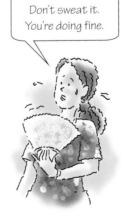

Don't sweat it. You're doing fine.

29. 4. Calorie-containing liquids can help maintain normal blood glucose levels as well as decrease the danger of dehydration. The child with diabetes mellitus should always take at least the usual dose of insulin during an illness, based on more frequent blood glucose checks. During an illness that involves vomiting or loss of appetite, NPH insulin may be lowered by 25% to 30% to avoid hyperglycemia, and regular insulin is given according to home glucose monitoring results. Minor illnesses usually do not require hospitalization. Giving increased amounts of clear liquids may prevent dehydration, but the child with diabetes mellitus should try to maintain caloric intake during illness.
CN: Safe, effective care environment; CNS: Management of care; CL: Apply

30. To increase the adolescent's compliance with treatment for diabetes mellitus, the nurse will attempt which strategy?
  1. Request a special diet in the high school cafeteria.
  2. Clarify the adolescent's values to promote involvement in care.
  3. Refer the adolescent to nutritional counseling.
  4. Educate the adolescent on long-term consequences of poor metabolic control.

30. **2.** Adolescent compliance with diabetes mellitus management may be hampered by "dependence versus independence" conflicts and ego development. Helping the adolescent clarify personal values fosters compliance and assists in psychosocial development. Providing for a special meal in the school cafeteria is not feasible and draws unwanted attention to the adolescent. The adolescent will be referred for nutritional counseling; however, the nurse would work with the adolescent too. An adolescent is usually concerned only with the present, not the future.
CN: Health promotion and maintenance; CNS: None; CL: Apply

31. The parent of a child with diabetes mellitus asks the nurse why blood glucose monitoring is needed. The nurse will base the reply on which premise?
  1. This is an easier method of testing.
  2. This is a less expensive method of testing.
  3. This allows children the ability to better manage their diabetes.
  4. This gives children a greater sense of control over their diabetes.

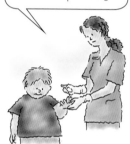

Teaching kids about their conditions and how to manage them can be empowering.

31. **3.** Blood glucose monitoring improves diabetes mellitus management and is used successfully by children from the onset of their diabetes. By testing their own blood, children can change their insulin regimen to maintain their glucose level in the normoglycemic range of 60 to 100 mg/dL (3.33 to 5.55 mmol/L). This allows them to better manage their diabetes mellitus. Glucose monitoring is the preferred method to monitor diabetes mellitus.
CN: Health promotion and maintenance; CNS: None; CL: Understand

32. Which criteria will the nurse use to measure good metabolic control in a child with diabetes mellitus?
  1. Fewer than eight episodes of severe hyperglycemia in 1 month
  2. Infrequent occurrences of mild hypoglycemic reactions
  3. Hemoglobin A1c values less than 12%
  4. Growth below the 15th percentile

32. **2.** Criteria for good metabolic control generally include few episodes of hypoglycemia or hyperglycemia, hemoglobin A1c values less than 8%, and normal growth and development.
CN: Health promotion and maintenance; CNS: None; CL: Apply

33. The nurse is preparing to discharge a school-age child with newly diagnosed diabetes mellitus. The parents express concern about the accommodations needed when the child returns to school. Which recommendation(s) will nurse include in discharge teaching? Select all that apply.
  1. A schedule for blood glucose testing with target ranges and interventions
  2. A written plan for the school to follow regarding insulin administration
  3. Home schooling to decrease the risk of complications
  4. No participation in physical education or recess
  5. Education for appropriate school staff about care that will be needed

33. **1, 2, 5.** It is important for the parents to feel confident the child will be safe in the school environment. The school care plan should include a schedule for when blood glucose testing should be done, what the target ranges are, and any interventions to be done for low or high blood sugars. If the child is to receive insulin injections at school, that aspect of the prescription should be specified. It is important for proper education of the school personnel who will be providing care at school. Home schooling is not recommended. It is important to keep the child's life as normal as possible. Regular exercise is an important part of the child's treatment plan, so physical activity is not restricted.
CN: Safe, effective care environment; CNS: Management of care; CL: Apply

34. The nurse is providing education regarding hypoglycemia to the parents of a child with diabetes mellitus. The nurse will inform the client and parents that which situation(s) can cause hypoglycemia? Select all that apply.
1. Taking less insulin than prescribed
2. Mild illness with a fever
3. Skipping a meal
4. Excessive exercise without a carbohydrate snack
5. Eating ice cream and cake to celebrate a birthday

34. **3, 4.** Excessive exercise without a carbohydrate snack could cause hypoglycemia. Skipping a meal can also result in hypoglycemia. The other conditions cause hyperglycemia.

CN: Health promotion and maintenance; CNS: None; CL: Analyze

35. Which assessment tool provides the **best** reflection of glycemic control of a child with diabetes mellitus during the preceding 2 to 3 months?
1. Fasting glucose level
2. Oral glucose tolerance test
3. Glycosylated hemoglobin level
4. The client's record of glucose monitoring

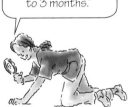

Looking for a clue to answer question #35? Focus on "2 to 3 months."

35. **3.** A glycosylated hemoglobin level provides an overview of a person's blood glucose level over the previous 2 to 3 months. Glycosylated hemoglobin values are reported as a percentage of the total hemoglobin to which glucose is bound within an erythrocyte. The time frame is based on the fact that the usual life span of an erythrocyte is 2 to 3 months; a random blood sample will theoretically give samples of erythrocytes for this same period. The other assessment factors will not provide a true picture of the person's blood glucose level over the previous 2 to 3 months.

CN: Health promotion and maintenance; CNS: None; CL: Apply

36. An adolescent client has received diet instruction as part of the treatment plan for diabetes mellitus type 1. Which statement by the adolescent indicates to the nurse the need for additional instruction?
1. "I will need a bedtime snack because I take an evening dose of NPH insulin."
2. "I can eat whatever I want as long as I cover the calories with sufficient insulin."
3. "I can have an occasional low-calorie drink as long as I include it in my meal plan."
4. "I should eat meals as scheduled, even if I am not hungry, to prevent hypoglycemia."

36. **2.** The goal of diet therapy in diabetes mellitus is to attain and maintain ideal body weight. Each pediatric client with diabetes mellitus will be prescribed a specific caloric intake and insulin regimen to help accomplish this goal.

CN: Physiological integrity; CNS: Basic care and comfort; CL: Apply

37. A child with diabetes mellitus is brought by the parents to the emergency department. The nurse observes a flushed face and drowsiness, and detects a fruity odor to the breath. The parents report the child has become progressively worse over the course of the day. The nurse suspects the child is experiencing which condition(s)? Select all that apply.
1. Hyperglycemia
2. Insulin overdose
3. Somogyi phenomenon
4. Ketoacidosis
5. Hypoglycemia

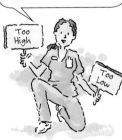

Remember: hyper means "too high" and hypo means "too low."

37. **1, 4.** In ketoacidosis, the blood glucose is markedly elevated. The child's skin is dry, and the face is flushed. The breath has a fruity odor. Insulin overdose produces hypoglycemia. Hypoglycemia is characterized by irritability, pallor, sweating, reports of hunger, and weakness. Somogyi phenomenon is rebound hyperglycemia in clients requiring fairly large doses of insulin. Hypoglycemia during the night with marked hyperglycemia in the morning is suggestive of Somogyi phenomenon.

CN: Physiological integrity; CNS: Physiological adaptation; CL: Analyze

38. The nurse is teaching an adolescent with diabetes mellitus how to mix regular and NPH insulins in the same syringe. Which action by the adolescent indicates the need for further instruction from the nurse?
1. Withdraws the NPH insulin first
2. Injects air into the NPH insulin bottle first
3. After drawing up the first insulin, removes air bubbles from the syringe
4. Injects an amount of air equal to the desired dose of insulin

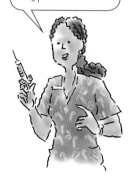

39. The nurse is caring for a child with excessive polyuria and polydipsia. Reviewing laboratory data reveals dehydration. Which medication will the nurse anticipate administering to this child?
1. Insulin
2. Desmopressin (DDAVP)
3. Levothyroxine
4. Propylthiouracil

40. When caring for a child with diabetes insipidus (DI), the nurse will question which prescription from the health care provider?
1. Administer desmopressin.
2. Increase dietary sodium intake.
3. Administer intravenous fluids.
4. Monitor urine output hourly.

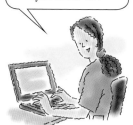

41. The nurse is providing education about home care to the parents of a child diagnosed with diabetes mellitus type 1. The nurse determines the education is successful when the parents make which statement(s)? Select all that apply.
1. "We can dispose of used lancets and insulin syringes in a puncture-proof container."
2. "I will be sure my child wears a medical alert bracelet."
3. "I should limit my child's exercise to prevent hypoglycemia."
4. "If my child takes insulin as prescribed, routine blood glucose checks are not needed."
5. "My child should receive immunizations for influenza and pneumonia."

42. An infant is diagnosed with diabetes insipidus (DI). The nurse will question the health care provider if which medication(s) is prescribed? Select all that apply.
1. NPH insulin
2. Glucose
3. Corticotropin
4. Aqueous vasopressin
5. Desmopressin

38. 1. Regular insulin is always withdrawn first so it will not become contaminated with NPH insulin. The adolescent with diabetes mellitus is instructed to inject air into the NPH insulin bottle equal to the amount of insulin to be withdrawn because there will be regular insulin in the syringe and the client will not be able to inject air when needing to withdraw the NPH. It is necessary to remove the air bubbles from the syringe to ensure a correct dosage before drawing up the second insulin.
CN: Physiological integrity; CNS: Pharmacological and parenteral therapies; CL: Apply

39. 2. The nurse would suspect the child has diabetes insipidus (DI). DDAVP is an antidiuretic used to treat DI. Insulin is used to treat diabetes mellitus type 1. Levothyroxine is synthetic thyroid hormone used to treat hypothyroidism. Propylthiouracil is an antithyroid used to treat hyperthyroidism.
CN: Health promotion and maintenance; CNS: None; CL: Analyze

40. 2. The nurse would question increasing dietary sodium for the client with DI. Increased sodium would lead to increased edema. Desmopressin is a synthetic antidiuretic hormone given to control polydipsia and polyuria. IV fluids are given to treat/prevent dehydration. It is important to frequently monitor urine output to gauge the status of the client.
CN: Safe, effective care environment; CNS: Management of care; CL: Apply

41. 1, 2, 5. Used lancets and syringes should be disposed of in a red biohazard container or a narrow, open, opaque, non-pierceable container like a bleach bottle. A medical alert bracelet identifying the child as having diabetes will be helpful in case of emergency. Prevention of influenza and pneumonia through immunization is important for the child's glycemic control and health. Exercise and regular monitoring of blood glucose levels are important components of the treatment program.
CN: Safe, effective care environment; CNS: Safety and infection control; CL: Apply

42. 1, 2, 3. The nurse would question insulin, glucose, and corticotropin in an infant diagnosed with DI. Aqueous vasopressin or desmopressin (DDAVP), which should alleviate the polyuria and polydipsia, are used to treat children with DI.
CN: Physiological integrity; CNS: Pharmacological and parenteral therapies; CL: Apply

CN: Client needs category   CNS: Client needs subcategory   CL: Cognitive level

43. Parents of a child prescribed growth hormone replacement ask the nurse, "When can our child stop taking this medicine?" Which statement will the nurse include when responding?
1. "The dosage of growth hormone will decrease as the child's age increases."
2. "The dosage will increase as the time of epiphyseal closure nears; then it is stopped."
3. "After giving growth hormone replacement for 1 year, your child can stop."
4. "The medication will be slowly tapered during the teenage years."

44. The nurse is providing education to an infant's parents about diagnostic testing for diabetes insipidus. The nurse knows which comment by the parents indicates an understanding of the teaching?
1. "Fluids will be offered every 2 hours."
2. "My infant's fluid intake will be restricted."
3. "My infant will be allowed to eat like normal."
4. "Formula will be restricted, but glucose water is okay."

45. The nurse is caring for a school-age client admitted for possible diabetes insipidus (DI). Which health care provider prescription will the nurse question?
1. Perform a 24-hour urine collection.
2. Assess serum electrolyte levels.
3. Check glycosylated hemoglobin (HbA1c) level.
4. Prepare client for a water deprivation test.

46. When providing information about treatment of diabetes insipidus to parents, a nurse explains the use of nasal spray and injections. The nurse understands which nasal spray requirement may deter the child's parent from choosing nasal spray treatment?
1. Applications must be repeated every 8 to 12 hours.
2. Urine testing is required weekly.
3. Nasal sprays can affect an infant's ability to smell.
4. Measuring the dose is difficult.

47. The nurse is providing education to parents of an infant newly diagnosed with diabetes insipidus. Which statement by the parent indicates an appropriate understanding of the nurse's teaching?
1. "When my infant stabilizes, I will not have to give hormone medication."
2. "I do not have to measure the amount of fluid intake that I give my infant."
3. "I realize that treatment for diabetes insipidus is lifelong."
4. "My infant will outgrow this condition by school age."

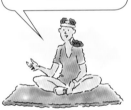

Feeling stressed? Close your eyes and take a deep breath. Everything is going to be fine.

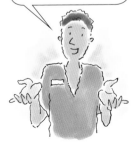

Unfortunately, diabetes insipidus is a condition that you don't outgrow.

43. 2. Dosage of growth hormone is increased as the time of epiphyseal closure nears to gain the most growth from the growth hormone. The medication is then stopped. There is no tapering of the dose.
CN: Physiological integrity; CNS: Pharmacological and parenteral therapies; CL: Apply

44. 2. The simplest test used to diagnose diabetes insipidus is restriction of oral fluids and observation of consequent changes in urine volume and concentration. A weight loss of 3% to 5% indicates severe dehydration, and the test should be terminated at this point. This test is done in the hospital while the infant is watched closely.
CN: Health promotion and maintenance; CNS: None; CL: Understand

45. 3. The nurse will question checking a HbA1c level because this is not related to DI. A HbA1c is performed on clients with diabetes mellitus type 1 or 2. To determine the type and severity of DI, the health care provider will assess electrolyte levels and urine, and may perform a water deprivation test.
CN: Safe, effective care environment; CNS: Management of care; CL: Apply

46. 1. Applications of nasal spray used to treat diabetes insipidus must be repeated every 8 to 12 hours; injections, although quite painful, last for 48 to 72 hours. The nasal spray must be timed for adequate night sleep. Nasal sprays have been used on infants with diabetes insipidus and are dispensed in premeasured intranasal inhalers, eliminating the need for measuring doses. Weekly urine testing is not required, and the sprays do not alter smelling.
CN: Physiological integrity; CNS: Pharmacological and parenteral therapies; CL: Apply

47. 3. Diabetes insipidus requires lifelong treatment. The amount of fluid intake is important and must be measured with the infant's output to monitor the medication regimen. The infant will not outgrow this condition.
CN: Safe, effective care environment; CNS: Management of care; CL: Apply

48. A child presents in the emergency department after being hit in the head by a baseball. The child begins to excrete extremely large amounts of urine and becomes dehydrated. Which prescription will the nurse question?
1. Administer intravenous fluids.
2. Administer hydrochlorothiazide.
3. Conduct neurologic checks hourly.
4. Administer desmopressin.

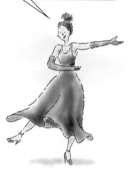

Spectacular! You've finished 48 questions already.

48. 2. The nurse suspects the child has central diabetes insipidus (DI), which can be acquired as the result of a head injury or tumor. The nurse would question hydrochlorothiazide; this is given to treat nephrogenic DI. All other prescriptions are expected in the treatment for central DI.
CN: Health promotion and maintenance; CNS: None; CL: Analyze

49. The nurse is providing education on injectable desmopressin to the parents of a child with diabetes insipidus. Which statement made by the parent indicates the need for further education from the nurse?
1. "I will hold the medicine under warm running water for 10 to 15 minutes before giving it."
2. "The medication must be shaken vigorously before being drawn up into the syringe."
3. "I will look in the suspension and expect to visualize small, brown particles."
4. "I will store this medication vial in the refrigerator."

49. 4. The medication should be stored at room temperature. When giving injectable desmopressin, it must be thoroughly resuspended in the oil by being held under warm running water for 10 to 15 minutes and shaken vigorously before being drawn into the syringe. If this is not done, the oil may be injected minus the drug. Small, brown particles, which indicate drug dispersion, must be seen in the suspension.
CN: Physiological integrity; CNS: Pharmacological and parenteral therapies; CL: Apply

50. Which assessment finding in a child receiving intranasal vasopressin will the nurse report to the health care provider?
1. Mucous membrane irritation
2. Severe coughing
3. Nosebleeds
4. Pneumonia

50. 1. Mucous membrane irritation caused by a cold or allergy renders the intranasal route of medication administration unreliable. Severe coughing, pneumonia, or nosebleeds should not interfere with the intranasal route of vasopressin administration.
CN: Physiological integrity; CNS: Pharmacological and parenteral therapies; CL: Analyze

51. Which action is appropriate for the registered nurse (RN) to delegation to the assistive personnel (AP)?
1. Determining the amount of insulin to give a child after checking glucose level
2. Decreasing the intravenous fluid rate of a child with diabetes insipidus
3. Applying oxygen via nasal cannula to a child with an oxygen saturation of 89%
4. Measuring the intake and output of a child experiencing ketoacidosis

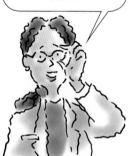

Can you spot which skill can be delegated in question #51?

51. 4. The RN would delegate measuring intake and output. The AP cannot evaluate a glucose level to determine how much insulin is needed, titrate IV rates, or apply oxygen.
CN: Safe, effective care environment; CNS: Management of care; CL: Analyze

52. The nurse will include which in-home management instruction for a child who is receiving intranasal desmopressin for symptomatic control of diabetes insipidus?
1. Give desmopressin only when urine output begins to decrease.
2. Clean the nares with soap and water before administering desmopressin.
3. Increase the desmopressin dose if polyuria occurs before the next scheduled dose.
4. Call the health care provider if the child has an upper respiratory infection or allergic rhinitis.

52. 4. Excessive nasal mucus associated with an upper respiratory infection or allergic rhinitis may interfere with intranasal desmopressin acetate absorption. Parents should be instructed to contact the health care provider for advice in altering the hormone dose during times when nasal mucus may be increased. To avoid overmedicating the child, the desmopressin acetate dose should remain unchanged, even if there is polyuria just before the next dose.
CN: Safe, effective care environment; CNS: Safety and infection control; CL: Apply

CN: Client needs category   CNS: Client needs subcategory   CL: Cognitive level

53. The nurse is caring for a child with hypopituitarism. Which finding(s) will **most** concern the nurse? Select all that apply.
1. Sleep disturbance
2. Polyuria
3. Delay in tooth development
4. Polydipsia
5. Short stature

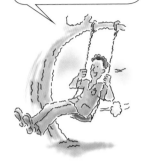

Now you've got some momentum! Keep pumping those legs.

54. Which statement made to the nurse by the parents of a child with hypopituitarism indicates the need for further education?
1. "My child will need to take growth hormone therapy."
2. "There is no genetic basis for this disorder."
3. "This disorder may be secondary to hypothalamic deficiency."
4. "My child may have other disorders related to pituitary hormone deficiencies."

55. The nurse is educating a class of fifth graders on personal health. Which statement related to growth will the nurse included?
1. "There is nothing that you can do to influence your growth."
2. "Intensive physical activity that begins before puberty might stunt growth."
3. "Children who are short in stature also have parents who are short in stature."
4. "You do not need to worry about calorie intake during puberty."

56. The nurse is providing education to the parents of an infant with hypopituitarism. Which statement(s) by the nurse is appropriate? Select all that apply.
1. "Without treatment, your child probably will not reach 4 feet (1.2 meters) in height."
2. "Your child's anterior fontanel may close sooner than normal."
3. "Without treatment, your child may experience delayed growth."
4. "Your child will take growth hormone therapy injections daily."
5. "A side effect of recombinant growth hormone (rhGH) is joint pain."

How am I measuring up?

57. When plotting height and weight on a growth chart, which finding indicates to the nurse a 4-year-old child has a growth hormone deficiency?
1. Upward shift of 1 percentile
2. Upward shift of 2 percentiles
3. Downward shift of 2 percentiles
4. Downward shift of 1 percentile

53. 1, 2, 4. Unexpected findings will most concern the nurse, such as sleep disturbance (may indicate thyrotoxicosis), polydipsia, and polyuria (both may indicate diabetes mellitus or diabetes insipidus). Expected findings in a client with hypopituitarism include short stature, high-pitched voice, and delayed tooth development.
CN: Safe, effective care environment; CNS: Management of care; CL: Apply

54. 2. There is a higher-than-average occurrence of hypopituitarism in some families, which indicates a possible genetic cause. The cause of idiopathic growth hormone deficiency is unknown. The condition is typically associated with other pituitary hormone deficiencies, such as deficiencies of thyroid-stimulating hormone and corticotropin, and thus may be secondary to hypothalamic deficiency. Growth hormone replacement therapy is the treatment.
CN: Physiological integrity; CNS: Physiological adaptation; CL: Apply

55. 2. Intensive physical activity (greater than 18 hours per week) that begins before puberty may stunt growth so that the child does not reach full adult height. During the school-age years, growth slows and does not accelerate again until adolescence. Children who are short in stature do not necessarily have parents who are short in stature. Nutrition and environment influence a child's growth.
CN: Health promotion and maintenance; CNS: None; CL: Apply

56. 1, 3, 4, 5. Hypopituitarism is a rare disorder where the pituitary does not produce any or enough of one or more hormones, which affects growth. Without treatment, children have a short stature and delayed growth. rhGH should be given daily at bedtime and a common side effect is joint pain. Anterior fontanel closure may be delayed.
CN: Physiological integrity; CNS: Physiological adaptation; CL: Apply

57. 3. When the health care provider evaluates the results of plotting height and weight, upward or downward shifts of 2 percentiles or more in children older than age 3 may indicate a growth abnormality.
CN: Health promotion and maintenance; CNS: None; CL: Understand

58. When assessing a 2-year-old child, which finding indicates to the nurse the possibility of growth hormone deficiency?
1. The child had normal growth during the first year of life but showed a slowed growth curve below the 3rd percentile for the second year of life.
2. The child fell below the 5th percentile for growth during the first year of life but, at this checkup, only falls below the 50th percentile.
3. There has been a steady decline in growth over the 2 years of this infant's life that has accelerated during the past 6 months.
4. There was delayed growth below the 5th percentile for the first year of life and below the 5th percentile for the second year of life.

59. The nurse is caring for a child with hyperthyroidism. Which prescription(s) from the health care provider will the nurse question? Select all that apply.
1. Propranolol
2. Atenolol
3. Methimazole
4. Levothyroxine
5. Calcitriol

60. The nurse will expect to find which characteristic(s) while assessing a child with growth hormone deficiency? Select all that apply.
1. Normal skeletal proportions
2. Crowded teeth
3. Appearing older than age
4. Difficulty keeping up with peers in play
5. Failure to show age-appropriate signs of puberty
6. Longer-than-normal upper extremities

61. When counseling the parents of a child with growth hormone deficiency, the nurse will encourage participation in which sport(s)? Select all that apply.
1. Swimming
2. Basketball
3. Field hockey
4. Football
5. Gymnastics

62. A single parent of a school-age child recently diagnosed with a growth hormone deficiency comments that the prescribed treatment plan seems very complicated. What is the **best** response from the nurse?
1. "Everyone feels that way at first."
2. "This must be a stressful time for you."
3. "Do not worry, it will get easier with time."
4. "I can teach you anything you need to know."

Well, bless my beta cells ... there's no deficiency in your knowledge of endocrine disorders.

58. 1. Children with growth hormone deficiency generally grow normally during the first year and then follow a slowed growth curve that is below the third percentile. Growth consistently below the 5th percentile may be an indication of failure to thrive.
CN: Health promotion and maintenance; CNS: None; CL: Apply

59. 4, 5. The nurse will question administering levothyroxine and calcitriol to a client with hyperthyroidism because these medications are used to treat hypothyroidism. Propranolol and atenolol are beta-blockers used to treat tachycardia and hypertension in clients with hyperthyroidism. Methimazole is an antithyroid agent used to treat hyperthyroidism.
CN: Safe, effective care environment; CNS: Management of care; CL: Apply

60. 1, 2, 4, 5. Skeletal proportions are normal for the age, but children with growth hormone deficiency appear younger than their chronological age. Their classmates appear to be growing faster than they do. They may have difficulty keeping up with other children of the same age in play. Parents report they are not outgrowing their clothes and shoes. Crowded teeth and a recessed mandible are common findings. There is failure to show signs of sexual development by 13 years of age in females and 15 years of age in males. However, later in life, premature aging is evident.
CN: Physiological integrity; CNS: Physiological adaptation; CL: Apply

61. 1, 5. Children with growth hormone deficiency can be no less active than other children if directed to size-appropriate sports, such as gymnastics, swimming, wrestling, or soccer.
CN: Health promotion and maintenance; CNS: None; CL: Apply

62. 2. The single parent appears to be overwhelmed trying to deal with the child's diagnosis and treatment plan. The best response is for the nurse to acknowledge the parent's stress. The other responses do not do that.
CN: Psychosocial integrity; CNS: None; CL: Apply

CN: Client needs category　CNS: Client needs subcategory　CL: Cognitive level

63. The parents of a child diagnosed with hypopituitarism tell the nurse they feel guilty because they should have recognized this disorder sooner. Which statement by the nurse about children with hypopituitarism is **most** appropriate?"
   1. "I understand and would feel the same way."
   2. "No reason to stress. You cannot go back in time."
   3. "They usually exhibit signs of this disorder soon after birth."
   4. "They are usually of normal size for gestational age at birth."

63. 4. Children with hypopituitarism are usually of normal size for gestational age at birth. Clinical features develop slowly and vary with the severity of the disorder and the number of deficient hormones. Stating "I understand" and "No reason to stress" are not therapeutic responses.
CN: Safe, effective care environment; CNS: Management of care; CL: Apply

64. When assessing a child with suspected growth hormone deficiency, the nurse is asked to measure the child's height and plot it on a growth chart. What is the **priority** action(s) of the nurse? Select all that apply.
   1. Remove the child's shoes and any hair ornaments prior to measurement.
   2. Have the child stand on a carpeted floor with only the shoulders against the wall.
   3. Measure either the height or the length, whichever is easier.
   4. Use the height as reported by the parent if the child is uncooperative.
   5. Select the appropriate growth chart based on age.

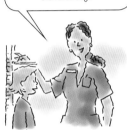

Accuracy counts when measuring the height of a client with growth hormone deficiency.

64. 1, 5. To accurately measure the child's height, remove the shoes, all hair ornaments, and bulky clothing. The child should stand on the uncarpeted surface with the feet flat and together. The head, back, buttocks, and heels should be flat against the wall. Use a flat headpiece to form a right angle with the wall and lower the headpiece until it firmly touches the crown of the head. For accuracy, the nurse cannot use a reported value. Use an age-appropriate chart so that growth can be properly reported.
CN: Health promotion and maintenance; CNS: None; CL: Apply

65. In explaining to parents the social behavior of children with hypopituitarism, the nurse will recognize which statement made by the parents as a need for further education?
   1. "I realize that my child might have school anxiety and low self-esteem. I will monitor my child for these complications."
   2. "Because my child is of short stature, people may expect less of my child than of peers the same age."
   3. "Because of my child's short stature, my child may not be pushed to perform at chronologic age."
   4. "My child's vocabulary is very well developed, so even though short in stature, no one will treat my child differently."

65. 4. Height discrepancy has been significantly correlated with emotional adjustment problems and may be a valuable predictor of the extent to which children with growth hormone delays will have trouble with anxiety, social skills, and positive self-esteem. Also, academic problems are not uncommon. These children are not usually pushed to perform at their chronologic age but are typically subjected to juvenilization (related to an infantile or childish manner).
CN: Psychosocial integrity; CNS: None; CL: Apply

66. The parents of a child who is going through testing for hypopituitarism ask the nurse what test results they should expect. The nurse's response will be based on which factor?
   1. Measurement of growth hormone will occur only one time.
   2. Growth hormone levels are decreased after strenuous exercise.
   3. There will be increased overnight urinary growth hormone concentration.
   4. Growth hormone levels are elevated 45 to 90 minutes following the onset of sleep.

66. 4. Growth hormone levels are elevated 45 to 90 minutes following the onset of sleep. Low growth hormone levels following the onset of sleep indicate the need for further evaluation. Exercise is a natural and benign stimulus for growth hormone release, and elevated levels can be detected after 20 minutes of strenuous exercise in normal children. Urinary growth hormone testing does not show an increase in concentration during overnight hours. Also, growth hormone levels need to be checked frequently related to the type of therapy instituted.
CN: Physiological integrity; CNS: Physiological adaptation; CL: Understand

67. Which comment made by a parent to the nurse indicates the possibility of hypopituitarism in the child?
1. "I can pass down my child's clothes to the younger sibling."
2. "Usually my child wears out clothes before the size changes."
3. "I have to buy larger-sized clothes for my child every few months."
4. "I have to buy larger shirts more frequently than larger pants for my child."

68. The nurse is providing education to parents who will be administering growth hormone to their child at home. Which time of day will the nurse instruct the parents to administer growth hormone to achieve optimal dosing?
1. At bedtime
2. After dinner
3. In the middle of the day
4. First thing in the morning

69. Which medication will the nurse anticipate administering to a male child newly diagnosed with hypopituitarism?
1. Desmopressin acetate
2. Pegvisomant
3. Testosterone
4. Somatropin

70. The nurse is educating parents of a child with hypopituitarism about realistic expectations of height for their child, who is successfully responding to growth hormone replacement. Which statement will the nurse include in the teaching?
1. "Your child will never reach a normal adult height."
2. "I have no idea how your child will grow."
3. "Your child will attain the eventual adult height at a slower rate."
4. "The rate of your child's growth will be the same as other children."

71. Which statement made by a parent of a child with short stature indicates to the nurse the need for further education?
1. "Obtaining blood studies will not aid in proper diagnosis."
2. "A history of my child's growth patterns should be discussed."
3. "X-rays should be included in my child's diagnostic procedures."
4. "A family history is important for me to share with my health care provider."

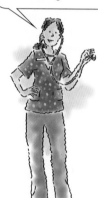
Is it true? Do kids really grow taller overnight?

67. 2. Parents of children with hypopituitarism usually comment that the child wears out clothes before growing out of them or that, if the clothing fits the body, it is typically too long in the sleeves or legs.
CN: Physiological integrity; CNS: Physiological adaptation; CL: Apply

68. 1. Optimal dosing is usually achieved when growth hormone is administered at bedtime. Pituitary release of growth hormone occurs during the first 45 to 90 minutes after the onset of sleep, so normal physiologic release is mimicked with bedtime dosing. Administering at any other time of day would not mimic the body's normal growth hormone release schedule.
CN: Physiological integrity; CNS: Pharmacological and parenteral therapies; CL: Apply

69. 4. The definitive treatment of growth hormone deficiency is replacement of growth hormone; it is successful in 80% of affected children. Desmopressin acetate is used to treat diabetes insipidus. Pegvisomant is a growth hormone antagonist used to treat hyperpituitarism. Testosterone may be given during adolescence for normal sexual maturation but is not the treatment for hypopituitarism.
CN: Physiological integrity; CNS: Pharmacological and parenteral therapies; CL: Apply

70. 3. Even when hormone replacement is successful, children with hypopituitarism attain their eventual adult height at a slower rate than their peers do; therefore, they need assistance in setting realistic expectations regarding height improvement. Stating "I have no idea" is not therapeutic.
CN: Health promotion and maintenance; CNS: None; CL: Apply

71. 1. A complete diagnostic evaluation should include a family history, a history of the child's growth patterns and previous health status, physical examination, physical evaluation, radiographic survey, and endocrine studies that may involve blood samples.
CN: Physiological integrity; CNS: Reduction of risk potential; CL: Apply

72. The nurse is assessing a school-age child recently diagnosed with growth hormone deficiency. Which finding will lead the nurse to suspect the child had been physically abused?
   1. Bruises and scrapes on both knees
   2. Small circular burns on the back
   3. A small soft tissue injury on the forehead
   4. Scratches on the forearms

73. The nurse will monitor a child with growth hormone deficiency for which associated metabolic alteration?
   1. Galactosemia
   2. Homocystinuria
   3. Hyperglycemia
   4. Hypoglycemia

74. When assessing a neonate diagnosed with diabetes insipidus, which finding concerns the nurse?
   1. Respiratory rate 58 breaths/minute
   2. Heart rate 150 beats/minute
   3. Sucking on hands and feet at feeding times
   4. Weight loss

75. A child is admitted to the hospital with weight loss and lack of energy. The child's ears and cheeks are flushed, and the nurse observes an acetone odor to the client's breath. The blood glucose level is 325 mg/dL (18 mmol/L), blood pressure is 104/60 mm Hg, pulse is 88 beats/minute, and respirations are 16 breaths/minute. Which prescription does the nurse expect the health care provider to prescribe **first**?
   1. Subcutaneous administration of glucagon
   2. Regular insulin by continuous infusion pump
   3. Regular insulin subcutaneously every 4 hours per sliding scale
   4. Administration of IV fluids in boluses of 20 mL/kg

76. In a child with diabetes insipidus, the nurse will expect which urine findings?
   1. Pale; specific gravity less than 1.006
   2. Concentrated; specific gravity less than 1.006
   3. Concentrated; specific gravity less than 1.030
   4. Pale; specific gravity more than 1.030

77. A child is on fluid restriction before diagnostic testing for diabetes insipidus. Which finding requires **immediate** nursing intervention?
   1. Pale urine
   2. Weight loss of 5%
   3. Increase in urine output
   4. Generalized edema

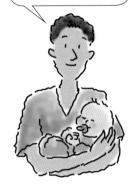

Just a few more questions … and then you can take a nap.

72. 2. Of the injuries described, circular burns to the back were the only injuries that could not have occurred inadvertently during play or been self-inflicted by the child.
CN: Psychosocial integrity; CNS: None; CL: Apply

73. 4. The development of hypoglycemia is a characteristic finding related to growth hormone deficiency. Galactosemia is a rare autosomal recessive disorder with an inborn error of carbohydrate metabolism. Homocystinuria is an indication of amino acid transport or metabolism problems. Hyperglycemia is not a problem in hypopituitarism.
CN: Physiological integrity; CNS: Physiological adaptation; CL: Understand

74. 4. Diabetes insipidus usually appears gradually. Weight loss from a large loss of fluid occurs. A normal neonate should gain weight as the neonate grows. The respiratory and heart rates are normal for a neonate. Sucking on hands and feet is expected due to the presence of the sucking reflex.
CN: Physiological integrity; CNS: Reduction of risk potential; CL: Analyze

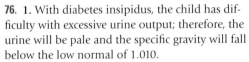

When urine output is increased, urine is more diluted, and thus pale.

75. 2. Weight loss, lack of energy, acetone odor to the breath, and a blood glucose level of 325 mg/dL (18 mmol/L) indicates diabetic ketoacidosis. Insulin is given by continuous infusion pump at a rate not to exceed a decrease in blood sugar greater than 100 mg/dL/hour (5.55 mmol/L/hour). Faster reduction of hypoglycemia could be related to the development of cerebral edema. Glucagon is administered for mild hypoglycemia. Sliding scale insulin is not as effective as the administration of insulin by continuous infusion pump in the treatment of diabetic ketoacidosis. Administration of IV fluids in boluses of 20 mL/kg is recommended for the treatment of shock.
CN: Safe, effective care environment; CNS: Management of care; CL: Analyze

76. 1. With diabetes insipidus, the child has difficulty with excessive urine output; therefore, the urine will be pale and the specific gravity will fall below the low normal of 1.010.
CN: Physiological integrity; CNS: Physiological adaptation; CL: Analyze

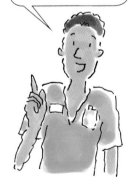

77. 2. A weight loss of 3% to 5% indicates significant dehydration and requires termination of fluid restriction. Pale urine is an expected finding with diabetes insipidus. Generalized edema does not occur with fluid restriction nor does increased urine output.
CN: Safe, effective care environment; CNS: Management of care; CL: Apply

CN: Client needs category   CNS: Client needs subcategory   CL: Cognitive level

78. In a child with diabetes insipidus, which characteristic will the nurse **most** likely find in the child's health history?
  1. Delayed closure of the fontanels, coarse hair, and hypoglycemia in the morning
  2. Gradual onset of personality changes, lethargy, and blurred vision
  3. Vomiting early in the morning, headache, and decreased thirst
  4. Abrupt onset of polyuria, nocturia, and polydipsia

79. When a child with diabetes insipidus has a viral illness that includes congestion, nausea, and vomiting, the nurse will instruct the parents to take which action?
  1. Make no changes in the medication regimen.
  2. Give medications only once per day.
  3. Obtain an alternate route for desmopressin acetate administration.
  4. Give medication 1 hour after vomiting has occurred.

80. The nurse is teaching an adolescent client how to draw up NPH insulin into an insulin syringe. The prescribed dose is 40 units. The client draws up the insulin in the syringe seen below. Which nursing action is **most** appropriate?

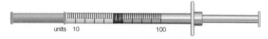

units 10   100

  1. Praise the client for the effort.
  2. Instruct the client on proper technique.
  3. Document the client's actions in the medical record.
  4. Provide additional teaching on drawing up insulin.

81. When providing care for a child with diabetes insipidus, the nurse recognizes which behavior might be difficult related to this child's growth and development?
  1. Taking the medication at school
  2. Taking the medication before bedtime
  3. Letting the parent administer the medication
  4. Self-administering vasopressin injection before school starts

82. The nurse cares for an infant diagnosed with congenital hypothyroidism. The parents state they administer levothyroxine to the infant once per week. Which finding(s) will the nurse expect to assess in this infant? Select all that apply.
  1. Irritability
  2. Fatigue
  3. Increased appetite
  4. Sleepiness
  5. Diarrhea
  6. Jitteriness

That's it! I think you got that one right.

SNAP

78. 4. Diabetes insipidus is characterized by deficient secretion of antidiuretic hormone leading to diuresis. Most children with this disorder experience an abrupt onset of symptoms, including polyuria, nocturia, and polydipsia. The other findings are symptoms of pituitary hyperfunction.
CN: Physiological integrity; CNS: Physiological adaptation; CL: Apply

79. 3. For a child with diabetes insipidus who has a viral illness, an alternate route for administration of desmopressin acetate would be needed for absorption due to nasal congestion. The other actions need to be prescribed by a health care provider.
CN: Physiological integrity; CNS: Pharmacological and parenteral therapies; CL: Apply

80. 4. The syringe shows the client drew up 50 units, which is 10 more units than is prescribed. The nurse must first intervene to ensure a medication error does not occur by providing additional teaching on how to draw up insulin. The nurse can praise the client for being willing to learn after intervening. The nurse would also document the client's actions and teach the client how to self-administer insulin once the client learns how to draw up the correct amount.
CN: Physiological integrity; CNS: Pharmacological and parenteral therapies; CL: Analyze

81. 1. Anything that singles out a child and makes the child feel different from peers will result in possible noncompliance with the medical regimen. It is important for the nurse to help the child schedule medication times for when the child is not in school.
CN: Health promotion and maintenance; CNS: None; CL: Apply

82. 2, 4. Signs of inadequate treatment in an infant with congenital hypothyroidism are fatigue, sleepiness, decreased appetite, and constipation. Levothyroxine should be administered daily on an empty stomach (about 30 minutes before the morning meal). Irritability and jitteriness are not signs noted with inadequate treatment.
CN: Physiological integrity; CNS: Reduction of risk potential; CL: Apply

CN: Client needs category   CNS: Client needs subcategory   CL: Cognitive level

83. The nurse is caring for a neonate with congenital hypothyroidism. Which assessment finding(s) will the nurse report to the health care provider? Select all that apply.
1. Hyperreflexia
2. Long forehead
3. Puffy eyelids
4. Small tongue
5. Umbilical hernia

84. Which nursing intervention is **priority** when working with a neonate suspected of having congenital hypothyroidism?
1. Early identification.
2. Promote bonding.
3. Allow rooming-in with the mother.
4. Encourage fluid intake.

85. The nurse has taught the parents of an infant diagnosed with hypothyroidism how to count the infant's pulse. Which intervention will the nurse teach the parents to complete if a high pulse rate is obtained in the infant?
1. Allow the infant to take a nap and then give levothyroxine.
2. Withhold levothyroxine and give a double dose the next day.
3. Withhold levothyroxine and call the health care provider.
4. Give levothyroxine and then consult the health care provider.

86. A 10-year-old child has been experiencing insatiable thirst, urinating excessively, and has serum glucose of 90 mg/dL (5 mmol/L). Which condition does the nurse suspect the child is experiencing?
1. Diabetes mellitus type 2
2. Diabetes mellitus type 1
3. Hyperthyroidism
4. Diabetes insipidus

87. The nurse is caring for a child newly diagnosed with diabetes mellitus type 1. Which assessment finding(s) will the nurse report to the health care provider? Select all that apply.
1. Polyuria
2. Weakness
3. Abdominal pain
4. Weight loss
5. Postprandial nausea
6. Orthostatic hypertension

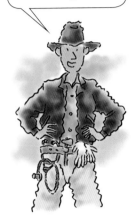

Time to break out your assessment tools. We have some assessing to do.

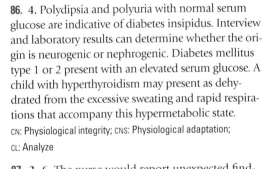

Hooray! You finished the test.

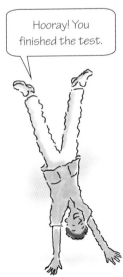

83. 1, 2, 4. The nurse would report hyperreflexia, a long forehead, and a small tongue because these findings are not associated with hypothyroidism. Expected assessment findings for a neonate with congenital hypothyroidism include depressed nasal bridge, short forehead, puffy eyelids, a large tongue; thick, dry, mottled skin that feels cold to the touch; coarse, dry, lusterless hair; abdominal distention; umbilical hernia; hyporeflexia; bradycardia; hypothermia; hypotension; anemia; and wide cranial sutures.
CN: Safe, effective care environment; CNS: Management of care; CL: Apply

84. 1. The most important nursing intervention is early identification of the disorder. Nurses caring for neonates must be certain screening is performed, especially in neonates who are preterm, discharged early, or born at home. Promoting bonding, allowing rooming-in, and encouraging fluid intake are all important but are less critical than early identification.
CN: Physiological integrity; CNS: Basic care and comfort; CL: Apply

85. 3. If parents have been taught to count the pulse of an infant diagnosed with hypothyroidism, they should be instructed to withhold the dose and consult their health care provider if the pulse rate is high. It is not appropriate to give after a nap, double the dose the next day, or continue with administration. The health care provider needs to assess the child.
CN: Physiological integrity; CNS: Reduction of risk potential; CL: Apply

86. 4. Polydipsia and polyuria with normal serum glucose are indicative of diabetes insipidus. Interview and laboratory results can determine whether the origin is neurogenic or nephrogenic. Diabetes mellitus type 1 or 2 present with an elevated serum glucose. A child with hyperthyroidism may present as dehydrated from the excessive sweating and rapid respirations that accompany this hypermetabolic state.
CN: Physiological integrity; CNS: Physiological adaptation; CL: Analyze

87. 3, 6. The nurse would report unexpected findings, which include abdominal pain and orthostatic hypertension. Polyuria, weakness, weight loss, and postprandial nausea are commonly seen in diabetes mellitus type 1.
CN: Safe, effective care environment; CNS: Management of care; CL: Apply

Chapter 33

Genitourinary Disorders

Pediatric genitourinary refresher

Glomerulonephritis (acute poststreptococcal glomerulonephritis)

Kidney disorder characterized by inflammatory injury in the glomerulus. Acute poststreptococcal glomerulonephritis occurs as an immune reaction to a group A beta-hemolytic streptococcal infection of the skin or throat

Key signs and symptoms
- Hematuria
- Mild periorbital or lower extremity edema with abrupt onset
- Hypertension
- Proteinuria
- Usually young school-age child

Key test results
- Urinalysis: RBCs, casts, small amounts of protein (0–3+)
- Altered electrolytes, elevated blood urea nitrogen (BUN) and creatinine levels
- Elevated antistreptolysin O (ASO) titer or streptozyme, decreased serum complement level

Key treatments
- Supportive
- Antihypertensives, corticosteroids, and diuretics; antibiotic treatment for active streptococcal infection
- Low salt diet
- Possible fluid restrictions

Key interventions
- Bed rest
- Strict intake and output (I&O)
- Frequent blood pressure monitoring
- Daily weight measurement
- Test urine frequently for protein and hematuria

Hypospadias and epispadias

Hypospadias
Congenital defect in which the urinary meatus is located on the underside of the shaft of the penis; may be accompanied by chordee, a downward curvature of the penis from a fibrous band of tissue

Epispadias
Congenital defect in which the urinary meatus is on the upper surface of the penis

Key signs and symptoms
- Altered angle of urination
- Meatus terminating at some point along lateral fusion line (hypospadias), ranging from the perineum to the distal penile shaft
- Meatus terminating on the upper surface of the penis (epispadias)

Key test results
- Observation confirms aberrant placement of the meatus; therefore, diagnostic testing is not necessary

Key treatments
- Avoid circumcision (the foreskin may be needed later during surgical repair)
- Analgesics: morphine or acetaminophen for postoperative pain relief
- Antispasmodic agent: propantheline prescribed postoperatively
- Surgery
- Meatotomy (surgical procedure in which the urethra is extended into a normal position); may initially be performed to restore normal urinary function
- When the child is age 12 to 18 months, surgery to release the adherent chordee (fibrous band that causes the penis to curve downward)
- Surgery possibly delayed until age 4 if repair is to be extensive
- Indwelling urinary catheter or suprapubic urinary catheter postoperatively

Key interventions
- Keep the area clean.
- Encourage parents to express feelings and concerns about changes in the child's body appearance or function; provide accurate information and answer questions thoroughly.
- Instruct parents in hygiene of uncircumcised penis.

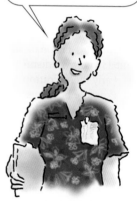

This chapter covers altered patterns of urinary elimination in children and includes glomerulonephritis, hypospadias, and—oh, a whole lot of other plumbing problems ... er, genitourinary disorders. Let's roll up our sleeves and get to work.

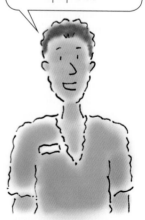

You can't just call a spadias a spadias. There are different types— like "hypospadias" and "epispadias."

638

- Provide postoperative care.
- Monitor for signs of infection.
- Leave the dressing in place for several days.
- Take care to avoid pressure on the child's catheter and avoid kinking the catheter.

Nephrotic syndrome (nephrosis)

Different types of kidney conditions distinguished by the presence of marked protein, edema, and hypoalbuminemia: idiopathic nephrosis is the most common type

Key signs and symptoms
- Severe proteinuria: frothy urine
- Edema: insidious onset, massive edema from shift into interstitial spaces, worsens during the day
- Hypovolemia
- Pallor, fatigue
- Usually toddler or preschool-age child

Key test results
- Protein in urine (3+ to 4+), possible microscopic hematuria
- Hypoalbuminemia (less than 2.5 g/dL [25 g/L]), elevated cholesterol and triglyceride, hemoglobin, hematocrit, and platelet levels

Key treatments
- Prednisone to initiate remission (0 to trace protein in the urine for 5 to 7 days)
- Diuretics, corticosteroids, possible albumin administration
- Diet with no added salt

Key interventions
- Prevent infection and skin breakdown.
- Monitor vital signs (temperature) every 4 to 8 hours.
- Assess weight daily.
- Assess edema and condition of the skin every 4 to 8 hours.
- Strict I&O.
- Adhere to "no added salt" diet and fluid restriction if prescribed; teach child and parents about no added salt diet.

Nephroblastoma (Wilms tumor)

Rare kidney cancer that primarily affects children. Most often occurs in one kidney, though sometimes found in both kidneys

Key signs and symptoms
- Associated congenital anomalies—microcephaly, intellectual disability, genitourinary tract problems

- Nontender mass, usually midline near the liver; usually detected by the parent while bathing or dressing the child

Key test results
- Excretory urography reveals a mass displacing the normal kidney structure
- Computed tomography (CT) scan or sonography reveals metastasis

Key treatments
- Nephrectomy within 24 to 48 hours of diagnosis because these tumors metastasize quickly
- Radiation therapy (following surgery)
- Chemotherapy (following surgery) with dactinomycin, doxorubicin, or vincristine

Key interventions
- Monitor vital signs and intake and output.
- Do not palpate the abdomen and prevent others from doing so.
- Handle and bathe the child carefully; loosen clothing around the abdomen.
- Prepare the child and family members for a nephrectomy within 24 to 48 hours of diagnosis.
- After nephrectomy:
  - monitor urine output and report output less than 30 mL/hour
  - assist with turning, coughing, and deep breathing
  - encourage early ambulation
  - provide pain medications, as necessary
  - monitor postoperative dressings for signs of bleeding
  - use aseptic technique for dressing changes.

Urinary tract infection

Infection in any structure of the urinary tract, especially the urethra and bladder

Key signs and symptoms
- Frequent urge to void with pain or burning on urination
- Lethargy
- Low-grade fever
- Urine that is cloudy and foul-smelling

Key test results
- Clean-catch urine culture yields large amounts of bacteria

Key treatments
- Cranberry juice to acidify urine
- Forced fluids to flush infection from the urinary tract
- Antibiotics: sulfamethoxazole-trimethoprim or ampicillin to prevent glomerulonephritis

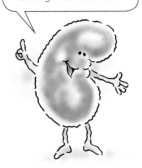

I kidney you not—this chapter will be easy. Just go with the flow.

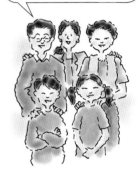

When a nephrectomy is required, educate the whole family on what to expect.

Key interventions

- Monitor intake and output.
- Evaluate toileting habits for proper front-to-back wiping and proper hand washing.
- Assist the child when necessary to ensure that the perineal area is clean after elimination.
- Encourage increased intake of fluids.
- Force fluids to achieve urine output of more than 2 L/day; however, discourage intake greater than 3 L/day.
- Teach the child and parents about:
  - refrigerating or culturing a urine specimen within 30 minutes of collection to prevent overgrowth of bacteria
  - completing the prescribed antibiotic therapy, even after symptoms subside
  - long-term follow-up care for high-risk children.

Sexually transmitted infections (STIs)

Diverse group of infections spread through sexual activity with an infected person. Besides AIDS, the most common STIs are chlamydia, gonorrhea, trichomoniasis, syphilis, genital herpes, and genital warts (human papillomavirus [HPV])

Key signs and symptoms

- Sores or lesions on the genitals or in the oral or rectal area
- Pain or burning on urination
- Discharge from the penis
- Unusual or foul-smelling vaginal discharge
- Pain during sex
- Sore, swollen lymph nodes, particularly in the groin, but sometimes more widespread
- Lower abdominal pain
- Rash over the trunk, hands, or feet

Key test results

- Culture of discharge from penis/vagina/rectum or oral cavity (gonorrhea, chlamydia)
- Scraping of lesion (genital herpes)
- Blood test (syphilis, HIV)

Key treatments

- Gonorrhea and chlamydia: oral or injectable antibiotics, partners should also be treated
- Gonorrhea: ceftriaxone 250 mg IM and azithromycin 1 g PO in a single dose
- Trichomoniasis: metronidazole, tinidazole
- Chlamydia: azithromycin 1 g in a single dose or doxycycline BID × 7 days
- Genital herpes: antiviral drugs (acyclovir, valacyclovir, famciclovir)
- Syphilis: penicillin G
- Genital warts: cryotherapy, trichloroacetic acid (TCA) or bichloroacetic acid application to remove warts. There is no cure for HPV.

Key interventions

- Gather health information, sexual history, and allergy history.
- Maintain nonjudgmental attitude.
- Teach methods for preventing STIs.
- Provide specific education that is appropriate for the particular STI.

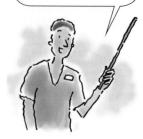

What are the signs of a urinary tract infection?

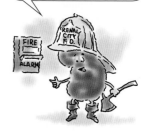

"Sound the alarm!" Some genitourinary disorders can cause serious complications.

the Point® You can download tables of drug information to help you prepare for the NCLEX®! View Generic Drug Names, Drug Classifications, Drug Actions, and Nursing Implications for the drugs discussed in this refresher at **http://thePoint.lww.com**

Genitourinary questions, answers, and rationales

1. The nurse is caring for a 5-year-old child, weighing 44 lb (20 kg) being treated for acute glomerulonephritis (AGN). Which assessment finding(s) indicates to the nurse improvement in the child's condition? Select all that apply.

1. A weight loss of 2.2 lb (1 kg)
2. Decreased urinary output over the last 24 hours
3. Lack of periorbital, facial, or body edema
4. A fluid intake of more than 2,000 mL in 24 hours
5. A blood pressure of 125/84 mm Hg

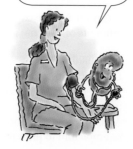

Hey—looks like you're back up to normal. The treatment must be working.

1.   1, 3. Weight loss indicates improvement in the condition. Weight gain is an early indication of excess fluid and occurs prior to visible edema. Diuretics cause excretion of excess fluid by preventing resorption of water and sodium. Sodium and water retention lead to edema. Increased urine output, not decreased output, and lack of edema indicate improved fluid balance and improvement in the condition. Normal fluid intake in a 44 lb (20 kg) child would be approximately 1,500 mL/day, not 2,000 mL/day. Often children with AGN are initially on a fluid restriction. Blood pressure drops as the child's condition improves.

CN: Health promotion and maintenance; CNS: None; CL: Analyze

CN: Client needs category   CNS: Client needs subcategory   CL: Cognitive level

2. When the nurse is caring for a child with acute glomerulonephritis, which nursing action(s) takes **priority**? Select all that apply.
1. Measure daily weight.
2. Increase oral fluid intake.
3. Provide sodium supplements.
4. Monitor the child for signs of hypokalemia.
5. Assess for periorbital or dependent edema.

3. A child has been diagnosed with acute glomerulonephritis. Based on the chart exhibit below, which component(s) does the nurse recognize as being consistent with this diagnosis? Select all that apply.

Laboratory Results

Urinalysis

Color	Cola
Appearance	Clear
Specific gravity	1.027
pH	5.5
Protein	Present
Blood	Present
RBC casts	Present
Crystals	Negative

1. Specific gravity
2. Protein
3. Blood
4. Red blood cell (RBC) casts
5. Color

4. Which statement by the nurse is the **best** response to parents who want to know the first indication their child's acute glomerulonephritis is improving?
1. Urine output will increase.
2. Urine will be protein-free.
3. Blood pressure will stabilize.
4. The child will have more energy.

5. The nurse is taking frequent blood pressure readings on a child diagnosed with acute glomerulonephritis. The parents ask the nurse why this is necessary. Which statement by the nurse is **most** accurate?
1. "Blood pressure fluctuations are a sign that the condition has become chronic."
2. "Blood pressure fluctuations are a common adverse effect of antibiotic therapy."
3. "Hypotension leading to sudden shock can develop at any time."
4. "Acute hypertension must be anticipated and identified early."

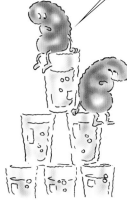

"Whoa!" It is important to achieve and maintain appropriate fluid balance.

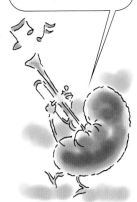

You're off to a great start! Let me toot my horn for you.

2. **1, 5.** The child with acute glomerulonephritis should be monitored for fluid imbalance, which is done through daily weights. Sodium and water retention lead to edema. Weight gain is an early sign of fluid retention. Increasing oral intake, providing sodium supplements, and monitoring for hypokalemia are not part of the therapeutic management of acute glomerulonephritis.
CN: Safe, effective care environment; CNS: Management of care; CL: Apply

3. **2, 3, 4, 5.** Urinalysis findings consistent with acute glomerulonephritis include the presence of RBC casts, hematuria, cola or tea color (from blood), and proteinuria. The specific gravity level is within the normal limits of 1.002 to 1.030.
CN: Physiological integrity; CNS: Physiological adaptation; CL: Analyze

4. **1.** One of the first signs of improvement during the acute phase of glomerulonephritis is an increase in urine output. It will take time for the urine to be protein-free. Antihypertensive drugs may be needed to stabilize blood pressure. Children generally do not have much energy during the acute phase of this disease.
CN: Physiological integrity; CNS: Physiological adaptation; CL: Analyze

5. **4.** Regular measurement of vital signs, including blood pressure, body weight, and intake and output, is essential to monitor the progress of acute glomerulonephritis and to detect complications that may appear at any time during the course of the disease. Hypertension is more likely to occur with glomerulonephritis than hypotension and should be anticipated. Blood pressure fluctuations do not indicate that the condition has become chronic and are not common adverse reactions to antibiotic therapy.
CN: Physiological integrity; CNS: Physiological adaptation; CL: Apply

CN: Client needs category   CNS: Client needs subcategory   CL: Cognitive level

6. When evaluating the urinalysis report of a child with acute glomerulonephritis, the nurse will expect which result?
1. Proteinuria and decreased BUN
2. Bacteriuria and increased creatinine
3. Hematuria and proteinuria
4. Bacteriuria and hematuria

7. Which statement regarding acute glomerulonephritis indicates the parents of a child with this diagnosis understand the education provided by the nurse?
1. "This disease occurs after a urinary tract infection."
2. "This disease is associated with renal vascular disorders."
3. "This disease occurs after a streptococcal infection."
4. "This disease is associated with structural anomalies of the genitourinary tract."

8. When obtaining a child's daily weight, the nurse notes the child has lost 6 lb (2.7 kg) after 3 days of hospitalization for acute glomerulonephritis. The nurse understands this is **most** likely the result of which factor?
1. Poor appetite
2. Reduction of edema
3. Decreased salt intake
4. Restriction to bed rest

9. The nurse is providing education about antihypertensive therapy to the parents of a child with glomerulonephritis. Which statement made by the parents indicates additional teaching is required?
1. "My child will need lifelong antihypertensive therapy."
2. "I should be sure to keep my child's regular appointments."
3. "I will monitor my child for dizziness and light-headedness."
4. "I will administer the medication at the same time each day."

10. A previously toilet-trained 4-year-old child begins wetting the bed after being hospitalized. Which statement will the nurse make to the parents?
1. "Children commonly show regressive behavior when hospitalized."
2. "Your child is just acting out to get attention from you."
3. "It is okay, sometimes 4-year-olds still have accidents."
4. "Let us try cutting back on fluids and see whether that helps."

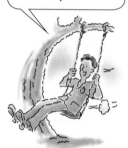

Hang on tight! We're flying through these questions.

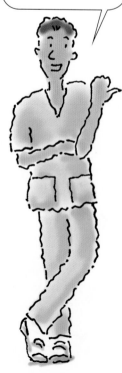

"Further teaching is required" is code for "the parent doesn't know what they're talking about."

6. 3. Urinalysis during the acute phase of glomerulonephritis characteristically shows hematuria, proteinuria, and increased BUN and creatinine levels.
CN: Physiological integrity; CNS: Physiological adaptation; CL: Analyze

7. 3. Acute glomerulonephritis is an immune-complex disease that occurs as a by-product of an antecedent streptococcal infection. Certain strains of the infection are usually beta-hemolytic streptococci.
CN: Physiological integrity; CNS: Physiological adaptation; CL: Understand

8. 2. When edema is reduced, the child will lose weight. This should normally occur after treatment for acute glomerulonephritis has been followed for several days. It will take longer for the child's appetite to improve, but this should not lead to such a dramatic weight loss in a child this age. Decreasing sodium intake will assist in decreasing edema; however, this alone would not result in such drastic weight loss in a child. Bed rest would not affect weight.
CN: Physiological integrity; CNS: Physiological adaptation; CL: Apply

9. 1. The child will be weaned off the antihypertensive drugs as blood pressure decreases and the condition improves. Regular appointments should be kept in order to monitor the child's blood pressure. Blood pressure should be rechecked 1 week after the antihypertensive has been discontinued. Dizziness and light-headedness can be a side effect. A daily antihypertensive should be given at the same time each day (as close to every 24 hours as possible).
CN: Physiological integrity; CNS: Pharmacological and parenteral therapies; CL: Apply

10. 1. Young children may exhibit regressive behaviors when they are under stress, such as occurs with hospitalization. The child may be acting out, but more likely, this is not voluntary bedwetting. Four-year-old children should be fully toilet trained. Restricting fluids as a first step in a hospitalized child is not appropriate; other causes of enuresis should be considered first.
CN: Psychosocial integrity; CNS: None; CL: Apply

CN: Client needs category   CNS: Client needs subcategory   CL: Cognitive level

11. The nurse will make which dietary recommendation to a child newly diagnosed with acute glomerulonephritis?
1. Reduce calories.
2. Increase potassium.
3. Limit calcium.
4. Moderately restrict sodium.

12. The nurse is evaluating a group of children for acute glomerulonephritis. The nurse will expect which child to **most** likely develop the disease?
1. A child who had pneumonia a month ago
2. A child who was bitten by a brown spider
3. A child who was born with a patent ductus arteriosus
4. A child who had a streptococcal infection 2 weeks ago

13. The nurse is assessing a child with acute glomerulonephritis. Which finding **immediately** concerns the nurse?
1. Cola-colored urine
2. Blurred vision
3. Albumin in the urine
4. Peripheral edema

14. Which comment made by a client's parent indicates to the nurse the need for further education about acute glomerulonephritis complications?
1. "Dizziness is expected, and I should have my child lie down."
2. "I will let the nurse know every time my child urinates."
3. "I need to ask my child about headaches every few hours."
4. "I should encourage my child to engage in quiet play activities."

15. The nurse is providing education to a client's parents about the treatment of acute glomerulonephritis. Which statement made by the parents reflects an understanding of the nurse's teaching?
1. "All children who have signs of glomerulonephritis are hospitalized for approximately 1 week."
2. "I should expect my child to have a normal energy level during the acute phase of glomerulonephritis."
3. "Children who have a normal blood pressure and a satisfactory urine output can generally be treated at home."
4. "Children with gross hematuria and significant oliguria should be seen by the health care provider every other day."

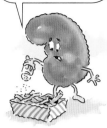

I know I shouldn't—I just can't resist.

Treat your kidneys well, and they'll keep trucking for many years to come.

11. 4. Moderate sodium restriction with a diet that has no added salt after cooking is usually effective. Reduced calories, increased potassium, and limited calcium consumption are not necessary because of the decrease in urine output.
CN: Physiological integrity; CNS: Basic care and comfort; CL: Apply

12. 4. A latent period of 10 to 14 days occurs between the streptococcal infection of the throat or skin and the onset of clinical manifestations. The peak incidence of disease corresponds to the incidence of streptococcal infections. Pneumonia is not a precursor to glomerulonephritis nor is a bite from a brown spider or patent ductus arteriosus. Children with cardiac anomalies are more susceptible to bacterial endocarditis, which can lead to glomerulonephritis.
CN: Health promotion and maintenance; CNS: None; CL: Analyze

13. 2. Visual disturbances can be an indication of rising blood pressure and should be investigated first. Presence of albumin in the urine, red blood cells (causing the cola-colored urine), and peripheral edema are common symptoms in acute glomerulonephritis.
CN: Physiological integrity; CNS: Reduction of risk potential; CL: Analyze

14. 1. Dizziness and headache are signs of encephalopathy, not glomerulonephritis, and must be reported to the nurse. Hypertensive encephalopathy, acute cardiac decompensation, and acute kidney failure are the major complications that tend to develop during the acute phase of glomerulonephritis. To maintain an accurate intake and output record, the parent should let the nurse know when the child urinates. Quiet play is encouraged to avoid overstressing the kidneys.
CN: Physiological integrity; CNS: Reduction of risk potential; CL: Analyze

15. 3. Children who have normal blood pressure and a satisfactory urine output can generally be treated at home. Those with gross hematuria and significant oliguria will probably be hospitalized for monitoring. Parents should expect children to have decreased energy during the acute phase of the disease.
CN: Physiological integrity; CNS: Reduction of risk potential; CL: Apply

16. Which nursing action(s) takes **priority** for a child with acute glomerulonephritis? Select all that apply.
1. Assess blood pressure every 4 hours.
2. Check urine specific gravity weekly.
3. Encourage daily fluid intake of 3,500 mL.
4. Weigh every morning using the same scale.
5. Provide a 2,500 mg sodium diet.

17. When instructing an 8-year-old child about obtaining a clean-catch urine specimen, which statement will be included by the nurse?
1. "You need to pee in the container in the bathroom right after a nap."
2. "The first time you pee after sleeping all night should be in the toilet first."
3. "When you go to the bathroom, start and end peeing in the container."
4. "It is alright if you touch the inside of the container you will pee in."

18. The nurse is caring for a child diagnosed with acute glomerulonephritis. Which food choice(s) is appropriate for a child with this diagnosis? Select all that apply.
1. Turkey sandwich with mayonnaise
2. Canned soup and crackers
3. Hot dog with ketchup and mustard
4. Tuna salad in a pita
5. Garden salad with grilled chicken
6. Apple with peanut butter

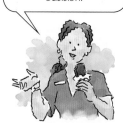

Did somebody mention food? I feel hungry all of a sudden.

19. Which therapy will the nurse expect to incorporate into the care of the child with acute glomerulonephritis?
1. Antiviral therapy
2. Dialysis therapy
3. Physical therapy
4. Play therapy

20. After the acute phase of glomerulonephritis is over, which discharge instruction will the nurse provide to the child's parents?
1. Every 6 months, a cystogram will be needed for evaluation of progress.
2. Weekly visits to the health care provider may be needed for evaluation.
3. It will be acceptable to keep the regular yearly checkup appointment for the next evaluation.
4. There is no need to worry about further evaluations by the health care provider.

16. 1, 4. Because hypertension is a complication of acute glomerulonephritis, the nurse should check the child's blood pressure every 4 hours. An increase in weight is the first sign of fluid retention, so the child should be weighed daily with the same scale to ensure accuracy. The urine specific gravity should also be monitored, but more frequently. The child may be placed on fluid or sodium restrictions.
CN: Physiological integrity; CNS: Reduction of risk potential; CL: Apply

17. 2. When collecting a clean-catch urine specimen, the first voided specimen of the day should never be used because of urinary stasis; this also applies after a nap. The specimen should be collected midstream, not at the beginning of urination. Touching the inside of the specimen container would contaminate the specimen.
CN: Physiological integrity; CNS: Reduction of risk potential; CL: Apply

18. 1, 4, 5, 6. Foods that are high in sodium should be eliminated from the child's diet. Snacks such as pretzels and potato chips should be discouraged. Because hot dogs contain a great deal of sodium, they should be eliminated from the child's diet. Canned foods and crackers are also high in sodium. Processed foods and restaurant foods typically contain large amounts of sodium. Any other foods that the child likes should be encouraged.
CN: Physiological integrity; CNS: Basic care and comfort; CL: Apply

19. 4. Play therapy is a very important aspect of care to help the child understand what is happening. It allows the child to express concerns and fears, so the child may avoid night terrors and growth and development regression. Antiviral and physical therapies are not treatments for acute glomerulonephritis. Dialysis therapy is appropriate for kidney failure.
CN: Health promotion and maintenance; CNS: None; CL: Apply

20. 2. Weekly or monthly visits to the health care provider will be needed for evaluation of improvement and will usually involve the collection of a urine specimen for urinalysis. A cystogram is not helpful in determining the progression of this disease; it is used to review the anatomical structures of the urinary tract.
CN: Physiological integrity; CNS: Reduction of risk potential; CL: Apply

21. The nurse is preparing to administer penicillin to a child with acute glomerulonephritis, weighing 55 lb (25 kg). The health care provider prescribes penicillin 500 mg by mouth every 8 hours. The recommended dose is 50 to 75 mg/kg/day by mouth every 6 to 8 hours. After reviewing the information, the nurse draws which conclusion?
   1. The prescribed dosage is larger than the maximum dosage recommended.
   2. The prescribe dosage is smaller than the minimum dosage recommended.
   3. The dose is safe to give and falls within the safe dose range for this child.
   4. It is not the nurse's responsibility to question the health care provider's prescription.

22. When providing discharge instructions to parents of an older child following hypospadias repair, which activity will the nurse encourage?
   1. Riding a bicycle
   2. Running on the playground
   3. Playing a game of cards
   4. Chasing the family pet

23. The parent of a neonate born with hypospadias is sharing feelings of guilt about this anomaly with a nurse. What is the **best** response by the nurse?
   1. "You should not feel guilty; there is nothing you could have done."
   2. "Maybe you need to talk to a specialist to see if it is hereditary."
   3. "Worrying is a waste of time; concentrate on taking care of your baby."
   4. "Do you want to talk about how you have been feeling?"

24. The nurse is preparing to administer penicillin 0.5 g to a child with glomerulonephritis. The nurse has available an oral solution of penicillin 250 mg/5 mL. How many milliliters will the nurse administer with each dose? Record your answer using a whole number.

_____ mL

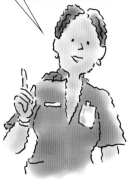

Careful. It's important to be accurate when calculating dosages. Your client's safety depends on it.

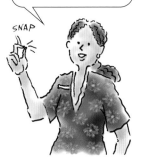

That was easy. I think you're getting the hang of this.

SNAP

21. **3.** The calculated safe dosage range for this child is 1,250 to 1,875 mg/day. The child will be receiving 1,500 mg/day (500 mg × 3 doses/day) which is within the recommended range, so it is safe to administer.
CN: Physiological integrity; CNS: Pharmacological and parenteral therapies; CL: Analyze

22. **3.** The child should not partake in potentially rough activities. Riding bicycles, running, and chasing animals should be avoided until allowed by the health care provider.
CN: Physiological integrity; CNS: Reduction of risk potential; CL: Analyze

23. **4.** The nurse should encourage the parent to talk about how the parent has been feeling and allow the parent to be heard. This defect is not hereditary. The other two options belittle the parent's feelings.
CN: Psychosocial integrity; CNS: None; CL: Apply

24. **10.**
The correct formula to calculate a drug dose is:

$$\frac{Dose\ on\ hand}{Quantity\ on\ hand} = \frac{Dose\ desired}{X}$$

The health care provider prescribes 0.5 g, which is the dose desired. The nurse has available 250 mg/5 mL, which is the dose on hand.

$$\frac{250\ mg}{5\ mL} = \frac{0.5\ g}{X}$$

$$\frac{250\ mg}{5\ mL} = \frac{500\ mg}{X}$$

$$250\ X = 2,500\ mL$$

$$X = 10\ mL$$

CN: Physiological integrity; CNS: Pharmacological and parenteral therapies; CL: Apply

CN: Client needs category   CNS: Client needs subcategory   CL: Cognitive level

25. The nurse is caring for an infant with hypospadias. The nurse will further assess the infant for which accompanying complication(s)? Select all that apply.
1. Undescended testes
2. Chordee
3. Ambiguous genitalia
4. Umbilical hernias
5. Inguinal hernias

26. The nurse is providing education about surgery to the parent of an infant with hypospadias. Which statement by the parent indicates an understanding of the education?
1. "Early surgery is to prevent separation anxiety."
2. "Doing the surgery in infancy helps prevent urinary complications."
3. "Infants are more accepting of hospitalization, so the surgery is done then."
4. "The surgery is done during infancy to promote development of normal body image."

27. A child is undergoing hypospadias repair. Which statement made by the child's parents about the principal objective of surgical correction implies a need for further education from the nurse?
1. "Surgery will improve the physical appearance of the genitalia for psychological reasons."
2. "The purpose of surgery is to enhance the child's ability to void in the standing position."
3. "Having this surgery will decrease our child's chance of future urinary tract infections."
4. "The purpose of our child having this surgery is to preserve a sexually adequate organ."

28. The nurse will counsel parents to postpone which action until after their son's hypospadias has been repaired?
1. Circumcision
2. Hearing test
3. Getting hepatitis B vaccine
4. Checking blood for inborn errors of metabolism

29. Which nursing intervention will be included when caring for a male infant following surgical repair of hypospadias?
1. Sterile dressing changes every 4 hours
2. Frequent inspection of the tip of the penis
3. Removal of the urethral stent on the second postoperative day
4. Urethral catheterization if the infant does not void within 8 hours

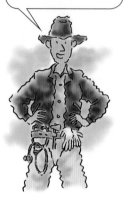

Assessing pediatric clients can be an adventure. Make sure you're fully equipped before you enter that exam room.

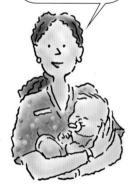

Remember the body part where hypospadias occurs? Keep that in mind when answering question #28.

25. 1, 2. Because undescended testes may also be present in hypospadias, the small penis may appear to be an enlarged clitoris. This should not be mistaken for ambiguous genitalia. If there is any doubt, more tests should be performed. Chordee, or ventral curvature of the penis, results from the replacement of normal skin with a fibrous band of tissue. It usually accompanies more severe forms of hypospadias. Hernias do not generally accompany hypospadias.
CN: Physiological integrity; CNS: Reduction of risk potential; CL: Apply

26. 4. Whenever there are defects of the genitourinary tract, surgery should be performed early to promote development of a normal body image, not acceptance of hospitalization. A child with normal emotional development shows separation anxiety at 7 to 9 months. Within a few months, the child understands the mother's permanence, and anxiety diminishes. Hypospadias does not put the child at a greater risk for urinary complications.
CN: Physiological integrity; CNS: Reduction of risk potential; CL: Apply

27. 3. A child with hypospadias is not at greater risk for urinary tract infections. The principal objectives of surgical corrections are to enhance the child's ability to void in the standing position with a straight stream, to improve the physical appearance of the genitalia for psychological reasons, and to preserve a sexually adequate organ.
CN: Physiological integrity; CNS: Reduction of risk potential; CL: Apply

28. 1. Circumcision should not be performed until after the hypospadias has been repaired. The foreskin might be needed to help in the repair of hypospadias. None of the other actions has any bearing on the repair of hypospadias.
CN: Physiological integrity; CNS: Reduction of risk potential; CL: Apply

29. 2. Following hypospadias repair, a pressure dressing is applied to the penis to reduce bleeding and tissue swelling. The penile tip should then be assessed frequently for signs of circulatory impairment. The dressing around the penis should not be changed as frequently as every 4 hours. The health care provider will determine when the urethral stent/catheter will be removed. The nurse would not catheterize the infant without notifying the health care provider first.
CN: Physiological integrity; CNS: Basic care and comfort; CL: Apply

30. After the nurse has provided discharge education to the parents of a child with hypospadias, which statement by the parent indicates additional education is needed?
1. "I will need to learn irrigation techniques."
2. "I should bathe my child in the tub daily."
3. "Proper catheter care helps prevent infection."
4. "I need to keep the catheter free of kinks."

31. Which task will the registered nurse (RN) delegate to the assistive personnel (AP)?
1. Obtain a sterile urine specimen from a child with vesicoureteral reflux.
2. Check the pain level of a child with a urinary tract infection.
3. Insert a Foley catheter in a child with nephrotic syndrome.
4. Assist a child with acute glomerulonephritis to the bathroom.

32. The nurse is preparing to calculate the safe dose range of a chemotherapy drug for a child with Wilms tumor. The drug is prescribed in mg/m². What information does the nurse need to calculate the body surface area (m²) of the child? Select all that apply.
1. The child's blood type
2. The child's weight
3. The child's height
4. The child's white blood cell count (WBC)
5. The child's birth weight

33. A 1-year-old underwent hypospadias repair yesterday and has a urethral catheter and IV in place. The nurse notes urinary drainage around the urethral catheter. Which nursing action is **best**?
1. Document the finding in the medical record.
2. Asses the child's vital signs.
3. Administer propantheline intravenously.
4. Notify the health care provider.

34. Which intervention by the nurse is **most** helpful when discussing hypospadias with the parents of an infant with this defect?
1. Refer the parents to a counselor.
2. Be there to listen to the parents' concerns.
3. Have the health care provider talk to the parents.
4. Suggest a support group to the parents.

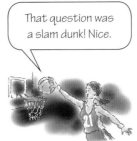

That question was a slam dunk! Nice.

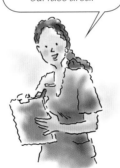

The long and the short of it is that you need to know the right dimensions to calculate body surface area.

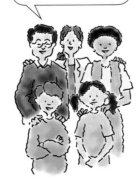

When working with pediatric clients, remember to care for the whole family.

30. 2. A tub bath should be avoided to prevent infection until the stent has been removed. Parents are taught to care for the indwelling catheter or stent and how to perform irrigation techniques if indicated. They need to know how to empty the urine bag and how to avoid kinking, twisting, or blockage of the catheter or stent.
CN: Physiological integrity; CNS: Reduction of risk potential; CL: Apply

31. 4. The RN would delegate assisting a client to the bathroom. APs cannot perform sterile procedures or assess clients.
CN: Safe, effective care environment; CNS: Management of care; CL: Analyze

32. 2, 3. Body surface area is calculated using a pediatric nomogram or by a formula. Both methods require knowledge of the height and weight of the child. The nurse does not need the child's blood type, WBC count, or birth weight to calculate the body surface area.
CN: Physiological integrity; CNS: Pharmacological and parenteral therapies; CL: Understand

33. 3. The child is showing signs of a bladder spasm. Propantheline is an antispasmodic that works effectively on children. It prevents bladder spasms while the catheter is in place. The nurse should do more than document the finding. The nurse does not need to assess vital signs or notify the health care provider because the child is not in distress or having signs of complications
CN: Physiological integrity; CNS: Pharmacological and parenteral therapies; CL: Apply

34. 2. The nurse must recognize that parents are going to grieve the loss of the normal child when they have a neonate born with a birth defect. Initially, the parents need to have a nurse who will listen to their concerns for their neonate's health. Suggesting a support group or referring the parents to a counselor might be helpful but would not be the initial action. The health care provider will need to spend time with the parents to discuss surgery, but the nurse is in the best position to allow the parents to vent their grief and anger.
CN: Psychosocial integrity; CNS: None; CL: Analyze

35. The nurse is assessing a 6-year-old child. The child reports dysuria and urgency. The parent reports the child has recently had enuresis. The nurse recognizes these as signs and symptoms of which condition?
1. Nephrotic syndrome
2. Urinary tract infection
3. Acute glomerulonephritis
4. Obstructive uropathy

35. 2. Frequency and urgency can lead to enuresis. All are symptoms of a urinary tract infection.

CN: Physiological integrity; CNS: Physiological adaptation; CL: Apply

36. Which teaching will the nurse provide to the child and parents regarding furosemide? Select all that apply.
1. It is best to take furosemide at bedtime.
2. Take the medication with food.
3. You can crush the tablets and add to food.
4. You should wear sunglasses while outside.
5. You need to change positions slowly.

36. 2, 3, 5. Furosemide is a diuretic medication. The child should change positions slowly due to orthostatic hypotension. Furosemide should be taken in the morning to prevent frequent urination during bedtime. Furosemide should be taken with food to limit gastrointestinal upset and can be crushed if needed. The child is at higher risk for sunburn, not photophobia, while taking furosemide.

CN: Physiological integrity; CNS: Pharmacological and parenteral therapies; CL: Apply

37. The nurse is preparing the parents of an infant with hypospadias for surgery. Which statement made by the parents indicates the need for further education?
1. "Skin grafting might be involved in my infant's repair."
2. "After surgery, my infant's penis will look perfectly normal."
3. "Surgical repair may need to be performed in several stages."
4. "My infant will probably be in some pain after the surgery and might need medication."

37. 2. It is important to stress to the parents that even after a repair of hypospadias the outcome is not a completely "normal-looking" penis. The goals of surgery are to allow the child to void from the tip of his penis, void with a straight stream, and stand up while voiding.

CN: Psychosocial integrity; CNS: None; CL: Apply

38. Which nursing action is **priority** when caring for a neonate with exstrophy of the bladder?
1. Monitor for a urinary tract infection.
2. Apply petroleum to the site.
3. Stress the importance of Kegel exercises.
4. Cover the site with moist, sterile gauze.

38. 4. It is priority for the nurse to protect the exposed bladder with a moist, sterile gauze or a film wrap to help prevent drying. The nurse will monitor for infection, but this is not the priority. Petroleum should not be applied to the site because this can harbor bacteria. Kegel exercises will be taught after the child is older.

CN: Safe, effective care environment; CNS: Management of care; CL: Apply

39. The nurse is preparing a presentation for a group of female adolescents about pelvic inflammatory disease (PID). Which information will the nurse include?
1. Poor hygiene practices increase the risk of PID.
2. The use of hormonal contraceptives decreases the risk of PID.
3. There are long-term complications related to PID.
4. There are risks of defects in future infants born to adolescents with PID.

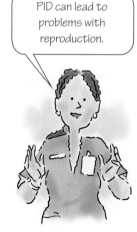

PID can lead to problems with reproduction.

39. 3. Long-term complications of PID include abscess formation in the fallopian tubes and adhesion formation leading to an increased risk of ectopic pregnancy or infertility. PID is not prevented by proper personal hygiene or by any form of contraception, even though some forms of contraception, such as the male or female condom, do help to decrease the incidence. PID does not increase the risk of birth defects in infants born to adolescents with PID.

CN: Health promotion and maintenance; CNS: None; CL: Apply

40. The nurse is providing education to the parent of a child with nephrosis being discharged on prednisone. In discussing prevention of infection, which statement(s) by the parent indicates a need for further teaching? Select all that apply.
1. "I will contact my child's health care provider if my child has a fever or a sore throat."
2. "We will all wash hands frequently, especially after using the bathroom."
3. "I should keep my child away from other people who are sick."
4. "I need to keep my house clean and prepare and store food properly."
5. "My child should be allowed to play with pets to aid in developing a healthy immune system."
6. "My child should receive all routine childhood immunizations."

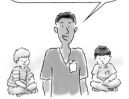

Make sure your client's parents have an accurate understanding of the condition and how to care for it.

40. 5, 6. Family members should be up-to-date on immunizations to prevent exposing the child; the immunocompromised child should not receive live-virus immunization. Immunocompromised children should not be around pets. Any signs and symptoms of infections should be reported for prompt treatment. Proper handwashing is the first line of defense against infection. The child should not be around anyone who is sick, especially someone with chicken pox or measles. Environmental cleanliness and handling and storing food properly decreases bacteria.
CN: Safe, effective care environment; CNS: Safety and infection control; CL: Apply

41. The nurse is educating a parent on how to care for the son's penis after hypospadias repair with a skin graft. Which statement made by the parent indicates the need for further education from the nurse?
1. "My infant can take baths after the repair has healed."
2. "I will change the dressing around his penis daily."
3. "I will make sure I change my infant's diaper often."
4. "I will notify the health care provider for penile color change."

41. 2. Dressing changes after a hypospadias repair with a skin graft are generally performed by the health care provider, but they are not performed every day because the skin graft needs time to heal and adhere to the penis. Changing the infant's diapers usually helps keep the penis dry. Baths are not given until postoperative healing has taken place. If the penis color changes, it might be evidence of circulation problems and should be reported to the health care provider.
CN: Physiological integrity; CNS: Reduction of risk potential; CL: Apply

42. After the nurse has completed discharge education, which statement made by the female adolescent treated for a sexually transmitted infection indicates discharge instructions were understood?
1. "I am not allergic to penicillin, so I will skip condoms and get a shot if infected."
2. "I will notify my sexual partners and not have unprotected sex from now on."
3. "I will be careful not to have intercourse with someone who is not clean."
4. "I am not worried because I do not think this will happen to me again."

42. 2. Goal achievement is indicated by the female adolescent's ability to describe preventive behaviors and health practices. The other statements indicate that she does not understand the need to take preventive measures.
CN: Health promotion and maintenance; CNS: None; CL: Apply

43. Which technique will the nurse consider when discussing sex and sexual activities with adolescents?
1. Break down all the information into scientific terminology.
2. Refer adolescents to their parents for sexual information.
3. Only answer questions that are asked; do not present any other content.
4. Present sexual information using the proper terminology and in a straightforward manner.

43. 4. Although many adolescents have received sex education from parents and school throughout childhood, they are not always adequately prepared for the impact of puberty. A large portion of their knowledge is acquired from peers, television, movies, and social media. Consequently, much of the sex information they have is incomplete, inaccurate, riddled with cultural and moral values, and not very helpful. The public perceives nurses as having authoritative information and being willing to take time with adolescents and their parents. To be effective teachers, nurses need to be honest and open with sexual information.
CN: Health promotion and maintenance; CNS: None; CL: Apply

44. The nurse is providing education to an adolescent diagnosed with chlamydia. Which statement by the adolescent indicates a correct understanding of the teaching?
1. "The preferred treatment for chlamydia is oral penicillin."
2. "I can stop taking my doxycycline after the discharge goes away."
3. "My sexual partners will also need to be treated."
4. "Since I have had chlamydia I am immune to it in the future."

45. Before an adolescent with syphilis can be treated, the nurse must determine which factor?
1. Portal of entry
2. Size of the chancre
3. Names of sexual contacts
4. Existence of medication allergies

46. The nurse is presenting a staff education workshop about preventing sexually transmitted infections (STIs) in adolescents. Which statement(s) will the nurse include? Select all that apply.
1. "Maintain a nonjudgmental attitude when dealing with adolescents that are sexually active."
2. "Educate adolescents about the specific behaviors that put them at risk for STIs."
3. "Being in a mutually monogamous relationship will decrease the risk of STIs for adolescents."
4. "Parents must be notified and give consent for an adolescent to be tested and treated for STIs."
5. "Abstinence is the only STI prevention strategy that should be discussed with adolescents."
6. "Sexually active adolescents should be taught to use condoms correctly and consistently."

47. An adolescent has been diagnosed with gonorrhea. The health care provider has prescribed ceftriaxone 250 mg to be administered prior to discharge from the clinic. Before preparing and administering the medication, which data will the nurse collect from the client? Select all that apply.
1. Allergy to penicillin
2. Previous history of treatment for gonorrhea
3. Allergy to cephalosporins
4. Names of sexual partners
5. Sites of sexual penetration

48. Which statement will the nurse include when educating an adolescent about gonorrhea?
1. "It is caused by *Treponema pallidum*."
2. "Treatment of sexual partners is an essential part of treatment."
3. "It is usually treated by multidose administration of penicillin."
4. "It may be contracted through contact with a contaminated toilet seat."

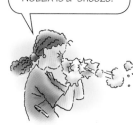
Achoo! Excuse me … practicing for the NCLEX is a "sneeze."

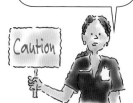
Medication administration requires a lot of questions.

44. 3. Sexual partners will need to be treated to prevent reinfection. The treatment of choice is doxycycline or azithromycin. When doxycycline is prescribed, the dosage is 100 mg by mouth, twice a day for 7 days. It is important to complete the full course of therapy even if symptoms subside. No immunity is conferred by exposure; it is possible to be infected multiple times if precautions are not taken.
CN: Health promotion and maintenance; CNS: None; CL: Apply

45. 4. The treatment of choice for syphilis is penicillin; clients allergic to penicillin must be given another antibiotic. The other information is not necessary before treatment can begin.
CN: Safe, effective care environment; CNS: Safety and infection control; CL: Apply

46. 1, 2, 3, 6. Many adolescents are reluctant to seek care because of concerns about judgmental attitudes of health care providers and confidentiality. Most states have laws that allow minors to receive STI and pregnancy services without the consent/knowledge of the parents. Abstinence is the only 100% effective strategy, but it is not the only strategy that should be discussed. Knowledge of specific behaviors that increase the risk of STIs, engaging in a mutually monogamous relationship, and correct and consistent condom use also reduce the risk of contracting STIs.
CN: Safe, effective care environment; CNS: Management of care; CL: Apply

47. 1, 3. Ceftriaxone is a third-generation cephalosporin and should not be administered if the client has an allergy to cephalosporins. Cephalosporins are also contraindicated if there has been a previous anaphylactic reaction to penicillin. The other information may be collected, but it does not relate to preparation or administration of the ceftriaxone.
CN: Safe, effective care environment; CNS: Safety and infection control; CL: Analyze

48. 2. Adolescents should be taught that treatment is needed for all sexual partners. *Treponema pallidum* is the causative organism of syphilis, not gonorrhea. The medication of choice is a single dose of IM ceftriaxone in males and a single oral dose of cefixime in females. Gonorrhea cannot be contracted from a contaminated toilet seat.
CN: Health promotion and maintenance; CNS: None; CL: Apply

49. When planning sex and contraceptive education for adolescents, which factor will the nurse consider?
1. Neither sexual activity nor contraception requires planning.
2. Most teenagers today are knowledgeable about reproduction.
3. Most teenagers use pregnancy to rebel against their parents.
4. Most teenagers are open about contraception but inconsistently use birth control.

50. A sexually active teenager seeks counseling from the school nurse about prevention of sexually transmitted infections (STIs). Which contraceptive measure will the nurse recommend?
1. Rhythm method
2. Withdrawal method
3. Prophylactic antibiotic use
4. Condom and spermicide use

51. The registered nurse (RN) and assistive personnel (AP) are rounding. The RN notes a child with nephrotic syndrome is experiencing dyspnea. What will the RN have the AP do **next**?
1. Put a non-rebreather mask on the child.
2. Listen to the lungs for adventitious breath sounds.
3. Call the child's health care provider.
4. Obtain the child's oxygen saturation level.

52. The nurse is preparing to administer 250 mg of ceftriaxone IM to an adolescent diagnosed with gonorrhea. Available is a vial of ceftriaxone 1 g powder for reconstitution. Instructions are to dilute with 3.6 mL of sterile water, 0.9% sodium chloride, or 1% lidocaine to make a solution of 1 g ceftriaxone per 4 mL of solution. How many milliliters will the nurse administer? Record your answer using a whole number.

_____ mL

53. Which statement by an adolescent will alert the nurse that more education about sexually transmitted infections (STIs) is needed?
1. "You always know when you have gonorrhea."
2. "The most common STI in kids my age is chlamydia."
3. "Most of the girls who have chlamydia do not even know it."
4. "Symptoms of gonorrhea may show up days or weeks after being infected."

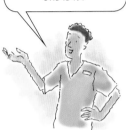

Only one answer to question #50 prevents STIs. Which one is it?

49. 4. Most teenagers today are very open about discussing contraception and sexuality, but they may get caught up in the moment of sexuality and forget about birth control measures. Adolescents receive most of their information on reproduction and sexuality from their peers, who generally do not have correct information. Teenagers generally become pregnant because they fail to use birth control for reasons other than rebelling against their parents. Contraception should always be part of sex education and requires planning.
CN: Health promotion and maintenance; CNS: None; CL: Apply

50. 4. Prevention of STIs is the primary concern of health care professionals. Barrier contraceptive methods, such as condoms with the addition of spermicide, seem to offer the best protection for preventing STIs and their serious complications. The other contraceptive choices do not prevent the transmission of an STI. Antibiotics cannot be taken throughout the life span.
CN: Health promotion and maintenance; CNS: None; CL: Apply

51. 4. The RN will have the AP obtain the child's oxygen saturation level. It is not appropriate for the AP to administer oxygen, assess lung sounds, or notify the health care provider.
CN: Safe and effective care environment; CNS: Management of care; CL: Analyze

52. 1.
The correct formula to calculate the drug dose is:
First, convert grams to milligrams. 1 gram = 1,000 mg.

$$dose\ ordered/dose\ on\ hand \times quantity = dose\ administered$$

$$\frac{250\ mg}{1,000\ mg} \times 4\ mL = 1\ mL$$

CN: Physiological integrity; CNS: Pharmacological and parenteral therapies; CL: Apply

53. 1. Gonorrhea can occur with or without symptoms. There are four main forms of the disease: asymptomatic, uncomplicated symptomatic, complicated symptomatic, and disseminated disease. All the other statements by the adolescent about STIs are accurate.
CN: Health promotion and maintenance; CNS: None; CL: Apply

54. A female adolescent with genital herpes has been taking acyclovir. Which statement by the adolescent is **most** concerning to the nurse?
1. "The lesions on my labia and rectum are painful."
2. "I am so glad this medication will cure me."
3. "I will never have unprotected sex again."
4. "Alcohol does not interfere with this medication."

54. 2. There is not a cure for genital herpes. Acyclovir is an antiviral medication that will help prevent outbreaks. Lesions are painful. Having protected sex will help prevent future STIs and pregnancy. While the nurse should investigate alcohol consumption by the adolescent, the statement does not prove the adolescent drinks, and is also a true statement.
CN: Health promotion and maintenance; CNS: None; CL: Analyze

55. Which statement is important for the nurse to include in discharge education for the adolescent taking metronidazole to treat trichomoniasis?
1. Sexual intercourse should stop.
2. Alcohol should not be consumed.
3. Milk products should be avoided.
4. Exposure to sunlight should be limited.

Be sure to explain all potential drug interactions to clients before discharge.

55. 2. While taking metronidazole to treat trichomoniasis, adolescents should not consume alcohol for at least 3 days following the last dose because the drug is similar to disulfiram and may lead to a psychotic reaction. Milk and sunlight have no effect on the adolescent while taking this medication. Sexual intercourse need not be avoided.
CN: Physiological integrity; CNS: Pharmacological and parenteral therapies; CL: Apply

56. When educating an adolescent about human immunodeficiency virus (HIV), which fact is **most** important for the nurse to include?
1. The incidence of HIV in the adolescent population has increased since 1995.
2. The virus can be spread through many routes, including sexual contact.
3. Knowledge about HIV transmission has led to an overall decrease of the virus.
4. Young women are contracting HIV at the fastest rate around the globe.

56. 2. HIV can be spread through many routes, including sexual contact and contact with infected blood or other body fluids. The other statements are true; however, adolescent education should be directed at the adolescent, not generalized. This age group does not associate themselves with being at risk simply due to statistics. Providing the adolescent with facts on how to prevent the spread of HIV is priority.
CN: Safe, effective care environment; CNS: Safety and infection control; CL: Analysis

57. The nurse is planning a program to educate adolescents about acquired immunodeficiency syndrome (AIDS). Which nursing action will lead to better acceptance of the program?
1. Survey the community to evaluate the level of education.
2. Obtain peer educators to provide information about AIDS.
3. Set up clinics in community centers and supply condoms readily.
4. Invite health care providers to host workshops in community centers.

57. 2. Peer education programs have shown that teens are more likely to pose questions to peer educators than to adults, and that peer education can change personal attitudes and the perception of the risk of HIV infection. The other approaches would be helpful but would not necessarily make the outreach program more successful.
CN: Health promotion and maintenance; CNS: None; CL: Analyze

If you can remember how AIDS is transmitted, question #58 will be easy.

58. Which adolescent does the nurse consider to be at greatest risk for developing acquired immunodeficiency syndrome (AIDS)?
1. A teen who lives in crowded housing with poor ventilation
2. A young, sexually active client with multiple partners
3. A homeless adolescent who lives in a shelter
4. A young, sexually active teen with one partner

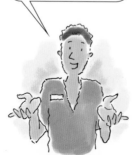

58. 2. The younger the client when sexual activity begins, the higher the incidence of human immunodeficiency virus and AIDS. Also, the more sexual partners, the higher the incidence of HIV and AIDS. Neither crowded living environments nor homeless environments by themselves lead to an increase in the incidence of AIDS.
CN: Health promotion and maintenance; CNS: None; CL: Analyze

CN: Client needs category   CNS: Client needs subcategory   CL: Cognitive level

59. When assessing an adolescent with pelvic inflammatory disease (PID), which finding(s) will the nurse expect? Select all that apply.
1. A hard, painless, red, defined lesion
2. Small vesicles on the genital area with itching
3. Cervical discharge with redness and edema
4. Lower abdominal pain
5. Urinary tract symptoms
6. Greenish-yellow discharge

59. **4, 5.** PID is an infection of the upper female genital tract most commonly caused by sexually transmitted infections. Initial symptoms in the adolescent may be generalized, with fever, abdominal pain, urinary tract symptoms, and vague, influenza-like symptoms. Small vesicles on the genital area with itching indicate herpes genitalis. Cervical discharge with redness and edema indicates chlamydia. A hard, painless, red, defined lesion indicates syphilis.
CN: Physiological integrity; CNS: Physiological adaptation; CL: Apply

60. After the nurse provides education to an adolescent about syphilis, which statement by the adolescent indicates the need for further education?
1. "The disease is divided into four stages: primary, secondary, latent, and tertiary."
2. "Affected persons are most infectious during the first year."
3. "Syphilis is easily treated with penicillin or doxycycline."
4. "Syphilis is rarely transmitted sexually."

60. **4.** About 95% of the cases of syphilis are transmitted sexually. There are four stages to syphilis, although some people may only experience the first three stages. Affected persons are most contagious in the first year of the disease. The drug of choice for treating syphilis is penicillin or doxycycline.
CN: Health promotion and maintenance; CNS: None; CL: Apply

61. In educating a group of parents about monitoring for urinary tract infections (UTIs) in preschoolers, which symptom(s) will the nurse state indicates a child needs to be evaluated? Select all that apply.
1. Voids only twice in any 6-hour period
2. Exhibits incontinence after being toilet trained
3. Has difficulty sitting still for more than 30 minutes at a time
4. Urine smells strongly of ammonia after standing for more than 2 hours
5. A fever with no other signs or symptoms

UTIs can make urination painful—so a lot of kids will hold it as long as they can.

61. **2, 5.** A child who exhibits incontinence after being toilet trained or has a fever with no other findings should be evaluated for UTI. Most urine smells strongly of ammonia after standing for more than 2 hours, so this does not necessarily indicate UTI. The other symptoms are not reasons for parents to suspect problems with their child's urinary system.
CN: Health promotion and maintenance; CNS: None; CL: Apply

62. The nurse is providing education to the parents of a child with recurrent urinary tract infections (UTIs). Which statement will the nurse include?
1. "Antibiotics should be discontinued 48 hours after symptoms subside."
2. "Recurrent symptoms should be treated by renewing the antibiotic prescription."
3. "Complicated UTIs are related to poor perineal hygiene practice."
4. "It is necessary for your child to have a follow-up urine culture."

62. **4.** A routine follow-up urine specimen is usually obtained 2 or 3 days after the completion of the antibiotic treatment. All of the antibiotic should be taken as prescribed and not stopped when symptoms disappear. If recurrent symptoms appear, a urine culture should be obtained to see whether the infection is resistant to antibiotics. Simple, not complicated, UTIs are generally caused by poor perineal hygiene.
CN: Health promotion and maintenance; CNS: None; CL: Apply

Be sure to tell clients all they need to know about us medications!

63. Which instruction will the nurse include in the education plan for the parents of a child receiving sulfamethoxazole-trimethoprim for a repeated urinary tract infection with *Escherichia coli*?
1. "Have your child drink at least a quart of cranberry juice per day."
2. "Make sure your child takes all of the medication."
3. "Return to the clinic in 3 days for another urine culture."
4. "Keep extra pills to give if the symptoms reappear within 2 weeks."

63. **2.** Discharge instructions for parents of children receiving an anti-infective medication should include taking all of the prescribed medication for the prescribed time. The child will not need to have a culture repeated until the medication is completed. Drinking highly acidic juices, such as cranberry juice, may help maintain urinary health but will not get rid of an infection already present.
CN: Physiological integrity; CNS: Pharmacological and parenteral therapies; CL: Apply

CN: Client needs category   CNS: Client needs subcategory   CL: Cognitive level

64. The nurse is monitoring a child with vesico-ureteral reflux. Which condition will the nurse be alert for as a potential complication?
1. Glomerulonephritis
2. Hemolytic uremia syndrome
3. Nephrotic syndrome
4. Kidney damage

65. The nurse reviewing a child's clean-catch urine specimen results understands that which result indicates a urinary tract infection (UTI)?
1. A specific gravity of 1.020
2. Cloudy color without odor
3. A large amount of casts present
4. 100,000 bacterial colonies per milliliter

66. The nurse is providing education to the parents of a child with a urinary tract infection. Which factor(s) will the nurse indicate contributes to urinary tract infections (UTIs)? Select all that apply.
1. Increased fluid intake
2. Short urethra
3. Ingestion of acidic juices
4. Constipation
5. Infrequent bladder emptying

67. The parent of a female child asks the nurse why the child seems to have so many urinary tract infections (UTIs). Which response by the nurse is **most** accurate?
1. "Vaginal secretions are too acidic."
2. "Girls cannot be protected by circumcision like boys."
3. "The urethra is in close proximity to the anus."
4. "Girls touch their genitalia more often than boys do."

68. A child has been sent to the school nurse for wetting her pants three times in the past 2 days. The nurse will recommend this child be evaluated for which complication?
1. School phobia
2. Emotional trauma
3. Urinary tract infection
4. Structural defect of the urinary tract

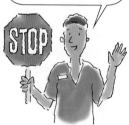

Hold up, there, partner. Remember to look for the **most** accurate answer in question #67.

64. 4. Reflux of urine into the ureters and then back into the bladder after voiding sets up the child for a urinary tract infection, which can lead to kidney damage due to scarring of the parenchyma. Glomerulonephritis is an autoimmune reaction to a beta-hemolytic streptococcal infection. Eighty percent of nephrotic syndrome cases are idiopathic. Hemolytic uremia syndrome may be the result of genetic factors.
CN: Health promotion and maintenance; CNS: None; CL: Analyze

65. 4. The diagnosis of UTI is determined by the detection of bacteria in the urine. Infected urine usually contains more than 100,000 colonies/mL, often of a single organism. The urine is usually cloudy, hazy, and may have strands of mucus. It also has a foul, fishy odor even when fresh. Casts and increased specific gravity are not specific to UTI.
CN: Physiological integrity; CNS: Physiological adaptation; CL: Analyze

66. 2, 4, 5. A short urethra contributes to infection because bacteria have to travel a shorter distance to the urinary tract. The risk of infection is higher in women than men because women have shorter urethras (0.75 in [1.9 cm] in young women, 1.5 in [3.8 cm] in mature women, 7.75 in [19.7 cm] in adult men). Urinary stasis contributes to bacterial growth. Constipation increases the risk of UTI. Increased fluid intake helps flush the urinary tract system, and frequent emptying of the bladder decreases the risk of urinary tract infection. Drinking highly acidic juices, such as cranberry juice, may help maintain urinary health. In addition to being acidic, cranberry juice is a healthy choice because studies suggest it helps prevent the bacteria from attaching to the bladder wall.
CN: Health promotion and maintenance; CNS: None; CL: Apply

67. 3. Girls are especially at risk for bacterial invasion of the urinary tract because of basic anatomical differences; the urethra is shorter and closer to the anus. Vaginal secretions are normally acidic, which decreases the risk of infection. Circumcision does not protect boys from UTIs. There is no documented research that supports that girls touch their genitalia more often than boys do.
CN: Health promotion and maintenance; CNS: None; CL: Apply

68. 3. Frequent urinary incontinence should be evaluated by the health care provider, and the nurse's first action should be to check the urine for infection. Children exhibit signs of school phobia by reporting an ailment before school starts and getting better after they are allowed to miss school. After infection, structural defect, and diabetes have been ruled out, emotional trauma should be investigated.
CN: Health promotion and maintenance; CNS: None; CL: Apply

CN: Client needs category   CNS: Client needs subcategory   CL: Cognitive level

69. Which intervention will the nurse recommend to parents of young girls to help prevent urinary tract infections (UTIs)?
1. Dress the child in cotton underwear.
2. Limit bathing as much as possible.
3. Increase fluids and decrease salt intake.
4. Educate the child about cleaning her perineum from back to front.

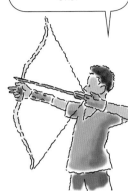

Bullseye! You really nailed that one.

69. 1. Cotton is a more breathable fabric than nylon and allows for dampness to be absorbed from the perineum. Dressing the child in cotton underwear helps prevent UTIs. Increasing fluids would be helpful, but decreasing salt is not necessary. Bathing should not be limited; however, the use of bubble bath or whirlpool baths should be avoided. If the child has frequent UTIs, taking a bath should be discouraged and taking a shower encouraged. The perineum should always be cleaned from *front to back*.
CN: Health promotion and maintenance; CNS: None; CL: Apply

70. The nurse is caring for a child with a urinary tract infection. The child weighs 46 lb (21 kg). The health care provider has prescribed amoxicillin 750 mg by mouth every 8 hours. The recommended pediatric dosage is 40 to 90 mg/kg/day in two to three divided doses. Which action will the nurse take?
1. Administer the medication in 4 ounces of juice.
2. Do not give the antibiotic until the culture and sensitivity results are final.
3. Hold the medication and notify the health care provider.
4. Give the medication after verifying the dosage with the charge nurse.

70. 3. The nurse should notify the health care provider that the prescribed dosage exceeds the recommended range for this child, which is 280 to 630 mg/dose.

$$recommended\ dosage \times doses\ per\ day \times weight$$
$$= mg\ per\ dose$$

$$\frac{40\ mg}{kg/day} \times \frac{1\ day}{3\ doses} \times 21\ kg = \frac{840}{3} = 280\ mg/dose$$

$$\frac{90\ mg}{kg/day} \times \frac{1\ day}{3\ doses} \times 21\ kg = \frac{1,890}{3} = 630\ mg/dose$$

Oral medication is not diluted in large volumes. Antimicrobial therapy is started after the cultures are collected, not until the results are obtained.
CN: Physiological integrity; CNS: Pharmacological and parenteral therapies; CL: Analyze

71. The nurse is caring for a child with a urinary tract infection. The health care provider has prescribed cephalexin 125 mg by mouth every 8 hours. Cephalexin is available 250 mg per 5 mL. How many milliliters will the nurse administer per dose? Record your answer using one decimal place.

_____ mL

71. 2.5.
The correct formula to calculate a drug dose is:

$$dose\ ordered/dose\ on\ hand \times quantity$$
$$= dose\ administered$$

$$\frac{125\ mg}{250\ mg} \times 5\ mL = 2.5\ mL$$

CN: Physiological integrity; CNS: Pharmacological and parenteral therapies; CL: Apply

72. When evaluating infants and young toddlers for signs of urinary tract infections (UTIs), a nurse understands which symptom is **most** common?
1. Abdominal pain
2. Feeding problems
3. Frequency
4. Urgency

72. 2. In infants and children younger than age 2, the signs of UTI are characteristically nonspecific, and feeding problems are usually the first indication. Symptoms more nearly resemble gastrointestinal tract disorders. Abdominal pain, urgency, and frequency are signs that would be observed in the older child with a UTI.
CN: Physiological integrity; CNS: Pharmacological and parenteral therapies; CL: Apply

73. When obtaining a urine specimen for culture and sensitivity from a child, the nurse understands which method of collection yields the **most** accurate results?
1. Bagged urine specimen
2. Clean-catch urine specimen
3. First-voided urine specimen
4. Catheterized urine specimen

73. 4. The most accurate tests of bacterial content are suprapubic aspiration (for children younger than age 2) and properly performed bladder catheterization. The other methods of obtaining a specimen have a high incidence of contamination not related to infection.
CN: Physiological integrity; CNS: Basic care and comfort; CL: Apply

CN: Client needs category   CNS: Client needs subcategory   CL: Cognitive level

74. After collecting a urine specimen for culture, which action by the nurse is **most** appropriate?
1. Take the specimen to the laboratory immediately.
2. Send the specimen to the laboratory on the scheduled run.
3. Take the specimen to the laboratory on the nurse's next break.
4. Keep the specimen in the refrigerator until it can be taken to the laboratory.

75. The nurse is providing education about fluid intake to the parents of a child with a urinary tract infection (UTI). Which statement by a parent indicates the need for further education?
1. "I will have my child drink 50 mL/lb (23 mL/kg) of body weight daily."
2. "Clear liquids should be the primary liquids that my child drinks."
3. "I should offer my child carbonated beverages about every 2 hours."
4. "My child should avoid drinking caffeinated beverages."

76. Which treatment will the nurse anticipate for a child who has a history of recurrent urinary tract infections (UTIs)?
1. Frequent catheterizations
2. Prophylactic antibiotics
3. Limited activities
4. Surgical intervention

77. The nurse is providing education to parents about administering medications to children for recurrent urinary tract infections. Which instruction will the nurse include?
1. Antibiotics should be given first thing in the morning.
2. Antibiotics should be given right before bedtime.
3. Antibiotics are generally given four times per day.
4. It does not matter when the antibiotic is given.

78. The nurse is providing education to a group of parents about urinary tract infections (UTIs). The nurse knows the education has been effective when the parents indicate which population is at **greatest** risk for progressive kidney injury after a UTI?
1. A school-age child who must get permission to go to the bathroom
2. An adolescent female who has started menstruation
3. A child who participates in competitive sports
4. A young infant who has an infection

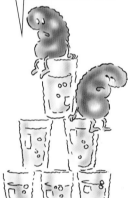

Whoa. This is a lot of water to process. It makes my nephrons hurt just thinking about it.

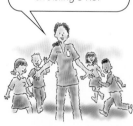

I believe the children are our future. Teach them well about avoiding UTIs.

74. 1. Care of urine specimens obtained for culture is an important nursing goal related to diagnosis. Specimens should be taken to the laboratory for culture immediately. If the culture is delayed, the specimen can be placed in the refrigerator, but storage can result in a loss of formed elements, such as blood cells and casts.
CN: Physiological integrity; CNS: Basic care and comfort; CL: Apply

75. 3. Carbonated or caffeinated beverages are avoided because of their potentially irritating effect on the bladder mucosa. Adequate fluid intake is always indicated during an acute UTI. It is recommended that a person drinks approximately 50 mL/lb (23 mL/kg) of body weight daily. The child should primarily drink clear liquids.
CN: Physiological integrity; CNS: Basic care and comfort; CL: Apply

76. 2. Children who experience recurrent UTIs may require antibiotic therapy for months or years. Recurrent UTIs would be investigated for anatomic abnormalities and surgical intervention may be indicated, but the child would also be placed on antibiotics before the tests. The child's activities are not limited. Frequent catheterization predisposes a child to infection.
CN: Physiological integrity; CNS: Physiological adaptation; CL: Apply

77. 2. Medication is commonly administered once per day, and the parents are advised to give the antibiotic before sleep because it is the longest period without voiding.
CN: Physiological integrity; CNS: Pharmacological and parenteral therapies; CL: Apply

78. 4. The hazard of progressive kidney injury is greatest when infection occurs in young children, especially those under age 2. A child who must get permission to go to the bathroom and an adolescent who has started menstruation might experience a simple UTI that would need to be treated. Competitive sports have no impact on UTI.
CN: Health promotion and maintenance; CNS: None; CL: Analyze

CN: Client needs category   CNS: Client needs subcategory   CL: Cognitive level

79. Which statement will the nurse make to help parents understand the recovery period after a child has had surgery to remove Wilms tumor?
   1. "Children will easily lie in bed and restrict their activities."
   2. "Recovery is usually fast in spite of the abdominal incision."
   3. "Recovery usually takes a great deal of time because of the large incision."
   4. "Parents need to perform the child's activities of daily living for about 2 weeks after surgery."

80. The nurse is caring for a toddler following a nephrectomy for Wilms tumor. The nurse has assessed the child's pain and is preparing to administer an oral opiate. Which method is the **best** choice for administering the medication?
   1. A one-ounce calibrated medicine cup
   2. A teaspoon
   3. An oral syringe
   4. An injectable syringe with the needle removed

81. When assessing a preschool child, which observation indicates to the nurse the client may have Wilms tumor?
   1. Pain in the abdomen
   2. Fever greater than 104°F (40°C)
   3. Blood pressure 86/52 mm Hg
   4. Swelling within the abdomen

82. When providing education to parents about administering sulfamethoxazole-trimethoprim to a child for treatment of a urinary tract infection, the nurse will include which instruction?
   1. Give the medication with food.
   2. Give the medication with water.
   3. Give the medication with a cola beverage.
   4. Give the medication one hour after a meal.

83. When the nurse is providing education about the diagnosis of Wilms tumor to a pediatric client's parents, which statement by a parent indicates the need for further education?
   1. "Wilms tumor usually involves both kidneys."
   2. "Wilms tumor is slightly more common in the left kidney."
   3. "Wilms tumor is staged during surgery for treatment planning."
   4. "Wilms tumor stays encapsulated for an extended time."

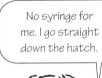

No syringe for me. I go straight down the hatch.

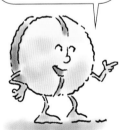

79. 2. Children generally recover very quickly from surgery to remove Wilms tumor, even though they may have a large abdominal incision. Children like to get back into the normalcy of being a child, which is through play. Parents need to encourage their children to do as much for themselves as possible, although some regression is expected.
CN: Psychosocial integrity; CNS: None; CL: Apply

80. 3. The most accurate and safest way to administer the medication is using an oral syringe. Using a medicine cup or teaspoon will lead to inaccurate measurement of the opiate, which needs to be carefully measured to ensure the child does not receive an overdose. The end of an injectable syringe is not appropriate for oral use.
CN: Physiological integrity; CNS: Pharmacological and parenteral therapies; CL: Apply

81. 4. The most common initial sign of Wilms tumor is a swelling or mass within the abdomen. The mass is characteristically firm, nontender, confined to one side, and deep within the flank. A high fever is not an initial sign of Wilms tumor. Blood pressure is characteristically increased, not decreased.
CN: Physiological integrity; CNS: Physiological adaptation; CL: Apply

82. 2. When giving sulfamethoxazole-trimethoprim, the medication should be administered with a full glass of water on an empty stomach. If nausea and vomiting occur, giving the drug with food may decrease gastric distress. Carbonated beverages should be avoided because they irritate the bladder.
CN: Physiological integrity; CNS: Pharmacological and parenteral therapies; CL: Apply

83. 1. Wilms tumor usually involves only one kidney and is usually staged during surgery so that an effective course of treatment can be established. Wilms tumor has a slightly higher occurrence in the left kidney, and it stays encapsulated for an extended time.
CN: Physiological integrity; CNS: Physiological adaptation; CL: Apply

84. Parents ask the nurse about the prognosis of their child diagnosed with Wilms tumor. The nurse will base the response on which factor?
1. Usually, children with Wilms tumor need only surgical intervention.
2. Survival rates for Wilms tumor are the lowest among childhood cancers.
3. Survival rates for Wilms tumor are the highest among childhood cancers.
4. Children with localized tumor have only a 30% chance of cure with multimodal therapy.

84. 3. Survival rates for Wilms tumor are the highest among childhood cancers. Usually, children with Wilms tumor who have a stage I or II localized tumor have a 90% chance of cure with multimodal therapy.
CN: Physiological integrity; CNS: Physiological adaptation; CL: Understand

85. The nurse is caring for a child with Wilms tumor involving both kidneys. The nurse will expect that treatment before surgery might include which method(s)? Select all that apply.
1. Peritoneal dialysis
2. Radiation
3. Chemotherapy
4. Abdominal gavage
5. Antibiotics
6. IV fluid therapy

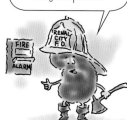

Wilms tumor is a true renal emergency. It requires a heavy-duty response.

85. 2, 3. If both kidneys are involved, the child may be treated with radiation therapy or chemotherapy preoperatively to shrink the tumor, allowing more conservative surgery. Peritoneal dialysis would be needed only if the kidneys were not functioning. Abdominal gavage is not indicated. Antibiotics are not needed because Wilms tumor is not an infection.
CN: Physiological integrity; CNS: Reduction of risk potential; CL: Apply

86. When the nurse is caring for a child with Wilms tumor preoperatively, which nursing intervention is **priority**?
1. Avoid abdominal palpation.
2. Monitor urinalysis results.
3. Prepare the child for long-term dialysis.
4. Educate the family on postoperative care.

86. 1. After the diagnosis of Wilms tumor is made, the abdomen should not be palpated. Palpation of the tumor might lead to rupture, which would cause the cancerous cells to spread throughout the abdomen. The nurse will monitor urinalysis results and provide education; however, it is priority to prevent the spread of cancerous cells. If surgery is successful, there will not be a need for long-term dialysis.
CN: Physiological integrity; CNS: Reduction of risk potential; CL: Analyze

87. A child is scheduled for surgery to remove Wilms tumor from one kidney. The parents ask the nurse what treatment, if any, they should expect after their child recovers from surgery. Which response by the nurse is **most** accurate?
1. "Your child will be monitored to determine what is needed."
2. "Kidney transplant is indicated eventually."
3. "No additional treatments are usually necessary."
4. "Chemotherapy with or without radiation therapy is indicated."

87. 4. Because radiation therapy and chemotherapy are usually begun immediately after surgery, parents need an explanation of what to expect. The child will be monitored; however, this statement does not fully disclose the course of treatment. Kidney transplant is not usually necessary.
CN: Physiological integrity; CNS: Physiological adaptation; CL: Apply

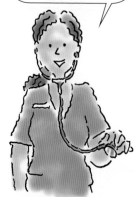

What substance is most likely to show up in your urine if you have nephrotic syndrome?

88. A toddler is admitted to the hospital with nephrotic syndrome. The nurse carefully monitors the toddler's fluid intake and output and checks urine specimens regularly with a reagent strip. Which finding is the nurse **most** likely to report?
1. Proteinuria
2. Glucosuria
3. Ketonuria
4. Polyuria

88. 1. In nephrotic syndrome, the glomerular membrane of the kidneys becomes permeable to proteins. This results in massive proteinuria, which the nurse can detect with a reagent strip. Nephrotic syndrome typically does not cause glucosuria or ketonuria. Because the syndrome causes fluids to shift from plasma to interstitial spaces, it is more likely to decrease urine output than to cause polyuria (excessive urine output).
CN: Physiological integrity; CNS: Reduction of risk potential; CL: Apply

89. The nurse is providing education about surgery to the parents of a child with Wilms tumor. Which statement by the nurse **best** explains the role of surgery for Wilms tumor?
1. "Surgery is not indicated in children with Wilms tumor."
2. "Surgery is usually performed within 24 to 48 hours of admission."
3. "Surgery is the least favorable therapy for the treatment of Wilms tumor."
4. "Surgery will be delayed until the child's overall health status improves."

89. 2. Surgery is the preferred treatment and is scheduled as soon as possible after confirmation of a renal mass, usually within 24 to 48 hours of admission, to make sure the encapsulated tumor remains intact.
CN: Physiological integrity; CNS: Physiological adaptation; CL: Understand

90. A 3-year-old child has had surgery to remove Wilms tumor. Which action will the nurse take **first** when the parent asks for pain medication for the child?
1. Get the pain medication ready for administration.
2. Ask the parents how they know the child is in pain.
3. Assess the child's pain using a smiley face pain scale.
4. Check for the last time pain medication was administered.

90. 3. The first action by the nurse should be to assess the child for pain. A 3-year-old child is too young to use a pain scale from 0 to 10 but can easily use the smiley face pain scale. Asking the parents about the child's pain is not appropriate. After assessing the pain, the nurse should then investigate the time the pain medication was last given and administer the medication accordingly.
CN: Physiological integrity; CNS: Pharmacological and parenteral therapies; CL: Analyze

91. The nurse is caring for a child diagnosed with Wilms tumor. Because of the parents' religious beliefs, they choose not to treat the child. Which statement by the nurse to a colleague indicates the need for further discussion?
1. "I know this is a lot of information for them to absorb in a short period of time."
2. "I do not think parents have the legal right to make these kinds of decisions."
3. "These parents just do not understand how easily treatable Wilms tumor is."
4. "I think the parents are in shock at this time about everything."

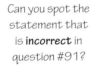

Can you spot the statement that is **incorrect** in question #91?

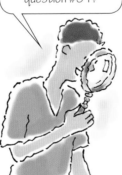

91. 2. Parents do have the legal right to make decisions regarding the health issues for their child. Religion plays an important role in many people's lives, and decisions about surgery and treatment for cancer are sometimes made that scientifically do not make sense to the health care provider. The parents are probably in a state of shock because a lot of information has been given, and this is a cancer that requires decisions to be made quickly, especially surgical intervention.
CN: Safe, effective care environment; CNS: Management of care; CL: Analyze

92. A child with nephrotic syndrome develops generalized edema as a result of nephrosis. Which action by the assistive personnel (AP) will cause the registered nurse (RN) to intervene?
1. Applying a moisturizer to the child's skin daily.
2. Changing the child's position every 2 hours.
3. Thoroughly drying the child after baths.
4. Having the child maintain continuous bed rest.

92. 4. Keeping the child on bed rest will promote skin breakdown and should be avoided. All other options will promote skin health.
CN: Safe, effective care environment; CNS: Management of care; CL: Analyze

93. A child with Wilms tumor has had surgery to remove a kidney and has received chemotherapy. The nurse will include which instruction at discharge?
1. Avoid contact sports.
2. Decrease fluid intake.
3. Decrease sodium intake.
4. Avoid contact with other children.

93. 1. Because the child is left with only one kidney, certain precautions, such as avoiding contact sports, are recommended to prevent injury to the remaining kidney. Decreasing fluid intake is not indicated; fluid intake is essential for renal function. The child's sodium intake should not be reduced. Avoiding other children is unnecessary, will make the child feel self-conscious, and may lead to regressive behavior.
CN: Physiological integrity; CNS: Reduction of risk potential; CL: Apply

CN: Client needs category   CNS: Client needs subcategory   CL: Cognitive level

94. The nurse is providing education to a parent of a preschool-age child with nephrosis who will be discharged on prednisone. Which statement(s) by the parent indicates the teaching has been effective? Select all that apply.
1. "My child should not receive any immunizations with live vaccines while on prednisone."
2. "Prednisone will prevent my child's kidneys from becoming infected."
3. "While on prednisone my child will be more susceptible to infections."
4. "Prednisone should never be discontinued abruptly."
5. "My child's appetite will be decreased, and weight loss may occur."

94. 1, 3, 4. Anyone receiving a systemic corticosteroid in high doses for longer than 2 weeks should wait at least 3 months before receiving a live-virus vaccine. Corticosteroids suppress the immune response, should not be discontinued abruptly due to the risk of acute adrenocortical crisis, and do not convey any infective protection. An initial weight gain may occur due to an increase in appetite.
CN: Physiological integrity; CNS: Pharmacological and parenteral therapies; CL: Apply

95. In providing psychosocial care to a 6-year-old child who has had abdominal surgery for Wilms tumor, which activity initiated by the nurse is **most** appropriate?
1. Allow the child to watch a 2-hour movie without interruptions.
2. Give the child a puzzle with five pieces to encourage movement while in bed.
3. Tell the child that medication can be given to prevent pain.
4. Provide the child with supplies and ask the child to draw how she feels.

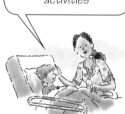

Effective nursing requires both physical and psychosocial activities

95. 4. A movie is a good diversion but giving supplies and encouraging the child to draw her feelings is a better outlet. Many procedures have been performed on this child since admission. The nurse probably cannot give enough pain medication so that a child who has had surgery will feel no pain. A puzzle with only five pieces is too basic for a 6-year-old and would not hold her interest.
CN: Psychosocial integrity; CNS: None; CL: Apply

96. When caring for a child after removal of Wilms tumor, which finding indicates to the nurse the need to notify the health care provider?
1. Fever of 100°F (37.8°C)
2. Absence of bowel sounds
3. Slight congestion in the lungs
4. Reports of pain when moving

96. 2. After tumor removal, the child is at risk for intestinal obstruction. Gastrointestinal abnormalities require notification of the health care provider. A slight fever following surgery is not uncommon; slight congestion in the lungs and reports of pain are also not uncommon.
CN: Physiological integrity; CNS: Reduction of risk potential; CL: Analyze

97. A parent reports her 6-year-old girl recently started wetting the bed and running a low-grade fever. A urinalysis is positive for bacteria and protein. A diagnosis of a urinary tract infection (UTI) is made, and the child is prescribed antibiotics. Which intervention(s) is appropriate? Select all that apply.
1. Limit fluids for the next few days to decrease the frequency of urination.
2. Assess the parent's understanding of UTIs and their causes.
3. Instruct the parent to administer the antibiotic as prescribed.
4. Provide instructions to the parent, not the child.
5. Discourage taking bubble baths or using bath bombs.
6. Advise wiping the perineum from the front to back after voiding and defecation.

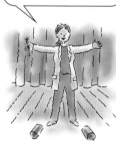

What a performance! You're really killing it on this test.

97. 2, 3, 5, 6. Assessing the parent's understanding of UTI and its causes provides the nurse with a baseline for education. The full course of antibiotics must be given to eradicate the organism and prevent recurrence, even if the child's signs and symptoms decrease. Bath additives can irritate the vulva and urethra and contribute to the development of a UTI. The child should wipe from the front to the back to minimize the risk of contamination after elimination. Fluids should be encouraged, not limited, to prevent urinary stasis and help flush the organism out of the urinary tract. Instructions should be given to the child at her level of understanding to help her better understand the treatment and promote compliance.
CN: Health promotion and maintenance; CNS: None; CL: Apply

98. The nurse is conducting a follow-up phone call with the parent of a child with nephrosis who was recently discharged. Which statement(s) by the parent indicates the discharge instructions are being followed correctly? Select all that apply.
1. "I am administering my child's prednisone once a day, every day."
2. "I have arranged for my child to be homeschooled."
3. "I am weighing my child every morning and keeping a logbook."
4. "If my child's morning urine has 2+ protein for 2 days, I will call the health care provider."
5. "My child is scheduled for his measles, mumps, and rubella (MMR) vaccine next week."

98. **1, 3, 4.** Initial therapy with prednisone is 60 mg/m²/day for 4 weeks. A single daily dose has fewer side effects. The child should avoid people who are ill, but there is no need to homeschool the child. Daily weights and urine protein checks should be measured and logged. Parents should notify the health care provider if the urine is 2+ for protein for 2 days in a row. A child on prednisone should not receive a live-virus vaccine like MMR.
CN: Safe, effective care environment; CNS: Management of care; CL: Analyze

99. The nurse has instructions to notify the health care provider if a 44 lb (20 kg) preschooler's urine output drops below 3 mL/kg/hour. The urine output for the previous hour was 30 mL. Which nursing intervention is **priority**?
1. Continue to monitor the child's urine output.
2. Encourage the child to drink more fluids.
3. Wait another 30 minutes and then notify the health care provider.
4. Notify the health care provider of the child's urine output.

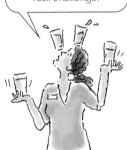

Maintaining proper fluid balance can be a real challenge.

99. **4.** The nurse should notify the health care provider of the child's urine output. The minimum urine output for this child is 3 mL × 20 kg = 60 mL/hour. Since the child had only a 30-mL urine output in the previous hour, it is crucial for the nurse to notify the health care provider. The nurse should continue to monitor the urine output after notifying the health care provider. Fluid should be encouraged as long as the child is not on fluid restrictions. The nurse should not wait another 30 minutes before notifying the health care provider because the lack of urine output could indicate a complication.
CN: Physiological integrity; CNS: Reduction of risk potential; CL: Analyze

100. A 6-year-old child's indwelling urinary catheter was removed at 0600. At 1200, the child still has not voided, appears uncomfortable, and the nurse palpates slight bladder distention. Which action will the nurse take **first**?
1. Insert a straight catheter, as prescribed, for urine retention.
2. Consult the health care provider about replacing the indwelling urinary catheter.
3. Wait a while longer to see whether the child can void independently.
4. Turn on the water faucet in the child's room and provide privacy.

100. **4.** Urine retention can result from many factors, including stress and use of opiates. Initially, the nurse should use independent nursing actions, such as providing the client with privacy, placing the client in a sitting or standing position to enlist the aid of gravity and increase intra-abdominal pressure, and turning on the water faucet. If these measures are unsuccessful and the health care provider has left a standing prescription for straight catheterization, the nurse can proceed with the catheterization. Consulting the health care provider would involve the use of a dependent nursing action; independent actions should be attempted first. Waiting longer will only increase the child's distention and pain.
CN: Physiological integrity; CNS: Basic care and comfort; CL: Analyze

101. The nurse is educating parents about Wilms tumor. Which statement made by a parent indicates the need for further education?
1. "My child could have inherited this disease."
2. "Wilms tumor can be associated with other congenital anomalies."
3. "This disease could have been a result of trauma to the baby in utero."
4. "There is no method to identify gene carriers of Wilms tumor."

101. **3.** Wilms tumor is not a result of trauma to the fetus in utero. Wilms tumor can be genetically inherited and is associated with other congenital anomalies. There is, however, no method to identify gene carriers of Wilms tumor.
CN: Psychosocial integrity; CNS: None; CL: Understand

CN: Client needs category   CNS: Client needs subcategory   CL: Cognitive level

102. When describing enuresis to a child's parents, which statement(s) will the nurse include in the description? Select all that apply.

1. "The child may experience involuntary urination after age 5."
2. "Episodes primarily occur when the child is awake and playing."
3. "The child may suffer feelings of shame and may withdraw from peers because of ridicule."
4. "The condition may respond to tricyclic antidepressants and antidiuretics."
5. "The condition may become permanent without appropriate intervention."

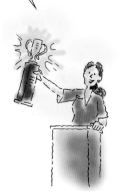

Outstanding! You really aced this test.

102. 1, 3, 4. Enuresis is a condition in which there is involuntary urination after age 5. It generally occurs while the child is sleeping. There can be long-lasting emotional trauma resulting from peer ridicule and feelings of shame and embarrassment. The condition may be treated with the use of tricyclic antidepressants and antidiuretics. With support and understanding, the condition generally resolves in time.

CN: Physiological integrity; CNS: Physiological adaptation; CL: Apply

Chapter 34

Integumentary Disorders

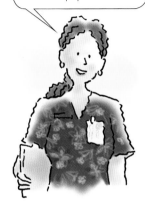

Skin diseases in children and teens are common and varied. This chapter covers common and uncommon skin disorders among these populations.

Pediatric integumentary refresher

Acne vulgaris

Overactive sebaceous glands that become plugged and inflamed

Key signs and symptoms

- Closed comedo or whitehead: acne plug not protruding from the follicle and covered by the epidermis
- Inflammation and characteristic acne pustules, papules, or, in severe forms, acne cysts or abscesses (caused by rupture or leakage of an enlarged plug into the dermis)
- Open comedo or blackhead: acne plug protruding from the follicle and not covered by the epidermis

Key treatments

- Exposure to ultraviolet light (but never when a photosensitizing agent, such as tretinoin, is being used)
- Oral tretinoin limited to those with nodulocystic or recalcitrant acne who do not respond to conventional therapy
- Systemic therapy: usually tetracycline to decrease bacterial growth; alternatively, erythromycin (tetracycline contraindicated during pregnancy and childhood because it discolors developing teeth)
- Topical medications: benzoyl peroxide, clindamycin, or erythromycin and benzoyl peroxide antibacterial agents, alone or in combination with tretinoin (retinoic acid)

Key interventions

- Identify predisposing factors.
- Instruct adolescent using tretinoin to apply it at least 30 minutes after washing the face and at least 1 hour before bedtime; warn against using it around the eyes or lips; after treatments, skin should look pink and dry.
- Advise adolescent to avoid exposure to sunlight or to use a sunblock; if prescribed regimen includes tretinoin and benzoyl peroxide, tell adolescent to use one preparation in the morning and the other at night.
- Instruct adolescent to take tetracycline on an empty stomach and not to take it with antacids or milk.
- Tell adolescent taking isotretinoin to avoid vitamin A supplements; discuss how to deal with the dry skin and mucous membranes that usually occur during treatment; the female should use 2 forms of birth control.
- Offer emotional support to the adolescent who is insecure about appearance.

Burns

Injuries to the tissues caused by heat, friction, chemical, electricity, or radiation

Key signs and symptoms

Superficial (first-degree) burn
- Dry, painful, red skin with edema
- Sunburn appearance

Superficial partial-thickness and deep partial thickness (second-degree) burn
- Moist, weeping blisters with edema
- Severe pain

Full-thickness (third-degree) burn
- Avascular site without blanching or pain
- Dry, pale, leathery skin

Key test results

- Many burn facilities use the Lund-Browder chart (body surface area chart that accounts for age) to determine the extent of injury

Key treatments

- IV fluids to prevent and treat shock; urine output maintained at 1 to 2 mL/kg/hour
- Protective isolation, depending on burn severity
- Tetanus toxoid according to child's immunization status

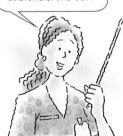

Tell your clients on tretinoin to make like a vampire and avoid the sun.

Key interventions

- Stop the burning in an emergency situation.
- Maintain a patent airway in the immediate postburn phase.
- Monitor vital signs, intake, and output.
- Prevent heat loss.
- Analgesia for pain.

Contact dermatitis

Irritation of the skin due to contact between the skin and a substance

Key signs and symptoms

- Characteristic bright red, maculopapular rash in the diaper area

Key treatments

- Cleaning affected area with mild soap and water
- Leaving affected area open to air

Key interventions

- Keep the diaper area clean and dry

Head lice

Tiny insects that live on the scalp

Key signs and symptoms

- Pruritus of the scalp
- White flecks attached to the hair shafts

Key test results

- Examination reveals lice eggs, which look like white flecks, firmly attached to hair shafts near the base

Key treatments

- Pyrethrin or permethrin shampoos, or lindane in resistant cases

Key interventions

- Explain the need to wash bed linens, hats, combs, brushes, and anything else that comes in contact with the hair

Impetigo

Acute, contagious staphylococcal or streptococcal skin disease

Key signs and symptoms

- Macular rash progressing to a papular and vesicular rash, which oozes and forms a moist, honey-colored crust

Key treatments

- Washing affected area with disinfectant soap

Key interventions

- Apply antibiotic ointment.
- Wash the area three times daily with antiseptic soap.

Rashes

Change of the skin which affects its color, appearance, or texture

Key signs and symptoms

Papular rash
- Raised solid lesions with color changes in circumscribed areas

Pustular rash
- Vesicles and bullae that fill with purulent exudate

Vesicular rash
- Small, raised, circumscribed lesions filled with clear fluid

Key test results

- Aspirate from lesions may reveal cause
- Patch test may identify cause

Key treatments

- Antibacterial, antifungal, or antiviral agent (depending on cause)
- Antihistamines if the rash is the result of an allergy

Key interventions

- Maintain standard precautions to prevent the spread of infection.
- Teach sanitary techniques.
- Cover weeping lesions.

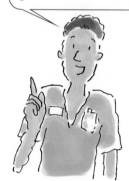

And coming in at number 1 on our top-ten list of least popular pets is … you guessed it … head lice.

Scabies

Contagious, itchy skin condition caused by mites

Key signs and symptoms

- Linear black burrows between fingers and toes and in palms, axillae, and groin

Key test results

- Drop of mineral oil placed over the burrow, followed by superficial scraping and examination of expressed material under a microscope, may reveal ova or mite feces

Key treatments

- Application of permethrin

Key interventions

- Teach the child and parents to apply permethrin from the neck down covering

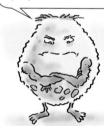

Hi. My name is Mr. Scabies. I get under people's skin—literally.

the entire body, wait 15 minutes before dressing, and avoid bathing for 8 to 12 hours.
- Explain the need to change bed linens, towels, and clothing after bathing and lotion application.

Lyme's disease

Inflammatory disease which is transmitted to humans via the deer tick

Key signs and symptoms
- Bull's eye rash is a classic symptom.
- Possible flu-like symptoms (e.g., fever, fatigue, headache)
- If not treated, can affect the heart and nervous system

Key test results
- Enzyme-linked immunosorbent assay test (ELISA)
- Western blot test

Key treatments
- Amoxicillin in children younger than 8 and doxycycline in children 8 and older, unless allergies make them contraindicated (cefuroxime given if penicillin allergy).

Key interventions
- DEET is an effective tick repellent but should be used on the child's clothes instead of the skin
- If child is outdoors often, long sleeves and pants should be worn and hair pulled back or under a hat

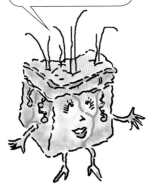

The skin's layers are the body's first line of defense against the outside world.

thePoint® You can download tables of drug information to help you prepare for the NCLEX®! View Generic Drug Names, Drug Classifications, Drug Actions, and Nursing Implications for the drugs discussed in this refresher at **http://thePoint.lww.com.**

Integumentary questions, answers, and rationales

1. A 3-year-old child gets a burn at the angle of the mouth from chewing on an electrical cord. Which finding will the nurse expect to observe 10 days after the injury?
1. Normal granular tissue
2. Contracture of the injury site
3. Ulceration with serous drainage
4. Profuse bleeding from the injury site

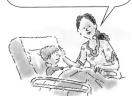

Yes— unfortunately, kids sometimes chew on electrical cords. That's why we have ERs.

2. An 18-month-old child is admitted to the hospital with full-thickness burns to the anterior chest. The parent asks how the burn will heal. Which statement will the nurse incorporate in the response?
1. "Surgical closure and grafting are usually needed."
2. "Healing takes 10 to 12 days, with mild scarring."
3. "Pigment will return to the injured area after a few months."
4. "Healing can take up to 6 weeks, with a high incidence of scarring."

3. A 7-year-old child is brought to the emergency department with burns to the back of the head and the back of the right thigh. Using the Lund-Browder classifications, which percentage of body surface area will the nurse document as affected?
1. 9.5%
2. 9.75%
3. 8.5%
4. 9%

1. 4. Ten days after oral burns from electrical cords, the eschar falls off, exposing arteries and veins. There will be profuse bleeding from the injury site. Burns to the oral cavity heal rapidly but with contractures and scarring. Although contractures are likely, they are not seen 10 days' postinjury. Ulcerations are not expected, nor would normal tissue be present already.
CN: Physiological integrity; CNS: Physiological adaptation; CL: Apply

2. 1. Full-thickness burns usually need surgical closure and grafting for complete healing. Deep partial-thickness burns heal in 6 weeks, with scarring. Healing in 10 to 12 days with little or no scarring is associated with superficial partial-thickness burns. With superficial partial-thickness burns, pigment is expected to return to the injured area after healing.
CN: Physiological integrity; CNS: Physiological adaptation; CL: Understand

3. 2. The back of the head in a 7-year-old is 5.5%. The back of the right thigh is 4.25%. Therefore, the total body surface area affected is 9.75%.
CN: Physiological integrity; CNS: Physiological adaptation; CL: Apply

CN: Client needs category   CNS: Client needs subcategory   CL: Cognitive level

4. The nurse is caring for a child in the burn unit who sustained partial-thickness burns to the lower extremities. The nurse determines which nutritional need is **most** appropriate?
1. The child needs 100 cal/kg daily.
2. The child needs increased protein daily.
3. The child should eat 4 to 5 meals a day.
4. The child needs to eat foods high in calcium.

5. Which finding(s) will the nurse expect to assess in a 9-year-old child with a deep partial-thickness burn? Select all that apply.
1. Erythema and pain
2. Minimal damage to the epidermis
3. Necrosis through all layers of skin
4. Tissue necrosis through most of the dermis
5. White, leathery appearance to the skin

6. When talking with the parents of a child with erythema infectiosum (fifth disease), the nurse will include which statement?
1. "There is a possible reappearance of the rash for up to 1 week."
2. "Your child should avoid contact with immunocompromised persons for 5 days."
3. "You need to keep your child away from pregnant women while contagious."
4. "Children with fifth disease are contagious only while the rash is present."

7. Parents are concerned their 3-year-old child has been exposed to erythema infectiosum (fifth disease). For which characteristic finding will the nurse instruct the parents to monitor?
1. A fine, erythematous rash with a sandpaper-like texture
2. Intense redness of both cheeks that may spread to the extremities
3. Low-grade fever, followed by vesicular lesions of the trunk, face, and scalp
4. A 3- to 5-day history of sustained fever, followed by a diffuse erythematous maculo-papular rash

8. A 4-year-old child is admitted to the burn unit with a circumferential burn to the left forearm. Which finding will the nurse report to the health care provider?
1. Numbness of fingers
2. +2 radial and ulnar pulses
3. Full range of motion and no pain
4. Bilateral capillary refill less than 2 seconds

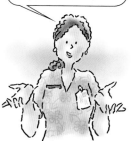

If you think fifth disease sounds bad, sixth, seventh, and eighth diseases will really blow your mind.

4. **2.** A burn injury causes a hypermetabolic state leading to protein and lipid catabolism, which affects wound healing. Caloric intake should be 1½ to 2 times the basal metabolic rate, with a minimum of 1.5 to 2 g/kg of body weight of protein daily. Increasing the number of meals or calcium intake is not required.
CN: Physiological integrity; CNS: Basic care and comfort; CL: Apply

5. **4, 5.** A client with a deep partial-thickness burn will have tissue necrosis to the epidermis and dermis layers. The appearance is usually white and leathery. Necrosis through all skin layers is seen with full-thickness injuries. Erythema and pain are characteristic of superficial injury. With deep burns, the nerve fibers are destroyed, and the client will not feel pain in the affected area. Superficial burns present with slight epidermal damage.
CN: Physiological integrity; CNS: Physiological adaptation; CL: Apply

6. **3.** There is a 3% to 5% risk of fetal death from hydrops fetalis if a pregnant woman is exposed during the first trimester. The cutaneous eruption of fifth disease can reappear for up to 4 months. A child with fifth disease is contagious during the first stage, not after the rash, when symptoms of headache, body aches, fever, and chills are present. The child should be isolated from pregnant women, immunocompromised clients, and clients with chronic anemia for up to 2 weeks.
CN: Safe, effective care environment; CNS: Safety and infection control; CL: Apply

7. **2.** The classic symptoms of erythema infectiosum begin with intense redness of both cheeks. An erythematous rash after a fever is characteristic of roseola. Children with varicella typically have vesicular lesions of the trunk, face, and scalp after a low-grade fever. An erythematous rash with a sandpaper-like texture is associated with scarlet fever, which is a bacterial infection.
CN: Physiological integrity; CNS: Physiological adaptation; CL: Apply

8. **1.** Circumferential burns can compromise blood flow to an extremity, causing numbness. Capillary refill less than 2 seconds indicates normal vascular blood flow. Absence of pain and full range of motion imply good tissue oxygenation from intact circulation. Presence of +2 pulses indicate normal circulation.
CN: Safe, effective care environment; CNS: Safety and infection control; CL: Apply

9. A family that recently went camping brings their child to the clinic with a report of a rash after a tick bite. Which finding **most** concerns the nurse?
  1. Erythematous rash surrounding a red lesion
  2. Bright rash with red outer border circling the bite site
  3. Onset of a diffuse rash over the entire body
  4. A linear rash of papules and vesicles that occurs 1 to 3 days after exposure

10. The nurse is educating a female adolescent on doxycycline. The nurse will instruct the client to avoid which situation(s)? Select all that apply.
  1. Taking with antacids
  2. Taking oral contraceptives
  3. Taking on an empty stomach
  4. Taking with milk
  5. Taking with food

11. Which prescription will the nurse question while caring for a child diagnosed with Kawasaki's disease?
  1. Obtain intravenous access
  2. IV immunoglobulin (IVIG)
  3. Erythromycin orally
  4. Acetylsalicylic acid orally

12. A child weighing 23 lb (10 kg) is diagnosed with Kawasaki's disease and started on gamma globulin therapy. The health care provider prescribes an IV infusion of gamma globulin, 2 g/kg, to run over 12 hours. How many grams will the nurse give the client per dose? Record your answer using a whole number.

_____ g

13. Parents are concerned because their child was exposed to varicella at day care. They ask the nurse about the disease. Which statement by the nurse is **most** accurate?
  1. "The rash is nonvesicular."
  2. "The treatment of choice is aspirin."
  3. "Varicella has an incubation period of 5 to 10 days."
  4. "A child is not contagious once the rash has crusted over."

14. The parents of a child diagnosed with varicella ask the nurse which medications are used to treat this virus. What medication(s) will the nurse include in the response? Select all that apply.
  1. Rimantadine
  2. Valacyclovir
  3. Oseltamivir
  4. Acyclovir
  5. Zanamivir

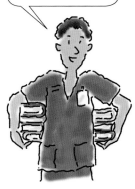

Doxycycline does not play well with others—best to take it all by itself.

9. 2. A bull's-eye rash is a classic symptom of Lyme's disease. In Lyme's disease, the rash is located primarily at the site of the bite and occurs almost immediately, not 2 months after exposure. Necrotic, painful rashes are associated with the bite of a brown recluse spider. A linear, papular, vesicular rash indicates exposure to the leaves of poison ivy.
CN: Safe, effective care environment; CNS: Management of care; CL: Apply

10. 1, 4, 5. Contraindications for doxycycline (a tetracycline) use are taking with antacids, milk, food, and pregnancy. The client should be instructed to take doxycycline on an empty stomach and to take her oral contraceptives to avoid pregnancy.
CN: Physiological integrity; CNS: Pharmacological and parenteral therapies; CL: Apply

11. 3. Kawasaki's disease is viral; therefore, the nurse would question administering an antibiotic. IV access is needed to administer IVIG. Aspirin, or acetylsalicylic acid, is the mediation of choice to relieve pain and prevent blood clots.
CN: Physiological integrity; CNS: Physiological adaptation; CL: Apply

12. 20.

$$dose\ desired \times client\ weight = dose\ administered$$

To calculate the dose, use the child's weight in kilograms.

$$2\ g/kg \times 10\ kg = 20\ g$$

CN: Physiological integrity; CNS: Pharmacological and parenteral therapies; CL: Apply

13. 4. When every varicella lesion is crusted over, the child is no longer considered contagious. The incubation period is 10 to 20 days. Use of aspirin has been associated with Reye's syndrome and is contraindicated in varicella. The rash is typically a maculopapular vesicular rash.
CN: Physiological integrity; CNS: Physiological adaptation; CL: Apply

14. 2, 4. In varicella, the medications used are acyclovir and valacyclovir. Rimantadine, zanamivir, and oseltamivir are used to treat influenza.
CN: Physiological integrity; CNS: Pharmacological and parenteral therapies; CL: Apply

CN: Client needs category   CNS: Client needs subcategory   CL: Cognitive level

15. Which statement(s) is appropriate when discussing frostbite with the parents of a child brought to the emergency department after an extended period of sledding? Select all that apply.
1. "Frostbit skin will appear white."
2. "Frostbit skin looks deeply flushed and red."
3. "Frostbite is helped by rubbing to increase circulation."
4. "The affected area may tingle and feel numb."
5. "The area should be gradually rewarmed with hot water."

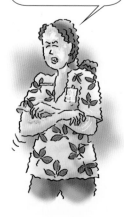

Brrr! My roommate keeps the thermostat so low I worry about getting frostbite.

15. 1, 4. Signs and symptoms of frostbite include tingling, numbness, burning sensation, and white skin. Treatment includes very gentle handling of the affected area. Rubbing is contraindicated as it can damage fragile tissue. Gradual rewarming by exposure to hot water can lead to more tissue damage.
CN: Physiological integrity; CNS: Physiological adaptation; CL: Apply

16. A parent brings a child to the health care provider's office because the child reports pain, redness, and tenderness of the left index finger. The child is diagnosed with paronychia. Which education will the nurse anticipate providing to the child and parents?
1. Apply cool compresses to the affected area.
2. Take all of the prescribed amoxicillin.
3. If a pus-filled blister develops, pop it.
4. Cut finger nails very short for prevention.

16. 2. Antibiotics are often prescribed for paronychia (infection in tissue around a nail). The client should take all of the antibiotic. Warm compresses promote healing. The client should notify the health care provider if a pus-filled blister develops. It may require incision and drainage. Popping the blister could lead to a worse infection. Cutting the nails too short places the client at risk for paronychia.
CN: Physiological integrity; CNS: Physiological adaptation; CL: Apply

17. The parent of a 5-month-old infant is planning a trip to the beach and asks for advice about sunscreen. Which instruction will the nurse incorporate into the education plan?
1. The sun protection factor (SPF) of the sunscreen should be at least 10.
2. Sunscreen should be applied to the exposed areas of the skin.
3. Sunscreen should not be applied to infants younger than age 6 months.
4. Sunscreen needs to be applied 30 minutes before going out in the sun.

Note the client's age in question #17. It's important.

17. 3. Sunscreen is not recommended for use in infants younger than age 6 months. These children should be dressed in cool, light clothes and kept in the shade. For children older than age 6 months, sunscreen should be applied evenly throughout the day and each time the child is in the water. The SPF for children should be 15 or greater. Sunscreen should be applied to all areas of the skin.
CN: Health promotion and maintenance; CNS: None; CL: Apply

18. The nurse is providing education about the treatment for paronychia. What will the nurse be sure to review with the parents?
1. Soak the affected finger in warm water.
2. Splint and put ice on the affected finger.
3. Allow the infection to resolve without treatment.
4. The child will need intravenous antibiotic therapy.

18. 1. Giving warm soaks is the treatment of choice for paronychia. Splinting and icing are not indicated. Untreated, the local abscess can spread beneath the nail bed, a condition called secondary lymphangitis. IV antibiotic therapy is not needed if the abscess is kept from spreading.
CN: Physiological integrity; CNS: Physiological adaptation; CL: Apply

19. The nurse is assessing a child and notes papules, pustules, and linear burrows of the finger and toe webs. What additional finding will the nurse expect?
1. Diffuse, pruritic wheals
2. Oval, white dots stuck to the hair shafts
3. Pain, erythema, and edema with an embedded stinger
4. The client to state the papules and pustules are pruritic

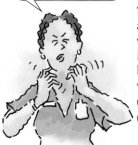

Grrr! Scabies really is as horrible as it sounds.

19. 4. Pruritic papules, vesicles, and linear burrows are diagnostic for scabies. Urticaria is associated with an allergic reaction of diffuse pruritic wheals. Nits, seen as white oval dots, are characteristic of head lice. Bites from honeybees are associated with a stinger, pain, and erythema.
CN: Physiological integrity; CNS: Physiological adaptation; CL: Apply

20. The nurse is performing a dressing change on a child when there is an announcement of a security situation. Which action will the nurse perform **first**?
1. Close the door and finish the procedure.
2. Go to the site of the security alert.
3. Report to the unit charge nurse.
4. Call the child's parents.

20. 1. A security alert notifies everyone in the hospital that there may be a dangerous situation occurring that indicates a trained show of force. The nurse should complete the dressing change, reassure the child, and then report to the charge nurse for further instructions. The nurse should not leave the room with the child's wound uncovered, nor would it be appropriate to leave the room without first reassuring the child. Notifying the child's parents is not the nurse's priority.
CN: Safe, effective care environment; CNS: Safety and infection control; CL: Analyze

21. An infant is being treated with antibiotic therapy for otitis media and develops an erythematous, fine, raised rash in the groin and suprapubic area. Which explanation will the nurse suspect?
1. The infant most likely has candidiasis.
2. The brand of diapers should be changed.
3. An over-the-counter cream is best to use.
4. Antibiotic therapy must be stopped.

21. 1. Candidiasis, caused by yeast-like fungi, can occur with the use of antibiotics. Changing the brand of diapers or suggesting the parent use an over-the-counter remedy would be appropriate for treating diaper rash, not candidiasis. The treatment for candidiasis is topical nystatin ointment. Antibiotic therapy should not be stopped.
CN: Physiological integrity; CNS: Physiological adaptation; CL: Apply

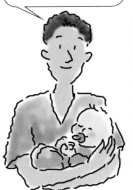

Increasing the frequency of diaper changes can help prevent diaper rash. Speaking of which …

22. The skin in the diaper area of a 6-month-old infant is excoriated and red. Which instruction(s) will the nurse give to the parent? Select all that apply.
1. Change the diaper more often.
2. Apply talcum powder with diaper changes.
3. Expose the infant's buttocks to air a few times a day.
4. Wash the area vigorously with each diaper change.
5. Decrease the infant's fluid intake to decrease saturating diapers.

22. 1, 3. Simply decreasing the amount of time the skin comes in contact with wet, soiled diapers will help heal the irritation. Allowing the skin to be exposed to air will also promote healing. Talcum is contraindicated in children because of the risks associated with inhalation of the fine powder. Gentle cleaning of the irritated skin should be encouraged. Infants should not have fluid intake restrictions.
CN: Safe, effective care environment; CNS: Safety and infection control; CL: Apply

23. A 9-year-old child is being discharged from the hospital after severe urticaria caused by an allergy to nuts. Which instruction is **priority** for the nurse to include in discharge education for the child's parents?
1. Keep the affected skin cool.
2. Apply prednisone topically for itching.
3. Administer diphenhydramine as needed.
4. How to use an epinephrine pen.

23. 4. Children who have urticaria in response to nuts, seafood, or bee stings should be warned about the possibility of anaphylactic reactions with future exposure. The use of epinephrine pens should be taught to the parents and to older children. The other treatment choices are acceptable; however, airway is priority.
CN: Physiological integrity; CNS: Reduction of risk potential; CL: Analyze

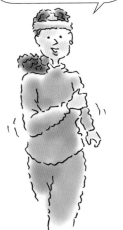

Way to go! You're running a good race.

24. The nurse is providing education about treatment options for the parent of a child with lice. Which adverse effect will the nurse teach regarding lindane shampoo?
1. Lindane can cause alopecia.
2. Lindane may lead to hypertension.
3. Lindane is associated with seizures.
4. Lindane increases liver function test results.

24. 3. Lindane is associated with seizures after absorption with topical use. Alopecia, hypertension, and increased liver function test results are not associated with the use of lindane.
CN: Physiological integrity; CNS: Pharmacological and parenteral therapies; CL: Apply

CN: Client needs category   CNS: Client needs subcategory   CL: Cognitive level

25. A 5-year-old is admitted to the emergency department with a broken clavicle. The nurse notices bruises in various stages of healing on the torso and extremities. The parent enters the room and angrily demands to take the child home. Which action is **most** appropriate?
1. Inform the parent the child has a broken bone and cannot leave.
2. Ask the parent whether it is known how the child received the bruises.
3. Step out of the room, notify the charge nurse, and then call security.
4. Take the child out of the room and call security.

26. Which instructions will the nurse include for a client's parents about the treatment of head lice?
1. The treatment should be repeated in 7 to 12 days.
2. Throw bed linen and hair accessories away.
3. Combing to remove eggs is not necessary with shampoo usage.
4. All contacts with the infested child should be treated.

27. The parents of a 4-year-old report their child has been scratching the rectum recently. About which infestation or condition will the nurse provide education?
1. Anal fissure
2. Lice
3. Pinworms
4. Scabies

28. While examining an adolescent with scabies, the nurse finds multiple contusions over the body in various stages of healing. Which nursing action(s) is appropriate? Select all that apply.
1. Privately ask the adolescent how the contusions were sustained.
2. Document the location, shape, and color of the contusions.
3. Notify the health care provider after completing an assessment.
4. Assess the adolescent's hemoglobin and platelet levels.
5. Inform the client how to use permethrin.

29. A parent tells the nurse, "I think my child has pinworms." Which response by the nurse is **best**?
1. Administer mebendazole to the client.
2. Bring your child to the emergency room.
3. Teach how to do the clear cellophane tape test.
4. Check the child's rectum at lunch.

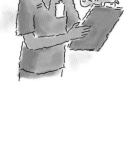

Don't try to worm your way out of answering question #27.

It is sad but true—humans can get worms too

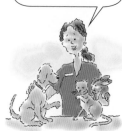

25. 3. To ensure the nurse's safety as well as the safety of the child, the best course of action would be to leave the room and immediately notify the charge nurse, and then call security. The nurse would not want to further anger the parent and create the potential for violence by taking the child out of the room. Asking for personal information and telling the parent the child cannot be taken are inappropriate actions.
CN: Psychosocial integrity; CNS: None; CL: Apply

26. 1. Treatment for head lice should be repeated in 7 to 12 days to ensure that all eggs are killed. Bed linen and hair accessories should be washed in hot, soapy water. Linens should be dried on high heat. Combing the hair thoroughly is necessary to remove the lice eggs. People exposed to head lice should be examined to assess the presence of infestation before treatment.
CN: Physiological integrity; CNS: Physiological adaptation; CL: Apply

27. 3. The clinical sign of pinworms is perianal itching that increases at night. Anal fissures are associated with rectal bleeding and pain with bowel movements. Lice are infestations of the hair. Scabies are associated with a pruritic rash characterized as linear burrows of the webs of the fingers and toes.
CN: Physiological integrity; CNS: Physiological adaptation; CL: Apply

28. 1, 2, 3, 5. The nurse would suspect the client is being abused. Asking the client about the injuries is appropriate. An accurate, precise examination must be properly documented as a legal document. The health care provider should be notified of the situation. The nurse would teach the client how to treat scabies with permethrin. Hemoglobin and platelet counts are not necessary when abuse is suspected.
CN: Psychosocial integrity; CNS: None; CL: Apply

29. 3. Detection is virtually 100% accurate with five cellophane tape tests. To determine if the child has pinworms, it is best to externally place cellophane tape near the rectum five times, at night. It needs to be determined if the client actually has pinworms before treatment is initiated. It is not necessary to bring the client to the emergency room based on the parent's statement, testing should occur at home first.
CN: Physiological integrity; CNS: Reduction of risk potential; CL: Apply

30. Each member of a family of a child diagnosed with pinworms is prescribed a single dose of mebendazole. Which statement will the nurse incorporate into the education plan?
1. The drug may stain the feces red.
2. The dose may be repeated in 2 weeks.
3. Fever and rash are common adverse effects.
4. The medicine will kill the eggs in about 48 hours.

30. **2.** Mebendazole is effective against the adult worms only (not eggs), so treatment should be repeated in 2 weeks to eradicate any emerging parasites. Staining the feces is not associated with mebendazole. Common adverse effects of mebendazole are reports of headaches and abdominal pain.

CN: Physiological integrity; CNS: Pharmacological and parenteral therapies; CL: Apply

31. A large dog bit the hand of a child. The nurse will expect to find which type of injury?
1. Abrasion
2. Crush injury
3. Fracture
4. Puncture wound

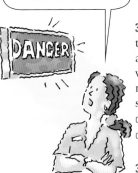

All those bacteria that live in a dog's mouth can enter the human body when a client is bitten.

DANGER

31. **2.** Although the bite of a large dog can exert pressure of 150 to 400 pounds per square inch (1,034 to 2,758 kilopascals), the bite causes crush injuries, not fractures. Abrasions are associated with friction injuries. Puncture wounds are associated with bites of smaller animals such as cats.

CN: Physiological integrity; CNS: Physiological adaptation; CL: Apply

32. The nurse is caring for a child who sustained a dog bite to the hand. Which intervention will the nurse incorporate **first**?
1. Give the rabies vaccine.
2. Administer antibiotics.
3. Clean and irrigate the wounds.
4. Assess the child's temperature.

32. **3.** Not every dog bite requires antibiotic therapy, but cleaning the wound is necessary for all injuries involving a break in the skin. Rabies vaccine is used if the dog is suspected of having rabies. Assessing the temperature will help diagnosis an infection, but not prevent one.

CN: Physiological integrity; CNS: Reduction of risk potential; CL: Analyze

33. When collecting data from a 6-year-old child with a 20% deep partial-thickness burn on the arms and trunk, the nurse determines the child has damage to what layer(s) of skin? Select all that apply.
1. Epidermis
2. Part of the dermis
3. All of the dermis
4. Subcutaneous tissue
5. Nerves and blood vessels

33. **1, 2.** A deep partial-thickness burn affects the epidermis and part of the dermis. A superficial (first-degree) burn affects the epidermis only. A full-thickness (third-degree) burn involves epidermis and all of the dermis as well as nerves and blood vessels in the skin.

CN: Physiological integrity; CNS: Physiological adaptation; CL: Apply

34. A child is brought to the health care provider's office for multiple scratches and bites from a kitten and is being evaluated for cat-scratch disease. Which symptom will the nurse expect to assess with cat-scratch disease?
1. Abdominal pain
2. Adenitis
3. Fever
4. Pruritus

Sometimes kids pick up more than toys when they're in day care.

34. **2.** Adenitis (inflammation of a gland or lymph node) is the primary feature of cat-scratch disease. Although low-grade fever has been associated with cat-scratch disease, it is present only 25% of the time. Pruritus and abdominal pain are not symptoms of cat-scratch disease.

CN: Physiological integrity; CNS: Physiological adaptation; CL: Apply

35. The nurse will monitor which child most closely for the development of giardiasis?
1. Child that rides a school bus
2. Child that plays on a playground
3. Child that plays football at school
4. Child that attends day care

35. **4.** Giardiasis is a very common intestinal parasitic infection, prevalent among children attending group day care or nursery school. Playgrounds, sporting events, and school buses do not present an unusual risk of giardiasis.

CN: Safe, effective care environment; CNS: Safety and infection control; CL: Apply

CN: Client needs category   CNS: Client needs subcategory   CL: Cognitive level

36. Which finding will the nurse expect to observe if a child has papules?
1. Palpable elevated masses
2. Loss of the epidermal layer
3. Fluid-filled elevations of the skin
4. Nonpalpable, flat changes in skin color

37. The nurse is caring for a child diagnosed with impetigo. Which prescription from the primary health care provider will the nurse complete **first**?
1. Assess the child for honey-colored crusts.
2. Administer erythromycin.
3. Wash lesions with soap and water.
4. Place on contact precautions.

38. A child is brought to the health care provider's office for treatment of a rash. Many petechiae are seen over the entire body. The nurse will suspect which condition?
1. Bleeding disorder
2. Scabies
3. Varicella
4. Vomiting

39. Which task will the registered nurse (RN) delegate to the assistive personnel (AP)?
1. Applying cream to the lesions of a child with impetigo
2. Teaching proper handwashing to a child with acne vulgaris
3. Checking a school-age child for head lice
4. Changing the diaper of a toddler with scabies

40. The registered nurse (RN) and assistive personnel (AP) are caring for a 5-year-old child who sustained full-thickness burns to the right upper extremity after tipping over a frying pan. The RN will **immediately** intervene if the AP is noted doing which action?
1. Wearing a mask while in the client's room
2. Applying an ice pack to the client's burn
3. Helping the child to the bathroom to void
4. Providing the client with a meal tray

41. Which statement will the nurse include when providing education to a parent about salmon patches (stork bites)?
1. "They are benign and usually fade in adult life."
2. "They are usually associated with syndromes of the neonate."
3. "They can cause mild hypertrophy of the muscle associated with the lesion."
4. "They are treatable with laser pulse surgery in late adolescence and adulthood."

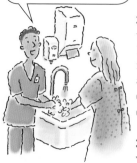

Hand washing is basic maintenance for your integument. Teach your clients to do it often.

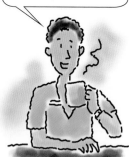

Hey—you've finished 40 questions. Nice going!

36. 1. Papules are palpable, elevated up to 0.5 cm. Nodules and tumors are elevated more than 0.5 cm. Erosions are characterized as loss of the epidermal layer. Fluid-filled lesions are vesicles and pustules. Macules and patches are described as nonpalpable, flat changes in skin color.
CN: Health promotion and maintenance; CNS: None; CL: Understand

37. 4. The nurse will first place the child on contact precautions to prevent spreading the disorder. Honey-colored crusts are expected in a child with impetigo. The nurse will administer erythromycin as prescribed and wash lesions daily.
CN: Safe, effective care environment; CNS: Management of care; CL: Analyze

38. 1. Petechiae are caused by blood outside a vessel, associated with low platelet counts and bleeding disorders. Petechiae are not found with varicella disease or scabies. Petechiae can be associated with vomiting, but in this case, they would be present on the face, not the entire body.
CN: Physiological integrity; CNS: Physiological adaptation; CL: Analyze

39. 4. The RN will delegate changing the diaper of a toddler with scabies to the AP. All other tasks require assessment or teaching by the RN.
CN: Safe, effective care environment; CNS: Management of care; CL: Analyze

40. 2. The RN should intervene if the AP is noted placing an ice pack on the burn. Applying an ice pack to the skin can further damage the area and increase the risk of hypothermia. Caretakers need to take caution not to cough or breathe directly on the affected area. A mask is required during dressing change sessions, not each time entering the room. However, it is more important to prevent additional damage. It is appropriate for the AP to assist the client to the bathroom and provide meals.
CN: Safe, effective care environment; CNS: Management of care; CL: Understand

41. 1. Salmon patches occur over the back of the neck in 40% of neonates and are harmless, needing no intervention. Laser pulse surgery is not recommended for salmon patches because they typically fade on their own in adulthood. Port-wine stains are associated with Sturge-Weber syndrome. Port-wine stains found on the face or extremities may be associated with soft tissue and bone hypertrophy.
CN: Health promotion and maintenance; CNS: None; CL: Apply

CN: Client needs category   CNS: Client needs subcategory   CL: Cognitive level

42. The nurse is assessing a toddler suspected of being a victim of abuse. Which finding by the nurse led to this suspicion?
 1. Multiple contusions of the shins
 2. Contusions of the back and chest
 3. Contusions at the same stages of healing
 4. Large contusion and hematoma of the forehead

43. When inspecting a neonate, the nurse observes a blue-black macular lesion over the lower lumbar sacral region. How will the nurse document this finding?
 1. Café au lait spots
 2. Mongolian spots
 3. Nevus of Ota
 4. Stork bites

44. The nurse is caring for a child who has experienced vomiting and diarrhea for 2 days. Which finding indicates to the nurse the child is experiencing severe dehydration?
 1. Gray skin and decreased tears
 2. Capillary refill less than 2 seconds
 3. Mottling and tenting of the skin
 4. Pale skin with dry mucous membranes

45. Clindamycin is being prescribed for a child diagnosed with severe acne. The nurse will educate the client on which adverse effect(s)? Select all that apply.
 1. Diarrhea
 2. Gram-negative folliculitis
 3. Teratogenesis
 4. Vaginal candidiasis
 5. Constipation

46. The nurse is providing acne education to a group of adolescents. Which statement by an adolescent indicates the teaching has been effective?
 1. "Diet is a cause of acne."
 2. "Gender is a cause of acne."
 3. "Poor hygiene is a cause of acne."
 4. "Hormonal changes are a cause of acne."

47. The nurse is caring for a child diagnosed with Kawasaki's disease. Which finding(s) will the nurse report to the health care provider? Select all that apply.
 1. Swollen lymph nodes in the neck
 2. Tonsillar exudate
 3. Vesicular lesions
 4. Dry, cracked lips
 5. Strawberry tongue
 6. Swollen red feet and hands

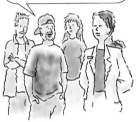

Word on the street is you're completely owning this test. Let me see your swagger.

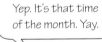

Yep. It's that time of the month. Yay.

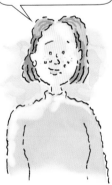

42. 2. Contusions of the back and chest are highly suggestive of abuse. Contusions at various stages of healing are red flags to potential abuse. Contusions of the shins and forehead are usually related to an active toddler falling and bumping into objects.
CN: Psychosocial integrity; CNS: None; CL: Apply

43. 2. Mongolian spots are large, blue-black macular lesions generally located over the lumbosacral areas, buttocks, and limbs. Café au lait spots occur between ages 2 and 16, not in infancy. Nevus of Ota is found surrounding the eyes. Stork bites, or salmon patches, occur at the neck and hairline area.
CN: Health promotion and maintenance; CNS: None; CL: Apply

44. 3. Severe dehydration is associated with mottling and tenting of the skin. Malnutrition is characterized by gray skin. Capillary refill less than 2 seconds is normal. Pale skin with dry mucous membranes is a sign of mild dehydration.
CN: Physiological integrity; CNS: Physiological adaptation; CL: Apply

45. 1, 2. Clindamycin is associated with both diarrhea and gram-negative folliculitis. Isotretinoin has been associated with severe birth defects. Most female clients are prescribed oral contraceptives while taking isotretinoin. Tetracycline is associated with yeast infections. Diarrhea is an adverse side effect of clindamycin, not constipation.
CN: Physiological integrity; CNS: Pharmacological and parenteral therapies; CL: Apply

46. 4. Acne is caused by hormonal changes in sebaceous gland anatomy and the biochemistry of the glands. These changes lead to a blockage in the follicular canal and cause an inflammatory response. Diet, hygiene, and the adolescent's gender do not cause acne.
CN: Health promotion and maintenance; CNS: None; CL: Apply

47. 2, 3. The nurse will report unexpected findings for further assessment and proper treatment as needed. Tonsillar exudate is consistent with pharyngitis caused by group A beta-hemolytic streptococci and vesicular lesions are associated with coxsackievirus, not Kawasaki's disease. Findings associated with Kawasaki's disease include a reddened pharynx; red, dry fissured lips and strawberry tongue; swollen lymph nodes in the neck; and swollen red feet and hands.
CN: Physiological integrity; CNS: Physiological adaptation; CL: Analyze

48. While caring for a 2-day-old neonate, a nurse notices the left side of the neonate reddens for 2 to 3 minutes. What nursing action is **most** appropriate?
  1. Notify the health care provider.
  2. Document the finding.
  3. Assess the oxygen saturation level.
  4. Change the infant's position.

48. 4. The nurse would suspect harlequin color change, which is a benign disorder related to the immaturity of the hypothalamic centers that control the tone of peripheral blood vessels. A newborn who has been lying on its side may appear reddened on the dependent side. The color fades on position change. If the neonate's color does not correct with repositioning, the nurse will implement the other actions.
CN: Health promotion and maintenance; CNS: None; CL: Analyze

49. When educating a client about tetracycline for severe inflammatory acne, how will the nurse instruct the client to take the drug?
  1. With or without meals.
  2. With milk or milk products.
  3. On an empty stomach with small amounts of water.
  4. 1 hour before or 2 hours after meals with large amounts of water.

49. 4. Tetracycline must be taken on an empty stomach to increase absorption and with ample water to avoid esophageal irritation. Milk products impede absorption.
CN: Physiological integrity; CNS: Pharmacological and parenteral therapies; CL: Apply

50. When advising parents about the prevention of burns from tap water, which instruction will the nurse include?
  1. Set the home water-heater temperature at 130°F (54.4°C) or less.
  2. Run the hot water first, then adjust the temperature with cold water.
  3. Before you put your infant in the tub, test the water with your hand.
  4. Supervise an infant in the bathroom, only leaving for a few seconds if needed.

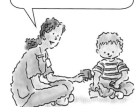

Babies and toddlers have particularly delicate skin.

50. 3. Instruct the parents to fill the tub with water first, then use the hands to test for hot spots in the water at different places in the tub. The cold water should be run first and then adjusted with hot water. Water heaters should be set at 120°F (48.9°C). The parents should never leave an infant alone in the bathroom, even for a second.
CN: Physiological integrity; CNS: Reduction of risk potential; CL: Apply

51. A 14-year-old adolescent is brought to the hospital with smoke inhalation because of a house fire. What is the nurse's **priority** intervention for this adolescent?
  1. Check the oral mucous membranes.
  2. Check for any burned areas.
  3. Obtain a medical history.
  4. Ensure a patent airway.

51. 4. The nurse's top priority is to make sure the airway is open and the adolescent is breathing. Checking the mucous membranes and burned areas is important but not as vital as maintaining a patent airway. Obtaining a medical history can be pursued after ensuring a patent airway.
CN: Safe, effective care environment; CNS: Management of care; CL: Apply

52. A 15-month-old child is diagnosed with pediculosis of the eyebrows. Which intervention by the nurse is **most** appropriate?
  1. Using lindane
  2. Using petroleum jelly
  3. Shaving the eyebrows
  4. Document the finding

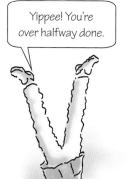

Yippee! You're over halfway done.

52. 2. Pediculosis must be treated and not just documented. Petroleum jelly should be applied twice daily for 8 days, followed by manual removal of nits. Lindane is contraindicated because of the risk of seizures. The eyebrow should never be shaved because of the uncertainty of hair return.
CN: Physiological integrity; CNS: Physiological adaptation; CL: Apply

53. A 13-year-old has received full-thickness burns over 20% of the body. When observing this client 72 hours after the burn, which finding will the nurse expect?
  1. Increased urine output
  2. Severe peripheral edema
  3. Respiratory distress
  4. Absent bowel sounds

53. 1. During the resuscitative-emergent phase of a burn, fluids shift back into the interstitial space, resulting in the onset of diuresis. Edema resolves during the emergent phase, when fluid shifts back to the intravascular space. Respiratory rate increases during the first few hours as a result of edema. When edema resolves, respirations return to normal. Absent bowel sounds occur in the initial stage.
CN: Physiological integrity; CNS: Physiological adaptation; CL: Apply

CN: Client needs category   CNS: Client needs subcategory   CL: Cognitive level

54. The clinic nurse is weighing a 3-month-old infant of Mediterranean descent during a routine examination. The nurse notes a bluish discoloration of the skin on the lower back of the infant? What will the nurse do **next**?
  1. Document the finding.
  2. Determine when the spot first appeared.
  3. See if the spot blanches.
  4. Notify the health care provider.

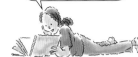

Can you spot the right answer in question #54?

54. 1. Bluish discolorations of the skin, which are common in babies of African, Native American, and Mediterranean races, are called Mongolian spots. Mongolian spots are caused by displaced pigment in a fetus and no treatment is needed. The nurse will document the finding. The other options are not necessary.
CN: Health promotion and maintenance; CNS: None; CL: Apply

55. Topical treatment with 2.5% hydrocortisone is prescribed for a 6-month-old infant with eczema. The nurse instructs the parent to use the cream for no more than 1 week based on which rationale?
  1. The medication loses its efficacy after repeated, prolonged use.
  2. Excessive use can have adverse effects, such as skin atrophy and fragility.
  3. If no improvement is seen, a stronger concentration will be prescribed.
  4. If no improvement is seen after 1 week, an antibiotic will be prescribed.

55. 2. Hydrocortisone cream should be used for brief periods to decrease adverse effects such as atrophy of the skin. The drug does not lose efficacy after prolonged use. A stronger concentration may not be prescribed, even if no improvement is seen. An antibiotic would be inappropriate in this instance.
CN: Physiological integrity; CNS: Pharmacological and parenteral therapies; CL: Apply

56. A 1-year-old infant is diagnosed with eczema during a well checkup. What will the nurse do **next**?
  1. Assess the skin for scaly patches with intense pruritus.
  2. Determine if there is a family history of asthma.
  3. Ask what kind of soap the family uses at home.
  4. Provide education on home care for eczema.

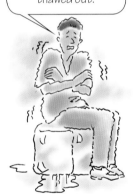

Brain freeze? Move on to another question and return to this one later, once your brain has thawed out.

56. 4. The nurse will provide education to the child's parents to help relieve the eczema. Scaly patches with itching are expected and properly noted for the diagnosis to be made. Children with a family history of asthma are at increased risk of developing eczema; however, the child is already diagnosed, making this irrelevant. Asking what type of soap is used limits the information the nurse will receive. Providing overall education would be much more effective.
CN: Physiological integrity; CNS: Physiological adaptation; CL: Analyze

57. A 4-year-old child had a subungual hemorrhage of the toe after a jar fell on the foot. Which nursing intervention is **most** appropriate?
  1. Check the child's hemoglobin level.
  2. Assess the child's pain level.
  3. Apply an adhesive bandage to the site.
  4. Prepare the child for electrocautery.

57. 4. The hematoma is treated with electrocautery to relieve pain and reduce the risk of infection. Checking hemoglobin is not necessary because the amount of blood loss would be negligible. The nurse would assess pain; however, pain is not the priority. Applying an adhesive bandage may increase pain from the pressure.
CN: Physiological integrity; CNS: Physiological adaptation; CL: Analyze

58. A 9-year-old child is brought to the emergency department with extensive burns received in a home fire. Which nursing intervention is **most** important?
  1. Administer antibiotics.
  2. Conduct wound management.
  3. Administer liquids orally.
  4. Administer frequent small meals.

Question #58 is asking for the **most** important aspect of care for the child.

58. 2. The most important aspect of caring for a burned child is wound management. The goals of wound care are to speed debridement, protect granulation tissue and new grafts, and conserve body heat and fluids. Antibiotics are not always administered prophylactically. Fluids are administered IV according to the child's body weight to replace volume. Enteral feedings, rather than meals, are initiated within the first 24 hours after the burn to support the child's increased nutritional requirements.
CN: Physiological integrity; CNS: Physiological adaptation; CL: Apply

CN: Client needs category   CNS: Client needs subcategory   CL: Cognitive level

59. The nurse is caring for a 12-year-old child with a diagnosis of eczema. Which nursing intervention is appropriate for this child?
1. Administer antibiotics as prescribed.
2. Administer antifungals as prescribed.
3. Pat dry the affected areas after bathing.
4. Use moisturizers immediately after a hot bath.

59. 3. The nurse will pat dry affected areas to prevent damaging the skin, which could lead to secondary infections. Tepid baths and moisturizers are indicated to keep the infected areas clean and minimize itching. Antibiotics are given only when superimposed infection is present. Antifungals are not administered in the treatment of eczema. Hot baths can exacerbate the condition and increase itching.
CN: Physiological integrity; CNS: Physiological adaptation; CL: Apply

60. The parent of a 4-month-old infant asks about the strawberry hemangioma on the infant's cheek. Which statement will the nurse include when responding to the parent?
1. "The lesion will continue to grow for 3 years, then it will be surgically removed."
2. "If the lesion continues to enlarge, referral to a pediatric oncologist is warranted."
3. "Surgery is indicated before 12 months of age, if the lesion is greater than 3 cm."
4. "It will continue to grow until 12 months of age, then will resolve by age 2 to 3 years."

60. 4. Hemangiomas are rapidly growing vascular lesions that reach maximum growth by age 1 year. The growth period is then followed by an involution period of 6 to 12 months. Lesions show complete involution by age 2 or 3 years. These benign lesions do not need surgical or oncologic referrals.
CN: Health promotion and maintenance; CNS: None; CL: Apply

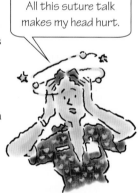

All this suture talk makes my head hurt.

61. A 3-year-old child is being discharged from the emergency department after receiving three sutures for a scalp laceration. Which discharge education is **most** appropriate?
1. Have the child take showers until the sutures are removed.
2. Tell the parent to take the child to the clinic in 5 to 7 days for suture removal.
3. Instruct the parent to apply antibiotic ointment to the site for 14 days.
4. Clean the suture site once a week with an alcohol or peroxide solution.

61. 2. The recommended healing time for a scalp laceration is 5 to 7 days. The child should take baths due to the location of the sutures (should keep them as dry as possible). Antibiotic ointment is not necessary. The site should be cleaned twice a day with soap and water to prevent excessive crusting and allow for easier removal.
CN: Physiological integrity; CNS: Physiological adaptation; CL: Apply

62. The nurse is providing discharge education for a 17-year-old on how to change a sterile dressing on the right leg. During the education session, the nurse observes redness, swelling, and induration at the wound site. What will the nurse do **next**?
1. Notify the health care provider.
2. Document the finding.
3. Send a specimen for culturing.
4. Discharge the client as prescribed.

62. 1. The nurse would suspect the wound has become infected and would notify the health care provider. The nurse will document the findings and any new prescriptions received after calling the health care provider. A culture may be prescribed. The nurse would not discharge the client before calling the health care provider.
CN: Safe, effective care environment; CNS: Management of care; CL: Analyze

63. When being examined, a 6-year-old child is noted to have a papulovesicular eruption on the left anterior lateral chest, with reports of pain and tenderness of the lesion. The nurse interprets this finding as which condition?
1. Contusion
2. Herpes zoster
3. Scabies
4. Varicella

63. 2. Herpes zoster is caused by the varicella zoster virus. It has papulovesicular lesions that erupt along a dermatome, usually with hyperesthesia, pain, and tenderness. Contusions are not found with papulovesicular lesions. Scabies appear as linear burrows of the fingers and toes caused by a mite. The papulovesicular lesions of varicella are distributed over the entire trunk, face, and scalp and do not follow a dermatome.
CN: Physiological integrity; CNS: Physiological adaptation; CL: Apply

64. During an examination of a 5-month-old infant, a flat, dull pink, macular lesion is noted on the infant's forehead. Which nursing action is **most** appropriate?
1. Check the infant's temperature.
2. Assess the body for other lesions.
3. Apply erythromycin ointment to the lesions.
4. Inform the parents the lesion will fade by 12 months.

65. The nurse is caring for a 15-year-old who has suffered full-thickness burns to 30% of the body. The health care provider has prescribed morphine 0.5 mg by mouth every 3 to 4 hours as needed for pain. The elixir comes in 2 mg/mL. How many milliliters will the nurse administer per dose? Record your answer using two decimal places.

_____ mL

66. A child's parents ask for advice on the use of an insect repellent that contains DEET. Which statement will the nurse incorporate in the response?
1. "Spray the child's clothing instead of the child's skin with DEET."
2. "The repellent works better as the outdoor temperature increases."
3. "The repellent is not effective against the ticks responsible for Lyme's disease."
4. "Apply insect repellent as you would sunscreen, frequently during the day."

67. Which pediatric client will the nurse assess **first** after receiving shift report?
1. A 1-year-old whose diaper area is beefy-red and tender.
2. A 3-year-old with eczema reporting intense pruritus.
3. A 5-year-old with impetigo needing the first dose of penicillin.
4. A 15-year-old needing education on isotretinoin usage.

68. When assessing a child with cellulitis, which symptom(s) will the nurse expect to find? Select all that apply.
1. Edema
2. Vesicular blisters
3. Temperature 102.4°F (39.1°C)
4. Tenderness
5. Warmth at the site
6. Redness with well-defined borders

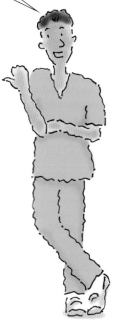
Something seems kind of fishy about question #64.

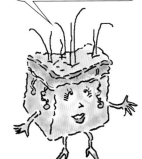
To succeed in learning these disorders, you'll need to get some skin in the game.

64. 4. The nurse knows this is a salmon patch, which is a common vascular lesion in infants. These patches appear as flat, dull-pink, macular lesions in various regions of the face and head. When they appear on the nape of the neck, they are commonly called *stork bites*. These lesions fade by the first year of life. The other options are not necessary.
CN: Safe, effective care environment; CNS: Management of care; CL: Apply

65. **0.25**
The correct formula to calculate a drug dose is:

$$\frac{Dose\ on\ hand}{Quantity\ on\ hand} = \frac{Dose\ desired}{X}$$

The health care provider prescribes 0.5 mg, which is the dose desired. The elixir is 2 mg/mL, which is the dose/quantity on hand.

$$\frac{2\ mg}{1\ mL} = \frac{0.5\ mg}{X}$$

$$X = 0.25\ mL$$

CN: Physiological integrity; CNS: Pharmacological and parenteral therapies; CL: Apply

66. 1. DEET spray has been approved for use on children. It should be used sparingly on all skin surfaces. By concentrating the spray on clothing and camping equipment, the adverse effects and potential toxic buildup are significantly reduced. Repellent is lost to evaporation, wind, heat, and perspiration. Each 10°F (5.5°C) increase in temperature leads to as much as a 50% reduction in protection time. DEET is very effective as a tick repellent.
CN: Physiological integrity; CNS: Reduction of risk potential; CL: Apply

67. 3. The nurse will first administer the antibiotic to the child with impetigo. This child must remain on contact precautions until 24 hours after antibiotic administration, making this child priority. The nurse will then assess each of the other clients accordingly.
CN: Safe, effective care environment; CNS: Management of care; CL: Analyze

68. 1, 3, 4, 5. Cellulitis is a deep, locally diffuse infection of the skin. It is associated with redness, fever, edema, tenderness, and warmth at the site of the injury. Vesicular blisters suggest impetigo. Cellulitis has no well-defined borders.
CN: Physiological integrity; CNS: Physiological adaptation; CL: Apply

CN: Client needs category   CNS: Client needs subcategory   CL: Cognitive level

69. Which statement about warts will the nurse incorporate when assisting with a community health education program on common skin problems?
1. "Cutting the wart is the preferred treatment for children."
2. "No treatment exists that specifically kills the wart virus."
3. "Warts are caused by a virus affecting the inner layer of skin."
4. "Warts are harmless and usually last 2 to 4 years if untreated."

70. A 2-year-old child has been diagnosed with cellulitis. The health care provider prescribes ceftriaxone 50 mg IM. The pharmacy sends 100 mg/2 mL. How many milliliters will the nurse administer? Record your answer using a whole number.

_____ mL

69. 2. The goal of treatment is to kill the skin that contains the wart virus. Cutting the wart is likely to spread the virus. The virus that causes warts affects the outer layer of the skin. Warts are harmless and last 1 to 2 years if untreated.
CN: Health promotion and maintenance; CNS: None; CL: Apply

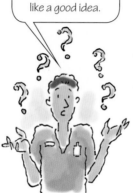

How will we tackle this dosage calculation? Setting up an equation sounds like a good idea.

70. 1.
The correct formula to calculate a drug dose is:

$$\frac{Dose\ on\ hand}{Quantity\ on\ hand} = \frac{Dose\ desired}{X}$$

The health care provider prescribes 50 mg, which is the dose desired. The pharmacy delivers 100 mg/2 mL, which is the dose/quantity on hand.

$$\frac{100\ mg}{2\ mL} = \frac{50\ mg}{X}$$

$$X = 1\ mL$$

CN: Health promotion and maintenance; CNS: None; CL: Apply

71. The nurse is working in a pediatric emergency department. Which client will the nurse assess **first**?
1. A 3-month-old with oral candidiasis
2. A 2-year-old with Lyme's disease
3. A 4-year-old with pinworms
4. A 5-year-old with orbital cellulitis

71. 4. The 5-year-old with orbital cellulitis should be seen first because significant damage to the optic nerve can occur, causing permanent vision problems or total loss of vision. The other clients would then be seen accordingly.
CN: Safe, effective care environment; CNS: Management of care; CL: Analysis

72. A child presents with a history of flu-like symptoms followed by a painful purplish rash that has blistered. Which additional finding(s) will the nurse expect to observe while assessing the child? Select all that apply.
1. Desquamation of the skin
2. Blisters on mucous membranes
3. Loose, green stools
4. Intermittent periods of vomiting
5. Photophobia

72. 1, 2. The nurse would suspect the child has Stevens-Johnson syndrome. Desquamation is characteristic of Stevens-Johnson syndrome, where the top layer of the skin is shed, followed by healing. Blisters are found on the skin and mucous membranes of the mouth, eyes, nose, and genitals. The other symptoms are not associated with Stevens-Johnson syndrome.
CN: Physiological integrity; CNS: Physiological adaptation; CL: Apply

73. Which instructions will the nurse include for the parents of a child who is to receive nystatin oral solution?
1. "Give the solution immediately after feedings."
2. "Give the solution first thing in the morning."
3. "Mix the solution with small amounts of food."
4. "Give half the solution before and half after meals."

73. 1. Nystatin oral solution should be swabbed onto the mouth after feedings to allow for optimal contact with mucous membranes. Administering nystatin before meals or with meals does not allow the best contact with the mucous membranes.
CN: Physiological integrity; CNS: Pharmacological and parenteral therapies; CL: Apply

74. An infant is examined and found to have a petechial rash. How will the nurse document this rash?
1. Purple, macular lesions larger than 1 cm in diameter.
2. Purple to brown bruises, macular or papular, of various sizes.
3. A collection of blood from ruptured blood vessels and larger than 1 cm in diameter.
4. Pinpoint, pink to purple, nonblanching, macular lesions that are 1 to 3 mm in diameter.

74. 4. Petechiae are small pinpoint, pink to purple, macular lesions 1 to 3 mm in diameter. Purple, macular lesions greater than 1 cm in diameter are defined as purpura. A bruise is defined as ecchymosis. A hematoma is a collection of blood.
CN: Physiological integrity; CNS: Physiological adaptation;
CL: Understand

75. While assessing a child, the nurse notes the rash below. Which nursing intervention is **priority**?

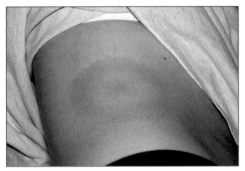

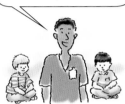

Which disease has a bull's-eye patter rash?

1. Place the child on contact precautions.
2. Give ibuprofen.
3. Administer amoxicillin.
4. Cover the site with sterile gauze.

75. 3. The nurse would suspect the child has Lyme's disease and administer amoxicillin. The nurse would follow standard precautions as this is not spread person-to-person. Ibuprofen may be given if the child reports pain or inflammation. The site does not need to be covered.
CN: Safe, effective care environment; CNS: Management of care;
CL: Analyze

76. Parents report their teenager is losing hair in small, round areas on the scalp. The nurse interprets this as suggesting which condition?
1. Alopecia
2. Amblyopia
3. Exotropia
4. Seborrhea dermatitis

76. 1. Alopecia is the correct term for thinning hair loss. Amblyopia and exotropia are eye disorders. Seborrhea dermatitis is cradle cap and occurs in infants.
CN: Physiological integrity; CNS: Physiological adaptation;
CL: Apply

77. When assessing a child with coxsackievirus, the nurse notes blisters on the child's palms and in the mouth. Which nursing intervention is appropriate?
1. Encourage the child to rupture the blisters.
2. Continue to monitor the child.
3. Apply oxygen at 2 L via nasal cannula.
4. Notify the health care provider.

77. 2. Symptoms of coxsackievirus include blisters on the palms, soles, and in the mouth. The nurse would continue to monitor the child as this is an expected finding. Rupturing the blisters could result in a secondary infection or scarring. Oxygen is not warranted at this time because the child has no symptoms of respiratory distress. The nurse would not notify the health care provider of stable, expected findings.
CN: Physiological integrity; CNS: Physiological adaptation;
CL: Apply

78. A parent of a toddler diagnosed with atopic dermatitis is concerned about how the child acquired the disease. The nurse will explain that atopic dermatitis is caused by which condition?
1. Fungal infection
2. Hereditary disorder
3. Sex-linked disorder
4. Viral infection

78. 2. Atopic dermatitis is a hereditary disorder associated with a family history of asthma, allergic rhinitis, or atopic dermatitis. Fungal and viral infections do not cause atopic dermatitis, nor is it sex-linked.
CN: Physiological integrity; CNS: Physiological adaptation;
CL: Apply

CN: Client needs category   CNS: Client needs subcategory   CL: Cognitive level

79. The parent of a 6-month-old infant with atopic dermatitis asks for advice on bathing the child. Which information will the nurse provide to the parent?
1. Bathe the infant twice daily.
2. Bathe the infant every other day.
3. Use bubble baths to decrease itching.
4. The frequency of the infant's baths is not important.

80. The nurse is providing discharge instructions to the parents of a child with atopic dermatitis. Which information will the nurse include? Select all that apply.
1. Keep the child's fingernails cut short.
2. Have the child wear loose, cotton clothing.
3. Use mild, fragrance-free laundry detergents.
4. Apply moisturizers two to three times a day and after bathing.
5. Keep the environment cool and humidified.

81. The nurse is caring for an 11-year-old child with cerebral palsy who has a pressure injury on the sacrum. When providing education for the parent about dietary intake, which food(s) will the nurse include? Select all that apply.
1. Quinoa
2. Whole grain products
3. Fruits and vegetables
4. Lean meats
5. Low-fat milk

82. A 10-year-old child is diagnosed with a common wart on the foot. What will the nurse do **next**?
1. Prepare the child for surgical removal of the wart.
2. Instruct the parent to apply ice to the wart three to four times a day.
3. Provide a protective boot for the child to wear on the left foot.
4. Tell the parent to return if the wart becomes painful or limits activity.

83. The nurse is explaining treatment to the parents of a child with hypertrophic scarring. Which method is **best** for the nurse to include?
1. Compression garments
2. Moisturizing creams
3. Physiotherapy
4. Splints

84. The nurse assesses a neonate and notes bruising on the scalp, along with diffuse swelling of the soft tissue that crosses over the suture line. What will the nurse do **next**?
1. Assess the neonate as prescribed.
2. Mark the swollen area.
3. Assess the neonate's glucose.
4. Check the neonate's bilirubin level.

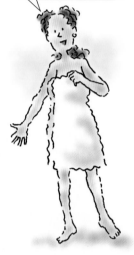

I'm so glad I don't have dermatitis—I love my hot baths.

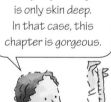

They say beauty is only skin deep. In that case, this chapter is gorgeous.

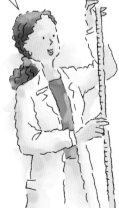

79. 2. Bathing removes lipoprotein complexes that hold water in the stratum corneum and increase water loss. Decreasing bathing to every other day can help prevent the removal of lipoprotein complexes. Soap and bubble bath should be used sparingly while bathing the child.
CN: Physiological integrity; CNS: Basic care and comfort; CL: Apply

80. 1, 2, 3, 4, 5. Each action would be included in teaching parents how to care for a child with atopic dermatitis at home. Interventions are aimed at controlling the itchy inflammation of the child's skin.
CN: Physiological integrity; CNS: Physiological adaptation; CL: Apply

81. 4, 5. Although the child should eat a balanced diet with foods from all food groups, the diet should emphasize foods that supply complete protein, such as lean meats and low-fat milk. Protein helps build and repair body tissue, which promotes healing. Legumes provide incomplete protein. Cheese contains complete protein but also fat, which should be limited to 30% or less of caloric intake. Whole grain products supply incomplete proteins and carbohydrates. Fruits and vegetables provide mainly carbohydrates.
CN: Physiological integrity; CNS: Basic care and comfort; CL: Apply

82. 4. Common warts generally require no treatment and self-resolve in a few weeks to months. The wart may need to be removed if the child reports pain, limited ability to be active, or becomes self-conscious. Ice or a boot should not be applied to the area.
CN: Safe, effective care environment; CNS: Management of care; CL: Apply

83. 1. Compression garments are worn for up to 1 year to control hypertrophic scarring. Moisturizing creams help decrease hyperpigmentation. Physiotherapy and splints help keep joints and limbs supple.
CN: Physiological integrity; CNS: Physiological adaptation; CL: Apply

84. 1. Caput succedaneum originates from trauma to the neonate while descending through the birth canal. It is usually a benign injury that spontaneously resolves over time. Marking the neonate's head is not necessary and would greatly concern the parents. Caput does not alter glucose or bilirubin levels.
CN: Physiological integrity; CNS: Physiological adaptation; CL: Apply

85. A 6-year-old child has had a recent diagnosis of Lyme's disease. Which medication will the nurse expect the health care provider to prescribe if the child has an allergy to penicillin?
1. Amoxicillin
2. Cefuroxime
3. Doxycycline
4. Clindamycin

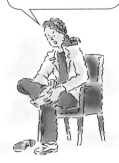

How can I have athlete's foot when I'm not even an athlete? No fair.

86. An adolescent reports feet that itch, sweat a lot, and have a foul odor. The nurse suspects which condition?
1. Candidiasis
2. Tinea corporis
3. Tinea pedis
4. Molluscum contagiosum

87. A child has a healed wound from a traumatic injury. A keloid has formed over the wound. How will the nurse describe the wound to the health care provider? Select all that apply.
1. Pink, thickened and smooth
2. Linear depressions of the skin
3. Rubbery in nature
4. Depressed vesicular lesion
5. Evulsion with eschar

88. An infant's parent gives a history of poor feeding for a few days. The nurse observes white plaques in the infant's mouth with an erythematous base. The plaques stick to the mucous membranes tightly and bleed when scraped. The nurse prepares to treat which condition?
1. Chickenpox
2. Herpes lesions
3. Measles
4. Oral candidiasis

89. The nurse notes the rash below on a child's upper arm. Which prescription by the health care provider will the nurse anticipate?

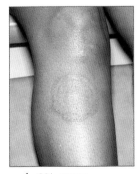

1. Ketoconazole 2% cream
2. Hydrocortisone 1% cream
3. Cover the site with sterile gauze
4. Apply alcohol to the site TID

CN: Client needs category   CNS: Client needs subcategory   CL: Cognitive level

85. **2.** In a child younger than 8 years of age, the treatment would be amoxicillin unless the child has an allergy to penicillin; in that case, cefuroxime would be used. In a child older than 8, the treatment would be doxycycline unless the client has a tetracycline allergy; in that case, the health care provider would prescribe amoxicillin or cefuroxime.
CN: Physiological integrity; CNS: Pharmacological and parenteral therapies; CL: Apply

86. **3.** Tinea pedis is a superficial fungal infection on the feet, commonly called athlete's foot. Candidiasis is a fungal infection of the skin or mucous membranes commonly found in the oral, vaginal, and intestinal mucosal tissue. Tinea corporis, or ringworm, is a flat, scaling, papular lesion with raised borders. Molluscum contagiosum is a viral skin infection with lesions that are small, red papules.
CN: Physiological integrity; CNS: Physiological adaptation; CL: Apply

87. **1, 3.** Keloids are an exaggerated connective tissue response to skin injury and can be described as pink, thickened, smooth, and rubbery in nature. Striae are linear depressions of the skin. An erosion is a depressed vesicular lesion. Evulsion with eschar formation is characteristic of a stage IV pressure ulcer.
CN: Physiological integrity; CNS: Physiological adaptation; CL: Apply

88. **4.** Oral candidiasis, or *thrush*, is a painful inflammation that can affect the tongue, soft and hard palates, and buccal mucosa. Chickenpox, or *varicella*, causes open ulcerations of the mucous membranes. Herpes lesions are usually vesicular ulcerations of the oral mucosa around the lips. Measles that form Koplik spots can be identified as pinpoint, white, elevated lesions.
CN: Physiological integrity; CNS: Physiological adaptation; CL: Apply

89. **1.** The nurse suspects the client has tinea corporis (ringworm), a fungal infection of the body. The nurse would expect an antifungal cream to be prescribed. The other treatments are not effective for tinea corporis.
CN: Physiological integrity; CNS: Physiological adaptation; CL: Apply

90. A school-age child was found unconscious at home and brought to the emergency department by the fire and rescue unit. During assessment, the nurse notes cherry-red mucous membranes, nail beds, and skin. What will the nurse do **next**?
1. Immediately notify the child's parents.
2. Assess the child's level of consciousness
3. Prepare the child for hyperbaric oxygen therapy
4. Administer oxygen via a facemask

90. 2. Cherry-red skin changes are seen when a child has been exposed to high levels of carbon monoxide. Immediate treatment involves administering oxygen to perfuse the child's tissue. The nurse would assess the child's level of consciousness, as this may be altered depending on the severity of carbon monoxide poisoning. The child's parents will be notified; however, stabilizing the child is the nurse's priority. Hyperbaric therapy may be prescribed.

CN: Safe, effective care environment; CNS: Management of care; CL: Analyze

91. A teenager asks advice about getting a tattoo. Which statement(s) made by the nurse about tattoos is correct? Select all that apply.
1. "Human immunodeficiency virus (HIV) is a possible risk factor."
2. "Hepatitis C is a possible risk factor."
3. "Tattoos are not easily removed with laser surgery."
4. "Allergic response to pigments is a possible risk factor."
5. "Hepatitis A is a possible risk factor."

91. 1, 2, 3, 4. Because of the moderate amount of bleeding with a tattoo, both hepatitis C and HIV are potential risks if proper techniques are not followed. Allergic reactions have been seen when establishments do not use pigments approved by the U.S. Food and Drug Administration for tattoo coloring. The removal of tattoos is not easily done, and most people are left with a significant scar. The cost is expensive and not covered by insurance. Hepatitis A is not a possible risk factor of tattoos.

CN: Health promotion and maintenance; CNS: None; CL: Apply

92. A toddler weighing 34 lb (15 kg) is started on amoxicillin and clavulanate therapy, 200 mg/5 mL, for cellulitis. The dose is 40 mg/kg over 24 hours given three times daily. How many milliliters will the nurse administer per dose? Record your answer using a whole number.

_____ mL

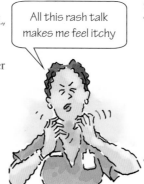

All this rash talk makes me feel itchy

92. 5.
The dose is first calculated by multiplying the weight and the milligrams and then dividing into three even doses.

$$weight \times mg = X \, mg$$

$$15 \, kg \times 40 \, mg = 600 \, mg$$

$$\frac{total \, mg}{number \, of \, does} = X \, mg \, per \, dose$$

The milligrams are then used to determine the milliliters based on the concentration of the medicine.

$$\frac{600 \, mg}{3} = 200 \, mg \, per \, dose$$

The concentration is 200 mg in every 5 mL.

CN: Physiological integrity; CNS: Pharmacological and parenteral therapies; CL: Apply

93. The nurse is assessing a 6-year-old child with a spiny projection from the skin suspended from a narrow stalk on the forehead. Which condition will the nurse suspect?
1. Filiform wart
2. Flat wart
3. Plantar wart
4. Venereal warts

93. 1. Filiform warts are long, spiny projections from the skin surface. Flat warts are flat-topped, smooth-surfaced lesions. Plantar warts are rough papules, commonly found on the soles of the feet. Venereal warts appear on the genital mucosa and are confluent papules with rough surfaces.

CN: Physiological integrity; CNS: Physiological adaptation; CL: Apply

94. A 4-year-old child has a tick embedded in the scalp. Which nursing action is appropriate?
1. Burn the tick at the skin surface.
2. Prepare the child for surgical removal of the tick.
3. Grasp the tick with tweezers and apply slow, outward pressure.
4. Apply ice over the tick until it spontaneously releases.

94. 3. Applying gentle outward pressure prevents injuring the skin and leaving parts of the tick in the skin. Surgical removal is indicated if portions of the tick remain in the skin. Burning the tick and applying ice for an extended time frame may injure the skin and should be avoided.
CN: Physiological integrity; CNS: Physiological adaptation; CL: Apply

95. An infant with hives is prescribed diphenhydramine 5 mg/kg over 24 hours in divided doses every 6 hours. The child weighs 18 lb (8 kg). How many milligrams will the nurse administer with each dose? Record your answer using a whole number.

_____ mg

95. 10.
Multiplying 5 mg by the weight (8 kg) gives the amount of milligrams for 24 hours.

$$5\,mg \times 8\,kg = 40\,mg$$

Divide this by the number of doses per day (4), giving milligrams/dose.

$$\frac{40\,mg}{4\,doses} = 10\,mg/dose$$

CN: Physiological integrity; CNS: Pharmacological and parenteral therapies; CL: Apply

The key to question #96 is the word **first**.

96. An 8-year-old child arrives at the emergency department with chemical burns to both legs. Which action will the nurse perform **first**?
1. Dilute the burns.
2. Apply sterile dressings.
3. Apply topical antibiotics.
4. Debride and graft the burns.

96. 1. Diluting the chemical is the first treatment. It will help remove the chemical and stop the burning process. The remaining treatments are initiated after dilution.
CN: Physiological integrity; CNS: Physiological adaptation; CL: Analyze

97. A 14-year-old diagnosed with acne vulgaris asks what causes it. Which factor(s) will the nurse identify for this client? Select all that apply.
1. Chocolates and sweets
2. Increased hormone levels
3. Growth of anaerobic bacteria
4. Caffeine
5. Heredity
6. Fatty foods

97. 2, 3, 5. Acne vulgaris is characterized by the appearance of comedones (blackheads and whiteheads). Comedones develop for various reasons, including increased hormone levels, heredity, irritation or application of irritating substances (such as cosmetics), and growth of anaerobic bacteria. A direct relationship between acne vulgaris and consumption of chocolates, caffeine, or fatty foods has not been established.
CN: Physiological integrity; CNS: Physiological adaptation; CL: Apply

98. A child has been admitted with a papular rash. Which illustration depicts this type of rash?

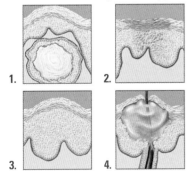

98. 3. A papular rash manifests with solid, raised lesions that are usually less than 1 cm in diameter. Option 2 depicts a small, discolored spot or patch on the skin called a macule. Option 4 depicts a pustule, which is a small, pus-filled lesion (a follicular pustule if it contains a hair). Option 1 depicts a cyst, which is a closed sac in or under the skin that contains fluid or semi-solid material.
CN: Physiological integrity; CNS: Physiological adaptation; CL: Apply

CN: Client needs category   CNS: Client needs subcategory   CL: Cognitive level

99. A 7-year-old child is admitted to the hospital for treatment of facial cellulitis. Which intervention(s) will the nurse initiate to help this child cope with the insertion of a peripheral intravenous (IV) line? Select all that apply.

1. Explain the procedure to the child immediately before the procedure.
2. Apply a topical anesthetic to the IV site before the procedure.
3. Determine which hand the child uses for drawing.
4. Explain the procedure to the child using abstract terms.
5. Avoid letting the child see the equipment before the procedure.
6. Tell the child that the procedure will not hurt.

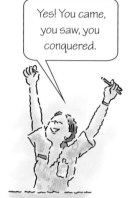

Yes! You came, you saw, you conquered.

99. 2, 3. Topical anesthetics reduce the pain of a venipuncture. The cream should be applied about 1 hour before the procedure and requires a health care provider's prescription. Asking which hand the child draws with helps to identify the dominant hand. The IV should be inserted into the opposite extremity so that the child can continue to play and to do homework with a minimum amount of disruption. Younger school-age children do not have the capability for abstract thinking. The procedure should be explained using simple words. Definitions of unfamiliar terms should be provided. The child should have the procedure explained well before it takes place so that he or she has time to ask questions. Although the topical anesthetic will relieve some pain, there is usually some discomfort involved in venipuncture, so the child should not be told otherwise.

CN: Psychosocial integrity; CNS: None; CL: Analyze

Part VI

Issues in Nursing

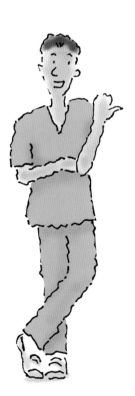

Chapter 35

Management & Leadership

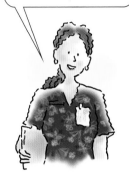

Knowing key concepts of management and leadership is just as important as your clinical knowledge for a successful nursing career. Test your knowledge of these concepts with the following questions.

Management & leadership refresher

Nurse manager role

- Assumes 24-hour accountability for the nursing care delivered in a specific nursing area

Management styles
- Autocratic: decisions made with little or no staff input; manager does not delegate responsibility; staff dependence is fostered; the autocratic leader excels in times of crisis
- Laissez-faire: little direction, structure, or support provided by manager; manager abdicates responsibility and decision making when possible; staff development is not facilitated; there is little interest in achieving the goals necessary for adequate client care
- Democratic: staff members are encouraged to participate in decision making when possible; most decisions are made by the group; staff development is encouraged; responsibilities are carefully delegated, and feedback is given to staff members to encourage professional growth
- Participative: problems are identified by the manager and presented to the staff with possible solutions; staff members are encouraged to provide input but the manager makes the decision; negotiation is the key; manager encourages staff advancement

Delegation

- Involves entrusting a task to another staff member
- Helps free the nurse of tasks that can be completed successfully by someone else

- Prepares staff member for career advancement

Discharge planning and client education

- Should be initiated on admission
- For clients with planned admissions, education should begin before hospitalization
- Should consider cultural and developmental needs

Clinical pathways
- Multidisciplinary guidelines for client care
- Documentation tool for nurses and other health care providers
- Provides sequences of multidisciplinary interventions that incorporate education, consultation, discharge planning, medications, nutrition, diagnostic testing, activities, treatments, and therapeutic modalities

Quality management

- System used to continually assess and evaluate the effectiveness of client care

Disaster management plan

- Must be able to be implemented quickly
- Must include measures to control resources, establish and maintain communication within the facility and with neighboring responders, protect as many lives as possible, protect property, provide resources for the community, and help the facility and staff recover after the disaster

I think you might be on the wrong clinical pathway.

687

Management & leadership questions, answers, and rationales

1. A medical–surgical nurse is assigned to work on the obstetrical–gynecological unit today. Which client will the charge nurse assign to the medical–surgical nurse?
1. A client who had a hysterectomy with a salpingo-oophorectomy 12 hours ago
2. A 26 weeks' gestation client on bed rest for preterm labor prescribed a non-stress test
3. A client who vaginally birthed a 2-lb (907-g) fetal demise yesterday
4. A 36 weeks' gestation client newly diagnosed with gestational hypertension

1. **1.** The charge nurse will assign the client who had a hysterectomy 12 hour ago to the medical–surgical nurse because this client is most similar to a medical–surgical client. The charge nurse should assign the medical–surgical nurse a stable client most like what the nurse cares for normally. All other clients are specific to obstetrics, not medical–surgical clients. The medical–surgical nurse would not be familiar with preterm labor care, assessing the fundus and lochia of a postpartum client, or assessing and educating an antepartum client newly diagnosed with gestational hypertension.
CN: Safe, effective care environment; CNS: Management of care; CL: Analyze

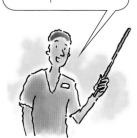

Which of these interventions is most appropriate for assistive personnel to perform?

2. The nurse is caring for a newly admitted client diagnosed with left-sided cerebrovascular accident (CVA), with expressive aphasia and right-sided weakness. When caring for this client, which intervention will the nurse delegate to the assistive personnel (AP)?
1. Accompanying the client to speech therapy
2. Initiating passive range of motion exercises
3. Begin educating the client on simple sign language phrases
4. Turning and positioning the client every 2 hours

2. **4.** Assistive personnel (AP) are taught proper positioning skills, although this activity should still be supervised. It is not necessary to accompany the client to speech therapy and would take the AP off the unit, reducing available help. Initiating passive range-of-motion exercise requires nursing judgment to determine the level of motion. It would not be necessary to teach the client sign language, as the speech therapist will be working with the client.
CN: Safe, effective care environment; CNS: Management of care; CL: Apply

3. The nurse finds a suicidal client trying to hang oneself with a belt. Which nursing action is **priority**?
1. Place the client in seclusion with intermittent checks.
2. Assign a nursing staff member to remain with the client.
3. Make the client stay with the group at all times.
4. Refuse to let the client back into his room.

3. **2.** Implementing a one-on-one staff-to-client ratio is the nurse's highest priority. This allows the client to maintain self-esteem and keeps the client safe. Seclusion may damage the client's self-esteem and does not provide adequate monitoring. Forcing the client to stay with the group or refusing to let the client in the room does not guarantee safety.
CN: Safe, effective care environment; CNS: Management of care; CL: Apply

4. While discussing a client's care with the licensed practice nurse (LPN), the nurse detects an odor of alcohol on the LPN's breath. Which nursing action is **priority**?
1. Monitor the LPN closely for the rest of the shift.
2. Tell the LPN it is not safe to drink while working.
3. Immediately report observations to the nurse manager.
4. Warn the LPN about potential loss of employment.

4. **3.** The nurse is obligated to report suspected substance use. Allowing the LPN to continue to work could jeopardize client care. Telling the LPN it is not safe to drink while working and warning the LPN of potential loss of employment does not address the issue of client safety.
CN: Safe, effective care environment; CNS: Management of care; CL: Apply

CN: Client needs category   CNS: Client needs subcategory   CL: Cognitive level

5. New evacuation procedures are being developed for the unit by a task committee at the long-term care facility but have not been approved. A bomb threat has occurred in the facility. Which action by the nurse manager is appropriate?
  1. Tell staff members to use personal judgment to determine which procedure to follow.
  2. Ask staff members to quickly meet among themselves and decide what procedure to follow.
  3. Have staff members assemble as a group to quickly offer their opinions about what to do.
  4. Inform staff that the procedure currently in place must be followed at this time.

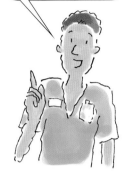

Now here's a question I know you can manage.

5. 4. In an emergency situation, the nurse manager must determine the best course of action for the safety and welfare of clients and staff. In this particular situation, there is no time for hesitation. Allowing staff members to do whatever they think is best will cause confusion and inefficient client evacuation because following different procedures will not allow them to function effectively as a team during this crisis. A meeting among the staff members and the nurse manager wastes valuable time during a life-or-death crisis.
CN: Safe, effective care environment; CNS: Management of care; CL: Apply

6. The assistive personnel (AP) reports to the registered nurse (RN) a client became short of breath while being bathed but is breathing better now. Which action will the RN take **first**?
  1. Tell the AP to observe the client for further shortness of breath.
  2. Go to the client's room and assess the client.
  3. Notify the health care provider about the client.
  4. Instruct the AP to complete the bath after the client rests.

6. 2. The nurse must assess the client to determine what caused the episode and obtain a pulse oximetry reading, if indicated. Instructing the AP to observe the client for further shortness of breath would be appropriate after the nurse has checked the client. The nurse needs to assess the client to determine if the health care provider needs to be notified. After checking the client, the nurse may ask the AP to complete the bath after allowing the client to rest.
CN: Safe, effective care environment; CNS: Management of care; CL: Analyze

7. The nurse manager will appropriately delegate which task to the unit charge nurse?
  1. Determine the staff assignments for the upcoming shift.
  2. Terminate the assistive personnel (AP) for insubordination.
  3. Decide the salary for a licensed practical nurse (LPN) following orientation.
  4. Tell a staff nurse to initiate disciplinary action against a peer.

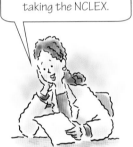

I wish I could delegate taking the NCLEX.

7. 1. Scheduling tasks may be safely and appropriately delegated to the unit charge nurse. Termination, disciplinary action, and salary should not be delegated to staff that do not have the authority to make such decisions.
CN: Safe, effective care environment; CNS: Management of care; CL: Apply

8. The registered nurse (RN) is concerned about the licensed practical nurse's (LPN's) relationship with the family of an ill preschooler. Which action by the LPN is **priority** for the RN to report to the unit nurse manager?
  1. The LPN tries to influence the family's decisions by giving personal thoughts and opinions.
  2. The LPN provides the family members with snacks and beverages labeled "client use only."
  3. The LPN allows the parents to give the child a bath during the unit's designated rest time.
  4. The LPN is heard speaking negatively about the way the family dresses.

8. 1. When a nurse attempts to influence a family's decision with personal opinions and values, the situation becomes one of inappropriate intrusion and a nontherapeutic relationship develops. This should be reported first. The other actions are not appropriate; however, they are not cause for immediate concern.
CN: Safe, effective care environment; CNS: Management of care; CL: Analyze

CN: Client needs category   CNS: Client needs subcategory   CL: Cognitive level

9. The nurse manager is appropriately using an autocratic method of leading the team. Which situation does the staff nurse determine demonstrates this form of leadership?
1. Planning vacation time for the staff on the unit
2. Directing staff activities if a client has a cardiac arrest
3. Evaluating a new medication administration process
4. Identifying strengths and weaknesses of an education video

10. A client is admitted for pneumonia secondary to human immunodeficiency virus (HIV). The registered nurse (RN) delegates giving the client oral medications to the licensed practical nurse (LPN). The LPN is hesitant to medicate the client for fear of contracting the virus. Which statement(s) is appropriate for the RN to include when responding to the LPN? Select all that apply.
1. "As an LPN, you should already know that there is little chance you will acquire HIV from administering medications."
2. "I know you are frightened, but by taking proper precautions, there is little to no risk of acquiring HIV."
3. "As the registered nurse, I am in charge. You need to go and do exactly what I have delegated to you."
4. "Personal protective equipment may prevent transmission of HIV if you come in contact with blood, body fluids, or secretions."
5. "If you do not give the medication to the child, I will write up an incident report and report you to the nurse manager."

11. Which client will the registered nurse (RN) assign to the licensed practice nurse (LPN) working on the obstetrical unit?
1. A 14-week-gestation client newly diagnosed with placenta previa
2. A 17-week-gestation client admitted with persistent nausea
3. A 20-week-gestation client following a cervical cerclage procedure
4. A 26-week-gestation client prescribed IV magnesium sulfate for preterm labor

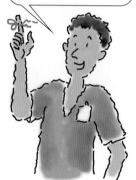

Remember—reserve the autocratic leadership approach for critical decisions that must be made rapidly.

9. **2.** In a crisis, the nurse manager should take command for the benefit of the client. Planning vacation time and evaluating procedures and client resources require staff input characteristic of a democratic or participative manager.
CN: Safe, effective care environment; CNS: Management of care; CL: Apply

10. **2, 4.** Recognizing the LPN is frightened and then clarifying information about the use of personal protective equipment provides guidance and education to alleviate fears. Telling the LPN he or she should already know there is little chance of acquiring HIV by administering medication is demeaning and does not encourage the LPN to take appropriate precautions. Statements such as "I am in charge" or "I will write up an incident report" are threatening and do not address the LPN's fears.
CN: Safe, effective care environment; CNS: Management of care; CL: Analyze

11. **2.** The RN should delegate the most stable client with predictable outcomes to the LPN. Of the clients, the 17 weeks' gestation client with persistent nausea is most stable. The 14 weeks' gestation client will require education on her newly diagnosed condition, which cannot be delegated to the LPN. The 20 weeks' gestation client will require frequent assessment for potential complications following the cerclage, which could include the onset of preterm labor. The 26 weeks' gestation client will also require frequent assessment while receiving IV magnesium sulfate. Along with frequent observation, these two clients will require frequent nursing judgment to determine stability.
CN: Safe, effective care environment; CNS: Management of care; CL: Analyze

12. The assistive personnel (AP) frequently disappears from the floor without telling anyone, and when returning to the floor, the AP's clothing smells strongly of smoke. The nurse must take steps to eliminate this behavior. Using the options below, place the steps in the chronologic order the nurse will complete them. Use each option once.

1.	Approach the AP privately to discuss the issue.

2.	Report the AP to the nurse manager if the behavior continues.

3.	Keep notes with dates and times this behavior is observed.

4.	Try to work with the AP to schedule daily breaks.

5.	Observe the AP's behavior for signs of improvement.

Congratulations! You managed this test amazingly well.

12. Ordered Response:

3.	Keep notes with dates and times this behavior is observed.

1.	Approach the AP privately to discuss the issue.

4.	Try to work with the AP to schedule daily breaks.

5.	Observe the AP's behavior for signs of improvement.

2.	Report the AP to the nurse manager if the behavior continues.

Keeping notes listing dates and times that the inappropriate behavior is observed will be helpful to verify facts. Then approach the AP privately and confidentially to discuss the issue. Work to schedule defined break times. The AP should contact the nurse before leaving the unit. Observe the AP's behavior for signs of improvement; bring the issue to the attention of the charge nurse for further action if the behavior continues.

CN: Safe, effective care environment; CNS: Management of care; CL: Analyze

CN: Client needs category   CNS: Client needs subcategory   CL: Cognitive level

Chapter 36

Ethical & Legal Issues

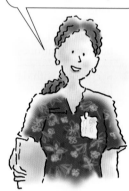

Ethical and legal issues are a daily challenge in nursing practice. Ace them on the NCLEX, and you'll be able to face each challenge with confidence! Let's go!

Ethical & legal refresher

Nurse practice acts

- State laws that are instrumental in defining the scope of nursing practice to protect the public
- Most important law affecting your nursing practice
- One for each state
- Designed to protect the nurse and public by defining the legal scope of practice and excluding untrained or unlicensed individuals from practicing nursing
- Outline conditions and requirements for licensure, such as passing the NCLEX-RN examination
- All states require completion of a board of nursing–approved educational program; your state may have additional requirements, including:
  - good moral character
  - good physical and mental health
  - minimum age
  - fluency in English
  - absence of drug or alcohol addiction.

Informed consent

- Agreement to do something or to allow something to happen only after all the relevant facts are disclosed
- The client's right to be adequately informed about a proposed treatment or procedure
- Responsibility for obtaining informed consent rests with the person who will perform the treatment or procedure (usually the health care provider)
- The client should be told he or she has a right to refuse a treatment or procedure without having other care or support withdrawn, and that consent can be withdrawn after giving it

Elements
- Description of the treatment or procedure
- Description of inherent risks and benefits that occur with frequency or regularity (or specific consequences significant to the given client or designated decision-maker)

- Explanation of the potential for death or serious harm (such as brain damage, stroke, paralysis, or disfiguring scars) or for discomforting adverse effects during or after the treatment or procedure
- Explanation and description of alternative treatments or procedures
- Name and qualifications of the person who will perform the treatment or procedure
- Discussion of possible consequences of not undergoing the treatment or procedure

Witnessing informed consent
- The client voluntarily consented
- The client's signature is authentic
- The client appears to be competent to give consent

Right to refuse treatment

- Any mentally competent adult may legally refuse treatment if fully informed about the medical condition and about the likely consequences of refusal
- Some clients may refuse treatment on the grounds of freedom of religion

Advance directives
- Living will: an advance care document that specifies a client's wishes about medical care if the client is unable to make the decision independently (in some states, living wills do not address the issue of discontinuing artificial nutrition and hydration)
- Durable power of attorney for health care: a document in which the client designates a person to make his or her medical decisions if the client becomes incompetent (differs from the usual power of attorney, which requires the client's ongoing consent and deals only with financial issues)

Grounds for challenging a client's right to refuse treatment
- Client is incompetent
- Compelling reasons exist to overrule client's wishes

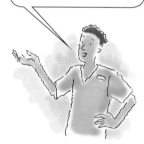

Consent must be informed and voluntary, and the client must be competent.

Living wills

- Living will laws generally include such provisions as:
  - who may execute a living will
  - witness and testator requirements
  - immunity from liability for following a living will's directives
  - documentation requirements
  - instructions on when and how the living will should be executed
  - under what circumstances the living will takes effect

Right to privacy

- Client has right of privacy regarding health information
- Privacy law allows disclosure of personal health information when needed for client care

Medication administration

- One of the most important and, legally, one of the riskiest tasks a nurse performs

Rights of administration

- Right drug
- Right client
- Right time
- Right dosage
- Right route

Negligence

- Failure to exercise the degree of care a person of ordinary prudence would exercise under the same circumstances

Four criteria for negligence claim

- A person owed a duty to the person making the claim
- The duty was breached
- The breach resulted in injury to the person making the claim
- Damages were a direct result of the negligence of the health care provider

Malpractice

- Specific type of negligence: a violation of professional duty or a failure to meet a standard of care or use the skills and knowledge of other professionals in similar circumstances

Documentation errors

- Complete, accurate, and timely documentation is crucial to the continuity of each client's care

Functions of well-documented record

- Reflects client care given
- Demonstrates results of treatment
- Helps plan and coordinate care contributed by each professional
- Allows interdisciplinary exchange of information about client
- Provides evidence of nurse's legal responsibilities toward client
- Demonstrates standards, rules, regulations, and laws of nursing practice
- Supplies information for analysis of cost-to-benefit reduction
- Reflects professional and ethical conduct and responsibility
- Furnishes information for continuing education, risk management, diagnosis-related group assignment and reimbursement, continuous quality improvement, case management monitoring, and research

Common documentation errors

- Omissions
- Personal opinions
- Vague entries
- Late entries
- Improper corrections
- Unauthorized entries
- Erroneous or vague abbreviations
- Illegible writing and lack of clarity

Abuse

- The nurse plays a crucial role in recognizing and reporting incidents of suspected abuse.
- If the nurse detects evidence of apparent abuse, the nurse must pass the information along to appropriate authorities.
- In many states, failure to report actual or suspected abuse constitutes a crime.

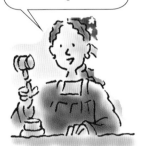

It would be malpractice to stop reading now.

Ethical & legal questions, answers, and rationales

1. A client with altered mental status fell out of bed while hospitalized and now the family wants to sue the facility stating the nurse is responsible. Which nursing action indicates professional negligence?
  1. The nurse went to the client's room 1 hour after the client asked for help.
  2. The nurse raised three of the four bedrails before leaving the client's room.
  3. The nurse placed the call bell within the client's reach before leaving the room.
  4. The nurse asked the client to call for help before attempting to get out of bed.

2. A client refused an injection, but the nurse administered it anyway. The client states, "I will sue you." Which nursing action is **most** appropriate?
  1. Wait to see if the client really does sue.
  2. Contact a personal attorney.
  3. Document exactly what happened.
  4. Explain to the client that it was an accident.

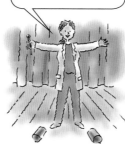

There's no statute of limitations on being awesome.

3. When giving medications to clients, the nurse fails to check the rights of medication administration. This results in the nurse giving penicillin to a client allergic to penicillin. The client experiences anaphylactic shock and dies. Which charge is **most** appropriate for the nurse's actions?
  1. Battery
  2. Negligence
  3. Collective liability
  4. Comparative negligence

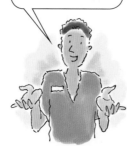

Don't let question #4 make you feel incompetent. There are many compelling reasons for you to succeed.

4. A client who is bleeding internally needs emergency surgery but refuses treatment. Which finding(s) is grounds for challenging a client's right to refuse treatment? Select all that apply.
  1. Client is incompetent.
  2. The nurse disagrees with the client's decision.
  3. Compelling reasons exist to overrule the client's wishes.
  4. The treatment would be more cost efficient.
  5. The health care provider does not want to be sued.

1. **1.** Any professional negligence action must meet certain demands to be considered negligence and result in legal action. They are commonly known as the four Ds: duty of the health care professional to provide care to the person making the claim, a dereliction (breach) of that duty, damages resulting from that breach of duty, and evidence that damages were directly due to negligence (causation). Waiting for an extended time to respond to a client's request for help indicates professional negligence. All other actions are appropriate for the nurse to complete.
CN: Safe, effective care environment; CNS: Management of care; CL: Analyze

2. **3.** The nurse should document exactly what happened. If the client does sue, the nurse's documentation will be vital. It is not appropriate for the nurse to contact someone outside the facility due to client confidentiality. Waiting is not appropriate. The nurse should document and notify the nurse manager. Attempting to rationalize the nurse's action to the client (accident) is not appropriate because this could make the client more uncomfortable with the situation.
CN: Safe, effective care environment; CNS: Safety and infection control; CL: Apply

3. **2.** Negligence is a general term that denotes conduct lacking in due care and is commonly interpreted as a deviation from the standard of care that a reasonable person would use in a given set of circumstances. Collective liability stems from cooperation by several manufacturers in a wrongful activity that by its nature requires group participation. Comparative negligence is a defense that holds injured parties accountable for their fault in the injury. Battery involves harmful or unwarranted contact with the client.
CN: Safe, effective care environment; CNS: Safety and infection control; CL: Analyze

4. **1, 3.** To challenge a client's right to refuse treatment, either the client must be incompetent or there must be compelling reasons to overrule the client's wishes. Even if the nurse disagrees with the client's decision or the treatment might be more cost efficient, the wishes of the client must be respected. The fact that the health care provider does not want to be sued should never interfere with care.
CN: Safe, effective care environment; CNS: Safety and infection control; CL: Apply

5. A client who is a member of the Jehovah's Witnesses refuses a blood transfusion based on religious beliefs and practices. Which ethical principle is the nurse following when honoring this client's wishes?
1. The right to die
2. Advance directive
3. The right to refuse treatment
4. Substituted judgment

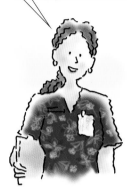

Never force a competent client to receive a treatment he or she doesn't want.

5. **3.** The right to refuse treatment is grounded in the ethical principle of respect for autonomy of the individual. The client has the right to refuse treatment as long as the client is competent and made aware of the risks and complications associated with refusal of treatment. The right to die involves whether to initiate or withhold life-sustaining treatment for a client who is irreversibly comatose, vegetative, or suffering with end-stage terminal illness. Substituted judgment is an ethical principle used when the decision is made for an incapacitated client based on what is best for the client. An advance directive is a document used as a guideline for starting or continuing life-sustaining medical care of a client with a terminal disease or disability who can no longer indicate personal wishes.
CN: Safe, effective care environment; CNS: Management of care; CL: Apply

6. A client falls while receiving care from the nurse. After assessment of the client, the nurse completes an incident report. What is the **next** anticipated step?
1. Sending the incident report to the state board of nursing
2. Documenting the incident in the nurse's personnel file
3. Suspending the nurse from the facility
4. Using the report to promote quality care and risk management

6. **4.** Unusual occurrences and deviations from care are documented on incident reports. Incident reports are internal to the facility and are used to evaluate the care, determine potential risks, and identify possible system problems that could have contributed to the error. This type of error would not result in suspension of the nurse or a report to the state board of nursing. Some facilities do trend and track the number of errors that take place on particular units, or by individual nurses, for educational purposes and as a way to improve the nursing process.
CN: Safe, effective care environment; CNS: Management of care; CL: Apply

7. The registered nurse knows a well-documented client's medical record serves which function(s)? Select all that apply.
1. Helps to ensure continuity of care for the client
2. Reflects what client care has been provided
3. Demonstrates results of treatment received
4. Supplies information for analysis of cost-to-benefit reduction
5. Allows a private way for only nurses to follow the care
6. Reflects professional and ethical conduct

7. **1, 2, 3, 4, 6.** A well-documented record performs the following functions: reflects client care given; demonstrates results of treatment; helps plan and coordinate care contributed by each professional; allows interdisciplinary exchange of information about client; provides evidence of nurse's legal responsibilities toward client; demonstrates standards, rules, regulations, and laws of nursing practice; supplies information for analysis of cost-to-benefit reduction; reflects professional and ethical conduct and responsibility; furnishes information for continuing education, risk management, diagnosis-related group assignment and reimbursement, continuous quality improvement, case management monitoring, and research. A well-documented client record is not private for only nurses; all members of the health care team are allowed to use the client record.
CN: Safe, effective care environment; CNS: Management of care; CL: Apply

8. Which item does the new nurse graduate correctly identify as defining the scope of nursing practice to protect clients?
1. Nursing process
2. Facilities' policies and procedures
3. Standards of care
4. Nurse Practice Act

8. 4. The Nurse Practice Act is a series of statutes enacted by each state to outline the legal scope of nursing practice within that state. State boards of nursing oversee this statutory law. Nurse practice acts set educational requirements for the nurse, distinguish between nursing practice and medical practice, and define the scope of nursing practice. Nursing process is an organizational framework for nursing practice, encompassing all major steps a nurse takes when caring for a client. Facility policies govern the practice in that particular facility. Standards of care are criteria that serve as a basis for comparison when evaluating the quality of nursing practice. Standards of care are established by federal, state, professional, and accreditation organizations.
CN: Safe, effective care environment; CNS: Management of care; CL: Apply

9. A new graduate nurse is working with the team that sets up organ donation. What is the **most** important concept the nurse must understand about organ or tissue donation before working with families?
1. It is done with a health care provider's approval and written prescription
2. The individual requesting does not have to believe in the benefits of organ donation
3. The individual requesting is knowledgeable about the basics of organ donation
4. The family is offered an opportunity to speak with an organ procurement coordinator

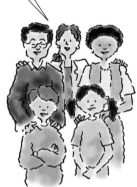

A big part of nursing is knowing when and to whom to refer a family for specialty assistance.

9. 4. The family should be offered an opportunity to speak with an organ procurement coordinator. An organ procurement coordinator is very knowledgeable about the organ donation process and dealing with grieving family members. Health care provider support in the process is desirable, but consent or written prescriptions are not necessary for a referral to the organ procurement organization. The individual requesting has to believe in the benefits of organ donation and support the process. Approaching the family should only occur when the family members are made aware of the client's condition and prognosis. Approaching a family member when he believes that there is still hope for recovery will only result in a negative outcome.
CN: Safe, effective care environment; CNS: Management of care; CL: Apply

10. The nurse observes a coworker administering a medication several hours after it had been scheduled. When confronted, the coworker simply makes a dismissive joke and then charts the medication as given at the scheduled time. Place the witnessing nurse's actions in ascending chronologic sequence. Use all options.

1.	Request a private meeting to discuss the incident.
2.	Encourage the nurse to take responsibility for these actions.
3.	Express concern and clearly inform the nurse that the behavior is unethical.
4.	Report the incident to the nurse manager if resistance is noted.
5.	Approach the coworker in a calm and professional manner.

10. Ordered Response:

5.	Approach the coworker in a calm and professional manner.
1.	Request a private meeting to discuss the incident.
3.	Express concern and clearly inform the nurse that the behavior is unethical.
2.	Encourage the nurse to take responsibility for these actions.
4.	Report the incident to the nurse manager if resistance is noted.

The nurse must maintain a calm and professional demeanor and talk with the coworker privately. It is important to discuss ethical concerns and encourage the coworker to take responsibility for these actions. The nurse manager should be informed of the incident if resistance by the offending nurse is noted.
CN: Safe, effective care environment; CNS: Management of care; CL: Analyze

11. There are reports that morphine has been missing from the medication room several times during the last 3 months. The nurse walks into the medication room and witnesses another nurse quickly slipping something into a pocket from the controlled substance drawer. Place the nurse's actions in ascending chronologic sequence. Use all options.

1. If directed, fill out a confidential incident report describing what was seen.

2. Approach the nurse manager privately and discuss the matter.

3. Do not share any observations with others on the unit.

4. Continue to observe the nurse in question for signs of unusual behavior.

5. Carefully review and document what was observed.

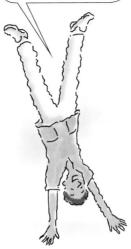

Hip, hip, hooray! Another test down.

11. Ordered Response:

5. Carefully review and document what was observed.

2. Approach the nurse manager privately and discuss the matter.

1. If directed, fill out a confidential incident report describing what was seen.

3. Do not share any observations with others on the unit.

4. Continue to observe the nurse in question for signs of unusual behavior.

A premature conclusion should not be drawn based on one suspicious incident. It is best to first review and carefully document in detail what was seen. Then speak with the nurse-manager privately and, if directed, fill out a confidential incident report describing what was observed. At this point, the charge nurse will follow through and further investigate the situation. It is important not to speak to others on the unit to maintain professionalism and to avoid spreading potentially unfounded rumors. The reporting nurse should remain alert for repeated suspicious behavior.

CN: Safe, effective care environment; CNS: Management of care; CL: Analyze

Appendices

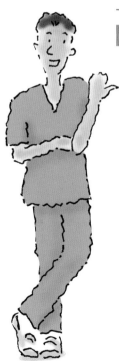

Comprehensive Test 1

This comprehensive test, the first of two, is just like the shortest NCLEX-RN test: 75 questions. It's a great way to practice!

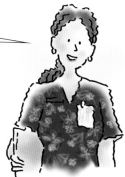

1. A client is experiencing cardiac tamponade after a chest trauma. Which finding(s) will the nurse expect to assess? Select all that apply.
1. Respiratory rate 42 breaths/minute
2. Dyspnea
3. Loss of consciousness
4. Blood pressure 72/42 mm Hg
5. Pale, sweaty skin
6. Increased urinary output

2. A victim of a motor vehicle accident with blunt chest trauma and no obvious signs of bleeding has a heart rate of 132 beats/minute, a blood pressure of 82/54 mm Hg, and muffled heart sounds. Which condition does the nurse suspect the client is experiencing?
1. Heart failure
2. Pneumothorax
3. Cardiac tamponade
4. Myocardial infarction (MI)

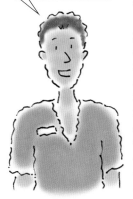

So, signs of shock + muffled heart sounds = what?

3. The nurse is caring for a client with cardiac tamponade. Which treatment will the nurse anticipate for this client?
1. Insertion of a stent
2. Infusion of dopamine
3. Blood transfusion
4. Pericardiocentesis

4. The nurse is providing education to a client about reducing risk factors for coronary artery disease. Which risk factor will the nurse inform the client is nonmodifiable?
1. Age
2. Hypertension
3. Personality
4. Smoking

1. 1, 2, 3, 4, 5. The nurse would suspect cardiogenic shock. Fluid accumulates in the pericardial sac, hindering motion of the heart muscle and causing it to pump inefficiently, resulting in signs of cardiogenic shock. Urinary output will be decreased with cardiogenic shock as the kidneys are not being perfused.
CN: Physiological integrity; CNS: Physiological adaptation; CL: Analyze

2. 3. Cardiac tamponade results in signs of obvious shock and muffled heart sounds. Heart failure results in inspiratory crackles, pulmonary edema, and jugular vein distention. Pneumothorax results in diminished breath sounds in the affected lung, respiratory distress, and tracheal displacement. In an MI, the client may report chest pain. An electrocardiogram could confirm changes consistent with an MI.
CN: Physiological integrity; CNS: Physiological adaptation; CL: Apply

3. 4. Pericardiocentesis, or needle aspiration of the pericardial cavity, is done to relieve tamponade. An opening is created surgically if the client continues to have recurrent episodes of tamponade. Dopamine is used to restore blood pressure in normovolemic individuals. Blood transfusions may be given if the client is hypovolemic from blood loss.
CN: Physiological integrity; CNS: Physiological adaptation; CL: Apply

4. 1. Age is a risk factor that cannot be changed. Hypertension, type A personality, and smoking factors can be controlled.
CN: Health promotion and maintenance; CNS: None; CL: Understand

5. The nurse is caring for a client suspected of having cardiac tamponade. For which diagnostic test will the nurse prepare the client?
1. Chest x-ray
2. Echocardiography
3. Electrocardiogram (ECG)
4. Pulmonary artery pressure monitoring

6. A client with a history of hypertension states, "I am stressed by my job but enjoy the challenge." What is the **best** response by the nurse?
1. "I feel the same way about my job."
2. "Take stress management classes."
3. "Spend more time with your family."
4. "Do not take your work home."

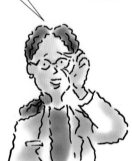

I keep looking for a way to modify my stress but haven't had much luck.

7. A client diagnosed with angina is being discharged from the hospital with a prescription for nitroglycerin. Which statement will the nurse include in the discharge teaching?
1. "If chest pain is experienced, immediately call the emergency response system."
2. "If chest pain is experienced longer than 1 hour, take a nitroglycerin."
3. "Store the nitroglycerin in the bathroom medicine cabinet."
4. "Take 1 tablet sublingually every 5 minutes, up to 3 doses, for chest pain."

8. A client with human immunodeficiency virus (HIV) is admitted to the hospital with flulike symptoms, dyspnea, and a cough. The client is placed on a 100% non-rebreather mask and arterial blood gases (ABGs) are drawn. The client's results are PaO$_2$, 70 mm Hg; PaCO$_2$, 55 mm Hg. Which nursing action is **most** appropriate?
1. Prepare the client for intubation.
2. Redraw ABGs in 1 hour.
3. Administer sodium bicarbonate.
4. Recheck the oxygen saturation level.

9. The nurse is discussing transmission of human immunodeficiency virus (HIV) to a group of high school students. Which substance does the nurse inform the students **most** commonly transmits the virus?
1. Blood
2. Feces
3. Saliva
4. Urine

5. **2.** Echocardiography measures pericardial effusion and can detect signs of right ventricular and atrial compression. Chest x-rays show a slightly widened mediastinum and enlarged cardiac silhouette. An ECG can rule out other cardiac disorders. Pulmonary artery pressure monitoring shows increased right atrial or central venous pressure and right ventricular diastolic pressure.
CN: Physiological integrity; CNS: Reduction of risk potential; CL: Apply

6. **2.** Stress management classes will educate the client on how to better manage the stress in one's life, after identifying the factors that contribute to the stress. Alternatives may be found to leaving the job, which the client enjoys. Not spending enough time with family and not taking the job home have not been identified as contributing factors to the client's stress.
CN: Physiological integrity; CNS: Reduction of risk potential; CL: Analyze

7. **4.** It is important to inform the client to take 1 tablet under the tongue every 5 minutes, up to 3 doses. If the pain is not relieved after 3 doses, the client should access the emergency medical system and go to the hospital. The client should not wait 1 hour to take the medication. The medication should not be stored in the bathroom medicine cabinet, because the moisture may render the medication inactive. The client should take the nitroglycerin before immediately going to the hospital, because the pain may be relieved by rest and nitroglycerin.
CN: Physiological integrity; CNS: Pharmacological and parenteral therapies; CL: Analyze

8. **1.** A decreasing partial pressure of arterial oxygen (PaO$_2$) and an increasing partial pressure of arterial carbon dioxide (PaCO$_2$) indicate poor oxygen perfusion. The nurse would prepare the client for intubation. Normal PaO$_2$ levels are 80 to 100 mm Hg and normal PaCO$_2$ levels are 35 to 45 mm Hg. No other action is appropriate for this client.
CN: Physiological integrity; CNS: Reduction of risk potential; CL: Analyze

9. **1.** HIV is most commonly transmitted by contact with infected blood. It exists in all body fluids, but transmission through feces, saliva, and urine is much less likely to occur.
CN: Safe, effective care environment; CNS: Safety and infection control; CL: Understand

CN: Client needs category CNS: Client needs subcategory CL: Cognitive level

10. A client with human immunodeficiency virus (HIV) has developed *Pneumocystis jiroveci* infection. Which prescription(s) will the nurse anticipate? Select all that apply.
1. Give sulfamethoxazole.
2. Administer trimethoprim.
3. Administer miconazole.
4. Monitor stool specimens.
5. Apply cardiac monitor.

11. A client with acquired immunodeficiency syndrome (AIDS) is intubated. Which nursing action is **most** appropriate for this client?
1. Use lubricant on the lips.
2. Provide oral care every 2 hours.
3. Suction the oral cavity every 2 hours.
4. Reposition the endotracheal (ET) tube every 24 hours.

12. The registered nurse (RN) observes the licensed practical nurse (LPN) apply a nasal cannula to a client requiring the highest possible concentration of oxygen. What will the RN do **next**?
1. Notify the nurse manager of the incident.
2. Call the health care provider.
3. Educate the LPN on oxygen delivery devices.
4. Remove the nasal cannula and apply a mask with reservoir bag.

13. A client is refusing all medications and is having difficulty breathing, with a respiratory rate of 34 breaths/minute and anxiety. What is the **priority** nursing action?
1. Notify the health care provider of the status of this client.
2. Withhold the medication until the next scheduled dose.
3. Encourage the client to take half of the prescribed medications.
4. Put the medicine in applesauce to give it without the client's knowledge.

14. The registered nurse (RN) and licensed practical nurse (LPN) are caring for a client with acquired immunodeficiency syndrome (AIDS). The RN notes the LPN does not assist with care of the client. Which action by the RN is appropriate?
1. Talk to the LPN.
2. Talk to the nurse manager.
3. Discuss the concern with a coworker.
4. Seek advice from the unit educator.

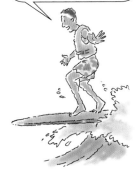

You're off to a great start! Ride that wave of momentum.

10. **1, 2.** *P. jiroveci* infection is caused by protozoa, which responds to antibiotics, not an antifungal. The treatment of choice is trimethoprim and sulfamethoxazole (TMP/SMX). Miconazole is used to treat fungal and yeast infections. Monitoring stool or applying cardiac monitors is not necessary.
CN: Physiological integrity; CNS: Physiological adaptation; CL: Analyze

11. **4.** Pressure causes skin breakdown. Repositioning the ET tube every 24 hours from one side of the mouth to the other (or to the center of the mouth) can relieve pressure. Extreme care must be taken to move the tube only laterally; it must not be pushed in or pulled out. The tape securing the tube must be changed daily. Two nurses should perform this procedure. Lubricant, oral care, and suctioning help keep skin clean and intact and reduce the risk of further infection; however, these actions do not prevent skin breakdown.
CN: Physiological integrity; CNS: Basic care and comfort; CL: Analyze

12. **4.** The nurse will first correct the error to facilitate the client's breathing. The RN would then educate the LPN. It is not necessary to inform the nurse manager or health care provider at this time.
CN: Physiological integrity; CNS: Physiological adaptation; CL: Analyze

13. **1.** The nurse should notify the health care provider of the client's condition and refusal to take the medications to allow the health care provider to decide what alternatives should be instituted. Withholding the medication does not improve the client's status. Even if the client takes some of the medications, the health care provider still needs to be notified. Giving medications in applesauce without the client's knowledge destroys trust between the nurse and client. The reason the client is refusing the medications needs to be explored.
CN: Physiological integrity; CNS: Pharmacological and parenteral therapies; CL: Analyze

14. **1.** The RN should approach the LPN first to determine feelings and experience in caring for a client with AIDS. The nurse manager and coworkers are not familiar with the LPN's abilities, but the unit educator may be approached if the RN cannot communicate with the LPN.
CN: Safe, effective care environment; CNS: Management of care; CL: Apply

15. A client's spouse is upset over the client's condition and lack of improvement. The spouse expresses feelings of powerlessness. Which response by the nurse is **best**?
1. "Yes, you are powerless to do anything about your spouse."
2. "There is nothing that can be done at this time."
3. "I completely understand what you are going through."
4. "Would you like to help with some comfort measures for your spouse?"

16. A client is admitted to the hospital with a diagnosis of respiratory failure. The client is intubated, placed on 100% FiO_2, and is coughing up copious secretions. Which nursing intervention is **priority**?
1. Get an x-ray.
2. Suction the client.
3. Restrain the client.
4. Obtain an arterial blood gas (ABG) analysis.

17. A client with an endotracheal tube has copious, brown-tinged secretions. Which nursing intervention is **priority**?
1. Obtain a sputum specimen.
2. Instill saline to break up secretions.
3. Notify the health care provider.
4. Administer a liquefying agent for the sputum.

18. A client's x-ray shows the endotracheal (ET) tube is 0.75 in (2 cm) above the carina, and there are nodular lesions and patchy infiltrates in the upper lobe. Based on this report, what will the nurse do **next**?
1. Place the client on airborne precautions.
2. Notify the health care provider.
3. Advance the ET tube.
4. Pulled back on the ET tube.

19. A client is placed in the negative pressure room for suspected tuberculosis (TB) upon admission. The nurse will prepare the client for which procedure?
1. Chest x-ray
2. Tracheostomy
3. Bronchoscopy
4. Mantoux tuberculin skin test

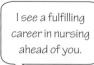

I see a fulfilling career in nursing ahead of you.

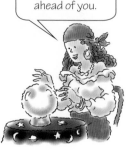

15. 4. The significant other expresses a need to help the client, and the nurse can encourage the spouse to do whatever the spouse feels comfortable with, such as putting lubricant on lips, a moist cloth on the forehead, or lotion on skin. The nurse may not understand the spouse's situation, and agreeing with a person does not diminish powerlessness. There are many ways the significant other can assist.
CN: Psychosocial integrity; CNS: None; CL: Analyze

16. 2. Suctioning the client is the priority because secretions can cut off the oxygen supply to the client and result in hypoxia. X-rays are the next priority; check placement of the endotracheal tube. Restraints are warranted only if the client is a threat to his or her safety. After the client has acclimated to the ventilator settings, ABG levels can be drawn.
CN: Physiological integrity; CNS: Reduction of risk potential; CL: Analyze

17. 1. Suspicious secretions should be obtained and sent for culture and sensitivity testing using sterile technique. Saline would dilute the specimen. The health care provider will be notified based on the test results. Various liquefying agents are available to help break up secretions; respiratory therapists can usually recommend the right agent, but this is not a priority.
CN: Safe, effective care environment; CNS: Safety and infection control; CL: Analyze

18. 1. The x-ray is conclusive and suggests tuberculosis. After placing the client on precautions to prevent further spreading, the health care provider will be notified. At 0.75 in (2 cm) above the carina, the ET tube is at an adequate level in the trachea and does not have to be advanced or pulled back.
CN: Physiological integrity; CNS: Reduction of risk potential; CL: Analyze

19. 3. Bronchoscopy can help diagnose TB and obtain specimens while clearing the bronchial tree of secretions. X-rays may be repeated periodically to determine lung and endotracheal tube status. Tracheostomy may be done if the client remains on the ventilator for a prolonged period. Mantoux tuberculin skin test only tells if the client has been exposed to TB.
CN: Physiological integrity; CNS: Reduction of risk potential; CL: Apply

CN: Client needs category   CNS: Client needs subcategory   CL: Cognitive level

20. A client comes to the clinic and informs the nurse of possible exposure to a family member with tuberculosis. The nurse administers the tuberculin skin test; 2 days later the test is positive. What does the nurse determine the results mean?

1. The client has an active disease.
2. The client had a recent infection.
3. The client has latent tuberculosis.
4. The client had presence of infection at some point.

21. A registered nurse (RN) notes a licensed practical nurse (LPN) applies a gown, gloves, and a respirator before entering the room of a client diagnosed with active tuberculosis. What will the RN do **next**?

1. Place the LPN in isolation.
2. Call the unit manager.
3. Continue monitoring the LPN.
4. Have the LPN put on a face shield.

22. A client has been diagnosed with tuberculosis (TB). Which pharmacologic therapy will the nurse question administering to this client? Select all that apply.

1. Theophylline
2. Penicillin
3. Rifampin
4. Isoniazid
5. Rifapentine
6. Pentamidine

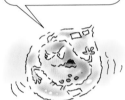

I'm one tough bug. It takes an arsenal of meds to take me down.

23. A client with a diagnosis of tuberculosis (TB) is being educated on treatment modalities. How long does the nurse inform the client that medications will be prescribed?

1. 2 to 4 months
2. 6 to 12 months
3. 18 to 24 months
4. More than 2 years

24. A client is diagnosed with tuberculosis (TB). Which action(s) by the nurse is appropriate? Select all that apply.

1. Inform the client about the need to be on isolation for 6 months.
2. Report the case to the required agencies.
3. Recommend skin testing for family members.
4. Report blood-tinged sputum to the health care provider.
5. Administer acetaminophen for a fever.

20. 4. A tuberculin skin test shows the presence of infection at some point; however, a positive skin test does not guarantee that an infection is currently present. Some people have false-positive results. Active disease may be viewed on a chest x-ray. Computed tomography scan or magnetic resonance imaging can evaluate the extent of lung damage.

CN: Safe and effective care environment; CNS: Safety and infection control; CL: Understand

21. 3. The RN will continue monitoring the LPN. The LPN applied correct personal protective equipment for a client on airborne precautions. The other actions are not appropriate.

CN: Safe, effective care environment; CNS: Safety and infection control; CL: Analyze

22. 1, 2, 6. Because TB has become resistant to many antibacterial agents, the initial treatment includes the use of multiple antitubercular or antibacterial drugs. The Centers for Disease Control and Prevention (CDC) recommends the use of rifampin, isoniazid, and rifapentine for use in treatment. The Public Health Agency of Canada recommends the use of isoniazid, rifampin, pyrazinamide, and ethambutol. Theophylline is a bronchodilator used to treat asthma and chronic obstructive pulmonary disease (COPD). Penicillins are used to treat *Staphylococcus aureus* infection—not TB. Pentamidine is used in the treatment of *Pneumocystis jiroveci* pneumonia.

CN: Physiological integrity; CNS: Pharmacological and parenteral therapies; CL: Apply

23. 2. Treatment for TB is usually continued for 6 to 12 months. Two to four months is not adequate time for treatment to be successful. More than 2 years or 18 to 24 months are treatment times that are beyond therapeutic value.

CN: Physiological integrity; CNS: Pharmacological and parenteral therapies; CL: Understand

24. 2, 3, 5. Required agencies must be informed of an outbreak of TB because it is a reportable disease. They, in turn, inform the Centers for Disease Control and Prevention or the Public Health Agency of Canada. Family members should be tested to determine if treatment is needed and to limit spreading the disease. Acetaminophen is appropriate for mild pain or fever. Isolation is needed until three negative cultures are achieved. Blood-tinged sputum is expected and does not require reporting.

CN: Safe, effective care environment; CNS: Safety and infection control; CL: Apply

CN: Client needs category   CNS: Client needs subcategory   CL: Cognitive level

25. A client tells the nurse, "I do not plan to take the prescribed tuberculosis medications." Which intervention by the nurse is **best**?
1. Have case management come speak with the client.
2. Tell the client the prognosis of untreated tuberculosis.
3. Call the client's primary health care provider.
4. Determine why the client does not want to take the medication.

26. The nurse is caring for a client at risk for skin impairment. Which nursing intervention is **best**?
1. Use a specialty mattress.
2. Position the client in alignment.
3. Reposition the client every 4 hours.
4. Massage bony prominences every shift.

27. A client admitted to the hospital with pneumonia has a history of Parkinson's disease, which is progressively worsening. Which clinical manifestation does the nurse anticipate assessing?
1. Impaired speech
2. Muscle flaccidity
3. Echolalia
4. Tremors in the fingers while sleeping

28. An older adult male client with Parkinson's disease is frequently incontinent of urine. Which intervention by the nurse is **most** appropriate?
1. Use adult briefs.
2. Apply a condom catheter.
3. Insert an indwelling urinary catheter.
4. Provide perineal care every 4 hours.

29. Family members report to the nurse they are exhausted and it is difficult taking care of a dependent family member. Which nursing action is **best**?
1. Determine if the client has the same perspective.
2. Tell the family members to discuss it among themselves.
3. Tell the family the client should go to a nursing care facility.
4. Call a family conference and ask social services for assistance.

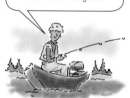
Having trouble with a question? Be patient. The answer will come to you.

25. 4. The nurse should determine why the client does not want to take the medications. This will guide the nurse to best care for the client. Notifying case management is not appropriate for this client. The client does need to understand the repercussion of forgoing treatment; however, knowing why will best direct the nurse. The primary health care provider may need to be notified, depending upon the rationale.
CN: Safe, effective care environment; CNS: Management of care; CL: Apply

26. 1. Specialty beds having fluid, air, and convoluted foam mattresses can protect pressure areas on the client. Pressure areas on the client should be padded to prevent skin breakdown. Positioning the client in alignment is important, but pressure areas still need to be protected. The client should be turned every 2 hours. Massaging bony prominences causes friction and may irritate tissues.
CN: Physiological integrity; CNS: Reduction of risk potential; CL: Apply

27. 1. In Parkinson's disease, dysarthria (impaired speech) is due to a disturbance in muscle control. Muscle rigidity results in resistance to passive muscle stretching. The client may have a masklike appearance. Tremors should decrease with purposeful movement and sleep. Echolalia is repeating a word that is heard and is usually experienced by clients with schizophrenia.
CN: Physiological integrity; CNS: Physiological adaptation; CL: Apply

28. 2. A condom catheter uses a condom-type device to drain urine away from the client. Applying a brief on the client may keep urine away from the body but may also be demeaning if the client is alert or the family objects. Because the client with Parkinson's disease is prone to urinary tract infections, an indwelling urinary catheter should be avoided because it may promote these infections. Skin care must be provided to prevent skin maceration and breakdown and should begin as soon as the client is incontinent.
CN: Physiological integrity; CNS: Basic care and comfort; CL: Analyze

29. 4. A family conference with social services can enlighten the family to all prospects of care available to them. The client should supply input if able, but this may not help solve the problems of exhaustion and care difficulties. The family may not be aware of alternative care measures for the client, so a discussion among themselves may not be helpful. The client may not qualify for a nursing care facility because of the need to meet stringent criteria.
CN: Safe, effective care environment; CNS: Management of care; CL: Apply

CN: Client needs category   CNS: Client needs subcategory   CL: Cognitive level

30. A primigravida at 22 weeks' gestation, with a history of rheumatic fever, tells the nurse her fingers feel tight and sometimes she feels as though her heart skips a beat. Which assessment finding **most** concerns the nurse?
1. Decreased urine output this trimester
2. Maternal heart rate 92 beats/minute
3. Bilateral crackles in the client's lungs
4. Fetal heart rate increases with fetal movement

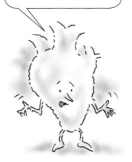

Listen up. The sounds I make can let you know when I'm in trouble.

31. A pregnant client is suspected of experiencing worsening mitral valve prolapse. The nurse will prepare the client for which procedure?
1. Stress test
2. Chest x-ray
3. Echocardiography
4. Cardiac catheterization

32. The nurse is caring for a client in labor with a history of rheumatic heart disease. Which intervention is **most** appropriate for the nurse to use to determine fetal well-being?
1. Urinalysis
2. Fetal heart tones
3. Maternal laboratory results
4. Nonstress test

33. The nurse is obtaining subjective data from a client who was recently admitted to the hospital. Which data does the nurse document as subjective?
1. Complete blood count
2. Vital signs
3. 2 × 2 cm sacral decubitus ulcer
4. Reports of nausea and abdominal pain

34. The nurse is caring for a pregnant client with cardiovascular disease. About which medication will the nurse anticipate educating the client?
1. Atenolol
2. Warfarin
3. Nifedipine
4. Furosemide

35. A client with placenta previa is hospitalized, and a cesarean birth is planned. In addition to the routine neonatal assessment, the nurse will assess the neonate for which condition?
1. Prematurity
2. Congenital anomalies
3. Respiratory distress
4. Aspiration pneumonia

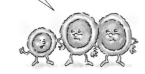

Wow. You guys are looking ancient. What are you, like, 116 days old?

30. **3.** Crackles should alert the nurse to cardiovascular compromise and heart failure. Pregnant clients should experience relief from urinary frequency as the fetus is off the bladder during this trimester. Maternal heart rate increase of 10 beats/minute is expected during pregnancy. The fetal heart rate described indicates accelerations.
CN: Health promotion and maintenance; CNS: None; CL: Analyze

31. **3.** Echocardiography is less invasive than x-rays and other methods; it provides the information needed to determine cardiovascular disease, especially valvular disorders. Cardiac catheterization and stress tests may be postponed until after birth.
CN: Physiological integrity; CNS: Physiological adaptation; CL: Apply

32. **2.** Fetal heart tones show how the fetus is responding to the environment. Assessing other signs and symptoms of the mother, including laboratory test results and urinalysis, can only determine the effect on the mother, not the fetus. A nonstress test may be indicated depending on the fetal heart tones.
CN: Health promotion and maintenance; CNS: None; CL: Apply

33. **4.** Subjective data, also known as symptoms or covert cues, include the client's own verbatim statements about health problems. Laboratory study results, physical assessment data, and diagnostic procedure reports are observable, perceptible, and measurable and can be verified and validated by others.
CN: Safe and effective care environment; CNS: Management of care; CL: Understand

34. **3.** Calcium channel antagonists, such as nifedipine may be used. Beta-blockers are generally safe to use, but not atenolol because it causes growth retardation. Prophylactic antibiotics are reserved for clients susceptible to endocarditis. If anticoagulants are needed, heparin is the drug of choice—not warfarin. Diuretics, such as furosemide, should be used with extreme caution, if at all, because of the potential for causing uterine contractions.
CN: Physiological integrity; CNS: Pharmacological and parenteral therapies; CL: Apply

35. **3.** Hypoxia, resulting in respiratory distress, is a potential risk due to decreased blood volume. The age of maturity of the neonate can be determined through established maternal dates. Congenital anomalies are not necessarily associated with placenta previa. Aspiration pneumonia is not considered a threat unless the amniotic fluid is meconium-stained.
CN: Physiological integrity; CNS: Reduction of risk potential; CL: Apply

CN: Client needs category   CNS: Client needs subcategory   CL: Cognitive level

36. The nurse is assisting a client with personal hygiene measures. The client has diabetes and is morbidly obese. The client states, "I have heard the other nurses and staff joking about me. Could you be my nurse tomorrow?" Which response by the nurse is **most** appropriate?
1. "I cannot promise that, but I will make sure those nurses know how you feel."
2. "I will check with the charge nurse to see if I can be your nurse."
3. "I will make sure the other nurses do not talk about you anymore."
4. "I am sorry. I will report your concerns to the nurse manager."

36. **4.** Telling the client that a nurse manager will be made aware of the inappropriate comments acknowledges the client's feelings and indicates care and concern. It is best to go through the proper chain of command and inform the nursing supervisor of this situation. Telling the client the nurse will make sure the others know how the client feels would only increase the client's embarrassment. Checking with the charge nurse is incorrect because assignments are based on experience and acuity. The nurse cannot guarantee the other nurses will not talk about the client.
CN: Safe, effective care environment; CNS: Management of care; CL: Apply

37. After the nurse assesses the vital signs and applies an external monitor to the client with suspected placenta previa, which nursing intervention is **priority**?
1. Insert an indwelling urinary catheter.
2. Plan for an immediate cesarean birth.
3. Place the client in Trendelenburg position.
4. Start IV catheters and obtain bloodwork.

37. **4.** The priority nursing intervention for a client with suspected placenta previa is to draw blood for hemoglobin analysis, hematocrit, type, and crossmatch and to insert IV catheters. Depending on the degree of bleeding and fetal maturity, a cesarean birth may be required. The nurse should not attempt Trendelenburg positioning or urinary catheterization. The client may be placed on her left side.
CN: Physiological integrity; CNS: Reduction of risk potential; CL: Apply

38. A pregnant client with vaginal bleeding asks the nurse how the fetus is doing. Which response by the nurse is **best**?
1. "I do not know for sure."
2. "I cannot answer that question."
3. "It is too early to tell anything."
4. "I will tell you what the monitors show."

38. **4.** The client deserves a truthful answer and the nurse should be objective without giving opinions. Relating what the monitors show is objective and truthful. Vague answers may be misleading and are not therapeutic.
CN: Psychosocial integrity; CNS: None; CL: Apply

39. The nursing staff is developing a care plan for a client who is receiving palliative care for end-stage leukemia. The client is experiencing breakthrough pain, rated as a 5 on a pain scale of 1 to 10. Which nursing action is **priority**?
1. Meet with the pain management team to devise a better plan to control pain.
2. Explain to the client that pain relief may not be possible.
3. Assess whether the client is misusing the pain medications.
4. Provide nonpharmacologic pain measures to the client.

39. **1.** Client comfort is top priority in palliative care. The nurse should meet with the pain management team to devise a plan to control the client's pain. Typically, palliative care doses are increased above the normal maximum doses to meet the client's needs. Clients who require opioids long term typically develop drug tolerance, so it is necessary to increase dosages. There is no need to assess the client for drug misuse. The nursing staff should also incorporate nonpharmacologic measures to relieve pain into the client's care plan, but these measures are not priority.
CN: Physiological integrity; CNS: Basic care and comfort; CL: Apply

40. The nurse working in the emergency department sees several pediatric clients arrive simultaneously. Which client will the nurse assess **first**?
1. A 2-month-old infant with stridor, sitting up in the mother's arms, and drooling
2. A 3-year-old child with a barking cough and flushed appearance
3. A 3-year-old child with Down syndrome who is pale and asleep in the mother's arms
4. A crying 4-year-old child with a laceration on the scalp

40. **1.** The 2-month-old infant with the airway emergency should be treated first because of the risk of epiglottitis. The 3-year-old with the barking cough and fever should be suspected of having croup and should be seen promptly, as should the child with the laceration. The nurse would need to gather more information about the child with Down syndrome to determine the priority of care.
CN: Safe, effective care environment; CNS: Management of care; CL: Analyze

CN: Client needs category   CNS: Client needs subcategory   CL: Cognitive level

41. The nurse is assessing a 2-year-old child with drooling, dysphagia, and dysphonia. Which primary health care provider prescription will the nurse question?
1. Place intubation equipment at bedside.
2. Get a throat culture.
3. Obtain a portable neck x-ray.
4. Administer antibiotic.

42. Which method is **best** for the nurse to use when approaching a 2-year-old client to auscultate breath sounds?
1. Tell the child it is time to listen to the lungs now.
2. Tell the child to lie down while the nurse listens to the lungs.
3. Ask the caregiver to wait outside while the nurse listens to the lungs.
4. Ask if the child would like the nurse to listen to the front or the back of the chest first.

43. A pregnant client being seen in the clinic reports increasing leg cramps. Which response by the nurse is **most** appropriate?
1. "Have you asked the health care provider to prescribe a muscle relaxant?"
2. "Sometimes gently stretching the legs helps relieve leg cramps."
3. "Relax. Everyone who is pregnant has leg cramps."
4. "Do not worry about them. They go away after you deliver."

44. Which immunization(s) will the nurse plan to administer to a healthy 2-year-old child in the winter? Select all that apply.
1. Diphtheria–tetanus–pertussis (DTaP)
2. Inactivated poliovirus (IPV) vaccine
3. Measles–mumps–rubella (MMR) vaccine
4. Pneumococcal vaccine (PCV) vaccine
5. *Haemophilus influenzae* type b (Hib) vaccine
6. Varicella vaccine
7. Influenza vaccine

45. The nurse is obtaining data on a child with epiglottitis. Which action by the nurse is appropriate?
1. Obtain a flashlight and tongue blade.
2. Obtain a sterile tongue blade and culture swab.
3. Ask the charge nurse to visualize the child's throat.
4. Wait for visualization to be done by the primary health care provider.

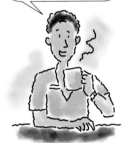
Feeling sleepy? Try some caffeine therapy.

41. 2. The child is exhibiting classic signs of epiglottitis. The nurse will question obtaining a throat culture because this action places the child at increased risk of having a laryngospasm, which would lead to airway loss. All other prescriptions are appropriate.
CN: Safe, effective care environment; CNS: Management of care; CL: Analyze

42. 4. The 2-year-old child needs to feel in control, and asking the client which side of the chest to listen to first best supports the child's independence. Giving the child no choice may make the child uncooperative. The child should be allowed to remain in the tripod position to facilitate breathing. The caregiver should be allowed to remain with the child because fear of separation is common in 2-year-olds.
CN: Health promotion and maintenance; CNS: None; CL: Apply

43. 2. Leg cramps are a common discomfort of pregnancy. Gentle stretching may be effective in relieving the cramps. Typically, muscle relaxants are not used for leg cramps associated with pregnancy. Telling the client to relax, not to worry, that every pregnant woman gets leg cramps, or that they go away after birth ignores the client's concern and dismisses the client's feelings.
CN: Physiological integrity; CNS: Basic care and comfort; CL: Apply

44. 7. Only the influenza vaccine would be needed at this age during the fall and winter. All other vaccines would be administered before or after this age according to the U.S. Centers for Disease Control and Prevention and the Public Health Agency of Canada.
CN: Health promotion and maintenance; CNS: None; CL: Apply

45. 4. Direct visualization of the epiglottis can trigger a complete airway obstruction and should only be done in a controlled environment by an anesthesiologist or a primary health care provider skilled in pediatric intubation. The nurse would not attempt to visualize the epiglottis; therefore, no equipment would be obtained and another nurse would not be approached.
CN: Physiological integrity; CNS: Basic care and comfort; CL: Apply

46. The mother of a 2-year-old child with epiglottitis states she has to leave to pick up another child from school. The 2-year-old child begins to cry, and the nurse notes increased stridor. Which intervention by the nurse is **best**?
1. Ask the mother how long she may be gone.
2. Tell the child everything will be all right.
3. Stay in the room and give the child a stuffed animal.
4. Tell the mother someone else needs to pick up the older child.

47. A client is being treated for gastrointestinal bleeding. On the fifth day of hospitalization, the client begins to have tremors, is agitated, and is experiencing hallucinations. Which condition does the nurse suspect the client is experiencing?
1. Alcohol withdrawal
2. Allergic response
3. Alzheimer's disease
4. Hypoxia

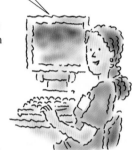

Woot woot! You've finished 48 questions already. Well done.

48. A client experiencing alcohol withdrawal reports itching everywhere from the bugs on the bed. Which action by the nurse is **most** appropriate?
1. Examine the client's skin.
2. Ask what kind of bugs are in the bed.
3. Tell the client there are no bugs on the bed.
4. Tell the client it is from tactile hallucinations.

49. A client experiencing alcohol withdrawal tells the nurse, "I see cockroaches on the ceiling." Which response by the nurse is **most** appropriate?
1. Ask the client to point to the cockroaches.
2. Ask the client if the cockroaches are still there.
3. Tell the client there are no cockroaches on the ceiling.
4. Tell the client it is dim in the room and turn on the overhead lights.

50. The nurse suspects a client is experiencing alcohol withdrawal. Which nursing action is **most** appropriate?
1. Verify with the family if the client has an alcohol use disorder.
2. Inform case management of the client's status.
3. Ask the client about alcohol consumption.
4. Tell the client everything will be all right.

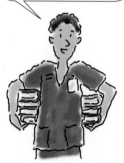

Check out that word "later" in question 51. It's important.

51. The nurse expects which finding in a client with later-stage cirrhosis?
1. Constipation
2. Diarrhea
3. Hypoxia
4. Vomiting

46. 4. Increased anxiety and agitation should be avoided in the child with epiglottitis to prevent airway obstruction. A 2-year-old child fears separation from parents, so the mother will need to stay. Other means of picking up the older child need to be found. Asking the mother how long she will be gone is not therapeutic because she should not leave. A 2-year-old cannot understand that all will be okay. Giving the child a stuffed animal and staying in the room will not comfort the child as much as the mother being there.
CN: Health promotion and maintenance; CNS: None; CL: Analyze

47. 1. Tremors, agitation, and hallucinations are signs of alcohol withdrawal, which can occur within 12 hours after the last drink or even 7 to 10 days later depending on the severity of alcohol use. An allergic reaction would cause labored breathing, skin rash, or edema as primary symptoms. Alzheimer's disease occurs in older individuals and has other psychosocial signs, such as a masklike face and altered mentation. Hypoxia would cause symptoms of respiratory distress.
CN: Psychosocial integrity; CNS: None; CL: Analyze

48. 1. The nurse first makes sure the client does not have a rash, skin allergy, or something on the skin (such as food crumbs) causing discomfort. Reality should then be presented to the client gently without being derogatory. The nurse should not support the client's hallucinations.
CN: Psychosocial integrity; CNS: None; CL: Apply

49. 4. The nursing goal for a client with alcohol withdrawal is to try to reorient the client to reality and minimize distortions. The nurse should not support the client's hallucinations or place the client on the defensive. The nurse should try to present reality gently without agitating the client.
CN: Psychosocial integrity; CNS: None; CL: Apply

50. 3. Confirming suspicions with the client is the most beneficial way to help in diagnosis and treatment of alcohol withdrawal. If the client is not cooperative, verification can be sought with the family. Case management is not required at this time but may be helpful in discharge planning. Giving false reassurance is not therapeutic for the client.
CN: Psychosocial integrity; CNS: None; CL: Apply

51. 3. In the later stage of cirrhosis, fluid in the lungs and weak chest expansion can lead to hypoxia. Constipation, diarrhea, and vomiting are early signs and symptoms of cirrhosis.
CN: Physiological integrity; CNS: Physiological adaptation; CL: Apply

CN: Client needs category   CNS: Client needs subcategory   CL: Cognitive level

52. A client with alcohol withdrawal will not stop pulling at the central venous catheter, saying, "I am swatting the spiders crawling over me." Which nursing intervention is **most** appropriate?
1. Encourage the client to rest.
2. Restrain the client's arms.
3. Tell the client there are no spiders.
4. Tell the client it is IV tubing, not spiders.

53. A client who experienced alcohol withdrawal is no longer having hallucinations nor tremors and states, "I would like to enter a rehabilitation facility to stop drinking." Which nursing intervention is **most** appropriate?
1. Determine if the client's employer will allow time off.
2. Have the client discuss this with family members.
3. Refer the client to Alcoholics Anonymous (AA).
4. Promote participation in a treatment program.

54. A client with cirrhosis is admitted to the hospital in a hepatic coma. Which assessment is the nurse's **priority**?
1. Perform a neurologic check.
2. Complete the client admission.
3. Turn the client every 2 hours.
4. Assess the client's respirations.

55. A client with cirrhosis is restless and continues to try to climb out of bed. The client fell earlier while trying to get out of the bed. Which nursing intervention is **priority**?
1. Move the client closer to the nurses' station.
2. Check on the client every hour.
3. Apply a vest restraint device.
4. Ensure no objects are on the client's floor.

56. A client with cirrhosis is jaundiced, edematous, and experiencing severe itching with dryness. Which nursing intervention is **most** appropriate for this client?
1. Put mittens on the hands.
2. Apply moisturizer to the skin daily.
3. Lubricate the skin with baby oil.
4. Wash the skin with soap and water.

52. 2. During periods of alcohol withdrawal, the nurse must take necessary measures to protect the client from self-harm, including preventing the dislodgment of the central venous catheter, which can cause a life-threatening embolus. Although encouraging the client to rest and presenting reality are important, the client may not heed the nurse's attempts to offer calm and reassurance in this situation. Client safety is the priority.
CN: Psychosocial integrity; CNS: None; CL: Analyze

53. 4. The client should be encouraged to enter a facility if it is in the client's best interest. Arrangements can be made and discussed with case management and the health care provider. The client can inform the family and employer, and support should be encouraged. Referral to AA should be considered after rehabilitation takes place.
CN: Psychosocial integrity; CNS: None; CL: Apply

54. 4. Priorities for the client in a coma include checking the airway, breathing, and circulation. After these are assessed, a neurologic check is needed to determine status. Completing the admission may require the help of family members. Turning the client is needed, but assessing the airway and breathing are priority.
CN: Physiological integrity; CNS: Reduction of risk potential; CL: Apply

55. 3. The client with cirrhosis may require gentle reminders not to get out of bed to prevent a fall. The vest restraint would help in this endeavor and ensure client safety. Moving the client and hourly rounding are appropriate interventions; however, the client has already fallen and continues to attempt to get out of bed. Clearing the client's floor is appropriate to prevent falls while the client is ambulatory, not while attempting to get out of bed.
CN: Safe, effective care environment; CNS: Management of care; CL: Apply

56. 2. Moisturizers applied to the skin are the best way to relieve dryness and are absorbed without oiliness. Mittens may help keep the client from scratching the skin open. Baby oil does not allow excretions through the skin and may block pores. Soap dries out the skin.
CN: Physiological integrity; CNS: Basic care and comfort; CL: Apply

CN: Client needs category   CNS: Client needs subcategory   CL: Cognitive level

57. A client with a spinal cord injury sustained in a previous motorcycle accident is hospitalized for renal calculi. The nurse will provider which education to the client regarding prevention of future renal calculi?
1. Eat yogurt daily.
2. Drink cranberry juice.
3. Eat more fresh fruits and vegetables.
4. Increase the intake of dairy products.

57. 2. Acidic urine decreases the potential for renal calculi. Most renal calculi form in alkaline urine. Cranberries, prunes, and plums promote acidic urine. Yogurt helps restore pH balance to secretions which can help with yeast infections. Fruits and vegetables increase fiber in the diet and promote alkaline urine. Dairy products may contribute to the formation of renal calculi.
CN: Physiological integrity; CNS: Reduction of risk potential; CL: Apply

58. A client with a spinal cord injury states difficulty recognizing the symptoms of a urinary tract infection (UTI). The nurse will educate the client to monitor for which early symptom(s) of a UTI? Select all that apply.
1. Lower back pain
2. Burning on urination
3. Urinary frequency
4. Elevated temperature
5. Change in the clarity of urine

58. 4, 5. The client with a spinal cord injury should recognize fever and change in the clarity of urine as early signs of UTI. Lower back pain is a late sign. The client with a spinal cord injury may not experience burning or frequency of urination.
CN: Physiological integrity; CNS: Reduction of risk potential; CL: Apply

59. A client tells the nurse, "I boil urinary catheters to keep them sterile." Which question asked by the nurse is **most** appropriate?
1. "What technique do you use for sterilization?"
2. "What temperature are the catheters boiled at?"
3. "Why don't you use prepackaged sterile catheters?"
4. "Are the catheters dried and stored in a clean, dry place?"

59. 1. The client should describe the procedure to make sure sterile technique is used. Water boils at 212°F (100°C), but the nurse should make sure the client is boiling the catheters for an appropriate amount of time. Catheters should be boiled just before use and allowed to cool before using. Prepackaged sterile catheters are not necessary if the proper sterilization techniques are used.
CN: Physiological integrity; CNS: Reduction of risk potential; CL: Apply

60. The nurse approaches a client who recently had a colostomy and finds the client crying. Which nursing action is **most** appropriate?
1. Leave and come back another time.
2. Ask the client if there is pain or discomfort.
3. Tell the client vital signs need to be obtained.
4. Sit down with the client and offer to talk.

60. 4. Asking open-ended questions and appearing interested in what the client has to say will encourage verbalization of feelings. Leaving the client may cause feelings of unacceptance. Asking closed-ended questions will not encourage verbalization of feelings. Ignoring the client's present state is not therapeutic for the client.
CN: Psychosocial integrity; CNS: None; CL: Apply

61. After a review of colostomy care, a client states, "I do not know if I can care for myself at home without help." Which nursing intervention is **most** appropriate?
1. Review care with the client again.
2. Provide written instructions for the client.
3. Ask the client if there is anyone who can help.
4. Arrange for home health care to visit the client.

61. 4. Although all of these interventions may benefit the client, home health care should be contacted to ensure continuity of appropriate care after discharge from the hospital.
CN: Safe, effective care environment; CNS: Management of care; CL: Apply

62. A client with a colostomy is experiencing mild diarrhea. Which instruction provided by the nurse is appropriate?
1. Eat prunes.
2. Drink apple juice.
3. Increase lettuce intake.
4. Increase intake of bananas.

62. 4. Bananas help make formed stool without irritating the bowel. Apple juice and prunes can increase the frequency of diarrhea. Lettuce acts as a fiber and can increase the looseness of stool.
CN: Physiological integrity; CNS: Basic care and comfort; CL: Apply

CN: Client needs category   CNS: Client needs subcategory   CL: Cognitive level

63. A postpartum client recovering from spinal anesthesia with morphine reports her nose itches. What will the nurse do **next**?
1. Assess the client's oxygen saturation level.
2. Document the client's statement.
3. Notify the primary health care provider.
4. Inform the client this is a normal response.

63. 4. Morphine causes a relatively high incidence of itching when used in spinal anesthesia. The itching usually begins at the tip of the nose, possibly becoming more generalized. Antipruritics, such as diphenhydramine or hydroxyzine hydrochloride, may be prescribed after the use of morphine. The other actions are not necessary.
CN: Physiological integrity; CNS: Pharmacological and parenteral therapies; CL: Analyze

64. A client reports a lot of gas in the colostomy bag. Which instruction is **best** for the nurse to provide this client?
1. Burp the bag.
2. Eat fewer beans.
3. Replace the bag.
4. Put a tiny hole in the top of the bag.

64. 1. Letting air out of the bag by opening it and burping it is the best solution. The client can be encouraged to note which foods are causing gas and to eat fewer gas-forming foods. Replacing the bag is costly. Putting a hole in the bag will cause fluids to leak out.
CN: Physiological integrity; CNS: Basic care and comfort; CL: Apply

65. A client recently diagnosed with prediabetes asks the nurse about risk factors for developing diabetes. The nurse will include which risk factors when responding to the client? Select all that apply.
1. Weight
2. Fat distribution
3. Family history
4. Ethnicity
5. Increased age
6. Sedentary lifestyle
7. Respiratory disease

65. 1, 2, 3, 4, 5, 6. Obesity, fat stored in the abdomen, inactivity, family history, ethnicity (African, Hispanic, Asian American, American Indian), increased age, having pre- or gestational diabetes, and polycystic ovarian syndrome are all risk factors for developing type 2 diabetes.
CN: Health promotion and maintenance; CNS: None; CL: Apply

66. Following gastric bypass surgery, a client is on nothing-by-mouth (NPO) status and reporting pain. The nurse administers morphine 4 mg intravenously. In 20 minutes, the client reports feeling nauseous. What will the nurse suspect as the **most** likely cause?
1. The surgery is causing the client's feelings of nausea.
2. Being NPO, the increase in gastric secretions is precipitating this symptom.
3. Morphine tends to cause feelings of nausea.
4. It is a reaction to blood remaining in the mouth after extubation.

66. 3. Although gastric bypass surgery may precipitate some feelings of nausea, the timing of this symptom after the administration of morphine is suspicious. Most likely, this client is experiencing nausea as a very common adverse effect of the analgesic morphine. The status of being NPO would not cause an increase in gastric secretions. It is possible that there may be some blood in the client's mouth after extubation, but the chances of this happening are minimal and less likely to be the cause of the client's nausea.
CN: Physiological integrity; CNS: Pharmacological and parenteral therapies; CL: Apply

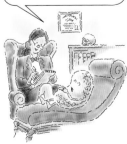

I feel like I always overthink things. Do you think I overthink things?

67. A client on a psychiatric unit asks the nurse about the medications another client takes. Which response by the nurse is **best**?
1. "Did you ask the client if I could share this information with you?"
2. "I cannot give you that information. I must protect all clients' privacy."
3. "Let me ask if it is okay for me to tell you about his condition and medications."
4. "The client is taking insulin for diabetes and digoxin for a heart condition."

67. 2. Revealing one client's medication to another client violates procedures of client confidentiality and directly violates the Health Insurance Portability and Accountability Act. Seeking the client's permission to release confidential information is an inappropriate action. Asking the client if he or she asked for permission is not appropriate. Assuring the client that the facility has an obligation to protect not all clients' confidentiality will provide the client with a sense of comfort.
CN: Safe, care environment; CNS: Management of care; CL: Apply

68. A health care provider prescribes a client amoxicillin 500 mg capsules × 2 PO now, followed by 500 mg PO every 6 hours. How many milligrams will the nurse administer the client for the initial dose? Record your answer as a whole number.

_____ mg

69. An older adult client fractured a hip after a fall in the home and surgical correction is not an option due to comorbid factors. The client tells the nurse, "How will I ever get better?" Which response by the nurse is **best**?
 1. "Do not stress; you are doing fine."
 2. "What is your biggest concern right now?"
 3. "Just give it some time and you will be okay."
 4. "You do not believe you are doing well?"

70. A client with a family history of diabetes asks the nurse which measures can be practiced to decrease the chance of developing the disease. Which response(s) by the nurse is **best**? Select all that apply.
 1. "Eat only poultry and fish."
 2. "Maintain optimal weight."
 3. "Omit carbohydrates from your diet."
 4. "Start a moderate exercise program."
 5. "Check blood glucose levels every month."

71. During a routine check, a client tells the nurse, "I slipped on a throw rug while going to the bathroom last night." Which nursing action is **priority**?
 1. Determine home safety.
 2. Prepare the client for x-rays.
 3. Assess the client's head.
 4. Obtain a urine specimen.

72. A client at 30 weeks' gestation is having contractions 5 minutes apart that began suddenly. The client is admitted directly to the obstetrics department. Which nursing intervention is **priority**?
 1. Call the health care provider.
 2. Have the client rate pain.
 3. Check fetal heart tones.
 4. Administer oxytocin.

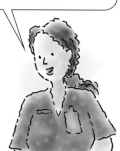

Keep your priorities in order when answering question #71. Which intervention will come first?

68. 1,000.
 The prescription states the nurse is giving two 500 mg capsules now, followed by 500 mg (0.5 g) every 6 hours. Therefore, the correct answer is 1,000 mg.
 CN: Physiological integrity; CNS: Pharmacological and parenteral therapies; CL: Apply

69. 2. Open-ended questions allow the client to control what is discussed and help the nurse determine care needs. Telling the client "you are fine" or "you just need more time" does not encourage verbalizing concern. A reiteration of the client's concerns may not be helpful in encouraging the client to verbalize feelings.
 CN: Health promotion and maintenance; CNS: None; CL: Apply

70. 2, 4. Exercise and weight control are the goals in preventing and treating diabetes. Red meat can be eaten along with poultry and fish but should be limited because it contributes to cardiovascular disease. Complex carbohydrates, especially whole grains, are necessary for a healthy diet. Fiber intake of 14 g/1,000 kcal is recommended. Checking blood glucose levels will help monitor the development of diabetes but will not prevent or decrease the chance of it occurring.
 CN: Physiological integrity; CNS: Reduction of risk potential; CL: Apply

71. 1. A safety assessment of the home can determine if changes need to be made to ensure the client does not fall again. The nurse might or might not determine if the client has experienced a head injury or confusion by asking how the injury occurred. Going to the bathroom at night is not necessarily a sign of a urinary tract infection, so a specimen may not be required.
 CN: Safe, effective care environment; CNS: Safety and infection control; CL: Apply

72. 3. The nurse should check fetal heart tones and assess the client's vital signs. The client should be placed on a monitor to check contractions and for continuous fetal monitoring. The health care provider should be notified as soon as possible. Pain is subjective and does not provide insight into labor progression. Oxytocin is given to augment labor, which is not indicated at this time.
 CN: Health promotion and maintenance; CNS: None; CL: Analyze

---

73. The nurse is caring for four clients. Which client's vital signs will the nurse report to the primary health care provider **first**?
1. A male client scheduled for elective surgery, blood pressure 120/72 mm Hg
2. A postoperative client with a pulse of 110 beats/minute on awakening at 0730
3. A female client scheduled for elective surgery with a blood pressure of 110/68 mm Hg
4. A client with a pulse of 120 beats/minute after 30 minutes of aerobic exercise

73. 2. The normal range for a pulse is 60 to 100 beats/minute and, in the morning, the rate is at its lowest. Blood pressures of 120/72 mm Hg for a healthy man and 110/68 mm Hg for a healthy woman are normal. Aerobic exercise increases the heart rate over the normal range of 60 to 100 beats/minute.
CN: Physiological integrity; CNS: Physiological adaptation; CL: Analyze

74. The nurse is assessing a 40-year-old client preparing to undergo elective facial surgery and notes a pulse rate of 130 beats/minute with a regular rhythm. What will the nurse do **next**?
1. Notify the health care provider.
2. Determine if the client is anxious.
3. Administer metoprolol.
4. Recheck the pulse in 30 minutes.

74. 2. The nurse will determine if the client is anxious because anxiety tends to increase heart rate, temperature, and respirations. The normal heart rate for a client this age is 60 to 100 beats/minute. More information is needed before determining if the health care provider needs notification or if medication is warranted. The nurse will continue to monitor the pulse rate.
CN: Physiological integrity; CNS: Physiological adaptation; CL: Apply

75. The nurse is assessing a client's arterial pulses. Which graphic displays the appropriate site for the nurse to use when palpating the dorsalis pedis pulse?

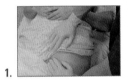

1.

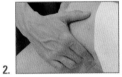

2.

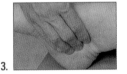

3.

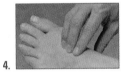

4.

You did it! Congratulations!

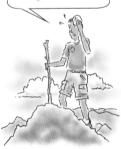

75. 4. To palpate the dorsalis pedis pulse, the nurse places the fingers on the medial dorsum of the foot while the client points the toes down. The first graphic shows palpation of the femoral pulse, located along the crease midway between the pubic bone and the anterior iliac crest. The second graphic shows palpation of the popliteal pulse in the popliteal fossa of the back of the knee. The third graphic shows palpation of the posterior tibial pulse, slightly below the malleolus of the ankle.
CN: Health promotion and maintenance; CNS: None; CL: Apply

Comprehensive Test 2

This second comprehensive test is just like the longest NCLEX-RN test: 265 questions. It's a great way to practice your endurance!

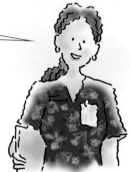

1. The nurse manager asks a nurse if the facility's rules of ethical conduct are understood. Which statement by the nurse indicates the need for further education?
1. "I make sure I do everything in my client's best interests."
2. "I do my best to maintain client confidentiality."
3. "I make sure clients know what to expect while in the hospital."
4. "I always serve as an advocate for clients in my care."

2. The nurse receives a medication prescription from the primary health care provider over the telephone. Which nursing intervention is **priority** when receiving a telephone prescription?
1. Inform the health care provider that medication prescriptions cannot be taken over the telephone.
2. Verify the prescription by repeating it back to the health care provider while on the phone.
3. Request a second health care provider repeat the prescription to the nurse over the telephone.
4. Inform the health care provider that the medication prescription must be signed in person within 1 hour.

3. The registered nurse (RN) and assistive personnel (AP) are caring for a group of clients. Which task will the RN appropriately delegate to the AP?
1. Apply a topical cream to the burns on a client's left leg.
2. Perform wet-to-dry dressing change for a postoperative client.
3. Turn a client every 2 hours who had a cerebrovascular accident.
4. Monitor a pressure injury on a client with muscular dystrophy.

1. 2. Nurses need to always act in the best interest of their clients, maintain confidentiality, serve as a client advocate, and ensure the clients know what to expect. It is not appropriate for the nurse to state, "I do my best" regarding maintaining client confidentiality. There are no reasons for a nurse to not maintain client confidentiality at all times.
CN: Safe, effective care environment; CNS: Management of care; CL: Apply

2. 2. When taking a medication prescription over the telephone, standard practice requires verbal verification of the prescription. Medication prescriptions taken over the phone are not prohibited. Having a second health care provider repeat the prescription opens another avenue for misinterpretation and error. Insisting the health care provider sign the prescription within 1 hour is unrealistic.
CN: Safe, effective care environment; CNS: Management of care; CL: Apply

3. 3. The RN can safely delegate the task of turning the client every 2 hours to the AP. The nurse must administer all medications; it is not within the scope of practice for AP to administer medication. The nurse must also perform dressing changes and document wound healing.
CN: Safe, effective care environment; CNS: Management of care; CL: Analyze

4. A client is provided two treatment options by the health care provider. During morning care, the client asks the nurse, "What is your opinion about which treatment I should do?" Which response by the nurse is **most** appropriate?

1. "If it were me, I would choose the least painful option."
2. "Which decision are you leaning towards at this time?"
3. "Why are you asking me? I have no idea what is best for you."
4. "Let us talk about the pros and cons of each choice."

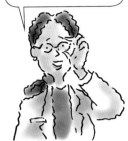

Sometimes the best intervention is to talk to your client.

4. **4.** Even though the client is asking, the nurse should not impose a personal opinion on the client. Instead, the nurse should discuss the options with the client and answer any questions; this will help the client make an informed decision. Asking which option the client is considering does not provide additional information or address the client's concern. Offering opinions about the least painful option imposes the nurse's opinion on the client. Brushing off the client's question with an angry retort is confrontational and offers the client no viable solution.
CN: Safe, effective care environment; CNS: Management of care; CL: Apply

5. A client with type 1 diabetes tells the nurse in the clinic, "I sometimes skip my insulin dose in the morning, so I will not gain back any of the weight I have lost." Which response by the nurse is **most** appropriate?

1. "Oh, I did not realize that holding off on insulin would keep the weight off."
2. "You are worried about your weight? There are safer ways to prevent weight gain."
3. "I just love when clients are able to find the good in a bad situation."
4. "You have lost a lot of weight. I am proud of you for wanting to be healthier overall."

5. **2.** The nurse needs to ask the client more questions about weight and begin instructing the client in healthy ways to avoid gaining weight. Making references that connect withheld insulin to weight loss encourage the client not to take the prescribed medication, which would be dangerous to the client's health. Stating "finding the good in a bad situation" does not address the issue.
CN: Safe, effective care environment; CNS: Management of care; CL: Apply

6. The nurse is caring for a client with a hemoglobin of 5.5 g/dL (55 g/L). The health care provider prescribes: Transfuse 2 units of packed bed blood cells stat. Upon entering the room with blood products in hand, the client tells the nurse, "I am a practicing Jehovah's Witness." What will the nurse do **next**?

1. Discuss the benefits of the transfusion.
2. Notify the health care provider.
3. Transfuse the blood product.
4. Obtain the client's vital signs.

6. **2.** The nurse would notify the health care provider to determine a new treatment plan. The administration of blood and blood products is forbidden for Jehovah's Witnesses. A person who receives blood products can be excommunicated. The nurse would not discuss benefits or proceed with the transfusion. Because the blood will not be administered, there is not a reason to obtain the client's vital signs.
CN: Safe, effective care environment; CNS: Management of care; CL: Analyze

7. The primary health care provider prescribes 60 mEq of potassium chloride liquid as a one-time dose. The pharmacy supplies a liquid containing 20 mEq/15 mL. How many milliliters will the nurse administer to the client? Record your answer using a whole number.

_____ mL

7. **45.**
The nurse can calculate the dose by setting up the following equation:

$$\frac{60\ mEq}{20\ mEq} = \frac{X\ mL}{15\ mL}$$

Then cross-multiply the fractions:

$$X \times 20\ mEq = 15\ mL \times 60\ mEq$$

Then solve for X:

$$X = 45\ mL$$

CN: Physiological integrity; CNS: Pharmacological and parenteral therapies; CL: Apply

CN: Client needs category   CNS: Client needs subcategory   CL: Cognitive level

8. The nurse enters a client's room at 0800 to administer a medication scheduled to be administered at 0730. The nurse notes the client is in the bathroom. Which nursing action is **most** appropriate?
1. Leave the medication on the bedside table for the client to take when done.
2. Enter the bathroom and administer the medication.
3. Return in 10 minutes and remain until the client takes the medication.
4. Ask the client to leave the bathroom to take the medication.

8. **3.** The nurse should return shortly to the client's room and remain there until the client takes the medication to verify that it was taken as directed. The nurse should never leave medication at a client's bedside. The nurse should provide privacy while the client is in the bathroom.
CN: Safe, effective care environment; CNS: Safety and infection control; CL: Apply

9. The nurse is caring for an infant with suspected transposition of the great arteries (TGA). The nurse will prepare the infant and family for which diagnostic test **first**?
1. Blood cultures
2. Cardiac catheterization
3. Chest x-ray
4. Echocardiogram

9. **3.** Chest x-ray would be done first to visualize congenital heart diseases such as TGA. Blood cultures will not diagnose TGA. Cardiac catheterization and an echocardiogram would be done after TGA is seen on the chest x-ray.
CN: Health promotion and maintenance; CNS: None; CL: Apply

10. The nurse is planning to administer the diphtheria, tetanus, pertussis (DTaP) vaccine to four infants. After assessing each infant, the nurse will administer the vaccine to which infant?
1. The child with a temperature of 103°F (39.4°C) and heart rate 140 beats/minute
2. The child diagnosed with a viral cold who has a runny nose and cough
3. The child taking prednisone for the treatment of acute lymphocytic leukemia
4. The child who experienced dyspnea after receiving the pervious DTaP vaccine

10. **2.** Children with cold symptoms can safely receive DTaP immunization. Children with a temperature more than 102°F (38.9°C), serious reactions to previous immunizations, or those receiving immunosuppressive therapy should not receive DTaP immunization.
CN: Health promotion and maintenance; CNS: None; CL: Analyze

11. The nurse is providing discharge instructions to the parents of a child who had a tonsillectomy. Which statement by the nurse is appropriate?
1. "Your child should drink extra milk."
2. "Your child should not drink from straws."
3. "Your child may resume a regular diet."
4. "Rinse the mouth with salt water daily."

When working with a pediatric client, remember the needs of the whole family.

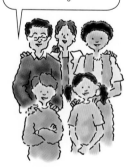

11. **2.** Straws and other sharp objects inserted into the mouth could disrupt the clot at the operative site. Extra milk would not promote healing and may encourage mucus production. For the first week after surgery, the child should eat soft foods. Rinsing with salt water will irritate the tissue at the operative site.
CN: Physiological integrity; CNS: Basic care and comfort; CL: Apply

12. A child with asthma uses a peak expiratory flow meter in school. The results indicate the peak flow is in the yellow zone. Which intervention by the school nurse is appropriate?
1. Follow the child's routine asthma treatment plan.
2. Monitor for signs and symptoms of an acute attack.
3. Activate the emergency medical response system.
4. Inform the child's parents to seek medical evaluation.

12. **2.** The routine treatment plan may be insufficient when the peak flow is in the yellow zone (50% to 80% of personal best). The child should be monitored to determine if an asthma attack is imminent, and the treatment plan should be reviewed to see if revisions are needed. There is no immediate need to see the health care provider if the child is asymptomatic. This is not an emergency situation.
CN: Physiological integrity; CNS: Reduction of risk potential; CL: Apply

CN: Client needs category   CNS: Client needs subcategory   CL: Cognitive level

13. The nurse is admitting a 2-year-old child diagnosed with respiratory syncytial virus (RSV) who is experiencing respiratory distress. The client's 8-year-old sibling is present. Which nursing action is **most** appropriate?
1. Administer palivizumab to the client.
2. Recommend the sibling be prescribed antibiotics.
3. Encourage the parents to take the sibling home.
4. Place the client on contact precautions.

14. A child comes to the school nurse reporting difficulty breathing. The nurse notes bilateral wheezing, prolonged expiration, dyspnea, and positioning. The child has a history of asthma. Which nursing action is **priority**?
1. Notify the child's parents of the findings.
2. Ask the morning results of the peak expiratory flow meter.
3. Administer the child a dose from the albuterol inhaler.
4. Tell the teacher the child cannot go play outside with the class.

15. A child is admitted to the pediatric unit newly diagnosed with type 1 diabetes. Which nursing action is **most** appropriate?
1. Assume the parents understand the treatment needed for diabetes.
2. Offer the parents opportunities to be involved in the child's care.
3. Give the parents time to adjust to the diagnosis before discussing care needed.
4. Inform the parents they will be shown how to care for the child prior to discharge.

16. The nurse is teaching child safety to the parents of a 6-month-old infant who is beginning to crawl. Which information will the nurse include in the education?
1. Keep furniture with sharp corners out of the area where the infant crawls.
2. Pad the infant's knees while crawling on wood and tile flooring.
3. Only allow the infant to crawl around on a blanket placed in the floor.
4. Place the infant in a baby walker to promote early walking.

17. The nurse is caring for a child with a fractured leg. The parents become concerned when their child begins sucking his thumb, a behavior previously given up. Which response by the nurse is **most** appropriate?
1. "Your child is likely feeling depressed."
2. "This indicates your child is in pain."
3. "Your child is seeking attention."
4. "Your child is responding to stress."

13. 4. The nurse would first place the child with RSV on contact precaution. The nurse would also encourage the parents take the sibling home (after initiating precautions) to limit the likelihood of transmission. Palivizumab, a monoclonal antibody, may be given to high-risk infants to prevent RSV.
CN: Safe, effective care environment; CNS: Safety and infection control; CL: Apply

14. 3. It is priority for the nurse to administer albuterol, a bronchodilator, to the child to maintain the airway. The nurse would perform the other options; however, they are not priority over airway.
CN: Safe, effective care environment; CNS: Safety and infection control; CL: Analyze

15. 4. The nurse would provide opportunities to involve the parents in the child's care. This will help the family be better prepared for home care and allow the nurse the opportunity to observe and provide additional teaching as needed. The nurse should never assume that the parents understand a disease. The parents may need time to adjust; however, this approach will limit the ability for the nurse to facilitate learning. The parents should be involved as soon as possible, not just at discharge.
CN: Safe, effective care environment; CNS: Management of care; CL: Apply

16. 1. Keeping furniture with sharp corners away from the infant who is beginning to crawl prevents injury. Padding the knees is not necessary. An infant will not remain on a blanket when crawling. Baby walkers are dangerous, have been associated with delayed ambulation, and use should not be encouraged.
CN: Safe, effective care environment; CNS: Safety and infection control; CL: Apply

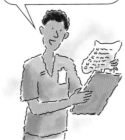

Dealing with mean clients makes me want to suck my thumb.

17. 4. Regression, or reverting back to a previously outgrown behavior, is a common response to stressful situations. The nurse should reassure the parents that thumb-sucking and other regressive behaviors should disappear after the stressful situation is resolved. Thumb-sucking is not a sign of depression or pain, or an attention-seeking behavior.
CN: Psychosocial integrity; CNS: None; CL: Apply

CN: Client needs category   CNS: Client needs subcategory   CL: Cognitive level

18. The nurse is providing education to a parent about how to administer antibiotics at home to a toddler with acute otitis media. Which statement by the parent indicates the nurse's teaching was successful?
  1. "I will give the antibiotics for the full 10-day course of treatment."
  2. "I will give the antibiotics until my child's ear pain is gone."
  3. "Whenever my child is cranky or pulls on an ear, I will give a dose of antibiotics."
  4. "I will pull my child's ear back and down when giving the antibiotic."

19. The nurse is providing education about injury prevention to the parents of a toddler. Which instruction is appropriate for the nurse to include?
  1. The toddler should wear a helmet when learning to walk.
  2. Place locks on all cabinets containing household cleaners.
  3. Allow the toddler to eat whole grapes with in a high chair.
  4. Do not allow the toddler to use pillows when sleeping.

20. The parents of a 15-month-old are concerned because their child says "no" to everything. Which response by the nurse is appropriate?
  1. "Saying 'no' is a normal part of toddler development."
  2. "Place your child in time-out when he tells you 'no.'"
  3. "Ignore the behavior and the child will grow out of it."
  4. "Explain to your child that saying 'no' all the time is bad."

21. A parent expresses concern over the toddler's eating habits, stating the toddler eats very little and consumes only a single type of food for weeks on end. Which response by the nurse is **most** helpful?
  1. "There is no need to be concerned. This is normal toddler behavior."
  2. "This behavior increases your child's likelihood of developing an eating disorder."
  3. "The health care provider will assess your child for a nutrient deficiency."
  4. "This feeding pattern is a form of control and indicates a behavioral pattern."

18. 1. Antibiotics must be given for the full course of therapy, even if the child feels well; otherwise, the infection will not be eradicated. Antibiotics should be taken at prescribed intervals to maintain blood levels and not as needed for pain. Antibiotics are given orally, not by the otic route. Otic solutions may also be administered if the client's tympanic membrane in not intact.
CN: Physiological integrity; CNS: Pharmacological and parenteral therapies; CL: Apply

19. 2. All household cleaners and poisons should be secured with childproof locks. The toddler's curiosity and the ability to climb and open doors and drawers makes poisoning a concern in this age-group. It is not appropriate for the toddler to wear a helmet while learning to walk. Instead, caregivers should omit dangerous objects from the environment, such as furniture with sharp corners. Pillows should not be placed in the crib of an infant to avoid suffocation; however, toddlers may use them.
CN: Safe, effective care environment; CNS: Safety and infection control; CL: Apply

20. 1. Saying "no" is normal at this age. The child is attempting to exert independence. Punishing the child with time-out is not appropriate because this is a normal stage of development. Ignoring the behavior is also inappropriate because the child needs to learn about limits. Children at this age will not fully understand rationales for this action being inappropriate.
CN: Health promotion and maintenance; CNS: None; CL: Apply

21. 1. Erratic eating is typical of toddlers. The physiologic need for food decreases at about age 18 months as growth declines from the rapid rate characteristic of infancy. The toddler also develops strong food and taste preferences, sometimes eating just one type of food for days or weeks and then switching to another. The child should not be forced to eat. Typically, the child switches to another food spontaneously after a while, correcting any nutritional imbalances. Parents may encourage the child to eat other foods by offering items from the various food groups at each meal. Erratic eating habits in toddlers are not characteristic of an eating disorder, a nutrient deficiency, or a behavioral problem.
CN: Health promotion and maintenance; CNS: None; CL: Apply

22. The nurse is teaching a group of parents about normal toddler development. Which information will the nurse include when discussing normal toddler play?
  1. Toddlers play with similar toys beside others rather than with them.
  2. Toddlers become interactive with children around them.
  3. Toddlers willingly share toys with other children.
  4. Toddlers prefer to play with one toy for a long period.

23. Parents bring their 13-month-old toddler to the clinic. The nurse notes erythema and small, oozing vesicles on toddler's buttock. Which instruction will the nurse give the parents?
  1. Change diapers frequently and expose the buttock to air when possible.
  2. Apply permethrin cream, leave it on for 8 hours, and then bathe the child.
  3. Wash the child's bed linens, clothing, and any stuffed animals with hot water.
  4. Use cloth diapers and rubber pants in place of disposable diapers until the rash heals.

24. When teaching the parents of a toddler with tetralogy of Fallot, the nurse will include which statement(s)? Select all that apply.
  1. "Reduce your child's caloric intake to decrease cardiac demand."
  2. "Relax discipline and limit-setting to limit your child's crying."
  3. "Make sure your child avoids contact with other small children."
  4. "Try to maintain a normal lifestyle to promote normal development."
  5. "Provide your child frequent rest periods when playing."

25. Which nursing intervention(s) is appropriate when caring for a neonate diagnosed with neonatal abstinence syndrome? Select all that apply.
  1. Monitor feeding patterns.
  2. Dim the lights in the room.
  3. Promote breastfeeding.
  4. Give phenobarbital.
  5. Swaddle in a blanket.

26. The nurse is caring for a client with a full-thickness burn. Before sending the client to hydrotherapy for a scheduled wound debridement, which nursing action is **priority**?
  1. Administer a 500 mL fluid bolus.
  2. Administer morphine sulfate.
  3. Initiate antibiotics as prescribed.
  4. Provide a high-protein drink.

22. 1. During the toddler stage, children typically engage in parallel play with others. They play side by side, usually with similar objects, without actually interacting. Preschool-age children become interactive with other children, and they have a better concept of sharing than toddlers do. Preschoolers may also play with toys for longer periods because they have longer attention spans than toddlers.
CN: Psychosocial integrity; CNS: None; CL: Apply

23. 1. The child shows signs of diaper dermatitis. Therefore, the nurse should instruct the parent to change the child's diapers frequently, expose to air when possible, and avoid rubber pants. Permethrin cream and washing all bed linens and clothing with hot water are indicated for the treatment of scabies, not diaper dermatitis.
CN: Physiological integrity; CNS: Reduction of risk potential; CL: Apply

24. 4, 5. Parents of a child with a congenital heart defect should treat the child normally and allow rest periods as needed. Reducing the child's caloric intake would not necessarily reduce cardiac demand. Altering disciplinary patterns and deliberately preventing crying or interactions with other children could foster maladaptive behaviors. Contact with peers promotes normal growth and development.
CN: Health promotion and maintenance; CNS: None; CL: Apply

25. 1, 2, 4, 5. The nurse would assess nutrition, decrease stimuli, administer medications, and swaddle the neonate. The neonate should be formula fed to prevent additional drug exposure.
CN: Psychosocial integrity; CNS: None; CL: Apply

26. 2. Because hydrotherapy is painful, the nurse should implement pain control measures before the treatment begins. Fluids and nutritional supplements can be given at any time and are not required specifically before hydrotherapy. Antibiotics should be administered according to a specified schedule without regard to treatment measures.
CN: Physiological integrity; CNS: Pharmacological and parenteral therapies; CL: Apply

CN: Client needs category   CNS: Client needs subcategory   CL: Cognitive level

27. A child is prescribed phenytoin, 5 mg/kg by mouth each day. When teaching the parents about the medication regimen, the nurse will use which approach?
   1. Conduct brief education sessions, provide written materials during each visit, and repeat information as appropriate.
   2. Ask the parents to spend an entire day at the facility so they can learn every detail about their child's care.
   3. Call the parents at home and explain everything, allowing time for them to ask questions.
   4. Send the parents the drug packaging inserts so they can become familiar with the medication.

28. When administering medication to a preschooler at 0900, which statement by the nurse is **best**?
   1. "It is time for you to take your medicine right now."
   2. "If you take your medicine now, you will go home sooner."
   3. "Here is your medicine. Would you like apple juice or water after?"
   4. "Do you want to take your morning medication now?"

29. A preschooler with a history of heart failure is prescribed digoxin. Which nursing intervention is **most** important to perform before administering this drug?
   1. Check apical heart rate for 1 minute.
   2. Obtain the blood pressure.
   3. Count the respiratory rate for 1 minute.
   4. Measure the urine output.

30. The nurse administers intravenous (IV) morphine to a client who sustained burns in a house fire. Which nursing action is **priority**?
   1. Give IV fluids.
   2. Monitor respirations.
   3. Administer bacitracin.
   4. Obtain blood pressure.

31. The nurse is evaluating a child with acute poststreptococcal glomerulonephritis (APSGN) for signs of improvement. Which early finding indicates to the nurse the child is improving?
   1. Increased urine output
   2. Increased appetite
   3. Increased energy level
   4. Decreased diarrhea

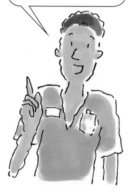

When teaching, remember parents often have short attention spans, too.

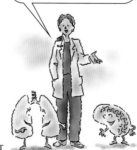

Morphine depresses the part of the brain that controls what essential function? Take a deep breath … it will come to you.

27. 1. Effective teaching methods include providing simple instructions in short sessions, providing written materials, repeating information, and allowing time for questions. The other options are ineffective teaching strategies that may be overwhelming for the parents and frustrating for the nurse.
CN: Health promotion and maintenance; CNS: None; CL: Apply

28. 3. Involving the child by offering a choice promotes cooperation and permits the child to make appropriate choices, enhancing a sense of control. Telling a child to take the medicine "right now" could provoke a negative response. Promising that the child will go home sooner could decrease the child's trust in nurses and health care providers. Asking a question with a potential "no" response is not the best approach.
CN: Psychosocial integrity; CNS: None; CL: Apply

29. 1. The child's apical pulse rate should be counted for 1 minute before digoxin administration. If the heart rate is below the specified rate in the health care provider's prescription (typically, 90 to 110 beats/minute for infants and young children), the dose should be withheld and the health care provider notified. Digoxin does not affect blood pressure, respiratory rate, or urine output.
CN: Physiological integrity; CNS: Pharmacological and parenteral therapies; CL: Apply

30. 2. Morphine depresses the brain's respiratory center; therefore, the nurse should assess the respirations to make sure breathing is not compromised. IV fluid replacement, antibiotics, and assessing blood pressure are also important, but these actions do not take priority over monitoring the respiratory status.
CN: Physiological integrity; CNS: Basic care and comfort; CL: Analyze

31. 1. Increased urine output, a sign of improving kidney function, typically is the first sign that a child with APSGN is improving. Increased appetite, an increased energy level, and decreased diarrhea are not specific to APSGN.
CN: Physiological integrity; CNS: Physiological adaptation; CL: Apply

CN: Client needs category   CNS: Client needs subcategory   CL: Cognitive level

32. A preschool-age child scheduled for surgery in the morning is admitted to the hospital for the first time. Which nursing action is appropriate to ease the child's anxiety?
1. Provide a video depicting the surgery for the child to watch.
2. Tell the child about being "put to sleep" for surgery.
3. Explain the surgical experience using dolls and medical equipment.
4. Explaining preoperative and postoperative procedures step by step.

33. Which client will the registered nurse (RN) assign to the licensed practical nurse (LPN)?
1. A client who just returned from surgery for an open cholecystectomy
2. A client newly diagnosed with diabetes with a glucose level 125 mg/dL (6.94 mmol/L)
3. A client with chronic iron-deficiency anemia prescribed an IV iron transfusion
4. A client who had a laparoscopic appendectomy yesterday requesting pain medication

34. The nurse is teaching a group of adolescent girls about personal hygiene. Which statement by an adolescent indicates the need for further education?
1. "It is important to bathe daily."
2. "It is unsafe to bathe during your period."
3. "I should not share my razor with anyone."
4. "I should not share my makeup with anyone."

35. When admitting an adolescent client, which strategy by the nurse is **most** appropriate?
1. Ask the client's caregivers to wait outside the room.
2. Document everything the client says in the medical record.
3. Ask the adolescent open-ended questions.
4. Discuss the nurse's own feelings about the situation.

36. Which nursing action is appropriate when discussing safe sexual practices with an adolescent?
1. Make sure the parent or legal guardian is present for the conversation.
2. Assess the adolescent's level of knowledge and concerns.
3. Only discuss options allowed by the adolescent's religious beliefs.
4. Obtain an informed consent from the parent before initiating the discussion.

32. 3. Explaining the surgical experience using dolls and medical equipment would ease anxiety and give the nurse an opportunity to clarify the child's misconceptions. Watching a video showing surgery is not appropriate for this age group. The nurse should avoid using such phrases as "put to sleep" because these may have a dual or negative meaning to a young child. Long explanations are inappropriate for the preschooler's developmental level and may increase anxiety.
CN: Psychosocial integrity; CNS: None; CL: Apply

33. 4. The RN would assign the most stable client with expected outcomes to the LPN. The postoperative client experiencing pain is stable and experiencing expected symptoms. The clients scheduled for surgery and newly diagnosed with diabetes will require extensive teaching and frequent assessments. The LPN should not initiate IV transfusions.
CN: Safe, effective care environment; CNS: Management of care; CL: Analyze

34. 2. Although some religious and cultural beliefs prohibit bathing during menses, there is no physical basis for this practice. Bathing daily is important because of the physical changes that occur during adolescence, including menstruation. Sharing of razors should be avoided to prevent the transmission of blood-borne pathogens. Makeup should not be shared because it may harbor bacteria.
CN: Health promotion and maintenance; CNS: None; CL: Apply

35. 3. Open-ended questions allow the adolescent to share information and feelings. The nurse should determine if the client prefers caregivers to be present during admission and assessments. Writing everything down can be a distraction and will not allow the nurse to observe how the adolescent behaves. Discussing the nurse's feelings may bias the assessment and is inappropriate when interviewing any client.
CN: Psychosocial integrity; CNS: None; CL: Apply

36. 2. Before proceeding with a discussion about safe sexual practices, the nurse should assess the adolescent's current level of knowledge and concerns. The adolescent has the right to discuss sexuality issues without knowledge or consent of parents. This discussion must remain confidential. The conversation does not have to remain within the confines of the adolescent's religious beliefs.
CN: Health promotion and maintenance; CNS: None; CL: Apply

CN: Client needs category   CNS: Client needs subcategory   CL: Cognitive level

37. The nurse is assessing a female client. Which statement(s) made by the client leads the nurse to suspect anorexia nervosa? Select all that apply.
1. "I have my menstrual period every 28 days."
2. "I jog three times per day for a total of 5 hours per day."
3. "I go out to eat with my friends at least three times per week."
4. "I keep my weight around 115 lb (52 kg), which is good for my height of 5 ft (1.52 m)."
5. "I generally eat a cup of fruit for breakfast, no lunch, and a protein bar for dinner."

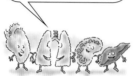

I love these organ recitals. Together we make some beautiful music.

37. 2, 5. Excessive exercise, consumption of very small amounts of food, and food rituals are all signs of anorexia nervosa. Menstruation commonly stops, and the client's weight is below normal. Going out to eat with friends is a common social event and is not a reliable indicator of anorexia nervosa. A weight of 115 lb (52 kg) is appropriate for someone who is 5 ft (1.52 m) in height.
CN: Physiological integrity; CNS: Reduction of risk potential; CL: Apply

38. A client has just undergone a bronchoscopy. Which intervention will the nurse perform **next**?
1. Assess level of consciousness (LOC).
2. Check airway patency.
3. Obtain vital signs.
4. Watch for bleeding.

38. 2. After a bronchoscopy, checking the client's airway patency is the most important nursing intervention. After checking airway patency, the nurse should monitor the client's breathing and check vital signs every 15 minutes until they are stable. After these initial interventions, the nurse should check LOC and monitor for bleeding.
CN: Physiological integrity; CNS: Reduction of risk potential; CL: Analyze

39. A client receiving long-term mechanical ventilation becomes very frustrated when trying to communicate. Which intervention will the nurse perform **next**?
1. Assure the client everything will be all right.
2. Ask a family member to interpret what the client is trying to say.
3. Ask the health care provider to wean the client off the mechanical ventilator.
4. Ask the client to write, use a picture board, or spell words with an alphabet board.

39. 4. If the client uses an alternative method of communication, the client will feel more in control and be less frustrated. Assuring the client that everything will be all right offers false reassurance. Telling the client not to be upset minimizes feelings. Neither of these methods helps the client to communicate. In a client with an endotracheal tube or tracheostomy tube, the family members are also likely to encounter difficulty interpreting the client's wishes. Making them responsible for interpreting the client's gestures may frustrate the family. The client may be weaned off a mechanical ventilator only when the physiologic parameters for weaning have been met.
CN: Psychosocial integrity; CNS: None; CL: Apply

40. After suctioning an adult client's tracheostomy, the nurse evaluates the client. Which findings indicate suctioning was effective?
1. A respiratory rate of 24 breaths/minute with accessory muscle use
2. Clear breath sounds and nonlabored respirations
3. Pulse rate 95 beats/minute and cyanosis of the skin and nail beds
4. Restlessness, pallor, and bubbling breath sounds

40. 2. Proper suctioning should produce a patent airway, as demonstrated by clear breath sounds and non-labored respirations. The other findings suggest ineffective suctioning. A respiratory rate of 24 breaths/minute and accessory muscle use may indicate mild respiratory distress. Increased pulse rate, rapid respirations, and cyanosis are signs of hypoxia. Restlessness, pallor, increased pulse and respiratory rates, and bubbling breath sounds indicate respiratory secretion accumulation.
CN: Physiological integrity; CNS: Reduction of risk potential; CL: Analyze

41. A client comes to the emergency department in status asthmaticus. Based on the chart exhibit below, how will the nurse interpret the client's arterial blood gas (ABG)?

Progress notes	
4/2	Client wheezing. Respiratory rate,
1830	44 breaths/minute; blood pressure,
	140/90 mm Hg; pulse 104 beats/minute;
	temperature, 98.4°F (36.9°C). ABG results
	show pH of 7.52; PaCO₂, 30 mm Hg
	(3.99 kPa); HCO3−, 26 mEq/L (26 mmol/L);
	and PO₂, 77 mm Hg (10.24 kPa).
	—C. Hill, RN

1. Respiratory acidosis
2. Respiratory alkalosis
3. Metabolic acidosis
4. Metabolic alkalosis

42. Which action(s) will the registered nurse include when caring for a client with emphysema? Select all that apply.
1. Reducing fluid intake to less than 850 mL per shift
2. Teaching diaphragmatic, pursed-lip breathing
3. Administering low-flow oxygen
4. Keeping the client in a supine position
5. Alternating activity with rest periods
6. Teaching the use of postural drainage and chest physiotherapy

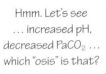

Hmm. Let's see … increased pH, decreased PaCO₂ … which "osis" is that?

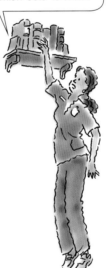

43. The nurse is caring for a client diagnosed with pulmonary edema. Which intervention is **best** for the nurse to use to monitor the client's respiratory status?
1. Arterial blood gas (ABG) analysis
2. Pulse oximetry checks
3. Skin color assessment
4. Auscultating lung sounds

41. 2. Following review of the nursing documentation, the nurse notes respiratory alkalosis related to alveolar hyperventilation. Respiratory alkalosis is marked by an increase in pH to more than 7.45 and a concurrent decrease in partial pressure of arterial carbon dioxide (PaCO₂) to less than 35 mm Hg (4.66 kPa). Metabolic alkalosis shows the same increase in pH but also an increased bicarbonate level and normal PaCO₂ (may be elevated also if compensatory mechanisms are working). Acidosis of any type means a low pH (below 7.35). Respiratory acidosis shows an elevated PaCO₂ and a normal-to-high bicarbonate level. Metabolic acidosis is characterized by a decreased bicarbonate level and a normal-to-low PaCO₂.
CN: Physiological integrity; CNS: Physiological adaptation; CL: Analyze

42. 2, 3, 5, 6. Diaphragmatic, pursed-lip breathing strengthens respiratory muscles and enhances oxygenation in clients with emphysema. Low-flow oxygen should be administered because a client with emphysema has chronic hypercapnia and a hypoxic respiratory drive. Alternating activity with rest allows the client to perform activities without excessive distress. If the client has difficulty mobilizing copious secretions, the nurse should teach the client and family members how to perform postural drainage and chest physiotherapy. Fluid intake should be increased to 3,000 mL/day, if not contraindicated, to liquefy secretions and facilitate removal. The client should be placed in high-Fowler's position to improve ventilation.
CN: Safe, effective care environment; CNS: Management of care; CL: Apply

43. 1. ABG analysis is the best measure for determining the extent of hypoxia caused by pulmonary edema and for monitoring the effects of therapy. The use of pulse oximetry is unreliable, especially in the case of severe vasoconstriction as is present in pulmonary edema. Although assessment of skin color and lung fields can be used to detect pulmonary changes, these options often are subject to interpretation by practitioners.
CN: Physiological integrity; CNS: Physiological adaptation; CL: Analysis

44. The nurse is caring for a client newly diagnosed with celiac disease. Which meal will the nurse order for this client?
1. Scrambled eggs, bacon, banana, and orange juice
2. Bagel with cream cheese, fresh pineapple, and tea
3. Cinnamon muffin, Canadian bacon, and water
4. Egg wrap in a wheat tortilla, cantaloupe, and apple juice

44. 1. Clients with celiac disease should avoid foods containing wheat, rye, and barley, such as bagel, muffin, and wheat wrap. The intestinal cells of individuals with celiac disease become inflamed when the child eats products containing gluten.
CN: Physiological integrity; CNS: Basic care and comfort; CL: Apply

45. An adult client ingests a large number of acetaminophen tablets in an attempt to commit suicide. Which laboratory result confirms an acetaminophen overdose?
1. Metabolic acidosis
2. Elevated liver enzyme levels
3. Increased serum creatinine level
4. Increased white blood cell (WBC) count

45. 2. Elevated liver enzyme levels, which could indicate liver damage, are associated with acetaminophen overdose. Metabolic acidosis is not associated with acetaminophen overdose. An increased serum creatinine level may indicate renal damage. An increased WBC count indicates infection.
CN: Physiological integrity; CNS: Pharmacological and parenteral therapies; CL: Apply

46. A client is undergoing a bedside thoracentesis. The nurse assists the client to an upright position with a table and pillow in front of the client, supporting the arms. Which rationale does the nurse give to the client for assuming this position?
1. To prevent fluid from accumulating at the base of the lung
2. There is less chance to injure lung tissue
3. It allows for better expansion of the lungs
4. It is less painful for the client in this position

46. 1. Fluids will drain and collect in the dependent positions. There is a risk of pneumothorax regardless of the client's position. The upright position does not allow for better expansion of the lung because the fluid in the pleural space is preventing this. Thoracentesis is done using local anesthesia, so it is not painful.
CN: Physiological integrity; CNS: Physiological adaptation; CL: Apply

47. The nurse is assessing an adolescent experiencing a sickle cell crisis. Which finding by the nurse is **most** significant to determine the state of hydration?
1. The adolescent has no bruises.
2. The adolescent has normal skin turgor.
3. The adolescent participates in exercise.
4. The adolescent maintains bladder control.

47. 2. Normal skin turgor indicates the adolescent is not severely dehydrated. Dehydration may cause sickle cell crisis or worsen a crisis. Bruising is not associated with sickle cell crisis. Bed rest is preferable during a sickle cell crisis. Bladder control may be lost when oral or IV fluid intake is increased during a sickle cell crisis.
CN: Physiological integrity; CNS: Physiological adaptation; CL: Analyze

48. The nurse is caring for a client with dyspnea who has a resting respiratory rate of 44 breaths/minute and dusky nail beds. Arterial blood gases are obtained, and the results are as follows: pH, 7.52; PaO_2, 50 mm Hg (6.65 kPa); $PaCO_2$, 28 mm Hg (3.72 kPa); HCO_3^-, 24 mEq/L (24 mmol/L). The nurse suspects which condition?
1. Metabolic acidosis
2. Metabolic alkalosis
3. Respiratory acidosis
4. Respiratory alkalosis

48. 4. A pH greater than 7.45 and a partial pressure of arterial carbon dioxide ($PaCO_2$) less than 35 mm Hg (4.66 kPa) indicate respiratory alkalosis. A pH less than 7.35 and a bicarbonate (HCO_3^-) less than 22 mEq/L (22 mmol/L) indicate metabolic acidosis. A pH greater than 7.45 and an HCO_3^- greater than 24 mEq/L (24 mmol/L) indicate metabolic alkalosis. A pH less than 7.35 and a $PaCO_2$ greater than 45 mm Hg (5.99 kPa) indicate respiratory acidosis.
CN: Physiological integrity; CNS: Reduction of risk potential; CL: Apply

49. A client diagnosed with alcohol use disorder is admitted to the hospital for detoxification. Later that day, the nurse notes the client's blood pressure has increased. The nurse administers lorazepam to prevent which complication?
   1. Stroke
   2. Seizure
   3. Fainting
   4. Anxiety reaction

50. Which action displayed by a grieving husband over his dying wife would cause the nurse to suggest counseling?
   1. He takes out wedding pictures and memorabilia to show to the staff.
   2. He refuses to acknowledge his wife's family and blames them for her health problems.
   3. He has already planned his wife's funeral arrangements.
   4. He is planning to give away his wife's treasured items to family members.

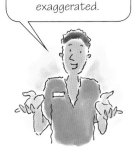

Many expressions of grief are normal. We're looking for ones that are excessive or exaggerated.

51. While the nurse is providing care, a client begins to exhibit signs of heightened anxiety. Which response by the nurse is **best**?
   1. "Everything will be fine. You do not need to worry."
   2. "Read this, then ask me any questions you may have."
   3. "Perhaps you should listen to the radio."
   4. "Let us talk about what is bothering you."

52. The nurse is providing discharge education to the parents of a school-age child with hemophilia. Which activity will the nurse recommend for the child? Select all that apply.
   1. Baseball
   2. Cross-country running
   3. Football
   4. Swimming
   5. Cheerleading
   6. Leisure walking

53. A client stepped on a piece of sharp glass while walking barefoot and comes to the emergency department with a deep laceration on the bottom of the foot. It is **most** important for the nurse to ask the client which question?
   1. "Was the glass dirty?"
   2. "Do you normally walk barefoot?"
   3. "When did you have your last tetanus shot?"
   4. "How many diphtheria-tetanus-pertussis (DTaP) shots have you received?"

49. 2. During detoxification from alcohol, changes in the client's physiologic status, especially an increase in blood pressure, may indicate an increased risk for seizure. Clients are treated with benzodiazepines to prevent this occurrence. Stroke, fainting, and anxiety are not the primary concerns when withdrawing from alcohol.
CN: Physiological integrity; CNS: Pharmacological and parenteral therapies; CL: Apply

50. 2. Abnormal grief may manifest itself as exaggerated or excessive expressions of normal grief reactions, such as anger, sadness, or depression. It is therapeutic to review a person's life with loved ones. Funeral planning can be therapeutic because it allows the individual to do one last thing for his loved one. It is therapeutic to share treasured items with staff and other family members.
CN: Physiological integrity; CNS: None; CL: Apply

51. 4. Anxiety may result from feelings of helplessness, isolation, or insecurity. This response helps reduce anxiety by encouraging the client to express feelings. The nurse should be supportive and develop goals together with the client to give the client some control over an anxiety-inducing situation. Because the other options ignore the client's feelings and block communication, they would not reduce anxiety.
CN: Psychosocial integrity; CNS: None; CL: Apply

52. 4, 6. Swimming is a noncontact sport with low risk of traumatic injury. Baseball, cross-country running, cheerleading, and football all involve a risk of trauma from falling, sliding, or contact. Leisure walking is a good low-impact activity that has a low risk of injury and promotes exercise.
CN: Physiological integrity; CNS: Physiological adaptation; CL: Apply

53. 3. Questioning the client about the date of the last tetanus immunization is important, because the booster immunization should be received every 10 years in adulthood (or at the time of the injury if the last booster immunization was given more than 5 years before the injury). Whether the client noticed dirt on the glass is immaterial because all deep lacerations require a tetanus immunization or booster. DTaP immunizations in childhood do not give lifelong immunization to tetanus. It is not important to ask if the client normally walks barefoot at this time.
CN: Safe, effective care environment; CNS: Safety and infection control; CL: Apply

CN: Client needs category   CNS: Client needs subcategory   CL: Cognitive level

54. The nurse is caring for a client suspected to have acute pancreatitis. Which assessment finding(s) indicate confirmation of this diagnosis to the nurse? Select all that apply.
1. Abdominal pain
2. Temperature 101.8°F (38.8°C)
3. Heart rate 110 beats/minute
4. Nausea
5. Vomiting
6. Unexplained weight loss
7. Steatorrhea

55. The primary health care provider prescribes acetaminophen 500 mg every 6 hours PRN for pain for a client in a long-term care facility. The pharmacy sends the concentration noted in the exhibit below. How many caplets will the nurse give? Record your answer using a whole number.

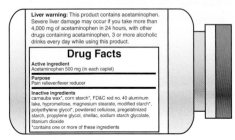

Liver warning: This product contains acetaminophen. Severe liver damage may occur if you take more than 4,000 mg of acetaminophen in 24 hours, with other drugs containing acetaminophen, 3 or more alcoholic drinks every day while using this product.

Drug Facts

Active ingredient
Acetaminophen 500 mg (in each caplet)

Purpose
Pain reliever/fever reducer

Inactive ingredients
carnauba wax*, corn starch*, FD&C red no. 40 aluminum lake, hypromellose, magnesium stearate, modified starch*, polyethylene glycol*, powdered cellulose, pregelatinized starch, propylene glycol, shellac, sodium starch glycolate, titanium dioxide
*contains one or more of these ingredients

_____ caplets

56. The nurse is educating a postmenopausal client on methods to prevent osteoporosis. Which statement by the client indicates teaching was successful?
1. "I need to take a multivitamin daily."
2. "I will drink at least two glasses of milk each day."
3. "I will start swimming three times per week."
4. "I will do weight-bearing exercises regularly."

57. A young adult client received the first chemotherapy treatment for breast cancer. Which statement by the client **most** concerns the nurse?
1. "I am thinking about joining a dance club."
2. "I do not think I am going to work tomorrow."
3. "I am not concerned about the adverse effects of the drugs."
4. "I really want to return to school for a college degree."

58. A client is diagnosed with prehypertension. Which treatment option(s) will the nurse expect to include in the client's care plan? Select all that apply.
1. Smoking cessation
2. Limiting alcohol consumption
3. Furosemide
4. Regular exercise
5. Metoprolol
6. Enalapril
7. Captopril

54. 1, 2, 3, 4, 5. Pancreatitis is accompanied by acute pain from autodigestion by pancreatic enzymes. Abdominal pain (upper, radiates to back, with touch, worse after eating), fever, tachycardia, nausea, and vomiting are findings associated with acute pancreatitis. Unexplained weight loss and steatorrhea are associated with chronic pancreatitis.
CN: Physiological integrity; CNS: Physiological adaptation; CL: Apply

55. 1.
Use the following equation:

$$\frac{dose\ desired}{dose\ per\ caplet} = number\ of\ caplets$$

$$\frac{500\ mg}{500\ mg/caplet} = 1\ caplet$$

CN: Physiological integrity; CNS: Pharmacological and parenteral therapies; CL: Apply

56. 4. Weight-bearing exercises are recommended for the prevention of osteoporosis. A multivitamin does not provide adequate calcium for a postmenopausal woman, and calcium alone will not prevent osteoporosis. Two glasses of milk per day do not provide the daily requirements for adult women. Swimming is not a weight-bearing exercise.
CN: Health promotion and maintenance; CNS: None; CL: Apply

57. 3. Adverse effects of chemotherapy may occur after treatment and should be discussed with the client; some can be treated, controlled, or prevented. The nurse needs to explore the client's meaning when indicating apathy about the adverse effects of chemotherapy drugs. The client may feel poorly after chemotherapy and may want to take time off from work until feeling better. Joining social clubs and returning to school is typical behavior for a young adult.
CN: Psychosocial integrity; CNS: None; CL: Apply

58. 1, 2, 4. Prehypertension signals the need for teaching about lifestyle modifications to prevent hypertension. Lifestyle modifications may include dietary changes, adopting relaxation techniques, regular exercise, smoking cessation, limiting intake of alcohol, and restricting sodium and saturated fat intake. Diuretics (furosemide), beta-adrenergic blockers (metoprolol), and angiotensin converting enzyme (ACE) inhibitors (enalapril and captopril) are used to treat hypertension.
CN: Health promotion and maintenance; CNS: None; CL: Apply

CN: Client needs category   CNS: Client needs subcategory   CL: Cognitive level

59. A client diagnosed with cardiomyopathy saw a posting on the Internet describing research about a new herbal treatment for the disorder. When the client asks the nurse about this treatment, which response by the nurse is **most** appropriate?

1. "Herbs are commonly used to treat cardiomyopathy."
2. "Cardiomyopathy can be treated only by heart surgery."
3. "The Internet is a reliable source of research, so try this treatment."
4. "You need to discuss this research with your health care provider."

59. 4. Although the Internet contains some valid medical research, there is no control over the validity of information posted. The research should be discussed with a health care provider, who can verify the accuracy of the information and determine if this is appropriate for this client. Herbs are not standard treatment for cardiomyopathy. Cardiomyopathy is treatable with drugs or surgery.

CN: Physiological integrity; CNS: Pharmacological and parenteral therapies; CL: Apply

60. The nurse is assessing a client 4 weeks after suffering a myocardial infarction (MI). The nurse is discussing cardiac rehabilitation with the client. Which statement by the client indicates additional education is needed?

1. "I perform relaxation exercises three times per day to reduce stress."
2. "My spouse and I are now following a low fat and low cholesterol diet."
3. "I will seek emergency help if my heart rate increases a lot while resting."
4. "I walk 4 miles (6.4 km) in 1 hour every single day."

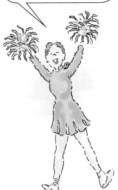

Hooray! You're doing great. Keep moving that ball down the field.

60. 4. Four weeks after an MI, a client's walking program should aim for a goal of 2 miles (3.2 km) in less than 1 hour. Walking 4 miles (6.4 km) in 1 hour is excessive and may induce another MI by increasing the heart's oxygen demands. Therefore, this client requires appropriate exercise guidelines and precautions. The other options indicate understanding of the cardiac rehabilitation program. The client should reduce stress, which speeds up the heart rate and thus increases myocardial oxygen demands. Reducing dietary fat and cholesterol intake helps lower the risk of atherosclerosis. A sudden rise in the heart rate while at rest warrants emergency medical attention because it may signal a life-threatening dysrhythmia and increase myocardial oxygen demands.

CN: Physiological integrity; CNS: Reduction of risk potential; CL: Analyze

61. The nurse is caring for a client experiencing dyspnea, dependent edema, hepatomegaly, crackles, and jugular vein distention. Which condition will the nurse suspect?

1. Pulmonary embolism
2. Heart failure
3. Cardiac tamponade
4. Tension pneumothorax

61. 2. A client with heart failure has decreased cardiac output caused by the heart's decreased pumping ability. A buildup of fluid occurs, causing dyspnea, dependent edema, hepatomegaly, crackles, and jugular vein distention. A client with pulmonary embolism experiences acute shortness of breath, pleuritic chest pain, hemoptysis, and fever. A client with cardiac tamponade experiences muffled heart sounds, hypotension, and elevated central venous pressure. A client with tension pneumothorax has a deviated trachea and absent breath sounds on the affected side as well as dyspnea and jugular vein distention.

CN: Physiological integrity; CNS: Physiological adaptation; CL: Apply

62. The nurse is performing an electrocardiogram (ECG) on a client with chest pain. The nurse will place the client in which position for this procedure?

1. Fowler's
2. Supine
3. Lateral
4. Prone

62. 2. The most appropriate position for a client undergoing an ECG is lying flat, as long as the client can tolerate being in a supine position. Otherwise, the client may be positioned with the head of the bed slightly elevated.

CN: Physiological integrity; CNS: Reduction of risk potential; CL: Understand

CN: Client needs category   CNS: Client needs subcategory   CL: Cognitive level

63. The nurse is caring for a client with a diagnosis of pericarditis. Which statement indicates a violation of client confidentiality?
1. The nurse discussed the client's diagnosis with another nurse at shift report.
2. The nurse discussed the client's medication therapy with the health care provider.
3. The nurse discussed the client's medication therapy with the hospital pharmacist.
4. The nurse discussed the client's diagnosis with a family friend over the telephone.

63. 4. Violation of confidentiality occurs when client information is discussed with nonmedical persons, such as family or friends, without the client's permission. It is appropriate to discuss a client's diagnosis with other members of the health care team.
CN: Safe, effective care environment; CNS: Management of care; CL: Analyze

64. The nurse administers furosemide to treat a client with heart failure. The nurse will **most** carefully assess the client for which adverse effect?
1. Increase in blood pressure
2. Increase in blood volume
3. Hypokalemia
4. Hypernatremia

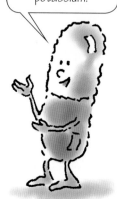

Be careful. I have a habit of getting wasted on potassium. Wait … I mean wasting potassium.

64. 3. Furosemide is a potassium-wasting diuretic. The nurse must monitor the serum potassium level and assess for signs of low potassium. As water and sodium are lost in the urine, blood pressure decreases, blood volume decreases, and urine output increases.
CN: Physiological integrity; CNS: Pharmacological and parenteral therapies; CL: Apply

65. A client is admitted to the emergency department after reporting acute chest pain radiating down the left arm. The client is anxious, dyspneic, and diaphoretic. The nurse will anticipate preparing the client for which laboratory study? Select all that apply.
1. Hemoglobin (Hgb) and hematocrit (Hct)
2. Serum glucose
3. Creatine kinase (CK)
4. Troponin T and troponin I
5. Myoglobin
6. Blood urea nitrogen (BUN)

65. 3, 4, 5. With myocardial ischemia or infarction, levels of CK, troponin T, and troponin I typically rise because of cellular damage. Myoglobin elevation is an early indicator of myocardial damage. Hgb, Hct, serum glucose, and BUN levels do not provide information related to myocardial ischemia.
CN: Physiological integrity; CNS: Reduction of risk potential; CL: Apply

66. The nurse administers sublingual nitroglycerin to a client reporting chest pain. Which statement by the client indicates to the nurse the treatment is effective?
1. "I have a bad headache."
2. "My chest pain is decreasing."
3. "I feel a tingling sensation around my mouth."
4. "I feel like my blood pressure must be up."

66. 2. Nitroglycerin, a vasodilator, increases the arterial supply of oxygen-rich blood to the myocardium, thus producing its intended effect: relief of chest pain. Headache is an adverse effect of nitroglycerin. The drug should not cause a tingling sensation around the mouth and it should lower, not raise, blood pressure.
CN: Physiological integrity; CNS: Pharmacological and parenteral therapies; CL: Analyze

67. The nurse is caring for a stable client with digoxin toxicity. Which treatment does the nurse anticipate for this client?
1. Activated charcoal
2. Symptomatic treatment
3. Hemodialysis
4. Atropine

67. 2. Stable clients with digoxin toxicity are best treated with time while their kidneys excrete the metabolites, and with symptomatic treatment for the rhythm disturbances or nausea resulting from the toxicity. Activated charcoal is effective only if the client has taken an overdose of digoxin and if a large amount of unabsorbed drug is in the gastrointestinal tract, before the serum level is elevated. Hemodialysis is reserved for clients who are extremely unstable despite symptomatic treatment or who have inadequate renal function to excrete the drug. Atropine might be used to treat the bradycardia that results from digoxin toxicity, but it is not necessarily used to treat the toxicity itself.
CN: Physiological integrity; CNS: Pharmacological and parenteral therapies; CL: Apply

CN: Client needs category   CNS: Client needs subcategory   CL: Cognitive level

68. A client newly diagnosed with heart failure is placed on bed rest and asks the nurse, "Why do I have to stay in bed?" Which response by the nurse is **best**?
1. "It will improve the heart's pumping action."
2. "It will enhance arterial oxygenation."
3. "It will decrease fluid volume in the heart."
4. "It will reduce the heart's workload."

68. **4.** Bed rest reduces the heart's workload by decreasing tissue demand for oxygen. Bed rest does not improve the heart's pumping action; medications such as digoxin are usually given to achieve this. Oxygen is administered to enhance arterial oxygenation. A diuretic, not bed rest, helps to decrease fluid volume.
CN: Physiological integrity; CNS: Physiological adaptation; CL: Apply

69. The nurse is caring for a client who suffered an acute myocardial infarction (MI). Which intervention is **most** appropriate for the nurse to include to assist the client with bowel elimination and prevent straining?
1. Maintain complete bed rest.
2. Limit fluid intake.
3. Give docusate as prescribed.
4. Provide a low-fat diet.

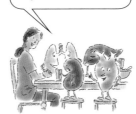

Remember to eat with your whole body in mind, not just your taste buds.

69. **3.** Administering a stool softener such as docusate will help the client pass stools without straining. Maintaining bed rest and limiting fluids may cause constipation and increase the client's need to strain with each bowel movement. A low-fat diet does not assist with elimination.
CN: Physiological integrity; CNS: Basic care and comfort; CL: Apply

70. The nurse is assessing a client who reports recent chest pain. Which statement by the client suggests angina pectoris to the nurse?
1. "The pain lasted about 45 minutes."
2. "The pain resolved after I ate a sandwich."
3. "The pain got worse when I took a deep breath."
4. "The pain occurred while I was mowing the lawn."

70. **4.** Angina pectoris is chest pain caused by a decreased oxygen supply to the myocardium. Lawn mowing increases the cardiac workload; this, in turn, increases the heart's need for oxygen and may precipitate angina. Anginal pain typically is self-limiting and lasts 5 to 15 minutes. Food consumption does not reduce this pain, although it may ease pain caused by a gastrointestinal ulcer. Deep breathing has no effect on anginal pain.
CN: Physiological integrity; CNS: Physiological adaptation; CL: Analyze

71. The nurse is caring for a client receiving oral digoxin 0.125 mg daily. The client develops sinus bradycardia with a heart rate of 50 beats/minute. Which action will the nurse take **first**?
1. Notify the health care provider.
2. Retake the vital signs in 30 minutes.
3. Discontinue the digoxin prescription.
4. Have the client turn on the left side.

71. **1.** Because bradycardia is an adverse effect of digoxin, the nurse should notify the health care provider and then follow the provider's prescription. Vital signs should be checked again, and the client's heart rate and rhythm should be monitored, but these would not be the first actions. The nurse cannot discontinue a medication prescription; only the health care provider can do so. Turning the client on the left side will not increase the heart rate.
CN: Safe, effective care environment; CNS: Management of care; CL: Apply

72. A client has a blockage in the proximal portion of a coronary artery. After learning about treatment options, the client decides to undergo percutaneous transluminal coronary angioplasty (PTCA). During this procedure, the nurse expects to administer which medication to the client?
1. An antibiotic
2. An anticoagulant
3. An antihypertensive
4. An anticonvulsant

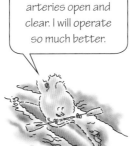

Please keep those arteries open and clear. I will operate so much better.

72. **2.** During PTCA, the client receives heparin, an anticoagulant, as well as calcium agonists, nitrates, or both to reduce coronary artery spasm. An antibiotic is not given routinely during this procedure; however, because the procedure is invasive, the client may receive prophylactic antibiotics afterward to reduce the risk of infection. An antihypertensive agent may cause hypotension, which should be avoided during the procedure. An anticonvulsant is not indicated because this procedure does not increase the risk of seizures.
CN: Physiological integrity; CNS: Pharmacological and parenteral therapies; CL: Apply

73. The nurse is discharging a client hospitalized for hypertension. Which statement from the client indicates an understanding of the nurse's discharge instructions?
1. "I should avoid eating meat and drinking milk."
2. "I should skip my medication dose if dizziness occurs."
3. "I will read labels to make sure I do not eat too much sodium."
4. "I will schedule a weekly appointment to check my blood pressure."

73. 3. The nurse must teach the hypertensive client how to modify the diet to restrict sodium and saturated fats. In addition, the nurse should explain the actions, dosages, and adverse effects of prescribed antihypertensives. A client receiving antihypertensives also may take a diuretic as part of the drug regimen, should eat a potassium-rich diet including meats and milk, and may require dietary potassium supplements and high-potassium foods to avoid electrolyte disturbances. Instead of skipping medication if dizziness occurs, the client should notify the health care provider of this symptom. The client can monitor blood pressure from home.

CN: Physiological integrity; CNS: Reduction of risk potential; CL: Apply

74. A client is admitted to the cardiac unit with a diagnosis of heart failure. The health care provider prescribes furosemide and digoxin. Which laboratory value will the nurse monitor while caring for this client?
1. Sodium
2. Potassium
3. Chloride
4. Calcium

74. 2. Digoxin may increase the risk of toxicity from furosemide-induced hypokalemia; therefore, potassium levels should be monitored closely. Concurrent administration of digoxin and furosemide does not affect sodium, chloride, or calcium levels.

CN: Physiological integrity; CNS: Pharmacological and parenteral therapies; CL: Understand

75. The nurse is assessing a new client at the cardiovascular clinic. When asking about the client's medical history, which finding will **most** concern the nurse?
1. Croup
2. Rheumatic fever
3. Severe staphylococcal infection
4. Medullary sponge kidney

75. 2. Childhood diseases and disorders associated with structural heart disease include rheumatic fever and severe streptococcal (not staphylococcal) infections. Croup—a severe upper airway inflammation and obstruction that typically strikes children ages 3 months to 3 years—may cause latent complications, such as ear infection and pneumonia. However, it does not affect heart structures. Likewise, medullary sponge kidney, characterized by dilation of the renal pyramids and formation of cavities, clefts, and cysts in the renal medulla, eventually may lead to hypertension but does not damage heart structures.

CN: Health promotion and maintenance; CNS: None; CL: Analyze

76. A disaster drill is in progress at the hospital. In preparation for potential admissions, the charge nurse on a cardiac step-down unit determines it is **best** to potentially discharge which client?
1. A 30-year-old client with recent episodes of ventricular tachycardia scheduled for electrophysiology studies
2. A 75-year-old client who had an inferior myocardial infarction yesterday and is receiving metoprolol
3. A 52-year-old client who had an endovascular graft placed for an abdominal aortic aneurysm 3 days ago
4. A 62-year-old client who was admitted this morning with new onset heart failure secondary to coronary artery disease

76. 3. Because endovascular grafting is a minimally invasive procedure for the repair of an abdominal aortic aneurysm, the client is usually discharged from the hospital in 1 to 3 days. It would be unsafe to recommend discharge for any of the other clients.

CN: Safe, effective care environment; CNS: Safety and infection control; CL: Analyze

CN: Client needs category   CNS: Client needs subcategory   CL: Cognitive level

77. A client reports generalized, steady abdominal pain with low back pain. Which finding indicates to the nurse the client is experiencing an abdominal aortic aneurysm?
1. Pulsating mass in the periumbilical area
2. Elevated cardiac enzymes
3. Positive Babinski's sign
4. Pink, frothy sputum

78. Which nursing interventions are **most** appropriate when caring for a client with acute thrombophlebitis of the left leg?
1. Wrap leg with a cool cloth and keep the extremity immobilized.
2. Increase the client's activity level and encourage leg exercises.
3. Administer nitroglycerin and oxygen at 2 L/min via nasal cannula.
4. Apply warm soaks and elevate the client's legs higher than the level of the heart.

79. The nurse is obtaining vital signs for a client who is receiving a heparin infusion to treat deep vein thrombosis. The client tells the nurse, "My gums bleed when I brush my teeth." What will the nurse do **first**?
1. Stop the heparin infusion.
2. Notify the health care provider.
3. Administer protamine sulfate.
4. Assess partial thromboplastin time level.

80. On a routine visit to the primary health care provider, a client with chronic arterial occlusive disease reports leg pain when exercising. Which recommendation(s) by the nurse is appropriate for this client? Select all that apply.
1. Taking daily walks
2. Engaging in aerobic exercise
3. Smoking cessation
4. Increasing daily fat intake
5. Avoiding foods that increase levels of high-density lipoproteins (HDLs)

77. 1. Signs of abdominal aortic aneurysm include gnawing, generalized, steady abdominal pain; lower back pain that is unaffected by movement; gastric or abdominal fullness; pulsating mass in the periumbilical area (if the client is not obese); systolic bruit over the aorta on auscultation of the abdomen; bruit over the femoral arteries; and hypotension (with aneurysm rupture). Elevated cardiac enzymes indicate heart muscle damage. Positive Babinski's sign indicates damage to the pyramidal tract of the central nervous system. Pink, frothy sputum is a sign of pulmonary edema.
CN: Physiological integrity; CNS: Physiological adaptation; CL: Apply

78. 4. To help treat thrombophlebitis, the nurse should prevent venostasis with measures such as applying warm soaks and elevating the client's legs. The client should remain on bed rest during the acute phase, after which the client may begin to walk while wearing antiembolism stockings. Treatment for thrombophlebitis may also include anticoagulants to prolong clotting time.
CN: Physiological integrity; CNS: Physiological adaptation; CL: Apply

79. 4. Because bleeding gums are an adverse effect of heparin that may indicate excessive anticoagulation, the nurse would evaluate the client's condition. Laboratory tests, such as partial thromboplastin time, should be performed before concluding that the client's bleeding is significant. The prescribed heparin dose may be therapeutic rather than excessive, so the nurse should not discontinue the heparin infusion unless the health care provider prescribes this after evaluating the client. Protamine sulfate is given to counteract heparin if indicated.
CN: Physiological integrity; CNS: Pharmacological and parenteral therapies; CL: Analyze

80. 1, 3, 5. The nurse would suspect the client is experiencing claudication. Taking daily walks relieves symptoms of intermittent claudication, although the exact mechanism is unclear. Aerobic exercise may make these symptoms worse. Smoking can lead to decreased blood flow and should be stopped. Clients with chronic arterial occlusive disease must reduce daily fat intake to 30% or less of total calories. The client should limit dietary cholesterol because hyperlipidemia is associated with atherosclerosis, a known cause of arterial occlusive disease. However, HDLs have the lowest cholesterol concentration, so this client should *eat*, not *avoid*, foods that raise HDL levels.
CN: Physiological integrity; CNS: Reduction of risk potential; CL: Analyze

81. The nurse is caring for a client receiving captopril for heart failure. Which finding(s) will the nurse highlight for the health care provider? Select all that apply.
1. Skin rash
2. Peripheral edema
3. Acute anorexia
4. Orthostatic hypotension
5. Nocturnal dyspnea

82. A client comes to the clinic for a skin assessment. Which finding is **most** concerning to the nurse?
1. A deep sunburn
2. A pruritic patch on the client's back
3. An irregular scar on the client's abdomen
4. An asymmetrical mole with blurred borders

83. A client with long-standing rheumatoid arthritis has frequent reports of severe joint pain. The nurse will plan to recommend the client take pain medication in which manner?
1. Conservatively
2. Intramuscular
3. On an as-needed basis
4. Regularly scheduled intervals

84. Which nursing intervention is appropriate for an adult client with chronic renal failure?
1. Weigh the client daily before breakfast.
2. Offer foods high in calcium and phosphorus.
3. Serve the client large meals and a bedtime snack.
4. Encourage the client to drink large amounts of fluids.

85. A client with a recent history of a stroke is being discharged from the rehabilitation facility with a walker. Which observation of the client's gait indicates to the nurse additional education regarding walker use is needed?
1. The client moves the weak leg forward with the walker.
2. The client moves the hands to the armrests of a chair before sitting in the chair.
3. The client's arms are fully extended when using the walker.
4. The client backs up to the chair until the legs touch the chair, then sits down.

86. The nurse is discussing with a parent the assessment of the child's behavior. The nurse recognizes which behavior as indicative of conduct disorder?
1. The child is wetting the bed at night.
2. The child has threatened suicide.
3. The child has purposely hurt animals.
4. The child has a fear of attending school.

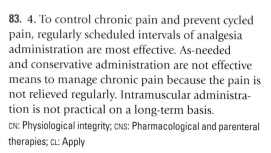

Remember, for the best results, clients should take pain medication as scheduled.

81. **2, 3, 5.** Peripheral edema, loss of appetite, and nocturnal dyspnea are signs of fluid volume overload and worsening heart failure. A skin rash and orthostatic hypotension are side effects to captopril.
CN: Physiological integrity; CNS: Pharmacological and parenteral therapies; CL: Analyze

82. **4.** The nurse is most concerned about the mole with findings indicative of skin cancer. A deep sunburn is a risk factor for skin cancer. A pruritic patch and an irregular scar are benign findings.
CN: Health promotion and maintenance; CNS: None; CL: Analyze

83. **4.** To control chronic pain and prevent cycled pain, regularly scheduled intervals of analgesia administration are most effective. As-needed and conservative administration are not effective means to manage chronic pain because the pain is not relieved regularly. Intramuscular administration is not practical on a long-term basis.
CN: Physiological integrity; CNS: Pharmacological and parenteral therapies; CL: Apply

84. **1.** Daily weights are obtained to monitor fluid retention. Calcium intake is encouraged, but clients with chronic renal failure have difficulty excreting phosphorus. Therefore, phosphorus must be restricted. To improve food intake, meals and snacks should be given in small portions. Fluids should be restricted for the client with chronic renal failure.
CN: Physiological integrity; CNS: Physiological adaptation; CL: Apply

85. **3.** When using a walker, the client's arms should be slightly bent at the elbow, allowing maximum support from the arms while ambulating. The weak leg is always moved forward first with the walker to provide the maximum support. The client should use the armrests of the chair for support because the armrests are more stable than the walker. When sitting, the client should always back up to the chair and feel the chair with his legs before sitting.
CN: Physiological integrity; CNS: Basic care and comfort; CL: Apply

86. **3.** Cruelty to animals is a symptom of conduct disorder. Enuresis and suicidal ideation are not usually associated with conduct disorder. Fear of going to school is school phobia.
CN: Psychosocial integrity; CNS: None; CL: Understand

87. The primary health care provider prescribes several medications for a client with hemorrhagic stroke. Which prescription will the nurse question?
1. Dexamethasone
2. Heparin sodium
3. Methyldopa
4. Phenytoin

Anticoagulants are a bad idea for clients at risk for bleeding.

88. A client has been admitted to the hospital with signs of mild dehydration. Which nursing intervention is **most** appropriate for this client?
1. Explain the need for increased fluid intake.
2. Place the client's preferred beverage at the bedside.
3. Serve small amounts of fluids at frequent intervals.
4. Administer an intravenous (IV) fluid bolus.

89. The registered nurse (RN) is caring for a client prescribed intravenous (IV) fluids. Which action(s) will the nurse perform while obtaining peripheral IV access? Select all that apply.
1. Wraps the elastic band loosely around the client's arm
2. Identifies the client prior to performing the procedure
3. Inspects multiple areas in the client's arm and hand before selecting a vein
4. Cleans the selected site with mild soap and warm water
5. Holds the IV catheter perpendicular to the client's vein when inserting
6. Secures the IV catheter in place with tape after removing the needle

90. The nurse is reviewing the proper technique for obtaining a urine specimen from an indwelling urinary catheter. When collecting the urine, which technique is **most** appropriate for the nurse to use?
1. Collect urine from the urinary drainage collection bag.
2. Disconnect the catheter from the drainage tubing to collect urine.
3. Remove the indwelling catheter and insert a sterile straight catheter to collect urine.
4. Clean the drainage port with alcohol and insert a sterile needle to collect the specimen.

87. 2. Administration of heparin, an anticoagulant, could increase the bleeding associated with hemorrhagic stroke. Therefore, the nurse should question this prescription to prevent additional hemorrhage in the brain. In a client with hemorrhagic stroke, dexamethasone may be used to decrease cerebral edema and pressure; methyldopa may be used to reduce blood pressure; and phenytoin may be used to prevent seizures.
CN: Physiological integrity; CNS: Pharmacological and parenteral therapies; CL: Analyze

88. 3. Fluids should be served in small amounts spread out at frequent intervals. Educating the client about the need for increasing fluids and including the client in the selection of beverages will aid in compliance. IV fluid boluses are not generally indicated for mild dehydration.
CN: Physiological integrity; CNS: Basic care and comfort; CL: Analyze

89. 2, 3, 6. The RN would identify the client, inspect carefully before selecting an appropriate site, and secure the IV catheter in place after insertion. The elastic band should be applied tightly around the arm, and the selected site cleaned with an antiseptic solution. The needle should be held at a 10 to 30 degree angle for insertion.
CN: Safe, effective care environment; CNS: Safety and infection control; CL: Apply

90. 4. The nurse should wear clean gloves, clean the drainage port with alcohol, and then obtain the specimen with a sterile needle to ensure the specimen and the closed urinary drainage system will not be contaminated. A urine specimen must collect new urine, and the urine in the bag could be several hours old and growing bacteria. The urinary drainage system must be kept closed to prevent microorganisms from entering. A straight catheter is used to relieve urine retention, obtain sterile urine specimens, measure the amount of postvoid residual urine, and empty the bladder for certain procedures. It is not necessary to remove an indwelling catheter to obtain a sterile urine specimen unless the health care provider requests that the whole system be changed.
CN: Safe, effective care environment; CNS: Safety and infection control; CL: Remember

CN: Client needs category   CNS: Client needs subcategory   CL: Cognitive level

91. Which outcome is appropriate for the nurse to set for a client admitted for depression and attempted suicide?
 1. The client will not feel suicidal again.
 2. The client will find a group home to live in.
 3. The client will remain hospitalized for about 6 months.
 4. The client will verbalize an absence of suicidal ideation, plan, and intent.

91. 4. An appropriate outcome is the client will verbalize no longer feeling suicidal. It is unrealistic to expect that the client will never feel suicidal again. There is no reason for a group home or 6 months of hospitalization for a client who says he or she no longer feels suicidal.
CN: Psychosocial integrity; CNS: None; CL: Apply

92. A registered nurse (RN) is supervising a licensed practical nurse (LPN). The LPN is caring for a client diagnosed with a terminal illness. Which statement by the LPN indicates to the RN teaching is needed?
 1. "Some clients write a living will indicating their end-of-life preferences."
 2. "I will make sure clients with terminal illnesses have a living will."
 3. "You can designate someone to make end-of-life decisions when you cannot yourself."
 4. "Some people do not desire to have cardio-pulmonary resuscitation."

92. 2. It is the client's decision to have a living will or not. The nurse cannot force a client to have a living will. A health care power of attorney can be designated to make health care decisions for the client in the event the client can no longer make decisions. Some clients do not want cardiopulmonary resuscitation (CPR) and this would be discussed and planned with the primary health care provider.
CN: Safe, effective care environment; CNS: Management of care; CL: Apply

93. An older adult client's husband tells the nurse he is concerned because his wife insists on talking about events that happened to her years ago. The nurse finds the client alert, oriented, and answering questions appropriately. Which statement by the nurse to the husband is **most** appropriate?
 1. "Your wife is reviewing her life."
 2. "I will consult the hospital's spiritual advisor."
 3. "Your wife should be discouraged from dwelling on the past."
 4. "Your wife is focusing on a more comfortable time."

93. 1. Life review or reminiscing is characteristic of older adults and the dying. A spiritual advisor might comfort the client but is not necessary for a life review. Discouraging the client from talking would block communication. Regression occurs when a client returns to behaviors typical of another developmental stage.
CN: Health promotion and maintenance; CNS: None; CL: Apply

94. The nurse is educating a client with a new colostomy. Which information will the nurse include in the teaching? Select all that apply.
 1. Limit daily fluid intake.
 2. Eat more fruits and vegetables.
 3. Empty the bag when it is about half full.
 4. Tape the end of the bag to the skin.
 5. Clean the bag with an alcohol solution.

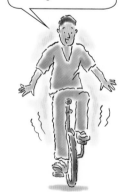

Impressive! You're really rolling through this test.

94. 2, 3. Emptying the bag when partially full prevents the bag from becoming heavy and detaching from the skin or skin barrier. Limiting fluids may cause constipation but will not prevent leakage. Increasing fruits and vegetables in the diet will help prevent constipation. Taping the bag to the skin will secure the bag to the skin but will not prevent detachment and could irritate the surrounding skin. If rinsing the bag, the client should use plain water, avoiding contact with the barrier.
CN: Physiological integrity; CNS: Basic care and comfort; CL: Apply

95. A client reports an inability to sleep while on the medical unit. Which nursing intervention is **most** appropriate for this client?
 1. Administer zolpidem at bedtime.
 2. Play relaxing music at bedtime.
 3. Question the client about sleeping habits.
 4. Move the client away from the nurses' station.

95. 3. Interviewing the client about sleeping habits may give more information about the causes of the inability to sleep. Sedatives should be given as a last option. Relaxing music may promote sleep but does not address this client's problem. Moving the client may not address the client's specific problem.
CN: Physiological integrity; CNS: Basic care and comfort; CL: Analyze

CN: Client needs category   CNS: Client needs subcategory   CL: Cognitive level

96. The nurse must obtain the blood pressure of a client in airborne isolation. Which method is **best** for the nurse to use when obtaining the client's blood pressure?
1. Dispose of the equipment after each use.
2. Wear gloves while handling the equipment.
3. Clean the equipment between client assessments.
4. Leave the equipment in the room for use only with that client.

96. 4. Leaving equipment in the room for use only with that client is appropriate to avoid organism transmission by inanimate objects. Disposing of equipment after each use prevents the transmission of organisms but is not cost-effective. Wearing gloves protects the nurse, not other clients. Cleaning the equipment is appropriate; however, best practice would be to leave the equipment in the room while the client is in the facility.
CN: Safe, effective care environment; CNS: Safety and infection control; CL: Apply

97. The nurse is providing education regarding the use of an incentive spirometer to a client who had abdominal surgery. Which statement made by the client demonstrates an adequate understanding of the use of the incentive spirometer?
1. "If I use this I will not have to ambulate as quickly after surgery."
2. "If I use this I will not have to take deep breaths to prevent my lungs from collapsing."
3. "Using the incentive spirometer will not hurt as bad as deep breathing exercises."
4. "It will help me to take slow, deep breaths to help prevent lung complications."

97. 4. Incentive spirometry helps the client take slow, deep breaths using floating balls, lights, or bellows. Early ambulation is still indicated for this client after abdominal surgery. Incentive spirometry is no more effective than deep breathing without equipment. Deep breathing and incentive spirometry cause equal discomfort during inspiration.
CN: Physiological integrity; CNS: Reduction of risk potential; CL: Understand

98. The nurse is assessing an adult client who is receiving intravenous gentamicin for the first time. Which finding(s) made by the nurse requires immediate intervention? Select all that apply.
1. Rash on the face, chest, and arms
2. Reports severe pruritus
3. Inspiratory wheezing
4. Heart rate of 65 beats/minute
5. Reports mouth is dry

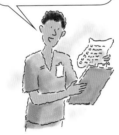

An allergic reaction to a medication demands immediate attention.

98. 1, 2, 3. Rash, inspiratory wheezes, and reports of severe itching indicate that the client is having an allergic reaction to the antibiotic. A heart rate of 65 beats/minute is within normal limits, and reports of mouth being dry are not indicative of an allergic reaction.
CN: Physiological integrity; CNS: Pharmacological and parenteral therapies; CL: Apply

99. The nurse is preparing to test a client's optic nerve (cranial nerve II) function. Which nursing action is appropriate?
1. Move finger back and forth in front of the client's face.
2. Shine a penlight in each of the client's eyes.
3. Cover one eye and have the client read a Snellen chart.
4. Have the client turn head from side to side.

99. 3. The Snellen chart is used to test the function of the optic nerve. Testing the cardinal fields assesses the oculomotor, trochlear, and abducens nerves. Corneal light reflex indicates the function of the oculomotor nerve. The accessory nerve is tested by moving the head side to side.
CN: Physiological integrity; CNS: Basic care and comfort; CL: Apply

100. The nurse is educating a client being discharged from the hospital with an indwelling catheter. Which statement made by the client demonstrates the education was effective?
1. "I will limit my fluid intake to 16 ounces per day."
2. "I will start taking showers instead of tub baths."
3. "I can open the drainage system to obtain a urine specimen."
4. "I will irrigate the catheter twice daily with sterile saline solution."

100. 2. A shower would prevent bacteria in the bath water from sustaining contact with the urinary meatus and the catheter, whereas a tub bath may allow easier transit of bacteria into the urinary tract. Increased—not limited—fluid intake is recommended for a client with an indwelling urinary catheter. Opening the drainage system would provide a pathway for the entry of bacteria. Catheter irrigation is performed only with a prescription from the health care provider to keep the catheter patent.
CN: Physiological integrity; CNS: Reduction of risk potential; CL: Apply

CN: Client needs category   CNS: Client needs subcategory   CL: Cognitive level

101. The nurse is caring for a client just placed in a vest restraint. Which nursing action is **priority**?
1. Have the assistive personnel (AP) check on the client hourly.
2. Notify the client's family of the change in the client's condition.
3. Assess the client's skin for breakdown each shift while in restraints.
4. Obtain vital signs every 15 minutes for the first hour following application.

102. One year after the death of an infant son, a client is diagnosed with dysfunctional grieving. Which statement **most** concerns the nurse?
1. "I go to my son's grave at least once a week."
2. "I still cannot talk about my son without crying."
3. "I still feel like it is my fault my son is not here."
4. "I am planning to go be with my son soon."

103. The nurse notices a client has been crying. Which nursing response is the **most** therapeutic?
1. "You will get through this illness and be okay."
2. "You seem sad. Would you like to talk?"
3. "Why are you crying and upsetting yourself?"
4. "It is hard being sick, but you must keep your chin up."

104. The nurse gives the wrong medication to a client. Which nursing action is **priority**?
1. Monitor the client for an interaction.
2. Complete an incident report.
3. Notify the facility's risk manager.
4. Administer the correct medication.

105. Which action places the nurse at risk for being charged with assault and battery by a client?
1. Taking a necklace that belonged to the client
2. Entering the client's room several times during the course of treatment
3. Performing a procedure without obtaining consent
4. Discussing the client's medical information with another nurse

106. A client newly diagnosed with breast cancer tells the nurse, "I know the lab made a mistake and I do not really have cancer." Which nursing response is **most** appropriate?
1. "Why are you in denial about having breast cancer?"
2. "You need to accept this and start treatment immediately."
3. "Let us talk about what it means to test positive for breast cancer."
4. "I know this is overwhelming, but you need to get it together."

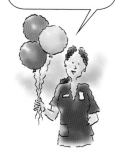

Way to go! You're rockin' this test.

101. 4. The registered nurse (not AP) should assess the client every 15 minutes for the first hour (vital signs, safety, restraint position, comfort, skin condition, need for toileting/food/drink), then at least every 4 hours for adults. The family should be notified of the change in the client's status, but this is not priority.
CN: Safe, effective care environment; CNS: Safety and infection control; CL: Apply

102. 4. The grieving parent reporting plans to be with the deceased son soon would most concern the nurse because this sounds like potential suicide. This comment should be further explored to determine the client's intent. Dysfunctional grieving can be debilitating, but client safety is priority. Visiting the son's grave, crying, and blame are all normal responses to the death of a loved one.
CN: Psychosocial integrity; CNS: None; CL: Apply

103. 2. Therapeutic communication is a primary tool of nursing. The nurse must recognize that the client's nonverbal behaviors indicate a need to talk. Asking "why" the client is crying might be interpreted as being judgmental. Giving opinions and advice are barriers to communication.
CN: Psychosocial integrity; CNS: None; CL: Apply

104. 1. It is priority for the nurse to monitor the client for an interaction (client safety). The nurse will complete an incident report and submit to the risk manager after ensuring the client is stable. The correct medication may be administer depending on the action of the incorrect medication administered.
CN: Safe, effective care environment; CNS: Management of care; CL: Analyze

105. 3. Performing a procedure on a client without informed consent can be grounds for charges of assault and battery. Fraud means to cheat, and harassment means to annoy or disturb. Breach of confidentiality refers to conveying information about the client.
CN: Safe, effective care environment; CNS: Management of care; CL: Apply

106. 3. The nurse should focus on the client's diagnosis in a therapeutic manner. Asking "why" may make the client defensive and not open up to the nurse. Telling a client to "accept this" and "get it together" are not therapeutic.
CN: Psychosocial integrity; CNS: None; CL: Apply.

CN: Client needs category   CNS: Client needs subcategory   CL: Cognitive level

107. At 34 weeks' gestation, a baby is born to a client who is single and lives alone. Which intervention will the nurse include in the client's care plan?
1. Schedule a postpartum visit for 2 weeks.
2. Request a referral to the health department.
3. Consult with case management.
4. Have a home health nurse visit the day after discharge.

108. A client who just gave birth is concerned about the neonate's Apgar scores of 7 and 8. The client says she was told scores lower than 9 are associated with learning difficulties later in life. Which response by the nurse is **most** appropriate?
1. "You should not worry so much, your infant is perfectly fine."
2. "You should ask about placing your infant in a follow-up diagnostic program."
3. "There are good special education programs available if your infant has issues."
4. "Apgar scores of 7 or above indicate your infant is transitioning well."

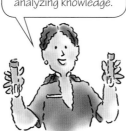

Don't think of this as a test … think of it as an experiment in applying and analyzing knowledge.

109. A primigravida at 25 weeks' gestation states she feels very anxious about not knowing what to expect during birth. Which intervention(s) by the nurse is **most** appropriate for this client? Select all that apply.
1. Provide information on labor and the birthing process.
2. Give the client a tour of the birthing unit.
3. Encourage the client to attend childbirth classes.
4. Have a 1-day postpartum woman talk with the client.
5. Ask the client if she has any questions regarding labor.

110. The nurse notes the fetal monitor strip exhibit below while caring for a 39-week-gestation client. Which action(s) by the nurse is appropriate? Select all that apply.

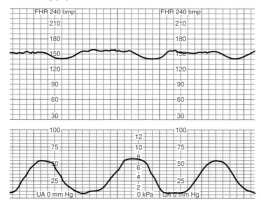

1. Place the client in the left lateral position.
2. Continue to monitor.
3. Increase the IV flow rate.
4. Apply oxygen.
5. Administer betamethasone.
6. Notify the health care provider.

CN: Client needs category   CNS: Client needs subcategory   CL: Cognitive level

107. 3. Because of the client's potential need for support and the premature condition of the neonate, a case manager consultation is appropriate. The case manager will determine if any referrals are needed. The mother has no physical indications for an early postpartum visit or need for a home visit.
CN: Safe, effective care environment; CNS: Management of care; CL: Analyze

108. 4. Apgar scores do not indicate future learning difficulties; they provide rapid assessment of the need for resuscitation. Apgar scores of 7 and 8 are normal and do not indicate a need for intervention. It is inappropriate to simply tell a client not to worry. There is no indication that follow-up and special education programs are needed.
CN: Health promotion and maintenance; CNS: None; CL: Apply

109. 1, 2, 3, 5. The nurse would attempt to relieve the client's anxiety by providing insight into the labor and birth process. Taking a tour of the unit, childbirth classes, and exploring the client's questions are all great ways to alleviate fears of the unknown. Talking with a hospitalized client is not appropriate.
CN: Health promotion and maintenance; CNS: None; CL: Apply

110. 1, 2, 3, 4, 6. Late decelerations indicate uteroplacental circulatory insufficiency and can lead to fetal hypoxia and acidosis if the underlying cause is not corrected. The client should be turned onto her side to increase placental perfusion and decrease contraction frequency. In addition, the IV fluid rate would be increased, and oxygen administered. The health care provider should be notified, and the nurse will continue to monitor the client and fetus. Betamethasone, a steroid, is given to preterm women to hasten fetal lung maturity.
CN: Physiological integrity; CNS: Reduction of risk potential; CL: Analyze

111. A client at 9 weeks' gestation reports always being tired. Which response by the nurse is **best**?
1. "Needs for rest and sleep typically increase during the first trimester of pregnancy."
2. "I will inform the health care provider to determine if you need additional testing."
3. "Did you stop drinking caffeine when you found out you were pregnant?"
4. "It is totally normal to feel tired and exhausted throughout your entire pregnancy."

111. 1. The nurse should allay the client's fears by informing her that needs for sleep and rest normally increase during the first trimester. The nurse should encourage the client to rest whenever possible. No follow-up testing is necessary since feeling tired during the first trimester of pregnancy is a normal occurrence. Asking "yes/no" questions is not therapeutic and limits gained insight. It is best to provide an explanation for the occurrence and not just state that it is normal.
CN: Physiological integrity; CNS: Basic care and comfort; CL: Apply

112. A parent is planning to enroll the 9-month-old infant in a daycare facility. The parent asks the nurse how to tell if a facility practices good infection control measures. Which information will the nurse include in the response? Select all that apply.
1. The facility keeps boxes of gloves in the director's office.
2. Soiled diapers are discarded in covered receptacles.
3. Toys are kept on the floor for the children to share.
4. Disposable papers are used on the diaper-changing surfaces.
5. Facilities for hand hygiene are located in every classroom.
6. Soiled clothing and cloth diapers are sent home in labeled paper bags.

112. 2, 4, 5. A parent can assess infection control practices by appraising steps taken by the facility to prevent the spread of disease. Placing soiled diapers in covered receptacles, covering the diaper-changing surfaces with disposable papers, and ensuring that hand sanitizers and sinks are available for personnel to wash their hands after activities are all indicators that infection control measures are being followed. Gloves should be readily available to personnel and, therefore, should be kept in every room—not in an office. Toys typically are shared by numerous children; however, this contributes to the spread of germs and infections. All soiled clothing and cloth diapers should be placed in a sealed plastic bag before being sent home.
CN: Safe, effective care environment; CNS: Safety and infection control; CL: Apply

113. A postpartum client tells the nurse she has not had a bowel movement in 3 days. Which action by the nurse is **most** appropriate?
1. Increase fluid intake.
2. Implement bed rest.
3. Add high-protein foods to her diet.
4. Manual removal of impacted stool.

113. 1. If a postpartum client has constipation, the nurse should recommend she drink plenty of fluids (1 to 2 qt [1 to 2 L] daily to replace fluids lost during labor and birth) and eat more *high-fiber* foods (such as fresh fruits and vegetables, bran, and prunes) to promote peristalsis. Activity and exercise also aid peristalsis. Bed rest decreases peristalsis. A high-protein diet will not help constipation. Manual removal of impacted stool is not required as there is no indication of impaction.
CN: Physiological integrity; CNS: Basic care and comfort; CL: Apply

114. A client received a new prescription for oral contraceptives. When providing education, which finding(s) will the nurse inform the client to report to the health care provider? Select all that apply.
1. Breast tenderness
2. Breakthrough bleeding within 3 months of use
3. Decreased menstrual flow
4. Blurred vision
5. Headache
6. Calf pain

114. 4, 5, 6. Some adverse effects of birth control pills, such as blurred vision and headaches, and pain in the calf with dorsiflexion of the foot, require a report to the health care provider. Because these effects in particular may result in cardiovascular compromise and embolus, the client may need to use another form of birth control. Breast tenderness, breakthrough bleeding, and decreased menstrual flow may occur as a normal response to the use of birth control pills.
CN: Physiological integrity; CNS: Pharmacological and parenteral therapies; CL: Apply

115. The nurse is monitoring the contractions of a client in the first stage of labor and notes increased bloody show. What will the nurse do **next**?
1. Notify the health care provider.
2. Continue to monitor the client.
3. Assess the client's cervix.
4. Insert an internal fetal scalp electrode.

116. The parent of a 3-day-old breastfed infant states the infant has had two recent diapers that contained a lot of loose, yellowish stool. Which response by the nurse is **best**?
1. "It is normal for breastfed infants to pass three or more loose, yellow stools per day."
2. "Please save the next diaper so the nurses can examine the stools."
3. "New parents tend to worry too much. Infants have frequent stools."
4. "Eliminating dairy products from your diet can help clear this up."

117. A client comes to the office for a routine prenatal visit. After reading the chart exhibit noted below, the nurse will prepare the client for which test?

Progress notes	
8/17 1520	Client is 11 weeks' pregnant; urine sample shows glycosuria. Client has a family history of diabetes.
	—June Gibson, RN

1. Maternal serum alpha fetoprotein
2. Indirect Coombs' test
3. Glucose tolerance test
4. Amniocentesis

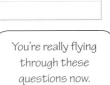

You're really flying through these questions now. Great job!

118. A client tells the nurse, "I do not want to sign the hepatitis B vaccination consent form because I heard that vaccinations can cause autism." Which nursing intervention is **most** appropriate?
1. Tell the client that such information has not been substantiated.
2. Support the client's decision because all vaccines have associated risks.
3. Encourage the client to discuss the issue with the health care provider.
4. Discuss the purpose of the vaccine and provide the vaccine information sheet.

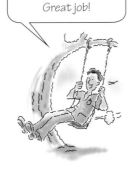

115. 2. The nurse will continue to monitor the client. Increased bloody show is an expected finding, indicating cervical dilation. The health care provider should not be notified. The nurse does not need to assess the cervix because the client is in early labor and frequent cervical assessment increases risk for infection. A fetal scalp electrode is not indicated because there are no signs of fetal distress.
CN: Health promotion and maintenance; CNS: None; CL: Apply

116. 1. Infants usually pass two to three stools daily, more if they are breastfed. By day 4, the stool of the bottle-fed infant is pasty and pungent; breastfed infants have stools that are sweet-smelling, loose, and yellow. It is not necessary for the mother to save the diaper to allow the nurses to assess the stool. Stating that new parents tend to worry too much is condescending. The mother should be instructed to report frequent, watery stools. Eliminating dairy products from the mother's diet will not change the quality of the infant's stools.
CN: Physiological integrity; CNS: Basic care and comfort; CL: Apply

117. 3. A glucose tolerance test is recommended to screen for gestational diabetes if the client is obese, has glycosuria, has a family history of diabetes, has lost a fetus for unexplained reasons, or has given birth to a large-for-gestational-age neonate. A maternal serum alpha fetoprotein tests for chromosomal abnormalities and spina bifida. The indirect Coombs' test screens maternal blood for red blood cell antibodies. Amniocentesis is used to detect fetal abnormalities.
CN: Physiological integrity; CNS: Reduction of risk potential; CL: Apply

118. 4. There are many misconceptions about vaccine safety and complications. The nurse should provide information about why the vaccine is given, the benefits and risks, and common adverse reactions. Health care providers provide a vaccine information sheet with all required information about the vaccine because informed consent requires full disclosure of available information. If the client still refuses after full disclosure, the nurse needs to support and document the decision. It is a nursing responsibility to complete client education first, then refer the client with additional questions and concerns to the health care provider.
CN: Safe, effective care environment; CNS: Management of care; CL: Apply

119. The nurse is providing education on how to perform perineal care to a postpartum client. Which activity indicates the client understands proper perineal care?
1. Using the peri-bottle bottle to clean the perineum after using the bathroom
2. Wiping the perineum from back to front after using the bathroom
3. Spraying water from peri-bottle into the vagina
4. Changing perineal pads every 8 hours

120. A neonate begins to gag and turns a dusky color. What will the nurse do **first**?
1. Alternate performing five chest thrusts and five back blows.
2. Notify the health care provider.
3. Provide oxygen via a facemask.
4. Suction the mouth then nose with a bulb syringe.

121. Just after birth, the nurse notes a neonate's axillary temperature is 94.1 °F (34.5 °C), pulse is 155 beats/minute, and respiratory rate is 58 breaths/minute. What will the nurse do **next**?
1. Place the neonate in a radiant warmer.
2. Obtain the neonate's blood pressure.
3. Assess the neonate for respiratory distress.
4. Place the neonate and mother skin-to-skin.

122. The nurse is assessing a 1-day-old neonate. Which finding(s) indicates possible asphyxia in utero? Select all that apply.
1. Grasps the nurse's finger when put in the palm of the neonate's hand
2. Stepping movements when held upright with the sole of the foot touching a surface
3. Toes do not curl downward when the soles of the feet are touched
4. The neonate does not respond when the nurse claps hands
5. Turning toward the nurse's finger when touching the cheek
6. The neonate displays weak, ineffective sucking

119. 1. Cleaning with a peri-bottle (squirt or spray bottle) should be performed after each voiding or bowel movement. The perineum should be cleaned from front to back, to avoid contamination from the rectal area. To keep the perineum clean, perineal pads must be changed when they are soiled. Water from the perineal irrigation bottle is not sterile and should never be directed into the vagina.
CN: Physiological integrity; CNS: Basic care and comfort; CL: Apply

120. 4. The nurse's first action should be to clear the neonate's airway with a bulb syringe. Chest thrusts and back blows are used when the infant is choking on a foreign object. After the airway is clear and the neonate's color improves, the nurse should comfort and calm the neonate. If the problem recurs or the neonate's color does not improve readily, the nurse should notify the health care provider. Administering oxygen when the airway is not clear would be ineffective.
CN: Physiological integrity; CNS: Reduction of risk potential; CL: Apply

121. 1. A neonate with a temperature of 94.1 °F (34.5 °C) is experiencing cold stress. The nurse must correct cold stress by placing the neonate under a radiant warmer. The nurse should rewarm the neonate gradually, observing closely and checking vital signs every 15 to 30 minutes. Obtaining a blood pressure or assessing for respiratory distress is not priority for this infant. While skin-to-skin contact does increase an infant's temperature, this infant is too cold for skin-to-skin contact.
CN: Safe, effective care environment; CNS: safety and infection control; CL: Apply

122. 3, 4, 6. Perinatal asphyxia is an insult to the fetus or newborn due to the lack of oxygen. If the neonate's toes do not curl downward when the soles of the feet are touched and the neonate does not respond to a loud sound, neurologic damage from asphyxia may have occurred. A normal neurologic response would be the downward curling of the toes when touched and extension of the arms and legs in response to a loud noise. Weak, ineffective sucking is another sign of neurologic damage. A neonate should grasp a person's finger when it is placed in the palm of the neonate's hand, do stepping movements when held upright with the sole of the foot touching a surface, and turn toward the nurse's finger when touching the cheek.
CN: Health promotion and maintenance; CNS: None; CL: Apply

123. Which nursing intervention is **priority** when caring for a neonate immediately after birth?
1. Completing a head-to-toe assessment
2. Giving the initial bath
3. Administering a vitamin K injection
4. Covering the neonate's head with a cap

124. The nurse is planning to administer erythromycin ointment to a neonate. Place the steps in the chronological order the nurse will compete them when administering erythromycin to the newborn's eyes. Use all options.

1. Gently raise the neonate's upper eyelid with the index finger and pull the lower eyelid down with the thumb.
2. Wash hands and put on gloves.
3. Close and manipulate the eyelids to spread the medication over the eye.
4. Shield the neonate's eyes from direct light and tilt the head slightly to the side that will receive the treatment.
5. Instill the ointment in the lower conjunctival sac.
6. Repeat the procedure for the other eye.

125. The nurse is caring for a neonate born at 38 weeks' gestation to a client with poorly controlled gestational diabetes. Which nursing intervention is **priority** for the infant during the first 24 hours of life?
1. Administer insulin subcutaneously.
2. Administer a bolus of dextrose IV.
3. Provide frequent feedings.
4. Monitor glucose levels.

123. 4. Covering the neonate's head with a cap helps prevent cold stress caused by excessive evaporative heat loss from the neonate's wet head. Initial baths are not given until the neonate's temperature stabilizes. A complete head-to-toe assessment should be completed within 2 hours of birth. Vitamin K can be administered within 4 hours after birth.

CN: Health promotion and maintenance; CNS: None; CL: Analyze

124. Ordered Response:

2. Wash hands and put on gloves.
4. Shield the neonate's eyes from direct light and tilt the head slightly to the side that will receive the treatment.
1. Gently raise the neonate's upper eyelid with the index finger and pull the lower eyelid down with the thumb.
5. Instill the ointment in the lower conjunctival sac.
3. Close and manipulate the eyelids to spread the medication over the eye.
6. Repeat the procedure for the other eye.

Ophthalmia neonatorum prophylaxis involves the instillation of 0.5% erythromycin or 1% tetracycline ointment into a neonate's eyes. This procedure is performed to prevent gonorrheal and chlamydial conjunctivitis, as well as to decrease the risk of permanent eye damage and blindness.

CN: Physiological integrity; CNS: Pharmacological and parenteral therapies; CL: Apply

125. 3. The neonate of a mother with gestational diabetes may be slightly hyperglycemic immediately after birth because of the high glucose levels that cross the placenta from mother to fetus. During pregnancy, the fetal pancreas secretes increased levels of insulin in response to this increased glucose amount that crosses the placenta from the mother. However, during the first 24 hours of life, this combination of high insulin production in the neonate coupled with the loss of maternal glucose can cause severe hypoglycemia. Frequent, early feedings given orally can prevent hypoglycemia. Insulin should not be administered because the neonate of a mother with gestational diabetes is at risk for hypoglycemia. A bolus of dextrose given IV may cause rebound hypoglycemia. If dextrose is given IV, it should be administered as a continuous infusion. Glucose levels should be monitored to determine if hypoglycemia is occurring; however, prevention is best and limits complications.

CN: Physiological integrity; CNS: Reduction of risk potential; CL: Apply

CN: Client needs category   CNS: Client needs subcategory   CL: Cognitive level

126. The nurse is moving a heavy object in a client's room. Which technique will the nurse use?
1. Bend from the waist.
2. Pull rather than pushing.
3. Stretch to reach an object.
4. Use large muscles in the legs for leverage.

127. A 36-year-old client reports dyspareunia to the nurse. Which statement by the client is **most** concerning to the nurse?
1. "I had sex a couple of times when I was 17."
2. "When I was 19 I had a spontaneous abortion."
3. "My second pregnancy was complicated with eclampsia."
4. "I had a human papillomavirus infection at age 32."

128. A 6-year-old child is newly diagnosed with type 1 diabetes. The nurse is preparing to provide education to the child and family. Which factor will the nurse consider when preparing education?
1. Another child with diabetes can educate the client
2. The child can educate the parents after the nurse educates the child
3. The child and parents should be educated together
4. Education should be directed to the parents, who then can educate the child

129. After delivering a neonate with a cleft palate and lip, the mother has minimal contact with the neonate and asks the nurse to provide most of the neonate's care. What is the **best** response by the nurse?
1. "You cannot stop caring for the child because of a deformity."
2. "I will take care of your baby while in the hospital, but it will be your job at home."
3. "I know you are nervous about caring for your baby. Let us go over some of the care."
4. "Do you have anyone that can take care of the baby for you while you are at home?"

130. The registered nurse (RN) and assistive personnel (AP) are caring for an older adult client who had a stroke and is paraplegic. Which task will the RN delegate to the AP?
1. Assess the client's emotional well-being.
2. Place the client on a cardiac monitor.
3. Give the client an aspirin.
4. Turn the client every 2 hours.

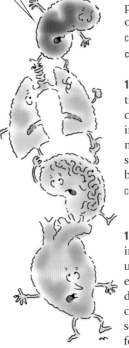

Keeping the whole body in balance can be challenging. Each system affects all the others.

126. **4.** Keeping the back straight and using the large muscles in the legs will help prevent back injury as the back muscles are relatively small compared with the larger muscles of the thighs. Bending from the waist can stress the back muscles, causing a potential injury. Pulling is not the best option and may cause straining. When feasible, an object should be pushed rather than pulled. Stretching to reach an object increases the risk of injury.
CN: Safe, effective care environment; CNS: Safety and infection control; CL: Understand

127. **4.** Like other viral and bacterial venereal infections, human papillomavirus is a risk factor for cervical cancer. Other risk factors for this disease include frequent sexual intercourse before age 16, multiple sex partners, and multiple pregnancies. A spontaneous abortion and pregnancy complicated by eclampsia are not risk factors for cervical cancer.
CN: Health promotion and maintenance; CNS: None; CL: Apply

128. **3.** The parents and child should participate in the nurse's education together to ensure an understanding and that the child has adult caregivers who are knowledgeable. Another child with diabetes should not be entrusted to educate this child, although that input would be valuable. The school-age child should not be the sole teacher for the parents. Parents should be included in the education plan but should not be responsible for educating their child.
CN: Health promotion and maintenance; CNS: None; CL: Apply

129. **3.** Talking to the mother in a nonjudgmental manner and making sure she understands that the nurse will help her with care during the hospital stay are therapeutic responses. Telling the mother that she cannot stop caring for the child is nontherapeutic and is giving advice. Taking over the care of the child while hospitalized and not allowing the mother to perform any care will not allow the nursing staff to determine if the child is being released into a safe home environment. Asking the client if someone else can perform the care is nontherapeutic and infers that the mother should not care for the child.
CN: Health promotion and maintenance; CNS: None; CL: Apply

130. **4.** The RN would delegate turning the client. Immobility can lead to severe physiologic problems such as skin breakdown, pressure injuries, pneumonia, and urinary tract infections. Therefore, frequent turning helps to minimize the effects of immobility. It is not appropriate for the RN to delegate assessing, medication administration, or placing the client on a cardiac monitor (which requires assessment to apply).
CN: Physiological integrity; CNS: Basic care and comfort; CL: Analyze

131. A client at 14 weeks' gestation tells the nurse, "I cannot believe I have mixed feelings about being pregnant. I tried for years to become pregnant." Which response by the nurse is **best**?
1. "You need to talk to your health care provider about these feelings."
2. "You are experiencing the normal ambivalence pregnant mothers feel."
3. "These feelings are expected in women who have had a spontaneous abortion."
4. "I am going to make you an appointment with a counselor to discuss your feelings."

131. 2. Conflicting, ambivalent feelings regarding pregnancy are normal for pregnant women. These feelings do not call for counseling or other professional interventions. Ambivalence is felt by most pregnant women, not exclusively mothers who had difficulty becoming pregnant.
CN: Psychosocial integrity; CNS: None; CL: Apply

132. A client with terminal cancer tells the nurse, "I have given up. I have no hope left. I am ready to die." Which response by the nurse is **most** therapeutic?
1. "You have given up hope?"
2. "You need to talk to a social worker."
3. "Do not let cancer win."
4. "There are cures for cancer found every day."

132. 1. The use of reflection invites the client to talk more about concerns. Deferring the conversation to a social worker or health care provider closes the conversation. Telling the client that cures for cancer are found every day gives false hope.
CN: Psychosocial integrity; CNS: None; CL: Apply

133. Three days after discharge, a client bottle-feeding her neonate calls the postpartum floor to ask what she can do for breast engorgement. Which instruction(s) by the nurse is **most** appropriate? Select all that apply.
1. "Wear a supportive bra during the day and night."
2. "Get under a warm shower and let the water flow on your breasts."
3. "Apply ice packs to your breast for 15 minutes at a time."
4. "Limit fluid intake because it contributes to breast engorgement."
5. "Contact your health care provider; you should not be engorged this late."

133. 1, 3. A supportive bra or breast binder is recommended for the client who is bottle-feeding her neonate to reduce engorgement. A warm shower will stimulate milk production; cold compresses may provide relief. It is normal to become engorged during the first few days after birth; drinking is not the cause. It is not necessary to contact the health care provider.
CN: Physiological integrity; CNS: Basic care and comfort; CL: Apply

134. A client with irritable bowel syndrome reports excessive flatulence. Which food(s) will the nurse recommend the client eat in moderation? Select all that apply.
1. Cauliflower
2. Lentil
3. Soybeans
4. Chickpeas
5. Cabbage
6. Milk
7. Onions

134. 1, 2, 3, 4, 5, 6, 7. All of the foods listed are common causes of flatulence.
CN: Physiological integrity; CNS: Basic care and comfort; CL: Apply

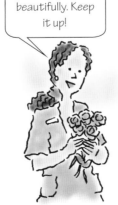

You're doing beautifully. Keep it up!

135. The registered nurse (RN) is making rounds to ensure airborne precautions are being observed while caring for clients with measles. Which action by the licensed practical nurse (LPN) indicates to the RN that further education is needed?
1. The nurse double-bags respiratory secretions.
2. The nurse dons a surgical isolation mask to enter the client's room.
3. The nurse gathers disposable client care items.
4. The client's meals are served on disposable trays.

135. 2. When entering the room of a client with measles, the nurse should wear an N95 particulate respirator mask because surgical isolation masks allow particles to pass through. All trash and waste should be disposed of as infectious waste, not just double-bagged. All client care items and meal trays should be disposable.
CN: Safe, effective care environment; CNS: Safety and infection control; CL: Apply

CN: Client needs category   CNS: Client needs subcategory   CL: Cognitive level

136. While assessing a client who just gave birth, the nurse notes: blood pressure, 110/70 mm Hg; pulse, 60 beats/minute; respirations, 16 breaths/minute; lochia, moderate rubra; fundus one fingerbreadth above the umbilicus and deviated to the side; and no calf tenderness. Which nursing intervention is **priority**?
1. Document the findings.
2. Ask the client to void.
3. Reassess the fundus in 15 minutes.
4. Massage the fundus.

136. 2. Placement of the fundus above the umbilicus and deviated to the side is not a normal finding. It indicates a full bladder. The client should empty the bladder and be rechecked. Lochia flow and vital signs are normal.
CN: Physiological integrity; CNS: Reduction of risk potential; CL: Analyze

137. A 9-lb, 6-oz (4,250 g) neonate is born to a client with diabetes. The nurse will monitor the neonate **most** closely for which complication(s)? Select all that apply.
1. Hyperbilirubinemia
2. Hypoglycemia
3. Caudal regression syndrome
4. Hypothermia
5. Polycythemia

137. 2, 3. Neonates of mothers with diabetes and large neonates are at risk for hypoglycemia related to increased production of insulin by the neonate in utero. Caudal regression syndrome (hypoplasia of lower extremities) occurs almost exclusively in neonates of mothers with diabetes. Hyperbilirubinemia, hypothermia, and polycythemia are not expected complications for this neonate. If the neonate becomes hypoglycemic, the client will then be at a higher risk for hypothermia.
CN: Physiological integrity; CNS: Reduction of risk potential; CL: Apply

138. The nurse is caring for a laboring client at 42 weeks' gestation who gained 6.6 lb (3 kg) during pregnancy. The nurse will anticipate caring for which complication(s)? Select all that apply.
1. Maternal hypoglycemia
2. A prolonged labor
3. Small-for-gestational-age neonate
4. Gestational hypertension
5. Cold stress in the neonate
6. Meconium aspiration in the neonate

138. 3, 5, 6. Women with limited weight gain are at higher risk for delivering low-birth-weight neonates. SGA and post-term neonates are at risk for cold stress due to a lack of brown fat. Post-term neonates are also at increased risk to release meconium, leading to aspiration. Weight is not associated with preventing a difficult birth, risk of gestational hypertension, or maternal hypoglycemia (which is a risk factor for neonatal hypoglycemia).
CN: Physiological integrity; CNS: Reduction of risk potential; CL: Analyze

139. The assistive personnel (AP) is preparing to bathe a client hospitalized for emphysema. Which action(s) will cause the registered nurse (RN) to intervene? Select all that apply.
1. Removing the oxygen and proceeding with the bath
2. Increasing the flow of oxygen to 6 L/minute by nasal cannula
3. Keeping the head of the bed slightly elevated during the bath
4. Placing the client supine to roll from side to side during the bath
5. Closing the door to the client's room while giving the client a bath

139. 1, 2, 4. The RN will intervene if the AP removes or adjusts the client's oxygen; this is beyond the AP's scope of practice. The elasticity of the lungs is lost for clients with emphysema. Therefore, these clients cannot tolerate lying flat because the abdominal organs compress the lungs making it appropriate to slightly elevate the head of the bed. The AP should provide privacy.
CN: Physiological integrity; CNS: Physiological adaptation; CL: Analyze

140. While removing a client's indwelling urinary catheter, the nurse gently pulls on the catheter after emptying the balloon. Which action will the nurse take **next**?
1. Reinsert the urinary catheter.
2. Document removal of the catheter.
3. Monitor the client for hematuria.
4. Have the unit charge nurse assess the client.

140. 2. The nurse would document the procedure. The nurse's action was appropriate; therefore, no additional intervention is needed.
CN: Safe, effective care environment; CNS: Safety and infection control; CL: Apply

CN: Client needs category   CNS: Client needs subcategory   CL: Cognitive level

141. A client at 38 weeks' gestation begins to choke on her food while eating at a restaurant. The nurse notes the woman coughing and holding the throat. Which action will the nurse complete **first**?
1. Stand behind the woman and give chest thrusts.
2. Administer back thrusts to the woman.
3. Stay with the woman and encourage her to keep coughing.
4. Activate the emergency response system.

142. A client with alcohol use disorder is being discharged from a mental health facility. Which information will the nurse include in the client's discharge teaching?
1. Provide the client a referral to a nutritionist.
2. Tell the client weekly urine testing is needed.
3. Instruct the client to come to the clinic for daily therapy.
4. Encourage participation in an alcoholism support group.

143. While at the clinic, a client tells the nurse, "You know, I am scheduled to retire next month, and I am really having a hard time coping." Which nursing response is **most** appropriate?
1. "Let us talk about your feelings."
2. "Do you have to retire?"
3. "I cannot wait to retire!"
4. "Let's talk about all the free time you will have."

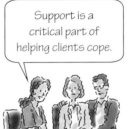

Support is a critical part of helping clients cope.

144. A client with a phobia is being treated with behavior modification therapy. The nurse will anticipate preparing the client for which treatment?
1. Dream analysis
2. Free association
3. Systematic desensitization
4. Electroconvulsive therapy (ECT)

145. A severely depressed client rarely leaves the chair. To prevent physiologic complications associated with psychomotor retardation, which nursing action is appropriate?
1. Restrict coffee from the client's diet.
2. Increase calcium and vitamin D intake.
3. Encourage resting in bed three times per day.
4. Have the client empty the bladder on a schedule.

146. During the termination phase of a therapeutic nurse–client relationship, which nursing intervention is **most** appropriate?
1. Tell the client there is no need for support groups now.
2. Address new issues with the client.
3. Review what has been accomplished during this relationship.
4. Avoid discussing the client's emotions.

141. 3. The nurse would stay with the woman and encourage her to continue coughing. If the woman was no longer about to cough or move air independently, the nurse would provide chest thrusts and activate the emergency response system as needed. Back thrusts are not done because they may dislodge the obstruction, further blocking the airway.
CN: Physiological integrity; CNS: Reduction of risk potential; CL: Analyze

142. 4. Support groups are essential for clients with alcohol use disorder after treatment. Membership is associated with relapse prevention. The client is probably experiencing nutritional deficits; however, a nutritionist is not required. The nurse can provide nutritional education. Weekly urine testing or day hospital treatment are not common.
CN: Safe, effective care environment; CNS: Management of care; CL: Apply

143. 1. The nurse would suspect the client is experiencing a maturational (developmental) crisis, which occurs at a predictable milestone during a life span, such as birth, marriage, or retirement. The nurse should talk to the client to determine the basis of the feelings to determine ways to facilitate coping with the life change, decrease anxiety, and determine if suicide is of concern.
CN: Health promotion and maintenance; CNS: None; CL: Apply

144. 3. Systematic desensitization is a behavior therapy used in the treatment of phobias. Dream analysis and free association are techniques used in psychoanalytic therapy. ECT is used with depression.
CN: Psychosocial integrity; CNS: None; CL: Understand

145. 4. To prevent bladder infections associated with stasis of urine, the client should be encouraged to routinely empty the bladder. Calcium, vitamin D, and coffee intake are not directly related to the psychological effects associated with this condition. Resting in bed is another form of psychomotor retardation.
CN: Health promotion and maintenance; CNS: None; CL: Apply

146. 3. Reviewing what has been accomplished is a goal of the termination phase of a therapeutic nurse-client relationship. It is appropriate to refer the client to support groups. During the termination phase, new issues should not be explored. Discussing the client's emotions during this phase is appropriate.
CN: Psychosocial integrity; CNS: None; CL: Apply

CN: Client needs category   CNS: Client needs subcategory   CL: Cognitive level

147. A hospitalized client becomes angry and belligerent toward the nurse after speaking on the phone with a friend. The nurse learns the friend cannot visit as expected. Which nursing intervention(s) is appropriate? Select all that apply.
1. Discuss the client's unmet needs.
2. Avoid the client until an apology is issued.
3. Suggest that the client direct the anger at the friend.
4. Invite the client to a quiet place to talk.
5. Help identify alternate ways of approaching the problem.

148. The nurse is caring for an 8-year-old child diagnosed with obsessive-compulsive disorder. Which behavior(s) will the nurse expect to assess when caring for this client? Select all that apply.
1. Checking and rechecking that the television is turned off before going to school
2. Repeatedly washing the hands before leaving the bathroom
3. Brushing teeth after each meal and snack throughout the day
4. Consistently climbing up and down a flight of stairs three times before leaving home
5. Feeding the dog the same meal every day at the same time
6. Wanting to play the same video game each night before taking a bath

149. The behavior of a client with borderline personality disorder causes the nurse to feel angry toward the client. Which nursing action is **most** appropriate?
1. Learn to ignore the client's frustrating behavior.
2. Have the client stay in their room until meal times.
3. Report personal feelings to the client's health care provider.
4. Tell the client how the behavior makes the nurse feel.

150. The nurse notes a client diagnosed with anxiety is having difficulty falling asleep. Which nursing intervention is **priority**?
1. Notify the client's primary health care provider.
2. Educate the client about relaxation techniques.
3. Allow the client to stay up and watch television.
4. Administer zolpidem 30 minutes before bed.

151. The nurse is caring for a client diagnosed with bipolar disorder receiving a maintenance dosage of lithium carbonate. The nurse notes the client is hyperactive and hyperverbal. Which nursing intervention is **most** appropriate?
1. Have the client sweep the floors on the unit.
2. Obtain lithium blood levels.
3. Send the client to a group therapy session.
4. Give the client a puzzle to work on.

147. 1, 4, 5. Feelings of displacement or directing anger toward the nurse need to be identified and understood by the client before the nurse can help guide the client to choose appropriate actions. Avoiding the client or having the anger directed at another person is inappropriate. Approaching the client in a calm manner and offering to assist in the problem-solving process allows the client to identify needs that are not being met and explore constructive ways of dealing with the anger.
CN: Psychosocial integrity; CNS: None; CL: Apply

148. 1, 2, 4. Compulsions involve symbolic rituals that relieve anxiety when they are performed. The disorder is caused by anxiety from obsessive thoughts, and acts are seen as irrational. Examples include repeatedly checking the television set, washing hands, or climbing stairs. An activity such as playing the same video game each night may be indicative of normal development for a school-age child. Frequent brushing of the teeth and feeding the dog a consistent meal are not abnormal actions.
CN: Psychosocial integrity; CNS: None; CL: Apply

149. 4. A nursing intervention used with personality disorders is to help the client recognize how one's behavior affects others. The nurse should tell the client the behavior is making the nurse angry. Ignoring the client, restricting the client, and reporting feelings to the health care provider are not therapeutic interventions.
CN: Psychosocial integrity; CNS: None; CL: Apply

150. 2. Relaxation techniques work very well with a client showing anxiety. If this does not help the client fall asleep, then pharmacologic interventions, diversion activities, and contacting the health care provider would be indicated.
CN: Psychosocial integrity; CNS: None; CL: Apply

151. 2. Hyperactive activity might indicate that the client's lithium levels are subtherapeutic; blood lithium levels will determine this. Providing distractions may be used after obtaining lithium levels.
CN: Physiological integrity; CNS: Pharmacological and parenteral therapies; CL: Analyze

CN: Client needs category   CNS: Client needs subcategory   CL: Cognitive level

152. A client with major depressive disorder has not responded to antidepressants. The nurse will plan to prepare the client for which intervention?
1. Electroconvulsive therapy (ECT)
2. Electroencephalography (EEG)
3. Electromyography (EMG)
4. Tranquilizer administration

152. 1. ECT is commonly used for treatment of major depressive disorder for clients who have not responded to antidepressants or who have medical problems that contraindicate the use of antidepressants. EEG is a tool used in the diagnosis and management of clients with anxiety, seizure disorder, sleep disorders, and degenerative disorders. EMG is used to assess muscles and the nerves that control them. Tranquilizers are used to treat schizophrenia or anxiety disorders.
CN: Physiological integrity; CNS: Physiological adaptation; CL: Understand

153. A client is receiving electroconvulsive therapy (ECT) for the treatment of major depressive disorder. Immediately following ECT, which nursing intervention is **priority**?
1. Assess the client's vital signs.
2. Let the client sleep undisturbed.
3. Allow the family to visit the client.
4. Darken the room for 1 hour.

Some treatments sound a lot worse than they actually are.

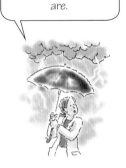

153. 1. Vital signs are monitored carefully for approximately 1 hour after ECT or until the client is stable. The client should not be restrained or left alone. Visitors should be allowed when the client is awake and alert. The room does not need to be darkened.
CN: Physiological integrity; CNS: Reduction of risk potential; CL: Apply

154. The nurse is looking at cardiac monitors from the nursing station and notes a client has a heart rate of 170 beats/minute with frequent premature ventricular contractions. Which action will the nursing take **first**?
1. Call the client's health care provider immediately.
2. Check the client and perform a full assessment.
3. Have an assistive personnel (AP) take the client's vital signs.
4. Obtain an electrolyte panel to review the client's potassium level.

154. 2. Because a change has occurred in the client's status, the nurse must assess the client first. This should not be delegated to the AP. Before the health care provider is notified or interventions are performed, a full assessment by the nurse must be made.
CN: Health promotion and maintenance; CNS: None; CL: Apply

155. The nurse is caring for a client that suddenly goes into cardiac arrest. Place the actions listed below in the ascending chronologic order the nurse will perform them. Use all options.

1.	Activate the emergency response system.
2.	Assess responsiveness.
3.	Call for a defibrillator.
4.	Provide two breaths.
5.	Assess pulse.
6.	Begin cycles of 30 compressions and 2 breaths.

155. Ordered Response:

2.	Assess responsiveness.
1.	Activate the emergency response system.
3.	Call for a defibrillator.
5.	Assess pulse.
4.	Provide two breaths.
6.	Begin cycles of 30 compressions and 2 breaths.

The nurse should first assess responsiveness. If the client is unresponsive, the nurse should activate the emergency response team and call for a defibrillator. Next, the nurse should assess the carotid pulse for no more than 10 seconds. If no pulse is present, the nurse should start cycles of 30 chest compressions and two breaths.
CN: Physiological integrity; CNS: Physiological adaptation; CL: Apply

156. A client on long-term mechanical ventilation tells the nurse, "I want the ventilator withdrawn." Which response by the nurse is **best**?
1. "Tell me how you are feeling."
2. "You need to talk to your family about this."
3. "Do you understand what that means?"
4. "You have been doing so well."

156. 1. Asking about the client's state of well-being is an open-ended response that encourages the client to express feelings. Asking if the client's family will agree with the decision is judgmental and inappropriate. Determining if the client understands the outcome of removing the ventilator is important; however, the nurse should explore the client's feelings and not ask a "yes/no" question. Telling the client, "You have been doing so well" to have the client continue the ventilator treatment is judgmental and dismisses the client's concerns.
CN: Safe, effective care environment; CNS: Management of care; CL: Apply

157. A client reports feelings of hopelessness, depression, poor appetite, insomnia, low self-esteem, and difficulty making decisions. The client tells the nurse the symptoms began at least 2 years ago and have been ongoing. The nurse suspects the client is suffering from which disorder?
1. Major depressive disorder
2. Dysthymic disorder
3. Cyclothymic disorder
4. Atypical affective disorder

157. 2. Dysthymic disorder is marked by feelings of depression lasting at least 2 years, accompanied by at least two of the following symptoms: sleep disturbance, appetite disturbance, low energy or fatigue, low self-esteem, poor concentration, difficulty making decisions, and hopelessness. Major depressive disorder is a recurring, persistent sadness or loss of interest or pleasure in almost all activities, with signs and symptoms recurring for at least 2 weeks. Cyclothymic disorder is a chronic mood disturbance of at least 2 years, marked by numerous periods of depression and hypomania. Manic signs and symptoms characterize atypical affective disorder.
CN: Psychosocial integrity; CNS: None; CL: Apply

158. The nurse is caring for a client who had abdominal surgery. When educating the client on coughing and deep breathing exercises, which information will the nurse include?
1. Sit upright, then splint the incision before coughing.
2. Splint the incision, take a deep breath, and then cough.
3. Lie prone, splint the incision, and then cough.
4. Lie supine, splint the incision, take a deep breath, and then cough.

158. 2. Splinting the incision with a pillow will protect the incision while the client coughs. Taking a deep breath will help open the alveoli, which promotes oxygen exchange and prevents atelectasis. Coughing and deep-breathing exercises are best accomplished in a sitting or semi-sitting position. Expectoration of secretions will be facilitated in a sitting position, as will splinting and taking deep breaths.
CN: Physiological integrity; CNS: Reduction of risk potential; CL: Apply

159. The health care provider prescribes a client 2 g cephalexin PO daily in equally divided doses of 500 mg each. How many times per day will the nurse administer this medication? Record your answer using a whole number.

_____ times per day

159. 4.

$$2\ g = 2{,}000\ mg$$

$$\frac{total\ daily\ dose}{amount\ per\ dose} = doses/day$$

$$\frac{2{,}000\ mg}{500\ mg} = 4\ doses/day$$

The nurse would administer the medication four times per day; 500 mg every 6 hours.
CN: Physiological integrity; CNS: Pharmacological and parenteral therapies; CL: Apply

CN: Client needs category   CNS: Client needs subcategory   CL: Cognitive level

160. Which symptom(s) reported by an adolescent's parents suggest to the nurse the adolescent is taking amphetamine and dextroamphetamine? Select all that apply.
1. Restlessness
2. Tachycardia
3. Excessive perspiration
4. Talkativeness
5. Mood swings
6. Excessive nasal drainage

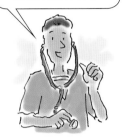

Remember that amphetamines are stimulants, and symptoms of use would reflect this.

160. 1, 2, 3, 4, 5. Amphetamine and dextroamphetamine are central nervous system stimulants. Symptoms of amphetamine use disorder include marked nervousness, restlessness, excitability, tachycardia, mood swings, talkativeness, and excessive perspiration.

CN: Health promotion and maintenance; CNS: None; CL: Analyze

161. The nurse is caring for an adult client receiving intravenous morphine sulfate for pain management. Which finding **most** concerns the nurse?
1. Voiding 350 mL of concentrated urine in 8 hours
2. Respiratory rate of 8 breaths/minute
3. Heart rate of 105 beats/minute
4. Pupils constricted and equal

161. 2. A respiratory rate of 8 breaths/minute is below normal and suggests respiratory depression, a common adverse effect of morphine. Voiding 350 mL of concentrated urine in 8 hours signals dehydration, and a heart rate of 105 beats/minute is slightly above normal for an adult and could be a result of pain. Constricted and equal pupils are an expected effect of opioids.

CN: Physiological integrity; CNS: Pharmacological and parenteral therapies; CL: Analyze

162. A client receiving chemotherapy is having difficulty deciding on a diversional activity due to decreased energy. Which statement by the client indicates to the nurse an understanding of appropriate activity options?
1. "I will play card games with my friends."
2. "I will take a long trip to visit my aunt."
3. "I will bowl with my team after discharge."
4. "I will eat lunch in a restaurant every day."

162. 1. During chemotherapy, playing cards is an appropriate diversional activity because it does not require a great deal of energy. To conserve energy, the client should avoid such activities as taking long trips, bowling, and eating in restaurants every day. However, the client may take occasional short trips and can dine out on special occasions.

CN: Physiological integrity; CNS: None; CL: Apply

163. The nurse is caring for a client who received chemotherapy 24 hours ago. Which precaution is necessary for the nurse to follow when caring for this client?
1. Wear sterile gloves before touching the client.
2. Place incontinence pads in the regular trash can in the client's room.
3. Wear personal protective equipment when handling blood, body fluids, or feces.
4. Have the client use a bedpan when needing to have a bowel movement.

163. 3. Chemotherapy drugs are present in the client's waste and body fluids for 48 hours after administration. The nurse should wear personal protective equipment, including a face shield, gown, and gloves when exposure to blood, body fluid, or feces is likely. Gloves alone offer minimal protection against exposure. Placing incontinence pads in the regular trash can and using a urinal or bed pan do not protect the nurse from exposure to chemotherapy drugs.

CN: Safe, effective care environment; CNS: Safety and infection control; CL: Apply

164. The registered nurse (RN) and assistive personnel (AP) are caring for a client who had a left modified radical mastectomy for breast cancer. Which action by the AP warrants intervening by the RN?
1. Assessing the blood pressure in the client's left arm
2. Having the client elevate the left arm as much as possible
3. Assisting the client while ambulating in the hallway
4. Assessing the client's temperature orally

164. 1. Lymphedema is a common postoperative adverse effect of modified radical mastectomy and lymph node dissection that occurs when lymph drainage is occluded, such as with blood pressure assessment. Elevation of the arm on the affected side will allow gravity to assist lymph drainage. It is appropriate for the AP to assist the client to ambulate and check temperatures orally in this client.

CN: Safe, effective care environment; CNS: Management of care; CL: Apply

165. The nurse is speaking to a group of high-risk women about the prevention of breast cancer. Which information will the nurse include in the teaching provided? Select all that apply.
1. Avoid smoking cigarettes.
2. Do not consume alcohol.
3. Remain physically active.
4. Breastfeed if possible.
5. Limit hormone therapy.

165. 1, 2, 3, 4, 5. There are steps women at high risk for breast cancer can take to decrease their chance of developing breast cancer. These steps include not smoking or drinking alcohol, being active and maintaining a healthy weight, breast-feeding children for as long as possible, limiting hormone therapy, and avoiding radiation exposure.
CN: Health promotion and maintenance; CNS: None; CL: Apply

166. The nurse is caring for a client admitted with rectal bleeding and suspected colorectal cancer. The nurse anticipates preparing the client for which diagnostic test?
1. Benzidine-based fecal occult blood test
2. Carcinoembryonic antigen (CEA)
3. Colonoscopy
4. Abdominal computed tomography (CT) scan

166. 3. Used to visualize the lower gastrointestinal tract, colonoscopy aids in detecting two-thirds of all colorectal cancers. Benzidine-based fecal occult blood test detects blood in the stool, which is a sign of colorectal cancer; however, the test does not confirm the diagnosis. CEA may be elevated in colorectal cancer but is not considered a confirming test. An abdominal CT scan is used to stage the presence of colorectal cancer.
CN: Health promotion and maintenance; CNS: None; CL: Apply

167. A client in the final stages of terminal cancer tells the nurse: "I wish I could just be allowed to die. I am tired of fighting this illness. I have lived a good life. I only continue my chemotherapy and radiation treatments because my family wants me to." What is the nurse's **best** response?
1. "Would you like to talk to a psychologist about your thoughts and feelings?"
2. "Would you like to talk to your minister about the significance of death?"
3. "Would you like to meet with your family and your health care provider together?"
4. "I know you are tired of fighting this illness, but death will come in due time."

167. 3. The nurse has a moral and professional responsibility to advocate for clients who experience decreased independence, loss of freedom of action, and interference with their ability to make autonomous choices. Coordinating a meeting between the health care provider and family members may give the client an opportunity to express his wishes and promote awareness of his feelings as well as influence future care decisions. All the other options are inappropriate.
CN: Psychosocial integrity; CNS: None; CL: Apply

168. A client with newly diagnosed testicular cancer asks the nurse, "Why me? I have always been a good person. What have I done to deserve this?" Which response by the nurse is **most** therapeutic?
1. "Do not worry. You will probably live longer than I will."
2. "I am sure a cure will be found soon."
3. "You seem upset. Let us talk about something happy."
4. "Would you like to talk about this?"

168. 4. Listening, responding quickly, and providing support promote therapeutic communication. Offering to talk about the client's feelings validates those feelings and allows the client to express them. Saying not to worry or that a cure will be found soon ignores the client's feelings. Saying "you seem upset" and then changing the subject identifies the client's feelings but does not follow through by exploring them.
CN: Psychosocial integrity; CNS: None; CL: Apply

169. The nurse is caring for a client currently experiencing pancytopenia. When reviewing the laboratory data, which value(s) does the nurse expect? Select all that apply.
1. White blood cell level 2000 μ/L (2×10^9/L)
2. Platelet level $100 \times 10^3/\mu$ L (100×10^9/L).
3. Red blood cell level $2.7 \times 10^3/\mu$ L (2.7×10^{12}/L
4. Hemoglobin 15.6 g/dL (156 g/L)
5. Hematocrit 46% (0.46)

169. 1, 2, 3. Pancytopenia is a deficiency of all blood cells, which includes a state of simultaneous leukopenia (decreased white blood cells), thrombocytopenia (decreased platelets), and anemia (decreased red blood cells). Pancytopenia has widespread effects on the body by leading to oxygen shortage and immune function. The hemoglobin and hematocrit levels are within normal limits.
CN: Physiological integrity; CNS: Physiological adaptation; CL: Analyze

CN: Client needs category   CNS: Client needs subcategory   CL: Cognitive level

170. A client tells the nurse, "I know that I am going to die." Which response by the nurse is **most** appropriate?
   1. "We have special equipment to monitor you."
   2. "We know what is wrong and you are not going to die."
   3. "Tell me why you think you are going to die."
   4. "Oh no, you are doing quite well considering your condition."

171. The pediatric nurse is working on the adult medical unit today. Which client will the charge nurse assign the pediatric nurse?
   1. A client diagnosed with congestive heart failure who has a heart rate of 125 beats/minute
   2. A client who had a laparoscopic appendectomy yesterday and is requesting pain medication
   3. A client newly diagnosed with type 1 diabetes whose glucose level is 375 mg/dL (20.81 mmol/L)
   4. A client experiencing intermittent chest pain scheduled to have a cardiac catheterization later today

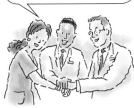

Health care is a team sport. Remember to communicate well with your teammates.

172. A client with acne vulgaris is seeking treatment. On which medication will the nurse anticipate educating the client?
   1. Minoxidil
   2. Tretinoin
   3. Zinc oxide gelatin
   4. Fluorouracil

173. A client has been admitted to the emergency department with severe right upper quadrant pain. Based on the data documented in the chart exhibit below, the nurse expects the client to have which diagnosis?

Progress notes	
6/10	Client admitted to the emergency department
0730	with severe right upper quadrant pain
	radiating to the back, nausea and
	vomiting, and fever. Laboratory results
	received via telephone as follows: glucose,
	462 mg/dL (25.6 mmol/L); white blood cells,
	14,000 cells/mm³ (14 × 10⁹ L); lipase, 214 u/L
	(3.57 μkat/L); and calcium, 6.5 mg/dL
	(1.63 mmol/L).
	—Sofia Nella, RN

   1. Peptic ulcer
   2. Crohn's disease
   3. Pancreatitis
   4. Irritable bowel syndrome

170. 3. A therapeutic approach would be to reflect on the client's comments, focusing on the specific words. Telling the client that special equipment is available, not to worry because nurses have training and knowledge to handle care, and that the client is doing quite well are nontherapeutic responses. Such statements offer false reassurance and ignore the client's needs.
CN: Psychosocial integrity; CNS: None; CL: Apply

171. 2. The pediatric nurse would be assigned a stable client, similar to clients the nurse normally cares for if possible. The charge nurse would assign the client who had an appendectomy yesterday (stable at this time) requesting pain medication. This is a common procedure performed on pediatric clients. The remaining clients are not stable.
CN: Safe, effective care environment; CNS: Management of care; CL: Analyze

172. 2. Tretinoin is a topical agent applied nightly to treat acne vulgaris. Minoxidil is used to promote hair growth. Zinc oxide gelatin is used for abrasions on the lower arms or legs; the affected area must be covered with a bandage for about 1 week. Fluorouracil is an antineoplastic topical agent used to treat superficial basal cell carcinoma.
CN: Physiological integrity; CNS: Pharmacological and parenteral therapies; CL: Understand

173. 3. The assessment findings combined with the laboratory results suggest pancreatitis. Signs and symptoms of pancreatitis include severe right upper quadrant pain, fever, nausea, and vomiting. Inflammation of the pancreas results in leukocytosis. Injured beta-cells are unable to produce insulin, leading to hyperglycemia, which may be as high as 500 to 900 mg/dL (22.75 to 49.95 mmol/L). Lipase and amylase levels become elevated as the pancreatic enzymes leak from injured pancreatic cells. Calcium becomes trapped as fat necrosis occurs, leading to hypocalcemia. Peptic ulcer, Crohn's disease, and irritable bowel syndrome do not cause amylase or lipase levels to increase.
CN: Physiological integrity; CNS: Reduction of risk potential; CL: Analyze

CN: Client needs category   CNS: Client needs subcategory   CL: Cognitive level

174. A client just diagnosed with terminal cancer is being transferred to home hospice care. The client's daughter tells the nurse, "I do not know what to say to my mother if she asks me if she is going to die." Which response(s) by the nurse is appropriate? Select all that apply.
1. "Tell your mother not to worry. She still has some time left."
2. "Let us talk about your mother's illness and how it will progress."
3. "You sound like you have questions about your mother dying."
4. "Do not worry, hospice will take care of your mother."
5. "Tell me how you are feeling about your mother dying."

174. 2, 3, 5. Talking about death is an uncomfortable situation. Conveying information clearly and openly can alleviate fears and strengthen the individual's sense of control. Encouraging verbalization of feelings helps build a therapeutic relationship based on trust and reduces anxiety. Advising the daughter not to worry, or having the daughter tell her mother that, ignores her feelings and discourages further communication.
CN: Psychosocial integrity; CNS: None; CL: Apply

175. The nurse notes a client's visitor looking at documentation for the client in the next bed. Which nursing action is **most** appropriate?
1. Notify hospital security.
2. Notify the charge nurse.
3. Move the documentation.
4. Tell the visitor to leave the room.

175. 2. The visitor was in violation of the other client's personal health information rights. Therefore, the nurse should notify the charge nurse of the breach in client confidentiality. The nurse should not call security. Moving the documentation or telling the visitor to leave is not appropriate.
CN: Safe, effective care environment; CNS: Management of care; CL: Analyze

176. The nurse is instructing a group of assistive personnel (AP) about client care. Which statement made by a AP concerns the nurse?
1. "I will turn clients who cannot turn themselves every 2 hours."
2. "I will cut food into small pieces for clients who have trouble chewing."
3. "I will provide 110°F (43.3°C) bath water for older adult clients."
4. "I will provide perineal care for clients while bathing or when the clients are soiled."

176. 3. Bath water should be about 102°F (39°C) to prevent burning an older adult client's skin. All other statements by the AP are appropriate.
CN: Safe, effective care environment; CNS: Management of care; CL: Apply

177. The nurse notes a rash on the chest and upper arms on a client during assessment. Which question(s) is appropriate for the nurse to ask this client? Select all that apply.
1. "When did the rash start?"
2. "Do you have any allergies?"
3. "How old are you?"
4. "What have you been using to treat the rash?"
5. "Have you recently traveled outside the country?"
6. "Do you smoke cigarettes or drink alcohol?"

177. 1, 2, 4, 5. The nurse should first find out when the rash began; this can assist with the correct diagnosis. The nurse should also ask about allergies; rashes can occur when a person changes medications, eats new foods, or contacts pollen. It is also important to find out how the client has been treating the rash; some topical ointments or oral medications may worsen it. The nurse should ask about recent travel; exposure to foreign foods and environments can cause a rash. The client's age, smoking, and drinking habits would not provide further insight into the rash or its cause.
CN: Physiological integrity; CNS: Physiological adaptation; CL: Analyze

CN: Client needs category   CNS: Client needs subcategory   CL: Cognitive level

178. The health care provider prescribes contact precautions for a client with a draining wound. Which action will the nurse take to initiate these precautions?
1. Pull the curtain to separate the client from the roommate.
2. Put a cart with gloves and gowns outside the client's room.
3. Place a box of masks outside the client's room.
4. Move the client to a negative pressure room.

179. The registered nurse (RN) and licensed practical nurse (LPN) are caring for a client. During assessment, the RN performs deep palpation. Which statement by the LPN indicates understanding of this assessment technique?
1. "Deep palpation is done to assess skin turgor."
2. "This technique is used to assess hydration."
3. "This allows the nurse to assess organs."
4. "Deep palpation assists in relaxing the client."

180. The nurse is caring for a client after surgical repair of a hip fracture. When preparing the client for discharge, which instruction(s) will the nurse include in the teaching? Select all that apply.
1. Do not flex the hip more than 90°.
2. Do not cross the legs.
3. Get help putting on shoes.
4. Keep feet flat on the floor.
5. Lean forward while sitting.

181. The nurse is caring for a client who is experiencing an exacerbation of gout. Which dietary modification(s) will the nurse instruct the client to follow? Select all that apply.
1. Eat a low-purine diet.
2. Limit fluid intake to no more than 1 L/day.
3. Eat a high-protein diet, with at least two servings of lean meat per day.
4. Eat a high-calcium diet.
5. Limit alcohol intake.

Remember to "select all that apply" in question #181.

182. A client at 32 weeks' gestation is admitted for prenatal testing. The client tells the nurse, "I am feeling a little faint." The nurse notes the client's skin is slightly diaphoretic to the touch. What will the nurse do **next**?
1. Turn the client to the left side.
2. Administer oxytocin intravenously.
3. Assess the client's blood pressure.
4. Monitor uterine contractions.

178. 2. Any type of transmission-based precaution requires that gloves be worn for client care, and a gown as well if soiling is possible. Placing an isolation cart outside the client's room makes isolation equipment readily available to those who must enter the client's room. Clients who require isolation precautions should be placed in a private room when possible. Masks or a negative pressure room are not required for clients on contact precautions.
CN: Safe, effective care environment; CNS: Safety and infection control; CL: Apply

179. 3. The purpose of deep palpation, in which the nurse indents the client's skin approximately 1.5 in (3.8 cm), is to assess underlying organs and structures, such as the kidneys and spleen. Skin turgor and hydration can be assessed using light touch or light palpation. This is not a relaxation technique.
CN: Health promotion and maintenance; CNS: None; CL: Understand

180. 1, 2, 3, 4. Discharge instructions should include not flexing the hip more than 90°, not crossing the legs, keeping feet flat on the floor, getting help to put on shoes, and sitting straight in a chair (at 90°). These restrictions prevent dislocation of the new prosthesis.
CN: Safe, effective care environment; CNS: Management of care; CL: Apply

181. 1, 5. Gout is characterized by an abnormal metabolism of uric acid. Individuals either produce too much uric acid or their body is unable to metabolize and excrete it. Purines are metabolized into uric acid. The client who suffers from gout should be placed on a low-purine diet with foods such as peanut butter, cherries, rice, pasta, fruits, and vegetables. Fluids do not have to be limited. A high-calcium diet will not affect the client. Alcohol intake should be limited as it is thought to trigger exacerbations.
CN: Physiological integrity; CNS: Basic care and comfort; CL: Apply

182. 1. The weight of the pregnant uterus is sufficiently heavy to compress the vena cava, which could impair blood flow to the uterus, possibly decreasing oxygen to the fetus. The client may experience supine hypotension syndrome (faintness, diaphoresis, and hypotension) from the pressure on the inferior vena cava. The side-lying position puts the weight of the fetus on the bed, not on the woman. It is not appropriate to administer oxytocin, assess blood pressure, or monitor contractions at this time, based on client findings.
CN: Physiological integrity; CNS: Reduction of risk potential; CL: Analyze

183. The nurse is caring for an older adult client with a cough. The client has a standing prescription for guaifenesin syrup 200 mg PO every 4 hours. The nurse has a dosage of 100 mg/5 mL. Mark on the medicine cup the amount of syrup the nurse will pour.

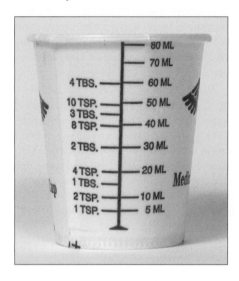

183. The correct formula to calculate a drug dosage is:

$$Dosage = \frac{Dose\ desired}{Dose\ on\ hand} \times Quantity$$

In this example, the equation is:

$$Dosage = \frac{200\ mg}{100\ mg} \times 5\ mL$$

$$Dosage = 10\ mL$$

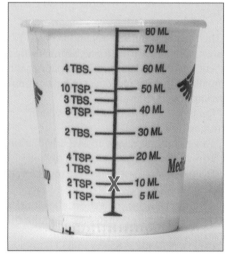

CN: Physiological integrity; CNS: Pharmacological and parenteral therapies; CL: Apply

---

184. The nurse is caring for a client in the fourth stage of labor. Based on the chart exhibit below, which postpartum complication does the nurse suspect the client has developed?

Progress notes	
7/30	Client's 24-hour blood loss is 600 mL. Uterus
1745	is soft and relaxed on palpation and client
	has a full bladder. Assisted client in emptying
	bladder and notified health care provider of
	findings. Vital signs stable at present.
	—Y. Jennings, RN

1. Postpartum hemorrhage
2. Puerperal infection
3. Deep vein thrombosis (DVT)
4. Mastitis

184. 1. Blood loss from the uterus that exceeds 500 mL in a 24-hour period is considered postpartum hemorrhage. If uterine atony is the cause, the uterus feels soft and relaxed. A full bladder can prevent the uterus from contracting completely, increasing the risk of hemorrhage. Puerperal infection is an infection of the uterus and structures above; its characteristic sign is fever. Two major types of DVT occur in the postpartum period: pelvic and femoral. Each has different signs and symptoms, but both occur later in the postpartum period (femoral, after 10 days' postpartum; pelvic, after 14 days). Mastitis is an inflammation of the mammary glands that disrupts normal lactation and usually develops 1 to 4 weeks' postpartum.

CN: Physiological integrity; CNS: Reduction of risk potential; CL: Analyze

Focus on the blood loss of "600 mL" and the uterus being "soft" in question #184.

185. A client has had an intravenous line in place for 3 days and begins to report discomfort at the insertion site. Based on the chart exhibit below, which nursing action is **priority**?

Progress notes	
3/11	IV site assessed and found to have
0730	blanching around the site, swelling, and
	coolness to the touch. Laboratory results:
	white blood cell count, 8500/µL (8.5 × 10⁹/L).
	—Keon Bradley, RN

   1. Remove the intravenous line.
   2. Notify the health care provider.
   3. Administer gentamicin.
   4. Apply an ice pack to the IV site.

186. The nurse is admitting a client with second-degree burns on the anterior and posterior portions of both legs. Based on the Rule of Nines, the nurse determines which percentage of the client's body is burned? Record your answer using a whole number.

_____ %

187. The nurse will expect which assessment finding(s) in a 9-month-old client? Select all that apply.
   1. Plays pat-a-cake
   2. Says "Dada" or "Mama"
   3. Walks independently
   4. Stands on tiptoes
   5. Builds a tower with blocks

185. 1. The assessment findings of pallor, swelling, skin that is cool to the touch at the IV insertion site, and a normal white blood cell count all indicate infiltration. The infusion should be discontinued and restarted in a different site. The nurse may apply ice to the site for discomfort, after removing the IV catheter.
CN: Physiological integrity; CNS: Physiological adaptation; CL: Analyze

186. 36.

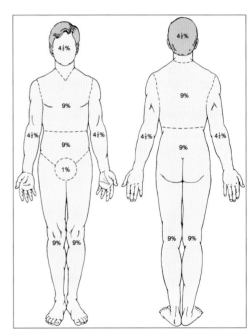

Using the Rule of Nines (see image), the anterior and posterior portions of one leg amount to 18%. Because both legs are burned, the total is 36%.
CN: Physiological integrity; CNS: Physiological adaptation; CL: Analyze

187. 1, 2. The nurse would expect a 9-month-old client to play pat-a-cake, say "dada" and/or "mama," respond to name, and may be beginning to pull up or stand alone. A toddler is expected to walk independently, stand on tiptoes, and build a block tower.
CN: Health promotion and maintenance; CNS: None; CL: Apply

188. The nurse is caring for an adolescent with diabetes brought to the emergency room with unusual behavior. The serum glucose level is 372 mg/dL (20.65 mmol/L). The health care provider prescribed the coverage schedule below:

150 to 200 mg/dL (8.32 to 11.1 mmol/L)—
  2 units of Humulin R
201 to 250 mg/dL (11.16 to 13.88 mmol/L)—
  4 units of Humulin R
251 to 300 mg/dL (13.93 to 16.65 mmol/L)—
  6 units of Humulin R
301 to 350 mg/dL (16.71 to 19.43 mmol/L)—
  8 units of Humulin R
351 to 399 mg/dL (19.48 to 22.14 mmol/L)—
  10 units of Humulin R
Over 400 mg/dL (22.2 mmol/L)—call the health care provider.
Mark the amount of insulin the nurse will draw into the insulin syringe.

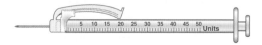

189. The nurse is caring for an infant who is irritable and has a high fever. Identify the **best** area for the nurse to palpate when assessing for increased intracranial pressure.

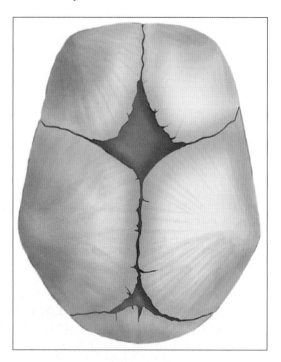

188. The adolescent's blood sugar is 372 mg/dL (20.65 mmol/L), thus falling within the 6-unit range. The nurse would draw up 6 units of Humulin R to administer.

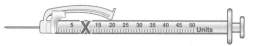

CN: Physiological integrity; CNS: Pharmacological and parenteral therapies; CL: Apply

189. The anterior fontanel is formed by the junction of the sagittal, frontal, and coronal sutures. It is shaped like a diamond and normally measures 4 to 5 cm at its widest point. The posterior fontanel closes during the first several months of life and the anterior fontanel closes around 2 years of age. A widened, bulging fontanel is a sign of increased intracranial pressure.

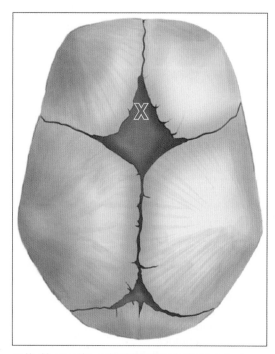

CN: Health promotion and maintenance; CNS: None; CL: Apply

CN: Client needs category   CNS: Client needs subcategory   CL: Cognitive level

190. The nurse is caring for a client who has been on prolonged bed rest. Based on the nursing documentation below, which procedure will the nurse implement **next**?

Progress notes	
2/19	Client instructed in contraction of back
1015	extensors, hip extensors, knee extensors,
	and ankle flexors and extensors. Client able
	to demonstrate correct technique without
	joint motion or muscle lengthening. Reports
	being p̄ a little tired s̄ after holding each
	contraction 5 seconds and repeating three
	times. Instructed to repeat exercises three
	times daily; client verbalized understanding
	of all information given.
	—Elana Lee, RN

1. Performing active range-of-motion exercises of the legs
2. Performing isometric exercises of the client's legs
3. Providing assistance walking the client to the bathroom
4. Performing passive range-of-motion exercises of the legs

190. **1.** Active range-of-motion exercises involve moving the client's joints through their full range of motion; they require some muscle strength and endurance. The client should have received passive range-of-motion exercises since admission to maintain joint flexibility and should have been taught isometric exercises to build strength and endurance for transfers and ambulation. Walking to the bathroom would be unsafe without the ability to first dangle the legs over the bedside and transfer from bed to chair.
CN: Physiological integrity; CNS: Reduction of risk potential; CL: Analyze

191. The nurse places electrodes on a collapsed client. The nurse notes the rhythm below.

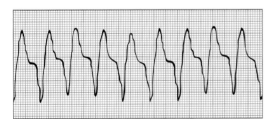

No pulse is noted. Which intervention will the nurse do **first**?
1. Apply oxygen to the client.
2. Perform a 12-lead electrocardiogram (ECG).
3. Begin chest compressions.
4. Prepare the client for cardioversion.

191. **4.** The rhythm the client is experiencing is ventricular tachycardia (VT). The nurse would anticipate the pulseless client in ventricular tachycardia needing cardioversion. The other options are incorrect.
CN: Physiological integrity; CNS: Reduction of risk potential; CL: Analyze

192. A client reports urinary frequency and burning. The primary health care provider diagnoses cystitis and prescribes sulfamethoxazole-trimoxazole. Which instruction will the nurse give the client?
1. "Expect your urine to be dark green in color for several days."
2. "Get some sun to help with vitamin D absorption."
3. "Discontinue the medication when your symptoms are gone."
4. "Take the medication with 6 to 8 oz (180 to 240 mL) of water."

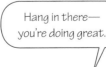
Hang in there— you're doing great.

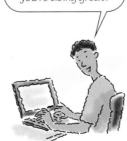

192. **4.** Adequate fluid intake is required with sulfa drugs to prevent crystalluria. The client's urine should not turn green from use of sulfamethoxazole-trimoxazole. The nurse should stress the importance of taking the entire prescription, warning that symptoms typically disappear before bacteria are eliminated from the system. The client should avoid prolonged sun exposure because sulfamethoxazole-trimoxazole may cause a photosensitivity reaction.
CN: Physiological integrity; CNS: Basic care and comfort; CL: Apply

CN: Client needs category   CNS: Client needs subcategory   CL: Cognitive level

193. At 0700, the nurse is assigned a client with an ascending colostomy. Which picture identifies the area where the nurse will assess the stoma?

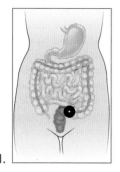
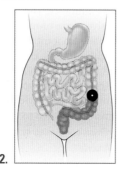

1.
2.

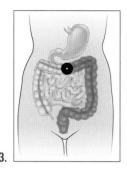
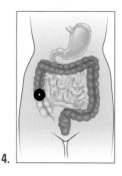

3.
4.

193. 4. A colostomy can be performed at any site of the colon. The location of an ascending colostomy is on the right side of the abdomen. An ostomy located in the ascending colon would likely produce continuous liquid output because feces in this section contain the most water and, therefore, have a liquid consistency. A sigmoid colostomy is located on the sigmoid colon and close to the location of a descending colostomy in the left side of the abdomen. The transverse colostomy is horizontal across middle abdomen or toward the right side of the body across the abdomen.

CN: Physiological integrity; CNS: Physiological adaptation; CL: Apply

194. The nurse is assessing a client with suspected right pyelonephritis. When teaching the client about the diagnosis, the nurse uses a diagram of the urinary structures. Mark the area the nurse will highlight as associated with the diagnosis.

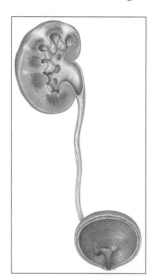

194. Pyelonephritis is a type of urinary tract infection that affects one or both kidneys. Right pyelonephritis is on the right side of the client's body but would be documented on the left in the anatomical position. Bacteria and viruses can move to the kidneys from the bladder or can be carried from other body systems through the bloodstream causing the disease process.

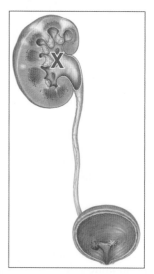

CN: Physiological integrity; CNS: Physiological adaptation; CL: Apply

195. The nurse assesses a client's lochia discharge on the first postpartum day and describes it in the chart exhibit noted below. What will the nurse do **next**?

Progress notes	
11/25	Perineal pad changed two times this shift
1645	for moderate amount of red discharge.
	—Alex Waters, RN

1. Perform fundal massage.
2. Administer oxytocin IM.
3. Assess the client's vital signs.
4. Document the findings.

195. 4. The nurse will document the expected findings. For the first 3 days after birth, the discharge is called lochia rubra. It consists almost entirely of blood, with only small particles of decidua and mucus. The other options are not appropriate for this client.

CN: Physiological integrity; CNS: Physiological adaptation; CL: Analyze

196. The clinic nurse is caring for a 12-year-old female client reporting dysuria. Which laboratory finding indicates to the nurse the client has a urinary tract infection?

Laboratory Results

Test: Urinalysis
Date: 12/15
Time collected: 1300

Parameter	Results
Color	Pale yellow
Turbidity	Clear
pH	7.8
Specific gravity	1.015
Protein	Negative
Glucose	Positive
Ketones	Positive
Red blood cells (RBCs)	<1 per high-power field
White blood cells (WBCs)	20 per high-power field
Casts	None

1. WBCs: 20 per high-power field
2. pH 7.8
3. Ketones: positive
4. Glucose: positive

Look for the result that is abnormal.

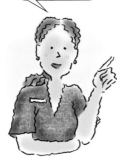

196. 1. A normal urinalysis would show less than 5 WBCs per high-power field. An elevated WBC count of 20 is an indication of bacteria and urinary tract infection. The normal range of urinary pH is 4.6 to 8.0. The presence of glucose or ketones in the urine does not indicate a urinary tract infection but may indicate diabetes mellitus.

CN: Physiological integrity; CNS: Reduction of risk potential; CL: Analyze

197. Which action will the nurse take when administering atenolol to a client for the first time?
1. Administer the medication to the client without explanation.
2. Inform the client of the new drug only if the client asks about it.
3. Inform the client of the new medication, its name, use, and the reason for the change.
4. Give it and tell the client the health care provider will explain the medication later.

197. 3. Informing the client about the medication, its use, and the reason for the change is important to the care of the client. Educating the client about the treatment regimen promotes compliance. The other responses are inappropriate.

CN: Safe, effective care environment; CNS: Safety and infection control; CL: Apply

CN: Client needs category   CNS: Client needs subcategory   CL: Cognitive level

198. A client exhibits signs of heightened anxiety. Which response by the nurse is **most** appropriate?
1. "I promise everything will be fine."
2. "Read this manual and let me know if you have questions."
3. "How about listening to the radio?"
4. "Let us talk about what is bothering you."

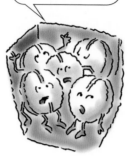

We hope the nurse's response gets us out of here and helping the client.

199. Which statement made by a client with a chlamydial infection indicates to the nurse the client understands potential complications?
1. "I am glad I am not pregnant; I would hate to have a malformed baby."
2. "I hope this medicine works before this disease destroys my kidneys."
3. "If I had known a diaphragm could cause this, I would have taken birth control pills."
4. "I need to treat this infection so it does not spread into my pelvis."

200. A client is injected with radiographic contrast medium and immediately shows signs of dyspnea, flushing, and pruritus. Which nursing intervention is **priority**?
1. Check the client's vital signs.
2. Assess breath sounds.
3. Apply a cold pack to the IV site.
4. Notify the code team.

201. A client is admitted to the medical-surgical unit with suspected acute myeloid leukemia. The nurse discusses the client's condition in the hallway. This action by the nurse jeopardizes which principle?
1. Plan of care
2. Client safety
3. Client's right to know
4. Confidentiality

202. The nurse is caring for a client with a postoperative wound evisceration. Which action will the nurse perform **first**?
1. Explain to the client what is happening and provide support.
2. Cover the protruding internal organs with moist, sterile gauze.
3. Place the client on nothing-by-mouth status.
4. Notify the health care provider of the finding.

198. 4. Anxiety may result from feelings of helplessness, isolation, or insecurity. This response helps reduce anxiety by encouraging the client to express feelings. The nurse should be supportive and develop goals together with the client to give the client some control over an anxiety-inducing situation. Because the other options ignore the client's feelings and block communication, they would not reduce anxiety.
CN: Psychosocial integrity; CNS: None; CL: Apply

199. 4. Chlamydia is a common cause of pelvic inflammatory disease and infertility. It does not affect the kidneys or cause birth defects. It can cause conjunctivitis and respiratory infection in neonates exposed to infected cervicovaginal secretions during birth. Use of a diaphragm is not a risk factor.
CN: Physiological integrity; CNS: Reduction of risk potential; CL: Apply

200. 2. The client is showing symptoms of an allergy to the iodine in the contrast medium. The first action is to make sure the client's airway is patent and breathing is effective. If compromised, call a cardiac arrest code. Checking vital signs and calling the code team are important nursing actions but not priority. A cold pack is not indicated.
CN: Physiological integrity; CNS: Physiological adaptation; CL: Analyze

201. 4. Discussing the client's condition in the hallway jeopardizes the client's right to confidentiality. This action should not jeopardize the plan of care. Statutory law and common law support the client's right to have information about his or her condition and treatment. Discussing the client's condition in the hallway does not jeopardize this right or client safety.
CN: Safe, effective care environment; CNS: Management of care; CL: Understand

202. 2. The nurse should first cover the wound with moistened gauze to prevent the organs from drying. Both the gauze and the saline solution must be sterile to reduce the risk of infection. The nurse should provide support that will reduce the client's anxiety, but covering the wound is the top priority. Evisceration requires emergency surgery; therefore, the nurse should place the client on nothing-by-mouth status and notify the health care provider immediately.
CN: Physiological integrity; CNS: Physiological adaptation; CL: Analyze

203. The clinic nurse is caring for a 12-year-old child with a diagnosis of eczema. Which nursing intervention(s) is appropriate for this child? Select all that apply.
1. Administer antibiotics as prescribed.
2. Give antifungals as prescribed.
3. Teach to take tepid baths.
4. Teach to use moisturizers immediately after bathing.
5. Discuss how to identify personal triggers.

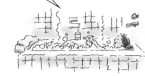

I'm glad I don't have eczema. I like my baths *hot*.

203. 3, 4, 5. Tepid baths and moisturizers are indicated for eczema to keep the infected areas clean and to minimize itching. The client needs to learn triggers to limit symptoms. Antibiotics are given only when superimposed infection occurs. Antifungals are not usually administered in the treatment of eczema. Hot baths can exacerbate the condition and increase itching.
CN: Physiological integrity; CNS: Physiological adaptation; CL: Apply

204. The nurse is caring for a wheelchair-bound client and notes the client has a ring pillow in the chair. Which nursing action is **priority**?
1. Instruct the client to remove the pillow.
2. Ask how long the client has been using a wheelchair.
3. Consult physical therapy for the client.
4. Request an egg crate mattress for the client.

204. 1. Rings or donuts are not to be used because they restrict circulation. It is not important for the nurse to determine how long a client has been in the wheelchair at this time. There is no provided information stating the client needs physical therapy or an egg mattress (prevent skin breakdown).
CN: Physiological integrity; CNS: Reduction of risk potential; CL: Apply

205. A client is prescribed clozapine 250 mg by mouth daily. How many tablets will the nurse administer when each tablet contains 100 mg? Record your answer using one decimal place.

_____ tablets

205. 2.5.
The correct formula to calculate a drug dosage is:

$$Dose\ on\ hand = \frac{Dose\ desired}{X}$$

In this example, the equation is:

$$100\ mg/tablet = \frac{250\ mg}{X}$$

$$X = 2.5\ tablets$$

CN: Physiological integrity; CNS: Pharmacological and parenteral therapies; CL: Apply

206. The nurse is caring for a client who had abdominal surgery and is reporting "gas pains." Which action by the nurse will **best** assist the client?
1. Encourage the client to ambulate.
2. Administer opioid analgesics.
3. Encourage the client to drink iced liquids.
4. Have the client turn to the right side.

206. 1. The nurse should encourage the client to ambulate to increase peristaltic movement of the bowel to alleviate gas and promote bowel function. Opioid analgesics often make the problem of gas worse by slowing motility. Hot liquids, not cold liquids, promote the elimination of gas. The client should lay on the left side to promote evacuation of gas.
CN: Physiological integrity; CNS: Reduction of risk potential; CL: Apply

207. The nurse monitoring a client's pulse notes it is easily palpable at 84 beats/minute and rhythmic. Which term will the nurse use in charting the pulse assessment?
1. Dysrhythmia
2. Bradycardia
3. Regular
4. Tachycardia

207. 3. The pulse is regular when it is rhythmic, easily palpable, and between the rate of 60 and 100 beats/minute. Tachycardia is a heart rate faster than 100 beats/minute. Dysrhythmia is a heart rate with either irregular rate or rhythm. Bradycardia is a heart rate slower than 60 beats/minute.
CN: Health promotion and maintenance; CNS: None; CL: Understand

CN: Client needs category   CNS: Client needs subcategory   CL: Cognitive level

208. The nurse is assessing a client's arterial pulses. Which graphic displays the site the nurse will use to palpate the client's dorsalis pedis pulse?

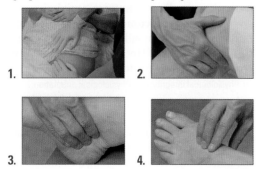

1. 2.

3. 4.

208. **4.** To palpate the dorsalis pedis pulse, the nurse places the fingers on the medial dorsum of the foot while the client points the toes down. The first graphic shows palpation of the femoral pulse, located along the crease midway between the pubic bone and the anterior iliac crest. The second graphic shows palpation of the popliteal pulse in the popliteal fossa of the back of the knee. The third graphic shows palpation of the posterior tibial pulse, slightly below the malleolus of the ankle.

CN: Health promotion and maintenance; CNS: None; CL: Apply

209. A client needs tracheal suctioning. Which nursing action(s) is correct when performing this procedure? Select all that apply.
1. Apply suction during insertion of the catheter.
2. Limit suctioning to 10 to 15 seconds duration.
3. Resterilize the suction catheter in alcohol after use.
4. Repeat suctioning intervals every 15 minutes until clear.
5. Oxygenate prior to suctioning.

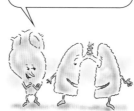

With his respiratory skills and my pumping power, our oxygen distribution system is second to none.

209. **2, 5.** The length of time a client should be able to tolerate the suction procedure is 10 to 15 seconds; any longer may cause hypoxia. Preoxygenation will help prevent hypoxia. Suctioning during insertion can cause trauma to the mucosa and removes oxygen from the respiratory tract. Suction catheters are disposed of after each use and are cleaned in normal saline solution after each pass. Suctioning, with supplemental oxygen between suctions, is performed in a minimum of 1-minute intervals to allow the client to rest.

CN: Physiological integrity; CNS: Physiological adaptation; CL: Apply

210. The nurse is preparing to insert a nasogastric tube. In which position will the nurse place the client in preparation for the procedure?
1. Fowler's
2. Prone
3. Side-lying
4. Supine

210. **1.** The upright Fowler's position is more natural for swallowing and protects against aspiration. Positioning the client on the back, stomach, or side places the client at risk for aspiration if the client should gag. It is also difficult to swallow in these positions.

CN: Physiological integrity; CNS: Basic care and comfort; CL: Understand

211. The nurse completes the intake and output record seen in the chart exhibit below for a client.

Intake	Output
4 oz of cranberry juice	1,300 mL of urine
½ cup of oatmeal	
2 slices of toast	
8 oz of black decaffeinated coffee	
tuna fish sandwich	
½ cup of fruit-flavored gelatin	
1 cup of cream of mushroom soup	
6 oz of 1% milk	
16 oz of water	

How many milliliters will the nurse document as the client's intake? Record the answer using a whole number.

_____ mL

211. **1,380.**
There are 30 mL in each ounce and 240 mL in each cup. The fluid intake for this client includes 4 oz (120 mL) of cranberry juice, 8 oz (240 mL) of coffee, ½ cup (120 mL) of fruit-flavored gelatin, 1 cup (240 mL) of cream of mushroom soup, 6 oz (180 mL) of milk, and 16 oz (480 mL) of water.

$$120\ mL + 240\ mL + 120\ mL + 240\ mL + 180\ mL + 480\ mL = 1,380\ mL$$

CN: Physiological integrity; CNS: Basic care and comfort; CL: Apply

212. The nurse is preparing to irrigate the right eye of a client who sustained a chemical burn in the eye. Which step(s) will the nurse use when performing the procedure? Select all that apply.
1. Tilt the client's head toward the left eye.
2. Place absorbent pads in the area of the client's shoulder.
3. Wash hands and put on gloves.
4. Place the irrigation syringe directly on the cornea.
5. Direct the solution onto the exposed conjunctival sac from the inner to outer canthus.
6. Irrigate the eye for 1 minute.

212. 2, 3, 5. The nurse should place absorbent pads on the client's shoulder area to prevent saturating the client's clothing and bed linens. The nurse should also wash his or her hands and put on gloves to reduce the transmission of microorganisms. The solution should be directed from the inner to outer canthus of the eye to prevent contamination of the unaffected eye. The head should be tilted toward the affected (right) eye to facilitate drainage and to prevent irrigating solution from entering the left eye. The irrigation syringe should be held about 1 in (2.5 cm) above the eye to prevent injury to the cornea. In a chemical exposure, the eye should be irrigated for at least 10 minutes.
CN: Physiological integrity; CNS: Reduction of risk potential; CL: Apply

213. The nurse is preparing to administer an iron dextran injection using the Z-track technique. Which diagram shows the correct technique the nurse will use when inserting the needle?

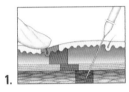
1.

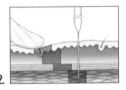
2.

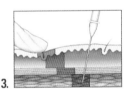
3.

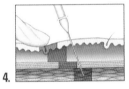
4.

213. 2. The correct Z-track technique shows the skin surface pulled about 0.5 in (1.25 cm) so the subcutaneous layers are moved out of alignment with the underlying muscle, allowing the needle to enter at a 90-degree angle. Option 1 is incorrect because the needle enters at a 45-degree angle. Option 3 is incorrect because the needle enters at a 60-degree angle. Option 4 is incorrect because the needle enters at a 120-degree angle.
CN: Physiological integrity; CNS: Pharmacological and parenteral therapies; CL: Apply

214. The nurse is caring for a client who sustained a severe burn to the face and neck. Which nursing intervention is **priority**?
1. Maintain a patent airway.
2. Start intravenous fluids.
3. Place ointment on the burned area.
4. Obtain data regarding the fire.

214. 1. The priority intervention in a client with a burned face and chest is to ensure the patency of the airway. The nurse should follow the ABCDE of care of a burned client. A is airway, B is breathing, C is circulation, D is disability, and E is expose and examine. Starting IV fluids would occur after patency of airway and breathing. Obtaining data would be part of the secondary survey. Ointment should not be applied to a burn until after being prescribed by the health care provider.
CN: Safe, effective care environment; CNS: Management of care; CL: Analyze

215. The nurse is caring for a 3-year-old client who sustained a buckle fracture of the radius after falling. Which nursing intervention is **priority**?
1. Assess the client's pain level.
2. Make the client NPO.
3. Prepare the client for a cast.
4. See if the client can move fingers.

215. 4. The nurse will first assess circulation by having the client move the fingers. The nurse would assess the client's pain after assessing circulation. Surgery is rarely needed for a buckle fracture; therefore, NPO status is not needed. The client will be placed in a sling or a cast for 3 to 4 weeks to heal.
CN: Safe, effective care environment; CNS: Management of care; CL: Apply

CN: Client needs category   CNS: Client needs subcategory   CL: Cognitive level

216. The nurse is caring for a client with peripheral vascular disease. When palpating for the dorsalis pedis pulse, where will the nurse place fingers for location of the pulse?

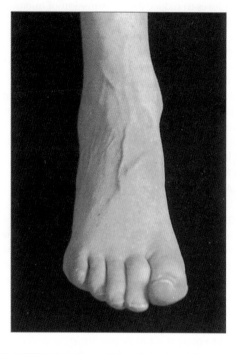

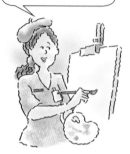

An eye for detail is a big asset in art and in test-taking.

216. The dorsalis pedis pulse is located on the dorsal surface of the foot.

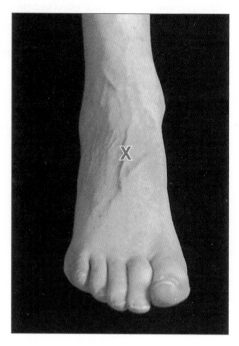

CN: Health promotion and maintenance; CNS: None; CL: Apply

217. While assessing a client, the nurse notes: temperature, 98.6°F (37°C); pulse, 80 beats/minute; and respirations, 30 breaths/minute. Which interpretation of these values does the nurse make?
1. Pulse is above normal range
2. Temperature is above normal range
3. Respirations are above normal range
4. Respirations and pulse are above normal range

217. 3. Normal vital signs for an adult client are: temperature, 96.6°F to 99°F (35.9°C to 37.2°C); pulse, 60 to 100 beats/minute; respirations, 16 to 20 breaths/minute.

CN: Health promotion and maintenance; CNS: None; CL: Apply

218. A client is scheduled for a surgical procedure for removal of a pancreatic tumor. The client tells the nurse, "I do not think I am going to live through the surgery. I am scared." What is the **best** response by the nurse?
1. "Well, it could happen. Not everyone makes it through surgery."
2. "If you feel like this, you should say goodbye to your family."
3. "Let us talk about your concerns and fears."
4. "When I had surgery, I felt the same way."

Best to keep an eye out for complications.

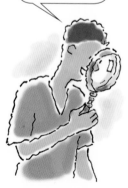

218. 3. The client is expressing concerns and fears related to having a serious surgical procedure; the most therapeutic response the nurse can give is to let the client know that she is not alone and someone is present to talk to about the feelings she is having. To tell the client that not everyone makes it through surgery is not addressing the fears that the client has and can make the anxiety about the procedure worse. Stating the client should say goodbye to her family also does not respond to the fears and lends finality to the situation. Discussing what the nurse felt when having surgery does not address the client's concern.

CN: Psychosocial integrity; CNS: None; CL: Apply

219. The nurse will teach the parents of a child with Kawasaki's disease the importance of keeping follow-up appointments to monitor and prevent which complication?
1. Encephalitis
2. Glomerulonephritis
3. Myocardial infarction
4. Idiopathic thrombocytopenic purpura (ITP)

219. 3. In Kawasaki's disease, inflammation of small and medium blood vessels can result in weakening of the vessels and aneurysm formation, especially in the heart. Blood flow through damaged vessels can cause thrombosis formation and myocardial infarction. Encephalitis, glomerulonephritis, and ITP are not associated with Kawasaki's disease.

CN: Health promotion and maintenance; CNS: None; CL: Apply

CN: Client needs category   CNS: Client needs subcategory   CL: Cognitive level

220. The nurse is working in the emergency room. Which client will the nurse assess **first**?
1. A 9-month-old infant with blood pressure 76/44 mm Hg, pulse 120 beats/minute, and respiratory rate 48 breaths/minute
2. A 5-year-old child with blood pressure 95/65 mm Hg, pulse 70 beats/minute, and respiratory rate 22 breaths/minute
3. A 10-year-old child with blood pressure 130/88 mm Hg, pulse 100 beats/minute, and respiratory rate 30 breaths/minute
4. A 30-year-old adult with blood pressure 114/78 mm Hg, pulse 80 beats/minute, and respiratory rate 15 breaths/minute

220. 3. The nurse will assess the 10-year-old client first because of the elevated blood pressure, pulse, and respiratory rate. All other clients' vital signs are within normal limits.
CN: Physiological integrity; CNS: Reduction of risk potential; CL: Analyze

221. The nurse is assessing a 1-day-old neonate and notes the skin and sclera appear yellow. Which action will the nurse complete **next**?
1. Place a biliblanket under the neonate.
2. Ensure the neonate is eating frequently.
3. Obtain the neonate's serum bilirubin level.
4. Review the prenatal history.

221. 3. The nurse will obtain a total bilirubin level to determine which course of action is needed, if any. Depending on the level, the neonate may need phototherapy with a biliblanket or bililight. Current recommendations are to begin phototherapy for levels at or above 15 mg/dL (257 mmol/L). Frequent feeding will assist with excreting excess bilirubin. The nurse should review the prenatal history when caring for a neonate; however, it is not needed at this time.
CN: Safe, effective care environment; CNS: Management of care; CL: Analyze

222. Which task will the registered nurse (RN) delegate to the assistive personnel (AP)?
1. Inserting an indwelling urinary catheter
2. Obtaining the first set of postoperative vital signs
3. Delivering meal trays to all clients on the unit
4. Giving subcutaneous insulin to a client

222. 3. The AP would be assigned to deliver trays to all clients on the unit. The RN cannot delegate sterile procedures, assessments (first set of postoperative vitals is an assessment of the client), or medication administration.
CN: Safe, effective care environment; CNS: Management of care; CL: Analyze

223. The nursery nurse notes greenish amniotic fluid while assisting with the birth of a neonate at 42 weeks' gestation. Which intervention will the nursery nurse perform **first**?
1. Auscultate lung bilaterally.
2. Check an axillary temperature.
3. Obtain the neonate's weight.
4. Perform an Apgar assessment.

223. 1. The nurse would first assess the neonate's airway and breathing by auscultating lungs, monitoring crying, and assessing for signs of respiratory distress (grunting, nasal flaring, retractions, tachypnea) due to suspicion of meconium aspiration syndrome. The nurse will check the temperature, obtain a weight, and complete an Apgar assessment; however, these are not priority over assessing airway and breathing.
CN: Safe, effective care environment; CNS: Management of care; CL: Analyze

224. The nurse is caring for a client recently diagnosed with congestive heart failure (CHF). Which finding will the nurse highlight for the health care provider to review?
1. Shortness of breath at night
2. Fatigue during the day
3. Nonpitting edema of the lower extremities
4. Reports of chest pain

224. 4. Chest pain should always be assessed by the health care provider. This can be an expected finding in CHF; however, complications such as myocardial infarction should be ruled out. All other symptoms are expected findings in a client with CHF.
CN: Physiological integrity; CNS: Reduction of risk potential; CL: Apply

CN: Client needs category   CNS: Client needs subcategory   CL: Cognitive level

225. Which neonate will the charge nurse assign to the licensed practical nurse (LPN)?
1. The neonate with a temperature 98.4°F (36.9°C), respirations 60 breaths/minute, and blood pressure 66/38 mm Hg
2. The neonate with a chest circumference 13 in (33 cm), heart rate 80 beats/minute, and weight 3,500 grams.
3. The neonate with a temperature 100.9°F (38.3°C), heart rate 112 beats/minute, and blood pressure 92/50 mm Hg.
4. The neonate with a head circumference 11 in (28 cm), length 17.7 in (45 cm), and weight 2,000 grams.

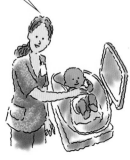

I enjoy working with neonates. Just be sure to measure them carefully.

226. While caring for a client diagnosed with congestive heart failure (CHF), the nurse will question which prescription from the health care provider?
1. Low sodium diet
2. 1,000 mL normal saline IV bolus
3. Furosemide orally
4. Influenza vaccine

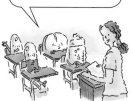

Medication education should include side effects, potential complications, and contraindications.

227. A 22-year-old client is prescribed desogestrel/ethinyl estradiol. On which potential complication(s) will the nurse educate the client? Select all that apply.
1. Rapid respirations
2. Difficulty walking
3. Iron deficiency anemia
4. Acne vulgaris
5. Blurred vision

228. Which finding will the nurse expect to assess in a small for gestational age (SGA) newborn?
1. Respiratory rate 22 breaths/minute
2. Hematocrit 78% (0.78)
3. Serum glucose 140 mg/dL (7.77 mmol/L)
4. Measured at 60th percentile for weight

229. A G1P0 client has been in active labor for 20 hours. The nurse performs a cervical assessment and determines the client is dilated to 4 cm/40% effaced/-3 station. The nurse will perform which intervention?
1. Insert an indwelling Foley catheter.
2. Prepare the client for a cesarean birth.
3. Intravenous oxytocin at 6 mU/minute.
4. Prepare the client for an amniotomy.

225. 1. The LPN should be given the most stable client. The neonate with no abnormal findings is most stable. Normal neonatal head circumference is 13 to 14 in (33 to 35.5 cm), chest circumference is 12 to 13 in (30.5 to 33 cm), length is 19 to 21 in (45 to 53 cm), weight is 2,500 to 4,000 g, temperature is 97.7°F to 99°F (36.5°C to 37.2°C), respirations are 30 to 60 breaths/minute, heart rate is 100 to 160 beats/minute, and blood pressure is 50 to 80 mm Hg systolic and 30 to 50 mm Hg diastolic.
CN: Physiological integrity; CNS: Reduction of risk potential; CL: Analyze

226. 2. CHF is a chronic condition where the heart is unable to effectively pump. The nurse would question giving this client an IV bolus because of the risk for fluid overload increasing symptoms. Clients may be placed on fluid restrictions. A low sodium diet and diuretics are recommended to limit fluid overload and edema. Influenza and pneumococcal vaccines are recommended to prevent infections which could exaggerate or worsen CHF.
CN: Physiological integrity; CNS: Reduction of risk potential; CL: Apply

227. 1, 2, 5. Potential complications include unusual bleeding, severe headache, dyspnea, changes in vision or coordination, and chest or leg pain. The nurse would inform the client to notify the health care provider if complications arise. Contraceptives can decrease anemia and acne.
CN: Physiological integrity; CNS: Pharmacological and parenteral therapies; CL: Apply

228. 2. The nurse would expect to assess an elevated hematocrit level due to presence of polycythemia. The nurse would not expect decreased respirations, hyperglycemia (would expect hypoglycemia), or normal weight. The expected percentile for weight would be below the 10th percentile.
CN: Physiological integrity; CNS: Reduction of risk potential; CL: Apply

229. 2. The nurse would anticipate the client undergoing a cesarean birth. The client has been in the active stage of labor for an extended time frame with minimal cervical change. No other intervention is appropriate for failure to progress.
CN: Health promotion and maintenance; CNS: None; CL: Analyze

230. A neonate is born at 41 weeks' gestation and weighs 2,250 g. The nurse determines the newborn's gestational size classification is small for gestational age (SGA). During the assessment, the nurse notes the following: red, ruddy skin color; blood pressure, 58/36 mm Hg; respiratory rate, 52 beats/minute; pulse, 148 beats/minute; axillary temperature, 97.9°F (36.6°C). Based on the assessment, which nursing action is **priority**?
1. Check rectal temperature.
2. Assess for hypoglycemia.
3. Notify the health care provider.
4. Obtain a hematocrit level.

231. The nurse is caring for a client diagnosed with acquired immunodeficiency syndrome (AIDS). Which finding will the nurse report to the health care provider **first**?
1. Dry cough
2. Watery diarrhea
3. Nausea
4. Sore throat

232. The nurse is caring for a client prescribed acetaminophen. Which finding warrants notification of the health care provider?
1. Takes one 500 mg tablet four times a day for pain
2. Takes the medication with milk
3. Has a rapid, weak pulse and dyspnea
4. Reports a cough for the past 2 days

233. The nurse determines a neonate's gestational size classification is average for gestational age. Which intervention will the nurse do **next**?
1. Obtain a glucose level.
2. Assess vital signs.
3. Document the finding.
4. Monitor for congenital anomalies.

234. A neonate born 3 days ago is experiencing tremors and difficulty feeding, and has a shrill, persistent cry. The serum glucose level is 90 mg/dL (5 mmol/L). The nurse will anticipate which prescription from the health care provider **first**?
1. Meconium drug toxicology screening
2. Insertion of a nasogastric tube
3. Methadone orally
4. Intravenous infusion of D10W

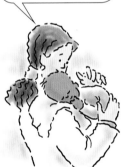

Feels about average. Then again, maybe I should use nursing science.

230. 4. Based on the findings, the nurse would assess the client for polycythemia (gestational age and red, ruddy skin). The vitals are within normal range. A rectal temperature is not needed. The client does not have signs of hypoglycemia. Assessments are needed before calling the health care provider.
CN: Safe, effective care environment; CNS: Management of care; CL: Analyze

231. 2. Each are expected findings in a client with AIDS. Watery diarrhea could lead to severe dehydration and needs immediate intervention as this would further compromise the client.
CN: Safe, effective care environment; CNS: Management of care; CL: Apply

232. 3. The nurse would report a rapid, weak pulse and dyspnea because these are signs of chronic overdose of acetaminophen. Taking 2000 mg per day for pain is acceptable. The medication can be taken with milk or food if gastrointestinal upset occurs. Reporting a cough for 2 days could indicate a multitude of conditions. This is too general to relate to acetaminophen overdosing.
CN: Physiological integrity; CNS: Pharmacological and parenteral therapies; CL: Apply

233. 3. The nurse will document the finding, because this is the expected finding in neonates and no complications are associated with average-for-gestational-size neonates. The other interventions are not necessary based on the gestational size classification.
CN: Health promotion and maintenance; CNS: None; CL: Apply

234. 1. The nurse would suspect the neonate is experiencing neonatal abstinence syndrome and would anticipate performing a drug screening. Meconium provides more detail regarding intrauterine drug exposure than a urine specimen. Once the underlying issue is determined, additional interventions may be prescribed, including assistive feeding and medication administration to combat withdraw effects.
CN: Safe, effective care environment; CNS: Management of care; CL: Analyze

235. The nurse is caring for a client reporting ringing in the ears and slow, difficult breathing. The client is taking ibuprofen and methotrexate for rheumatoid arthritis. Which prescription will the nurse complete **first**?
1. Giving intravenous fluids
2. Administering activated charcoal
3. Preparing for intubation
4. Performing urinalysis

236. A 36-hour postpartum client with a second-degree perineal laceration is experiencing perineal pain. Which nursing intervention(s) is appropriate for this client? Select all that apply.
1. Apply an ice pack to the client's perineum.
2. Give 600 mg ibuprofen every 8 hours PRN.
3. Administer 100 mg docusate BID.
4. Increase the client's intravenous fluid.
5. Apply a warm compress to the perineal area.

237. A client is admitted to the hospital with suspected bacterial meningitis. Which prescription will the nurse complete **first**?
1. Administer antibiotics as prescribed.
2. Send specimen to the laboratory for culture.
3. Monitor client for seizure activity.
4. Administer morphine as needed.

238. The nurse is preparing to perform fundal massage on a postpartum client. Place the steps for performing a fundal massage in the order the nurse will complete them. Use each option once.

1. Place the client in supine position.
2. Explain the procedure to the client.
3. Place one hand around the top of the fundus.
4. Place one hand on the abdomen just above the symphysis pubis.
5. Rotate the upper hand to massage the fundus.

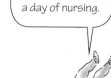
Yoga helps me calm up after a day of nursing.

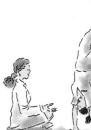

239. The clinic nurse is educating an older client diagnosed with shingles on acyclovir administration. Which statement by the client indicates the nurse's teaching is effective?
1. "I can crush the capsules and take with food."
2. "If I have a headache, I will immediately report it."
3. "I do not need to take this medication with food or water."
4. "My kidney function will need to be monitored."

235. 3. The nurse suspects the client is experiencing ibuprofen toxicity and would prepare the client for intubation first, due to the difficulty breathing. Activated charcoal would be administered. IV fluids are given, and renal function is monitored. Airway is priority.
CN: Physiological integrity; CNS: Pharmacological and parenteral therapies; CL: Apply

236. 2, 3, 5. The nurse would administer ibuprofen for inflammation and docusate to soften stools (limiting straining with bowel movements which increase pain). The nurse would also apply a warm compress or administer a sitz bath to promote healing. Ice is applied in the first 24 hours' postpartum to decrease inflammation. It is not appropriate to increase IV fluids for pain management.
CN: Health promotion and maintenance; CNS: None; CL: Apply

237. 2. First, the nurse would obtain and send a specimen for cultures. This should be done before administering antibiotics, which need to be given as soon as possible to limit symptoms and transmission to others. The nurse will monitor for seizures and administer pain medication as needed.
CN: Safe, effective care environment; CNS: Management of care; CL: Analyze

238. Ordered Response:
2. Explain the procedure to the client.
1. Place the client in supine position.
4. Place one hand on the abdomen just above the symphysis pubis.
3. Place one hand around the top of the fundus.
5. Rotate the upper hand to massage the fundus.
CN: Health promotion and maintenance; CNS: None; CL: Apply

239. 4. Acyclovir is an antiviral medication that can affect renal function. The capsules cannot be broken, crushed, or chewed. A headache is a common side effect that does not need to be reported unless headaches become chronic or debilitating. The client should take acyclovir with a full glass of water.
CN: Physiological integrity; CNS: Pharmacological and parenteral therapies; CL: Apply

240. The nurse is caring for four pediatric clients. Which client will the nurse assess **first**?
1. A 10-day-old client recently diagnosed with pulmonary stenosis with a systolic murmur
2. A 3-year-old client who had valve replacement surgery with a temperature of 102°F (38.9°C)
3. A 6-year-old client with tonsillitis scheduled to have surgery tomorrow who needs to void
4. A 4-year-old client, 1 day after tubal myringotomy surgery, with purulent tympanic drainage

241. The nursing team consists of a registered nurse (RN) and a licensed practical nurse (LPN). Which client will the RN assign to the LPN?
1. A 2-day-old client with a tracheoesophageal atresia scheduled for surgery today
2. A 10-month-old client who had a circumcision 3 days ago
3. A 13-year-old client newly admitted with respiratory rate 32 breaths/minute
4. A 17-year-old client admitted for diabetes experiencing fruity breath

242. The nurse is caring for an older adult client who had a left hip replacement yesterday. Which assessment finding **most** concerns the nurse?
1. Right calf tenderness
2. Decreased intake at meals
3. Pain 7 of 10 on numeric scale
4. Heart rate 75 beats/minute

243. A client is receiving magnesium sulfate intravenously to prevent seizure activity. Which nursing intervention is **priority**?
1. Have calcium gluconate readily available.
2. Monitor deep tendon reflexes.
3. Insert an indwelling urinary catheter.
4. Assess serum magnesium levels.

244. A client is prescribed nifedipine for hypertension and angina. Which information will the nurse include when educating the client about nifedipine administration? Select all that apply.
1. Do not drink grapefruit juice.
2. Avoid St. John's wort.
3. Monitor blood pressure.
4. Do not change positions quickly.
5. Do not suddenly stop taking medication.

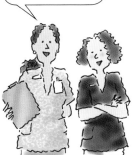

Teamwork helps us give all clients the care they need.

240. **2.** The nurse will assess the client with a fever first. This client is at increased risk of endocarditis and may need antibiotic therapy started. All other clients are stable with expected findings.
CN: Safe, effective care environment; CNS: Management of care; CL: Analyze

241. **2.** The LPN would be assigned the 3-day postoperative client with no complications listed. The RN would need to care for the remaining clients. The client scheduled for surgery will require education and frequent assessments after surgery. The newly admitted client will require education. The client with fruity breath is not stable.
CN: Safe, effective care environment; CNS: Management of care; CL: Analyze

242. **1.** The nurse would be most concerned about calf tenderness. This could indicate a deep vein thrombus (DVT) and requires immediate intervention. Decreased intake and pain need to be addressed; however, they are not priority over a potential DVT. The heart rate is within normal range.
CN: Physiological integrity; CNS: Reduction of risk potential; CL: Apply

243. **1.** It is priority for the nurse to have the antidote, calcium gluconate, readily available for toxicity. Toxicity can be life-threatening and requires immediate intervention. The nurse will monitor level of consciousness, respirations, reflexes, urinary output, and serum magnesium levels (therapeutic range is 5 to 8 mg/dL).
CN: Physiological integrity; CNS: Pharmacological and parenteral therapies; CL: Analyze

244. **1, 2, 3, 4, 5.** The nurse would include each option in the client's teaching. Taking nifedipine with grapefruit juice can cause hypotension. St. John's wort may decrease the effectiveness of nifedipine. The client's blood pressure should be monitored to assess effectiveness of dosage. Changing positions quickly can lead to orthostatic hypotension. Abruptly stopping can cause rebound angina.
CN: Physiological integrity; CNS: Pharmacological and parenteral therapies; CL: Apply

245. The nurse is caring for a client with celiac disease. Which meal will the nurse order this client for breakfast?
1. Scrambled eggs with cheese, orange slices, and fat-free milk
2. Bagel with cream cheese, bacon, and decaffeinated coffee
3. Boiled egg, sausage, blueberry muffin, and orange juice
4. Oatmeal with brown sugar, strawberry yogurt with granola, and whole milk

246. The nurse is caring for a client taking oral ketoconazole. Which assessment finding will the nurse **immediately** report the primary health care provider? Select all that apply.
1. Nausea
2. Left upper quadrant pain
3. Temperature 101.8°F (38.8°C)
4. Clay-colored stool
5. Increased appetite
6. Yellow sclera

247. A client prescribed fentanyl states, "I take phenelzine daily." Which nursing action is **most** appropriate?
1. Administer the fentanyl.
2. Notify the health care provider.
3. Monitor the client for constipation.
4. Document the client's home medications.

248. The nurse is caring for a client diagnosed with pneumonia. Which finding(s) will the nurse expect to assess in this client? Select all that apply.
1. Cough with phlegm
2. Skin breakdown
3. Bradycardia
4. Sharp chest pain
5. Dehydration.
6. Capillary refill less than 2 seconds.

249. The nurse is providing discharge education to a client with pneumonia. Which statement by the client indicates additional teaching is needed?
1. "I will take all of my antibiotic."
2. "I will continue to drink a lot."
3. "I will take acetaminophen for fever and pain."
4. "I can go back to work before my fever is gone."

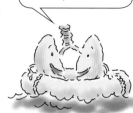

I hate pneumonia ... at least we have this inner tube to keep afloat.

245. 1. A client with celiac disease must follow a gluten-free diet. Gluten is found in wheat, rye, and barley. These are found in many pastas, noodles, breads, pastries, baked goods, crackers, cereals, granola, beers, thickened sauces and gravies, and any other food made with wheat flour. Eggs, non-processed meats, oatmeal, fruits, vegetables, beans, seeds, low-fat dairy, and nuts are naturally gluten free.
CN: Physiological integrity; CNS: Basic care and comfort; CL: Analyze

246. 1, 2, 3, 4, 6. Ketoconazole is an antifungal medication that should only be used when other antifungal medications cannot be used or are not effective because it can cause serious liver damage. The primary health care provider should be notified immediately for any signs of liver damage, which includes nausea, vomiting, jaundice, stomach pain, fever, fatigue, anorexia, dark urine, clay-colored stool, and elevated liver function tests.
CN: Physiological integrity; CNS: Pharmacological and parenteral therapies; CL: Apply

247. 2. The nurse would notify the health care provider. Phenelzine is a monoamine oxidase inhibitor (MAOI) and should not be taken with fentanyl to avoid complications such as serotonin syndrome. The nurse would not administer the medication. Constipation is a side effect of phenelzine; however, this is not priority. The nurse will document home medications in the medical record.
CN: Physiological integrity; CNS: Pharmacological and parenteral therapies; CL: Apply

248. 1, 4, 5. The nurse would expect the client to have a productive cough, fever, chills, difficulty breathing, pain (in chest from coughing), dehydration, fatigue, and tachycardia. Skin breakdown, bradycardia, and decrease capillary refill are not associated with pneumonia.
CN: Physiological integrity; CNS: Reduction of risk potential; CL: Apply

249. 4. The client should not return to work until the fever has subsided and cough is nonproductive. All other statements are correct.
CN: Physiological integrity; CNS: Reduction of risk potential; CL: Apply

250. The nurse is caring for a client prescribed ferrous sulfate. Which information will the nurse include when educating this client?
1. Take with meals.
2. Do not take with orange juice.
3. Crush and add to food.
4. Do not take with dairy.

251. Which client will the medical-surgical nurse assess **first**?
1. Client with pneumonia coughing up mucus
2. Client with nephrolithiasis reporting pain at 2 out of 10 on pain scale
3. Client whose chest pain was relieved by nitroglycerin
4. Client who had a cholecystectomy reporting bloody stool

252. The nurse is caring for a client who just had a laparoscopic cholecystectomy. Which finding will the nurse **immediately** report to the health care provider?
1. Pain rated a 6 of 10 on pain scale
2. Left calf swelling and warmth
3. Temperature 100.6°F (38.1°C)
4. 0.5-in (1.25-cm) bloody stain on adhesive dressing

253. The registered nurse (RN) and assistive personnel (AP) are caring for a client receiving magnesium sulfate. Which task will the RN delegate to the AP?
1. Document urine output.
2. Check reflexes.
3. Auscultate breath sounds.
4. Determine level of consciousness.

254. A child presents to the emergency department with a fractured tibia. During the assessment the child tells the nurse, "My mom pushed me down the stairs." Which nursing intervention is appropriate?
1. Ask the child to state what happened again in 1 hour.
2. Move the child to an undisclosed location in the hospital.
3. Restrict the parents from entering the child's room.
4. Document the subjective findings in the medical record.

255. The nurse is caring for a client in labor receiving oxytocin intravenously. Which finding will cause the nurse to stop the infusion?
1. Late fetal heart rate decelerations
2. Urine output 120 mL in 4 hours
3. Respiratory rate 20 breaths/minute
4. Uterine contractions every 4 minutes, lasting 45 seconds

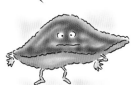

"Immediately" is another way asking about the top priority.

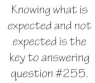

Knowing what is expected and not expected is the key to answering question #255.

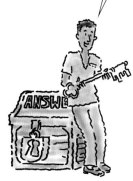

250. 4. The nurse will inform the client not to take ferrous sulfate with dairy products or antacids or to consume them within an hour of taking medication. For best absorption, ferrous sulfate should not be taken with meals and should be taken with orange juice or something acidic. It should not be crushed. CN: Physiological integrity; CNS: Pharmacological and parenteral therapies; CL: Apply

251. 4. The nurse would assess the client with bloody stool because this could indicate internal hemorrhage, a complication from surgery. The nurse would expect a productive cough with pneumonia, mild pain with nephrolithiasis indicates improvement, and relieved chest pain indicates effective treatment. CN: Safe, effective care environment; CNS: Management of care; CL: Analyze

252. 2. The nurse would immediately report signs of a deep vein thrombus to the health care provider. Pain is not a priority for this client. Increased temperature should be reported, but this is not priority over a DVT. Scant drainage is expected following surgical procedures. CN: Safe, effective care environment; CNS: Management of care; CL: Analyze

253. 1. The nurse would appropriately delegate documenting urine output to the AP. The AP cannot assess reflexes, breath sounds, or level of consciousness; each requires nursing judgment. CN: Safe, effective care environment; CNS: Management of care; CL: Analyze

254. 4. The nurse will document subject findings and client statements in the record. The nurse does not need to repeatedly ask the child what happened. This could lead to mistrust from the child. The nurse cannot hide the child or restrict the parents from entering the child's room. CN: Psychosocial integrity; CNS: None; CL: Apply

255. 1. The nurse would stop the transfusion if late decelerations were noted because this indicates placental insufficiency. All other findings are within normal range for a laboring client. CN: Physiological integrity; CNS: Pharmacological and parenteral therapies; CL: Analyze

CN: Client needs category   CNS: Client needs subcategory   CL: Cognitive level

256. The nurse is caring for a pediatric client receiving digoxin. Which finding(s) will the nurse report to the health care provider? Select all that apply.
1. Nausea
2. Vomiting
3. Diarrhea
4. Double vision
5. Heart rate 45 beats/minute

256. 1, 2, 3, 4, 5. The nurse would report all the listed findings. Nausea, vomiting, diarrhea, and visual disturbances indicate toxicity. A heart rate less than 60 beats/minute warrants holding the medication, and the health care provider should be notified.
CN: Physiological integrity; CNS: Pharmacological and parenteral therapies; CL: Apply

257. The nurse is educating a client diagnosed with asthma on albuterol inhaler usage. Which statement by the client indicates additional teaching is needed?
1. "This medication will help me breath better."
2. "I will shake my inhaler before each use."
3. "The effects of this medication last 30 minutes."
4. "I should keep my inhaler with me at all times."

257. 3. Additional teaching is needed if the client states the effects last 30 minutes. The effects generally last 4 to 6 hours. All other statements regarding albuterol inhaler usage are correct.
CN: Physiological integrity; CNS: Pharmacological and parenteral therapies; CL: Apply

258. The nurse observes the neonate feeding, as shown in the image below. Which action will the nurse perform **next**?

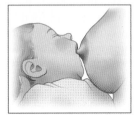

1. Educate the mother on how to remove the neonate from the breast.
2. Ask the mother if she wants to continue breastfeeding.
3. Provide encouragement for the mother to continue breastfeeding.
4. Listen to determine if any audible swallowing or gulping can be heard.

258. 1. The nurse will educate the mother on removing the neonate to limit nipple trauma. The neonate is not properly latched to the breast. The bottom lip is turned inward and should be flanged outward. The nurse would not allow the mother to continue feeding the neonate, provide encouragement to continue, or listen for swallowing because allowing the neonate to stay latched will lead to breast tissue trauma.
CN: Health promotion and maintenance; CNS: None; CL: Apply

259. The nurse is caring for a client diagnosed with an autoimmune disorder who is prescribed oral prednisone. Which statement by the client indicates additional teaching is needed?
1. "If this medicine makes me feel bad, I will stop taking it."
2. "It is okay if I take prednisone with food or milk."
3. "This medication makes me at more risk to get sick."
4. "I may have an increased appetite while taking prednisone."

259. 1. Prednisone should not be abruptly stopped or the client could experience withdrawal symptoms (severe fatigue, aches, nausea, lightheadedness). All other statements regarding prednisone are correct.
CN: Physiological integrity; CNS: Pharmacological and parenteral therapies; CL: Apply

260. The registered nurse (RN) and assistive personnel (AP) are providing client care. Which task will the RN delegate to the AP?
1. Selecting a meal for a client with phenylketonuria (PKU)
2. Assisting a client with influenza to the bathroom
3. Placing a client with epiglottitis on precautions
4. Giving an enema to a client with rectal prolapse

260. 2. The RN would delegate assisting the client to the bathroom. Clients with PKU must limit the intake of phenylalanine, which requires proper understanding of amounts in various foods. Education is needed when placing a client on precautions. The client with a rectal prolapse would require assessment.
CN: Safe and effective care environment; CNS: Management of care; CL: Analyze

CN: Client needs category   CNS: Client needs subcategory   CL: Cognitive level

261. A 9-year-old client with hemophilia presents with hematuria, bruising, and joint pain that started suddenly after falling on the playground. Which nursing action is **priority**?
1. Administer desmopressin.
2. Administer fresh frozen plasma.
3. Auscultate the lung sounds.
4. Place the child on fall precautions.

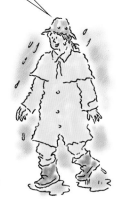

An injury can be like a rainfall for clients with hemophilia.

261. 2. The nurse will first administer plasma to the client with hemophilia experiencing active bleeding. Hemophilia is a disorder of the blood-clotting system. The plasma will allow the child the ability to clot. Desmopressin is a synthetic hormone that stimulates the body to release clotting factors. This method is not as quick acting as administering plasma. The nurse would assess the child and place the child on fall precautions after bleeding is controlled.
CN: Safe, effective care environment; CNS: Management of care; CL: Analyze

262. Which child will the pediatric charge nurse assign to the licensed practical nurse (LPN)?
1. A child with hyperthyroidism who has a thyroxine (T4) level of 10 µg/dL (128.7 nmol/L)
2. A child with phenylketonuria who has a serum phenylalanine level of 11 mg/dL (666 µmol/L)
3. A child whose white blood cell (WBC) count is 28,000 mm³ (28 × 10⁹/L) and platelets 31,000 mm³ (31,000 × 10⁹/L)
4. A child whose serum glucose is 456 mg/dL (25.31 mmol/L) with pH, 7.30; CO₂, 35 mEq/L (35 mmol/L); HCO₃⁻, 20 mEq/L (20 mmol/L); PaO₂, 78 mm Hg (10.37 kPa)

262. 1. The charge nurse will assign the most stable client to the LPN. The child with hyperthyroidism has a normal T4 level. All other clients are unstable. The phenylalanine level is elevated, indicating problems with the child's diet that need to be addressed. The WBC count is greatly elevated and platelet level seriously low, placing the child at risk for bleeding. The glucose level is elevated, and the child is experiencing metabolic acidosis.
CN: Safe, effective care environment; CNS: Management of care; CL: Analyze

263. The nurse is caring for a 4-year-old child with gastroenteritis who has a history of sickle cell disease. During assessment the nurse notes: temperature, 97.7°F (36.5°C); heart rate, 124 beats/minute; respiratory rate, 25 breaths/minute; blood pressure, 70/40 mm Hg; and pale skin. Which action will the nurse complete **first**?
1. Administer morphine sulfate.
2. Provide oxygen via a facemask.
3. Initiate IV access and give fluids.
4. Cover the child with warm blankets.

263. 3. The nurse recognizes the client is dehydrated and would first administer fluids to restore what has been lost and attempt to prevent a sickle cell crisis. There is no indication that the child is in pain. The child's respirations are on the high end of normal and no other signs of distress are noted. The child's temperature does not warrant a warm blanket.
CN: Safe, effective care environment; CNS: Management of care; CL: Analyze

264. Which client with diabetes will the pediatric nurse assess **first**?
1. A preschooler whose glucose level is 90 mg/dL (5 mmol/L)
2. An adolescent eating pepperoni pizza and cake for lunch
3. A school-aged client needing education on a new insulin pump
4. A toddler who just received aspart insulin and is refusing to eat

264. 4. The nurse will assess the child who received aspart insulin (fast-acting) and is refusing to eat. This child is at great risk for developing hypoglycemia. A glucose level of 90 mg/dL (5 mmol/L) is within normal range. The adolescent needs education on proper diet, but this is not priority. The school-aged child needs education on a new pump, but this is not priority over preventing hypoglycemia.
CN: Safe, effective care environment; CNS: Management of care; CL: Analyze

265. The nurse is caring for a client with phenylketonuria (PKU). Which meal will the nurse order for this client?
1. Strawberry and almond salad, buttered toast, and fat-free milk
2. Ham and cheese sandwich, potato chips, applesauce, and tea
3. Egg salad sandwich, corn, beef jerky strip, and grape juice
4. Salad, pear and mango slices, carrot sticks, watermelon, and apple juice

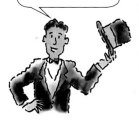

Bon travail! You are ready for the NCLEX-RN.

265. 4. The best meal for a client with PKU is low in phenylalanine. Foods low in phenylalanine include fruits, select vegetables, juices, and low-protein breads and pastas. Foods highest in phenylalanine are protein-rich foods such as milk, ham, eggs, steak, pork chops, cheese, and peanut butter.
CN: Physiological integrity; CNS: Basic care and comfort; CL: Analyze

CN: Client needs category   CNS: Client needs subcategory   CL: Cognitive level

Credits

Chapter 1

Hot spot sample   Surface Anatomy Photography Collection.

Chapter 3

Question 38:   Weber, J., Kelley, J. *Health Assessment in Nursing,* 2nd ed. Philadelphia: Wolters Kluwer, 2003.

Question 121:   Adapted from Timby, B.K. *Fundamental Nursing Skills and Concepts,* 10th ed. Philadelphia: Wolters Kluwer, 2012.

Chapter 5

Question 128:   Adapted from Moore, K.L., Dalley, A.F., Agur, A.M.R. *Clinically Oriented Anatomy,* 7th ed. Baltimore: Wolters Kluwer, 2013.

Chapter 6

Question 92 (options 1–3):   Carter, P. J. *Lippincott's Textbook for Nursing Assistants,* 4th ed. Philadelphia: Wolters Kluwer, 2015.

Question 92 (option 4):   Moore, L. W., ed. *NCLEX-PN Q&A plus! Made Incredibly Easy,* 2nd ed. Philadelphia: Wolters Kluwer, 2018.

Question 135:   Anatomical Chart Company. *Brain Anatomical Chart.* Philadelphia: Wolters Kluwer, 2000.

Chapter 7

Question 62:   *Rapid Review Anatomy Reference Guide,* 3rd ed. Ambler: Anatomical Chart Company, 2009.

Question 72:   *Illustrated Pocket Anatomy: The Muscular & Skeletal Systems Study Guide.* Ambler: Anatomical Chart Company, 2007.

Question 78:   LifeART image copyright (c) 2020 Lippincott Williams & Wilkins. All rights reserved.

Chapter 8

Question 10:   Craven, R.F., Hirnle, C.J. *Fundamentals of Nursing: Human Health and Function.* Philadelphia: Wolters Kluwer, 2009.

Question 59:   Carter, P.J., Lewsen, S. *Lippincott's Textbook for Nursing Assistants.* Philadelphia: Wolters Kluwer, 2004.

Chapter 10

Question 80:   Adapted from Carter, P.J. *Lippincott's Textbook for Nursing Assistants,* 2nd ed. Philadelphia: Wolters Kluwer, 2008.

Chapter 21

Question 30:   Adapted from Stephenson, S.R., ed. Diagnostic medical sonography. *Obstetrics and Gynecology,* 3rd ed. Baltimore: Wolters Kluwer, 2012.

Chapter 22

| Question 40: | *Maternal-Neonatal Nursing Made Incredibly Easy!* 2nd ed. Ambler: Wolters Kluwer, 2007. |

Chapter 24

| Question 71: | Lisko, S., ed. *NCLEX-RN Questions and Answers Made Incredibly Easy!* 7th ed. Philadelphia: Wolters Kluwer, 2017. |
| Question 72: | Nath, J.L. *Using Medical Terminology*, 2nd ed. Baltimore: Wolters Kluwer, 2013. |

Chapter 25

| Question 6: | Weber, J., Kelley, J. *Health Assessment in Nursing*, 2nd ed. Philadelphia: Wolters Kluwer, 2003. |

Chapter 26

| Question 122: | Lisko, S., ed. *NCLEX-RN Questions and Answers Made Incredibly Easy!* 7th ed. Philadelphia: Wolters Kluwer, 2017. |

Chapter 27

| Question 89: | Adapted from *Skeletal System Anatomical Chart*. Ambler: Anatomical Chart Company, 2000. |

Chapter 34

Question 75:	Goodheart, H.P. *Goodheart's Photoguide of Common Skin Disorders*, 2nd ed. Philadelphia: Lippincott Williams & Wilkins, 2003.
Question 89:	Goodheart, H.P. *Goodheart's Photoguide of Common Skin Disorders*, 2nd ed. Philadelphia: Lippincott Williams & Wilkins, 2003.
Question 98:	*Visual Nursing: A Guide to Diseases, Skills, and Treatments*, 2nd ed. Philadelphia: Wolters Kluwer, 2012.

Comprehensive Test 1

| Question 75: | Jensen, S. *Nursing Health Assessment: A Best Practice Approach*. Philadelphia: Wolters Kluwer, 2011. |

Comprehensive Test 2

Question 183:	Buchholz, S. *Henke's Med-Math: Dosage Calculation, Preparation & Administration*, 8th ed. Philadelphia: Wolters Kluwer, 2016.
Question 186:	Rosdahl, C.B. *Textbook of Basic Nursing*, 11th ed. Philadelphia: Wolters Kluwer, 2017.
Question 188:	Buchholz, S. *Henke's Med-Math: Dosage Calculation, Preparation & Administration*, 7th ed. Philadelphia: Wolters Kluwer, 2012.
Question 189:	Adapted from Jensen, S. *Nursing Health Assessment: A Best Practice Approach*. Philadelphia: Wolters Kluwer, 2011.
Question 191:	LifeART image copyright (c) 2020 Lippincott Williams & Wilkins. All rights reserved.
Question 193:	Adapted from Timby, B.K., Smith, N.E. *Introductory Medical-Surgical Nursing*, 10th ed. Philadelphia: Wolters Kluwer, 2010.
Question 194:	*Urinary Tract Anatomical Chart*. Ambler: Anatomical Chart Company, 2000.
Question 208:	Jensen, S. *Nursing Health Assessment: A Best Practice Approach*. Philadelphia: Wolters Kluwer, 2011.
Question 213:	Adapted from *Nursing Procedures*, 4th ed. Ambler: Lippincott Williams & Wilkins, 2004.
Question 216:	Adapted from Bickley, L.S., Szilagyi, P. *Bates' Guide to Physical Examination and History Taking*, 8th ed. Philadelphia: Lippincott Williams & Wilkins, 2003.

Appendices

Heart Sounds	Adapted from Jensen, S. *Nursing Health Assessment: A Best Practice Approach*. Philadelphia: Wolters Kluwer, 2011.
Breath Sounds	Adapted from Jensen, S. *Nursing Health Assessment: A Best Practice Approach*. Philadelphia: Wolters Kluwer, 2011.

Commonly Used Abbreviations

kg = kilogram

g = gram

mg = milligram

mcg = microgram

mEq = milliequivalent

l = liter

dl (deciliter) = 100 milliliters

ml = milliliter

mm = millimeter

mm Hg = millimeters of mercury

mmol = millimole

fl = fluid liter

fmol = fluid mole

pg = picogram

kPa = kilopascal

Commonly Used English to Metric Conversion Equations

1 inch (in) = 2.5 centimeters (cm)

$d_{(in)} = d_{(cm)}/2.54$

$d_{(cm)} = d_{(in)} \times 2.54$

1 pound (lb) = 0.45 kilogram (kg)

$m_{(lb)} = m_{(kg)}/0.45359237$

$m_{(kg)} = m_{(lb)} \times 0.45359237$

1 ounce (oz) = 28 grams (g)

$m_{(oz)} = m_{(g)}/28.34952$

$m_{(g)} = m_{(oz)} \times 28.34952$

Temperature (Fahrenheit, Celsius)

$T_{(°C)} = (T_{(°F)} - 32) \times 5/9$

$T_{(°F)} = T_{(°C)} \times 9/5 + 32$

Normal Adult Laboratory Values*

Determination	Conventional Unit	Reference Range, SI
Hematologic Values (Complete Blood Count)		
Hematocrit	Male: 42%–50% Female: 35%–48%	Male: 0.42–0.52 Female: 0.35–0.48
Hemoglobin	Male: 13–18 g/dl Female: 12–16 g/dl	Male: 8.1–11.2 mmol/l Female: 7.4–9.9 mmol/l
Leukocyte count	5,000–10,000/mm^3	$4.3–10.8 \times 10^9$/l
Erythrocyte count	4.2 million–5.9 million/mm^3	$4.2–5.9 \times 10^{12}$/l
Mean corpuscular volume (MCV)	80–94 mcm^3	80–94 fl
Mean corpuscular hemoglobin (MCH)	27–32 pg	1.7–2.0 fmol
Mean corpuscular hemoglobin concentration (MCHC)	33%–38%	19–22.8 mmol/l
Erythrocyte sedimentation rate (Zeta Centrifuge)	41%–54%	Male: 1–13 mm/h Female: 1–20 mm/h
Hematologic Values (Hemoglobin Studies)		
Platelet count	150,000–450,000/mm^3	$150–450 \times 10^9$/l
Blood, Plasma, or Serum Values		
Carbon dioxide content	24–32 mEq/l	24–30 mmol/l
Chloride	95–105 mEq/l	100–106 mmol/l
Cholesterol	<200 mg/dl	Same
Creatinine	0.7–1.4 mg/100 ml	60–130 mcmol/l
Glucose	Fasting: 60–100 mg/dl	3.9–5.6 mmol/l
Glycated hemoglobin (HbA1c)	4.0%–6%	Same
Lipids, total	400–1,000 mg/dl	3.10–5.69 mmol/l
Magnesium	1.5–2.4 mEq/l	0.7–1.3 mmol/l
Oxygen saturation (arterial)	95%–100%	0.96–1.00 l
PCO$_2$	35–45 mm Hg	4.7–6.0 kPg
pH	7.35–7.45	Same
PO$_2$	95–100 mm Hg (dependent on age while breathing room air) >500 mm Hg while on 100% O$_2$	10.0–13.3 kPa
Phosphorus (inorganic)	3.0–4.5 mg/100 ml	1.0–1.5 mmol/l
Potassium	3.5–5.0 mEq/l	3.5–5.0 mmol/l
Albumin	3.5–5.0 g/100 ml	33–50 g/l
Sodium	135–145 mEq/l	135–145 mmol/l
Urea nitrogen (BUN)	10–20 mg/100 ml	2.9–8.9 mmol/l
Urine Values		
Calcium	150 mg/day or less	3.8 mmol/day or less
Creatine	0–200 mg/24 hr	<0.75 mmol/day

*Laboratory values may vary according to techniques used in different laboratories.

Normal Pediatric Laboratory Values*

Vital Sign	Infant 0 to 12 months	Child 1 to 11 years	Pre-Adolescent/Adolescent 12 and Older
Heart Rate	100–160 bpm	85–110 bpm	Female: 55–85 bpm Male: 50–85
Respiration (breaths)	30–60 bpm	17–30 bpm	15–20 bpm
Blood Pressure (systolic/ diastolic)	50–80/30–50 mm Hg	90–120/55–75 mm Hg	110–120/65–80 mm Hg
Temperature	97.5–99.9°F 36.4–37.7°C	95.9–99°F 35.5–37.2°C	96.4–99.6°F 35.8–37.6°C

*Laboratory values may vary according to techniques used in different laboratories.

Erikson's Stages of Psychosocial Development

Approximate Age	Virtues	Psychosocial Crisis
0–1 years	Hope	Basic trust vs. mistrust
1–3 years	Will	Autonomy vs. shame and doubt
3–6 years	Purpose	Initiative vs. guilt
6–12 years	Competence	Industry vs. inferiority
12–19 years	Fidelity	Identity vs. role confusion
19–40 years	Love	Intimacy vs. isolation
40–65 years	Care	Generativity vs. stagnation
65 to death	Wisdom	Ego integrity vs. despair

From Erikson, E.H. *Identity and the Life Cycle.* New York: International Universities Press, 1959.

Heart Sounds

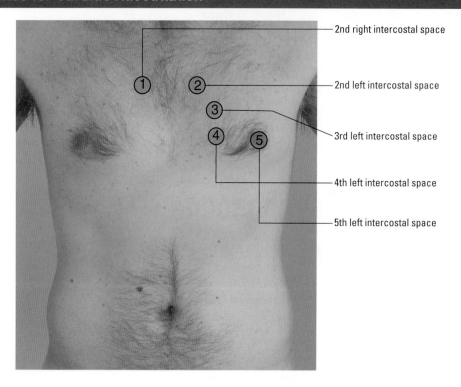

- 2nd right intercostal space
- 2nd left intercostal space
- 3rd left intercostal space
- 4th left intercostal space
- 5th left intercostal space

Breath Sounds

Sites and Sequence for Posterior Auscultation

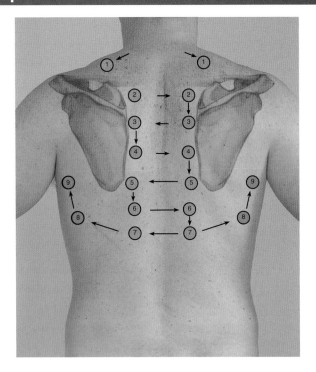

Sites for Anterior Chest Palpation, Percussion, and Auscultation

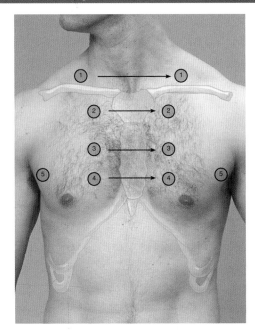